GAMSAT-Prep.com

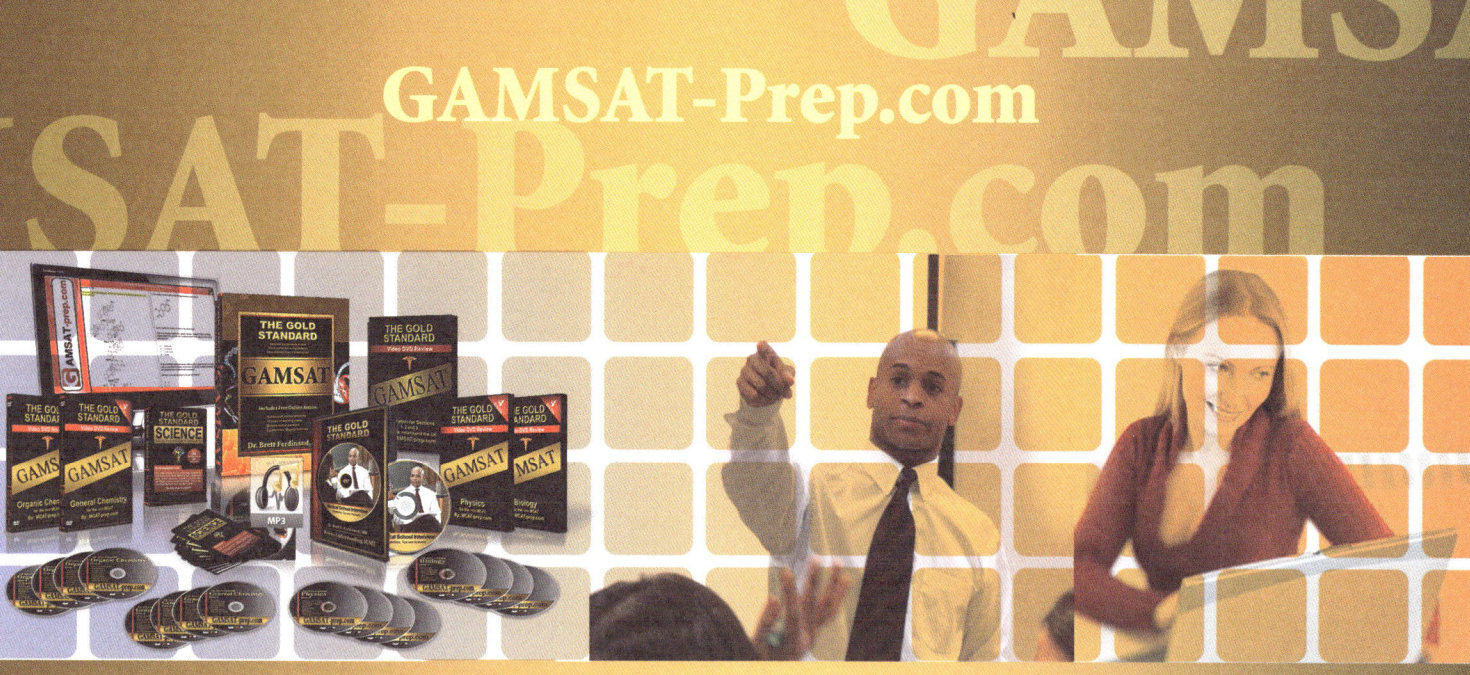

The Gold Standard textbook is a critical component of a multimedia experience including live courses on campus, DVDs, MP3s, smartphone apps, online videos and interactive programs, practice GAMSATs and a lot more.

GAMSAT-Prep.com

The only prep you need.™

SAVE MONEY!

This coupon can be used to save $50 AUD or £30 or €35 off the Live Gold Standard Complete GAMSAT Course OR $50 AUD or £30 or €35 off our online teaching course: The Platinum Program.

To learn more about these programs, go to GAMSAT-prep.com, click on GAMSAT Courses in the top Menu and then scroll down to see "Complete GAMSAT Course".

Expiry Date: August 30, 2018   **Coupon Code: 839XVC9839**

Not redeemable for cash. Not valid in conjunction with another discount offer, non-refundable and not for re-sale. This coupon is governed by the Terms of Use found at GAMSAT-prep.com.

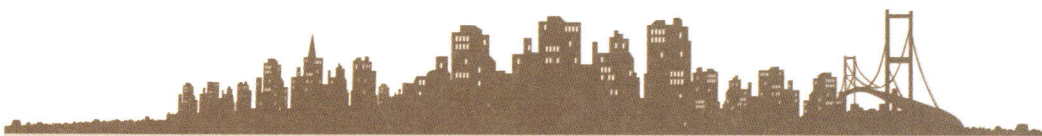

Gold Standard Live GAMSAT Courses are held in the following cities:
Sydney • Melbourne • Dublin • London • Brisbane • Perth • Adelaide • Cork

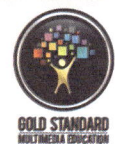

* GAMSAT is administered by ACER which does not endorse this study guide.

THE GOLD STANDARD

GAMSAT

Editor and Author

Brett Ferdinand BSc MD-CM

Contributors

Lisa Ferdinand BA MA
Sean Pierre BSc MD
Kristin Finkenzeller BSc MD
Ibrahima Diouf BSc MSc PhD
Charles Haccoun BSc MD-CM
Timothy Ruger BA MA
Jeanne Tan Te

Illustrators

Daphne McCormack
Nanjing Design
 • Ren Yi, Huang Bin
 • Sun Chan, Li Xin

RuveneCo inc

Free Online Access Features*

Chapter Review Questions
Worked Solutions for the GS-1 Exam
10 Hours of Teaching Videos from our GS Video Library
Organic Chemistry Summary (cross-referenced)
Physics Equation List (cross-referenced)

*One year of continuous access for the original owner of this textbook.

Be sure to register at www.GAMSAT-prep.com by clicking on Register in the top right corner of the website. Once you login, click on GAMSAT Textbook Owners in the right column and follow directions. Please Note: benefits are for 1 year from the date of online registration, for the original book owner only and are not transferable; unauthorized access and use outside the Terms of Use posted on GAMSAT-prep.com may result in account deletion; if you are not the original owner, you can purchase your virtual access card separately at GAMSAT-prep.com.

Visit The Gold Standard's Education Center at www.gold-standard.com.

Copyright (c) 2015 RuveneCo (Worldwide), 5th Edition

ISBN 978-1-927338-28-5

THE PUBLISHER AND THE AUTHORS MAKE NO REPRESENTATIONS OR WARRANTIES WITH RESPECT TO THE ACCURACY OR COMPLETENESS OF THE CONTENTS OF THIS WORK AND SPECIFICALLY DISCLAIM ALL WARRANTIES, INCLUDING WITHOUT LIMITATION WARRANTIES OF FITNESS FOR A PARTICULAR PURPOSE. NO WARRANTY MAY BE CREATED OR EXTENDED BY SALES OR PROMOTIONAL MATERIALS. THE ADVICE AND STRATEGIES CONTAINED HEREIN MAY NOT BE SUITABLE FOR EVERY SITUATION. THIS WORK IS SOLD WITH THE UNDERSTANDING THAT THE PUBLISHER IS NOT ENGAGED IN RENDERING LEGAL, ACCOUNTING, MEDICAL, DENTAL, CONSULTING, OR OTHER PROFESSIONAL SERVICES. IF PROFESSIONAL ASSISTANCE IS REQUIRED, THE SERVICES OF A COMPETENT PROFESSIONAL PERSON SHOULD BE SOUGHT. NEITHER THE PUBLISHER NOR THE AUTHORS SHALL BE LIABLE FOR DAMAGES ARISING HEREFROM. THE FACT THAT AN ORGANIZATION OR WEBSITE IS REFERRED TO IN THIS WORK AS A CITATION AND/OR A POTENTIAL SOURCE OF FURTHER INFORMATION DOES NOT MEAN THAT THE AUTHORS OR THE PUBLISHER ENDORSES THE INFORMATION THE ORGANIZATION OR WEBSITE MAY PROVIDE OR RECOMMENDATIONS IT MAY MAKE. READERS SHOULD BEWARE THAT INTERNET WEBSITES LISTED IN THIS WORK MAY HAVE CHANGED OR DISAPPEARED BETWEEN WHEN THIS WORK WAS WRITTEN AND WHEN IT IS READ.

All rights reserved. No part of this book may be reproduced, stored in a retrieval system, or transmitted in any form or by any means, electronic or mechanical, including photocopying, recording, or otherwise, without permission in writing from the publisher. Images in the public domain: Brandner, D. and Withers, G. (2013). The Cell: An Image Library, www.cellimagelibrary.org, CIL numbers 197, 214, 240, 9685, 21966, ASCB.

Material protected under copyright in Section I and Section III of The Gold Standard GAMSAT Exams were reproduced with permission; credits follow each passage.

Address all inquiries, comments, or suggestions to the publisher. For Terms of Use go to: www.GAMSAT-prep.com

The reviews on the back cover represent the opinions of individuals and do not necessarily reflect the opinions of the institutions they represent.

Gold Standard GAMSAT Product Contact Information

Distribution in Australia, NZ, Asia	**Distribution in Europe**	**Distribution in North America**
Woodslane Pty Ltd	Central Books	RuveneCo Publishing
10 Apollo Street Warriewood	99 Wallis Road	334 Cornelia Street # 559
NSW 2102 Australia	LONDON,	Plattsburgh, New York
ABN: 76 003 677 549	E9 5LN, United Kingdom	12901, USA
learn@gamsat-prep.com	orders@centralbooks.com	buy@gamsatbooks.com

RuveneCo Inc. is neither associated nor affiliated with the Australian Council for Educational Research (ACER) who has developed and administers the Graduate Australian Medical School Admissions Test (GAMSAT) nor The University of Sydney. Printed in China.

PREFACE

No science background in university? Great in the sciences but little experience reading from the humanities or writing essays? Had a bad experience with a high-school physics teacher? Full-time arts student? Full-time mom? Part-time job? It's OK. The Gold Standard has you covered. This is not just a textbook, it is a multimedia learning experience.

The Gold Standard has integrated textbook reading with many free features including online problem solving with worked solutions; essays for you to review in the book and online; 10 hours of online videos with clear teaching from our extensive video library; online equation lists and organic reaction summary; a full-length paper practice test with online detailed explanations, score converter and a forum thread to discuss every individual question - for free - and much more.

Frankly, I wanted the revisions to end there but your predecessors kept demanding more. For 5 years, I have been teaching monthly GAMSAT webinars, teaching science review GAMSAT courses on campuses in Australia, the UK and Ireland, as well as producing over 100 YouTube videos giving step-by-step worked solutions to the official (ACER's) practice materials for the GAMSAT. The result of those experiences is this new edition of the Gold Standard GAMSAT. All content was revised and we added in excess of 50% more pages and 100% more practice questions.

Everywhere you turn in this textbook, I hope you will be able to hear the voice of someone who is genuinely trying to help you learn, and to keep you on a path that is relevant to this particular exam. The nature of GAMSAT-level questions will likely surprise you. It is unlike any exam you have experienced. Preparing for this exam requires that you build a certain foundation of knowledge, explore an incredible array of concepts, practice answering basic questions to confirm your understanding, as well as experiencing GAMSAT-level practice questions and practice exams under timed conditions.

Your formula for success comes in 3 parts: content review, practice problems and full-length testing. We will guide you through the process.

Let's begin . . .

– B.F., MD

GAMSAT-Prep.com

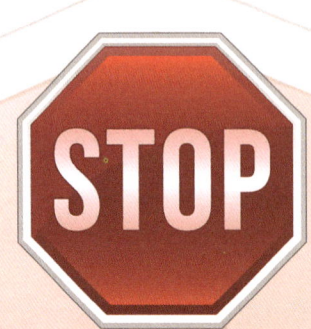

GAMSAT SCORE!

Good, we have your attention! We just want to be sure that you understand that not every student needs the same Section 3 (science) score in order to be admitted to medical school. Some science students must ace Section 3 to be admitted while some non-science students can gain admittance with an average Section 3 score because of an exceptional performance in the non-science sections. This book is for all students. This means that there may be some science chapters that might not be "worth it" for the non-science student. So we have colour-coded the importance of chapters in providing pertinent background information based on our experience.

HIGH   MEDIUM   LOW

Now you can use your own judgement based on how much time you have to study and our assessment of the **importance** of that chapter. You will find this coding system particularly helpful when studying Biology. Also, if you have no science background in any of the subjects then we highly recommend taking advantage of the 10 hours of online video time that comes with this textbook. In addition, we suggest that all students complete the non-science problem sets in this textbook as well as the science chapter review questions with worked solutions that are online. Reviewing content only provides the background needed for science reasoning. In order to move to the next level, you must do problem sets followed by timed full-length practice beginning with the GS-1 test which is at the back of this textbook. Review, practice and full-length testing can help you obtain an exceptional GAMSAT score.

As of the publication date of this textbook, calculators are no longer permitted.

To further discuss any of the issues above: gamsat-prep.com/forum.

Preface v
Introduction 1

Part I: MEDICAL SCHOOL ADMISSIONS

  1. Improving Academic Standing 5
  2. The Medical School Interview 10
  3. Autobiographical Materials and References 18

Part II: UNDERSTANDING THE GAMSAT

  1. The Structure of the GAMSAT 25
  2. The Recipe for GAMSAT Success 33

A. Review for Section 1

  3.1. Overview 39
  3.2. How to Improve Your Section I Score 40
  3.3. Style of Questions 44
  3.4. Online Help 45
  3.5. Types of Questions 45
  3.6. Warm-up Exercises 60
  3.7. Short Test and Analysis 66
  3.8. Section 1 Mini Tests 77
      Verbal Reasoning Exercise 1 (Humanities and Social Sciences) 78
      Verbal Reasoning Exercise 2 (Science-based Passages) 105
      Poetry Test 131
      Cartoon Test 144
      Graphs and Tables Test 160

B. Review for Section 2

  4.1. Overview 174
  4.2. Key Skills to Develop for Section II 177
  4.3. Building Your Vocabulary 213
  4.4. Practice Materials 232
  4.5. Advice on How to Generate Ideas 232
  4.6. Exercises for Developing a Logical Response 240
  4.7. The Scoring Key 261
  4.8. Sample Corrected Essays 263
  4.9. Frequently Asked Questions 270
  4.10. Common Grammatical Errors 274
  4.11. Section II Practice Worksheets 285
  4.12. Samples of Excellent Essays 289

REVIEW FOR SECTION 3: THE SCIENCES

PROLOGUE

- Common Root Words of Scientific Terms P-1
- Prefixes P-1
- Suffixes P-4
- The Natural Order to Study the Sciences P-6

MATH

1. Numbers and Operations GM-03
2. Scientific Measurement GM-33
3. Algebra GM-45
4. Geometry GM-77
5. Trigonometry GM-97
6. Probability and Statistics GM-109
7. Chapter Review Solutions GM-123

PHYSICS

1. Translational Motion PHY-03
2. Force, Motion and Gravitation PHY-11
3. Particle Dynamics PHY-19
4. Equilibrium PHY-25
5. Work and Energy PHY-33
6. Fluids and Solids PHY-39
7. Wave Characteristics and Periodic Motion PHY-49
8. Sound PHY-61
9. Electrostatics and Electromagnetism PHY-67
10. Electric Circuits PHY-77
11. Light and Geometrical Optics PHY-89
12. Atomic and Nuclear Structure PHY-99

GENERAL CHEMISTRY

1. Stoichiometry CHM-03
2. Electronic Structure and the Periodic Table CHM-15
3. Bonding CHM-31
4. Phases and Phase Equilibria CHM-45
5. Solution Chemistry CHM-61
6. Acids and Bases CHM-75
7. Thermodynamics CHM-91
8. Enthalpy and Thermochemistry CHM-99
9. Rate Processes in Chemical Reactions CHM-113
10. Electrochemistry CHM-131

GAMSAT-Prep.com

ORGANIC CHEMISTRY

1. Molecular Structure of Organic Compounds ORG-03
2. Stereochemistry.. ORG-13
3. Alkanes ORG-29
4. Alkenes ORG-37
5. Aromatics ORG-51
6. Alcohols ORG-61
7. Aldehydes and Ketones ORG-71
8. Carboxylic Acids ORG-81
9. Carboxylic Acid Derivatives ORG-89
10. Ethers and Phenols ORG-101
11. Amines ORG-107
12. Biological Molecules ORG-115
13. Separations and Purifications ORG-139
14. Spectroscopy ORG-147

BIOLOGY

1. Generalized Eukaryotic Cell BIO-03
2. Microbiology BIO-29
3. Protein Synthesis BIO-41
4. Enzymes and Cellular Metabolism BIO-51
5. Specialized Eukaryotic Cells and Tissues BIO-65
6. Nervous and Endocrine Systems BIO-81
7. The Circulatory System BIO-103
8. The Immune System BIO-115
9. The Digestive System BIO-121
10. The Excretory System BIO-131
11. The Musculoskeletal System BIO-139
12. The Respiratory System BIO-147
13. The Skin as an Organ System BIO-153
14. Reproduction and Development BIO-159
15. Genetics BIO-173
16. Evolution... BIO-189

GOLD STANDARD GAMSAT EXAM

1. The Gold Standard GAMSAT 1057
2. Practice Test GS-1 .... GS-1

ANSWER KEY AND ANSWER DOCUMENTS

1. Cross-referenced Answer Keys AK-3
2. Answer Documents AK-5

GAMSAT-Prep.com
THE GOLD STANDARD

The Graduate Australian Medical School Admissions Test (GAMSAT) is a paper-based test (no calculators are allowed) and consists of 2 essay writing tasks and 185 multiple-choice questions. This exam requires approximately 5.5 hours to complete and is comprised of 3 Sections. There is no break between Section I and II. There is a lunch break between Section II and III. The following are the three subtests of the GAMSAT exam:

1. **Section I: Reasoning in Humanities and Social Sciences - 75 questions; 100 min.**

   - Interpretation and understanding of ideas in socio-cultural context. Source materials: written passages, tabular or other visual format.

2. **Section II: Written Communication - 2 essays; 60 min.**

   - Ability to produce and develop ideas in writing. Task A essay: socio-cultural issues, more analytical; Task B more personal and social issues.

3. **Section III: Reasoning in Biological and Physical Sciences - 110 questions, 170 min.**

   - Chemistry (40%), Biology (40%), Physics (20%). First-year undergraduate level in Biology and Chemistry and Year 12 in Physics.

> The overall GAMSAT score is calculated using the following formula*:
>
> Overall Score = (1 x Section I + 1 x Section II + 2 x Section III) / 4

* Note: the formula applies to all medical schools that require the GAMSAT in Australia, the UK and Ireland except for the University of Melbourne which currently weighs all 3 sections equally.

Common formula for acceptance:

GPA + GAMSAT score + Interview = Medical School Admissions

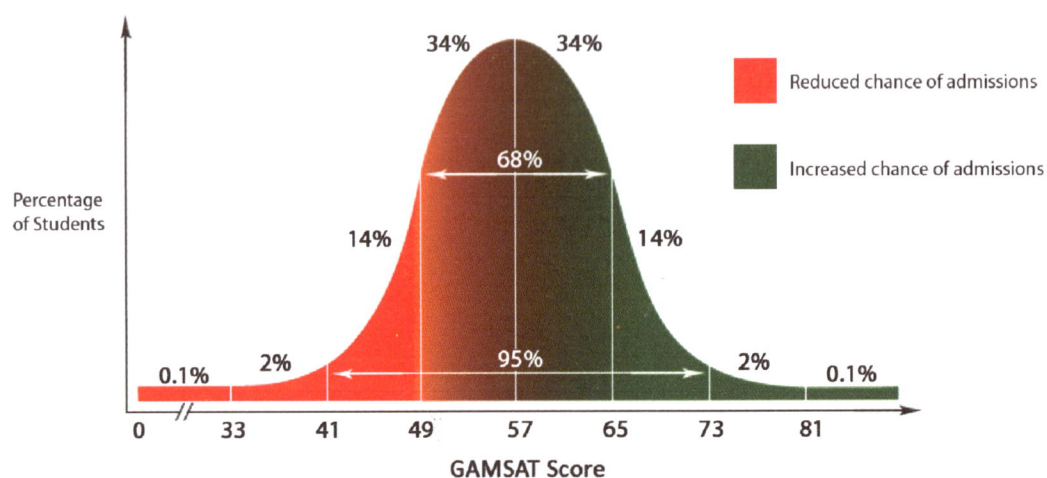

Typical Overall GAMSAT Score Distribution (Approx)

INTRODUCTION

==The GAMSAT is challenging, get organised.==

gamsat-prep.com/free-GAMSAT-study-schedule

1. How to study:
1. Study the Gold Standard (GS) textbook and videos to learn
2. Do GS Chapter review practice questions
3. Consolidate: create and review your personal summaries (= Gold Notes) daily

2. Once you have completed your studies:
1. Full-length practice test
2. Review mistakes, all solutions
3. Consolidate: review all your Gold Notes and create more
4. Repeat until you get beyond the score you need for your targeted medical/dental school

Recommended GAMSAT Communities:
- All countries (mainly Australia): pagingdr.net
- Mainly UK: newmediamedicine.com/forum/gamsat/
- Mainly Ireland: boards.ie

Is there something in the Gold Standard that you did not understand? Don't get frustrated, get on-line: gamsat-prep.com/forum

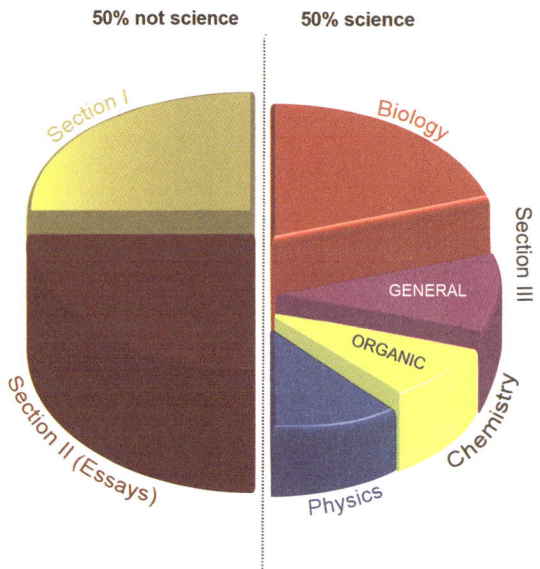

GAMSAT Scores
50% not science | 50% science
Section I, Section II (Essays), Biology, General, Organic, Chemistry, Physics, Section III

3. Full-length practice tests:
1. ACER practice exams
2. Gold Standard GAMSAT exams
3. Other sources if needed

4. How much time do you need?
On average, 3-6 hours per day for 3-6 months; depending on life experiences, 2 weeks may be enough and 8 months could be insufficient.

To make the content easier to retain, you can also find aspects of the Gold Standard program in other formats such as:

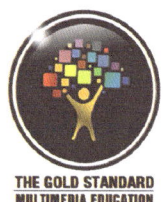  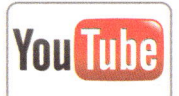 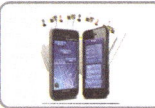 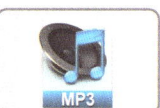 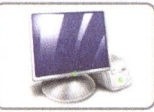

Good luck with your studies!

Gold Standard Team

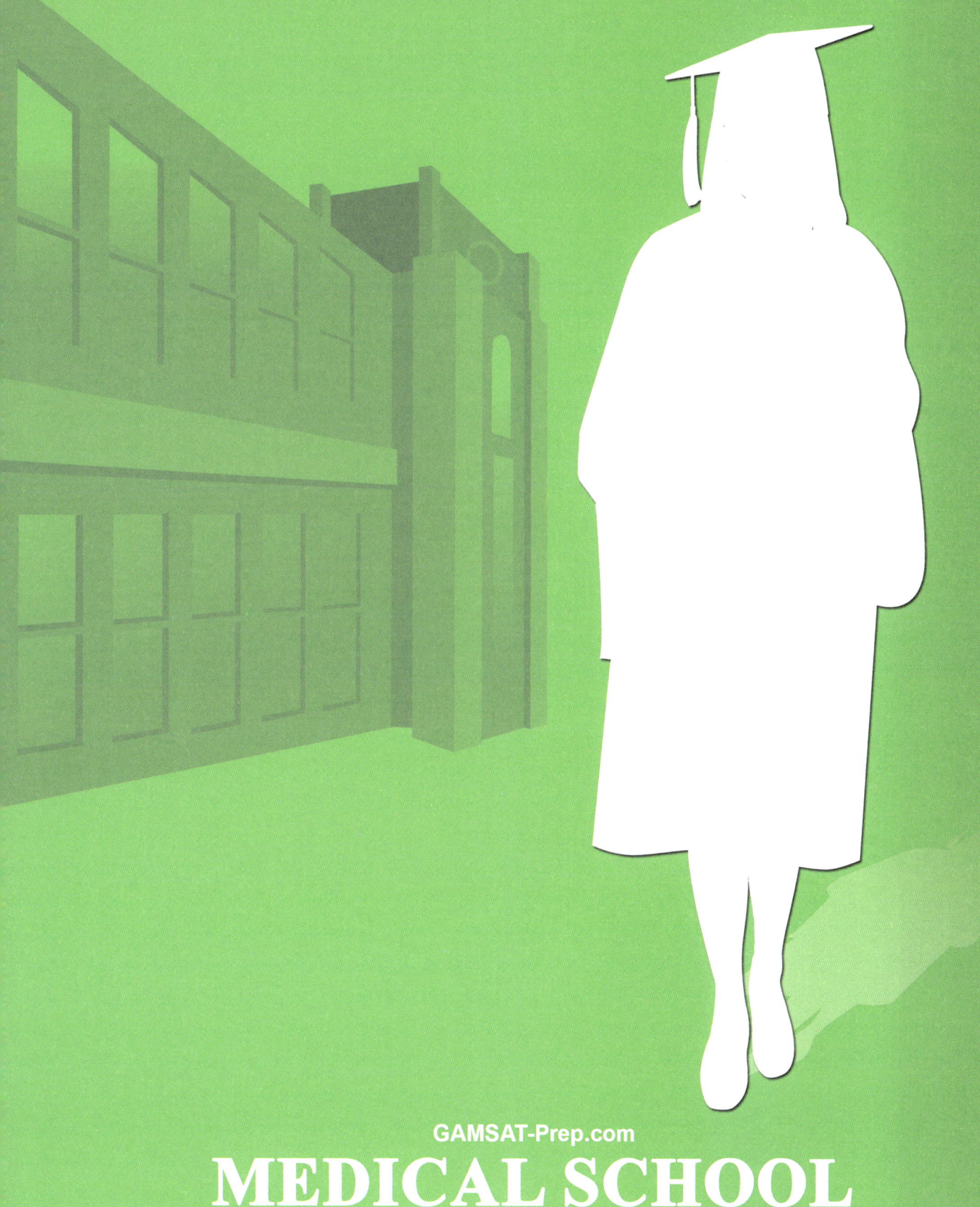

GAMSAT-Prep.com
MEDICAL SCHOOL ADMISSIONS
PART I

GAMSAT-Prep.com
THE GOLD STANDARD

IMPROVING ACADEMIC STANDING

1.1 Lectures

Before you set foot in a classroom you should consider the value of being there. Even if you were taking a course like 'Basket-weaving 101', one way to help you do well in the course is to consider the value of the course to **you**. The course should have an *intrinsic* value (i.e. 'I enjoy weaving baskets'). The course will also have an *extrinsic* value (i.e. 'If I do not get good grades, I will not be accepted...'). Motivation, a positive attitude, and an interest in learning give you an edge before the class even begins.

Unless there is a student 'note-taking club' for your courses, your attendance record and the quality of your notes should both be as excellent as possible. Be sure to choose seating in the classroom which ensures that you will be able to hear the professor adequately and see whatever she may write. Whenever possible, do not sit close to friends!

Instead of chattering before the lecture begins, spend the idle moments quickly reviewing the previous lecture in that subject so you would have an idea of what to expect. Try to take good notes and pay close attention. The preceding may sound like a difficult combination (esp. with professors who speak and write quickly); however, with practice you can learn to do it well.

And finally, do not let the quality of teaching affect your interest in the subject nor your grades! Do not waste your time during or before lectures complaining about how the professor speaks too quickly, does not explain concepts adequately, etc... When the time comes, you can mention such issues on the appropriate evaluation forms! In the meantime, consider this: despite the good or poor quality of teaching, there is always a certain number of students who **still** perform well. You must strive to count yourself among those students.

1.2 Taking Notes

Unless your professor says otherwise, if you take excellent notes and learn them inside out, you will *ace* his course. Your notes should always be up-to-date, complete, and separate from other subjects.

GAMSAT-Prep.com
THE GOLD STANDARD

To be safe, you should try to write everything! You can fill in any gaps by comparing your notes with those of your friends. You can create your own shorthand symbols or use standard ones. The following represents some useful symbols:

|·|	between
=	the same as
≠	not the same as
∴	therefore
Δ	difference, change in
cf.	compare
c̄ or w	with
c̄out or w/o	without
esp.	especially
∵	because
i.e.	that is
e.g.	for example

Many students rewrite their notes at home. Should you decide to rewrite your notes, your time will be used efficiently if you are paying close attention to the information you are rewriting. In fact, a more useful technique is the following: during class, write your notes only on the right side of your binder. Later, rewrite the information from class in a complete but condensed form on the left side of the binder (*this condensed form should include mnemonics which we will discuss later*).

Some students find it valuable to use different color pens. Juggling pens in class may distract you from the content of the lecture. Different color pens would be more useful in the context of rewriting one's notes.

1.3 The Principles of Studying Efficiently

If you study efficiently, you will have enough time for extracurricular activities, movies, etc. The bottom line is that your time must be used efficiently and effectively.

During the average school day, time can be found during breaks, between classes, and after school to quickly review notes in a library or any other quiet place you can find on campus. Simply by using the available time in your school day, you can keep up to date with recent information.

You should design an individual study schedule to meet your particular needs. However, as a rule, a certain amount of time every evening should be set aside for more in depth studying. Weekends can be set aside for special projects and reviewing notes from the beginning.

On the surface, the idea of regularly reviewing notes from the beginning may sound like an insurmountable task which would take forever! The reality is just the opposite. After all, if you continually study the information, by the time mid-terms approach you would have seen the first lecture so many times that it would take only moments to review it again. On the other hand, had you not been reviewing regularly, it would be like reading that lecture for the first time!

You should study wherever you are comfortable and effective studying (i.e. library, at home, etc.). Should you prefer studying at home, be sure to create an environment which is conducive to studying.

Studying should be an active process to memorize and understand a given set of material. Memorization and comprehension are best achieved by the **elaboration** of course material, **attention, repetition,** and practising **retrieval** of the information. All these principles are borne out in the following techniques.

1.4 Studying from Notes and Texts

Successful studying from either class notes or textbooks can be accomplished in three simple steps:

- **Preview the material**: read all the relevant headings, titles, and sub-titles to give you a general idea of what you are about to learn. You should never embark on a trip without knowing where you are going!

- **Read while questioning**: **passive studying** is when you sit in front of a book and just read. This can lead to boredom, lack of concentration, or even worse - difficulty remembering what you just read! **Active studying** involves reading while actively questioning yourself. For example: how does this fit in with the 'big picture'? How does this relate to what we learned last week? What cues about these words or lists will make it easy for me to memorize them? What type of question would my professor ask me? If I was asked a question on this material, how would I answer? Etc...

- **Recite and consider**: put the notes or text away while you attempt to **recall** the main facts. Once you are able to recite the important information, **consider** how it relates to the entire subject.

N.B. if you ever sit down to study and you are not quite sure with which subject to begin, always start with either the most difficult subject or the subject you like least (usually they are one in the same!).

1.5 Study Aids

The most effective study aids include practice exams, mnemonics and audio MP3s.

Practice exams (*exams from previous semesters*) are often available from the library, upper level students, online or directly from the professor. They can be used like maps which guide you through your semester. They give you a good indication as to what information you should emphasize when you study; what question types and exam format you can expect; and what your level of progress is.

One practice exam should be set aside to do one week before 'the real thing.' You should time yourself and do the exam in an environment free from distractions. This provides an ideal way to uncover unexpected weak points.

Mnemonics are an effective way of memorizing lists of information. Usually a word, phrase, or sentence is constructed to symbolize a greater amount of information (i.e. LEO is A GERC = Lose Electrons is Oxidation is Anode, Gain Electrons is Reduction at Cathode). An effective study aid to active studying is the creation of your own mnemonics.

Audio MP3s can be used as effective tools to repeat information and to use your time efficiently. Information from the left side of your notes (*see 1.2 Taking Notes*) including mnemonics, can be dictated and recorded. Often, an entire semester of work can be summarized into one 90 minute recording.

Now you can listen to the recording on an iPod while waiting in line at the bank, or in a bus or with a car stereo on the way to school, work, etc. You can also listen to recorded information when you go to sleep and listen to another one first thing in the morning. You are probably familiar with the situation of having heard a song early in the morning and then having difficulty, for the rest of the day, getting it out of your mind! Well, imagine if the first thing you heard in the morning was: "Hair is a modified keratinized structure produced by the cylindrical down growth of epithelium..."! Thus MP3s become an effective study aid since they are an extra source of repetition.

Some students like to **record lectures**. Though it may be helpful to fill in missing notes, it is not an efficient way to repeat information.

Some students like to use **study cards** (flashcards) on which they may write either a summary of information they must memorize or relevant questions to consider. Then the cards are used throughout the day to quickly flash information to promote thought on course material.

MEDICAL SCHOOL ADMISSIONS

1.5.1 Falling Behind

Imagine yourself as a marathon runner who has run 25.5 km of a 26 km race. The finishing line is now in view. However, you have fallen behind some of the other runners. The most difficult aspect of the race is still ahead.

In such a scenario some interesting questions can be asked: Is now the time to drop out of the race because 0.5 km suddenly seems like a long distance? Is now the time to reevaluate whether or not you should have competed? Or is now the time to remain faithful to your goals and give 100%?

Imagine one morning in mid-semester you wake up realizing you have fallen behind in your studies. What do you do? Where do you start? Is it too late?

Like a doctor being presented with an urgent matter, you should see the situation as one of life's challenges. Now is the worst time for doubts, rather, it is the time for action. A clear line of action should be formulated such that it could be followed.

For example, one might begin by gathering all pertinent study materials like a complete set of study notes, relevant text(s), sample exams, etc. As a rule, to get back into the thick of things, notes and sample exams take precedence. Studying at this point should take a three pronged approach: i) a regular, consistent review of the information from your notes from the beginning of the section for which you are responsible (i.e. *starting with the first class*); ii) a regular, consistent review of course material as you are learning it from the lectures (*this is the most efficient way to study*); iii) regular testing using questions given in class or those contained in sample exams. Using such questions will clarify the extent of your progress.

It is also of value, as time allows, to engage in extracurricular activities which you find helpful in reducing stress (i.e. sports, piano, creative writing, etc.).

THE MEDICAL SCHOOL INTERVIEW

2.1 Introduction

The application process to most medical schools includes interviews. Only a select number of students from the applicant pool will be given an offer to be interviewed. The medical school interview is, as a rule, something that you *achieve*. In other words, after your school grades and GAMSAT scores (and/or references and autobiographical materials for international schools) have been reviewed, you are offered the ultimate opportunity to put your foot forward: a personalized interview.

Depending on the medical school, you may be interviewed by one, two or several interviewers. You may be the only interviewee or there may be others (i.e., *a group interview*). There may be one or more interviews lasting from 20 minutes to two hours. And, of course, there is the increasingly popular multiple mini-interview (MMI) which includes many short assessments in a timed circuit.

Despite the variations among the technical aspects of the interview, in terms of substance, most medical schools have similar objectives. These objectives can be arbitrarily categorized into three general assessments: (i) your personality traits, (ii) social skills, and (iii) knowledge of medicine.

Personality traits such as maturity, integrity, compassion, sincerity, honesty, originality, curiosity, self-directed learning, intellectual capacity, confidence (*not arrogance!*), and motivation are all components of the ideal applicant. These traits will be exposed by the process of the interview, your mannerisms, and the substance of what you choose to discuss when given an ambiguous question. For instance, bringing up *specific* examples of academic achievement related to school and related to self-directed learning would score well in the categories of intellectual capacity and curiosity, respectively.

Motivation is a personality trait which may make the difference between a high and a low or moderate score in an interview. A student must clearly demonstrate that they have the enthusiasm, desire, energy, and interest to survive (typically) four long years of medical school and beyond! If you are naturally shy or soft-spoken, you will have to give special attention to this category.

Social skills such as leadership, ease of communication, ability to relate to others and work effectively in groups, volunteer work, cultural and social interests, all constitute skills which are often viewed as critical for future physicians. It is not sufficient to say in an interview: "I have good social skills"! You must display such skills via your interaction with the interviewer(s) and by discussing specific examples of situations which clearly demonstrate your social skills.

Knowledge of medicine includes <u>at least</u> a general understanding of what the field of medicine involves, the curriculum you are applying to, and a knowledge of popular medical issues like abortion, euthanasia, AIDS, the health care system, etc. It is striking to see the number of students who apply to medical school each year whose knowledge of medicine is limited to headlines and popular TV shows! It is not logical for someone to dedicate their lives to a profession they know little about.

Doing volunteer work in a hospital is a good start. Alternatively, getting a part-time job in a hospital or having a relative who is a physician can help expose you to the daily goings-on in a hospital setting. An even better strategy to be informed is the following: (i) keep up-to-date with the details of medically related controversies in the news. You should also be able to develop and support opinions of your own; (ii) skim through a medical journal at least once; (iii) read the medical section of a popular science magazine (i.e. Scientific American, Discover, etc.); (iv) keep abreast of changes in medical school curricula in general and specific to the programs to which you have applied. You can access such information at most university libraries and by writing individual medical schools for information on their programs; (v) do a First-Aid course.

2.2 Preparing for the Interview

If you devote an adequate amount of time for interview preparation, the actual interview will be less tense for you and <u>you</u> will be able to control most of the content of the interview.

Reading from the various sources mentioned in the preceding sections would be helpful. Also, read over your curriculum vitae and/or any autobiographical materials you may have prepared. Note highlights in your life or specific examples that demonstrate the aforementioned personality traits, social skills or your knowledge of medicine. Zero in on qualities or stories which are either important, memorable, interesting, amusing, informative or "all of the above"! Once in the interview room, you will be given the opportunity to elaborate on the qualities you believe are important about yourself.

Email or call the medical school and ask them about the structure of the interview (i.e., one-on-one, group, MMI, etc.) and ask them if they can tell you who will interview you. Many schools have no qualms volunteering such information. Now you can determine the person's expertise by either asking or looking through staff members of the different faculties or medical specialties

GAMSAT-Prep.com
THE GOLD STANDARD

at that university or college. A cardiac surgeon, a volunteer from the community, and a medical ethicist all have different areas of expertise and will likely orient their interviews differently. Thus you may want to read from a source which will give you a general understanding of their specialty.

Choose appropriate clothes for the interview. Every year some students dress for a medical school interview as if they were going out to dance! Medicine is still considered a conservative profession, you should dress and groom yourself likewise. First impressions are very important. Your objective is to make it as easy as possible for your interviewer(s) to imagine you as a physician.

Do practice interviews with people you respect but who can also maintain their objectivity. Let them read this entire chapter on medical school interviews. They must understand that you are to be evaluated *only* on the basis of the interview. On that basis alone, one should be able to imagine the ideal candidate as a future physician.

2.3 Strategies for Answering Questions

Always remember that the interviewer controls the *direction* of the interview by his questions; you control the *content* of the interview through your answers. In other words, once given the opportunity, you should speak about the topics that are important to you; conversely, you should avoid volunteering information which renders you uncomfortable. You can enhance the atmosphere in which the answers are delivered by being polite, sincere, tactful, well-organized, outwardly oriented and maintaining eye contact. Motivation, enthusiasm, and a positive attitude must all be evident.

As a rule, there are no right or wrong answers. However, the way in which you justify your opinions, the topics you choose to discuss, your mannerisms and your composure all play important roles. It is normal to be nervous. It would be to your advantage to channel your nervous energy into a positive quality, like enthusiasm.

Do not spew forth answers! Take your time - it is not a contest to see how fast you can answer. Answering with haste can lead to disastrous consequences as happened to a student I interviewed:

Q: *Have you ever doubted your interest in medicine as a career?*
A: *No!*
   Well,...ah...I guess so. Ah ... I guess everyone doubts something at some point or the other...

MEDICAL SCHOOL ADMISSIONS

Retractions like that are a bad signal but it illustrates an important point: there are usually no right or wrong answers in an interview; however, there are right or wrong ways of answering. Through the example we can conclude the following: <u>listen carefully to the question</u>, <u>try to relax</u>, and <u>think before you answer</u>!

Do not sit on the fence! If you avoid giving your opinions on controversial topics, it will be interpreted as indecision which is a negative trait for a prospective physician. You have a right to your opinions. However, you must be prepared to defend your point of view in an objective, rational, and informative fashion. It is also important to show that, despite your opinion, you understand both sides of the argument. If you have an extreme or unconventional perspective and if you believe your perspective will not interfere with your practice of medicine, <u>you must let your interviewer know that</u>.

For example, imagine a student who was against abortion under *any* circumstance. If asked about her opinion on abortion, she should clearly state her opinion objectively, show she understands the opposing viewpoint, and then use data to reinforce her position. If she felt that her opinion would not interfere with her objectivity when practising medicine, she might volunteer: "If I were in a position where my perspective might interfere with an objective management of a patient, I would refer that patient to another physician."

Carefully note the reactions of the interviewer in response to your answers. Whether the interviewer is sitting on the edge of her seat wide-eyed or slumping in her chair while yawning, you should take such cues to help you determine when to continue, change the subject, or when to stop talking. Also, note the more subtle cues. For example, gauge which topic makes the interviewer frown, give eye contact, take notes, etc.

Lighten up the interview with a well-timed story. A conservative joke, a good analogy, or anecdote may help you relax and make the interviewer sustain his interest. If it is done correctly, it can turn a routine interview into a memorable and friendly interaction.

It should be noted that because the system is not standardized, a small number of interviewers may ask overly personal questions (i.e., about relationships, religion, etc.) or even questions which carry sexist tones (i.e., *What would you do if you got pregnant while attending medical school?*). Some questions may be frankly illegal. If you do not want to answer a question, simply maintain your composure, express your position diplomatically, and address the interviewers <u>real</u> concern (i.e. *Does this person have the potential to be a good doctor?*). For example, you might say in a non-confrontational tone of voice: "I would rather not answer such a question. However, I can assure you that whatever my answer may have been, it would in no way affect either my prospective studies in medicine nor any prerequisite objectivity I should have to be a good physician."

2.4 Sample Questions

There are an infinite number of questions and many different categories of questions. Different medical schools will emphasize different categories of questions. Arbitrarily, ten categories of questions can be defined: ambiguous, medically related, academic, social, stress-type, problem situations, personality oriented, based on autobiographical material, miscellaneous, and ending questions. We will examine each category in terms of sample questions and general comments.

Ambiguous Questions:

- *Tell me about yourself.*
  How do you want me to remember you?
  What are your goals?
  There are hundreds if not thousands of applicants, why should we choose you?
  Convince me that you would make a good doctor.
  Why do you want to study medicine?

COMMENTS: These questions present nightmares for the unprepared student who walks into the interview room and is immediately asked: "Tell me about yourself." Where do you start? If you are prepared as previously discussed, you will be able to take control of the interview by highlighting your qualities or objectives in an informative and interesting manner.

Medically Related Questions:

What are the pros and cons to our health care system?
If you had the power, what changes would you make to our health care system?
Do doctors make too much money?
Is it ethical for doctors to strike?
What is the Hippocratic Oath?
Should fetal tissue be used to treat disease (i.e. Parkinson's)?
If you were a doctor and an under age girl asked you for the Pill (or an abortion) and she did not want to tell her parents, what would you do?
Should doctors be allowed to 'pull the plug' on terminally ill patients?
If a patient is dying from a bleed, would you transfuse blood if you knew they would not approve (i.e. Jehovah Witness)?

COMMENTS: The health care system, euthanasia, cloning, abortion, and other ethical issues are very popular topics in this era of technological advances, skyrocketing health care costs, and ethical uncertainty. A well-informed opinion can set you apart from most of the other interviewees.

MEDICAL SCHOOL ADMISSIONS

Questions Related to Academics:

Why did you choose your present course of studies?
What is your favorite subject in your present course of studies? Why?
Would you consider a career in your present course of studies?
Can you convince me that you can cope with the workload in medical school?
How do you study/prepare for exams?
Do you engage in self-directed learning?

COMMENTS: Medical schools like to see applicants who are well-disciplined, committed to medicine as a career, and who exhibit self-directed learning (i.e. such a level of desire for knowledge that the student may seek to study information independent of any organized infrastructure). Beware of any glitches in your academic record. You may be asked to give reasons for any grades they may deem substandard. On the other hand, you should volunteer any information regarding academic achievement (i.e. prizes, awards, scholarships, particularly high grades in one subject or the other, etc.).

Questions Related to Social Skills or Interests:

Give evidence that you relate well with others.
Give an example of a leadership role you have assumed.
Have you done any volunteer work?
What would you do as Prime Minister with respect to the trade imbalance with China?
Is the monarchy a legitimate institution?
What are the prospects for a lasting peace in Afghanistan? Iraq? the Sudan? the Middle-East?
What do you think of the regional free-trade agreements?

COMMENTS: Questions concerning social skills should be simple for the prepared student. If you are asked a question that you cannot answer, say so. If you pretend to know something about a topic in which you are completely uninformed, you will make a bad situation worse.

Stress-Type Questions:

How do you handle stress?
What was the most stressful event in your life? How did you handle it?
The night before your final exam, your father has a heart-attack and is admitted to a hospital, what do you do?

COMMENTS: The ideal physician has positive coping methods to deal with the inevitable stressors of a medical practice. Stress-type questions are a legitimate means of determining if you possess the raw material necessary to cope with medical school and medicine as a career. Some interviewers go one step further. They may decide to introduce stress <u>into</u> the interview and see how you handle it. For example, they may decide to ask you a confrontational question or try to back you into a corner (i.e. *You do not know anything about medicine, do you?*). Alternatively, the interviewer might use silence to introduce stress into the interview. If you have completely and confidently answered a question and silence falls in the room, <u>do not</u> retract previous statements, mutter, or fidget. Simply wait for the next question. If the silence becomes unbearable, you may consider asking an intelligent question (i.e. a specific question regarding their curriculum).

MMI-Type Problem Situations:

A 68 year-old married woman has a newly discovered cancer. Her life expectancy is 6 months. How would you inform her?
A 34 year-old man presents with AIDS and tells you, as his physician, that he does not want to tell his wife. What would you do?
You are playing tennis with your best friend and the ball hits your friend in the eye. What do you do?
A 52 year-old female diabetic comes to your ER in a coma but dies almost immediately. You are the physician who must now inform her husband and daughter. Enter the room and talk to them.
Your best friend in med-school has a part-time job to support herself. She has been unable to make it to some compulsory seminars because of her job and has asked you to mark her name present on the roll. What do you do and why?

COMMENTS: Some programmes have a few MMI stations with an actor in the room or other students. As for the other questions, listen carefully (or in the case of MMI, read the question posted on the door carefully) and take your time to consider the best possible response. Keep in mind that the ideal physician is not only knowledgeable, but is also <u>compassionate</u>, <u>empathetic</u>, <u>honest</u> and is objective enough to understand <u>both sides</u> of a dilemma. Be sure such qualities are clearly demonstrated.

Personality-Oriented Questions:

If you could change one thing about yourself, what would it be?
How would your friends describe you?
What do you do with your spare time?
What is the most important event that has occurred to you in the last five years?
If you had three magical wishes, what would they be?
What are your best attributes?

COMMENTS: Of course, most questions will assess your personality to one degree or the other. However, these questions are quite direct in their approach. Forewarned is forearmed!

Question Based on Autobiographical Materials:

COMMENTS: Any autobiographical materials you may have provided to the medical schools is fair game for questioning. You may be asked to discuss or elaborate on any point the interviewer may feel is interesting or questionable.

MEDICAL SCHOOL ADMISSIONS

Miscellaneous Questions:

Should the federal government reinstate the death penalty? Explain.
What do you expect to be doing 10 years from now?
How would you attract physicians to rural areas?
Why do you want to attend our medical school?
What other medical schools have you applied to?
Have you been to other interviews?

COMMENTS: You will do fine in this grab-bag category as long as you stick to the strategies previously iterated.

Ending Questions:

What would you do if you were not accepted to a medical school?
How do you think you did in this interview?
Do you have any questions?

COMMENTS: The only thing more important than a good first impression is a good finish in order to leave a positive lasting impression. They are looking for students who are so committed to medicine that they will not only re-apply to medical school if not accepted, but they would also strive to improve on those aspects of their application which prevented them from being accepted in the first attempt. All these questions should be answered with a quiet confidence. If you are given an opportunity to ask questions, though you should not flaunt your knowledge, you should establish that you are well-informed. For example: "I have read that you have changed your curriculum to a more patient-oriented and self-directed learning approach. I was wondering how the medical students are getting along with these new changes." Be sure, however, not to ask a question unless you are genuinely interested in the answer.

2.5 The Interview: Questions, Answers and Feedback

Specific interview questions can be found online for free at futuredoctor.net. Dr. Ferdinand reproduced and captured the intense experience of a medical school interview on video to be used as a learning tool. "The Gold Standard Medical School Interview: Questions, Tips and Answers" DVD was filmed live in HD on campus in front of a group of premedical students - most of whom were invited for medical school interviews. A volunteer is interviewed in front of the class and the entire interview is conducted as if it were the real thing. After the interview, an analysis of each question and the mindset behind it is discussed in an open forum format. If you are not sure that you have the interviewing skills to be accepted to medical school, then it is a must-see video.

Whenever Dr. Ferdinand is conducting his live Medical School Interview seminar in Sydney, London or Dublin, the dates will be posted at GAMSAT-prep.com.

AUTOBIOGRAPHICAL MATERIALS AND REFERENCES

3.1 Autobiographical Materials

Autobiographical materials include resumes, CVs, personal statements, questionnaires and other written materials that may be required when applying to medical school or a graduate program. In general, these materials and letters of reference are required by almost all institutions in the US and Canada but relatively few institutions in Australia, Ireland and the UK. Consult individual institutions regarding their requirements. Just in case the information can serve you well, we have included it. Autobiographical materials are a sort of *written interview*. Thus the same objectives, preparation, and strategies apply as previously mentioned for interviews. However, there are some unique factors.

For example, you can begin writing long in advance of the deadline. The ideal way to prepare is to use your computer or to have a few sheets of paper at home where you continually write any accomplishments or interesting experiences you have had anytime in your life! By starting this process early, months later you should, hopefully(!), have a long list from which to choose information appropriate for the autobiographical materials. Your resume or curriculum vitae may also be of value.

Be sure to write rough drafts and have qualified individuals proofread it for you. Spelling and grammatical errors should not exist.

The document should be written on the appropriate paper and/or in the format as stated in the directions. Do not surpass your word and/or space limit. Usually the submission is online but if they require it on paper, ideally, it would be laser printed on business paper. The document should be so pretty that your parents should want to frame it and hang it in the living room! Handwritten or typed material with 'liquid paper' or 'white-out' is simply not impressive.

Your document must be clearly organized. If you are given directive questions then organization should not be a problem. However, if you are given open-ended questions or if you are told, for example, to write a 1000 word essay about yourself, adequate organization is key. There are two general ways you can organize such a response: *chronological* or *thematic*. However, they are not mutually exclusive.

In a **chronological** response, you are organized by doing a systematic review of important events through time. In writing an essay or letter, one could start with an interesting or amusing story from childhood and then highlight important events chronologically and in concordance with the instructions.

In the **thematic** approach a general theme is presented from the outset and then verified through examples at any time in your life. For example, imagine the following statement somewhere in the introduction of an autobiographical letter/essay:

My concept of the good physician is one who has a solid intellectual capacity, extensive social skills, and a creative ability. I have strived to attain and demonstrate such skills.

Following such an introduction to a thematic response, the essayist can link events from anytime to the general theme of the essay. Each theme would thus be examined in turn.

And finally, keep in mind the advice given for interviews since much of it applies here as well. For example, the appropriate use of an amusing story, anecdote, or an interesting analogy can make your document an interesting one to read. And, as for interviews, specific examples are more memorable than overly generalized statements.

3.2 Letters of Reference

Letters of reference (a.k.a. *assessments* which are written by *referees*) are required by most medical schools in North America. It provides an opportunity for an admissions committee to see what other people think of you. Consequently, it is often viewed as an important aspect of your application package.

Choose the people who will submit your letter of reference in accordance with instructions from the medical schools to which you are applying. If no such instructions are given, then construct a list of possible referees. Choose from this list individuals who: (i) you can trust; (ii) are reliable; (iii) can write, at least, reasonably well; (iv) understand the importance of your application; and (v) can present with some confidence attributes you have which are consistent with those of a good physician. A good balance would be to have one referee who is a professor, another a physician and a third who has experience with your social skills or achievements.

Often students either want or are told to have someone as a referee who they do not know well (i.e. a professor). In such a case choose your referee prudently. If they agree to give you a recommendation, give them your resume, curriculum vitae, or any other autobiographical materials you may have. Alternatively, you may ask to arrange a mini-interview. Either way, you would have armed your referee with information which can be used in a specific and personal manner in the letter of reference.

People are not paid to write you a letter of reference! Therefore, make it as easy as possible for them. Give them an ample amount of time before the deadline for submission. Also, supply them with a stamped envelope with the appropriate address inscribed. Besides being the polite thing to do, they may also be impressed by your organization. And finally, once the letter of reference has been sent, do not forget to send a "Thank-you" card to your referee.

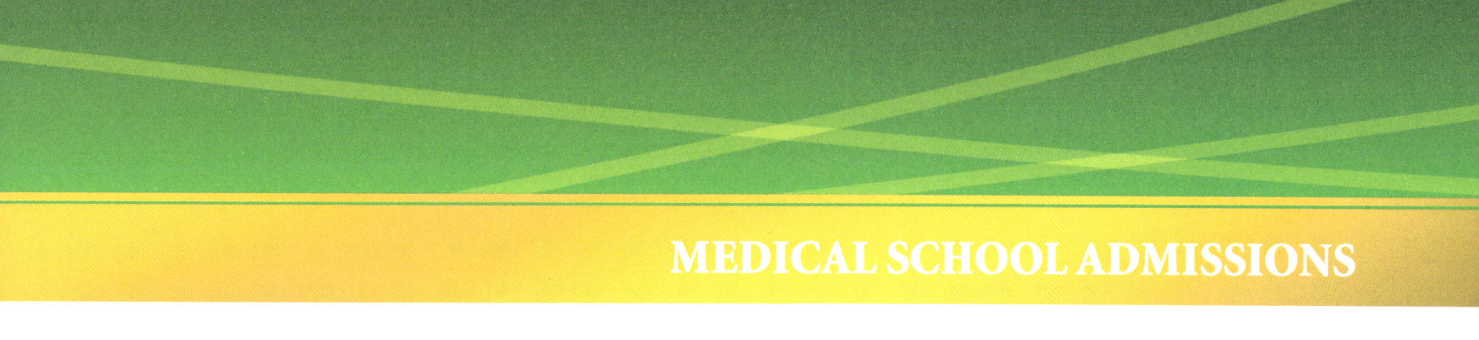

$\mathcal{A} + \mathcal{B} = ?$

GAMSAT-Prep.com

UNDERSTANDING THE GAMSAT

PART II

UNDERSTANDING THE GAMSAT

THE STRUCTURE OF THE GAMSAT

1.1 Introduction

The Graduate Australian Medical School Admissions Test (GAMSAT) is a prerequisite for admission to participating medical and dental schools in Australia, Ireland and the UK. Each year thousands of applicants submit GAMSAT test results to medical, dental and graduate schools as well as other programmes (i.e. pharmacy, optometry, veterinary science, etc.). While the actual weight given to GAMSAT scores in the admissions process varies from school to school, often they are regarded in a similar manner to your university GPA (i.e. your academic standing).

The GAMSAT is available to any student who has already completed a bachelor's degree, or who will be enrolled in their penultimate (second to last) or final year of study for a bachelor's degree, at the time of sitting the test. The test is administered as follows: test dates in Australia and Ireland are conventionally in March; the test date in the UK is usually in September. Students can sit the GAMSAT twice in one year. As examples, in Australia: GAMSAT Australia (March) then GAMSAT UK in Melbourne (September); in the UK: GAMSAT UK (September) and then GAMSAT Ireland (March).

GAMSAT results are generally valid for 2 years. There is no restriction on the number of times you may sit the GAMSAT. Currently, results from sitting the GAMSAT in any one country can be used in applying to any other country that requires the GAMSAT.

To access the most up to date information and to register for the GAMSAT, consider visiting one of the following websites:

> **Australia:** www.gamsat.acer.edu.au
> **Ireland:** www.gamsat-ie.org
> **UK:** www.gamsatuk.org

1.1.1 The *new* MCAT for International Applicants or for US/Canada

The new Medical College Admission Test (MCAT) is a prerequisite for admission to nearly all the medical schools in North America. Each year, over 50,000 applicants to American and English Canadian medical schools submit MCAT test results.

The MCAT is a computer based test (CBT) administered on a Saturday or a weekday, more than 20 times per year. To register for the MCAT, you should consult your undergraduate adviser and register online: www.aamc.org.

GAMSAT-Prep.com
THE GOLD STANDARD

The MCAT can be used by international students applying to medical schools that accept GAMSAT scores. Only international students have the option of sitting the MCAT instead of the GAMSAT. Consult individual programmes for confirmation.

1.2 The Format of the GAMSAT

The GAMSAT aims to test your skills in problem solving, critical thinking, writing as well as mastery and application of concepts in the basic sciences. The exam is divided into three sections. All questions, save for Section II, are multiple choice with 4 options per question. Ten minutes reading time is given for Sections I and III, and five minutes for Section II. The following is your schedule for the test day:

Section I	
Reasoning in the Humanities and Social Sciences	
Questions	75
Time	100 minutes

Section II	
Written Communication	
Questions	2
Time	60 minutes
Lunch	60 minutes

Section III	
Reasoning in Biological and Physical Sciences	
Questions	110
Time	170 minutes

Biological and Physical Sciences collectively include biology, general and organic chemistry at the introductory university level, and physics at essentially the Grade 12 level. Overall, the subject material is weighted as follows:

Biology	40%
Chemistry	40%
Physics	20%

The layout of Section I and Section III are similar with separate "Units" containing stimulus material followed by multiple choice questions. Section I may use excerpts from poems, novels, articles, a cartoon, etc. However, for Section III, the stimulus material can also include a passage, graph, equation(s), text, data, etc.

1.2.1 GAMSAT vs MCAT

UNDERSTANDING THE GAMSAT

The MCAT's most recent incarnation began in 2015. Besides the subjects that the MCAT traditionally covered, which were the same as the GAMSAT, the new MCAT now includes biochemistry, psychology and sociology. It is a computer-based exam with 230 questions and there is no longer an essay section. The total test time is now about 7 h, 30 min. The value of understanding the differences and similarities between the two exams is as follows: (1) some students who are citizens of Australia, Ireland or the UK may choose to also sit the MCAT in order to apply to one of the majority of medical schools in the US and Canada that require the MCAT; (2) currently, international students have the option to sit either the GAMSAT or MCAT in order to submit applications to Australia, Ireland or the UK, some choose to sit the MCAT (or both tests) in order to

Table 1: Comparing the two standardized tests for medical school admissions.

	GAMSAT	**MCAT (before 2007)**	**MCAT (2007-2014)**
Testing method	Paper	Paper	Computer
Total test time	5½ hours	8 hours	5½ hours
Name of Verbal Section	Section 1	Verbal Reasoning	Verbal Reasoning
# Questions; Time	75 questions; 100 min.	65 questions; 85 min.	40 questions; 60 min.
Writing Section	Section 2	Writing Sample	Writing Sample
# Questions; Time	2 questions; 60 min.	2 questions; 60 min.	2 questions; 60 min.
Physical and Biological Sciences*	Section 3	1) Physical Sciences 2) Biological Sciences	1) Physical Sciences 2) Biological Sciences
# Questions; Time	110 questions; 170 min.	154 questions (total); 200 min. (total)	104 questions (total); 140 min. (total)
Breaks	• None between Section I and II • 1 hour for lunch	• 5 min. between sections • 1 hour for lunch	• 5 min. between sections • Lunch optional (max. 1 hour)
Countries	Australia, Ireland, UK	US, Canada	US, Canada
Test Frequency	Once or twice annually per country	Twice annually per country	More than 20 test dates annually
Official Practice Materials	4 booklets (e-books)	10 booklets	1 manual, 8 CBTs (practice tests #3 to #11)

* Physical Sciences includes physics and general or inorganic chemistry. Biological Sciences includes biology and organic chemistry. This table was used with permission from GAMSATtestpreparation.com.

also apply to North American medical programmes.

The 2 tests have both significant similarities and significant differences. The GAMSAT makes it possible for a student with little science background to learn independently and, with strong reasoning skills, succeed. Whereas, the MCAT requires formal training in the sciences because of the number of equations and facts that are considered 'presumed knowledge'.

Thus the GAMSAT leans on reasoning while the MCAT contains more memorization (though nowhere near as much memorization as required for an average introductory level university science course). It is the issue of presumed knowledge that makes some students say that the MCAT is more difficult but clearly that depends on your pre-exam reading history and learning experiences.

1.2.2 English as a Second Language (ESL)

Many ESL students will need to pay extra attention to Section I and Section II of the GAMSAT. Specific advice for all students will be presented in the chapters that follow. This advice should be taken very seriously for ESL students.

Having said that, GAMSAT scores are subjected to a statistical analysis to check that each question is fair, valid and reliable. Test questions in development are scrutinized in order to minimize gender, ethnic or religious bias, in order to affirm that the test is culturally fair.

Candidates whose native language is not English are permitted to bring a printed bilingual dictionary on test day for use in Section I and Section II only. The pages must be unmarked and all paper notes removed. Any candidate using this option must submit the dictionary to the Supervisor for inspection before the test begins.

Depending on your English skills, you may or may not benefit from an English reading or writing summer course. Of course, you would have the option of deciding whether or not you would want to take such a course for credit. GAMSAT-prep.com also offers an online speed reading/comprehension program with extra practice questions.

1.3 How the GAMSAT is Scored

The GAMSAT is scored for each of the three sections individually. The sections consisting of multiple choice questions are first scored right or wrong resulting in a raw

UNDERSTANDING THE GAMSAT

score. Note that wrong answers are worth the same as unanswered questions so ALWAYS ANSWER ALL THE QUESTIONS even if you are not sure of certain answers. The raw score is then converted to a scaled score ranging from 0 (lowest) to 100 (highest). Essentially, the scores are scaled to ensure that the same proportion of individual marks within each section are given from year to year (using Item Response Theory). The scaled score is neither a percentage nor a percentile. It is not possible to accurately replicate this scoring system at home.

Section II is marked by three independent markers from each zone. A scale of 10 points is used. Should there be a difference of 5 or more in two scores then an additional marker will be used. Ultimately, the three closest scores are totaled for the Section II raw score which is then converted to a scaled score.

You will receive a score for each of the three sections, together with an Overall GAMSAT Score. The Overall Score is a weighted average of the three component scores.

The Overall GAMSAT Score is determined using the following formula:

Overall Score = (1 × Section I + 1 × Section II + 2 × Section III) ÷ 4

Standards for interviews or admissions may vary for both Sectional Scores and the Overall GAMSAT Score. For example, one particular medical school may establish a cutoff (minimum) of 50 for any given section and 60 for the Overall GAMSAT Score. Contact individual programmes for specific score requirements.

The GAMSAT may include a small number of questions which will not be scored. These questions are either used to calibrate the exam or were found to be either too ambiguous or too difficult to be counted or are trial questions which may be used in the future. So if you see a question that you think is off the wall, unanswerable or inappropriate for your level of knowledge, it could well be one of these questions so never panic! And of course, answer every question because guessing provides a 25% chance of being correct while not answering provides a 0% chance of being correct!

1.3.1 GAMSAT Scores in Different Countries

GAMSAT scores are interchangeable and can be used to apply to any university that requires the GAMSAT. You may sit GAMSAT UK, Australia or Ireland to apply to universities in any of these countries.

You must ensure that your scores have not expired if you are using a score from a previous sitting of the GAMSAT (i.e. GAMSAT scores cannot be more than two years old). Otherwise, you choose the GAMSAT score

GAMSAT-Prep.com
THE GOLD STANDARD

that you wish to submit for consideration for admissions.

Since there is no limit to the number of times you can sit the GAMSAT, you may even choose to sit the exam twice in one year: for example, GAMSAT Australia or Ireland in March and then GAMSAT UK in September.

Any two tests on different examination dates will have, essentially, the same format; however, the questions are (for the most part) different for each exam.

How many times did you sit the GAMSAT?	
Once	67%
Twice	27%
3 Times	6%
2010 Gold Standard GAMSAT survey at the University of Sydney (Usyd Medical Science Society), n>100, average reported GAMSAT score (most recent): 62.2.	

1.3.2 Average, Good and High GAMSAT Scores

Please keep in mind that the percentile rank indicates your test performance relative to all the students who sat the same test on the same day. It records the percentage of students whose scores were lower than yours.

Score	Percentile	Score
56-58	50th	average
61-63	75th	usually good*
73 or higher	98th	very high

*Please note, a "good" score may be good enough for admittance to one particular medical school but below the cutoff of another. Consult the websites of the medical institutions to which you intend to apply. Click on your national icon at the following webpage to get a summary of scores required at institutions near you: www.gamsat-prep.com/GAMSAT-scores.

30   THE STRUCTURE OF THE GAMSAT

UNDERSTANDING THE GAMSAT

An average GAMSAT score is often around 56-58 and a high GAMSAT score is over 63. Please keep in mind when evaluating the statistics provided and the graphic: this data is meant to give you a general idea of the process. The numbers can vary somewhat from one exam sitting to another. And as mentioned previously, you cannot replicate the scoring system at home since there is no formula provided to convert raw scores into official GAMSAT scores.

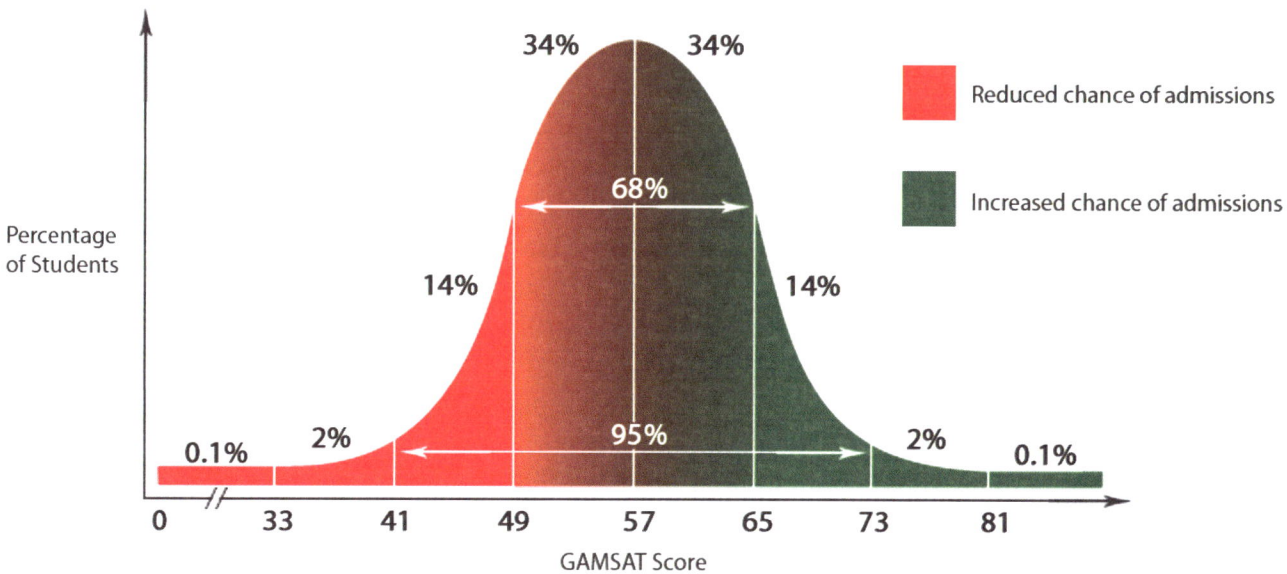

Figure 1: Typical Overall GAMSAT Score Distribution (Approx.)

1.3.3 When are the scores released?

The test date in Australia and Ireland is traditionally in March while it is usually in September for the UK. GAMSAT results are released within 2 months of sitting the exam. Candidates are emailed login information to access their personal results report. Should there be any changes to the exam dates or any other modifications, get the up to date information online at one of the ACER websites listed in Section 1.4.

1.4 ACER

The GAMSAT has been developed by the Australian Council for Educational Research (ACER) with the Consortium of Graduate Medical Schools to help in the selection of students to graduate-entry programmes. ACER administers the GAMSAT and publishes several important sets of materials which are available on their website: i) GAMSAT Practice Questions; ii) GAMSAT Sample Questions; and iii) GAMSAT Practice Test and GAMSAT Practice Test 2 which are released operational full-length tests. GAMSAT Practice Test 2 was released in 2010 for the very first time.

These materials can be obtained online:

Australia: www.gamsat.acer.edu.au
Ireland: www.gamsat-ie.org
UK: www.gamsatuk.org

Some students purchase commercially available simulated GAMSAT exams without ever having seen the materials from ACER. This is often a serious mistake. If you are looking to sit an actual GAMSAT, you go to the source. The source of the GAMSAT is ACER. Once you have been exposed to their style of questions and stimulus material, you will be in a better position to accurately assess other simulated practice material should you require it.

There are some students who feel that their experience with the real GAMSAT was not well represented by ACER's practice materials. Usually, this is not a problem with the materials; rather, it is a problem with the technique used in preparation. We will discuss this in detail in the next chapter.

Did you feel the ACER practice tests accurately represented the real exam?	
YES	63%
NO	37%

2010 Gold Standard GAMSAT survey at the University of Sydney (Usyd Medical Science Society), n>100, average reported GAMSAT score (most recent): 62.2.

UNDERSTANDING THE GAMSAT

THE RECIPE FOR GAMSAT SUCCESS

2.1 The Important Ingredients

- Time, Motivation
- Read from varied sources
- The Gold Standard GAMSAT DVD
- A review of the 4 basic GAMSAT sciences

GAMSAT-Specific Information
- The Gold Standard GAMSAT textbook
- *optional:* The Gold Standard DVDs, MP3s or online programs (GAMSAT-prep.com)
- *optional:* GS Essay Correction Service or GAMSAT University online.

- *AVOID:* textbooks (too much detail), upper level courses for the purpose of improving GAMSAT scores

GAMSAT-Specific Problems
- Free chapter review problems
- The Gold Standard GAMSAT test (GS-1)
- Official ACER practice materials and full-length tests
- *optional:* more full-length GAMSAT practice tests (GAMSAT-prep.com)

If you could prepare all over again, what would you do differently?	
Top 5 Responses	
1	Study more
2	More practice essays
3	Newspapers, current events
4	More multiple choice questions
5	More science review
2010 Gold Standard GAMSAT survey at the University of Sydney (Usyd Medical Science Society), n>100, average reported GAMSAT score (most recent): 62.2.	

GAMSAT-Prep.com
THE GOLD STANDARD

2.2 The Proper Mix

1) Study regularly and start early. There is a lot of material to cover and you will need sufficient time to review it all adequately. Creating a study schedule is often effective. Starting early will reduce your stress level in the weeks leading up to the exam and may make your studying easier. Depending on your English skills and the quality of your science background, a good rule of thumb is: 3-6 hours/day of study for 3-6 months.

2) Keep focused and enjoy the material you are learning. Forget all past negative learning experiences so you can open your mind to the information with a positive attitude. Given an open mind and some time to consider what you are learning, you will find most of the information tremendously interesting. Motivation can be derived from a sincere interest in learning and by keeping in mind your long term goals.

3) Section I and II preparation: Begin by reading the advice given in Chapters 3 and 4 in this textbook as well as The Gold Standard GAMSAT DVD. Time yourself and practice, practice, practice with various resources for Section I as needed at GAMSAT-prep.com and of course the ACER materials. You can also review free corrected Section II essays at GAMSAT-prep.com/forum.

For Section I, you should be sure to understand each and every mistake you make as to ensure there will be improvement. For Section II, you should have someone who has good writing skills read, correct, and comment on your essays. Have the person read Chapter 4 for guidance on what they should be evaluating. And finally, you also have the option of having your essays corrected, scored and returned to you with personal advice (GAMSAT-prep.com). ACER has introduced a program to automatically correct practice essays which you should seriously consider.

4) Section III preparation: The Gold Standard is not associated with ACER in any way; however, contained herein is each and every topic that you are responsible for in the Biological and Physical Sciences, as evidenced by past testing patterns. Thus the most directed and efficient study plan is to begin by reviewing - not memorizing - the science sections in this textbook. While doing your science survey, you should take notes specifically on topics that are marked Memorize or Understand on the first page of each chapter. Your notes, we call them Gold Notes (!!), should be very concise (no longer than one page per chapter). Every week, you should study from your Gold Notes at least a few times.

As you are incorporating the information from the science review, do the Biological and Physical Sciences problems included in the free chapter review questions online at GAMSAT-prep.com. This is the best way to more clearly define the depth of your understanding and to get you accustomed to the most challenging of the questions you can expect on the GAMSAT.

UNDERSTANDING THE GAMSAT

5) **Sit practice exams.** Ideally, you would finish your science review in The Gold Standard text and/or the science review online videos (or DVDs) at least a couple of months prior to the exam date. Then each week you can sit a practice exam under simulated test conditions and thoroughly review each exam after completion. Scores in practice exams should improve over time. Success depends on what you do between the first and the last exam. You can start with ACER's "GAMSAT Practice Questions" then continue with The Gold Standard (GS) practice exams and then complete the practice materials from ACER.

You should sit practice exams as you would the actual test: in one sitting within the expected time limits. Doing practice exams will increase your confidence and allow you to see what is expected of you. It will make you realize the constraints imposed by time limits in completing the entire test. It will also allow you to identify the areas in which you may be lacking.

Some students can answer all GAMSAT questions quite well if they only had more time. Thus you must time yourself during practice and monitor your time during the test. On average, you will have 1.3 minutes per question in Section I and 1.5 minutes per question for Section III. In other words, every 30 minutes, you should check to be sure that you have completed approximately 23 questions (Section I) or 20 questions (Section III). If not, then you always guess on "time consuming questions" in order to catch up and, if you have time at the end, you return to properly evaluate the questions you skipped.

Set aside at least the equivalent of a full day to review the explanations for EVERY test question. Do NOT dismiss any wrong answer as a "stupid mistake." You made that error for a reason so you must work that out in your mind to reduce the risk that it occurs again. You can reduce your risk by testproofing answers (a technique first described in the GAMSAT DVD: spending 5-10 seconds being critical of your response) and by considering the questions in the table below.

1. Why did you get the question wrong (or correct)?
2. What question-type or passage-type gives you repeated difficulty?
3. What is your mindset when facing a particular passage?
4. Did you monitor your time during the test?
5. Are most of your errors at the beginning or the end of the test?
6. Did you eliminate answer choices when you could and actually cross them out?
7. For Section I, what was the author's mindset and main idea for each passage?
8. Was your main problem a lack of content review or a lack of practice?
9. In which specific science content areas do you need improvement?
10. Have you designed a study schedule to address your weaknesses?

GAMSAT-Prep.com
THE GOLD STANDARD

6) Big on concepts, small on memorization: Remember that the GAMSAT will primarily test your understanding of concepts. The GAMSAT is not designed to measure your ability to memorize tons of scientific facts and trivia, but both your knowledge and understanding of concepts are critical.

Evidently, some material in this textbook must be memorized; for example, some very basic science equations (i.e. weight W = mg, Ohm's Law, Newton's Second Law, etc.), rules of logarithms, trigonometric functions, the phases in mitosis and meiosis, naming organic compounds and other basic science facts. Based on past testing patterns, we will guide you. Nonetheless, ==for the most part, your objective should be to try to understand, rather than memorize== the biology, physics and chemistry material you review. This may appear vague now, but as you immerse yourself in the science review chapters and practice material, you will more clearly understand what is expected of you.

7) Relax once in a while! While the GAMSAT requires a lot of preparation, you should not forsake all your other activities to study. Try to keep exercising, maintain a social life and do things you enjoy. If you balance work with things which relax you, you will study more effectively overall.

2.3 It's GAMSAT Time!

1) On the night before the exam, try to get a good night sleep. The GAMSAT is physically draining and it is in your best interest to be well rested when you sit the exam.

2) Avoid last minute cramming. On the morning of the exam, do not begin studying ad hoc. You will not learn anything effectively, and noticing something you do not know or will not remember might reduce your confidence and lower your score unnecessarily. Just get up, eat a good breakfast, consult your Gold Notes (the top level information that you personally compiled) and go do the exam.

3) Eat breakfast! It will make it possible for you to have the food energy needed to go through the first two parts of the exam.

4) Pack a light lunch. Avoid greasy food that will make you drowsy. You do not want to feel sleepy for the afternoon section. Avoid sugar-packed snacks as they will cause a 'sugar low' eventually and will also make you drowsy. A chocolate bar or other sweet highly caloric food could, however, be very useful during the last section when you may be tired. The 'sugar low' will hit you only after you have completed the exam when you do not have to be awake!

5) Make sure you answer all the questions! You do not get penalized for incorrect answers, so always choose something even if you have to guess. If you run out of time, pick a letter and use it to answer all the remaining questions. ACER performs statistical

analyses on every test so no one letter will give you an unfair advantage so just choose your "lucky" letter and move on!

6) Pace yourself. Do not get bogged down trying to answer a difficult question. If the question is very difficult, make a mark beside it, guess, move on to the next question and return later if time is remaining.

7) Remember that some of the questions may be thrown out as inappropriate, used solely to calibrate the test or trial questions. If you find that you cannot answer some of the questions, do not despair. It is possible they could be questions used for these purposes.

8) Do not let others psyche you out! Some people will be saying between exam sections, 'It went great. What a joke!' Ignore them. Often these types may just be trying to boost their own confidence or to make themselves look good in front of their friends. Just focus on what you have to do and tune out the other examinees.

9) Do not study at lunch. You need the time to recuperate and rest. Eat, avoid the people discussing the test sections and relax! At most, you can review your Gold Notes.

10) Before reading the "stimulus material" of the problem (the passage, article, etc.), some students find it more efficient to quickly read the questions first. In this way, as soon as you read something in the stimulus material which brings to mind a question you have read, you can answer immediately (this is especially helpful for Section I). Otherwise, if you read the text first and then the questions, you may end up wasting time searching through the text for answers.

11) Read the text and questions carefully! Often students leave out a word or two while reading, which can completely change the sense of the problem. ==Pay special attention to words in italics, CAPS, bolded, or underlined.== Underline or circle anything you believe might be important in the passage.

12) You must be both diligent and careful with the way you fill out your answer document because you will not be given extra time to either check it or fill it in later.

13) If you run out of time, just do the questions. In other words, only read the part of the passage which your question specifically requires in order for you to get the correct answer.

14) Expel any relevant equation onto your exam booklet! Even if the question is of a theoretical nature, sometimes equations contain the answers and they are much more objective than the reasoning of a nervous pre-medical student! In physics, it is often helpful to draw a picture or diagram. Arrows are valuable in representing vectors.

15) Consider having the following on test day: a watch (mobile phones are not permitted in the exam room) and layers of clothes so that you are ready for too much heat or an overzealous air conditioning unit.

GAMSAT-Prep.com
THE GOLD STANDARD

16) Solving the problem may involve algebraic manipulation of equations and/or numerical calculations. Be sure that you know what all the variables in the equation stand for and that you are using the equation in the appropriate circumstance.

In chemistry and physics, the use of **dimensional analysis** will help you keep track of units <u>and</u> solve some problems where you might have forgotten the relevant equations. Dimensional analysis relies on the manipulation of units and is the source of many easy GAMSAT marks every year. For example, if you are asked for the energy involved in maintaining a 60 watt bulb lit for two minutes you can pull out the appropriate equations <u>or</u>: i) recognize that your objective (unknown = energy) is in joules; ii) recall that a watt is a joule per second; iii) convert minutes into seconds. {note that minutes and seconds cancel leaving joules as an answer}

$$60 \frac{\text{joules}}{\text{second}} \times 2 \text{ minutes} \times 60 \frac{\text{seconds}}{\text{minutes}}$$

$$= 7200 \text{ joules} \quad \text{or} \quad 7.2 \text{ kilojoules}$$

17) The final step in problem solving is to ask yourself: *is my answer reasonable*? For example, if you would have done the preceding problem and your answer was 7200 kilojoules, intuitively this should strike you as an exorbitant amount of energy for an everyday light bulb to remain lit for two minutes! It would then be of value to recheck your calculations. {'intuition' in science is often learned through the experience of doing many problems}

18) Whenever doing calculations, the following will increase your speed: (i) manipulate variables but plug in values only when necessary; (ii) avoid decimals, use fractions wherever possible; (iii) square roots or cube roots can be converted to the power (*exponent*) of 1/2 or 1/3, respectively; (iv) before calculating, check to see if the possible answers are sufficiently far apart such that your values can be approximated (i.e. 19.2 ≈ 20, 185 ≈ 200). Since 2012, calculators ceased being permitted for the GAMSAT. We added over 100 pages of GAMSAT Math to this new edition to help you to become quick and efficient with your calculations.

19) Are you great in biology and organic chemistry but weak in the physical sciences? Since biology and organic chemistry represent more than 1/2 your science score, you should attack those problems from the outset to ensure that you have fully benefitted from your strengths. Now you can go back and complete the physics and general chemistry. This is just an example of 'examsmanship': managing the test to maximize your performance.

20) Learn to relax or at least you must learn to manage your anxiety. Channel that extra energy into acute awareness of the information being presented to you. If you have a history of anxiety during exams to the extent that you feel that it affected your score, then you should start learning relaxation techniques now. You can search online regarding various methods such as visualization, deep breathing and other techniques that can even be used during the exam if needed.

UNDERSTANDING THE GAMSAT

REVIEW FOR SECTION I

3.1 Overview

Section I of the GAMSAT is, for many applicants, the most difficult section to do well. This can be explained by the absence of an overall set of facts to study in order to prepare. Some applicants, due to the lack of review material, neglect to prepare for this section.

While the best preparation is regular reading from a variety of sources throughout your high school and undergraduate studies, it is also possible to improve your ability to do well in this section as you approach the test date. You should not neglect to prepare for this section as it accounts for one of your final GAMSAT numerical scores!

Section I is called "Reasoning in Humanities and Social Sciences." You are provided 100 minutes to complete 75 questions. This section consists of a number of "Units" where each Unit presents stimulus material and a number of multiple choice questions (4 options per question).

The stimulus material in Section I can be anything from a poem, a cartoon, a picture, an extract from a play, novel, song, instructional manual or magazine. Essentially anything that involves words or symbols and thinking is fair game. There is no specific presumed knowledge required to answer any of the questions. Reasoning, analysis, timing and pacing are all key components to success.

Which GAMSAT section was the easiest?	
Section I	5%
Section II	54%
Section III	41%
2010 Gold Standard GAMSAT survey at the University of Sydney, n>100, <5% with a non-science background; average reported GAMSAT score (most recent): 62.2.	

3.2 How to Improve Your Section I Score

3.2.1 One Year or More Before the GAMSAT

Read! Be known as a "voracious reader"! Read any novel that interests you. Read editorials from national, international and local newspapers (among your options: the reference section of the library or online).

For those of you with a short attention span: Ted.com. With Ted.com you will have short, powerful lectures on a great range of topics - many of which will stick to you and create new tools in your use of language: analogies, examples, stories which span the globe as well as time. Ted.com is a free website. We will always update further suggestions on GAMSAT-prep.com which you can find by clicking on FREE GAMSAT in the top menu. Please do note that Section 1 is not a test about pre-existing knowledge but about reasoning based on the given stimulus. Hence you should go through these materials with the purpose of identifying the main ideas or arguments of the speakers or writers.

At least once per week, for 1-3 hours, you should read among the following (all of which are available in a university library or online):

- **Novels**
- **Philosophy** (i.e. The Meaning of Things by AC Grayling)
- **Local Newspapers** Most popular conservative and liberal national newspapers: editorials (because they tend to be argumentative) and newspaper cartoons since they use a style of humour and presentation that is fair game for the GAMSAT.
- **The Economist**
- **The New York Times**

Your exposure to knowledge outside of the sciences, creativity, culture, poetry, current affairs, political cartoons and more will have a significant impact on your performance in Section I and Section II. The added benefit - which you may only appreciate later - will be your improved performance in the medical school interviews and possibly even less obvious at the moment - an increased well-roundedness.

Be sure that when you are reading, especially opinion pieces, you are reading actively. Continually ask questions …

1) How would you summarise or simplify what is being presented?
2) Identify the main points.
3) How would you describe the author's attitude to the topic?

UNDERSTANDING THE GAMSAT

3.2.2 One Year or Less Before the GAMSAT

Read section 3.2.1 one more time! Even at this point in your preparation, being a voracious reader - with all that it entails - should be your goal. Besides reading, you need to practice. The best strategy is to take ACER's GAMSAT Practice Questions (it is not a full-length test) and sit Section I as a timed exam and then review your mistakes. This should be done as soon as you commence your preparation. The ACER booklets are the closest that you will get to the real exam.

Using one of the shorter practice tests as a baseline of your test performance under timed conditions will help you understand what is expected. Take note of the type of passages and questions that give you the most difficulty (e.g., poetry, cartoon, prose, commentaries). This will enable you to slowly build on your weaknesses and target particular problem areas.

The two full-length ACER practice exams should be completed later in the preparation process to further measure your performance while providing enough time to continually address your weaknesses.

If you performed well and understood the source of your errors then you will only require ACER and the Gold Standard (GS) GAMSATs in order to complete your preparation for Section I.

If, on the other hand, you struggled in the test or struggled to understand your mistakes then you may need additional work on strategies, practice or, as mentioned previously, a formal course for or without credit. An optional Section I GAMSAT program can be found at GAMSAT-prep.com.

Practice Problems
• ACER materials
• GS book and online

Practice Exams
• ACER materials
• GS book and online

Additional Practice Options
• GAMSAT-prep.com

3.2.3 Exam Strategies

1) You will be allotted 10 minutes reading time before Section I begins. Though writing must not commence until signalled, you should use your reading time to begin working through questions, and answering them in your mind. If you 'browse', there should be a purpose; for example, you are seeking your favourite question type, like poetry or drama, to read and to mentally construct answers.

2) Read carefully and annotate. The test is yours. You paid for it so do not be afraid to strike-out, circle or more rarely, to make notes. Doing so helps you to read actively and then later, to find keywords or points without having to search aimlessly.

3) Always try to identify the main points of each paragraph, the idea behind the text and the structure of the passage as you read. Doing this will make it easier for you to answer the questions. Some students find it helpful to do the following: just before you read from each Unit, imagine someone young that you know - for example, a younger brother, sister, cousin, etc. Imagine that once you finish reading the stimulus material, you will have to explain it to them in words that they understand. Keep that imagery during your evaluation of the material so you have a heightened sense of awareness and responsibility for what you are reading.

4) The "Questions First, Passage Once Technique": some applicants like to quickly scan the questions prior to reading the text. Then they read the passage and answer questions as they read the information (usu. the questions are placed in the same order as you would find the answers in the passage). You may find it more efficient to work in that way. Try one of the practice exams this way and, if you find it easier to answer the questions correctly, you should use this method on the actual GAMSAT.

5) Pace yourself. A major problem in this section is that test takers run out of time. Read at a reasonable speed. You want to read carefully but quickly. You will have about 1.3 minutes per question in Section I. Every 30 minutes, you should check your watch to be sure that you have completed approximately 23 questions. Of course, you can judge time in any way you want (20, 25, 30 minute intervals, etc.). But decide on a system when you are practicing then stick to that system on exam day. Of course, if you have not completed the desired number of questions in the interval that you have set for yourself, then you consistently guess on time-consuming questions in order to catch up and, if you have time at the end, you return to properly evaluate the questions you skipped or marked.

6) 'Examsmanship': Play to your strengths. The following can be quite effective for both Section I and Section III. During your reading time, identify the locations of your favourite content and begin to consider your answers. When the exam begins, answer all the question types that you are most comfortable with and then go back to answer the rest of the questions. Fill out your answer sheet as you go along but be very diligent to ensure you are always answering the correct question. As always, keep an eye on the time. By playing to your strengths, you can maximise your score.

7)   Do not skim through the stimulus material. Ideally, you only want to read through once in order to answer the questions correctly. This way you will be able to finish in the allotted time. Of course, referring back to material that you annotated is not the same as having to re-read a passage because you read too quickly the first time.

8)   We have already established that reading diverse material in the period leading up to the exam will be useful since the stimulus material will be from a variety of sources. Use this reality to help you create a mindset that, in the exam, you are prepared for "edutainment." You are ready to learn interesting, vibrant material which sometimes borders on a form of entertainment (novels, poems, cartoons, some articles, etc.). After completing a Unit, look forward to what you can learn and discover in the next Unit. Having properly prepared and then to sit the exam with the right attitude will give you an edge.

3.2.4 Question and Answer Techniques

1)   Process of Elimination (PoE): cross out any answers that are obviously wrong. Oftentimes, after crossing out clearly wrong answers, you will find yourself in a dilemma between two closely similar options. In this case, you should choose the more encompassing answer. For instance, if you cannot discriminate between options A and B, ask yourself: Does A include and speak for B? Does B include or speak for A? Choose the option that incorporates the idea of the other.

2)   Beware of the Extreme: words such as *always, never, perfect, totally*, and *completely* are often (but not always) clues that the answer choice is incorrect.

3)   Comfortable Words: moderate words such as *normally, often, at times*, and *ordinarily* are often included in answer choices that are correct.

4)   Mean Statements: mean or politically incorrect statements are highly unlikely to be included in a correct answer choice. For example, if you see any of the following statements in an answer choice, you can pretty much guarantee that it is not the correct answer:
   Parents should abuse their children.
   Poor people are lazy.
   Religion is socially destructive.
   Torture is usually necessary.

5)   Never lose sight of the question. By the time students read answer choices **C**. and **D**., some have forgotten the question and are simply looking for "true" sounding statements; you can then fall into the next trap:

True but False and False but True: for example,

Answer Choice D.: Most people are of average height. → This is a true statement.

However, the question was: What is the weight of most people?

Therefore, the true statement becomes the incorrect answer!

Continually check the question and check or cross out right and wrong answers.

6) Be on the lookout for qualifiers such as NOT. These may or may not be emphasised in the question stem or the options. They can also come in the form of double negatives in an attempt to confound the exam candidate.

3.3 Style of Questions

i) **Knowledge:** Simply put, you will not be asked questions based on prior knowledge. The very simplest of GAMSAT questions may ask you to recall information from a passage; however, this is rare. Most questions will require a higher level of reasoning and analysis.

ii) **Comprehension:** Identify key concepts and/or facts in a passage. This will require the candidate to infer, summarise and translate from the information presented.

iii) **Application:** Use the information presented in the passage to solve problems. This involves applying knowledge to new or existing problems presented in the stimulus/questions.

iv) **Analysis:** These types of questions require a holistic view of the stimulus and questions; they ask the candidate to organise ideas based on patterns and trends.

v) **Synthesis:** Use current information to create new ideas. Synthesis-style questions build further upon the inferences made in more basic comprehension questions, and often come after comprehension questions within a unit. These questions ask candidates to make greater, more difficult inferences.

vi) **Evaluation:** These are the most cognitively challenging questions and require candidates to evaluate, judge and consider ideas or facts at a much higher and nuanced resolution. Often, many of the answer options will appear correct thus higher logic must be used to develop the answer in a process of elimination. Look out for words such as 'least', 'closest', 'most' as they tend to be used in this style of question.

UNDERSTANDING THE GAMSAT

3.4 Online Help

You can get Section 1 help online including over 20 mini-tests through GAMSAT University at GAMSAT-prep.com. You can find general advice for written verbal skills at About.com.

To access our latest suggestions for all GAMSAT sections including Section 1, go to GAMSAT-prep.com and click FREE GAMSAT in the top menu.

3.5 Types of Questions

Before we address the particular types of questions that you may be asked, it is useful to understand the nature of GAMSAT questions in general, and Section 1 questions in particular. Bloom's Taxonomy is an educational tool used to categorise questions that may be asked within an academic context. The levels of Bloom's model ascend according to the level of cognition required to answer particular questions. GAMSAT questions require candidates to exercise the levels leading towards the top of this model. Essentially, you will not be asked to simply recall or comprehend information you have read. Rather, the great majority of questions will require you to carry out complex cognitive tasks such as inferring, organising and evaluating.

Please note that the styles of questions discussed in Section 3.3 correspond to the different levels of thinking skills in Bloom's Taxonomy, namely:

- Knowledge
- Comprehension
- Application
- Analysis
- Synthesis
- Evaluation

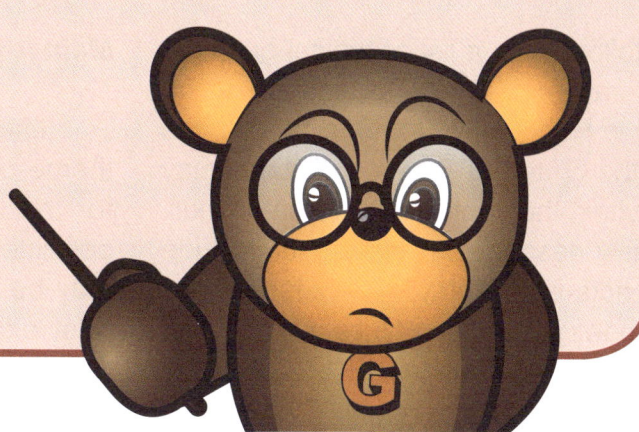

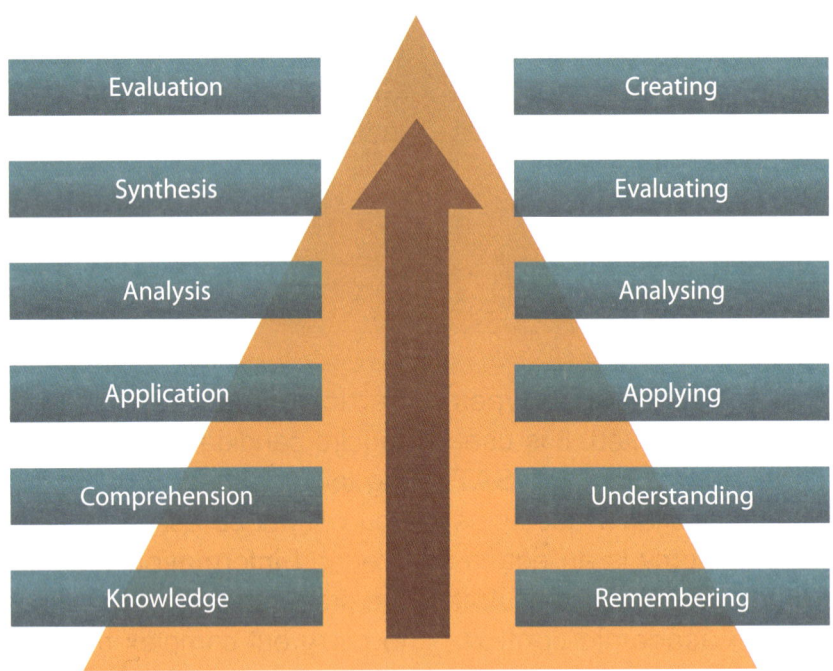

Figure 2: Bloom's original taxonomy on the left and revised taxonomy on the right (Anderson, Krathwohl 2002; Adapted from Tangient LLC 2014).

The following is a list of typical question types you can expect to find as part of the Reasoning in Humanities and Social Sciences section of the GAMSAT. These questions may be asked within the context of different stimuli. As previously described, these stimuli include prose (extracts from literature, academic journals etc.), poetry and song lyrics, graphs and figures, cartoons and images, etc.

Main Idea Questions

These test your comprehension of the theme of the article. Questions may ask you for the main idea, central idea, purpose, a possible title for the passage, and so on. You may be asked to determine which statement best expresses the author's arguments or conclusions.

Inference Questions

These require you to understand the logic of the author's argument and then to decide what can be reasonably inferred from the article and what cannot be reasonably inferred. Occasionally, you will be asked to link like arguments/statements together into groups.

Analysis of Evidence Questions

These ask you to identify the evidence the author uses to support his/her argument. You may be required to analyse relationships between given and implied information. You may be asked not only to understand the way the author uses different pieces of information but also to evaluate whether the author has built sound arguments.

Implication Questions

You may be asked to make judgments about what would follow if the author is correct in his/her argument or what a particular discovery might lead to. You may be given new information and then asked how this affects the author's original argument.

Tone Questions

You may be asked to judge the attitude of the author towards the subject. The ability to understand tone also extends to comprehension of humour in its various guises including satire, lampoon, irony, hyperbole and parody among others (section 3.5.5).

Hybrid Questions

Often more than one question type is used in the same instance. An "implication" question can be answered through the "tone" or "evidence" which is presented within the material. In addition, an assessment of material such as a "main idea" often includes "an analysis of evidence." There may be a number of "hybrid" type questions, which include one or more of all the question types discussed. In logically deducing and ruling out answers, two central ideas are very helpful: the most "encompassing" of the answers, and which of the answers has the most "explanatory power" in relation to the others. This will become more clear as we do some exercises.

3.5.1 Main Idea Questions

According to Bloom's Taxonomy, main idea questions ask candidates to utilise the intermediate skill of analysis which involves recognising and organising ideas into a hierarchy. These are therefore not the most difficult questions you will face in Section 1, yet they are very important as they are quite prevalent.

We will do some exercises to ensure that you can successfully deal with these question types. Please take a piece of paper (i.e. Post-it note) to cover the answers while you are responding to the questions. The worked solutions and/or answers are upside down when appropriate. To find the main idea, ask

GAMSAT-Prep.com
THE GOLD STANDARD

the following three questions.

> 1. What is this passage about (the topic)?
> 2. What is the most important thing the author says about the topic (the main idea)?
> 3. Do all of the other ideas in the passage support this main idea?

Read the following passage and find the main idea.

For most immigrants, the journey to America was long and often full of hardships and suffering. The immigrants often walked the entire distance from their villages to the nearest seaport. There the ships might be delayed and precious time and money lost. Sometimes ticket agents or ship captains fleeced the immigrants of all they owned.

The most important idea in this paragraph is:
A. immigrants had to walk long distances to get to seaports.
B. ship schedules were very irregular.
C. ship captains often stole all the possessions of immigrants.
D. the journey of immigrants to America was very difficult and often painful.

1. What is this passage about?
   _____
   _____

2. What is the most important thing the author says about the topic (the main idea)?
   _____
   _____

3. Do all of the other ideas in the passage support this main idea?
   _____
   _____

1. This paragraph is about the immigrants' journey to America. This is the topic of the paragraph.
2. The author says that the immigrants' journey "was long and often full of hardships and suffering." This is the main idea of the paragraph.
3. To be absolutely sure that this is the main idea, ask yourself: Do all of the other ideas in the passage support this main idea? There are other ideas in the paragraph, but each one is an example of some kind of hardship suffered by the immigrants. Thus, the correct choice is D.

The Main Idea at the Beginning of a Passage

Did you notice that the main idea was contained in the first sentence? Often the main idea is in the first sentence. The main idea may also be contained in the title of a passage.

Read the following passage and find the main idea.

Working conditions in the factories were frequently unpleasant and dangerous. A workday of 14 or 16 hours was not uncommon. The work was uncertain. When the factory completed its orders, the men were laid off. Often the pay was inadequate to feed a man's family. This meant that often an entire family had to work in factories in order to sur-

48 REVIEW FOR SECTION I

vive.

This paragraph is most concerned with:
A. unfavourable and difficult working conditions in factories.
B. the passage of child-labour laws.
C. the lack of job security in early factories.
D. the low pay scale of early factories.

1. What is this passage about?
   _____
   _____

2. What is the most important thing the author says about the topic (the main idea)?
   _____
   _____

3. Do all of the other ideas in the passage support this main idea?
   _____
   _____

> 1. The topic of the passage is working conditions in the factories.
> 2. Working conditions in the factories were frequently dangerous and unpleasant.
> 3. All of the other sentences give examples of dangerous or unpleasant working conditions. The correct choice is A.
>
> Notice that all answer choices have an element of truth. However, the most encompassing, and therefore relevant, answer is A. Answer choices B, C and D are all specific examples of conditions that are included in A. In Section 1, you may often be able to narrow your answer choices to two options. In these cases, always ensure you choose the most encompassing answer.

UNDERSTANDING THE GAMSAT

The Main Idea in the Middle of a Passage

Sometimes the main idea is stated somewhere in the middle of a paragraph. That is why the three questions about the main idea are so helpful.

What is this passage about? → will help you focus on the main idea.

What is the most important thing the author says about the topic? → will point out the main idea.

Do all of the other ideas in the passage support this main idea? → will help you to be sure you have chosen the most important idea rather than one of the less important ideas.

If you can answer these three questions, you will find the main idea no matter where it is placed in the paragraph.

Read the following passage carefully and ask yourself the three key questions. Then answer the question following the passage.

Many who had left the Catholic Church during the Protestant upheaval eventually returned to their original faith. However, the religious struggle of the sixteenth century destroyed the unity of Western Christendom. No longer was there one Church, nor one people, or one empire.

UNDERSTANDING THE GAMSAT   49

GAMSAT-Prep.com
THE GOLD STANDARD

The main point the author makes in this paragraph is that:

A. the Protestant Reformation destroyed the Catholic Church.
B. the Protestant Reformation did not affect the Catholic Church.
C. some Protestants rejoined the Catholic Church.
D. Western Christendom was never again unified after the Protestant Reformation.

1. What is this passage about?
   _____
   _____

2. What is the most important thing the author says about the topic (the main idea)?
   _____
   _____

3. Do all of the other ideas in the passage support this main idea?
   _____
   _____

The topic is the Protestant upheaval. The most important thing the author says about the Protestant upheaval is that it destroyed the unity of Western Christendom. The first sentence gives an example of unity. The second sentence points out that this example of unity was of very minor importance compared to the disunity. The third sentence expands this idea of disunity and tells how extensive the disunity was. The main idea is contained in the second sentence. All of the other ideas support that sentence. Thus, the correct choice is D.

Answer choice A is close, however, it fails to address the specific notion of unity. Answer choice C is true, however, it is not the main idea. Answer choice B is simply incorrect.

The Main Idea in Several Sentences

The main idea is not always contained in a single sentence. Sometimes it takes more than one sentence to express a complex idea. Then you must piece together ideas from two or more sentences to find the main idea. The three questions are particularly helpful with paragraphs like this one:

Locke, of course, was no lone voice. The climate was right for him. He was a member of the Royal Society, and was thus intimately concerned with the work of the great seventeenth-century scientists. He argued that property, the possession of land and the making of money was a rational consequence of human freedom. This promise linked him to other great developments of the period: the formation of the powerful banks, the agricultural revolution, the new science, and the Industrial Revolution.

UNDERSTANDING THE GAMSAT

The main idea of this paragraph is:

A. John Locke believed that property was a product of human freedom.
B. John Locke was linked to the agricultural and industrial revolutions as well as to the new science and the formation of banks.
C. Property is the possession of land and the making of money.
D. John Locke's views on property linked him to all the other great developments of the seventeenth century.

1. *What is this passage about?*
   _____
   _____

2. *What is the most important thing the author says about the topic (the main idea)?*
   _____
   _____

3. *Do all of the other ideas in the passage support this main idea?*
   _____
   _____

You probably took a little more time to piece together the main idea. Notice that all of the choices are true statements. All of them are found in the passage. But now you are asked to judge which is the most important.

1. The topic is John Locke. More precisely, the passage is about how John Locke was linked to the great events of the seventeenth century.

2. What is the most important thing the author says about John Locke and the events of his time? Locke's idea that property was a natural result of human freedom linked him to the great developments of his period.

3. The first sentence says that Locke was not "a lone voice"; the second sentence says that the "climate was right for him." These sentences support the idea that Locke was linked to the developments of his period. The third sentence states explicitly that Locke was "intimately concerned with the work of seventeenth-century scientists." The fourth sentence states Locke's ideas on property (part of the main idea). The last sentence links Locke with the great developments of his period (part of the main idea) and it lists those developments. Since all of the sentences in the paragraph support your statement of the main idea, you may be confident that you have the complete main idea. All of the other statements support the main idea, but they do not state it completely. Choice D is therefore correct.

The Main Idea in Several Paragraphs

So far, you have learned to find the main idea of paragraphs. To find the main idea of passages consisting of several paragraphs, first find the main idea of each paragraph. In the passage below, the main idea of each paragraph has been underlined.

Americans have long believed that George Washington died of injuries he received from a fall from a horse. <u>We now know that his doctors killed him.</u> Oh, it was

UNDERSTANDING THE GAMSAT 51

no political assassination. They killed him by being what they were; physicians practicing good eighteenth-century medicine (which prescribed bleeding for every disease and injury). Washington, was bled of two quarts of blood in two days.

It is commonly thought that the practice of blood-letting died with the eighteenth century, but even today leeches are sold in every major city in the United States. <u>These blood-sucking little worms are still used by ignorant people to draw off "bad blood,"</u> the old-world treatment for every disease of body and spirit.

The cities of America are infested with an even worse kind of bloodsucker than the leech. Like the leech, he is not a cure-all, but a cure-nothing. Like the leech, he transmits diseases more dangerous than those he is supposed to cure. And like his brother, the primordial worm, he kills more often than he cures. His name is "pusher". <u>His treatment is not blood-letting, but addiction.</u>

The purpose of the passage is to:
A. explain how George Washington died.
B. describe the eighteenth-century practice of using leeches to treat diseases.
C. denounce the practice of blood-letting.
D. make a comparison between leeches and drug pushers.

Re-read only the underlined portions of the passage. These sentences can be used to form a summary of the passage:

George Washington died of bleeding. Leeches are still used by ignorant people for treating diseases.

The cities of America are infested with an even worse kind of bloodsucker than the leech. His name is "pusher."

Now ask yourself the same questions you used to find the main idea of a single paragraph.

1. *What is this passage about?*
   _____
   _____

2. *What is the most important thing the author says about the topic (the main idea)?*
   _____
   _____

3. *Do all of the other ideas in the passage support this main idea?*
   _____
   _____

---

1. The topic is leeches, blood-letting, and drug pushers.
2. Drug pushers are worse than leeches and do more harm than blood-letting.
3. The first paragraph explains that leeches were used in the eighteenth century and could kill people. The second paragraph explains that ignorant people still use leeches. The third paragraph compares leeches and drug pushers and stresses that drugs are the more harmful.
The answer is D.

In addition to asking the three questions, you could also ask whether each of the answer choices is too narrow or too broad. For example, in the previous question choices A, B, and C are all too narrow to be the main idea.

3.5.2 Inference Questions

Some questions ask you to make inferences. An inference is a conclusion not directly stated in the text, but implied by it. Referring back to Bloom's Taxonomy, inferences is a high-level cognitive skill considered to be a component of Synthesis in the original taxonomy, and a component of Creating in the revised taxonomy. Inferring may also extend to extrapolating upon a particular idea, or sentiment. These types of questions can be complex.

Read the following passage. The topic is not directly stated, but you can infer what the paragraph is about.

Dark clouds moved swiftly across the sky blotting out the sun. With no further warning, great cracks of thunder and flashes of lightning disturbed the morning's calm. Fortunately, the deckhands had already tied everything securely in place and closed all portholes and hatches or we would have lost our gear to the fury of wind and water.

1. This passage most likely describes:
    A. a storm during an African safari.
    B. a storm at sea.
    C. an Antarctic expedition.
    D. a flash flood.

2. Which of the following statements is false?
    A. The storm was unexpected.
    B. The storm came suddenly.
    C. It was windy.
    D. It was cloudy.

Nowhere in the paragraph are the words "sudden storm at sea" but, obviously, that is what the paragraph is about. The words dark clouds, thunder, lightning, wind, and water all suggest a storm. The words deckhands and portholes suggest a ship at sea. Several other words give you the feeling of the suddenness of the storm. You are justified in inferring that the writer was caught in a sudden and terrible storm at sea. The answer to question 1 is B.

Are you justified in concluding that the storm was unexpected? You know that things that happen suddenly are often unexpected. Was that the case with this storm? The last sentence tells you that the deckhands had already tied everything down and closed all portholes and hatches. That sentence indicates the storm was expected. The answer to question 2 is A.

Note that Answer A is a false statement and that's why it is the correct answer. Students often make mistakes with double negative questions (i.e. the question is asking for something false and the answer has "unexpected"). Process of elimination (3.2.4) and annotating your exam paper (i.e. putting x's or check marks next to answer choices) will reduce the chance that you will make a mental error.

Read the following paragraph. You will be asked to examine the cause-effect relationships implied by it later.

Effect of Position on Valsalva Maneuver: Supine vs. 20 Degree Position

Blood pressure (BP) changes in response to the Valsalva manoeuvre (VM), which reflect the integrity of the baroreflex that regulates BP. Performing this manoeuvre in the standard supine position often prevents adequate venous preload reduction, resulting in a rise rather than a fall in BP, the "flat top" Valsalva response. We determined whether performing the Valsalva Maneuver (VM) at a 20 degree angle of head up tilt improves preload reduction, thereby reducing the frequency of flat top responses, improving reflex vasoconstriction, and increasing the Valsalva ratio (VR). 130 patients were evaluated in a prospective study. Each patient performed the VM in both supine and 20 degree positions.

Flat top responses were present in 18% of subjects when supine. Twenty degree position reduced the flat top response by 87%. The components of the response that are dependent on preload reduction also showed significant improvement with the 20 degree position.

A 20 degree angle of tilt is sufficient to reduce venous preload, decreasing flat top response rate and improving the VR and the morphology of the VM. We recommend this modification for laboratory evaluation of the VM, whenever a "flat-top" response is seen.

(PMC2729588; 2009)

3. The "flat top" response is triggered by:
   A. a high preload reduction.
   B. a rise in blood pressure.
   C. supine performance of the VM.
   D. performance of the VM with 20 degree head tilt.

In this case, there are many concepts that are likely to be foreign to the candidate. Rest assured, you do not require prior knowledge of such concepts to answer such questions. In this case, the correct answer is C. A is incorrect because it is actually a low preload reduction that causes the flat top response. B is incorrect as a rise in blood pressure is in fact what constitutes the flat top response. Finally, D is incorrect as the 20 degree head tilt is the method that the study shows reduces the prevalence of the "flat top" response.

Read the following paragraph. The question following it is concerned with the relationships between the main idea and supporting details.

Do we live in a revolutionary age? Our television and newspapers seem to tell us that we do. The late twentieth century has seen the governments of China and Cuba, among others, overthrown. The campuses of

UNDERSTANDING THE GAMSAT

our universities erupted into violence; above the confusion of voices could be heard slogans of social revolution. We are constantly reminded that we live in a time of scientific and technological revolution. Members of militant racial groups cry for the necessity and inevitability of violent revolution. Even a new laundry detergent is described as "revolutionary!" Many causes, many voices, all use the same word.

4. Revolutionary ages are generally marked by:
    A. violence, slogans, science.
    B. violence, television coverage, governments overthrown.
    C. peace, science, technology.
    D. violence, confusion, governments overthrown.

Notice that the author does not answer his own question in the first sentence (the main idea). All of the other sentences give illustrations or examples of "revolution." The question asks you to make a generalisation about the nature of revolution from these examples. Choices A and B include examples from a particular revolution (if one does exist). They are not true generalisation. Choice C is patently contrary to the ideas of the passage. Choice D is correct.

3.5.3 Analysis of Evidence Questions

Some questions ask you to check back in the text to see if the passage confirms or refutes a particular detail. This is the easiest kind of question to answer. In fact, the answer may be so obvious, you may be tempted to feel that some kind of trick is involved. Relax! If you can find the answer in the passage, you are almost certainly right.

While it will not be as simple as just comprehending a particular fact, often only basic insight is required. The trick here may be to watch for double negatives, or the understanding of particular or sophisticated vocabulary.

Do not worry if you learn new words during your GAMSAT preparation. That's normal! The majority of students will learn many new words and expressions while studying for Section 1. If you don't, then you are probably not practicing enough (or you have unusually advanced English skills). Be sure to take notes for your Section 1 preparation just as you would for Section 2 and Section 3. Review your notes often.

Attempt the following questions relating to the poem Beat! Beat! Drums! by Walt Whitman.

Beat! Beat! Drums! by Walt Whitman

Beat! beat! drums!—Blow! bugles! blow!
Through the windows—through the doors—burst like a force of armed men,
Into the solemn church, and scatter the congregation;
Into the school where the scholar is studying;
Leave not the bridegroom quiet—no happiness must he have now with his bride;
Nor the peaceful farmer any peace plowing his field or gathering his grain;
So fierce you whirr and pound, you drums—so shrill you bugles blow.

Beat! beat! drums! Blow! bugles! blow!
Over the traffic of cities—over the rumble of wheels in the streets;
Are beds prepared for sleepers at night in the houses? No sleepers must sleep in those beds;
No bargainers' bargains by day—no brokers or speculators. Would they continue?
Would the talkers be talking? would the singer attempt to sing?
Would the lawyer rise in the court to state his case before the judge?
Then rattle quicker, heavier drums—and bugles wilder blow.

Beat! beat! drums! Blow! bugles! blow!
Make no parley—stop for no expostulation;
Mind not the timid—mind not the weeper or prayer;
Mind not the old man beseeching the young man;
Let not the child's voice be heard, nor the mother's entreaties. Recruit! recruit!
Make the very trestles shake under the dead, where they lie in their shrouds awaiting the hearses.
So strong you thump, O terrible drums—so loud you bugles blow.

5. The poem relates an instance of which of the following?
   A. Conscription for war
   B. Propaganda dictated by authority
   C. Commercial infiltration of daily life
   D. Spawning of a social revolution

6. In the context of the poem, which of the following is closest in meaning to 'expostulation'?
   A. Confirmation
   B. Remonstration
   C. Exclamation
   D. Negotiation

7. The author uses many persons to emphasise his point. Which of these combinations is not used by the author?
   A. Clergy, fathers and children
   B. Mothers, children and those who perished
   C. Businessmen, farmers and physicians
   D. Brides, mothers and the judiciary

Question 5 clearly relates to war, thus the answer is A. The words bugle (the small trumpet often used for military signals), recruit and references to the dead on trestles (eventually, hearses) all support this notion. Note that the instruments are "loud" and "terrible" like war itself. Answer choices B, C and D could be assumed, but are not supported by evidence in the passage.

Question 6 asks you to define the term expostulation in context. Given the careless, relentless and advancing nature of the piece, B is the correct answer. Expostulation, or remonstration in this context, refers to disagreeing or arguing about something. Answer choices A and D are close, but fail to encompass the sentiment of the use of the word. Answer choice C can be ruled out easily as incorrect.

Question 7 is a basic comprehension question. All combinations within answer choices A, B and D are used by Whitman in the poem. Answer choice C is the correct answer as the author makes no reference to physicians while stressing the undiscriminating recruitment drive for war.

3.5.4 Implication Questions

Sometimes you will have to apply one of the ideas in a passage to another situation. Sometimes this type of question takes a broad generalisation from the passage and asks you to apply it to a specific situation. In the context of Bloom's Taxonomy, this involves the higher cognitive skill of synthesis. Attempt the passage below.

In December 1946, full-scale war broke out between French soldiers and Viet Minh forces. The people tended to support the Viet Minh. Communist countries aided the rebels, especially after 1949 communist regime came to power in China. The United States became involved in the struggle in 1950, when the United States declared support of Vietnamese independence, under Bao Dai.

Finally, in 1954, at the battle of Dien Bien Phu, the French suffered a shattering defeat and decided to withdraw. The 1954 Geneva Conference, which arranged for a cease-fire, provisionally divided Vietnam into northern and southern sectors at the 17th parallel. The unification of Vietnam was to be achieved by general elections to be held in July 1956 in both sectors under international supervision. In the north, the Democratic Republic of Vietnam was led by its president, Ho Chi Minh, and was dominated by the Communist party.

In the south, Ngo Dinh Diem took over the government when Bao Dai left the country in 1954. As the result of a referendum held in 1955, a republic was established in South Vietnam, with Diem as President.

8. A good title for this passage would be (main idea question):
   A. "The United States and Vietnam"
   B. "The Geneva Conference"
   C. "The Vietnamese Fight for Independence"
   D. "The Career of Bao Dai"

9. In the second paragraph the word "provisionally" means (implication question):

   A. temporarily.
   B. permanently.
   C. with a large, outfitted army.
   D. helplessly.

10. Bao Dai was in 1950 (implication question):

    A. a possible Vietnamese independence leader.
    B. the leader of the French.
    C. the brother of Dien Bien Phu.
    D. the President of South Vietnam.

11. The tone of this passage is (tone question):

    A. objective.
    B. partial to the French.
    C. partial to the North Vietnamese.
    D. cynical.

12. From the passage, we might assume that in 1946, the Viet Minh were (implication question):

    A. South Vietnamese.
    B. Vietnamese rebels.
    C. North Vietnamese.
    D. French-supporting Vietnamese.

Answers (upside down):
8. C
9. A
10. D
11. A
12. B

3.5.5 Tone Questions

An author may express his feelings or attitudes toward a subject. This expression of emotion imparts a tone to the writing. To determine the tone of a passage, think of the emotions or attitudes that are expressed throughout the passage. Below are some terms used to describe tone.

Term	Meaning
Admiring	respectful, approving
Belittling	making small, depreciating

Term	Meaning
Cynical	unbelieving, sneering
Denigrating	blackening, defamatory
Didactic	instructive, authoritarian
Ebullient	exuberant, praising
Hyperbolic	overstated, exaggerating
Ironic	incongruous, contrasting
Lampooning	satirical, making fun of
Laudatory	praising

UNDERSTANDING THE GAMSAT

Term	Meaning
Mendacious	untruthful, lying
Objective	factual
Optimistic	hopeful
Praising	commending, laudatory
Reverential	exalted, regarding as sacred
Ridiculing	deriding, mocking, scornful
Saddened	sorrowful, mournful
Sanguine	confident, hopeful
Sarcastic	bitter, ironic
Sardonic	mocking, bitter, cynical
Satiric	ridiculing, mocking
Tragic	sad

A tragic tone reflects misfortune and unfulfilled hopes. A satiric tone mocks and ridicules its subject. An author may use an ironic tone to develop a contrast between (1) what is said and what is meant, (2) what actually happens and what appears to be happening, or (3) what happens and what was expected to happen. These are just a few of the emotions or attitudes that influence the tone.

Words themselves, statements and the general sentiment of the author all contribute to tone. Thus when attempting any Section 1 question, ensure you maintain awareness of the tone of the author. Even if there are no questions directly asking about tone, tone is likely to have a bearing upon how you approach other questions, especially when the stimulus is poetry, literature, or journalistic.

Attempt the questions below.

A certain rugby team won a regional championship for the first time in many years. Different people reacted differently.

13. "Wow! I can't believe it! This is the best thing that could have happened in this city!" The tone of this remark is:
    A. serious.
    B. excited.
    C. sarcastic.
    D. amazed.

14. "Ah! This is like it was when I was a boy. It makes my chest swell with pride again and brings tears to my eyes."
    The tone of this remark is:
    A. sentimental.
    B. excited.
    C. sarcastic.
    D. amazed.

15. "The team's manager and coach have had a lot of influence throughout the season. They deserve a lot of credit for this victory."
    The tone of this remark is:
    A. serious.
    B. excited.
    C. sarcastic.
    D. amazed.

16. "What!? They won!? And they started off so poorly this season. I just can't believe it!"
    The tone of this remark is:
    A. serious.
    B. excited.
    C. sarcastic.
    D. amazed.

17. "It couldn't have been skill since they don't have that. It couldn't have been bribery, since they don't have any money. The other team must all have been sick. It's the only way they could have won."
    The tone of this remark is:
    A. serious.
    B. excited.
    C. sarcastic.
    D. amazed.

Answers:
13. B
14. A
15. A
16. D
17. C

3.6 Warm-up Exercises

These short, relatively easy passages will help consolidate the principles and techniques explained in Section 3.5.

Passage 12

As the mid-century approached, the women of America were far from being acclimated to their assigned dependent role. In fact, leaders of the growing suffrage movement were seeking equality under the law. Incredible as it seems now, in early nineteenth-century America a wife, like a black slave, could not lawfully retain title to property after marriage. She could not vote, and she could legally be beaten by her master.

18. One of the goals of the suffrage movement was:
    A. dependence on a master.
    B. equality with men.
    C. recognition of divorce.
    D. abolition of slavery.

19. Which sentence describes American women of the early 19th century?
    A. They were against marriage.
    B. They were satisfied with their role in society.
    C. They were victims of a male-dominated society.
    D. They had many slaves to do their work.

Answers:
18. B
19. C

Passage 13

No dwelling in all the world stirs the imagination like the tipi of the Plains Indian. It is without doubt one of the most picturesque of all shelters and one of the most practical movable dwellings ever invented. Comfortable, roomy, and well ventilated, it was ideal for the roving life these people led in following the buffalo herds up and down the country. It also proved to be just as ideal in a more permanent camp during the long winters on the prairies.

20. What is a tipi?
    A. A buffalo
    B. An Indian
    C. A prairie
    D. A residence

21. What kind of life did the Plains Indians lead?
    A. They wandered with the buffaloes.
    B. They led comfortable and ideal lives.
    C. They spent their lives in one place.
    D. They lived in large, airy caves.

Passage 14

A dozen years ago, Thornton Wilder and I made the happy discovery that we were both invited to a White House dinner for the French Minister of Culture, Andre Malraux. We decided at once to go together. He was to pick up my wife and me at our hotel, and specified that I should have a double old-fashioned ready for him. Thornton did justice to the drink. He also delighted my wife. She was nervous about the dress she was wearing, and he told her it reminded him of the black swan of Tasmania and was so graceful that it danced almost by itself. He illustrated in long, slow undulations, his arms waving. My wife was ham all evening.

22. Who is the narrator of the passage?
    A. Andre Malraux
    B. Thornton Wilder
    C. The passage does not say.
    D. Tasmania

23. What does "happy" mean in the expression "happy discovery"?
    A. Fortunate
    B. Contented
    C. Optimistic
    D. Clever

24. What delighted the narrator's wife?
    A. The invitation to the White House
    B. Wilder's compliment
    C. A double old-fashioned
    D. Attending the dinner with Wilder

Passage 15

Nobody knows with certainty how big a proportion of the world's population is suffering from the basic problem of chronic undernourishment. But the commonly quoted United Nations estimate of 460 million sufferers is, if anything, on the low side. This represents 15 percent of the global population. Many more suffer from other deficiencies, making global totals even more difficult to calculate.

25. The paragraph indicates that:
    A. malnutrition is the number one problem in modern society.
    B. relatively few people suffer from malnutrition.
    C. the United Nations is supplying food to those suffering from malnutrition.
    D. it is not easy to count the number of people in the world who are undernourished.

25. D

Passage 16

Another way to fight insomnia is to exercise every day. Muscular relaxation is an important part of sleep. Daily exercise leaves your muscles pleasantly relaxed and ready for sleep.

26. What is insomnia?
    A. Muscular relaxation
    B. Inability to sleep
    C. Exercise
    D. Sleep

27. According to the passage, daily exercise:
    A. helps a person fall asleep more readily.
    B. is harmful for the muscles.
    C. prepares a person for fighting.
    D. is unnecessary.

26. B
27. A

Passage 17

The decade was erected upon the smoldering wreckage of the 60's. Now and then, someone's shovel blade would strike an unexploded bomb; mostly the air in the 70's was thick with a sense of aftermath, of public passions spent and consciences bewildered. The American gaze turned inward. It distracted itself with diversions trivial or squalid. The U.S. lost a President and a war, and not only endured those unique humiliations with grace, but showed enough resilience to bring a Roman-candle burst of spirit to its Bicentennial celebration.

28. What image is used to describe the 70's?
    A. A celebration
    B. A race
    C. A postwar period
    D. A long movie full of passion

29. What is the author's attitude regarding the events of the 70's?
    A. He is pessimistic.
    B. He is bewildered.
    C. He is optimistic.
    D. He is afraid.

Passage 18

One bright spot in the U.S. economy in 1979 was the surprising decline in gasoline use. Rising fuel costs are finally prodding Americans to cut back on consumption, and the need for this becomes more acute all the time.

30. How does the author view the decline in gas consumption?
    A. He is indifferent.
    B. He thinks it is a good sign.
    C. He doesn't see the need for it.
    D. He is unhappy about it.

31. Why are Americans using less gasoline?
    A. The economy is good.
    B. They do not need as much.
    C. They want to spend more time at home.
    D. Gasoline is becoming very expensive.

Passage 19

During the early part of the colonial period, living conditions were hard, and people had little leisure time for reading or studying. Books imported from abroad were expensive and were bought mainly by ministers, lawyers, and wealthy merchants. The only books to be found in most homes were the Bible and an almanac, a book giving general information about such subjects as astronomy, the weather, and farming.

32. The early colonists did not do much reading because:
    A. they did not know how to read.
    B. the Bible told them that reading was sinful.
    C. they did not have time.
    D. they were not interested in reading.

33. Books were bought primarily by:
    A. the nobility.
    B. professional and wealthy people.
    C. the lower class.
    D. sellers of almanacs.

Passage 20

Never before in history have people been so aware of what is going on in the world. Television, newspapers, radio keep us continually informed and stimulate our interest. The sociologist's interest in the world around him is intense, for society is his field of study. As an analyst, he must be well acquainted with a broad range of happenings and must understand basic social processes. He wants to know what makes the social world what it is, how it is organised, why it changes in the way that it does. Such knowledge is valuable not only for those who make great decisions, but also for you, since this is the world in which you live and make your way.

34. The passage chiefly concerns:
    A. the work of a sociologist.
    B. the news media.
    C. modern society.
    D. decision-makers.

35. It can be inferred that a good sociologist must be:
    A. persistent.
    B. sensitive.
    C. objective.
    D. curious.

36. According to the passage, modern society is more aware of world events than were previous societies because:
    A. the news media keep us better informed.
    B. travel is easier and faster.
    C. there are more analysts.
    D. today's population is more sociable.

34. A
35. D
36. A

Passage 21

Whatever answer the future holds, this much I believe we must accept: there can be no putting the genie back into the bottle. To try to bury or to suppress new knowledge because we do not know how to prevent its use for destructive or evil purposes is a pathetically futile gesture. It is, indeed, a symbolic return to the methods of the Middle Ages. It seeks to deny the innermost urge of the mind of men; the desire for knowledge.

37. The author believes that:
    A. new ideas should not be encouraged.
    B. we should return to the methods of the Middle Ages.
    C. new knowledge is always used for evil purposes.
    D. to suppress knowledge is a useless act.

38. What is the meaning of "no putting the genie back into the bottle"?
    A. Once new discoveries have been made, it is impossible to deny their existence and to control the consequences which might result from them.
    B. We cannot be sure that knowledge will be used for humanitarian purposes.
    C. The desire for knowledge was not strong during the Middle Ages.
    D. We cannot answer tomorrow's questions today.

39. According to the author, man's most basic desire is:
    A. to know the future.
    B. to prevent destruction and evil.
    C. to become less ignorant.
    D. to avoid useless activity.

40. The passage was written:
   A. to convince us that the Middle Ages contributed little to modern society.
   B. to inspire us to meet challenges wisely.
   C. to persuade us to mistrust new ideas.
   D. to show us what we can expect in the future.

42. The author understands "language" to mean:
   A. the totality of the way a given people expresses itself.
   B. the giving or receiving of a message.
   C. the exchange of words between two people.
   D. the written works of a population.

> 37. D
> 38. A
> 39. C
> 40. B This answer remains after eliminating the others.

> 41. C
> 42. A

Passage 22

It is important to distinguish among communication, language, and speech. These terms may, of course, be used synonymously, but strictly speaking, communication refers to the transmission or reception of a message, while language, which is usually used interchangeably with speech, is here taken to mean the speech of a population viewed as an objective entity, whether reduced to writing or in any other form.

41. According to the author, which word could be best used to replace "speech"?
   A. Communication
   B. Transmission
   C. Language
   D. Reception

Passage 23

The long, momentous day of John Glenn began at 2:20 a.m. when he was awakened in his simple quarters at Cape Canaveral's hangars by the astronauts' physician, Dr. William K. Douglas. Glenn had slept a little over seven hours. He shaved, showered, and breakfasted. Outside, the moon was obscured by fleecy clouds; the weather, responsible for four of the nine previous postponements, looked rather ominous.

43. At approximately what time did Glenn go to sleep?
   A. 5 p.m.
   B. 7 p.m.
   C. 9 a.m.
   D. 7 a.m.

44. Which statement about the weather is true?
   A. It was perfect for the occasion.
   B. It was cloudy and rainy.
   C. It had caused delays in the past.
   D. The passage does not say.

45. Who is John Glenn?
  A. A doctor
  B. A weatherman
  C. A spaceman
  D. A sailor

43. B
44. C
45. C

3.7 Short Test and Analysis

The multiple choice Section I of the GAMSAT, as described before, is organised into Units. Now that you have worked through all the warm-up exercises, you can proceed to test yourself with GAMSAT-style Units with appropriate stimulus material. We will work through the answers when you are finished.

There are 7 Units with 15 questions: choose the best answer for each question. You have 20 minutes. Please time yourself.

BEGIN ONLY WHEN TIMER IS READY

Unit 1

Questions 1–2

The Global Economy

Marked by a rise of technology, the global economy can be thought of as a complex international system, interlinked through the flow of goods, services, and information. Geographically, there are spatial changes, in labour and production, and the global economy is marked by a lifting of trade barriers and restrictions. Globalisation has to some extent levelled out the competitive labour between major industrial countries and emerging countries. While prior to globalisation, the United States dominated the global economy to a great extent, with the advent of information technologies, such as computers, the internet and the Web, the relocation of jobs from high wage to low wage countries, the emergence of economic blocs, such as NAFTA, and the nascent beginning of industrialisation in Southeast Asia, the U.S. is purportedly dwindled to roughly one quarter of the global economy's flow of goods, services and information.

UNDERSTANDING THE GAMSAT

1. The best metaphor listed below used in describing the global economy would be?
    A. Medium
    B. River
    C. Network
    D. Hypertext

2. One can make the inference that the spatial changes in labour and production, are not only due to the lifting of trade barriers and restrictions, but also because of:
    A. the production of goods and services in the US only.
    B. the advent of information technologies, such as the internet.
    C. the rise of the minimum wage in the United States.
    D. the displacement of labour due to economic factors.

Unit 2

Question 3

Oxymorons are literary devices, which bring two contradictory terms together, to establish a nuance of meaning, or use, for effect. The rhetorical term oxymoron, made up of two Greek words meaning "sharp" and "dull", is itself oxymoronic. "cheerful pessimist", "wise fool", and "sad joy," are all examples of oxymorons. This device is used in literary classics, but also in everyday speech. "The true beauty of oxymorons," says Richard Watson Todd, "is that, unless we sit back and really think, we happily accept them as normal English." Todd illustrates his point in the following passage:

> *It was an open secret that the company had used a paid volunteer to test the plastic glasses. Although they were made using liquid gas technology and were an original copy that looked almost exactly like a more expensive brand, the volunteer thought that they were pretty ugly and that it would be simply impossible for the general public to accept them. On hearing this feedback, the company board was clearly confused and there was a deafening silence. This was a minor crisis and the only choice was to drop the product line.*

(Much Ado About English. Nicholas Brealey Publishing, 2006)

3. Given the description about oxymorons, which of the following phrases could LEAST be considered an oxymoron?
   A. Unbiased opinion
   B. Devout atheist
   C. Eloquent apathy
   D. Idiot savant

Unit 3

Questions 4–5

Morning at the Window (T.S. Eliot)

They are rattling breakfast plates in basement kitchens,
And along the trampled edges of the street
I am aware of the damp souls of housemaids
Sprouting despondently at area gates.

The brown waves of fog toss up to me
Twisted faces from the bottom of the street,
And tear from a passer-by with muddy skirts
An aimless smile that hovers in the air
And vanishes along the level of the roofs.

4. After reading this poem, one could make a general comparison based on which of the following elements or attributes?
   A. Vapor
   B. Liquid
   C. Shadow
   D. Light

5. After studying the verbs, adverbs, and adjectives in this poem, one could make the general assessment that the tonality of the poem indicates a sense of:
   A. a detached observation of randomness.
   B. involved despair but superior attitude.
   C. quiet desperation, yet engaged.
   D. distanced and disconnected reception.

Unit 4

Questions 6–10

Cyberterrorism

Cyberterrorism, simply defined, is a convergence of computers, the internet, and terrorism. A specialist in cyberterrorism, Dorothy Denning, defines cyberterrorism as, "unlawful attacks and threats of attack against computers, networks, and the information stored therein when done to intimidate or coerce a government or its people in furtherance of political or social objectives." Further, to qualify as cyberterrorism, an attack should result in violence against persons or property, or at least cause enough harm to generate fear.

To some extent, differentiation is made between cyber crimes, such as phishing and cyber sapping from cyberterrorism, but the line of demarcation becomes less accurate when major corporations are being hacked into.

The line between the two usually focusses on the "level of danger" or "threat" which is usually not an individual hacker, but a "premeditated use of disruptive activities, or the threat thereof, against computers and/or networks, with the intention to cause harm or further social, ideological, religious, political or similar objectives, or to intimidate any person in furtherance of such objectives." This definition is a merger of cyber and definitions of terrorism by the United States Department of Defense. The line between cyber crime and cyberterrorism becomes quite arbitrary when considering that such a "cyber crime" as "identity theft" could be used by a terrorist to establish another identity, or multiple identities. The use of bots, malware, spy ware, viruses, and worms, provides another example, in which one must distinguish whether the purported use on computer networks is by an alienated teenager, or a terrorist.

Many countries (U.S., U.K., and India) will admit to "hacking" or internet intrusions from the same suspects: China and/or Russia, and admit that the internet must be thought of as a utility, in the same manner, as water, power, and possibly vulnerable to cyber-attack. There have been other "intrusions" in the past few years. The U.S. Power grid was invaded by software (by China or Russia), Estonia, Chechnya and Kyrgyzstan have all come under cyber attack, an estranged employee dumped massive amounts of sewage in Australia through a rigged computer program, air control traffic in Alaska was hacked, causing a partial shutdown of the airport. These are notable examples that are quite real to those who would proclaim that cyberterrorism is a myth. "Hackers" theorise an attack on vulnerable businesses and corporations within the infrastructure of countries, instead of government "intrusions." One has to admit that the private sector and government sector are intertwined, interdependent, and possibly vulnerable to cyberterrorism.

6. According to the passage, the difference between "cyber crime" and "cyberterrorism" seems to be:
   A. categorical and convincing.
   B. academic and undefined.
   C. unsubstantial and congruent.
   D. tenuous, yet well-defined.

7. From your reading of the passage, we can surmise that the author is:
   A. strongly opposed to hacking and cyber crime.
   B. just sticking to the facts.
   C. opinionated yet professionally restrained.
   D. striving to be impartial and objective.

8. From your reading of the passage, why do you surmise the internet must be thought of as a public utility, much the same as water or power?
   A. Because it is run by both public and private companies
   B. Because governments and the internet are connected
   C. Because it could be a likely target by terrorists
   D. Because most of the developed countries have access to the internet

9. What would be the best argument listed below to formulate the opinion that cyberterrorism is a myth?
   A. There is no real war being fought on the internet.
   B. Terrorism is marked by violence and fear.
   C. Real terrorism blows up buildings and kills people.
   D. There is a difference between cyber crime and cyberterrorism.

10. What does the author mean by "infrastructure" in line 28, paragraph 3?
    A. The vulnerable aspects of digital networks
    B. The digital networks of private enterprise
    C. The digital networks of private and public enterprise
    D. The digital networks of public enterprise

Unit 5

Question 11

Two very short stories by Franz Kafka

The Wish to be a Red Indian

If one were only an Indian, instantly alert, and on a racing horse, leaning against the wind, kept on quivering jerkily over the quivering ground, until one shed one's spurs, for there needed no spurs, threw away the reins, for there needed no reins, and hardly saw that the land before one was smoothly shorn heath when horse's neck and head would be already gone.

The Trees

For we are like tree trunks in the snow. In appearance they lie sleekly and a little push should be enough to set them rolling. No, it can't be done, for they are firmly wedded to the ground. But see, even that is only appearance.

11. A wise literary critic remarked that the whole point of reading Kafka was to re-read. Indeed, he presents us with an abstract world of images which almost seem to operate on their own volition. After re-reading these two very short stories, which of the following abstract terms, by way of ratio, would best describe the stories, respectively?
    A. Initiation – Naturalisation
    B. Transformation – Simulation
    C. Alienation – Perception
    D. Being - Becoming

Unit 6

Questions 12–14

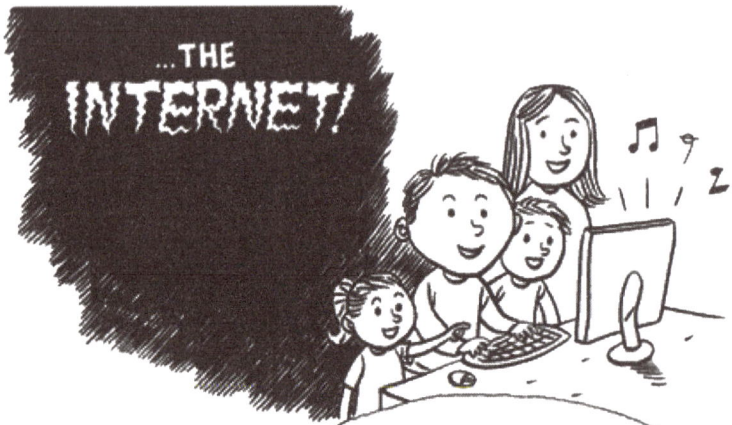
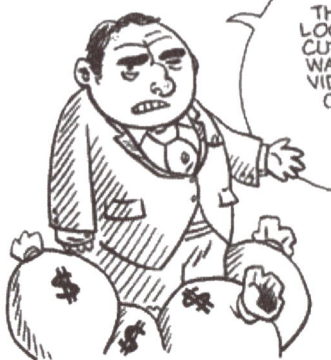

12. Undoubtedly biased for the free exchange of copyrighted material, which of the following groups of subjects would most adequately represent the contentious ideas presented within the cartoon?
    A. Popular Media, Hypertextuality, File-Sharing
    B. Intellectual Property, The Internet, Piracy
    C. Corporate Greed, Data Transfer, Representation
    D. Human Rights, Copyrights, Media

13. In the cartoon, the following line is stated by the corporate character with the bags of money: "That's why we need to ban you from the internet..." This style or figure of speech could be best described as:
    A. litotes.
    B. rhetoric.
    C. hyperbole.
    D. cliché.

14. Comparing the use of the Internet to other forms of media historically, is an argument by:
    A. definition.
    B. synthesis.
    C. induction.
    D. analogy.

Unit 7

Question 15

Nietzsche quote: "Without chaos, how could one create a dancing star?"

After reading the above aphorism from the philosopher Nietzsche, one immediately notices the existence of two seemingly asymmetrical terms; namely chaos and the ability to create, or the functioning of the act of creation. Given this odd pairing, one can make certain assumptions and inferences about Nietzsche's beliefs. Which of the following would not be a highly likely inference to be drawn?
    A. Nietzsche does not view the term 'chaos' with the same negative connotations of modern times.
    B. Creativity and chaos are interlinked.
    C. Chaos is necessary for creation.
    D. Chaos precludes creativity.

> If time remains, you may review your work. If your allotted time (20 minutes) is complete, please proceed to the Answer Key.

3.7.1 Units 1–7 Answer Key and Explanations

1.	C	4.	A	7.	D	10.	C	13.	C
2.	B	5.	D	8.	C	11.	B	14.	D
3.	C	6.	B	9.	D	12.	B	15.	D

1. A controlling metaphor can be thought of as a "Main Idea" type of question, in relation to section 3.5. In addition, this metaphor must be "inferred" based on the logic presented within the paragraph. (C) A metaphor can be inferred through the main idea within the first sentence. In describing the global economy, it can "be thought of as a complex international system, interlinked through the flow of goods, services, and information." The two terms "interlinked" and "flow" particularly stand out, indicating the metaphor of a "network." While (A) "Medium" and (D) "Hypertext" are certainly related, they do not encompass the complexity of the global economy. The metaphor of (B) "River" indicates the general notion of a flow and the possibilities of interlinkage, but is limited by one direction –that is a river is linear, while a complex network would have a flow, in many different directions.

2. This is most certainly an "analysis of evidence" type of question in relation to section 3.5. We are asked to make logical connections in relation to the evidence, as an example is being presented and extended. The correct choice (B) "The evolution of digital technologies," would effect the spatial redistribution of labour and production – communication and the flow of information could be accomplished with relative ease on a global level. This line of thought follows logically from the first sentence, in terms of a "flow of... information," i.e. not only the "outsourcing" of labour and production to different companies. Since information is also a commodity, in many instances, this would be the correct choice. (A) can be ruled out as a non-sequiter. Although (C) "the rise of the minimum wage" and (D) "the displacement of labour due to economic factors" may have consequential effects on the rise of the global economy geographically, the more encompassing influence adhering to the idea of "global" would most certainly be advances in technology and digital communications.

3. The answer is (C). (A) is easily excluded since an opinion is, by definition, subjective and therefore biased. (D) is also easily excluded as a savant is defined as one with unusually high mental capacity. (B) is more difficult as it could be argued that an atheist is devout to their beliefs about nothing as a subject. However, (C) is least oxymoronic because to be apathetic is to be emotionless – this does not preclude eloquency.

4. (A) Vapor is the correct choice, as indicated by "the brown waves of fog" which enters and controls the imagery of the poem, in the second stanza, which also "toss," "tear," "hover," and finally "vanish" as a vapor. (C) "Shadow" and (D) "Light" are certainly implied by the title, but are not referred to within the internal composition of the poem. (B) "Liquid" is evidently in line with "the damp souls" which are "sprouting" but a vapor would be a more encompassing idea which is also inclusive of a sense of liquidity. This question is a "tone" type of question, in which assessments must be made logically on the basis of how and what images are presented. Usually when doing analysis of poetry, imagery is paramount to interpretation. Keep this in mind, when reviewing and analysing poetry since poems are

a regular feature of GAMSAT Section I. The images not only control the tonality of the poetry, but contribute to the overall main idea as well.

5. As evidenced in the above analysis, this question concerns "tone" and on the basis of these verbs, adverbs and adjectives, we can infer the correct choice of (D). There is a remote, "distanced and disconnected reception" as evidenced by the words, "rattled," "trampled," "despondently," and "aimless." Within the poem, there is nothing to suggest (A) "detached observation" (which would be more in line with "the scientific method") because the speaker is "aware," and subjectively involved and perceptive, nor is there anything suggesting (B) "despair" or superiority, or (C) desperation which can be ruled out.

6. (B) "Academic and undefined" is the correct answer. Much of the discussion is of a theoretical nature and focusses on "definitions." The discussion is certainly not (A), (C), or (D), but the answers require a certain level of understanding in terms of vocabulary and the terminology used. This question is certainly an "analysis of evidence" question. Defining the terms is a tactful way of presenting evidence and used often to provide clarity in an exposition, as well as necessary qualifications, reservations concerning the topic, and limits and controls the discussion.

7. (D) The author is striving to be impartial and objective, not sticking to just the facts (B) for certain value judgments are inferred and assumed within the assessment. The author is not (C) very opinionated, for generalisations concerning the subject is supported with evidence in the use of examples and testimony. Though the author (A) may be strongly against hacking and cyberterrorism, as activities which he or she may find reprehensible, there are no calls to action for countermeasures, nor is the language used emotionally-charged. For these reasons, this is a hybrid question which corresponds to both "analysis of evidence" and the general "tone" of the argument in relation to section 3.5.

8. Even though (A), (B),& (D) are all true to some extent, the concepts do not necessarily relate to both of the ideas advanced in the question: the internet as a public utility within the context of terrorism; so by way of deduction, we find that (C) is the correct answer in that the internet shared by many, such as a public utility, is a likely, easily accessible, and vulnerable target to terrorist attacks. This is an "analysis of evidence" type of question as presented in section 3.5. One makes assessments in a logical and deductive manner, by ruling out certain choices based on the evidence presented and its logical extension.

9. (D) "There is a difference between cyber crime and cyberterrorism" is the correct choice. Many have argued that the inflated cyber crimes have been unnecessarily associated with terrorism, and have lacked many of the defining characteristics of a terrorist attack. Following this line of reasoning, (A) could be inferred, and very close to being the correct answer, but only as inclusive of answer (D). The two other choices can be easily ruled out, as too general (B) to be applicable or (C) much too specific. This question also corresponds to "an analysis of evidence," most notably in how both are "defined" as mentioned above in relation to question 6. On another level, it hints of an "implication question" because it questions the reader not only to assess the evidence, but implies that the author may or may not be correct in his evaluation of the subject.

10. The answer is (C). Although line 28 is non-specific, lines 29-30 go on to define an interdependency between both the private and public sectors. This is also implicit given the theme of interconnectivity throughout the stimulus. (A) is too specific and is implied in the other three options. (B) and (D) are also implied in (C).

11. This is probably one of the most difficult questions presented in this section - due to Kafka's writings, the issues of interpretation, and the abstract ratios given as answers. (B) "Transformation-Simulation" is the correct answer. Undoubtedly, a transformation is occurring in the first passage, and an association of a tree's appearance with a representation, or in more general terms, simulation, simulacra, and simulacrum. It does help to know Latin and Greek etymological roots in this instance. Answer (D) would be a close answer if the ratio was reversed to Becoming-Being, but not as it is respective to the order of the passages. Though there may or may not be an (A) Initiation, within the passage, and the term Naturalisation, though having connections to Nature – the tree - is vague and lacks specificity, so this is not correct. (C) Alienation-Perception is also very close, but the term "Alienation" carries negative connotations, when in fact the first passage, is a "wish" that results in a sense of liberated freedom and movement. Perception would be quite correct, in assessing Kafka's 2nd passage, since perception is so interlinked with appearance. But given the ratio, (C) can be ruled out as not as qualified or encompassing as (B). This is also a hybrid type of question, which presents abstract terms to define a main idea based on tone. So not only is the reader asked to relate an abstract term to a "main idea" type of question, but also review the "tone" of the passage by examining the dominant images.

12. All of the answer choices are at least partially correct. The most encompassing and specific in relation to the cartoon's contentions is (B). Through "an analysis of evidence" in assessing the "main ideas" presented within the material, this answer can be deduced. Again, we must determine what the most encompassing answer choice is while possessing the most explanatory power.

13. The answer is (C). (A) is incorrect as litotes is a form of understating something in an attempt to actually emphasise the opposite – this is clearly not the case here. (B) Rhetoric is employed, yet it is too general. (D) Cliché is a red herring as the character itself is a cliché, yet what he says is a (C) hyperbole.

14. These comparisons are certainly an argument by "analogy" (D) by contrasting different forms of media throughout the years with the internet. (A) "Definition" is not correct, because the internet is not being defined or interpreted as a specific media or medium. (C) An argument from "synthesis" would be a clash of ideas, in proper terms, dialectic and the result of this clash. This can be ruled out as well in relation to the cartoon. (C) "Induction" is close but not as encompassing as (D) analogy. As such, this question is "an analysis of evidence" type of question as referred to in section 3.5.

15. All of the answers in relation to the Nietzsche quote can be inferred to some extent except (D), the correct choice. A certain degree of familiarity with vocabulary, particularly the term "precludes" is assumed and necessary to make the correct choice in (D). This phrase essentially would be antipodal – in opposition to the other assessments, meaning Chaos limits or rules out Creativity. This is an "inference" type of question, as presented in section 3.5. We infer that all of the choices are correct, in relation, to the quote except for (D), which negates, instead of affirms a relation between the two: chaos and creativity.

UNDERSTANDING THE GAMSAT

3.8 Section 1 Mini Tests

We work hard to continually improve each new edition of the Gold Standard GAMSAT. This current edition contains hundreds of new non-science pages as well as hundreds of new science pages. Adding brand new content to textbooks is always exciting because of the prospect of enhancing the learning experience; however, it can be a bit hazardous because the content has not had the same level of exposure as 'older' content.

Nonetheless, we have tested our practice questions with hundreds of students prior to publication. As with the entire book, we have carefully edited the content. However, if you have any questions or concerns about any content in these new sections, please go to gamsat-prep.com/forum to find the Gold Standard GAMSAT Textbook Section 1 thread.

The following sections contain 5 mini tests that are grouped according to specific types of passages:

- Verbal Reasoning Exercise 1 (Humanities and Social Sciences)
- Verbal Reasoning Exercise 2 (Science-based Passages)
- Poetry Test
- Cartoon Test
- Graphs and Tables Test

The objective is to help build your Section 1 reasoning skills one area at a time. We strongly suggest that you ALWAYS time yourself for every practice test. Otherwise, you would be eliminating one of the major components of your preparation making it more difficult to get a top GAMSAT Section 1 score. On the other hand, in the case that you are not pressured for time, do not assume that a specialty test is the same as a full-length exam. Just consider this experience as just another step in your training.

At the end of each mini test, you should work through the answers and explanations. Keep notes of your wrong answers and then go back to the specific section(s) in this chapter, reviewing and analysing how you can still improve for your next attempts. Naturally, as you progress with your review, you should also consider full-length practice tests (i.e. Section 1, Section 2 and Section 3 in one sitting) including those from ACER and Gold Standard.

Olympic athletes go to the gym to improve strength and fitness. The gym is not the sport. These mini tests are part of your Section 1 gym. Train well and it will be reflected in your performance.

GAMSAT-Prep.com
THE GOLD STANDARD

3.8.1 Verbal Reasoning Exercise 1 (Humanities and Social Sciences)

The following is a sample mini test, aimed at developing your skills in reading and answering passages that contain arguments within the humanities or social science context. There are 7 Units with 40 questions. Choose the best answer for each question. You have 50 minutes. Please time yourself.

BEGIN ONLY WHEN TIMER IS READY

Unit 1

Questions 1 - 6

I can honestly say that I had no idea that the National Wildlife Federation came into being because of one cartoonist. Ding Darling used his cartoons to promote conservation ethics as far back as 1930 and was instrumental in creating the government agency that used the practice of scientific management for fish and wildlife. As an interesting note, Mr. Darling also led the development of the federal duck stamp that is still the primary source of revenue for waterfowl management and has to be purchased by all waterfowl hunters to this day. Darling pointed out that while several people cared about wildlife conservation, there was no organised fashion to advocate or influence policy decisions. His work and input valued the importance of multiple stakeholder participation, accepting attitudes, values, and beliefs of many groups. And his dream came true in 1936 when he "convinced President Franklin Roosevelt to invite over 2,000 hunters, anglers, and conservationists from across the country to the first North American Wildlife conference in Washington D.C." This is where the General Wildlife Federation, later changed to National Wildlife Federation, was formed with the idea of uniting all outdoor and wildlife enthusiasts behind a common goal of conservation, and Ding Darling became the first president of the organisation.

Darling's quest to unite all voices concerning conservation was the basis for many laws and policies that are present today at the national level. The National Wildlife Federation returns every year to Washington D.C. to provide governance, vision, and grassroots needed to achieve joint conservation goals.

The National Wildlife Federation is one of the nation's largest conservation organisations and there are approximately 4,000,000 supporters that are committed to sustaining the nature of America for the benefit of people and of wildlife. Joining their family of wildlife supporters only takes a gift of $30 or more, and member benefits include a one-year subscription to National Wildlife magazine, NWF membership card and decal, nature travel opportunities that include exclusive invitations to see wildlife in their natural habitat with NWF Expeditions, plus a 10% discount off all NWF catalog merchandise.

I have discovered that the National Wildlife Federation covers 47 state affiliates along with their 4,000,000 supporters and partners in many communities across the country to help protect and restore wildlife habitat, confront global warming, and connect with nature. NWF works diligently to be "the voice of conservation for diverse constituencies, which include hunters, anglers, gardeners, birdwatchers, scientists, and families raising the next generation of habitat stewards."

National Wildlife Federation has the professional expertise and grassroots power to make a difference for wildlife and our children's future. None of these happened by chance from climate change to mining reform, from the wilderness to energy development, from backyard habitats to connecting people to nature. What started out as a cartoonist's dream became one of the largest grassroots conservation organisations in the country.

Natural Wildlife Federation demands strategic planning that can accommodate change. There has to be acceptance of varying attitudes, values, and beliefs, while encouraging a collaborative approach to conservation and at the same time, promoting lifelong learning and growth. With cooperation from state affiliates, the National Wildlife Federation today continues in the quest for strict change and equally positioning national conservation leaders. Some of the benefits of assimilating an integrated stakeholder-based information model include strong state affiliate-constituents and gross effective engagement of members over a broad constituent base.

Darling's original ideas are still a mainstay of conservation imperatives, goals, and objectives. So without a concerned citizen who happened to be a cartoonist, there would probably not be an organisation like the National Wildlife Federation in today's society.

1. What is the main idea of the passage?
    A. Ding Darling dedicated his craft to advance his environmental cause.
    B. Ding Darling is the seminal force behind the creation of the National Wildlife Federation.
    C. The National Wildlife Federation became one of the most influential conservationist groups in the United States.
    D. The National Wildlife Federation seeks to unite all outdoor enthusiasts and wildlife supporters for a common cause of saving the environment.

2. Which of the following is the National Wildlife Association involved in?
   I. Organising groups and communities to advance wildlife and habitat conservation goals
   II. Spearheading government agencies that promote respect for diverse constituencies
   III. Facilitating activities that bring people closer to nature

   A. I
   B. I and II
   C. I and III
   D. I, II, and III

3. Based on passage information, which of the following would have Ding Darling MOST probably considered as a theme for one of his cartoons?
   A. The pleasure of birdwatching
   B. Condemnation of smuggling rare species of birds in the Amazon
   C. The Native Americans' honour and respect for the buffalo
   D. Call for organised civic action to combat global warming

4. What is the author's purpose for writing the passage?
   A. To trace the history of the National Wildlife Association and its activities
   B. To stress the importance of Ding Darling and his cartoons
   C. To illustrate the influential role of Darling in helping establish the National Wildlife Federation
   D. To promulgate pro-hunting cartoons for the average hunter belonging to the National Wildlife Association

5. Based on passage information, which of the following could have Ding Darling LEAST likely done?
   A. Published cartoons that condemned the destruction of the waterfowl habitat
   B. Organised a conference attended by environmental advocates from diverse backgrounds
   C. Served in a government agency involved in studies and management of wildlife and their habitats
   D. Rallied against the National Rifle Association's fund-raising agenda on encouraging ownership of hunting rifles

6. The author of the passage would MOST likely support a civic cause that:
   A. encourages artists to use their talents in influencing sociopolitical movements.
   B. advocates the restoration of a polluted river.
   C. urges government legislation of stricter environmental protection laws.
   D. calls for the participation of ordinary citizens in advancing social change.

Unit 2

Questions 7 - 12

To the romantic poets, poetry was an instrument of emotion and feeling intended to reconnect man with the natural world, and in general, the poet was viewed as a person uniquely equipped to guide the layman to this reconnection.

Romanticism as a movement appeared following a period in history when great importance was put on scientific discovery and formal education. In the eyes of the romantic poets, mankind had become so swept up in the pursuit of knowledge and innovation that they had disconnected from both the natural world, and their deeper, natural selves. Though the philosophies of the individual poets differed, in general romantic poetry focussed on and lauded primitivism and emotion while minimising (but not discounting) the importance of reason and logic. The ultimate goal of romantic poetry was the attainment of the sublime, the ultimate, transcendental connection with the natural self.

Samuel Taylor Coleridge, one of the pioneers of the Romantic Movement, believed that the creative imagination was the key to man achieving his connection to the sublime. This caused much difficulty though, as the source of creative imagination was impossible to trace and because creative inspiration was quite fickle. Coleridge struggled with this conundrum throughout his life but felt that as a poet and as one who understood the importance of the creative imagination, it was his right and responsibility to better mankind through his poetry. William Wordsworth was, along with Coleridge, another leader in the early Romantic Movement.

Wordsworth believed that beauty and inspiration was to be found in the most rudimentary and common things and was not something that could only be found in the high and lofty. It was the role of the poet to extract and explain that beauty. In his preface to "Lyrical Ballads," Wordsworth describes a poet as a man speaking to men, but ensures that he differentiates the poet as a man ". . . endowed with more lively sensibility, more enthusiasm and tenderness, who has a greater knowledge of human nature, and a more comprehensive soul, than are supposed to be common among mankind. . ." Thus, while rustic man could be privy to the sublime, it took the unique soul of a poet to make the sublime accessible to all. Like Coleridge, Wordsworth believed that creative imagination was the source of poetry and the avenue to the sublime. He was also of the belief that poetry was the result of the "spontaneous overflow of powerful feelings."

Percy Shelley not only believed that poets were charged with reconnecting man with nature, he believed poets were the "unacknowledged legislators of the world." He stated as much in "A Defence of Poetry," an essay in which he explained the importance of poetry in reconnecting man with feeling and emotion, and the importance of the poet as a person who could influence the course of mankind through this reconnection. However, unlike Coleridge and Wordsworth who sought out recognition and importance, Shelley recognised the role of the poet as one who affects mankind from the shadows of obscurity.

Though Coleridge, Wordsworth and Shelley may have differed in their individual poetic philosophies, the three poets, along with their Romantic colleagues, each strove to the same end. Each of these poets recognised great value in the natural feelings and emotions of man, and the connection sparked by man's place in the natural world. Each strove to capture and explain that connection through creative imagination and ultimately, through poetry.

7. The author suggests that the Romantic poets:
   A. attempted to attain the sublime and ultimate connection with one's natural self.
   B. believed they had the unique task of showing and reconnecting man with the natural world.
   C. thought science was diminishing man's creative imagination.
   D. were against Victorian morals and ways of thinking.

8. According to the passage, the problem with creative inspiration was that it was:
   A. something that could only be found in the high and lofty.
   B. to be found in the most unsophisticated things.
   C. impossible to trace.
   D. capricious.

9. Which of the following assertions is NOT made in the passage regarding Romanticism?
   A. It was a reaction to the burgeoning trend towards scientific and formal knowledge.
   B. It sought to reconnect man to his natural self through creative imagination.
   C. It challenged the use of reason and logic over emotion.
   D. It emphasised feelings and emotions as the key to man's reconnection with the natural world.

10. What is the author's purpose for writing the passage?
    A. To point out the differences in the Romantic poets and their philosophies
    B. To show that despite differences in their philosophies, the Romantics had the same end in mind
    C. To illustrate Romantic tendencies in juxtaposition to the idealism of the poets involved
    D. To capture the essence of Romanticism through the eyes of the various philosophers

11. The "sublime" is a concept that many critics and scholars would generally refer as indescribable but can take various forms such as a mountain, a landscape, a poem, a good meal, a heroic deed or a state of mind. Given the information on Coleridge and Wordsworth's Romantic principles, the sublime is considered:
    A. a form of spontaneous powerful emotion.
    B. attainable through creative imagination.
    C. ephemeral in the natural world.
    D. an inspired connection with one's natural self.

12. The more popular notion of the word "romantic" is that which is associated with love or strong affection and at times, irrationality. Which of the following assertions in the passage would be confused to be of the same concept as those advanced by the Romantic Movement?
    A. The works of the Romantic poets such as the lyrical ballads often dealt with love.
    B. Romantic poets are also known for their typical temper and passion.
    C. The Romantic poets emphasised the importance of natural feelings and emotions in preference to reason and logic.
    D. Wordsworth claims that poetry is a result of the "spontaneous overflow of powerful feelings."

Unit 3

Questions 13 - 18

   Gauguin's attitude toward art marked a break from the past and a beginning to modern art. He was from the start preoccupied with suggestion rather than description. Gauguin considered naturalism an error to be avoided, and he sought to render images in their purest, simplest and most primitive form. He wanted to portray the essence of things rather than the exterior form, which could only be achieved through simplification of the form. The beginning of his modern tradition lay in his rejection of Impressionism. He firmly believed throughout his life that "art is an abstraction" and that "this abstraction [must be derived] from nature while dreaming before it." One must think of the creation that will result rather than the model, and not try to render the model exactly as one sees it. Like all Post-Impressionist artists, he passed through an Impressionist phase but became quickly dissatisfied with the limitations of the style, and went on to discover a new style that had the directness and universality of a symbol and that concentrated on impressions, ideas and experiences. It was the birth of "Synthetism" or rather Synthetist-Symbolic, as Gauguin referred to it, using the term "symbolic" to indicate that the forms and patterns in his pictures were meant to suggest mental images or ideas and not simply to record visual experience.

Symbolism flourished around the period of 1885 to 1910 and can be defined as the rejection of direct, literal representation in favour of evocation and suggestion. Painters tried to give a visual expression to emotional experiences, and therefore the movement was a reaction against the naturalistic aims of Impressionism. Satisfying the need for a more spiritual or emotional approach in art, Symbolism is characterised by the desire to seek refuge in a dream-world of beauty and the belief that colour and line in themselves could express ideas. Stylistically, the tendency was towards flattened forms and broad areas of colour, and features of the movement were an intense religious feeling and an interest in subjects of death, disease, and sin.

Similarly, "Synthetism" involved the simplification of forms into large-scale patterns and the expressive purification of colours. Form and colour had to be simplified for the sake of expression. This style reacted against the "formlessness" of Impressionism and favoured painting subjectively and expressing one's ideas rather than relying on external objects as subject matters. It was characterised by areas of pure colours, very defined contours, an emphasis on pattern and decorative qualities, and a relative absence of shadows.

Gauguin's new art form merged these two movements and succeeded in freeing colour, form, and line, bringing it to express the artists' emotions, sensibilities, and personal experiences of the world around them. His style created a break with the old tradition of descriptive naturalism and favoured the synthesis of observation and imagination. Gauguin sustained that forms are not discovered in nature but in one's wild imagination, and it was in himself that he searched rather than in his surroundings. For this reason, he scorned the Impressionists for their lack of imagination and their mere scientific reasoning. Furthermore, Gauguin used colour unnaturalistically for its decorative or emotional effect and reintroduced emphatic outlines. "Synthetism" signified for him that the forms of his pictures were constructed from symbolic patterns of colour and linear rhythms and were not mere scientific reproductions of what is seen by the eye.

13. What is the author's purpose for writing the passage?
    A. To define Synthesism in contrast to Impressionism
    B. To illustrate the methods of Gauguin in relation to Symbolism
    C. To define Gauguin's art form and principles
    D. To give a biographical account of Gauguin

14. What could be inferred to be the best title for this passage?
    A. Gauguin's Rejection of Impressionism
    B. Gauguin: From Expressionist to Symbolist
    C. Gauguin's New Art Form: Synthetism
    D. An Overview of Gauguin's Theories and Applications of Art

15. Which of the following hypothetical evidences would diminish the author's opinion of Gauguin?
    A. Gauguin's style of painting was copied from Van Gogh.
    B. Gauguin made a clean break from the aesthetic tenets of Impressionism.
    C. Gauguin modified many of the symbolic ideals in his painting.
    D. Gauguin's style of painting was representative of a move away from realism.

16. What dualism or dichotomy is NOT presented in the passage?
    A. Suggestion and Description
    B. Naturalism and Expressionism
    C. Observation and Imagination
    D. Impressionism and Expression

17. According to the passage, Gauguin rejected Impressionism for a number of reasons. Which of the following reasons CANNOT be inferred as a motive of this rejection?
    A. Limitations of the style of Impressionism
    B. Lack of intense feelings and emotions in Impressionism
    C. Universality of symbols in Impressionism
    D. Lack of imagination in Impressionism

18. According to the passage, Symbolism is associated or represented by:
    I. a rejection of literal and direct representation.
    II. disfavoured evocation and suggestion.
    III. the time period of 1885 to 1910.

    A. I only
    B. I and II
    C. II only
    D. I and III

Unit 4

Questions 19 - 25

Human conduct and belief are now undergoing transformations profounder and more disturbing than any since the appearance of wealth and philosophy put an end to the traditional religion of the Greeks.

It is the age of Socrates again: our moral life is threatened, and our intellectual life is quickened and enlarged by the disintegration of ancient customs and beliefs. Everything is new and experimental in our ideas and our actions; nothing is established or certain any more. The rate, complexity, and variety of change in our time are without precedent, even in Periclean days; all forms about us are altered, from the tools that complicate our toil, and the wheels that whirl us restlessly about the earth, to the innovations in our sexual relationships and the hard disillusionment of our souls.

The passage from agriculture to industry, from the village to the town, and from the town to the city has elevated science, debased art, liberated thought, ended monarchy and aristocracy, generated democracy and socialism, emancipated woman, disrupted marriage, broken down the old moral code, destroyed asceticism with luxuries, replaced Puritanism with Epicureanism, exalted excitement above content, made war less frequent and more terrible, taken from us many of our most cherished religious beliefs and given us a mechanical and fatalistic philosophy of life. All things flow, and we seek some mooring and stability in the flux.

In every developing civilisation, a period comes when old instincts and habits prove inadequate to altered stimuli, and ancient institutions and moralities crack like hampering shells under the obstinate growth of life. In one sphere after another, now that we have left the farm and the home for the factory, the office and the world, spontaneous and "natural" modes of order and response break down, and intellect chaotically experiments to replace with conscious guidance the ancestral readiness and simplicity of impulse and wonted ways. Everything must be thought out, from the artificial "formula" with which we feed our children, and the "calories" and "vitamins" of our muddled dietitians, to the bewildered efforts of a revolutionary government to direct and coordinate all the haphazard processes of trade. We are like a man who cannot walk without thinking of his legs, or like a player who must analyse every move and stroke as he plays. The happy unity of instinct is gone from us, and we flounder in a sea of doubt; amidst unprecedented knowledge and power, we are uncertain of our purposes, values and goals.

From this confusion, the one escape worthy of a mature mind is to rise out of the moment and the part and contemplate the whole. What we have lost above all is total perspective. Life seems too intricate and mobile for us to grasp its unity and significance; we cease to be citizens and become only individuals; we have no purposes that look beyond our death; we are fragments of men, and nothing more.

No one (except Spengler) dares today to survey life in its entirety; analysis leaps and synthesis lags; we fear the experts in every field and keep ourselves, for safety's sake, lashed to our narrow specialties. Everyone knows his part, but is ignorant of its meaning in the play. Life itself grows meaningless and becomes empty just when it seemed most full.

Let us put aside our fear of inevitable error, and survey all those problems of our state, trying to see each part and puzzle in the light of the whole. We shall define philosophy as "total perspective," as mind overspreading life and forging chaos into unity. Perhaps philosophy will give us, if we are faithful to it, a healing unity of soul. We are so slovenly and self-contradictory in our thinking; it may be that we shall clarify ourselves and pull ourselves together into consistency and be ashamed to harbour contradictory desires or beliefs. And through this unity of mind may come that unity of purpose and character which makes a personality and lends some order and dignity to our existence. Philosophy is harmonised knowledge making a harmonious life; it is the self-discipline which lifts us to security and freedom. Knowledge is power, but only wisdom is liberty.

Our culture is superficial today, and our knowledge dangerous, because we are rich in mechanisms and poor in purposes. The balance of mind which once came of a warm religious faith is gone; science has taken from us the supernatural bases of our morality and all the world seems consumed in a disorderly individualism that reflects the chaotic fragmentation of our character.

We move about the earth with unprecedented speed, but we do not know, and have not thought, where we are going, or whether we shall find any happiness there for our harassed souls. We are being destroyed by our knowledge, which has made us drunk with our power. And we shall not be saved without wisdom.

19. What could be inferred as the best title for this passage?
    A. What is Philosophy?
    B. The Age of Uncertainty
    C. The Dualities of Wisdom
    D. How We can Progress

20. The tone of the author is:
    A. bleak.
    B. hopeful.
    C. existential.
    D. cautious.

21. Which of the following statements would most likely contradict the author's thesis?
    A. Inconsistency is the key to flexibility.
    B. Values and morals are essentially socially-constructed.
    C. A given culture's development of wisdom in relation to the world's fragmentation is determined by symbolic behaviour.
    D. There is progress in technology in relation to a higher sense of spiritual development.

22. How does the author define philosophy?
    I. As a "total perspective"
    II. As mind overspreading life and forging chaos into unity
    III. As the essential balance between mind and matter
    A. I only
    B. II only
    C. I and II
    D. I, II, and III

23. Based on passage information, philosophy is based according to which of the following notions?
    A. A synthesis of opposites
    B. A struggle for progress
    C. A reaching for goodness
    D. Harmony

24. In the passage, the author assigns knowledge and wisdom to particular representations. Which of the following best exemplifies this ratio?
    A. Power-Liberty
    B. Essence-Existence
    C. Being-Becoming
    D. Static-Active

25. The author claims that the movement from agriculture to industry gave people a fatalistic and mechanical view of life. Within the post-industrial age we currently live in, the movement to the digital world has given people a view of life, which is:
    A. disconnected and shallow.
    B. connected and hopeful.
    C. simultaneously interconnected yet disassociated.
    D. a network of linear lines of information affecting humanity globally.

Unit 5

Questions 26 - 32

The Sick Rose by William Blake

O Rose thou art sick.
The invisible worm,
That flies in the night
In the howling storm:

Has found out thy bed
Of crimson joy:
And his dark secret love
Does thy life destroy.

Here the title encapsulates the essential dynamic of the poem. The rose is an archetypal symbol, which means that it has been seized on by all cultures which have known roses as symbolising very much the same range of human experience, and is spontaneously recognised as doing so even by those who do not know what a symbol is.

Archetypes contain the ability to release a certain range of meanings with peculiar depth and power. Things become symbols because of characteristics evident in ordinary life, and these remain the primary elements in the symbol however much it might have been elaborated in the literary tradition. We are all aware of the rose as a queen of flowers, beautiful, rich in colour (especially the red rose), heady in perfume, sensuous in texture, incurved, enfolding erotic promise. The rose activates all the senses like the body of a desired woman. Rose metaphors are part of our common language. Rosy cheeks signify health; rosy lips are asking to be kissed. Few men have never sent a woman a bunch of red roses; and even when there is no verbal message, the woman has no difficulty knowing what that means. Burns wrote: 'My love is like a red, red, rose'. In giving a woman a red rose, a man is giving her an image of herself, or herself as he would wish her to be, rich with sexual passion.

As a primary female sexual symbol, the rose in the ancient world was attributed to Aphrodite/Venus, goddess of sexual love. The book which distilled and defined the courtly love invented by the medieval troubadours was called the Roman de la Rose, where the rose symbolises a woman's awakening to sexual love.

If we add together all the associations of the word rose, those we supply from our own experience, those common in our culture, and those we happen to be familiar with in the literary tradition, we have a very strong sense of youth, health, beauty and joy, of the feminine at its most desirable, of vitality and creativity, of the gratification of erotic desires. The last adjective we anticipate is 'sick'. Sickness, disease, corruption, are not only contrary to all the primary meanings of 'rose', but strike us as a violation of them, a sacrilege. The two words cancel each other out, leaving a void, a chaos. The title enacts linguistically the degradation of the rose the poem then dramatises. Blake was by no means the first poet to exploit this shock effect. In A Midsummer Night's Dream Shakespeare, needing to convey what happens when the natural progression of the seasons is violated and Great Creating Nature made sterile, writes: 'heavy-headed frosts / Fall in the fresh lap of the crimson rose'. And in Lycidas Milton wrote 'as killing as the canker to the rose'.

The poets Blake was most familiar with and most respected were Shakespeare and Milton, and he expected his readers to know them well. 'The Sick Rose' draws so heavily on both of them that it can hardly be read, or loses half its force, if the reader is unaware of the power and quite specific meanings flowing into this poem from Twelfth Night, Hamlet and Paradise Lost.

In Book IX of Paradise Lost, Satan, having crossed the howling storm of chaos, 'with meditated guile' flies 'as a mist by night' into Eden, where he enters the serpent, the fittest creature to communicate his 'dark suggestions' to Eve. (The first meaning of 'worm' in the Oxford English Dictionary is 'serpent, snake, dragon'.) Satan views Eve " . . . so thick the roses bushing round about her glowed" to which she is compared to, with a "storm so nigh" given as a background context from where Satan has come from. His avowed purpose is 'all pleasure to destroy' since he has lost his own capacity for joy. When Eve tells Adam what has happened, he describes her as 'deflowered': From his slack hand the garland wreathed for Eve, down dropped, and all the faded roses shed.

Nakedness and sex become for both of them a cause for shame, which they had never known before. This story, with its memorable imagery of the invisible tempter flying through a howling storm, becoming a worm, and desecrating the joy of the marriage bed for both man and woman, clearly looms behind 'The Sick Rose' and feeds it with potent suggestions. These suggestions mingle with others from Shakespeare. The worm which destroys the beauty of a young woman must remind us of Viola's story of an imaginary sister: She never told her love,

But let concealment, like a worm i' the bud, Feed on her damask cheek: she pin'd in thought. The examples lend their credence that "The Sick Rose" is remarkably influenced by Milton and Shakespeare.

26. Given that the rose is an archetype recognised by all cultures as a symbol, it can be inferred that:
    A. poetry, as an aspect of culture, is an archetype which is created through symbolisation.
    B. the archetype is understood through language and interpretation of the referent.
    C. things are symbolised through evidentiary and ordinary characteristics representing the same elements.
    D. symbols are a generalised and universal aspect of all cultures as evidenced through archetypes.

27. By linking the contrary meanings of "sick and rose," the poem itself displays:
    A. an oxymoron throwing the reader into an abyss of chaos.
    B. a juxtaposition between romantic and destructive imagery.
    C. a tonality and effect which contradict each other linguistically.
    D. an explosion of multiple meanings and effects on the reader.

28. The author's attitude towards archetypes can be characterised as:
    A. telescopic.
    B. critical.
    C. focussed.
    D. encompassing.

29. The commentator refers to Milton in Paradise Lost in order to emphasise the beginning of:
    A. sin.
    B. the fall from Grace.
    C. shame.
    D. dualism.

30. Within the passage, it can be reasonably noted that the meaning of archetypes in culture have:
    A. profound reflections of man's common consciousness.
    B. associations with a certain range of intention.
    C. influences on the literary tradition.
    D. interrelations with linguistic structures.

31. Based on the author's discussions, if a reader is unfamiliar with Blake's allusions to Milton and Shakespeare:
    A. the rose will be overlooked as an essential archetype in the poem.
    B. the meaning of the poem loses half its force and power.
    C. the meaning of the poem will be lost in superficial interpretation.
    D. the worm will be misinterpreted within the scope of the poem's imagery.

32. The characterisation of Blake's poem with Milton can be reasonably described as:
    A. redundant.
    B. irrevocable.
    C. inharmonious.
    D. uncanny.

Unit 6

Questions 33 - 35

The "Theatre of the Absurd" is a term coined by Hungarian-born critic Martin Esslin, who made it the title of his 1962 book on the subject. The term refers to a particular type of play which first became popular during the 1950s and 1960s and which presented on stage the philosophy articulated by French philosopher Albert Camus in his 1942 essay, "The Myth of Sisyphus", in which he defines the human condition as basically meaningless. Camus argued that humanity had to resign itself to recognising that a fully satisfying rational explanation of the universe was beyond its reach; in that sense, the world must ultimately be seen as absurd.

Esslin regarded the term "Theatre of the Absurd" merely as a "device" by which he meant to bring attention to certain fundamental traits discernible in the works of a range of playwrights. The playwrights loosely grouped under the label of the absurd attempt to convey their sense of bewilderment, anxiety, and wonder in the face of an inexplicable universe. According to Esslin, the five defining playwrights of the movement are Eugène Ionesco, Samuel Beckett, Jean Genet, Arthur Adamov, and Harold Pinter, although these writers were not always comfortable with the label and sometimes preferred to use terms such as "Anti-Theatre" or "New Theatre". Other playwrights associated with this type of theatre include Tom Stoppard, Arthur Kopit, Friedrich Dürrenmatt, Fernando Arrabal, Edward Albee, N.F. Simpson, Boris Vian, Peter Weiss, Vaclav Havel, and Jean Tardieu. The most famous, and most controversial, absurdist play is probably Samuel Beckett's **Waiting for Godot**. The characters of the play are strange caricatures who have difficulty communicating the simplest of concepts to one another as they bide their time awaiting the arrival of Godot. The language they use is often ludicrous, and following the cyclical patter, the play seems to end in precisely the same condition it began, with no real change having occurred. In fact, it is sometimes referred to as "the play where nothing happens." Its detractors count this a fatal flaw and often turn red in the face fomenting on its inadequacies. It is mere gibberish, they cry, eyes nearly bulging out of their head - a prank on the audience disguised as a play. The plays supporters, on the other hand, describe it is an accurate parable on the human condition in which "the more things change, the more they are the same." Change, they argue, is only an illusion. In 1955, the famous character actor Robert Morley predicted that the success of **Waiting for Godot** meant "the end of theatre as we know it." His generation may have gloomily accepted this prediction, but the younger generation embraced it. They were ready for something new - something that would move beyond the old stereotypes and reflect their increasingly complex understanding of existence.

Whereas traditional theatre attempts to create a photographic representation of life as we see it, the Theatre of the Absurd aims to create a ritual-like, mythological, archetypal, allegorical vision, closely related to the world of dreams. The focal point of these dreams is often man's fundamental bewilderment and confusion, stemming from the fact that he has no answers to the basic existential questions: why we are alive, why we have to die, why there is injustice and suffering. Ionesco defined the absurdist everyman as "Cut off from his religious, metaphysical, and transcendental roots … lost; all his actions become senseless, absurd, useless." The Theatre of the Absurd, in a sense, attempts to reestablish man's communion with the universe. Dr. Jan Culik writes, "Absurd Theatre can be seen as an attempt to restore the importance of myth and ritual to our age, by making man aware of the ultimate realities of his condition, by instilling in him again the lost sense of cosmic wonder and primeval anguish. The Absurd Theatre hopes to achieve this by shocking man out of an existence that has become trite, mechanical and complacent. It is felt that there is mystical experience in confronting the limits of human condition."

-Adapted from J. Crabb, Theatre of the Absurd; 2006

33. The author's tone is:
    A. analytical.
    B. persuasive.
    C. definitional.
    D. historical.

34. One can infer from the passage information, that the characteristics of the "Theatre of the Absurd":
  I. follows literary conventions of meaning.
  II. attempts to restore the importance of myth and ritual to our present age.
  III. represents an imitative representation of reality.

  A. I and III
  B. I, II, and III
  C. III only
  D. II only

35. Based on passage information, it can be inferred that in Samuell Beckett's play *Waiting for Godot*:
  A. the characters are caught up in the absurdity of their existence.
  B. the plot is a strange mimic of reality.
  C. old stereotypes are shattered, as new role models emerge.
  D. mythic and ritualised archetypes are explored within the postmodern context.

Unit 7

Questions 36 - 40

Jacques Marie Émile Lacan (April 13, 1901 – September 9, 1981) was a French psychoanalyst and psychiatrist who made prominent contributions to psychoanalysis and philosophy, and has been called "the most controversial psychoanalyst since Freud". Lacan's foci usually centre on language and the creation of subjectivity-objectivity, yet language itself is problematic.

Terry Eagleton puts it this way: "for Lacan all discourse is, in a sense, a slip of the tongue: if the process of language is as slippery as he suggests, we can never mean precisely what we say, or say precisely what we mean. Meaning is always in some sense an approximation, a near-miss, a part failure, mixing non-sense and non-communication into sense and dialogue. We can certainly never articulate the truth in some 'pure' unmediated way: Lacan's own notoriously sybilline style, a language of the unconscious all in itself, is meant to suggest that any attempt to convey a whole unblemished meaning in speech or script is a pre-Freudian illusion."

In a web article on the "Cult of Lacan," Richard Webster analyses a paragraph from one of Lacan's early works. Referring to his "mirror" stage of childhood development, trying to pin down this oracular or prophetic style of writing, Lacan writes, "This jubilant assumption of his specular image by the child at the infant stage, still sunk in his motor incapacity and nursing dependence, would seem to exhibit in an exemplary situation the symbolic matrix in which the I is precipitated in a primordial form, before it is objectified in the dialectic of identification with the other, and before language restores to it, in the universal, its function as a subject."

Webster explains how the rhetoric works:

"The passage, regarded by many Lacanians as a crucial formulation, is an interesting example of Lacan's expository style. The dominant register is a scientific one; we are told that the 'I' is 'precipitated' as though what is being described is a chemical experiment. 'Primordial form' is a phrase with a similar scientific resonance although this time the field evoked is that of geology or evolutionary biology. In both cases something called the 'I' is referred to as though it were a solid object with physical properties which can be both transformed and described. When Lacan goes on to refer to the stage 'before the "I" is objectified in the dialectic of identification with the other' and to the power of language to restore to the I 'its function as a subject' he writes as if he were referring to a theory of human development which is widely understood and commonly held to be true. Yet, apart from the Hegelian or Marxist resonance of the word 'dialectic,' no information is offered as to what this theory might be or where any exposition of it might be found."

Yet the crucial passage from Lacan makes more sense when accompanied by Lacan's prior remarks concerning the "mirror" stage in relation to the chimpanzee:

The child, at an age when he is for a time, however short, outdone by the chimpanzee in instrumental intelligence, can nevertheless already recognise as such his own image in a mirror. This recognition is indicated in the illuminative mimicry of the Aha-Erlebniss, (Eureka, or Sudden Insight) which is the expression of situational apperception, an essential stage of the act of intelligence.

This produces the split subject – look at me, which is not me, as well as the dialectic of self and other, as well as self and the outside world: subject-object. Lacan continues:

This act, far from exhausting itself, as in the case of the monkey, once the image has been mastered and found empty, immediately rebounds in the case of the child in a series of gestures in which he experiences in play the relation between the movements assumed in the image and the reflected environment, and between this virtual complex and the reality it reduplicates - the child's own body, and the persons and things, around him.

We can then infer, that the "symbolic matrix" of discourse – language mediates a "dialectic" between Self and Other, Subject and Object, mediated or "restored" as the "I" through language, a part of and a part from Other and Object learned in "the mirror stage" according to Lacan.

36. For Lacan, "meaning" is:
    A. never unmediated, always in some sense symbolic and loose.
    B. always unmediated through language, and the dominant discursive structure or mode.
    C. partially mediated through the acquisition of language in the "mirror stage".
    D. partially unmediated through the acquisition of language in the "mirror stage".

37. From passage information, what would "sibylline" mean within the context of the passage?
    A. Simplistic
    B. Complex
    C. Prophetic
    D. Misunderstood

38. Which of the following notions would NOT represent how Webster addresses the style of Lacan?
    A. Lacan uses different sorts of scientific languages, from chemistry and biology.
    B. Lacan uses Marxist terminology and the notion of a "dialectic" between Self and Other.
    C. Lacan's style has an apparent lack of obscurity in the use of terms we are familiar with.
    D. Lacan has an oracular style of writing, as if it is common sense.

39. Based on passage information, which of the following notions BEST represents Lacan's "mirror stage of development"?
    A. The infant recognises himself as Other through language.
    B. The infant recognises Self as a "part of and apart from" the mirror and language.
    C. The infant becomes a split subject (Self and Other) from recognition as Other, yet as Self also, within the "mirror" while acquiring language.
    D. The infant becomes a subject as "I" in relation to the Other, through language.

40. Based on passage information, what could one infer to be Lacan's main theoretical weakness?
    A. Use of jargon
    B. Use of ambiguous phrases
    C. Faulty comparisons between chimpanzees and infants
    D. Over-reliance on language to describe subjectivity

> If time remains, you may review your work. If your allotted time (50 minutes) is complete, please proceed to the Answer Key.

UNDERSTANDING THE GAMSAT

3.8.2 Verbal Reasoning Exercise 1 (Humanities and Social Science) Answer Key and Explanations

1.	B	9.	C	17.	C	25.	C	33.	C
2.	C	10.	B	18.	D	26.	C	34.	D
3.	C	11.	B	19.	A	27.	B	35.	B
4.	C	12.	C	20.	C	28.	D	36.	A
5.	D	13.	C	21.	D	29.	C	37.	C
6.	D	14.	C	22.	C	30.	A	38.	C
7.	B	15.	A	23.	D	31.	B	39.	C
8.	D	16.	D	24.	A	32.	D	40.	B

1. **Correct Answer: B**
Identifying the main idea of this passage can be tricky if the main subject is not clarified as well: is it Ding Darling or the National Wildlife Federation? The passage starts with Ding Darling and goes on to discuss the specifics of his actions; and then, for a while centres on the NWF because this is Darling's biggest achievement ever since he started using his cartoons for his environmental cause. NWF is, therefore, used merely as a vehicle to demonstrate Darling's achievement and how he was able to succeed in promoting his cause. This would then eliminate answer choices C and D.
On the other hand, the author highlights Darling's efforts to "unite all outdoor and wildlife enthusiasts behind a common goal of conservation," resulting to the founding of the NWF. This makes B as most representative of the passage's central point.
Although A is also true, this only forms part of Darling's driving motives in forming the General Wildlife Federation, which was eventually changed to the National Wildlife Federation.

2. **Correct Answer: C**
This is a question that tests your ability to differentiate the accomplishments of Ding Darling from the organisation that he helped establish.
(I) This is indicated in the last sentence of Paragraph 1:
"This is where the General Wildlife Federation, later changed to National Wildlife Federation, was formed with the idea of uniting all outdoor and wildlife enthusiasts behind a common goal of conservation, and Ding Darling became the first president of the organisation."
Paragraph 4 likewise supports this claim.
(II) Qualifying this answer entails separating the works of the NWF from Ding Darling's. P1 S2 indeed indicates that Darling "was instrumental in creating the government agency that used the practice of scientific management for fish and wildlife." On the other hand, although the NWF is mentioned in the passage as annually returning to Washington D.C. to "to provide governance, vision, and grassroots needed to achieve joint conservation goals," this does not clearly indicate spearheading any government agency. Hence, statement II cannot accurately pertain to one of the activities in which the NWF is involved.
(III) This is clearly implied in P4 S1 and P5 S2.

3. **Correct Answer: C**
This question requires clearly identifying Darling's conservation principles and the nature of his works. These can be inferred in P1 S5:
"His work and input valued the importance of multiple stakeholder participation, accepting attitudes, values, and beliefs of many groups."
(A) This primarily describes what NWF would promote, not Darling's. (P3 Last Sentence)
(B) Although this involves conservation ethics, Darling's work is only limited within North America. The Amazon is a South American territory. This is an off-tangent answer.
(C) This corresponds to the statement of P1 S5; therefore, the correct answer.
(D) Darling's work are all related to the preservation of wildlife and natural habitats. Global warming is an issue confronted by NWF. This is likewise off-tangent.

4. **Correct Answer: C**
This passage is an example of the main idea and the author's purpose being practically the same. Answering this question thus also involves identifying the main idea of the passage, i.e. the influential role of Ding Darling in the creation of the NWF. The explanation has already been discussed in Question 1.
This is also supported by the author's repeated mention of Darling's contributions to the association and to conservationist goals in general:
"Darling's quest to unite all voices concerning conservation was the basis for many laws and policies that are present today at the national level. The National Wildlife Federation returns every year to Washington D.C. to provide governance, vision, and grassroots needed to achieve joint conservation goals." (P2)
"What started out as a cartoonist's dream became one of the largest grassroots conservation organisations in the country." (P5 Last Sentence)
"Darling's original ideas are still a mainstay of conservation imperatives, goals, and objectives.

So without a concerned citizen who happened to be a cartoonist, there would probably not be an organisation like the National Wildlife Federation in today's society." (Last Paragraph)

5. **Correct Answer: D**
This is another question that is closely related to the main idea and likewise highly requires clearly understanding the nature and extent of Darling's involvements.
(A) This is supported by P1 S2 and S3.
(B) This is indicated in P1 Last Two Sentences.
(C) This is also mentioned in P1 S2.
(D) This is a rather illogical answer since owning a hunting rifle does not necessarily prove to cause any anti-conservationist objectives or activities. Likewise, the passage does not indicate that Darling has criticised or rallied against other organised groups. This is, therefore, the least likely that Darling could have done.

6. **Correct Answer: D**
This question requires delineating the author's views apart from those of Darling's and NWF's. These are indicated in the following lines:
"What started as a cartoonist's dream became one of the largest grassroots conservation organisations in the country." (P5 Last Sentence)

7. **Correct Answer: B**
This question requires differentiating the author's view and statements about the Romantic poets in general, from those of the three Romantic poets referred in the passage:
"To the romantic poets, poetry was an instrument of emotion and feeling intended to reconnect man with the natural world, and in general the poet was viewed as a person uniquely equipped to guide the layman to this reconnection." (P1)
"Each of these poets recognised great value in the natural feelings and emotions of man, and the connection sparked by man's place in

the natural world. Each strove to capture and explain that connection through creative imagination and ultimately, through poetry." (Last paragraph)

(A) This option is a misreading of the information found in the last sentence of Paragraph 2 pertaining to the goal of Romantic poetry - not poets.

(C) This is another misreading of the idea that "In the eyes of the romantic poets, mankind had become so swept up in the pursuit of knowledge and innovation that they had disconnected from both the natural world, and their deeper, natural selves." The Romantic poets saw the scientific discoveries diminishing man's connection with the natural selves and the world – not creative imagination. In fact, they also valued reason and logic as indicated in P2 S3:

"Though the philosophies of the individual poets differed, in general romantic poetry focussed on and lauded primitivism and emotion while minimising (but not discounting) the importance of reason and logic."

(D) This answer is an anachronism, i.e., the Victorian era comes after the Romantic age temporally.

8. **Correct Answer: D**
This is another question that calls for differentiating the concepts and perspectives presented in the passage. The trick in this question lies in the use of the terms "creative inspiration" and "creative imagination," which can get incorrectly interchanged and thus easily misinterpreted because they are being used in various details and concepts.

The answer can be readily found in P3 S3:
"This caused much difficulty though, as the source of creative imagination was impossible to trace and because creative inspiration was quite fickle."

This opposes Wordsworth's belief that inspiration is derived from the most basic and simplest of things:

"Wordsworth believed that beauty and inspiration was to be found in the most rudimentary and common things and was not something that could only be found in the high and lofty." (P4 S1)

(A) This is in contradiction to Wordsworth's view of beauty and inspiration.

(B) The passage does not imply that this is a problem of creative inspiration, as indicated in P4 S1.

(C) This refers to creative imagination - not inspiration.

9. **Correct Answer: C**
Although Romanticism as a movement was formed during the height of scientific discoveries, it did not essentially (C) challenge the use of reason and logic, but rather of man's tendency to be consumed by "the pursuit of knowledge and innovation" as indicated in P2:

"In the eyes of the romantic poets, mankind had become so swept up in the pursuit of knowledge and innovation that they had disconnected from both the natural world, and their deeper, natural selves. Though the philosophies of the individual poets differed, in general romantic poetry focussed on and lauded primitivism and emotion while minimising (but not discounting) the importance of reason and logic."

(A) The Romantic movement is thus in response, indeed, (though not necessarily a challenge) to the scientific and formal knowledge at that time. (P2 S2)

(B) This is supported in the last sentence of Paragraph 2 and the last paragraph. Beliefs of the three Romantic poets mentioned also emphasise this idea. (P3 S1, P4 S5, P5 S2)

(D) This is clearly stated in the second sentence of the last paragraph.

10. **Correct Answer: B**
The essay does not focus on just (A) differences, so this option can be ruled out. Nor does the essay focus on (D) "philosophers." C men-

GAMSAT-Prep.com
THE GOLD STANDARD

tions "tendencies," which is ambiguous as this statement neither specify poetic tendencies nor does the passage involve "juxtaposition" which implies difference. This leaves B as the most inclusive and general of the answer choices.

11. **Correct Answer: B**
    The question specifies an answer that involves identifying a common view between Coleridge and Wordsworth pertaining to the "sublime." These can be found in the following lines:
    "Samuel Taylor Coleridge, one of the pioneers of the Romantic Movement, believed that the creative imagination was the key to man achieving his connection to the sublime." (P3 S1)
    "Like Coleridge, Wordsworth believed that creative imagination was the source of poetry and the avenue to the sublime." (P4 S5)
    The rest are decoys that are meant to sound like commonly used terms in the passage and could be mistaken as relevant concepts. They are really just off-tangent concepts.

12. **Correct Answer: C**
    This question requires recognising similarities between new information introduced and a significant concept discussed in the passage. The question specifies the ideas associated with the layman's term "romantic": love, affection, irrationality. These serve as the bases in relating with the Romantic Movement's own concept.
    A and B are decoys that use outside knowledge and not discussed in the passage.
    (C) This is discussed in the passage, particularly in P2 S3.
    (D) This would sound highly relevant. However, this is only specific to Wordsworth's principle, not to Romanticism in general. Likewise, Wordsworth's claim does not address the concept of "irrationality."

13. **Correct Answer: C**
    A, B, and D are either too specific, too general, or impartial in relation to passage information. This leaves C as the correct answer in relation to the author's general purpose.

14. **Correct Answer: C**
    A, B, and D are either too specific, too general, or impartial in relation to passage information, leaving C as the BEST title that embodies the main idea of the passage.

15. **Correct Answer: A**
    B, C, and D are all partially correct, in terms of passage information. A may or may not be true yet would function "hypothetically" as going against the author's argument, making this the BEST choice option.

16. **Correct Answer: D**
    A, B, and C are all presented as "dichotomies" or dualisms within the passage information. They reflect either-or modes of thinking. Only D is not presented, making this the best choice option.

17. **Correct Answer: C**
    A, B, and D can all be inferred to be a "motive" based on passage information and by re-reading. Only C, which is not correct as an assessment of "Impressionism," can be considered the best choice option.

18. **Correct Answer: D**
    A simple re-read or re-scan will affirm (D) I and III as correct, ruling out the other answers/options.

19. **Correct Answer: A**
    This type of question focusses on a general assessment of the passage as a whole and its main purpose. We must consider that all of the answers are partially correct, therefore the answer that is most inclusive will be correct. By doing this we can assess that (A) encompasses all the others mentioned in (B), (C), and (D), as evidenced in the introductory sentence and Paragraph 7 in its entirety.

20. **Correct Answer: C**
    This is a complex-sounding question, which requires a process of deduction. Again, we must look for the lateral distinction of inclusion to indicate the answer to this tone question. All the answers are partially correct, yet one will stand out from the others and include the other answers. There are passages which are (A) bleak, as well as (D) cautious, yet these are relatively too focussed to be general assessments of the "tone of the author." There are also indications of (B) some hope in the author's suggestions about wisdom and liberty, yet we cannot define the entire passage as "hopeful." (C) Existential is the most inclusive of the others, because "existence will carry with it moments of caution, hope, as well as bleakness and despair." Despite its "absurdist" ring, the reflections of existential thought, found in Camus, Sartre, Ionesco, and others run the full range and gamut of human emotions and actions. The term existentialism has often been compared to a "tragic optimism" view of life, which this passage certainly suggests.

21. **Correct Answer: D**
    This is a complex-sounding question and the answers are full of abstractions, which one must be very careful, while ruling out answers.
    A simply does not make sense – a created sort of joke and certainly does not go against the thesis.
    B is a tangent and not really related to the author's thesis.
    C is also a tangent and not really related to the author's thesis.
    D would go against the author's "entropic" view of humankind. If this is considered to be true, even hypothetically, it would qualify as the best choice, given the other options.

22. **Correct Answer: C**
    This detail-oriented question can be answered by a close reading particularly in Paragraph 6:
    We shall define philosophy as "total perspective," as mind overspreading life and forging chaos into unity.

23. **Correct Answer: D**
    This is a best option type of question, in which all of the answers may be partially correct or inferred and/or implicative of passage information. Only D answers the question directly and can be found in Paragraph 7:
    Philosophy is harmonised knowledge making a harmonious life.

24. **Correct Answer: A**
    This is a detail-oriented question based on a distinction which the author makes within the passage. The best ratio is A while the other answers are created distractions. This idea is reflected in the following statement, from the passage:
    Knowledge is power, but only wisdom is liberty.
    (B) A distraction – philosophical babble of existentialism
    (C) Babble of philosophy in general
    (D) Never mentioned

25. **Correct Answer: C**
    This is an inference question based on modern affiliations of people with the internet. To answer this question, one must find the best choice based on a "generalisation." We must also rule out certain options at the same time.
    A is too generalised. We cannot proclaim we all feel disconnected and shallow.
    B is also too generalised; we cannot all proclaim we feel connected and hopeful.
    (C) When on the internet, we feel interconnected, yet disassociated. This is a generalisation but also a bit of paradox, because the context of face-to-face communication is not there. It is similar to Derrida's idea of "absent presence" therefore the correct answer.
    D is too generalised, and the metaphor of a network is faulty. If there is a metaphor for the

internet – the rhizome would be descriptive. Linear suggests one-way, we know that is untrue for the internet. There are multiple connections, going in multiple ways simultaneously constituting a quite complex assemblage of information and communication.

26. **Correct Answer: C**
    Given the complexity of this question, which is based on detail and close reading or re-scan, one must be very careful because of the way terms are being emplaced together.
    (A) This is too obvious and is somewhat tautological in reasoning (circular argument). If read carefully, it really does not answer the question.
    (B) This is never really mentioned within the passage; this answer concerns linguistics.
    (C) This is a summation of P2 S2 and answers the question.
    (D) This is too obvious also and tautological, not really answering the question.

27. **Correct Answer: B**
    This is an associative type of question where the answer must be the BEST choice or inference given the range of options:
    A is partially true, yet "the abyss of chaos" is too extreme.
    (B) This is the correct answer: the romantic imagery of the rose versus the destructive imagery of a worm flying through the storm making the rose sick.
    (C) Linguistically, a real rose can be sick – infected with disease, bug-ridden, etc. This is an incorrect option.
    (D) This answer is too general. Yes, there are multiple meanings and effects upon a reader, but that is a condition of most poetry.

28. **Correct Answer: D**
    This question is another best option type given the range of answers, in which one must deduce through a process of elimination (PoE) to arrive at the correct answer.
    (A) Telescopic is vague and similar to C, which is also incorrect. It suggests nothing of the author's attitude towards archetypes.
    (B) Critical is also vague. This could be translated in a number of different ways – serious and analytical, which suggests more of an approach rather than an "attitude."
    (C) This can be ruled out for a similar reason as A.
    (D) Archetypes as encompassing can be inferred to be correct because it is the theoretical framework of which the poem is analysed. Given the statements in P2, this idea can easily be supported.

29. **Correct Answer: C**
    This is a detail-oriented question, which must be drawn from the passage itself because all of the answers may be implicative of the passage or inferred to be at least partially correct. Within the passage itself A and B may be implied, yet never directly mentioned as in C - Last Paragraph, S1. D is indicative of Blake yet overly complex and not mentioned within the passage.

30. **Correct Answer: A**
    This type of question is also detail-oriented, which must be solved by close reading, rescan and deduction through the process of elimination (PoE).
    A is implied in Paragraph 2.
    (B) This answer is a created distraction – intention is never mentioned within the passage.
    C and D are either too obvious or too literal to be correct yet lacks specificity.

31. **Correct Answer: B**
    This type of question is also detail-oriented, which must be solved by close reading, rescan and deduction through the process of elimination (PoE).
    A and C are tangential and unfocussed, therefore, incorrect. D is too specific yet likewise tangential and unfocussed. B can be affirmed by Paragraph 5 in general and thus correct.

32. Correct Answer: D

This complex-sounding question must proceed to be answered by the comparison of the poem with Milton:

A is partially true. The stories are the same, yet the language and style is quite different.

B is incorrect and a created tangent distraction amounting to nonsense, which means cannot be recovered(?).

C is also incorrect: the general theme of both poem and the Milton excerpt is quite similar.

D is correct. The similarities of the two almost border on weirdness given the general thematic, which is almost mirror-like based on the interpretation.

33. Correct Answer: C

Answering this question requires understanding that the purpose of the author is to define and explicate the main subject. To define means to describe something by stating its characteristics. First, the passage tells us where the term 'theatre of the absurd' came from. Next, it tells us it was taken from Albert Camus' ideas which were expressed in his novel 'Le Mythe de Sisyphe'. Next it tells us that many playwrights have been classified as belonging to this movement. In addition, the passage tells us one characteristic that defines all the plays that are classified under the term: they all express a profound inability to make sense of the universe and life on earth. Then it goes on to describe one play which best showcases the movement: Beckett's Waiting for Godot. It briefly describes what the play is all about so that we can understand what 'theatre de l'absurde' is.

A is wrong because the writer does not analyse the movement (it does not compare or contrast it; it does not evaluate it either).

(B) The author does not try to persuade the readers to do anything about the literary movement (to oppose or support it). Hence option B cannot be the answer.

(D) This passage does not strictly give a narrative of a historical development (the passage does not focus on the when and where, dates and places). It focusses on ideas and it attempts to describe something to us for us to understand what it is : it (C) defines it.

34. Correct Answer: D

I and III go against the whole grain, warp and woof of the passage. Only II mentioned in the concluding paragraphs in additional commentary, and a direct paraphrase can be ascertained as correct. Therefore the correct answer is D.

"Dr. Jan Culik writes, 'Absurd Theatre' can be seen as an attempt to restore the importance of myth and ritual to our age, by making man aware of the ultimate realities of his condition, by instilling in him again the lost sense of cosmic wonder and primeval anguish."

35. Correct Answer: B

A, C, and D are used to describe the "theatre of the absurd" as a whole, but by simply going back to the paragraph that discusses "Waiting for Godot", it is clear that B is correct: ". . .describe it is an accurate parable on the human condition in which 'the more things change, the more they are the same'."

When words like "best support", "infer", "essentially", or "come up", the answer will involve a definite logical leap. A "logical leap" is using the facts from a first premise and choosing to go toward a direction of thinking that can be directly related to the first premise.

A first premise is like a diving board on a swimming pool. The logical leap is when you jump off that diving board and reach the general area that is marked on the tiles (you know, that coloured patch of tile) that indicates that your jump was good (it's on the deep part of the pool where you are expected to land).

When you grasp what the first premise says and means, you can choose which idea should naturally follow. The next thought or idea is not given to you, you are supposed to find it yourself (infer), supply it yourself (hypothesise), or in this case, choose it from a set of options.

36. **Correct Answer: A**
    This is a similar pair question based on definition and interpretation. C and D are similar pair that can be deduced to be incorrect. Although the mirror stage is mentioned later, the passage does not link this up to the "meaning" of "meaning." In the dichotomy of A, the correct choice, and B, always unmediated - which contradicts itself, the following excerpt from the passage explains language as unmediated:
    Terry Eagleton puts it this way: "for Lacan all discourse is, in a sense, a slip of the tongue: if the process of language is as slippery as he suggests, we can never mean precisely what we say, or say precisely what we mean. Meaning is always in some sense an approximation, a near-miss, a part failure, mixing non-sense and non-communication into sense and dialogue.

37. **Correct Answer: C**
    This is an inference of definition type of question based on context.
    "Lacan's own notoriously sibylline style, a language of the unconscious all in itself, is meant to suggest that any attempt to convey a whole unblemished meaning in speech or script is a pre-Freudian illusion."
    In a web article on the "Cult of Lacan," Richard Webster analyses a paragraph from one of Lacan's early works. Referring to his "mirror" stage of childhood development, trying to pin down this oracular or prophetic style of writing.

38. **Correct Answer: C**
    (C) To state that Lacan is not obscure, of which can hardly be said, is far from being true. The other notions of A, B, and D are all passage excerpt ideas discussed by Webster.

39. **Correct Answer: C**
    Lacan's "mirror stage" is most adequately, and paradoxically, expressed in C based on the passage's last paragraph:
    We can then infer, that the "symbolic matrix" of discourse – language mediates a "dialectic" between Self and Other, Subject and Object, mediated or "restored" as the "I" through language, a part of and a part from Other and Object learned in "the mirror stage" according to Lacan.

40. **Correct Answer: B**
    (A) Jargon usually refers to specialised languages of the arts and sciences so can be ruled out.
    (C) Comparisons between mammalia are not the main weakness. Such comparisons are done all the time in the sciences.
    (D) Subjectivity - or being a subject - is not a notable weakness since a human has much to do with the acquisition of language.
    (B) The use of ambiguous phrases - analysed by Webster is quite specific and applicable to Lacan, in terms of his main theoretical weakness, making B the best choice.

UNDERSTANDING THE GAMSAT

3.8.3 Verbal Reasoning Exercise 2 (Science-based Passages)

The following is a sample mini test which is designed to aid in developing your skills in reading and answering passages that are related to science or medicine. These types of passages are known to appear in Section 1 of recent GAMSATs.

There are 7 Units with 40 questions. Choose the best answer for each question. You have 50 minutes. Please time yourself.

BEGIN ONLY WHEN TIMER IS READY

Unit 1

Questions 1 - 5

Gold was first discovered at Summitville mine in Colorado in 1870. Significant gold production from underground workings occurred prior to 1900. In 1903, the Reynolds adit (entrance for access, drainage, and ventilation) was driven to drain the underground workings and serve as an ore haulage tunnel. Production occurred sporadically through the 1950s. The district received some exploration attention in the 1970s as a copper prospect, but no mining for copper was pursued.

Similar to many historic gold mining districts in the western United States, Summitville received renewed interest in the early 1980s due to technological advances that allow extraction of low-grade ores with cyanide heap leach techniques. In 1984, Summitville Consolidated Mining Company, Inc. (SCMCI), initiated open pit mining of gold ore from rocks surrounding the historic underground workings, where gold concentrations had been too low to be economic for the underground mining operations. Ore from the pit was crushed and placed on a heap leach pad overlying a protective liner. Cyanide solutions were sprinkled onto the heap and trickled down through the crushed ore, dissolving the gold. The processing solutions were then collected from the base of the heap leach pile, and the gold was chemically extracted from the solutions.

Environmental problems developed soon after the initiation of open-pit mining. Acidic, metal rich drainage into the Wightman Fork of the Alamosa River increased significantly from numerous sources on site, including the Reynolds adit and the Cropsy waste dump. Cyanide-bearing processing solutions began leaking into an underdrain system beneath the heap leach pad, where they then mixed with acid ground waters from the Cropsy waste dump. Cyanide solutions also leaked from transfer pipes directly into the Wightman Fork several times over the course of mining.

    SCMCI had ceased active mining and had begun environmental remediation when it declared bankruptcy in December 1992 and abandoned the mine site. The bankruptcy created several immediate concerns. Earlier in 1992, the company had brought a water treatment plant on line to begin treating the estimated 150 to 200 million gallons of spent cyanide processing solutions remaining in the heap; however, treatment was proceeding so slowly relative to influx of snowmelt waters that the waters were in danger of overtopping a containment dike and flowing directly into the Wightman Fork. In addition, piping carrying the processing solutions to the treatment plant would have frozen within several hours, releasing cyanide solutions and stopping water treatment.

    At the request of the State of Colorado, the U.S. Environmental Protection Agency (EPA) immediately took over the site under EPA Superfund Emergency Response authority and increased treatment of the heap leach solutions, thereby averting a catastrophic release of cyanide solutions from the heap. Summitville was added to the EPA National Priorities List in late May, 1994. Ongoing remediation efforts include decommissioning of the heap leach pad, plugging of the Reynolds and Chandler adits, backfilling of the open pit with acid-generating mine waste material, and capping of the backfilled pit to prevent water inflow. The total cost of the cleanup has been estimated to be from US $100 million to $120 million.

    The environmental problems at Summitville have been of particular concern due to the extensive downstream use of Alamosa River water for livestock, agricultural irrigation, and wildlife habitat. Increased acid and metal loadings from Summitville are suspected to have caused the 1990 disappearance of stocked fish from Terrace Reservoir and farm holding ponds along the Alamosa River. The Alamosa River is used extensively to irrigate crops in the southwestern San Luis Valley. Important crops include alfalfa (used for livestock feed), barley (used in beer production), wheat, and potatoes; there has been concern about potential adverse effects of the increased acid and metal loadings from Summitville on the metal content and viability of these crops. The Alamosa River also feeds wetlands that are habitat for aquatic life and migratory water fowl such as ducks and the endangered whooping crane; there are concerns about Summitville's effects on these wetlands and their associated wildlife.

- U.S. Department of the Interior | U.S. Geological Survey

1. What is the main idea of the passage?
   A. Open pit mining has disastrous effects.
   B. Open pit mining in Summitville has caused pending environmental hazards.
   C. There is a need for stricter controls and regulations governing open pit mining.
   D. Open pit mining typically affects the environment.

2. What is the author's purpose of the passage?
   A. To demonstrate and warn of the potential harmful effects left by Summitville mining to environment, particularly the Alamosa River
   B. To illustrate the environmental need for legislation for all open pit mining areas
   C. To demonstrate and suggest that similar efforts in other areas should follow the Summitville mining "cleanup" protocol and agenda
   D. To rally support for environmental groups and their political eco-green proposals and agenda

3. What evidence would MOST STRONGLY support the author's argument?
   A. Cyanide toxins can contaminate wetlands downstream in typical mining areas.
   B. The disappearance of certain species has been noted due to open pit mining.
   C. There are neither regulatory controls in place for monitoring of toxins nor clean-up planning in case of emergencies.
   D. Open pit mining threatens all life in as much as it threatens the general ecosystem of the area.

4. According to passage information, which of the following were NOT potentially affected by the runoff into the Alamosa River?
   I. Wildlife habitat
   II. Potable drinking water
   III. Livestock

   A. I and III
   B. II only
   C. III only
   D. II and III

5. What are the dominant kinds of evidence or support used by the author to strengthen his or her thesis?
   A. Real examples and statistics
   B. Hypothetical examples and statistics
   C. Expert testimony and current regulations
   D. Emotional appeals and green reasoning

Unit 2

Questions 6 - 11

    The appearances in the heavens have from earliest historic ages filled men with wonder and awe; then they gradually became a source of questioning, and thinkers sought for explanations of the daily and nightly phenomena of sun, moon and stars. Scientific astronomy, however, was an impossibility until an exact system of chronology was devised. Meanwhile, men puzzled over the shape of the earth, its position in the universe, what the stars were and why the positions of some shifted, and what those fiery comets were that now and again appeared and struck terror to their hearts.

    In answer to such questions, the Chaldean thinkers, slightly before the rise of the Greek schools of philosophy, developed the idea of the seven heavens in their crystalline spheres encircling the earth as their center. This conception seems to lie back of both the later Egyptian and Hebraic cosmologies, as well as of the Ptolemaic. Through the visits of Greek philosophers to Egyptian shores, this conception helped to shape Greek thought and so indirectly affected western civilisation. Thus our heritage in astronomical thought, as in many other lines, comes from the Greeks and the Romans reaching Europe (in part through Arabia and Spain), where it was shaped by the influence of the schools down to the close of the Middle Ages when men began anew to withstand authority in behalf of observation and were not afraid to follow whither their reason led them.

    But not all Greek philosophers, it seems, either knew or accepted the Babylonian cosmology. According to Plutarch, though Thales (640?-546? B.C.) and later the Stoics believed the earth to be spherical in form, Anaximander (610-546? B.C.) thought it to be like a "smooth stony pillar, "Anaximenes (6th century) like a "table." Beginning with the followers of Thales or perhaps Parmenides (?-500 B.C.), as Diogenes Laërtius claims, a long line of Greek thinkers including Plato (428?-347? B.C.) and Aristotle (384-322 B.C.) placed the earth in the centre of the universe. Whether Plato held that the earth "encircled" or "clung" around the axis is a disputed point; but Aristotle claimed it was the fixed and immovable center around which swung the spherical universe with its heaven of fixed stars and its seven concentric circles of the planets kept in their places by their transparent crystalline spheres. "The sense for beauty is obviously an attribute of the human mind, merely one phase of intellectuality, nothing less, nothing more."

    The stars were an even greater problem. Anaximenes thought they were "fastened like nails" in a crystalline firmament, and others thought them to be "fiery plates of gold resembling pictures." But if the heavens were solid, how could the brief presence of a comet be explained? Among the philosophers were some noted as mathematicians whose leader was Pythagoras (c. 550 B.C.). He and at least one of the members of his school, Eudoxus (409?-356? B.C.), had visited Egypt, according to Diogenes Laërtius, and had in all probability been much interested in and influenced by the astronomical observations made by the Egyptian priests. On the same authority, Pythagoras was the first to declare the earth was round and to discuss the antipodes. He too emphasised the beauty and perfection of the circle and of the sphere in geometry, forms which became fixed for 2000 years as the fittest representations of the perfection of the heavenly bodies.

6. The opening statement of the passage suggests that the human desire for knowledge is:
   A. profound.
   B. empirical.
   C. innate.
   D. referential.

7. One can infer that our knowledge of astronomy has been acquired:
   A. indirectly from the Chaldeans.
   B. from the birth of trigonometry.
   C. directly from the Greeks.
   D. from eclectic sources.

8. By declaring the Earth round, Pythagoras was:
   A. devising a system of chronology.
   B. stressing the exactitude of the sphere.
   C. linking astronomy to trigonometry.
   D. redefining earlier beliefs.

9. By placing the Earth at the centre of the universe, Plato and Aristotle can be inferred to be:
   A. ethnocentric.
   B. heliocentric.
   C. anthropocentric.
   D. geopocentric.

10. According to passage information, only until an exact system of chronology was established was:
    A. scientific astronomy a possibility.
    B. the temporal exactness of astronomy created.
    C. the spatial exactness of astronomy created.
    D. the fusion of trigonometry and astronomy possible.

11. The writer's main focus on astronomy is:
  A. analytical.
  B. historical.
  C. deductive.
  D. inductive.

Unit 3

Questions 12 - 16

In the natural sciences, enquiry is concerned with uncovering or discovering that which exists. "Invention" is not considered to be a feature of scientific enquiry and is perhaps not compatible with the dispassionate relationship with knowledge that scientists have traditionally claimed. Design, by contrast, claims invention (and personal ownership of it) as a central principle so it is difficult at first to see where the two traditions can overlap.

A central problem of science is how to recognise and define worthwhile subjects for investigation. For one thing, we may be faced with a myriad of opportunities and no means to decide which are going to be fruitful. On the other hand, our environment may limit our ability to recognise scientific problems and possibilities, especially the ones which could lead to significant changes in our understanding. To illustrate this second problem, philosophers have speculated on the science and culture of imaginary worlds which have fundamentally different and more restricted conditions than ours. If you and your environment consist of gases with no solid objects to reflect on, then you may not be able to conceive of geometry as we know it. If you lived in a 1- or 2-dimensional world you would have a very different set of concepts from us and, no doubt, people living in a 5-dimensional world would see us as conceptually impoverished in much the same way. Artists also engage with these issues, often in stimulating and accessible forms. For example, science fiction writers explore imaginary worlds which shape their civilisations in ways that may inform us about our own experience. Brian Aldiss described a world where each season lasted for many lifetimes, including a harsh winter which few people and institutions survived, effectively cutting people off from their history and most of the knowledge acquired during the previous summer. This fictional device provided a fresh perspective for the examination of individuals and societies confronted with difficult circumstances.

These abstracted questions have their parallels in everyday life and more mundane enquiries. Michael Polanyi describes the 'logical gap' between existing knowledge and any significant discovery or innovation. No matter how thorough our factual knowledge of the situation that we inhabit, the pursuit of logical reasoning or iterative development of existing concepts would not, on its own, allow us to cross this gap. There must be also some kind of leap of 'illumination' by which the scientist imagines a new concept and proposes it as a worthwhile subject for investigation. As Polanyi says "Illumination. ...is the plunge by which we gain a foothold in another shore of reality. On such plunges the scientist has to stake, bit by bit, his entire professional life."

Polanyi was concerned with what he called the "tacit dimension" in our knowledge. In particular he wished to give proper value to the process of recognising, and making a commitment to, ideas or hypotheses, which may result from a rich understanding and knowledge but cannot be explained by explicit reasoning, in order to carry out the enquiry that will lead to them being more widely understood and accepted. I have used the term "accepted" rather than "proved" (itself shorthand for Karl Popper's concept of a falsifiable hypothesis that has proved so far to be reliable) because Polanyi held that all scientific knowledge is a question of "passionate belief" rather than dispassionate proof, requiring us to take account of the methods, competence, judgement and integrity of scientists, and the knowledge and principles that we already hold, before we accept the knowledge which they offer us. This seems much more reasonable today, when more people appreciate the limitations of science, than 50 years ago when Polanyi was developing his ideas.

12. The crux of the problem, which the author specifically focusses on is:
    A. developing protocol for what scientific endeavours are advisable to pursue.
    B. how scientific invention is related to discovery.
    C. the idea that scientific knowledge is a question of passionate belief.
    D. the idea that scientific knowledge is a question of dispassionate proof.

13. The relevance or significance of the passage, in relation to scientific invention and discovery, concerns:
    A. knowledge.
    B. criteria.
    C. instrumentation.
    D. measurement.

14. According to passage information, Polyani makes a distinction between tacit knowledge and what can be inferred as knowledge which is:
    A. socially constructed.
    B. hypothetically determined.
    C. explicit reasoning.
    D. deductively reasoned.

15. According to passage information, for Polyani, "illumination" is:
    I. the key to invention and discovery in scientific endeavour.
    II. the bridge over the logical gap of theory and application.
    III. the connection between innovation and what is already known.

    A. I only
    B. II only
    C. II and III
    D. I and III

16. The author pursues the notion of which central problem that may limit our ability to recognise scientific problems and possibilities?
    A. Instrumentation designed to measure phenomena
    B. Knowledgeable processes involved in research
    C. Methodologies which are employed in measurement
    D. Environment or setting surrounding us

Unit 4

Questions 17 - 23

The politicisation of science is the manipulation of science for political gain. It occurs when government, business, or advocacy groups use legal or economic pressure to influence the findings of scientific research or the way it is disseminated, reported or interpreted. The politicisation of science may also negatively affect academic and scientific freedom. Historically, groups have conducted various campaigns to promote their interests in defiance of scientific consensus, and in an effort to manipulate public policy.

In August 2003, United States, Democratic Congressman Henry A. Waxman and the staff of the Government Reform Committee released a report concluding that the administration of George W. Bush had politicised science and sex education. The report accuses the administration of modifying performance measures for abstinence-based programs to make them look more effective. The report also found that the Bush administration had appointed Dr. Joseph McIlhaney, a prominent advocate of abstinence-only program, to the Advisory Committee to the director of the Centre for Disease Control. According to the report, information about comprehensive sex education was removed from the CDC's website.

The Union of Concerned Scientists (UCS) also issued a report indicating that the Bush administration delayed for nine months an EPA report (eventually leaked) that indicated that 8 percent of women between the ages of 16 and 49 have blood mercury levels that could lead to reduced I.Q. and motor skills in their offspring. When new rules of mercury emissions were finally released by the EPA, at least 12 paragraphs were transferred, sometimes verbatim, from a legal document prepared by industry attorneys.

According to the Waxman Report, other issues considered for removal from government sponsored programs included agricultural pollution, the Arctic National Wildlife Refuge and breast cancer; the report found that a National Cancer Institute website has been changed to reflect the administration view that there may be a risk of breast cancer associated with abortions. The website was updated after protests and now holds that no such risk has been found in recent, well-designed studies. In addition, proponents for "Intelligent Design" (ID) over "Evolution" have government-spearheaded efforts to be entered into the public schools and with success.

The overwhelming majority of the scientific community, which supports theories that are testable by experiment or observation, oppose treating ID, which is neither, as scientific theory. A 1999 report by the National Academy of Sciences states, "Creationism, intelligent design, and other claims of supernatural intervention in the origin of life or of species are not science because they are not testable by the methods of science." Public officials have supported public schools teaching intelligent design alongside evolution in science curricula.

In January 2007, the House Committee on Science and Technology announced the formation of a new subcommittee, the Science Subcommittee on Investigations and Oversight, which handles investigative and oversight activities on matters covering the committee's entire jurisdiction. The subcommittee has authority to look into a whole range of important issues, particularly those concerning manipulation of scientific data at Federal agencies.

In an interview, subcommitte chairman Rep. Brad Miller pledged to "look into. . . scientific integrity issues under the Bush Administration. There have been lots of reports in the press of manipulating science to support policy, rigging advisory panels, and suppressing research by federal employees or with federal dollars. I've written about that here before, and you interviewed me a year ago about the manipulation of science. In addition to the published reports, the committee staff has been collecting accounts, some confidential, of interference by political appointees." Yet the promised reports were far from adequate (two educational reports) or not released completely to the public, quite possibly due to bipartisan politics and mutual scratch-back negotiations concerning other political agendas.

The issue is far from over. Patrick Michaels, as recently as April 2011, had written (CATO Institute), covering the climate change controversy, that "The conflation of political agendas with science is destroying the credibility of academia, with the complicity of the editors of our major scientific journals," noting a recent SCIENCE article which attempted to revive a 19th Century idea of "climatic determinism" - people do good things when things get warmer, bad things when cold – obviously, politically motivated.

17. Paragraph 1 mentions that "historically, groups have conducted various campaigns to promote their interests in defiance of scientific consensus, and in an effort to manipulate public policy." What is weak in this statement?
    A. Too generalised in terms of "various campaigns"
    B. Unspecific in terms of "what groups"
    C. Misleading in terms of the statement "defiance of scientific consensus"
    D. Misleading in the statement "manipulate public policy"

18. What does "abstinence based programs" imply within the context of the paragraph?
    A. That the fundamental choice of such programs is clearly part of a democratic "agenda"
    B. That some ideological assumptions are carried along with such a choice
    C. That this was the educational program, which was wanted by the people
    D. That the choice precludes programs such as diseases, teen pregnancy and contraception

19. What is particularly weak in terms of evidence or support of the thesis with the following passage commentary: "In addition, proponents for 'Intelligent Design' (ID) over 'Evolution' have government-spearheaded efforts to be entered into the public schools and with success"?
    A. The statement is ambiguous (success).
    B. The statement is non-referential (efforts).
    C. The statement is too specific (proponents).
    D. The statement does not follow reasoning (in addition).

20. What is particularly weak or lacking in the following statement: "Public officials have supported public schools teaching intelligent design alongside evolution in science curricula"?
    A. The statement is politically motivated.
    B. The statement lacks concrete reference.
    C. The statement is too specific.
    D. The statement is circular reasoning.

21. According to passage information, Rep. Miller stated that there were "scientific integrity issues" under the Bush administration, which included:
    I. suppressing research.
    II. rigged advisory panels.
    III. blatant disregard of scientific methodology.

    A. I
    B. I and II
    C. II and III
    D. I and III

22. The author's political or ideological tone is:
    A. impartial.
    B. conservative.
    C. right of center.
    D. liberal.

23. What is weak or lacking in the second part of the statement: "Yet the promised reports were far from adequate (two educational reports) or not released completely to the public, quite possibly due to bipartisan politics and mutual scratch-back negotiations concerning other political agendas"?
    A. The statement undermines the main thrust of the argument.
    B. The statement uses unfamiliar terminology and colloquial jargon.
    C. The statement is too specific - does not generalise sufficiently.
    D. The statement is assumptive and inferential – too much of an argumentative leap.

Unit 5

Questions 24 - 28

It has become more and more common to link together the once disparate concepts of biology and morality. One such way of doing this, which some sociobiologists have advocated, is by introducing the idea of "epigenetic rules". Epigenetic rules mean something like the following: there are certain genetically based processes that are realised in chemically and structurally similar ways in all (or most) humans. For example, there are specific patterns of neurotransmitters and organisational features of fibres and brain tissue that develop in more or less the same fashion in all humans, and this development is somehow regulated, though not determined, by our genes. By influencing and shaping the physical and consequently cognitive processes of the brain, genes affect, but do not determine, the range of possibilities humans possess. Epigenetic rules, then, are the sorts of processes that both constrain and predispose humans to behave and think within a certain range of options. Often cited as examples are certain phobias that transcend cultural boundaries; people tend to fear the dark, high places, snakes, etc.

These epigenetic constraints and dispositions are not limited to simple behaviours and perceptions, but also to our moral sense; epigenetic rules provide a boundary for what humans consider moral. For example, epigenetic rules may predispose us to consider altruism a virtue, since there is an evolutionary advantage (or so some geneticists claim) for altruism; from a genetic point of view, altruistic acts often involve sacrificing the genes of one organism for the furthering of the gene pool of the entire population.

While this is unquestionably a provocative perspective, there are many points with which to take issue. It first seems that this thesis runs the risk of claiming that any common behaviour that transcends cultures and time periods may now be easily attributable to epigenetic rules. As one opponent of this view proposed, there are certain truths about humans, such as 'all humans have a tendency to throw spears pointy-end first'. This behaviour is observed in most cultures ('spears' can be replaced with 'pointy-edged object'), yet it is not at all clear that such behaviour is evidence that humans are genetically predisposed toward this. Rather, it seems that given a certain amount of intelligence and interaction with our environment, many different cultures will reach similar conclusions about which end of a spear proves the most effective. At the least, it is a very open question why humans exhibit similar behaviour patterns. In some cases our intuitions side more with genetics, in others, such as the example above, it seems that other factors are at work.

Further, merely knowing that a particular moral inclination has a genetic basis does not indicate how wrong it is to kill innocent people, so even if it could be shown that this sentiment has a genetic basis, it is possible to override or at least temper it. To put it more generally, just because morality has a basis in our genes (if it in fact does), it does not follow that we should look to our genes to generate, or even help out with, a theory of morality. As the philosopher Friedrich Nietzsche pointed out, explaining the origin of something like morality does not explain why it is successful, nor does the origin necessarily hold the key to explaining or furthering or even affecting its success.

24. The central point of the passage is that:
    A. epigenetic rules exist; now it is just a matter of carefully researching their content.
    B. epigenetic rules may exist but sociobiologists have been too hasty in claiming that they do.
    C. epigenetic rules probably exist but sociobiologists should focus on different behaviours to determine the content of the rules.
    D. epigenetic rules do not exist.

25. The author's statement, "epigenetic rules may predispose us to consider altruism a virtue, since there is an evolutionary advantage to altruism", assumes that:
    A. epigenetic rules favour evolutionary advantages.
    B. epigenetic rules are themselves evolutionary advantages.
    C. altruism is an evolutionary advantage.
    D. what was considered an evolutionary advantage in the past may not be considered to be one currently.

26. Based on the information in the last paragraph, the author would most likely agree with which of the following statements?
    A. The fields of science and morality should remain separate.
    B. The fact that most humans do not condone killing innocent people indicates the existence of epigenetic rules.
    C. Genetic discoveries should not be strongly relied on to provide solutions to moral dilemmas.
    D. Until research has unquestionably proven that there are relevant connections, we should not look to science to provide answers to moral dilemmas.

27. Which of the following is a claim made by the author but NOT supported in the passage by evidence, explanation, or example?
    A. Epigenetic rules transcend cultural and historical boundaries.
    B. Epigenetic rules influence conceptions of morality.
    C. Not all similarities between humans have a genetic basis.
    D. Explaining the origin of something does not explain why it is successful.

28. A recent study suggests that people living in rural areas fear snakes much more than gunshots while people living in urban areas fear gunshots more than snakes. These findings:
    A. support the author's views.
    B. support the sociobiologists' views.
    C. indicate that neither is correct.
    D. indicate that both are correct.

Unit 6

Questions 29 - 34

An "ethics of science" refers to ethical problems involved with scientific research, discoveries, and inventions. In scientific research and invention, experiments on humans, invention of biological weapons, etc., are scientific issues that assume ethical importance. In the field of medicine, ethical problems are associated with issues such as medical research, genetic manipulation, abortion, and euthanasia. In the field of environmental concerns, environmental ethics assumes an important place, as well.

The general issues that give rise to ethical questions concern scientific research and invention. In 1964, an experiment was carried out by the American psychologist Stanley Milgram that involved fooling people into thinking they were inflicting increasingly severe electric shocks on unseen but protesting victims. This experiment raised the ethical issue of whether it was morally right for a scientist to encourage people to inflict pain on others for experimental purposes. The issue of the invention of biological weapons that could affect civilians is an ethical one in the sense that it concerns the rightness or wrongness of harming civilians in war. The whole issue revolves around the concept of crime against humanity. One other issue related also to medicine is the issue of cloning, in which humans prescribe the genes of clones. How would a cloned child see his individuality after knowing that he was a clone? Wouldn't he feel his individuality as forever compromised? What if things go awry in the cloning process? Would that constitute crime against a human? Who would be held responsible if things go awry?

Medical ethics is the study of moral standards in relation to the field of medicine. The ultimate issues underlying medical ethics are issues such as the definition of life and the value of life that are seen in perspective of ethical theories regarding what differentiates good acts and principles from evil. Two of the problems, viz., medical research and embryo research will be discussed here. Research in medicine has the objective of alleviating human pain. However, this requires a study of how the human body works and what new drugs could be safely used to alleviate human pain. Things like experiments with embryos and test of drugs on humans assume ethical character when considering issues such as the value of life and the moral aim of medicine. For instance, during the 1980s there was a widespread debate about the ethics of research using human embryos. In such research, the embryos used were destroyed after 14 days from fertilisation. The argument that ended the debate in UK leading to the legitimising of such research, up to the 14-day limit, was that a pre-14-day embryo was not in a state to be treated as an individual person since its cells were not differentiated to fulfill specific functions along with the possibility that the embryo was still in a condition to split into two identical twins. The 14-day limit assumed that since the nervous system begins to develop at about the 15th day from fertilisation, there was nothing ethically wrong in destroying it on the 14th day, since the embryo doesn't know that it is a person. This also justifies abortion before the 14th day and provides a kind of ethical basis for research in human cloning.

The several assumptions behind the legalising of embryo research are that ethics is related to persons and not to potential persons, that personality is a matter of the nervous system and not the organism housing such a system, that humans are not accountable to anyone other than humans for what they do with any phenomenon of life; in other words, since God or some absolute judicial system doesn't exist, humans can decide what is to be done with humans. Such assumptions, however, cannot be accepted as axiomatic; they are philosophical issues, of course, but also crucial as pertaining to human life itself. In their ultimate development, such issues are settled according to the religious or anti-religious mindset of the political or judicial system in which the issues are raised.

29. What is the main idea of the passage?
    A. An ethics of science concerns different disciplines and fields.
    B. Scientific ethics, particularly in the medical field, is marked by controversy.
    C. The ethics of science is a philosophical, not scientific, issue.
    D. Ethical questions basically concern research and invention.

30. How is the main idea, or thesis, mainly supported within the passage?
    A. Real examples
    B. Hypothetical examples
    C. Real and hypothetical examples
    D. Emotional appeals

31. In the second paragraph, the author uses many rhetorical questions to emphasise cloning's ethical issues. How does this BEST function in terms of providing evidence?
    A. It lets the reader know that the questions are essentially unsolved.
    B. The questions propel the reader to contemplate certain issues, thus becoming more involved.
    C. It augments the support of the other forms of support used in the argument.
    D. It is a stylistic device, which really does not function in argumentation.

32. What does the term "axiomatic" mean within the context of the last paragraph?
    A. Biased or prejudiced
    B. Set in stone
    C. Needing further elaboration
    D. Passive or redundant

33. Certain assumptions are carried along implicitly with the passage argument. Which of the following would NOT be an implicit assumption in the passage?
    A. Human life is valuable, ethics concerns this as a paramount principle.
    B. People should follow good morals and conduct, including scientists and researchers.
    C. All life is valuable, and proper ethics should apply to all life.
    D. Ethics is largely subjective, a reflection of the dominant political ideology of society.

34. Which of the following statements from the passage seems particularly weak in supporting the author's argument?
    I. ". . . such issues are settled according to the religious or anti-religious mindset of the political or judicial system in which the issues are raised."
    II. ". . . that humans are not accountable to anyone other than humans for what they do with any phenomenon of life . . ."
    III. " . . . issues underlying medical ethics are issues such as the definition of life and the value of life that are seen in perspective of ethical theories regarding what differentiates good acts and principles from evil."

    A. I
    B. I and II
    C. III
    D. I, II, and III

Unit 7

Questions 35 - 40

Some would argue that with capitalism came the notion that society is best understood as the autonomous actions of individuals. This idea has its biological correlate in Darwin's theory of natural selection where evolution takes place at the level of the reproduction of individuals in a species. In science, in general, we find it in the reductionist assumption that the whole is best understood in terms of its parts, and the more minute the level one goes to, the better the explanation.

This way of conceptualising the world also has the effect of breaking up the world into autonomous domains: internal and external. Views of causation are also affected in that causes become referred to as either internal or external. Internal factors (genes) cause organisms to be the way they are and the external environment causes some organisms to be selected for and thereby to survive into the next generation.

One might assert that this is the way in which biology has been conceived since Darwin, and that it is a terribly impoverished way of viewing biology, and that our understanding of nature would be richer if we moved away from our reductionist tendencies and instead recognised the complex interaction of the organism with the environment it creates. We would also be more effective in solving our problems if we moved away from the tendency to focus merely on the proximal physiological causes of disease, for example, focusing on the bacteria or viruses associated with disease instead of social factors.

These proposals to avoid pure reductionism and to take into account causes other than physiological ones are well founded. But by implying that the traditional focus on physiological causes is merely an intricate way of masking the social cause behind the disease, one ignores the more innocuous motivations for picking physiological causes before social ones.

First, it must be said that no legitimate medical scientist or physician would claim that there is merely one cause - the cause - for nearly any disease. When it is said in science textbooks that something is the cause of something else what is really being said is something is the proximal physiological cause of something else. It is proximal because it is the nearer to the effect (disease process) and physiological because it itself is some biological or chemical agent (i.e. not social agent). People may be troubled by western medicine's overemphasis of these causes as opposed to social ones. However, there seem to be very good, socially unproblematic reasons for often choosing to put the emphasis on the proximal physiological causes of disease.

Second, there is a logical reason. Consider bacteria and viruses. Wherever there is tuberculosis there is tubercle bacillus bacteria. The bacteria are a necessary condition for someone having the disease. The same cannot be said of sweat shops or unregulated, industrialised capitalism. In fact, individuals in the upper class and rural areas, as well as individuals in nonindustrial Marxist countries have also become infected by tubercle bacillus bacteria and come down with tuberculosis. This is not to say that for something to be labelled a cause of disease it must be a necessary condition, but the logical relationship of necessity helps us understand the claim that something is the cause of something else.

In addition, giving a necessary condition of disease does not limit one to saying that the cause of disease must be a proximal physiological one. Chewing tobacco releases toxic chemicals, which may be the cause of a specific form of gum disease in the chewer. Wherever this form of gum disease is found so is a user of chewing tobacco. In this case, it would seem perfectly appropriate to say that chewing tobacco is a cause of the disease, although not the proximal physiological one.

Finally, a reformed orientation toward science and medicine will yield a more fruitful way of doing investigations. Short-sighted causal explanation allows for the social structure to go unexamined for its deleterious effects on the community, but physiological explanations are important in determining the cause and potential solutions, both physiological and social.

35. What does the author mean by "capitalism . . . has its biological correlate in Darwin's theory of evolution"?
    A. Both focus on complex relationships between groups of organisms and their surroundings.
    B. Both are of the opinion that the more detailed level one goes to, the better the explanation.
    C. Both hold a 'survival of the fittest' framework, e.g., the most successful organism will survive and reproduce.
    D. Both hold the view that explanations are most effective when looking at individual entities.

36. Based on Paragraph 3, it appears that reductionist accounts of causation typically focus on which of the following causes?
    A. Social causes, because they are directly related to effects
    B. Physiological causes, more assignable to effects, in general
    C. Both social and physiological causes – simultaneous causes
    D. Either; the point is that reductionist accounts attempt to break down general causes into more specific ones

37. Based on the passage, an assumption made by those who argue against physiological accounts of causation is that:
    A. physiological accounts of causation tend to disregard the potential existence of harmful social agents.
    B. physiological accounts of causation are often incorrect by neglecting the social causes.
    C. social accounts of causation can replace physiological accounts of causation.
    D. explanations can be reductionist without being physiological.

38. The author mentions individuals in non-industrialised Marxist countries to make which of the following points?
    A. Post-industrial capitalism is not a necessary precondition for tuberculosis.
    B. Regardless of one's location, tubercle bacillus bacteria is the actual cause of tuberculosis.
    C. Living in an industrialised capitalist country is not a cause of tuberculosis.
    D. The best causal explanations are those which specify necessary conditions.

39. The central point of the passage is that:
    A. while the social accounts of causation are important, the physiological level provides better causal explanations.
    B. though some are suspicious, there are good reasons for including physiological accounts of causation along with social accounts of causation.
    C. people arguing against reductionist accounts of causation will most likely endorse the social accounts of causation.
    D. people arguing against physiological accounts of causation do not realise their importance.

40. Which of the following is NOT mentioned in the passage as a reason why proximal physiological explanations of causation are as desirable as social ones?
    A. They generally share more in an important logical relationship.
    B. They are important in determining both causes and potential solutions.
    C. They are, in some cases, necessary preconditions for a particular disease.
    D. They are more effective in getting at the actual cause of a disease than social explanations of causation.

> If time remains, you may review your work. If your allotted time (50 minutes) is complete, please proceed to the Answer Key.

GAMSAT-Prep.com
THE GOLD STANDARD

3.9.1 Verbal Reasoning Exercise 2 (Science-based Passages) Answer Key and Explanations

1.	B	9.	D	17.	B	25.	A	33.	D
2.	B	10.	A	18.	D	26.	C	34.	B
3.	A	11.	B	19.	A	27.	D	35.	D
4.	B	12.	A	20.	B	28.	A	36.	B
5.	A	13.	B	21.	B	29.	B	37.	A
6.	C	14.	C	22.	D	30.	C	38.	A
7.	D	15.	D	23.	D	31.	B	39.	B
8.	C	16.	D	24.	B	32.	B	40.	D

1. **Correct Answer: B**
   A, C, and D are all too general and lack the specific focus of the passage, which is adequately expressed in B.

2. **Correct Answer: B**
   A and D, similar to the preceding question are too general. C is a statement of policy - marked by the word "should" and a call to action, which is never addressed within the passage. This leaves B, which possesses the specificity of "purpose" and reflects the passage information, as the best option.

3. **Correct Answer: A**
   D is too encompassing, and not really addressed adequately within the passage. C may or may not be true but also never addressed adequately within the passage, except for brief references to clean-up acts. B assumes a causal link not adequately established within the passage - there may be other factors involved. The statement needs more support within the passage to qualify as the best answer. A is specific enough to qualify as the BEST choice option in terms of significance and relevance, i.e. one can assume that cyanide toxins will have an "effect" on wildlife within a wetland. This would also be encompassing of the probability or possibility of B.

4. **Correct Answer: B**
   II is never mentioned within the passage while a rescan will confirm that I and III are addressed.

5. **Correct Answer: A**
   D can quickly be ruled out due to the phrase "green reasoning," which is essentially meaningless. B can be ruled out, for there is little evidence which follows a hypothetical line of thought, such as "If this were to happen . . ." or "suppose that . . . then this would follow". C can be ruled out because there is no testimony used as support within the passage, such as "noted biologist Dr. Smith" or "the U.S. Geological Survey states that. . ." This leaves A as the correct answer, and both examples are used within the passage to support the main idea or thesis.

6. **Correct Answer: C**
   This is an inference question, which must seek out and understand the underlying idea or motivation behind humankind's quest for knowledge.
   A is incorrect because it is too general and has no specific basis within the passage.
   B is a decoy that seems descriptive of the early thinkers' method for establishing a scientific study of astronomy. On the other hand, the question is actually asking for a characteristic that will describe the human desire for knowledge.

C is correct because "filling men with awe and wonder" and "daily source of questioning" suggest that the tendency is already within us – to seek out knowledge, or in Kantian terms, "a priori".
D is incorrect because it lacks specificity and is somewhat tautological (circular argument) – the notion of desiring knowledge because "something is there" is partially true but lacks the human element.

7. **Correct Answer: D**
This is a best option question where the other questions must be ruled out by the process of a unilateral distinction – which finds the most inclusive of the other answers or options. All the answers are partially true, yet only D is inclusive of A, B and C, which can all be considered as an "eclectic (or diverse) source."

8. **Correct Answer: C**
This is another "best option" type of question, where one must infer the best answer in relation to the others. This question is also based on close reading.
A is incorrect because the passage never mentions chronology in relation to Pythagoras.
B is partially correct yet not as inclusive of C.
C is correct and inclusive of B and D.
D is partially correct, yet not accepted by the vast majority.
"By linking astronomy to trigonometry, Pythagoras was redefining earlier beliefs."

9. **Correct Answer: D**
This is a complex-sounding question type, which requires inferring the meaning of the terms within the text. All the words contained "centric," which can be understood by their etymology as "centred."
(A) "ethno" pertains to an ethnic culture. Despite being derived from the Greek culture, one cannot make the inference or link between the two. This answer is incorrect.

(B) "helio" pertains to the idea that positions the Sun as the center of the solar system – later by Copernicus.
(C) "anthropo" pertains to man, such as anthropology – this can obviously be ruled out.
(D) "geopo" pertains to the Earth such as geography, geo-logy and is correct.

10. **Correct Answer: A**
This is a detail-oriented question which can be assessed by a close reading or re-scan. P1 S2 states "Scientific astronomy, however, was an impossibility until an exact system of chronology was devised." Thus the question posed is a reversed statement making A as the correct answer.
B is a distractor – linguistics is never mentioned in the passage. C is another distractor - the spatial exactness would of course be later with Thales and Pythagoras, where (D) trigonometry was fused with astronomy. Chrono means "time" as well.

11. **Correct Answer: B**
This is a general idea question about the passage relating to the methodology or focus of the writing. This requires assessing how the passage proceeds and develops its thesis or main idea. The numerous facts, figures, and dates – although not temporally correct, are united by general themes of belief about the heavens. The title "The Gradual Acceptance . . ." also gives clues that the writer is writing within a temporal framework. One must also note that Paragraphs 1 and 2 are largely written within this same temporality.
A is incorrect. While analysis is within the passage, it is certainly not the main focus.
(C) The term "deduction" belongs to logic and functions as a distractor.
(D) "Induction" is also a term belonging to logic and functions as a distractor.

GAMSAT-Prep.com
THE GOLD STANDARD

12. **Correct Answer: A**
All answers (B) (C) and (D) are not "problems" per se, but theoretical issues - worth pursuing in their own terms, but not related to the question. (A) can be inferred to be the "crux" of the problem, indicated by the following passage information: "A central problem of science is how to recognise and define worthwhile subjects for investigation. For one thing, we may be faced with a myriad of opportunities and no means to decide which are going to be fruitful. On the other hand, our environment may limit our ability to recognise scientific problems and possibilities, especially the ones which could lead to significant changes in our understanding."

13. **Correct Answer: B**
(C) and (D) represent technological and/or verifiability issues in relation to theory, as such both answers can be deduced to be incorrect. (A) knowledge is too broad a subject to be warranted as the correct answer, and in line with question 24, one can infer (B) criteria - the means by which the two are assessed, to be the best choice option.

14. **Correct Answer: C**
This detail-oriented question can be answered as (C) from the following passage information: "Polanyi was concerned with what he called the "tacit dimension" in our knowledge. In particular he wished to give proper value to the process of recognising, and making a commitment to, ideas or hypotheses, which may result from a rich understanding and knowledge but cannot be explained by explicit reasoning, in order to carry out the enquiry that will lead to them being more widely understood and accepted."

15. **Correct Answer: D**
Only I and III can be inferred to be correct in this detail-oriented question, these concepts are within the passage as follows:
These abstracted questions have their parallels in everyday life and more mundane enquiries. Michael Polanyi describes the 'logical gap' between existing knowledge and any significant discovery or innovation. No matter how thorough our factual knowledge of the situation that we inhabit, the pursuit of logical reasoning or iterative development of existing concepts would not, on its own, allow us to cross this gap. There must be also some kind of leap of 'illumination' by which the scientist imagines a new concept and proposes it as a worthwhile subject for investigation. As Polanyi says "Illumination. ...is the plunge by which we gain a foothold in another shore of reality. On such plunges the scientist has to stake, bit by bit, his entire professional life."

16. **Correct Answer: D**
This is one of the main ideas (the second problem) of Paragraph 2, and illustrated and expanded upon in Paragraphs 3 and 4.

17. **Correct Answer: B**
The weakest evidence in the statement would be not naming the groups, especially after a statement implying this is done historically. The second best weakness would be the ambiguous "various campaigns". These are not listed or referred to, especially historically. C and D are relatively weak only insofar as they are generalisations.

18. **Correct Answer: D**
The best implication is clearly D, which is the most specific. A is politically incorrect. B is true or untrue, but a generalisation. C is not referential to the question being asked.

19. **Correct Answer: A**
Deduction - B is referential, so incorrect. C is also incorrect because it is not specific, and also particularly weak in the statement. (D) The statement does follow the reasoning of the passage information, yet (A) the term "success" is

ambiguous - one immediately wishes to know "to what degree." Statistics and other data would strengthen this phrase.

20. **Correct Answer: B**
    The statement is not necessarily (A) politically motivated; it seems impartial to a certain extent, as a statement of fact (true or untrue). (C) The statement is not too specific - this begs for an answer, which leads one to infer B as the best option - lack of concrete evidence such as what public officials, what schools, etc. D is not tautological, thus not circular reasoning. Such reasoning would base the evidence on the thesis, and the thesis on the evidence such as "intelligent design should be taught in public schools because it is intelligent design".

21. **Correct Answer: B**
    This detail-oriented question supports I and II, based on passage data. This can be affirmed by a close reading or re-scan of Paragraph 7, which has no mention of (III) scientific methodology.

22. **Correct Answer: D**
    The passage is obviously (D) liberal, critical of conservative politics.

23. **Correct Answer: D**
    This is an assumption question which requires deduction. (A) The statement is not necessarily contradictory, or (B) unfamiliar yet at the same time, popular (colloquial). Nor is it (C) too specific, AND does not generalise sufficiently (which would be somewhat of a contradiction). The statement is assumption-based (quite possibly) and inferential - the reader is required to make too much of an argumentative leap from the first passage to the second - in question. The correct answer is D.

24. **Correct Answer: B**
    Options A and D cannot be correct because epigenetic rules are debated throughout the passage without a conclusion on their existence. Answer choice C is wrong because it is not the main idea of the passage to "focus on different behaviours to determine the content of the rules"; rather, the passage mentions specific behaviours to question the concept of such rules in the first place.

    While the passage does not mention that the sociobiologists are hasty, the entire passage implies that the notion of epigenetics has been embraced even if there is, as yet, no evidence that it does. Epigenetics is simply an inference that sociobiologists have made since there are several behaviours that are common to most humans.

    The passage begins with a premise: genes determine how our brains and neurotransmitters develop. Therefore, according to the sociobiologists, there are common behaviours among humans (fear of the dark, for example). The sociobiologists then jump to include 'morality' in the common behaviours (altruism, for example). From this, the sociobiologists argue that our genes determine our morality. This is a very wide jump from one point to another - it is a too sweeping a generalisation. These all mean that the claim was made even before there is evidence for it. That is why it is 'hasty'. Option B, which is the correct answer, is also found in the second sentence of Paragraph 1.

25. **Correct Answer: A**
    Option C is true, but that is not the point being made by the author. Option D is an opinion, which is not part of the quote. Option B cannot be confirmed. This leaves A as the best option.

26. **Correct Answer: C**
    In the final paragraph, the author never objects to the linkage between science and morality. He seems to be suspicious at the linkage and then he objects strongly about using genes as a source of a theory of morality. However, he does not say that the genes, which may be linked,

should not be sought.

On the other hand, consider the validity of the following statement given the author's assertions: "Genetic discoveries should not be strongly relied on to provide solutions to moral dilemmas." That makes C the best answer.

27. **Correct Answer: D**

    This question is quite straightforward. It asks you to choose which statement is a claim made in the passage that is not supported by any evidence. To answer the question, you just need to scan the passage for the four statements to see which one was claimed but was unsupported by any evidence or example.

    Options A, B and D would need proof from the passage to be considered and are therefore incorrect. Option C is found in sentence 4 of Paragraph 1.

28. **Correct Answer: A**

    This question requires differentiating the argument of the author from those of the sources or references cited in his or her article.

    The author presents the sociobiologist perspective in the first 2 paragraphs (epigenetic rules, behaviour has a basis in our genes) and then in Paragraph 3, he begins to make his case for environment/experience being understated by epigenetic rules.

    If, in the question, it stated that everyone in the world has a near equal fear of snakes, that would support the idea of a human gene (or genes) being responsible for behaviour. However, the question suggests that where you live has an impact on what you fear which is more in line with the (A) author's perspective.

29. **Correct Answer: B**

    A is unfocussed and too general. C is related, but it only relates to the issue of legalising the embryo research as discussed in the passage. Therefore, it is not the main idea. D is also obliquely related in as far as the passage is concerned. B can be inferred to be the best choice, having the most encompassing idea.

30. **Correct Answer: C**

    The passage is largely supported by (C) real and hypothetical examples. The use of "what if" questions function more as hypothetical examples rather than as emotional appeals. But mostly, the author draws from actual events to support the article's main idea.

31. **Correct Answer: B**

    In the case of this passage, rhetorical questions stimulate the reader with "what if" questions, to become more involved on a critical thinking level.

    A is not necessarily true. Closure of these questions are of a hypothetical nature and does not, at least on the surface level, require a response. C is true, but not the BEST option in terms of function. D is partially true because the questions can be considered as stylistic devices; therefore, they DO serve a function in the argumentation. This makes statement D incorrect.

32. **Correct Answer: B**

    The meaning of the term "axiomatic" can be inferred from the context of the last paragraph (as suggested in the question). The "fill in the blank" trick works here as well:

    "Such assumptions, however, cannot be accepted as (axiomatic); they are philosophical issues, of course, but also crucial as pertaining to human life itself." Now try replacing the word "axiomatic" with any of these:

    (A) biased or prejudice - not really related; therefore, deduced as incorrect.

    (B) set in stone - seems to make sense. (This is the best choice.)

    (C) needing further elaboration - contradicts the basic essence of the sentence. Incorrect.

    (D) passive or redundant does not make sense.

33. **Correct Answer: D**
The meaning of implicit is implied, it is not obviously stated. A, B and C can all be inferred to be implied within the passage's argument. D is certainly not implied, and the statement itself is a bit of a contradiction between self and society/ideology, making this the best option.

34. **Correct Answer: B**
I is weak because it makes an arbitrary association of religion or non-religion (mindset) to political and judicial systems. II is weak because it is contradictory to the passage argument and its inferred assumptions (if a sense of ethics is applied). III seems fairly logical and sequential. Therefore, B represents the best choice.

35. **Correct Answer: D**
The answer to the question can be deduced from the following: "This idea has its biological correlate in Darwin's theory of natural selection where evolution takes place at the level of the reproduction of individuals in a species."
Option B gives the definition of reductionist thinking but it does not state what capitalism and Darwinism have in common - which is, (D) both go down to the level of the individuals.

36. **Correct Answer: B**
The answer to the question can be deduced from the following:
"We would also be more effective in solving our problems if we moved away from the tendency to focus merely on the proximal physiological causes of disease, for example, focusing on the bacteria or viruses associated with disease instead of social factors."

37. **Correct Answer: A**
The answer to this question is briefly implied in the last paragraph of the passage: "Short-sighted causal explanation allows for the social structure to go unexamined for its deleterious effects on the community. . ." This makes B somewhat inaccurate. At the most, the author would simply consider that focusing on physiological causes alone is "a terribly impoverished way of viewing biology," but not entirely incorrect. After all, "physiological explanations are important in determining the cause and potential solutions."
C is out scope.
D can be a tempting option. However, this statement would imply that even explanations within a social context is reductionist as well.

38. **Correct Answer: A**
This is a question of why and then an example is used. The answer to this question can be found in Paragraph 6:
"In fact, individuals in the upper class and rural areas, as well as individuals in nonindustrial Marxist countries have also become infected by tubercle bacillus bacteria and come down with tuberculosis. This is not to say that for something to be labeled a cause of disease it must be a necessary condition, but the logical relationship of necessity helps us understand the claim that something is the cause of something else."
A is why industrialisation is mentioned at all - to illustrate how it is not required. This is the correct answer.
B would be mistakenly selected if one does not get the point of the author.
C is the opposite of the point being made.
D is a vague and irrelevant choice that could be tempting.

39. **Correct Answer: B**
Option C is found in Paragraph 4. It is a true statement, but it is not the main argument of the passage. D is slightly discussed in Paragraph 5 but it is not a valid argument. A is also wrong because the whole passage talks about both social and physiological accounts; not about how one is better than another. This leaves B as the correct answer.
The central point of the passage can be followed this way: First, it explains what it means

when we say that something causes disease. The passage asserts that when doctors say that a bacteria causes disease, the doctor is simply saying that the immediate physiological cause is the presence of the bacteria. It is the most precise and measurable way of finding out what causes disease.

The passage also asserts that these physiological causation do not take into account social agents that may cause disease. Because it is difficult to precisely and accurately pinpoint which social agents cause disease, people are suspicious about social agents causing disease.

40. **Correct Answer: D**
This question asks you to choose which of the options was NOT mentioned in the passage.

Option D is the best answer because it states that physiological causes are more effective in determining the actual cause of the disease that social causes. This is NOT mentioned in the passage. What the passage actually states is that we would be more effective if we focussed not only on the physiological causes but also on the social causes.

This part of the passage directly contradicts statement D:

"We would also be more effective in solving our problems if we moved away from the tendency to focus merely on the proximal physiological causes of disease, for example, focussing on the bacteria or viruses associated with disease instead of social factors."

3.8.5 Poetry Test

Units with poems or song lyrics appear two to three times in Section 1 of the GAMSAT. This Poetry mini test is composed of 5 units with 20 questions. They are designed to get you used to interpreting themes, patterns, and symbolisms in poems and songs, among others.

Please choose the best answer for each question. You have 25 minutes. Please time yourself.

BEGIN ONLY WHEN TIMER IS READY

Unit 1

Questions 1 - 4

Chemin De Fer

Alone on the railroad track
I walked with pounding heart.
The ties were too close together
or maybe too far apart.

The scenery was impoverished: 5
scrub-pine and oak; beyond
its mingled gray-green foliage
I saw the little pond

where the dirty old hermit lives,
lie like an old tear   10
holding onto its injuries
lucidly year after year.

The hermit shot off his shot-gun
and the tree by his cabin shook.
Over the pond went a ripple   15
the pet hen went chook-chook.

"Love should be put into action!"
Screamed the old hermit.
Across the pond an echo
Tried and tried to confirm it.   20

Elizabeth Bishop

1. The emotions expressed by the speaker walking with a "pounding heart" (line 2) and the dirty old hermit "holding onto its injuries" (line 11) suggest that:
   A. both characters suffer from insecurity.
   B. the speaker is in a state of flight while the hermit, of entrapment.
   C. both characters are experiencing pain.
   D. the speaker's present mood is positive while the hermit's, negative.

2. "Chemin De Fer" is a French word for railroad. The title of the poem and the meaning evoked by the last two lines represent:
   A. indifference.
   B. an unwelcomed rebound.
   C. stagnation.
   D. an inescapable cycle.

3. The poet's use of the image of the pond (line 8) and her reference to the echo (lines 19 - 20) imply that:
   A. the hermit represents the pond; and the speaker, the echo.
   B. both characters similarly feel isolated.
   C. the hermit is an outcast and the speaker is a fugitive.
   D. the speaker and the hermit represent one and the same person.

4. Which of the following insights about Elizabeth Bishop's poetic style best describe the quality of "Chemin De Fer"?
   A. Too much intellectualisation of the poetic images results to obliquity.
   B. Heavily using extended metaphors creates a mask of the poet's persona.
   C. Using an outsider's perception to view another outsider's circumstance is an effective means of identifying perceptions and consciousness.
   D. To identify one's self as an outcast and to try to live, and love, in two worlds, is to dream of the impossible safe place.

Unit 2

Questions 5 - 7

Driving to Town Late to Mail a Letter

It is a cold and snowy night. The main street is deserted.
The only things moving are swirls of snow.
As I lift the mailbox door, I feel its cold iron.
There is a privacy I love in this snowy night.
Driving around, I will waste more time.   5

Robert Bly

5. Based on the images described in the first 3 lines, what is the atmosphere of the poem?
    A. Melancholic
    B. Austere
    C. Stark
    D. Desolate

6. The irregular rhythm and metre of the poem helps create which effect that accurately suggests the poem's overall scenario?
    A. An attempt to break away from monotony
    B. An aimless disposition
    C. A relaxed atmosphere
    D. Disinterest in important matters

7. The last 2 lines of the poem imply that the speaker:
    A. perceives life as lacking in purpose.
    B. considers solitude to be a waste of time.
    C. ends his ambivalent mood with a final choice to "waste more time".
    D. welcomes the chance, brought about by the weather, to commune with nature and the self.

Unit 3

Questions 8 - 12

The Waking

I wake to sleep, and take my waking slow.
I feel my fate in what I cannot fear.
I learn by going where I have to go.

We think by feeling. What is there to know?
I hear my being dance from ear to ear.   5
I wake to sleep, and take my waking slow.

Of those so close beside me, which are you?
God bless the Ground! I shall walk softly there,
And learn by going where I have to go.

Light takes the Tree; but who can tell us how?   10
The lowly worm climbs up a winding stair;
I wake to sleep, and take my waking slow.

Great Nature has another thing to do
To you and me, so take the lively air,
And, lovely, learn by going where to go.   15

> This shaking keeps me steady. I should know.
> What falls away is always. And is near.
> I wake to sleep, and take my waking slow.
> I learn by going where I have to go.

Theodore Roethke

8. The line "I wake to sleep, and take my waking slow. . ." has generated various interpretations from several critics, the most predominant of which is in reference to "dying". Which of the following lines would reinforce this interpretation?
    A. Light takes the Tree; but who can tell us how?
    B. This shaking keeps me steady.
    C. Great Nature has another thing to do. . .
    D. God bless the Ground! I shall walk softly there

9. Which tone does the repeating, heavily end-stopped lines of the poem create?
    A. Shortness of breath
    B. Cycle and Stability
    C. Interrupted thoughts
    D. Emphasis and Confidence

10. The paradox introduced in the first line is further reinforced in several succeeding lines of the poem (lines 2, 11, 16, 17) in order to:
    A. emphasise the contrast between life and death.
    B. indicate a peaceful acceptance of the inevitable and life's ironies.
    C. illustrate opposing forces in life.
    D. reflect the speaker's confusion.

11. Another interpretation of the poem is that the theme revolves around its rejection of the intellect as the way to "enlightenment". What would support this interpretation?
    A. The repeated use of words based on feelings rather than reason
    B. The poem's constant use of paradoxes
    C. The poet's romantic references to Nature
    D. The predominance of irrational lines

12. "What falls away is always. And is near" suggests:
    A. resignation to one's fate.
    B. a fast approaching death.
    C. the inseparability of life and death.
    D. fear of the uncertain.

Unit 4

Questions 13 – 16

One Flesh

Lying apart now, each in a separate bed,
He with a book, keeping the light on late,
She like a girl dreaming of childhood,
All men elsewhere - it is as if they wait
Some new event: the book he holds unread,   5
Her eyes fixed on the shadows overhead.

Tossed up like flotsam from a former passion,
How cool they lie. They hardly ever touch,
Or if they do, it is like a confession
Of having little feeling - or too much.   10
Chastity faces them, a destination
For which their whole lives were a preparation.

Strangely apart, yet strangely close together,
Silence between them like a thread to hold
And not wind in. And time itself's a feather   15
Touching them gently. Do they know they're old,
These two who are my father and my mother
Whose fire from which I came, has now grown cold?

Elizabeth Jennings

13. What does "chastity" mean in the second stanza?
    - A. Abstinence
    - B. Isolation
    - C. Virtue
    - D. Mortality

14. The different meanings of "touch" in lines 8 and 16, respectively, equate:
    - A. passion and time.
    - B. youth and old age.
    - C. truth and evanescence.
    - D. action and imagination.

15. The thread (line 14) signifies:
    - A. union.
    - B. spiritual isolation.
    - C. absence of communication.
    - D. lifeline.

16. "Flotsam" (line 7) symbolises:
- **A.** spent passion.
- **B.** impotence.
- **C.** uselessness.
- **D.** deterioration.

Unit 5

Questions 17 - 20

Gift

O my love, what gift of mine
Shall I give you this dawn?
A morning song?
But morning does not last long -
The heat of the sun   5
Wilts like a flower
And songs that tire
Are done.

O friend, when you come to my gate.
At dusk   10
What is it you ask?
What shall I bring you?
A light?

A lamp from a secret corner of my silent house?
But will you want to take it with you   15
Down the crowded street?
Alas,
The wind will blow it out.

Whatever gifts are in my power to give you,
Be they flowers,   20
Be they gems for your neck
How can they please you
If in time they must surely wither,
Crack,
Lose lustre?   25
All that my hands can place in yours
Will slip through your fingers
And fall forgotten to the dust
To turn into dust.

Rather, 30
When you have leisure,
Wander idly through my garden in spring
And let an unknown, hidden flower's scent startle you
Into sudden wondering-
Let that displaced moment 35
Be my gift.
Or if, as you peer your way down a shady avenue,
Suddenly, spilled
From the thick gathered tresses of evening
A single shivering fleck of sunset-light stops you, 40
Turns your daydreams to gold,
Let that light be an innocent
Gift.

Truest treasure is fleeting;
It sparkles for a moment, then goes. 45
It does not tell its name; its tune
Stops us in our tracks, its dance disappears
At the toss of an anklet
I know no way to it-
No hand, nor word can reach it. 50
Friend, whatever you take of it,
On your own,
Without asking, without knowing, let that
Be yours.
Anything I can give you is trifling - 55
Be it a flower, or a song-

Rabindranath Tagore

17. The beginning stanza of the poem depicts:
    A. sadness.
    B. confusion.
    C. a quest.
    D. affection.

18. "Displaced moment" (line 35) means:
    A. an unguarded moment.
    B. a rare opportunity.
    C. a gift.
    D. random.

19. "Shady avenue" (line 37) connotes:
    A. danger.
    B. obstacle.
    C. desperation.
    D. chaos.

20. The speaker regards the "gift" as something that is:
    A. trifling.
    B. elusive.
    C. spontaneous.
    D. surprising.

If time remains, you may review your work. If your allotted time (25 minutes) is complete, please proceed to the Answer Key.

UNDERSTANDING THE GAMSAT

3.8.6 Poetry Test Answer Key and Explanations

1.	B	6.	B	11.	A	16.	B
2.	D	7.	D	12.	C	17.	D
3.	D	8.	D	13.	D	18.	B
4.	C	9.	B	14.	C	19.	B
5.	D	10.	B	15.	A	20.	C

1. **Correct Answer: B**
   This poem is often identified by various critics as one of Bishop's medium in obliquely expressing her own fears and feelings of alienation in reference to her gender identity.
   The poet successfully portrays two polarised emotions in this piece: fear resulting to an urge to escape, and frustrations resulting to a refusal to move on. In line 2, being alone on a railroad track and having unstable perceptions of one's path with "ties (being) too close together or... too far apart" connote a sense of danger and of fear. On the other hand, an image of seclusion in the character of the hermit, a ripple, and an echo that bounces back to the hermit's point, suggests containment.
   This is a "hybrid" type of question that can be answered through a correct interpretation of the emotions depicted in the poem and the "evidence" found within their contexts.
   A is merely a general statement on a common feeling experienced by the two characters. The question stem specifically points at two emotions cited in the poem. In C, pain is apparent in the hermit's character but not necessarily in the speaker's. D is a misreading of the tones presented in the poem.

2. **Correct Answer: D**
   This question specifically refers to "Chemin De Fer" (railroad) and the last two lines of the poem: "Across the pond an echo / Tried and tried to confirm it." Railroads operate on a recurring schedule, so to speak. The same recurring action is stated in the repeated sound of the echo. Recurrence denotes a cycle. In addition, the general atmosphere of isolation suggests something inescapable.
   A is an out-of-context interpretation of the title and the final lines of the poem. B is a misinterpretation of the final lines of the poem and is not congruent with a railroad's symbolism. C is another aspect of the poem's imagery. However, this is more appropriately represented by the pond – NEITHER the railroad NOR the echo.

3. **Correct Answer: D**
   This question requires analysis and relating concepts to the following "evidences" provided in the poem: (1) Pond contains water. Water mirrors whatever is placed parallel to it; (2) An echo reflects sounds. The poem starts with a premise of escapism. The speaker, therefore, avoids facing his/her own issues by reflecting these on an "invented" character.
   A is too direct, yet does not provide a substantial answer. B describes what the two characters may possibly feel but does not answer what the images of the pond and the echo imply. C seems plausible; however, this is not the best answer. The question asks: which among the options can identify what is being implied by

UNDERSTANDING THE GAMSAT 139

the poet's use of the image of the pond and her reference to the echo? This requires an answer that will present an insight into the poem's symbolism. D is the best option because it offers a considerable interpretation parallel to what the question asks.

4. **Correct Answer: C**
This is an implication question that requires determining two things: the overall idea that the poet tries to communicate in her poem; and, the means or technique that the poet employs in order to get her thoughts across to the readers. This poem speaks about fear and frustration, and flight and confrontation on love. The poet uses images that symbolise the "act of mirroring".
A is wrong because the poem is emotionally charged rather than objective or "intellectualised". B is halfway true in stating that the extended metaphors hide or indirectly portray the truth. However, the term "persona" distorts the concept of the statement. "Persona" refers to a person's facade, not the inner personality or thinking. C is more accurate in presenting an insight into the poem's quality. D states the poem's possible theme, NOT an insight about the poem's quality.

5. **Correct Answer: D**
This is a tone question that entails a careful consideration of specific images presented in the poem's first 3 lines. "Swirls of snow" (line 2) calls to mind some sort of a ghost town or deserted place. "Deserted (street)" (line 1) sets such an atmosphere. These two images are powerful enough to connote a desolate – solitary - mood in the first part of the poem.
(A) Although sadness is a possible aspect that comes with a desolate atmosphere, it is not established in the first 3 lines. B or apathy is usually associated with "cold", but this option takes the interpretation of the poem out of context. C offers a synonym of "laziness", which can likewise be associated to cold weather. Again, this option takes the mood of the poem out of context.

6. **Correct Answer: B**
This is another tone question that involves recognising the overall attitude or mood of the poem's speaker in relation to the poem's structure. The irregularity in poetic structure combines with the images in depicting a scenario of being adrift or aimless: "swirls of snow" suggests a movement without a definite direction; so does "driving around" with the intention of wasting time.
A is an out-of-context interpretation. C is a more general view of the poem's atmosphere compared to B. D is not established in the poem. In fact, the speaker has just performed an errand of mailing a letter amid the difficult weather.

7. **Correct Answer: D**
This implication question requires judging the attitude projected by the speaker of the poem in lines 4 and 5. Line 4 reveals the speaker's outlook towards the rather unfriendly weather by stating, "There is a privacy I love in this snowy night." "Wasting time" then, in the poem's essence is not a negative endeavour but an opportunity to enjoy one's private moment.
A is an incomplete interpretation of the poem that disregards the speaker's remark in line 4. B is a misreading of lines 4 and 5. C is wrong because there is no indication in the poem where the speaker is expected to decide or choose.

8. **Correct Answer: D**
In order to understand this seemingly complicated poem, careful consideration of the accompanying details of each line is required. The word "Ground" in the line, (D) "God bless the Ground! I shall walk softly there" reinforces the idea of death.
(A) Line 10 implies enlightenment rather than

death. The image following the line depicts the "lowly worm" climbing to take the light.
(B) Line 16 is a paradox of finding stability out of chaos.
(C) Line 13 is ambiguous. If taken within the context of its stanza, it could mean that the author tells the reader to enjoy what Nature has to offer.

9. **Correct Answer: B**
The lines "I wake to sleep, and take my waking slow" and "I learn by going where I have to go" are alternately repeated in every stanza, either linking the thought of the preceding lines or reasserting a dominant idea of the poem. In effect, this (B) cycle keeps the general context of the poem within the perspectives of these 2 lines.
A is not possible because all the lines have complete thoughts. Shortness of breath could have comprised unrelated, broken thoughts. C is also wrong because no separate idea is inserted in between the sentences within a single stanza.
(D) Emphasis is a possible effect of the repetitions. Confidence, however, is not obvious in the poem.

10. **Correct Answer: B**
In order to arrive at the best answer, the specified lines must first be interpreted.
Line 2: "I feel my fate in what I cannot fear." Instead of fearing the unknown, the line suggests a brave acceptance of one's fate.
Line 11: "The lowly worm climbs up a winding stair." The UPWARD action of climbing to take the light, in contrast to the LOWLY state of a small worm, indicate a slow and quiet determination to elevate ones' self from the "dark" despite the twists ("winding") of life.
Line 16 "This shaking keeps me steady. I should know." Shaking implies the uncertain and unforeseen in life. It can also indicate a sign of a fatal illness. In any case, the speaker expresses a calm ("steady") acknowledgement of such circumstances.
Line 17 "What falls away is always. And is near." This line recognises the fact that "falling away", i.e. opposing forces, is always a part of life.
Lines 2, 11, 16, and 17 altogether convey a positive recognition about certain facts of life. The question asks for a correlation of this shared idea to the first line of the poem, "I wake to sleep, and take my waking slow." Sleeping is as essential as waking, and vice versa. As indicated by the speaker's statement to "take" i.e. "accept" his waking slow, the opposing states of waking and sleeping do not signify a contrast but of inevitability. Hence, it can be inferred that paradoxes are used in the poem to reconcile seemingly unlike states – to be more specific, to accept the inevitable (line 2), the ironies (lines 11 and 17), and the uncertain (line 16) in life.
A and C, therefore, are wrong. D is a misinterpretation.

11. **Correct Answer: A**
The answer to this question can be deduced from the following:
"I FEEL my fate in what I cannot FEAR." (line 2);
"We think by FEELING." (line 4);
" LIVELY air" (line 14); and,
"LOVELY, learn by going where to go." (line 15)
Feel, fear, feeling, lively and lovely are subjective words spread in the different stanzas of the poem. In lines 4 and 15, the subjective words are used as a means to thinking and learning, as opposed to using the mind.
B is wrong because paradoxes are mainly used in this poem in order to illustrate the innate but inevitable contrast of life, not a rejection of intellect. C is debatable because although "Nature" is regarded in romanticism as a contrast to scientific rationalism, "Nature" is usually presented as a work of art itself.
(D) The lines are seemingly irrational at initial reading. However, further analysis reveals that these are meant to show the inherent duality of life.

12. **Correct Answer: C**

"What falls away is always" indicates a condition that lingers. The fact that it "is near" means that it is inescapable too. In other words, death will always come with life.

A does not point to the essence of the line being referred in the question. B is only applicable to the second statement: "And is near." However, a fast approaching death happens only once, not "always". D is not implied in the line or within the context of the stanza.

13. **Correct Answer: D**

The message of this poem is best understood by the logical interpretation of the symbolisms and expressions presented in the poem. These can be inferred from the context of the lines or stanzas specified.

The second stanza alludes to the lack of marital relations between the old couple. The death of sexual desire accompanying old age can be said to equate (D) death, which is everyone's destination and part of life's preparation.

(A) Abstinence and (B) isolation are not exactly regarded as things that everyone prepares for in later life. (C) Virtue may be hoped for but this necessitates being morally good or righteous. This is neither implied anywhere in the poem nor is the poem about morality. This leaves D as the correct answer.

14. **Correct Answer: C**

This question is specifically confined to lines 8 and 16. Respectively, touch is likened to confession and time as fleeting in these lines. This makes C correct.

A is literal but does not correctly answer the question. B and D are mentioned in other parts of the poem but not in response to the lines specified.

15. **Correct Answer: A**

The meaning of this word is taken from the following: "Strangely apart, yet strangely close together, / Silence between them like a thread to hold / And not wind in. And time itself's a feather / Touching them gently." This implies that despite the absence of spoken communication, the couple is still connected by their marital union and by the memories of the time that they have spent together.

B and D are not implied in the stanza. C is a literal reference to the "silence" mentioned in the same line.

16. **Correct Answer: B**

The symbolism of this word can be derived from the following: "Tossed up like flotsam from a former passion, / How cool they lie. They hardly ever touch, / Or if they do, it is like a confession / Of having little feeling - or too much." The general thought of these lines directs to the incapacity of the couple to effectively demonstrate passionate feelings or sexual desires. This makes B as the correct answer.

A is wrong because the question asks what the word symbolises, not what it means in the context of its sentence or line. C would refer to the general function of weak, old people. However, "flotsam" was referred in the poem in relation to passion; hence, C is a remote option. D is also wrong because the word is not associated with just a failing capacity but a sexual INcapacity.

17. **Correct Answer: D**

The reference to a loved one in the beginning line suggests that the poem has an affectionate tone. Therefore, D answers this simple inference question. A is wrong because the succeeding lines must not be misinterpreted to be depressing but the speaker's way of showing that material things fade through time. B is also a misinterpretation. C may sound like a possible option because of the line, "what ... / Shall I give you this dawn?" However, the speaker is able to rationalise and answer his own question in the succeeding lines. Therefore, C is a weak choice.

18. **Correct Answer: B**
    This question calls for an "analysis of evidence", which can be construed from: "...let an unknown, hidden flower's scent startle you" (line 33). This means that a "displaced moment" is rare not only because it is unexpected but also it is beautiful; extraordinary in its occurrence and extraordinary in that it is not so easily noticed or yearned for.
    Although A is true, this answer is encompassed by B. C is what "displaced moment" is being paralleled with by the speaker. The question asks for what the phrase means, NOT to what it is being equated. D is not explicitly mentioned in the stanza.

19. **Correct Answer: B**
    This is an inference question that requires contextual interpretation of the stanza. The answer can be deduced from lines 37 to 41. The speaker's reference to a darkness enlightened by a realisation of a dream indicates that "shady avenue" implies the hardships or "obstacles" undergone by a person.
    A and C are not suggested in the stanza. D is wrong because the stanza does not mention a circumstance too forceful to constitute chaos.

20. **Correct Answer: C**
    The speaker details his idea of a "gift" in the last stanza. He regards gifts that are material and man-made to be insignificant. Instead, he mentions of "displaced moment" and "whatever you take of it, / on your own, / without asking, without knowing" - things and instances that come at the spur-of-the-moment – to be the "truest treasures". This makes C as the most apt choice.
    A refers to the material gifts. B is wrong because the speaker only mentions the "unexpected" gifts among everyday matters, not those that are hard to find. D is a component of being spontaneous, but this choice offers a limited response compared to C.

GAMSAT-Prep.com
THE GOLD STANDARD

3.8.7 Cartoon Test

Units with cartoon interpretation usually appear once or twice during the real exam. This mini test presents 11 units with 20 questions. Choose the best answer for each question. You have 25 minutes. Please time yourself accordingly.

BEGIN ONLY WHEN TIMER IS READY

Unit 1

Questions 1 - 2

Cartoon 1

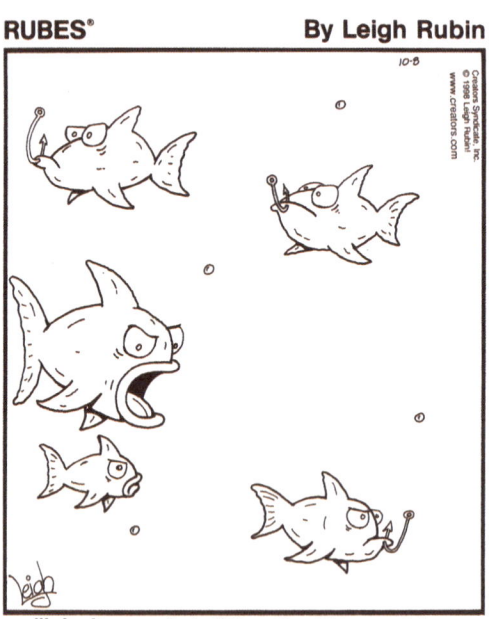

Reprinted with permission from Creators Syndicate.

1. The humour portrayed in the cartoon is a form known as:
    A. satire.
    B. analogy.
    C. double entendre.
    D. juxtaposition.

2. The dialogue in the cartoon can be paralleled to a real-life situation wherein:
   A. adolescents tend to imitate fashion trends to the dislike of their parents.
   B. parents constantly nag on their children about being too radical.
   C. parents and children tend to be at odds when it comes to social conformity.
   D. the young generation often ignores the wisdom of the elders.

Unit 2

Questions 3 - 4

For questions 3 and 4, consider the following quotation and analyse the cartoon.

The Internet will help achieve "friction free capitalism" by putting buyer and seller in direct contact and providing more information to both about each other.

Bill Gates

Cartoon 2

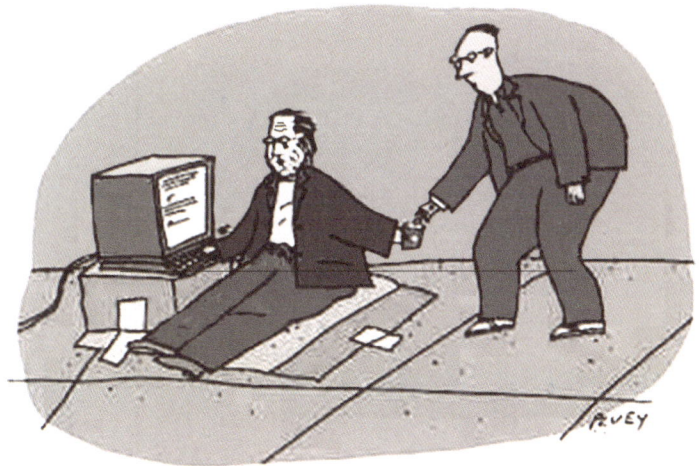

"Thanks pal, let me put you on my mailing list."

Cartoon by P.C. Vey. Reproduced with permission.

3. The statement of Bill Gates is MOST suggestive of:
   A. a growth in commerce due to digital technology.
   B. a positive development in information systems.
   C. good leadership in E-Commerce.
   D. the important role of information technology in marketing strategies.

4. This cartoon contains a typical theme in British humour that speaks about:
   A. the impoverished working class trying to 'beat the system'.
   B. making fun of social stereotypes.
   C. the ironic humour of everyday life.
   D. black humour.

Unit 3

Questions 5 - 6

For questions 5 and 6, consider the following comment and analyse the cartoon.

Global warming is too serious for the world any longer to ignore its danger or split into opposing factions on it.

Tony Blair

Cartoon 3

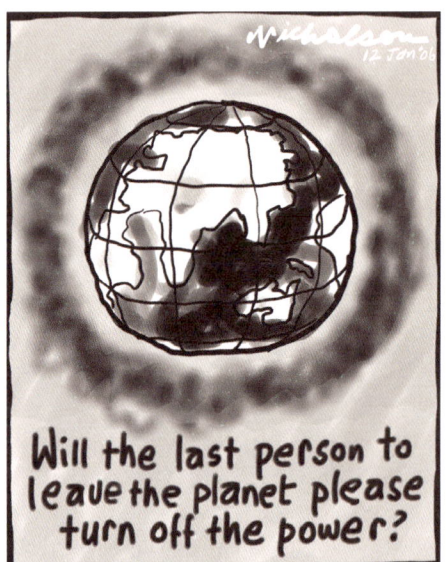

Cartoon by Nicholson from "The Australian" www.nicholsoncartoons.com.au.
Printed with permission.

5. The comment of Tony Blair connotes:
   A. an appeal to emotions.
   B. an appeal for immediate action.
   C. a warning against passivity.
   D. a contempt for passivity.

6. The statement in the cartoon signifies a:
- A. positive vision of the future.
- B. bleak vision of the future.
- C. remote possibility.
- D. warning.

Unit 4

Questions 7 - 8

Cartoon 4

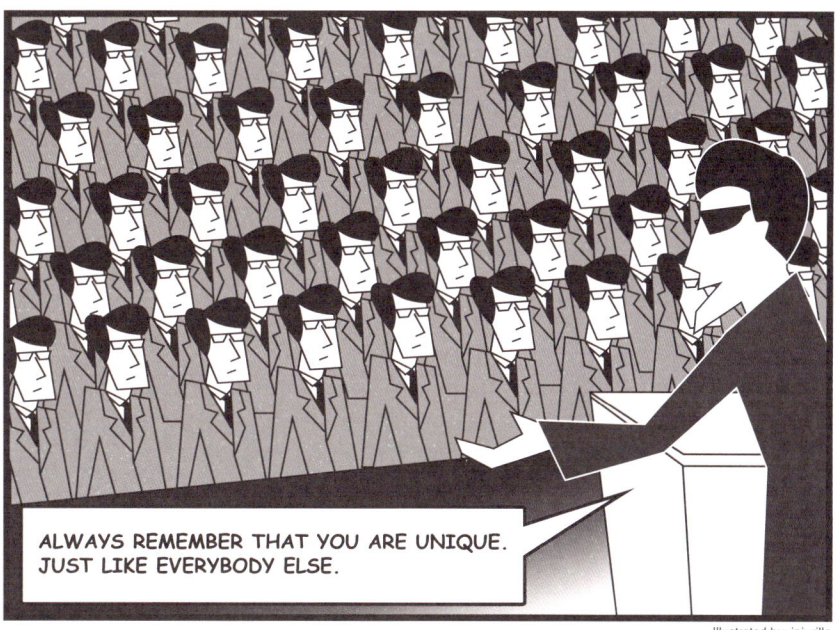

Printed with permission from Jonathan P. Jurilla

7. The cartoon is humorous because:
- A. of the analogy between individuality and the audience in the cartoon.
- B. of the irony expressed in both the textual and graphical messages.
- C. as a matter of fact, individuality is difficult to attain.
- D. of the way the message is delivered by the speaker.

8. The cartoon is an example of:
    A. graphic art with an erroneous text.
    B. a social commentary.
    C. irony.
    D. quip.

Unit 5

Questions 9 - 11

For questions 9 to 11, consider the following quotation and analyse the cartoon.

> *A soul mate is someone who has locks that fit our keys, and keys to fit our locks. When we feel safe enough to open the locks, our truest selves step out and we can be completely and honestly who we are; we can be loved for who we are and not for who we're pretending to be. Each unveils the best part of the other. No matter what else goes wrong around us, with that one person we're safe in our own paradise.*
>
> Richard Bach

Cartoon 5

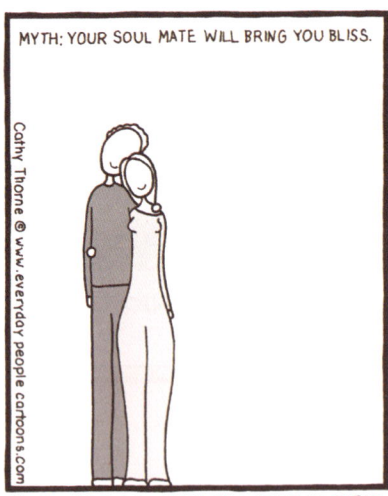

Printed with permission from Cathy Thorne.

9. The statement of Richard Bach describes:
    A. a universal truth about love.
    B. a lesson learned in finding true love.
    C. an aspiration to find true love.
    D. an ideal about love and romantic relationships.

10. The statements in the cartoon express:
    A. a disbelief in soul mates.
    B. a disenchantment with soul mates.
    C. the truth about soul mate.
    D. an accismus*.
       *Accismus: expressing the want of something by denying it.

11. The cartoon could be best described as:
    A. a metaphorical illustration of the quotation.
    B. a satirical interpretation of the quotation.
    C. a cliché.
    D. an alternative interpretation of the quotation.

Unit 6

Question 12

Cartoon 6

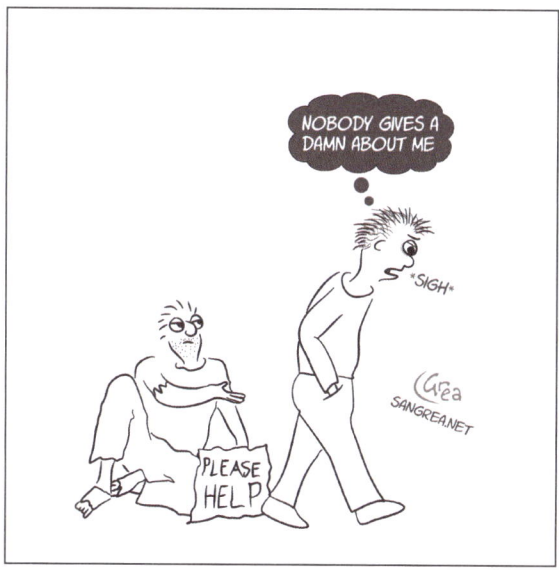

Printed with permission from Grea Korting www.sangrea.net

12. The joke in the cartoon mostly stems from:
    A. the similarity in the characters' situations.
    B. the juxtaposition of the characters' concerns.
    C. the paradox in the speaker's situation.
    D. the irony of the characters' situations.

Unit 7

Question 13

The following relate to the importance of good communication skills.

Communication is said to be a vehicle in transferring knowledge and fostering cooperation and understanding in society. Of course, this is not limited to the verbal medium. Nonverbal expressions such as gestures, facial reactions, and signs all form part of the communication process.

Cartoon 7

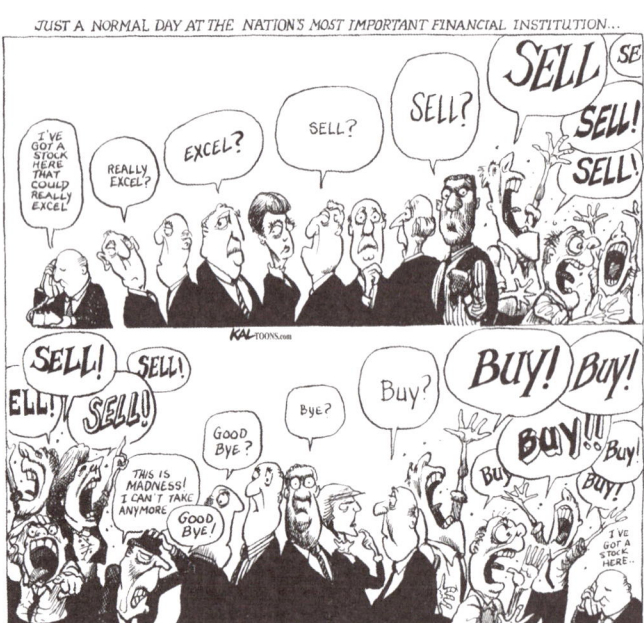

Printed with permission from Kevin Kallaugher.

The following are views of famous writers about communication:

I. I quote others only in order the better to express myself.
   - Michel de Montaigne
II. When people talk, listen completely. Most people never listen.
   - Ernest Hemingway
III. After all, when you come right down to it, how many people speak the same language even when they speak the same language?
   - Russell Hoban
IV. It seemed rather incongruous that in a society of supersophisticated communication, we often suffer from a shortage of listeners.
   - Erma Bombeck

13. Which of the views coincide with the way communication is portrayed in the cartoon?
   A. I and II
   B. III and IV
   C. II, III and IV
   D. II and IV

Unit 8

Question 14

Cartoon 8

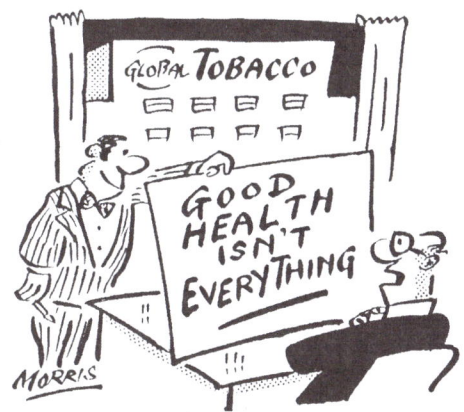

"That's a crazy idea but it might work."
Printed with permission from CartoonStock Ltd.

14. The cartoon reflects a commentary about certain scenarios that resulted from the anti-smoking bans.

   Study the following comments:
   I. Tobacco companies have sought new and creative ways of getting "around the law" as advertisements have been increasingly regulated with certain bans in print, radio and television media.
   II. Health warnings will remain as part of anti-smoking campaigns.
   III. Tobacco companies use alternative campaigns that do not necessarily look like tobacco advertisements but have an effect of promoting smoking.
   IV. Anti-smoking laws leave tobacco companies with limited marketing alternatives.

   Which of these comments would apply to the cartoon?
   A. Comment I only
   B. Comments II and IV only
   C. Comment IV only
   D. Comments I and III only

Unit 9

Questions 15 - 16

Cartoon 9

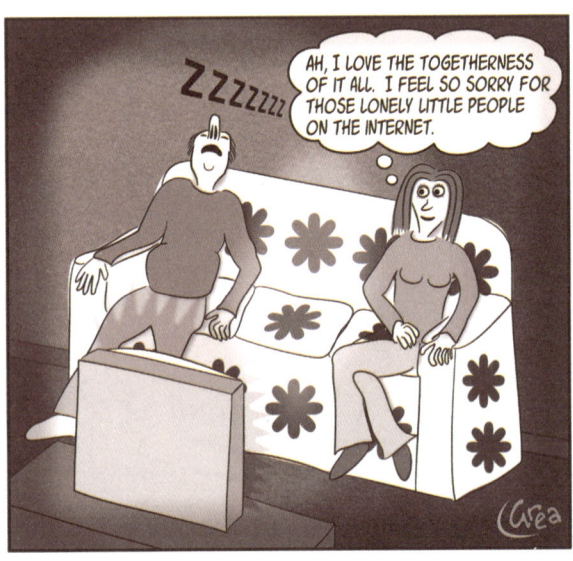

Printed with permission from Grea Korting www.sangrea.net

15. The thought expressed by the wife in the cartoon is an example of:
    A. subliminal perception.
    B. denial.
    C. psychological repression.
    D. a metaphor.

16. Based on the cartoon, the best advice on marriage would then be:
    A. "A successful marriage requires falling in love many times, always with the same person." (Mignon McLaughlin, The Second Neurotic's Notebook, 1966)
    B. "In every marriage more than a week old, there are grounds for divorce. The trick is to find, and continue to find, grounds for marriage." (Robert Anderson, Solitaire & Double Solitaire)
    C. "Never feel remorse for what you have thought about your wife; she has thought much worse things about you." (Jean Rostand, Le Mariage, 1927)
    D. "I have learned that only two things are necessary to keep one's wife happy. First, let her think she's having her own way. And second, let her have it." (Lyndon B. Johnson)

UNDERSTANDING THE GAMSAT

Unit 10

Questions 17 - 18

In February 2008, former Prime Minister Kevin Rudd read an apology that particularly addressed the "stolen generations" of Aborigines in Australia. Part of the momentous speech was the Parliament's recognition that the indigenous people were indeed mistreated in the past, and that the families suffered severe impacts from the forced removal of the children.

Compensation claims followed and were filed in the courts. However, not all claims were granted because many of the removals were done with consent and in accordance to specific legal acts of the Australian law.

Cartoon 10

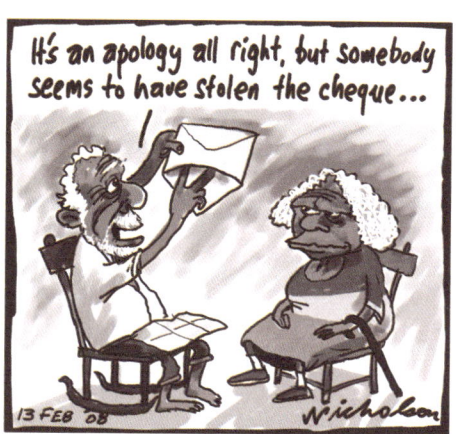

Cartoon by Nicholson from "The Australian" www.nicholsoncartoons.com.au.
Printed with permission.

17. The statement of the speaker in the cartoon:
    A. shows that the Aborigines doubted the sincerity of the government's apology.
    B. stresses that the Aborigines should be entitled to a monetary compensation from the government.
    C. shows that some Aborigines possibly did not understand the legal conditions of deserving a payout.
    D. stresses that the Aborigines expected a compensation to accompany the verbal apology.

18. The word "apology" is used in the cartoon to equate:
    A. hypocrisy.
    B. vindication.
    C. indemnity.
    D. profit.

GAMSAT-Prep.com
THE GOLD STANDARD

Unit 11

Questions 19 - 20

Cartoon 11

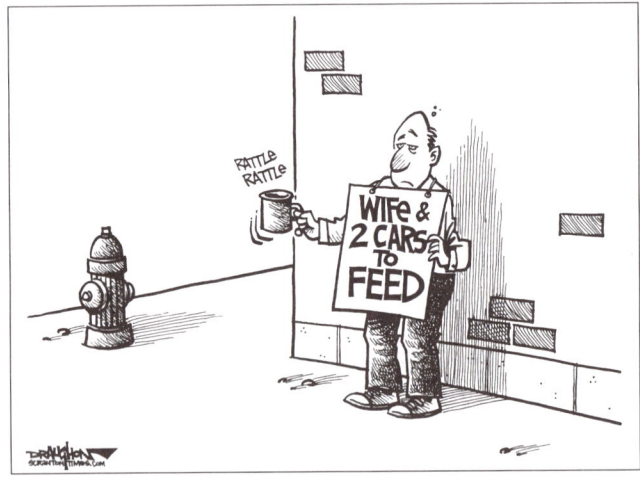

Printed with permission.
(Copyright 2004) Dennis Draughon & The Scranton Times (PA)

19. The cartoon is a reaction to:
    A. an economic depression.
    B. the unbearable rising prices of petrol.
    C. a pretentious lifestyle.
    D. social indifference towards the needy.

20. The type of humour found in the cartoon is:
    A. a pastiche.
    B. an understatement.
    C. a parody.
    D. a hyperbole.

If time remains, you may review your work. If your allotted time (25 minutes) is complete, please proceed to the Answer Key.

3.8.8 Cartoon Test Answer Key and Explanations

1.	C	6.	D	11.	B	16.	B
2.	C	7.	B	12.	D	17.	C
3.	D	8.	B	13.	D	18.	C
4.	B	9.	D	14.	D	19.	B
5.	B	10.	B	15.	B	20.	D

1. **Answer: C**

    Choices A and D are similar to each other in their use of contrasts. (A) Satire uses irony as a form of contrast in order to achieve humour with the intent of criticising society. However, irony in satires must be strongly charged to the point of being socio-political. Clearly, the dialogue in the cartoon merely connotes a joke on everyday family life issues.

    (D) Juxtaposition is also a form of contrast by placing two elements, which could be objects or texts in an art form, next to each other. In the cartoon, the parent-fish is portrayed to be asserting a parental rule against the child-fish who has already committed the "violation" of this same rule. It would, then, seem that the possible answer in this question would be (D). However, while there is clear contrast here, another option – (C) – also poses a more appropriate representation of the cartoon's humour.

    (C) Double entendre is a type of humour that connotes a "double meaning". The cartoon can be interpreted as either a joke about the plight of fishes or as a creative comparison of parent-child conflict in real-life. C then becomes the best choice of answer.

    (B) Analogy must be expressed in a statement that would sound ridiculous. For example, "Her face was a perfect oval, like a circle that had its two sides gently compressed by a ThighMaster." The dialogue in the cartoon does not come close to this form of humour.

2. **Answer: C**

    Choice A offers a very literal interpretation of what the cartoon may be trying to portray.

    Choices B, C, and D are closely similar. However, (B) mentions the word "radical". The term mostly connotes political leanings. The cartoon only shows a fashion trend among youngsters. (D) requires a much profound dialogue or illustration. The best choice is (C) because it embraces a more general interpretation of both the text and the cartoon illustration by using the term "social conformity".

3. **Answer: D**

    Although choices A, B, and D all have something to do with information or identity management, D makes an inclusion of the effect of information technology in business. Bill Gates' quote uses the term buyer and seller, and these are clearly common terms used in business. C merely speaks of Bill Gates' status in the internet industry.

UNDERSTANDING THE GAMSAT 155

4. **Answer: B**

The cartoon satirises a reversal of attitudes and a duality of roles between the beggar and the middle class. In a way, the cartoon does distort the way society generally perceives these two stereotypes. The correct answer is B.

A is easily negated as the correct answer because, as already mentioned, the cartoon tends to create a duality of roles between a beggar (i.e. accepts a donation) and a member of the working class (i.e. wears an office suit). One couldn't really tell for sure unless the cartoon would be given a literal interpretation.

(C) The cartoon may be portraying an "everyday life" scenario, but the joke doesn't necessarily qualify as an irony of daily life. (D) Black humour is usually grotesque and portrays a much darker plight such as death. The humour contained in this cartoon is a bit light for black humour.

5. **Answer: B**

"Too serious for the world any longer to ignore" provides the clue that the comment is not just a statement of (C) warning or (D) opinion but a call for (B) urgency of action. A would be a contentious choice.

6. **Answer: D**

A is wrong because the cartoon shows the earth on its final days. "The last person to leave the planet" suggests an exodus, which is not exactly a positive thing. (B) Although the cartoon projects humour and witticism, the idea being hinted is rather unwelcoming and terrifying. The statement likewise requests an involvement ("please turn off the power") from the reader ("the last person"), this makes the cartoon, not just a mere presentation of the artist's vision of the future but, more of a (D) warning of a fast coming reality. In other words, option D includes the idea in option B. (C) The accompanying quotation provides the idea of a serious threat or reality, not impossibility.

7. **Answer: B**

Answering this question requires evaluating the relevance of the text to the graphical illustration. A and D mislead the examinee to pay primary attention to the image. C is a profound interpretation of the cartoon but it is not the device used to make the cartoon humorous. This leaves D as the best answer.

8. **Answer: B**

A and B are the farthest choices because no obvious errors in spelling and grammar can be found nor is there any references about social or political justice. D is close but then again, while quip may sometimes require a certain degree of sarcasm, it has to depict witticism, first and foremost. C is the best choice because both the illustration and the textual message expresses subtle wit and contrasts.

9. **Answer: D**

The quotation simply describes the author's model of a compatible partner in a relationship referred as soul mate. "Soul mates" are what many hope to find as expressed in C. However, the kind of relationship described in the quotation does not always apply in every relationship. Therefore, it is not (A) a universal truth. Obviously, it is not (B) a lesson or wisdom being imparted either. This leaves D as the best answer.

10. **Answer: B**

A is incorrect as the cartoon acknowledges the existence of soul mates. The second statement "Your soul mate will bring up every one of your unresolved issues" is just the artist's opinion about soul mates - not a (C) universal truth. D is a red herring – there is no evidence to suggest the author of the cartoon/statements is demonstrating a desire for a soul mate via repression. Therefore, B is the correct answer.

A little more about answer choice D: do not expect to find a definition among answer choices during the real GAMSAT, nor during your practice full-length exams. We were just trying to be polite during your training!

11. **Answer: B**

Since the cartoon portrays an opposite view of the quotation, A and D can be eliminated from the choices. (B) Taking the quotation into context, it should be noted that there is mention of the line "Each unveils the best part of the other." One should recall that satire uses humour by highlighting the irony or contrast of a situation or, in this case, the quotation. This is the correct answer. C is quite subjective depending on the reader's point of view.

12. **Answer: D**

The cartoon shows both a (A) similarity and (B) contrast between the beggar and the passerby. Both characters are in a depressed situation. The beggar seeks financial help yet the passerby overlooked his plight. Ironically, the passerby expresses a need for emotional attention and feels too aggrieved by his own problem that he fails to see the beggar's worse condition. Therefore, the answer is D as it encompasses choices A and B. C is a ruse: the paradox would have applied between the two characters' situations - not in the speaker's situation.

13. **Answer: D**

The cartoon is about the distortion of information as words get passed on to the next receiver. In general, the cartoon depicts miscommunication and its source is a failure to listen fully. Quote I is about improving one's communication skills through imitating others. Quote II is an advice to listen and focus as poor listening can be a cause of miscommunication. Quote III implies that miscommunication is common even among people who speak the same language - they don't listen to each other. Quote IV also implies miscommunication even with advanced technology - again, the source is not listening. Choice D is the correct answer.

14. **Answer: D**

Comment I: The line, "That's a crazy idea but it might work," implies entertaining an idea that has not been thought of before – therefore new and creative - but is hoped to pass a certain scrutiny (e.g., an anti-smoking regulation).

Comment II: "Good health isn't everything" is not a health warning.

Comment III: "Good health isn't everything" is another way of saying that there are benefits in vices that cannot be found in a healthy lifestyle. In a way, this is the kind of advertisement described in Comment III.

Comment IV: The cartoon shows a presentation of a novel idea in an advertising campaign. This doesn't show a limitation of options.

15. **Answer: B**

Of the four choices, (D) metaphor is the easiest to eliminate. A metaphor is an analogy or a parallelism of the resemblance of two things. The statement of the wife expresses a contrast between her situation and those of "the people on the internet".

(A) Subliminal perception requires a stimulus that is unnoticeable but perceived anyway. In the illustration, the wife may look like she doesn't notice her husband falling asleep, but her thoughts in the cartoon tells that she chooses not to recognise it either.

(B) Denial and (C) repression are both forms of defence mechanism. Their main difference is that denial is a refusal to accept a pressing or unbearable problem while repression, against a desire that might result to a problem or cause a suffering if that desire is satisfied. The wife is clearly refusing to recognise a lack of "together"-ness with her husband despite spending their time in the same place.

16. Answer: B
A can be easily confused as the correct answer. The advice would relate more to extra-marital temptations as opposed to falling in love "with the same person". This situation is not illustrated in the cartoons.

C proposes an advice from a husband's standpoint only. The cartoon, however, presents only the wife's perspectives.

(D) This cartoon does not depict a power struggle between husband and wife. Hence, advice D is not applicable.

This leaves (B) as the best answer: the wife is finding a way to cope - albeit in an unfavourable light - with their failing communication.

17. Answer: C
(A) The line "It's an apology all right..." indicates that the speaker does acknowledge the apology. What he is only suspicious of is having been cheated in the monetary proceeds due him.

(B) This tone of suspicion in the speaker's statement, however, does not necessarily echo an assertion or a call to grant the compensation.

(C) What can be conveyed from the cartoon is the speaker's expectation of receiving some monetary benefit. This expectation hence illustrates his misunderstanding that all Aborigines will receive a claim. As stated in the descriptive paragraph, NOT ALL Aborigines were granted a payout because others were taken into government guardianship under reasonable circumstances.

(D) Indeed, the cartoon clearly implies that the Aborigines expected to be automatically compensated. This expectation therefore highlights the reason why C is the correct answer.

18. Answer: C
A is not implied anywhere in the cartoon. B and D sound plausible but not accurate enough in relation to the graphic illustration as well as in the given descriptive paragraph. (C) Indemnity refers to payment made to someone in order to compensate for damages. This is indicated by the speaker's immediate reaction upon receiving an envelope.

19. Answer: B
While there is an absence of sympathisers and donors in the cartoon, such lack fails to show a discernible portrayal of social indifference either. (D) can be therefore eliminated as the answer.

Having two cars indeed speaks of a high-profiled lifestyle. However, resorting to begging does not necessarily show pretence as it does a decline in one's financial state. Therefore, (C) is not a definite answer.

The cartoon indeed shows either poverty or economic scarcity. The sign bearing the words "2 cars to feed" specifically pinpoints the cause of poverty. Between choices (A) and (B), the one that has a link to "cars", i.e. "petrol" is (B).

20. Answer: D
(A) Pastiche is a form of a lampoon. The cartoon is not taken from a famous work. Hence, it does not qualify for a pastiche.

(B) An understatement is an extreme diminution of an otherwise important characteristic or topic in order to achieve humour. The cartoon does not reduce the problem implied by the cartoon but rather exaggerates it. A hyperbole exactly does that. The answer is D.

C is wrong because it is not an imitation of another art work.

GAMSAT-Prep.com
THE GOLD STANDARD

3.8.9 Graphs and Tables Test

The following mini test aims to help you focus on interpreting graphs and tables. These types of stimuli usually appear in two to six Section 1 units of the GAMSAT.

There are 6 units with 20 questions in this mini test. Please choose the best answer for each question. You have 25 minutes. Please time yourself.

BEGIN ONLY WHEN TIMER IS READY

Unit 1

Questions 1 - 4

Study the following abstract on medical consultation and the computer, and the accompanying consultation (hermeneutic) circle.

Abstract

Objective: Studies of the doctor–patient relationship have focussed on the elaboration of power and/or authority using a range of techniques to study the encounter between doctor and patient. The widespread adoption of computers by doctors brings a third party into the consultation. While there has been some research into the way doctors view and manage this new relationship, the behaviour of patients in response to the computer is rarely studied. In this paper, the authors use Goffman's dramaturgy (theatrical approach: scene, actor, stage, script, act) to explore patients' approaches to the doctor's computer in the consultation and its influence on the patient–doctor relationship.

Design: Observational study of Australian general practice. 141 consultations from 20 general practitioners were videotaped and analysed using a **hermeneutic framework.***

*Hermenuetics is an old term which refers to the interpretation of biblical, literary, and mythical texts. This process of interpretation (assigning meaning) gathered more momentum in philosophical and social science studies particularly, as how meaning is developed between the text and the subject – that each mutually defines the other. In as much as we question a given text, it will question or influence us in a co-creation of meaning.

Results: Patients negotiated the relationship between themselves, the doctor, and the computer demonstrating two themes: dyadic (dealing primarily with the doctor) or triadic (dealing with both computer and doctor). Patients used three signalling behaviours in relation to the computer on the doctor's desk (screen watching, screen ignoring, and screen excluding) to influence the behaviour of the doctor. Patients were able to draw the doctor to the computer and used the computer to challenge doctor's statements.

Conclusion: This study demonstrates that in consultations where doctors use computers, the computer can legitimately be regarded as part of a triadic relationship. Routine use of computers in the consultation changes the doctor–patient relationship, and is altering the distribution of power and authority between doctor and patient.

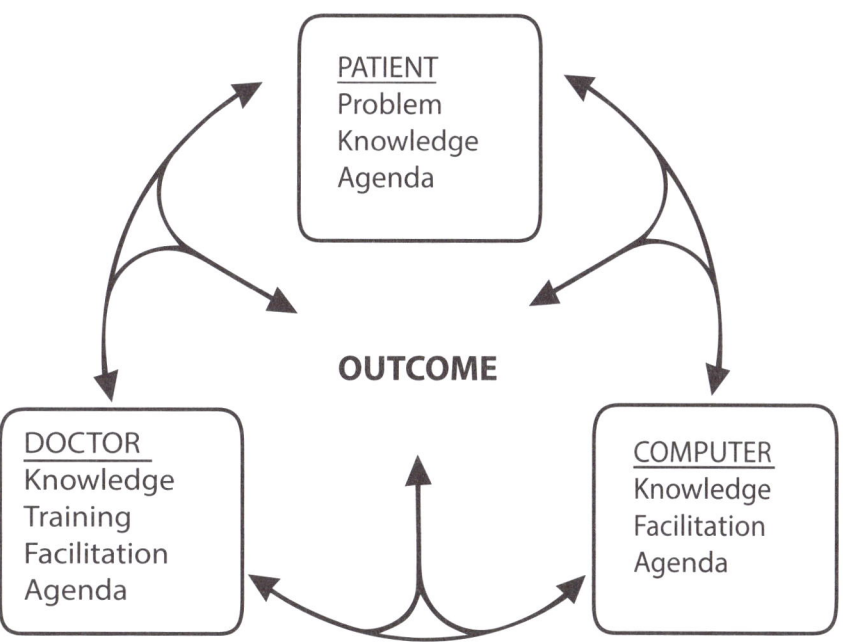

1. The main focus of the study according to the abstract and diagram is:
    A. to document the influence of the computer on the dyadic patient-doctor relationship.
    B. to understand the patient's influence on the doctor's use of the computer in medical consultations.
    C. to explore the patient's behaviour in response to the influence of doctors' use of a computer.
    D. to assess the use of computers in the triadic doctor-patient-computer relationship.

2. Based on the abstract, note, and diagram, which statement can be said to be the least congruent with the meaning of "hermeneutic"?
   A. The use of a computer in consultations transforms doctor-patient relationships and interactions.
   B. The outcome of the consultation is created by mutual interactions between doctor, patient, and the use of a computer.
   C. The patient's perception of the doctor-computer usage influences the outcome of the consultation.
   D. Doctor-patient relationships and interactions are facilitated by a computer in the consultation.

3. The commentary and graph imply that interactions between patient, doctor, and computer comprise a:
   A. group relationship with mutual definition.
   B. triadic relationship with mutual facilitation.
   C. dyadic relationship with mutual agendas.
   D. processual relationship with mutual knowledge.

4. The metaphor used to approach this research is a:
   A. network.
   B. theatre.
   C. system.
   D. machine.

UNDERSTANDING THE GAMSAT

Unit 2

Questions 5 - 8

When viewing the chart below, assume that the first score (Judge's) is correct. **There are errors in the chart in the other ordinal scores.** *First, find the inconsistencies in the scores to answer the questions.*

CHART (with errors)

	Judge's score x	Score minus 8 $x-8$	Tripled score $3x$	Cubed score x^3
Alice's cooking ability	10	2	300	1000
Bob's cooking ability	9	1	27	792
Claire's cooking ability	8.5	0.5	25.5	614.125
Dana's cooking ability	8	0	24	521
Edgar's cooking ability	5	3	15	150

5. From the cooks in the chart, who has a correct score in all representational summaries?
   - A. Edgar
   - B. Bob
   - C. Dana
   - D. Claire

6. The order of the scores, if calculated correctly, can be described to decrease:
   - A. steadily.
   - B. exponentially.
   - C. parsimoniously.
   - D. regressively.

7. If there were any discrepancies in the tripled score, and they were corrected, the average correct tripled score would be:
   - A. 24.3
   - B. 135.3
   - C. 13.53
   - D. 23.4

8. What would be the cubed score of the average judge's score?
   - A. 664.125
   - B. 531.441
   - C. 512
   - D. 614.125

GAMSAT-Prep.com
THE GOLD STANDARD

Unit 3

Questions 9 - 11

The following are charts measuring oil production and consumption from the years of 1990 – 2009 for both countries: Australia and the U.K. Take note that certain numerical estimates or assumptions are listed below the graphical representations. Study these carefully for certain questions will be based on these estimates.

Australia and UK Oil Production and Consumption

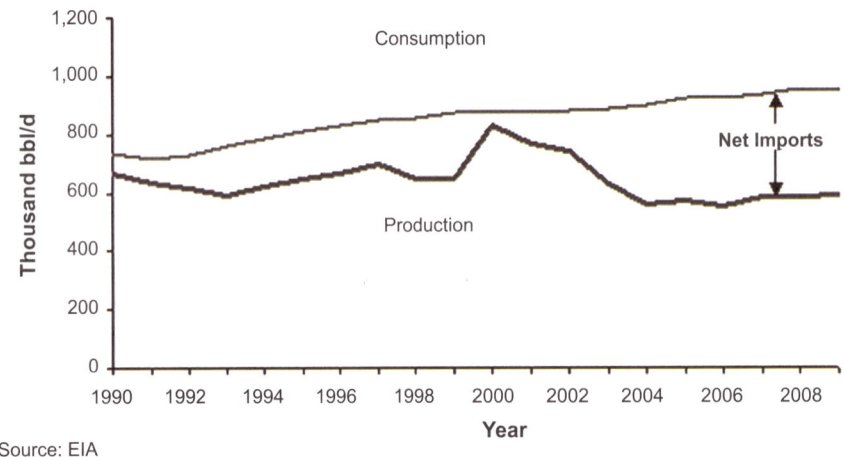

Bbl. /d = barrels per day

Estimates and assumptions based on graphical data:
Population – Australia (2000) – 19,153,000 +/-
Consumption Assumed 820,000 (2000)
23.35 barrels per day per citizen (2000)

UNDERSTANDING THE GAMSAT

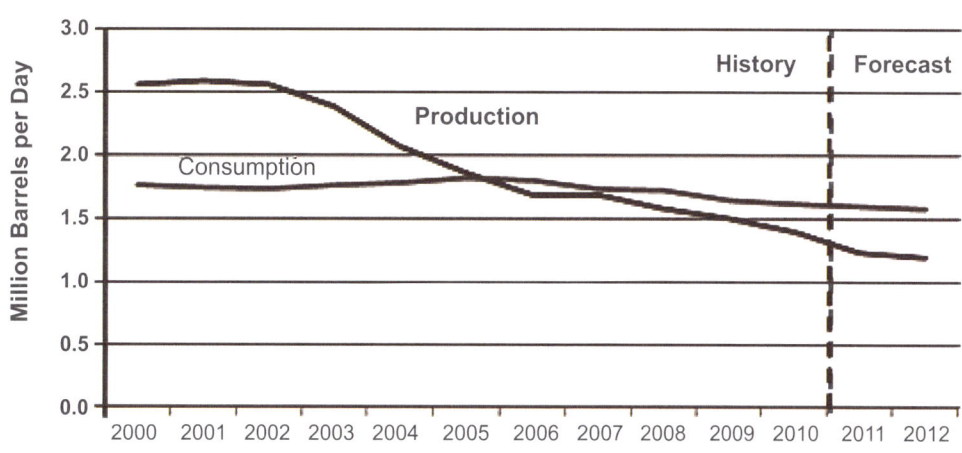

Source: U.S. Energy Information Administration

Estimates and Assumptions based on graphical data:

Population – UK (2000) – 58,893, 000 +/-

Consumption Assumed 1,750,000 (2000)

33.65 Barrels per day per citizen (2000)

9. Assuming in 2000 that the consumption level of oil per barrel per day for the UK was 1,750,000 and Australia was 820,000, based on the population for that year, what is the rough difference of bbl/d per citizen between each country in that year?

   A. 33
   B. 23
   C. 10
   D. 13

10. The net imports in Australia in 2008 were roughly:

    A. 300,000 bbl/d.
    B. 400,000 bbl/d.
    C. 350,000 bbl/d.
    D. 450,000 bbl/d.

11. What has been the most consistent variable from both graphs?

    A. Production
    B. Net Imports
    C. Consumption
    D. Barrels per day

Unit 4

Questions 12 – 15

Carefully read the following commentary and study the accompanying graph.

The PRECEDE-PROCEED planning system or framework is from the National Cancer Institute for communication strategies in health education.

Once health communications planners identify a health problem, they can use a planning framework such as the two described: social marketing and PRECEDE-PROCEED. These planning systems can help identify the social science theories most appropriate for understanding the problem or situation. Thus planners use the theories and models described below within the construct of a planning framework. Using planning systems like social marketing and PRECEDE-PROCEED increases the odds of program success by examining health and behaviour at multiple levels. Planning system perspectives emphasise changing people, their environment, or both.

The PRECEDE-PROCEED framework is an approach to planning that examines the factors contributing to behavior change. These include:

- Predisposing factors - the individual's knowledge, attitudes, behaviour, beliefs, and values before intervention that affect willingness to change

- Enabling factors - factors in the environment or community of an individual that facilitate or present obstacles to change

- Reinforcing factors - the positive or negative effects of adopting the behaviour (including social support) that influence continuing the behaviour

These factors require that individuals be considered in the context of their community and social structures, and not in isolation, when planning communication or health education strategies.

UNDERSTANDING THE GAMSAT

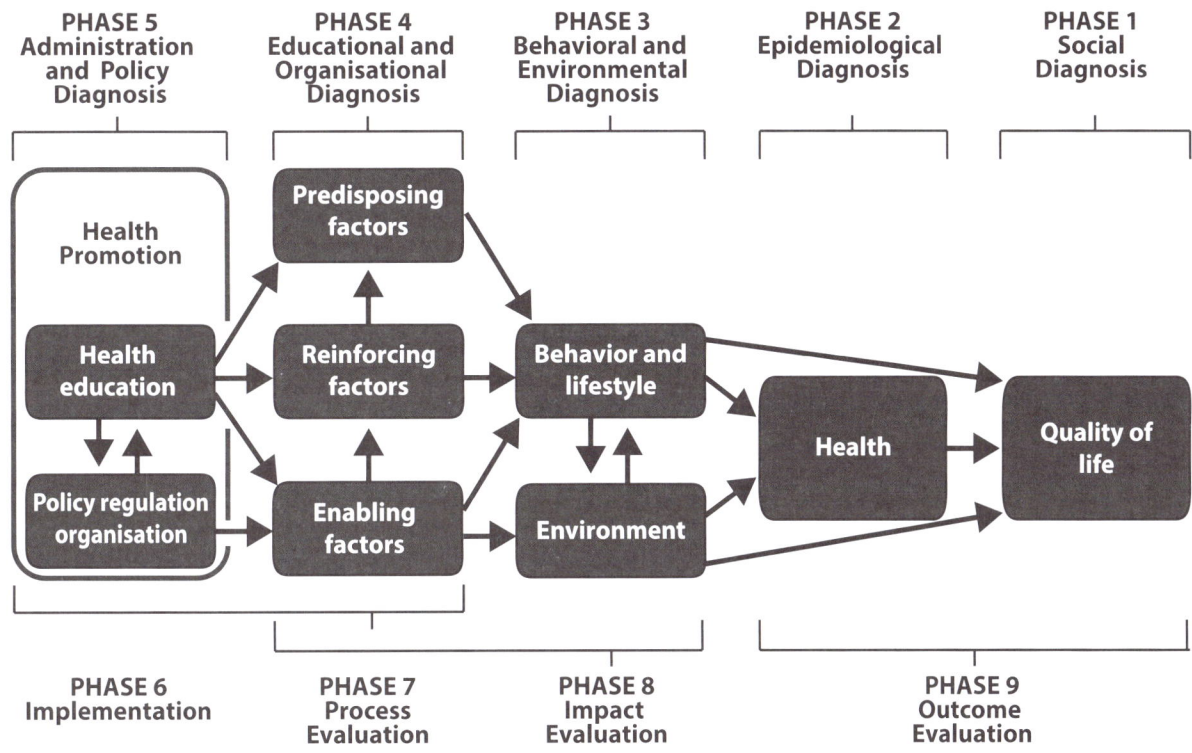

12. The most crucial phases as illustrated in the diagram are phases:
    A. 3 and 8.
    B. 4 and 7.
    C. 5 and 6.
    D. 1 and 5.

13. How are phases 3 and 8 related (Behavioural and Environmental Diagnosis and Impact Evaluation, respectively)?
    A. Through predisposing, reinforcing and enabling factors
    B. Through process evaluation and educational diagnosis
    C. Through examining impact evaluation and behavioural/environmental diagnosis
    D. Through implementation of the process and epidemiological diagnosis

14. The relationship between Phases 5 and 6 can be described as:
    A. linear orientation.
    B. mutual reciprocity.
    C. branching influence.
    D. symbiotic or commensal.

15. According to the commentary and diagram, why are the "factors" considerably important?

    A. They are the foundational basis for behavioural change.
    B. They are interlinked with impact modification.
    C. They are the hub of activity within the graph itself.
    D. They are the required phase or level for changes in administration and policy.

Unit 5

Questions 16 - 17

Venn diagrams or set diagrams are diagrams that show all possible logical relations between finite collections of sets (aggregation of things). Venn diagrams were conceived around 1880 by John Venn. They are used to teach elementary set theory, as well as illustrate simple set relationships in probability, logic, statistics, linguistics and computer science. The number of shared areas, according to symbolic logic, is represented by n. These shared areas are logical connections.

Intersections of the Greek, Latin, and English Alphabets – Venn Diagram.

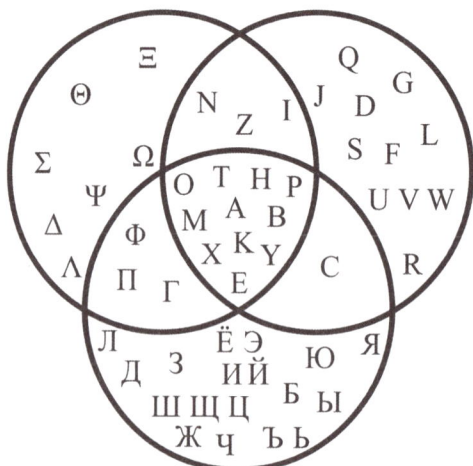

16. Which of the following conclusions cannot be supported by the Venn diagram?

    A. The Greek alphabet does not share C with English and Latin.
    B. Z is shared only by Greek and English alphabets.
    C. Greek, Latin, and English alphabets share more vowels than consonants.
    D. R is exclusively English.

UNDERSTANDING THE GAMSAT

17. Which pair of words can be made using the combination of Greek-English alphabets, but not the combination of Latin-English alphabets?

    A. Home, path
    B. Ozone, cable
    C. Bait, biome
    D. None of the above

Unit 6

Questions 18 - 20

Reptiles are popular as pets in the United States: an estimated 7.3 million pet reptiles are owned by approximately three percent of households. Because the most popular reptile species will not breed if closely confined, most reptiles are captured in the wild and imported. The number of reptiles imported into the U.S. has increased dramatically since 1986 and primarily reflects importation of iguanas.

A high proportion of reptiles are asymptomatic carriers of Salmonella. Fecal carriage rates can be more than 90 percent; attempts to eliminate Salmonella carriage in reptiles with antibiotics have been unsuccessful and have led to increased antibiotic resistance. A wide variety of Salmonella serotypes (over 4400) has been isolated from reptiles, including many that rarely are isolated from other animals (reptile-associated serotypes). Serotype refers to distinct variations within a subspecies of bacteria or viruses. These microorganisms, viruses, or cells are classified together based on their cell surface antigens. Reptiles can become infected through transovarial transmission or direct contact with other infected reptiles or contaminated reptile feces. High rates of fecal carriage of Salmonella can be related to the eating of feces by hatchlings - a typical behaviour for iguanas and other lizards - which can establish normal intestinal flora for hindgut fermentation.

During the early 1970s, small pet turtles were an important source of Salmonella infection in the United States; an estimated four percent of families owned turtles, and 14 percent of salmonellosis cases were attributed to exposure to turtles. In 1975, the Food and Drug Administration prohibited the distribution and sale of turtles with a carapace smaller than four inches; many states prohibited the sale of such turtles. These measures resulted in the prevention of an estimated 100,000 cases of salmonellosis annually. However, since 1986, the popularity of iguanas and other reptiles that can transmit infection to humans has been paralleled by an increased incidence of Salmonella infections caused by reptile-associated serotypes.

GAMSAT-Prep.com
THE GOLD STANDARD

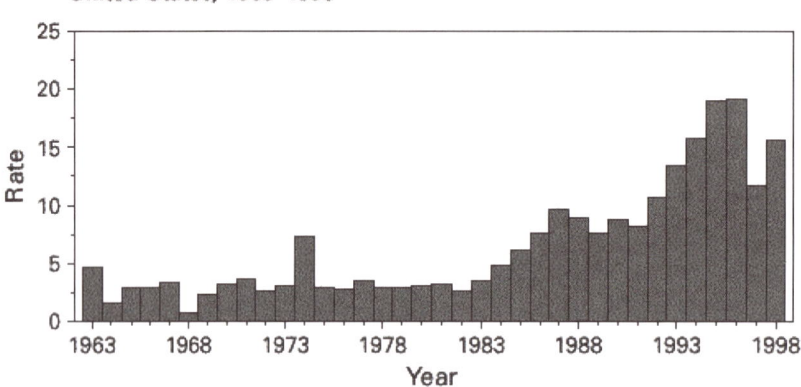

18. The highest rate of reptile-associated serotypes isolated from humans occurred in:
    A. 1994.
    B. 1995.
    C. 1996.
    D. 1997.

19. The largest decline in the rate, by a single year, of reptile-associated serotypes isolated from humans was roughly:
    A. 40,000,000.
    B. 5,000,000.
    C. 20,000,000.
    D. 75,000,000.

20. The most dramatic increase in rate occurred from:
    A. 1968 - 1974.
    B. 1997 - 1998.
    C. 1991 - 1996.
    D. 1978 - 1984.

If time remains, you may review your work. If your allotted time (25 minutes) is complete, please proceed to the Answer Key.

UNDERSTANDING THE GAMSAT

3.8.10 Graphs and Tables Test 1 Answer Key and Explanations

1. C	5. D	9. C	13. C	17. D
2. D	6. A	10. C	14. B	18. C
3. B	7. A	11. C	15. A	19. D
4. B	8. B	12. B	16. C	20. C

1. **Correct Answer: C**
   As stated in the abstract objective: "to explore patients' approaches to the doctor's computer in the consultation, and its influence on the patient–doctor relationship", this clearly confirms **C** as the correct answer.

2. **Correct Answer: D**
   This question asks you to choose the LEAST correct option. The diagram demonstrates that (A) doctor-patient relationships are certainly influenced by the use of computers. The note and diagram explain that (B) hermeneutics are based on a mutual definition. The abstract results explain why **C** agrees with the meaning of hermeneutics.

   The answer is **D**. The use of a computer was part of the study's methodology and the doctor-patient interaction can be said to have been facilitated by a computer to a certain extent. However, this statement does not coincide with the concept of hermeneutics, which concerns the co-creation of meanings (i.e. the facilitation needs to be reciprocal).

3. **Correct Answer: B**
   "Patients negotiated the relationship between themselves, the doctor, and the computer demonstrating two themes: dyadic (dealing primarily with the doctor) or triadic (dealing with both computer and doctor)." This quote from the results overview confirms **B** as the correct answer.

4. **Correct Answer: B**
   The reference to Goffman's dramaturgy indicates (**B**) theatre as the correct answer: "*In this paper, the authors use Goffman's dramaturgy (theatrical approach: scene, actor, stage, script, act) to explore patients' approaches to the doctor's computer in the consultation, and its influence on the patient–doctor relationship.*"

5. **Correct Answer: D**
   First, using a scratch pad, this would represent the corrected table - corrected scores are highlighted.

   There are no errors in Claire's scores, indicating **D** as the correct answer.

	Judge's score x	Score minus 8 $x-8$	Tripled score $3x$	Cubed score x^3
Alice's cooking ability	10	2	**30**	1000
Bob's cooking ability	9	1	27	**729**
Claire's cooking ability	8.5	0.5	25.5	614.125
Dana's cooking ability	8	0	24	**512**
Edgar's cooking ability	5	**-3**	15	**125**

6. **Correct Answer: A**
   The scores decrease steadily with Alice's scores to be the highest and Edgar's scores to be the lowest, indicating **A** as the correct answer. **(B)** Exponentially is incorrect because the decrease of scores would be in large quantitative amounts. **(C)** Parsimoniously is nonsense, while **D** regressively refers to best fit, smallest size decreases of numerical relations, more properly suited to statistical analysis techniques – this answer is a bit of a red herring or distraction. Also, the question stem already states that the scores are supposed to decrease (i.e. regress).

7. **Correct Answer: A**
   To find the average, total the 5 scores and divide by 5. 30+27+25.5+24+15 = 121.5/5 = 24.3
   This indicates **A** as the correct answer.

8. **Correct Answer: B**
   First, find the average judge's score:
   10 + 9 + 8.5 + 8 + 5 = 40.5
   40.5/5 = 8.1 (Average Judge's Score)

   To find the cubed score x3 (8.1 x 8.1 x 8.1). This results to 531.441 indicating **B** as the correct answer.

9. **Correct Answer: C**
   A quick scan of the estimates and assumptions based on graphical data (33.65 bbl/d per citizen in the UK in 2000 and 23.35 bbl/d per citizen in Australia in 2000) indicates a rough difference of 10 bbl/d confirming **C** as the correct answer.

10. **Correct Answer: C**
    Net imports refer to the difference between consumption and production. A trick for these kinds of questions is using a straight edge, like a ruler or piece of paper aligned across the graph. This alignment will roughly show the difference between 600,000 and 950,000 indicating **(C)** 350,000 bbl/d as the correct answer.

11. **Correct Answer: C**
    A quick glance will affirm that **(C)** consumption has varied the least - making it the most consistent variable.

12. **Correct Answer: B**
    (B) Phases 4 and 7 are central hubs of activity within the diagram connecting 3 and 5, as well as 6 and 7. The whole gist of the last paragraph, concerning the factors, stresses this importance in terms of behaviour change and its relation to health education strategies.

13. **Correct Answer: C**
    This easy detail-oriented quick scan question is transparently **C**.

14. **Correct Answer: B**
    One can infer within the rubric of Health Promotion, of which both phases 5 and 6 are associated with. There is mutual dynamism occurring between "health education" and "policy regulation and organisation". The arrows are pointing to each other indicating a mutually defining, modifying or changing process. For these reasons, **(B)** mutual reciprocity is the correct answer. The other answers are incorrect because **(A)** linear orientation stresses a one-way, unidirectional flow of information. **C** applies to the arrows moving into phases 4 and 7, yet this does not address the internal relationship between 5 and 6 while **D** is plain bio-babble distraction.

15. **Correct Answer: A**
    Considering that the commentary and diagram are essentially concerned with health education in relation to behavioural change, **A** is the correct answer. The other answers are holistically related to the diagram itself but do not reflect the essential focus of behavioural change. Without these contextually defining factors, the diagram would be meaningless. The whole framework of the analysis is based on the factors as can be inferred from the commentary excerpt:

    The PRECEDE-PROCEED framework is an approach to planning that examines the factors contributing to behaviour change. . . These factors require that individuals be considered in the context of their community and social structures, and not in isolation, when planning communication or health education strategies.

16. **Correct Answer: C**
A quick perusal of the Venn diagram will confirm that all propositions **A**, **B**, and **D** are true while **C** the correct answer cannot be supported by the Venn diagram.

17. **Correct Answer: D**
A scrabble-type question will reveal that **(D)** none from the given pairs of words can be created exclusively from the Greek-English alphabets combination.

18. **Correct Answer: C**
Hints to these types of questions:
1. Use a straight edge to determine numerical approximations, differences, and estimates.
2. In this particular graph, determine the mid-points between numeric data, which roughly corresponds to 2.5.

Using the straight edge trick or method, we find that 1996 is the highest rate at about 19.5 (per 10,000,000 population) slightly higher than 1995, making C the correct answer.

19. **Correct Answer: D**
Occurring and noticeable from 1996 to 1997, again we find, using the straight edge method a difference of between 19.5 and 12.0 indicating a difference of 7.50. This makes **D** the correct answer.

20. **Correct Answer: C**
A straight edge will confirm the following differences corresponding to the years listed, indicating **C** as the correct answer:

(A) 1968 – 1974 = 6.0 difference +/-
(B) 1997 – 1998 = 3.0 difference +/-
(C) 1991 – 1996 = 9.0 difference +/-
(D) 1978 – 1984 = 7.5 difference +/-

GAMSAT-Prep.com
THE GOLD STANDARD

REVIEW FOR SECTION II

4.1 Overview

GAMSAT Section II, or "Written Communication," is comprised of 2 writing tasks, which should be completed within a 60-minute time limit. Each writing task has four to five quotations that appertain to a common theme.

Additionally, candidates will be given 5 minutes to read through the instructions and quotations before the actual test starts. This short reading time should allow you to start examining the two writing tasks carefully and begin to plan a response to each. Take note that you are not allowed to write or make any notes during your 5 minutes reading time. Also note that the reading time allotted to sections I and III is 10 minutes, each.

Why write an essay?

In the early 1990s, the essay was included in the MCAT following complaints from the deans of various medical schools concerning the communication skills of medical students. Subsequently, it was included in the inaugural GAMSAT in 1995 and, of course, has continued to this day. Ironically, the new MCAT no longer has an essay section.

Section II will measure your ability to:

1) articulate your perspective on a given topic
2) synthesise ideas and concepts
3) express ideas in a logical and cohesive way
4) write clearly, using standard English and appropriate grammar, spelling and punctuation.

Being the only non-multiple choice section of the GAMSAT, this section requires two handwritten essays that must respond to two different themes. The first essay "Task A" is supposed to address a socio-cultural theme and the second essay "Task B", personal and social themes. You may use 1 or more of the given quotations as the basis for your written response. In selecting topics, ACER makes an effort to minimise factors which might disadvantage candidates from non-English speaking backgrounds.

You are not expected to write a short polished essay of final draft quality. The people grading your exam are aware that you only had 30 minutes to write the essay. Nevertheless, you will be expected to come up with a 'good' essay expressing your well-considered view of the ideas or themes presented in each writing task. Please refer to Section 4.7 for a scoring key. You may also consult Section 4.8 and GAMSAT-prep.com for examples of what a 'good' essay is in the eyes of the markers.

UNDERSTANDING THE GAMSAT

	Writing Task A	Writing Task B
Writing style	• persuasive • argumentative	• reflective • discursive/ argumentative
Theme	• socio-cultural • philosophical • political	• interpersonal/personal • social
Topics (examples)	• affirmative action • censorship • democracy • education • human nature • intelligence • meritocracy • politics • progress • space exploration • wealth	• conformity • family • friendship • humour • love • marriage • self-confidence • self-discovery • wisdom • youth • hatred

Several years ago, GAMSAT required a different writing format of response to the socio-political theme of Task A from the personal theme of Task B. However, in recent years, no mention of a particular essay style has been made in any of ACER's official materials, and many candidates have scored well using the same writing style in both Tasks A and B. In fact, some candidates find it much easier to practice and follow one format.

Of course, those who possess significant skills in prose should work to their strengths. A word of caution though: personal essays can be difficult to control at times, and can attract the disapproval of essay markers if they become ill-structured or overly sentimental. In this case, using the more objective style of argumentative-persuasive would be a better option.

GAMSAT-Prep.com
THE GOLD STANDARD

4.1.1 General Pointers for Section II

While you do not need any specific knowledge to do well in this section, you should read from varied sources (see Section 3.2.1) to familiarise yourself with current political and social concerns.

You are expected to write a first draft quality essay. A few grammatical, punctuation or spelling errors will not affect your mark greatly. However, a large number of such errors to the extent that your ideas become difficult to follow, will harm you. You are allowed to cross out words, sentences or passages. Do not try to recopy your essay. You are not expected to and you will not have the time to do this. However, please be sure that your writing is legible.

A title is not mandated but it could be helpful especially if it were catchy or intriguing. A good title should grab the reader's attention and - having crystallised the essay's thesis - orient the reader to the literary feast that is about to unveil. Both Tasks must have at least 3 paragraphs: an introduction, the body and the conclusion.

The use of creativity can be great. For example, some students choose to write the essay (especially Task A) as though it is a conversation between two people. Other students use metaphors. For example, you can use a video camera as a metaphor of an objective observer that switches from scene to scene. In the final scene (the conclusion or resolution), one could begin by saying: "And now, the camera is truly in focus" as one describes how the conflict is resolved.

Though such creative expressions can be quite powerful, they cannot make up for the following basic fact: you must address the needs of the essay. You must clearly deal with the concerns of ACER which includes: (1) addressing the central theme clearly; (2) applying at least one of the quotations to your essay; (3) demonstrating logical thinking; and to a lesser extent, (4) organisation and technical issues. Of course, being "overly" creative could have its own risks (i.e. inappropriate distraction). Creativity is best left to those with significant literary ability. It is crucial that candidates become expert at their essay structure and develop a strong body of knowledge and arguments for GAMSAT-style issues. Without a practiced writing style, strong structure, and an eclectic body of knowledge, no amount of gloss or ingenuity will score well – markers will see your essays for the mere veneer they are.

For Writing Task A, since this is formal writing, minimise your use of contractions as well as first-person and second-person pronouns ("I," "me," "you"). For both tasks, consider avoiding using contracted words such as "can't", "don't" or "won't". Finally, attempt to expand your vocabulary by avoiding the use of negating prefixes such as 'not', 'in' or 'un'. For example, instead of saying "not complete" use the positive form of the word, which is "partial". Another example might be using the word "vague" instead of 'unclear'. The use of positive terms will elevate the quality of your essay.

Specific examples can be powerful from history or from current affairs. Both will be greatly bolstered with the advice in Sections 3.2.1 and 3.2.2 of the previous chapter - irrespective of your academic background.

> Typically, the most interesting ideas will get the most marks.

4.2 Key Skills to Develop for Section II

It must be noted that assessment in Section II largely focusses on a candidate's ability to form an opinion and validate it as a logical response to the task's theme. In other words, you are to write about what you think, NOT how much knowledge you have, about the topic. The ideas that you will discuss must be highly relevant to what the quotations are talking about, and they must demonstrate careful reasoning. Your ideas must be supported by evidence. You cannot simply state an idea without detailing supporting examples and theory; or in the case of personal essays, relevant anecdotes. Keep in mind that your essay will not be marked for having the most correct idea but for having a logical point of view. Having said that, you must still keep in mind that a real person is marking your essay. Unsavoury or politically incorrect ideas are unlikely to score well. While remaining objective, generally distasteful ideas will likely have negative implications for how this person views your work.

> **A Section II response:**
> - must be relevant to the theme of the writing task
> - must express a well-thought-out opinion
> - must demonstrate logical thinking
> - must be supported by evidence

GAMSAT-Prep.com
THE GOLD STANDARD

4.2.1 Generating the Response

Forming a response for a Section II writing task starts with two important skills - identifying the theme and stating your thesis.

- Identifying the Theme

While you will be asked to generate a written response to only one or two of the given quotations - referred in the exam as "comments", a particular set will noticeably talk about a common topic. Some comments will offer contradicting views; hence, the theme is presented as a debatable issue. In other cases, the comments will convey varying definitions of the same subject.

Your initial task is to determine what the comments, when taken together, are trying to say about an idea. This is different from merely identifying the topic. Finding the theme means answering the question: "What is it about this topic that the comments are saying?" Even if you choose to develop an essay based on just one or two comments, you still need to consider the general context within which an idea is discussed.

Still, some students make the mistake of either reacting to the topic alone or choosing one of the comments and discussing a point that may be true within the quotation's context but so far off from the main idea (i.e. the theme) of all the comments. Let's take the following as an example:

* * * * *

Comment 1

Justice is justly represented blind, because she sees no difference in the parties concerned.

William Penn

* * * * *

Comment 2

Justice cannot be for one side alone, but must be for both.

Eleanor Roosevelt

* * * * *

Comment 3

It is better that ten guilty persons escape than one innocent suffer.

William Blackstone

* * * * *

Comment 4

It is more important that innocence be protected than it is that guilt be punished, for guilt and crimes are so frequent in this world that they cannot all be punished.

John Adams

* * * * *

Comment 5

Justice consists not in being neutral between right and wrong, but in finding out the right and upholding it, wherever found, against the wrong.

Theodore Roosevelt

As an aside, it is recommended that you learn about important historical figures such as William Blackstone or Theodore Roosevelt. Although the recent GAMSATs have not credited the sources of their quotes in the stimulus, this has been common practice in the past. If you understand the biography of a famous figure, you are likely to have a better insight into his or her statement. In general, historical biographies are great repositories of ideas and can serve as evidence for your arguments.

Going back to our sample quotations, the word "justice" is mentioned repeatedly, so this must be the topic. Now here's an example of an incorrect response: you recognise that the topic of this writing task is justice, so you open your essay with another quote by Abraham Lincoln: "I have always found that mercy bears richer fruits than strict justice." Then you proceed to cite the arguments between strictly enforcing justice and balancing it with mercy.

Or, you pick the fourth comment and talk about how punishment can leave a negative mark on a person's life. Then you cite an example about a young offender who was sent to prison for shoplifting. While in prison, he was exposed to cruelty and violence. This traumatic experience became an impetus for him to resent the justice system and become a ruthless criminal.

While the discussion in both cases may be very interesting, the general topic of this writing task does not really pertain to justice vs mercy or crime and punishment, but to justice being nondiscriminatory. So how can you mine the five comments for a main idea?

Here is a good procedure that you can follow to determine a theme:

First, read all the comments and note the words or phrases that are often mentioned. Repetition of words and phrases means that these are being emphasised. In our example, the words "justice", "guilt" or "guilty" and "innocence" or "innocent" are mentioned the most.

Second, observe how each comment either discusses the repeated words in a positive or a negative light. Note that the comments highlight facets of meaning or aspects of a given topic.

The first two comments speak of justice as making no distinction between different parties or sides. The next two comments place more importance in the protection of the innocent rather than punishing the guilty. The last comment views justice as upholding what is right.

Third, synthesise the ideas from all the comments. This is what you should react to. Your essay will either support or contradict this idea in the comments.

Again from our example, we were able to sift three ideas: that justice does not discriminate between two parties; that justice can only be achieved if the innocent is protected; and justice should always seek for what is right. We can then phrase this as a debatable issue: Should justice remain impartial or should justice ensure that the innocent is protected and uphold what is right?

Now you can decide which side to take and defend. The stand you choose will help formulate your thesis statement.

Let's take another set of quotations and apply the three-step approach that we just discussed:

* * * * *

Comment 1

Parents are always more ambitious for their children than they are for themselves.

* * * * *

Comment 2

We never know the love of a parent till we become parents ourselves.

Henry Ward Beecher

* * * * *

Comment 3

Parents can only give good advice or put them on the right paths, but the final forming of a person's character lies in their own hands.

Anne Frank

* * * * *

Comment 4

Some mothers are kissing mothers and some are scolding mothers, but it is love just the same, and most mothers kiss and scold together.

Pearl S. Buck

* * * * *

Comment 5

A father's goodness is higher than the mountain, a mother's goodness deeper than the sea.

Japanese Proverb

First, the most repeated word in this writing task is "parents".

Second, the first comment says that parents want their children to have a better life or future than their own. The second comment says children will only appreciate their parents when they become one. The third comment says parents can only guide their children but their children will still decide for themselves. The last two comments basically express the same view - every parent shows his or her love in different ways.

Third, we are now aware that while there are four thoughts on "parents" in this writing task, they all have to do with how parents show love or provide guidance to their children. This should now become the backdrop of your essay's discussion.

You can choose to agree or disagree with the idea that no matter the parenting style, parents want what's best for their children. Alternatively, you can expound on the issue of parents being overprotective and whether or not this is justifiable. Whichever perspective you choose, it needs to be expressed in the form of a thesis statement.

- Stating the Thesis

Whether your essay takes the form of a discursive or a reflective piece, the thesis statement has to be apparent. The thesis statement serves as your main response because it embodies the overall point of your essay. It answers the question, "What is it that I will try to prove in this piece?" Now, there are important points that you should take into account when composing your thesis statement.

1. **The thesis statement should be ideally written within the first paragraph; it is usually placed in the last sentence.** Because you are writing a 30-minute piece, you will not have the luxury of time to beat around the bush. Communicate the premise of your essay early on.

   Of course, there are essays where the thesis statement is declared in the last paragraph. Should you take this path, you have to ensure that you will hold the interest of your reader all throughout the piece or that your arguments are organised to fit this kind of structure. Nevertheless, this is only advisable if you are a skilled writer who has used this technique effectively in many practice attempts.

2. **The thesis statement should be clearly stated in the declarative format.** In some cases, an essay might pose a question; for example, "Should justice stay blind and impartial in all instances?" This is not exactly a thesis statement. The answer to this question IS the thesis statement. Hence you need to present your thesis in the declarative (e.g., "This essay will prove that justice cannot remain blind if the protection of the innocent is compromised.")

   Again, because this is a 30-minute writing task, you cannot waste time posing several questions because you will need to answer all of them. Otherwise, your essay will feel unresolved and indecisive. Remember that your task is to provide a definite standpoint - not just raise questions.

3. **A thesis statement should be a debatable claim to be proven using logical reasoning.** It should not be a statement about a generally accepted idea or fact. If you choose to make a generally accepted idea, your essay will fail to be a dialectic as you will likely struggle to present a sound antithesis. A failure to do so will naturally lead to a lower mark.

4. **A good thesis statement should cover a narrow scope of the topic.** If you embark on a very broad premise such as justice or parenting in general, you will either run out of time or overwhelm yourself with a plethora of evidences to offer in order to persuade your reader that your position is valid. The narrower the scope of your thesis, the more effective your argument will be. Again, the more general your thesis, the more difficult it will be to develop and respond to an antithesis.

Example of a factual statement: It is every parent's duty to guide his or her children onto the right path.

Example of a debatable and narrow thesis: Parents should refrain from becoming too close with their children if they want to develop emotionally resilient and responsible adults.

4.2.2 Writing an Interesting Introduction

"The beginning is the most important part of the work," according to Plato. How you write your essay's introduction is indeed critical. You either impress and arouse the markers' interest or you forewarn them that this is going to be a difficult read. This makes beginning the essay quite intimidating for some candidates. For others, generating the initial ideas itself is a struggle.

The good news is that you can remedy a scriptophobia of introductions by following an outline for writing your first paragraph. You can choose to adopt a logical introduction or a creative and catchy one.

- The Logical Introduction

Most discussion essays follow this type of introduction. Your main aim will be to set a logical connection between the main idea, which the comments express and the viewpoint you are taking.

It is also important to introduce the quote at this stage. This may seem redundant, however, it will give you an opportunity to demonstrate that you understand the idea being quoted. You will also be required to define the key term/s, especially if you are responding to them through a particular assumption. Do not be scared to address any parameters in the initial paragraph. For instance, you may decide to limit the discussion about justice to a particular area. By doing this, you are demonstrating to the marker that you have recognised the breadth of the theme, and you are choosing to thoroughly examine one aspect.

Sentence 1: state your interpretation of the comments' theme.

You can choose to write a summation of the comments' core idea or a paraphrase of one or two of the given comments. Alternatively, you can interlace a restatement of your selected quote.

Example:

A point of debate about the essence of justice is whether justice should remain unbiased or advocate for what is right.

Sentences 2 to 3: introduce the quote, and then define what the theme means in this context. Alternatively, expound the idea of the first sentence by citing the two sides of the argument.

A good formula to use for these two sentences would be to write something to this effect: *"Some say that . . . (quote or paraphrase one of the comments). Others say that . . . (quote or paraphrase another one of the comments)."*

Example 1:

Some say that justice cannot choose who it should favour. Others say that it should prompt one to always choose the right thing to do.

Example 2:

As Eleanor Roosevelt once said, "Justice cannot be for one side alone, but must be for both." On the other hand, proponents against this view will argue that justice cannot sacrifice the truth and the protection of the innocent.

Sentence 4: state which point of view you are taking. This is essentially your thesis statement.

Example:

Justice needs to be dispensed by going through the process of the legal system even if the end result does not suit everyone's ideal of justice.

Now let's put everything together and see if the introduction makes sense:

A point of debate about the essence of justice is whether justice should remain unbiased or advocate for what is right. Some say that justice cannot choose who it should favour. Others say that it should prompt one to always choose the right thing to do. Nevertheless, I believe that justice needs to be dispensed by going through the process of the legal system even if the end result does not suit everyone's ideal of justice.

- The Catchy Introduction

Another way to open your essay is by making it unique or striking. In an exam where thousands of papers are being marked, novelty and freshness of ideas can give your piece an edge. Uniqueness may also refer to presentation style. There are several creative devices to help you bait the markers' attention. We will discuss five of the most effective ones, namely: <u>surprising facts or statistics, dramatic anecdotes, analogies or metaphors, thought-provoking questions, and powerful quotations.</u>

However, please keep in mind that no matter which style you choose, you should not deviate from the main purpose of your introduction: to link the ideas between the comments and your own.

1. Surprising fact or statistics

This approach requires adequate research and reading from various sources such as history, published research and the news.

Example 1:

In 16th century England, an otherwise loyal subject of Henry VIII uttered, "I like not the proceedings of this realm". For this, he was imprisoned.

Example 2:

On June 11, 1963, a Vietnamese Mahayana Buddhist monk named Thích Quang Duc burned himself to death in Saigon to protest the predominantly Catholic South Vietnamese government's persecution of Buddhists.

Example 3:

An article in The Economist in 2013 reported that ten people were killed in a fire in a factory used by famous foreign clothes retailers in the Bangladeshi capital. Bangladesh is the world's second largest supplier of clothes, yet three-fifths of its factories are far from being a risk-free work environment.

Example 4:

It takes 2400 litres of water to make one hamburger.

Example 5:

Every year, three times as much garbage is being dumped in oceans as the weight of fish caught.

2. Dramatic anecdote

If you perceive yourself as someone with unique stories to tell, then this style might work for you. Basically, you begin your essay with an engaging narrative. It could be about a personal experience or an imagined scenario that depicts the essence of your response to the writing task.

If you do decide to adopt this introductory device, make sure to expose yourself to as many creative narrative styles. Practice regularly so that you develop the following key skills:

- Use of vivid, descriptive language
- Keeping the narrative concise yet entertaining

Creative introductions still follow the conventions of a standard introductory paragraph.

Example 1:

By the time I was five years old, I learnt all of The Beatles songs as my parents would always play their albums at home. One song particularly stood out to me - "Help!" In times of need during my five years in the world, I always had my friends to lend a helping hand, whether it be help to colour in my new art book or help to keep me from boredom when I played alone with my Barbie dolls. I could not imagine my life without help from my friends. After listening to John Lennon's song longing for friendship, I took it upon myself to respond. I proceeded to write an appealing letter to John letting him know that I would be delighted to be his friend - I would help him with his interest in music and he could voice my Ken dolls when we played my favourite game.

Example 2:

As I laid eyes on the tray of fresh fruits on our breakfast table this morning, I imagine a not-so-distant future when fruits take the form of morning shots instead. Natural food consumption would have become a luxury, reserved only for the privileged and moneyed. Farms and plantations would have all dried up and devoid of soil nutrients. Rain would have been only spoken in fairy tales. Earth would have been deprived of its once abundant blessings from Mother Nature; and so we have to create an artificial environment somewhere in space for plants to grow. Such are possibilities that I envision as I look at my morning fruits with global warming in the background.

3. Analogy, metaphor, simile

Analogies and metaphors are creative tools for thinking about a concept. They are usually effective in making a complicated idea or a very broad theme simpler to understand. You may also use this stylistic device if you want to give an old and tired concept a fresh treatment.

Basically, you have to choose a symbol or an equivalent situation that will embody the central point of your essay. Then you discuss it with an "as if" perspective. The trick is to use this symbol as a main reference throughout your paper. Refer back to it in the body as well as in the conclusion of your essay.

Reading creative literature frequently is a great way of honing the skillful use of analogies, metaphors and similes in an essay.

Example 1:

People attempt love like climbers attempt Mt. Everest. You struggle upward and end whenever and wherever you grow weary. If you do make it to the top to see the view, it is amazing; but most people will die trying. Love's dual nature . . .

Example 2:

A democratic government is like a boarding school. The lawmakers and public officials take the role of housemasters or mistresses in keeping the house and in overseeing its day-to-day running while you go on with your personal endeavours. You pay your taxes just like you would pay the boarding school fees; otherwise, the services will cease to fully operate. Citizens are also called to vote much like parents would be invited in a meeting for consultations on key issues. If you fail to show up in such a referendum, then you forfeit your opportunity to be heard. The balancing system in a democratic government is such that . . .

4. Thought-provoking question

Sometimes, an idea becomes all the more powerful when you inject some intrigue or controversy into it. This is what you intend to do when you pose a thought-provoking question at the start of your essay. But as already discussed, make sure to provide a clear answer to your own question during your main discussion. Remember that a question is only used here in order to emphasise a point. It is not up for the markers to answer or think about.

Examples:

Would you break the law to keep your country safe?

What will you say at your parents' funeral?

Is doing something wrong acceptable if no one is harmed anyway?

If money cannot buy happiness, can you be truly happy even without money?

5. Powerful quotation

"I quote others only in order to better express myself," DeMontaigne once said. A properly placed quotation can have a powerful effect on your Writing Task. If used improperly, you will have inadvertently confirmed that you misunderstood the statement provided.

You can choose to use a quotation to support your position or to provide the opposite point of view. But remember: the quotation must parallel the theme of the writing task, and a quote must be written word for word. Markers will not be impressed if you misquote John F. Kennedy or The Constitution. If you only forgot the name of someone who is not well-known, you can get away with saying something like: "It has been said that..."

Don't forget that even with creative introductions, responding to the comments' theme is still the central objective. You may also still need to expound on the idea brought forward by the surprising fact, the dramatic anecdote, the analogy, the thought-provoking question or the powerful quotation that you used. Basically, all of the ingredients of the logical introduction must remain while you add the extra creativity using the latter methods. Finally, the introductory paragraph must also be concluded by a strong thesis statement.

Here is an example of an introduction, which employs a dramatic anecdote in response to our previous quotes on parents:

My mother and I never really got along. I think it started when I was about five. My mother was suffering from palpitations and she kept telling me that my misbehaviours would aggravate her condition. Whenever she saw me, she noticed something wrong with what I wore or with what I was doing. She never told me she loved me, and she never hugged or kissed me - and to think that I was an only child. Surprisingly, the events following my mother's death would prove that par-

ents do need to distance themselves from their children if it means teaching them to be emotionally resilient and to live responsibly.

The next sample introduction uses one of the interesting historical facts that we featured earlier. It is a response to the following comments:

* * * * *

Comment 1

A people which is able to say everything becomes able to do everything.

Napoleon Bonaparte

* * * * *

Comment 2

Freedom of Speech is ever the Symptom, as well as the Effect of a good Government.

Cato's Letters

* * * * *

Comment 3

To have a right to speak about something is not the same as to be in the right mind and position in saying it.

* * * * *

Comment 4

Free speech includes the right to not speak.

Jimmy Wales

* * * * *

Comment 5

Freedom of speech is a principal pillar of a free government.

Benjamin Franklin

In 16th century England, an otherwise loyal subject of Henry VIII uttered, "I like not the proceedings of this realm". For this, he was imprisoned. It is hard to imagine a time when people can be put to death for speaking their minds. Yet history has taught us that despite adverse consequences, free speech proves to be one of the most powerful indicators of democracy and a vehicle of positive change. Therefore, for a country like Australia to be considered a truly free society, it must amend its constitutional declaration of rights to include free speech or the freedom to express one's opinion publicly without fear of censorship or punishment.

If you want to practice formulating your own initial paragraph in response to a given set of comments, you can jump to the end of this chapter (Section 4.11) to find the Section II practice worksheet for writing an introduction.

4.2.3 Supporting Your Thesis

After you have established your view on the overall idea of the various comments, your next task is to provide reasons why you are choosing a particular stand (thesis). Each reason must be discussed in one paragraph and supported by an evidential example.

Consider the markers to be educated yet skeptically, neutral readers. They may not be hostile to your point of view. They may not also agree with all your assumptions and conclusions; but they certainly need to be convinced that your claim has logical bases. You must be able to show them that you can very well defend your views in an intelligent and systematic manner.

Hence the primary purpose of using examples is to strengthen your point. Do not enumerate an aimless list of events and all sorts of examples just to interpret a quote or define the theme. Every assertion you make in the essay must be substantiated, placed in concrete scenarios and logically argued in defence of your main thesis. **The key is in sifting the strongest and most relevant supporting examples.**

● Qualities of Effective Examples

The following is a list of factors to consider when choosing which examples to use in your supporting arguments.

1. Relevance

Everything you include in your essay should be about backing up the thesis statement. Stay on track. Always keep that thesis statement in mind when you discuss your examples. In addition, remember that whatever points you make in the body of your essay are meant to be synthesised in the concluding paragraph. If you discuss a number of unrelated ideas, this will result in a conclusion which is disorganised or characterised by redundant statements.

2. Balance

The evidence you present must include a full range of opinions about the issue. Your argument must not only be convincing but must also be well-rounded. Choose the strongest possible refutation to your thesis. However, do not say outright how the opposing views are wrong. Rather, examine one or two counterpoints and explain why you disagree with them. It could be because those views are biased or outdated. Be firm but maintain tact.

When done properly, including a counterargument gives your paper credibility. It means that you have thoroughly considered all possible assertions about the subject before arriving at an informed decision. It may seem counter-intuitive to detail arguments in refutation of your thesis; however, there exists sound reason to do so. Inclusion of an antithesis demonstrates critical thinking; it shows that you have thought about the weaknesses of your thesis, and it then allows you to defend your thesis in a new context. It is not enough to state your thesis and supporting examples, nor is it enough to simply discuss the "for" and "against" of your argument – the best essays will address one or more arguments in support of the thesis, an argument supporting the antithesis and then also address the shortcomings of this antithesis.

3. Accuracy

If necessary, cite data that are accurate and up-to-date. Include your sources. These will make your claims all the more real and valid.

● Different Types of Supporting Examples

There are several types of examples that you can use to build your argument, but it is important to understand how you can use them in conjunction with the three levels of appeals in reasoning:

Logos - is an appeal to the reader's mind and sense of reason because it employs factual and quantifiable evidence. Examples are drawn from research and wide reading hence they are predominantly objective. They become even more convincing when interpreted in the light of your thesis. This is the most common appeal used in argumentative essays.

The following are forms of factual evidence:

> **Real examples** drawn from history or current events

> **Statistics** such as those cited in surveys and case studies

> **Published research** from reputable journals and books

> **News Report**

Ethos - makes use of the writer's credibility or 'ethical appeal'. For example, if the theme speaks about environmental issues and you happen to have experience working in a climate change organisation, you might want to mention it in your essay. Just make sure that it is highly relevant in your discussion.

A usual form of evidence used in this level of appeal is an expert testimony:

> **Expert testimony** or opinion coming from a reputable source in a specialised field

In this case, the quality of evidence is just as important as the credibility of the source. Would you believe information cited in The Economist rather than from a student newsletter?

Ethos can also be achieved through the use of an authoritative tone, as well as sophisticated language.

Pathos - appeals to the reader's emotions and imagination. One of the most effective means to convey pathos is through a narrative in which the reader can sympathise and even identify with the writer's point of view. It should be evident by now that an argument can take the form of a narrative or a reflective essay if your main objective is to prove a point. Pathos, when appropriately used in conjunction with ethos, can be quite powerful.

> **Narrative** drawn from first-hand experience

Take note that a personal example is only material in an argumentative piece if it is able to illustrate the main assertion that you want to make. Moreover, this type of justification would be ideal to use when more objective and more logical sources of evidence are not available. In this instance, the validity of an argument cannot be easily questioned because it is based on a "lived experience". Further, a personal narrative must be emotionally, psychologically or spiritually poignant.

● Forming Opinions

The importance of reading a wide range of topics cannot be stressed enough. Your choice of reading materials should include opinion articles from reputable newspapers and magazines, books on political theories and even philosophical essays. However, do not just take note of possible supporting examples, which you can get from these sources. Aside from reading for the purpose of exposing yourself to different issues and concepts, you also need to develop the habit of forming your own judgement based on what the writers are saying. This second purpose is the essence of the Section II writing tasks.

Some successful candidates in the past reveal that they engage in journal writing as part of their Section II preparation. If you have the time to emulate this strategy, you can keep a notebook where you can write out your thoughts about certain events, debates, and other writer's opinions on current issues. Do you agree with them? Why or why not? What do these issues mean to you? How do these issues affect you or members in your community?

4.2.4 Organisation and Structure

Keeping a logical organisation of your thoughts is another important element in building an argument. It allows the marker to have a clear vision of your reasoning process. Moreover, an orderly, sound explanation of each argued point adds weight to your claims.

It is also essential to keep in mind that Section II is a timed writing test. Following a prepared format for your writing tasks will save you time in planning what to do. Instead, you can just focus on developing quality content and still maintain coherence throughout the piece. We will discuss this further in the next sections.

Of course, you have to practice using an essay template as many times as you can prior to the actual sitting. The earlier you practice using a certain template, the better chance for you to get so used to writing in an organised manner such that you would become confident enough to experiment injecting your own style.

Nevertheless, do not forget that **structure precedes style**. A reader will be less likely to appreciate a stylish but disorganised essay. One idea must flow smoothly to the next. You have to be able to indicate properly if you are about to shift your line of argument or extend it with a detailed discussion.

There are "transitional cues" that you can use depending on your purpose in the different paragraphs. The following usually apply, although they are not limited to the first paragraph and its supporting paragraphs:

To place what you just said in a particular context: in this connection, in relation to, in this perspective

To give an example or an illustration: for example, for instance, in this case, to illustrate, as an illustration, take the case of, to take another example, namely, that is, as shown by, as illustrated by, as expressed by

To offer a similar point: similarly, in other words, likewise, in a similar manner, like, in the same way

The following are commonly found in the paragraph that offers a counterargument:

UNDERSTANDING THE GAMSAT

To show contrast: however, nevertheless, rather, whereas, on the other hand, on the contrary, but, yet, although, conversely, meanwhile, in contrast, otherwise, one may object that . . .

To compare: by comparison, compared to, balanced against, vis a vis, alternatively

The next transitional cues are mostly used towards the concluding paragraphs:

To refer back to an earlier point: as I have said, in brief, as I have noted, as indicated earlier, as has been noted

To express a resolution: granted, naturally, of course, in any case

To prove your point: for the same reason, obviously, evidently, indeed, in fact

To show cause and effect: as a result, consequently, hence, therefore, due to, for this reason

To conclude: on the whole, to sum up, to conclude, in conclusion, as I have shown, as I have said

The next list of transitional cues are used in any part of an essay as deemed necessary:

To add something: further, furthermore, equally important, moreover, in addition, not only . . . but also

To introduce a new idea: furthermore, moreover, in addition

To emphasise an idea: indeed, definitely, extremely, undeniably, absolutely, obviously, surprisingly, without a doubt, certainly

The last paragraph is your last shot at convincing the markers that your essay deserves a high score. Summarise the major points discussed in the preceding paragraphs so that your ideas follow a logical conclusion. Never introduce any new ideas or another example. Instead, address any questions posed in the essay. Then restate your thesis using different words and in the light of the various arguments presented.

The next two sections will now focus on the format of the two writing tasks (A and B).

4.2.5 Focussing on Task A

Let "A" be Argumentative!

In the current GAMSAT, there is no strict imposition coming from ACER that candidates should adhere to a certain style. However, the argumentative (thesis – antithesis – resolution) or discursive (pro – con – resolution) formats prove to be the most effective in dealing with socio-cultural topics.

GAMSAT-Prep.com
THE GOLD STANDARD

Moreover, as a candidate seeking admission to a medical education (a science-based degree!), you should be able to display an ability to be objective in weighing the pros and cons of various arguments.

An argumentative essay has three tasks. These tasks are summarised below:

Gold Standard Structure for Writing Test A

1. **Thesis:** the first paragraph should provide an explanation or an interpretation of the theme. You may also include one or two quotations that you have chosen, followed by an expression of your position on the point of issue. The second paragraph (and sometimes a 3rd) provides an example, real or hypothetical, that supports your thesis.

2. **Antithesis:** the next paragraph or paragraphs evaluate opposing views to the one presented in the Thesis.

3. **Synthesis:** the final paragraph concludes with a way for the conflict between the viewpoint expressed in the Thesis and the one presented in the Antithesis to be reconciled.

These three tasks should keep you quite busy for approximately 30 minutes that you have to write the essay. The tasks, however, once you are familiar with them, will help you by structuring your essay automatically.

Alternatively, you can follow a detailed outline, which can serve as either a Writing Task A template or a checklist to make sure that the essay meets all the requirements. In any case, having a framework of presentation allows you to actually think of the substance as the form has already been prepared.

Gold Standard Detailed Structure (Test A)

Paragraph 1: Open with a thesis statement.

a. Paraphrase the comment you are responding to. You can state it as a regular statement or you may use a creative device.

b. Explain what the comment means to you in light of the overall theme.

c. State your agreement or disagreement with this main idea. This is your expression of the thesis statement.

Paragraph 2: Provide support for your thesis.

a. Give the reason why you agree or disagree with the comments.

b. Explain what your argument is and provide an example or examples to support them.

c. Explain how the examples relate to the arguments.

Paragraph 3: Discuss an antithesis to your main idea.

a. Cite the strongest argument against your main idea.

b. Discuss it so that you can show the marker that you are capable of 'reasoning' through objections and observations that may put your arguments in jeopardy.

c. Provide an illustration of the counter-argument.

Paragraph 4: Explain why you stay firm with your thesis.

a. Demolish the antithesis by showing its weaknesses against your arguments in support of the thesis.

b. Alternatively, you can cite situations in which your thesis best applies and in which instances the antithesis can be appreciated.

Paragraph 5: Conclude your essay.

a. Tie up all the ideas and present it for the consideration of the reader.

b. You may propose a plan of action or a course of action so that the reader can act upon your ideas.

c. You can also invite the reader to agree with you.

You may also want to use Section II Practice Worksheet III (Task A Template) found in Section 4.11 as a guide every time you practice writing your Task A responses.

Why not the expository format?

The Written Communication section assesses your thinking process in forming your views on the given themes. An expository essay simply explains an idea, a theme or an issue. Explanations may show your vast knowledge on a subject but not necessarily your ability to form judgments.

An argumentative or discursive essay, on the other hand, involves the process of establishing a claim (your thesis statement) and then proving it with the use of logical reasoning, examples, and research.

The following are two sample responses to the quotations on justice. The sample responses were both written by students within the prescribed time limit. Just as an additional exercise, after reading the instructions and quotations, you should try completing an essay in 30 minutes prior to reviewing the two sample responses.

Note: There does not exist one essay format that everyone should use. We are presenting formats that would optimise the score of most candidates.

Confidence and skill level may lead you to apply your own approach with or without creativity. The key is to practice your chosen approach and improve with time.

Writing Task A

Read the following statements and write a response to any one or more of the ideas presented.

Your essay will be evaluated on the value of your thoughts on the theme, logical organisation of content and effective articulation of your key points.

* * * * *

Comment 1

    Justice is justly represented blind, because she sees no difference in the parties concerned.

William Penn

* * * * *

Comment 2

    Justice cannot be for one side alone, but must be for both.

Eleanor Roosevelt

* * * * *

Comment 3

    It is better that ten guilty persons escape than one innocent suffer.

William Blackstone

* * * * *

Comment 4

    It is more important that innocence be protected than it is that guilt be punished, for guilt and crimes are so frequent in this world that they cannot all be punished.

John Adams

* * * * *

Comment 5

    Justice consists not in being neutral between right and wrong, but in finding out the right and upholding it, wherever found, against the wrong.

Theodore Roosevelt

Sample Response 1 (Discursive Essay)

The Net of Justice: Selective or Unselective?

Even if guilty men walk free, justice is done provided the innocent avoid punitive measures. This was the notion expressed by judge and author of the Commentaries on the Laws of England William Blackstone when he declared, "It is better that ten guilty persons escape than one innocent suffer." From this perspective one can define justice to be served only when the guilty are punished, and the innocent unaffected. While some proponents of Blackstone's view argue that this is the only way justice can be achieved, there are those who advocate that justice necessitates castigating some of the innocent. The following dialectic will urge that justice can only be achieved if the innocent remain unscathed in the pursuit of justice.

When the guilty and innocent fail to be differentiated, injustice occurs. It is reasonable to hold this view because the innocent are necessarily punished for crimes that they have not committed. If society does not discriminate between the guilty and the innocent, it either grants freedom to all or freedom to none, and it is clear that both situations fail to amount to justice. For example, the sexual abuse scandals in the Catholic Church over the last few decades have been cause for great communal debate. Initially the heinous crimes against children had been ignored by senior figures from within the church. At this point, justice was not affected upon the individual perpetrators, and this has primed the contemporary state. Today, it has become very difficult to prosecute the perpetrators of sexual abuse due to the amount of time that has passed. The result of this injustice and constant revelation of new scandal from the past has led to an undercurrent of hatred and anger for the Catholic Church that is perhaps unwarranted when one considers that only very few of their congregation actually committed crimes. This notion is also evident in the newly enacted laws restricting the associative activities of motorcycle clubs in Queensland. Though members may not be criminals themselves, they are treated as such due to their association with gangs labelled 'outlaws'. In these instances, one can see that the failure to sequester the guilty and the innocent can lead to great injustice as either the guilty are free, or the innocent are punished.

Conversely, there exists merit for countervailing arguments, especially given the complexity of the subject that is justice. Some argue that in some instances it is necessary to prosecute both the guilty and the innocent in pursuit of justice. This notion might be exemplified in areas such as sport where athletes are forced to endure mandatory drug testing at any hour of the day or night. In this situation, all are considered guilty before they have even laid step onto their respective sporting arenas. Though this view is understandable, the example of drugs in sport is more an anomaly than a rule, and the damages to the innocent are rather insignificant when the higher purpose is considered. The invalidity of this greater argument becomes apparent when one applies this rule to subjects such as the mandatory detention of asylum seekers. All asylum seekers whether legitimate or fraudulent are processed through the same means: off shore, within a dangerous penitentiary and with a long wait. Asylum seekers legitimately seeking refuge from the flames and bullets of their homelands find no sanctuary due to these inappropriate processes and the plight of those afflicted by this unjust process exemplifies the shortcoming inherent in the notion that it is acceptable to punish the innocent in the pursuit of the guilty.

Thus, justice can only be achieved when the guilty are differentiated and prosecuted. When this fails to occur, so does justice as exhibited by the current plight of the Catholic Church and Queensland motorcycle clubs. Though there are anomalous instances where it may be acceptable to net the innocent with the guilty, this rule usually applies to instances where the imposition is insignificant and is not applicable across greater society. Therefore, it is difficult to find difference with Blackstone's view.

Sample Response 2 (Persuasive Essay)

The Justice System

Justice depends upon fallible humans applying imperfect laws, thus, justice is imperfect. But without the justice system, without the laws and the rules, society will break down and anarchy will reign.

We call it a "system" because dispensing justice involves several steps, several procedures and several people. There are legislators who make laws that define what behaviours are deemed to be criminal acts. There are police officers who enforce these criminal laws and apprehend persons thought to be violating the law. Then there are prosecutors who weigh the availability of evidence as well as the admissibility of the evidence gathered by the police. The prosecutors decide if there is enough evidence to obtain a conviction and file indictments based on the evidence gathered. The accused are afforded the right to retain their own lawyer so that they can put up a defence. The accused are given their day in court to face their accusers. The judge decides what pieces of evidence can be considered by the court or by the jury. The jury decides if the evidence presented gives them a moral certainty that a crime was indeed committed by the person accused of it.

Justice is not simple. There are concepts such as "innocent until proven guilty" and the "right against self-incrimination" that ensure that each accused person is afforded due process of law before he is found guilty. Ultimately, justice is practical: is there enough evidence to prove that a crime has been committed and that the accused committed the crime? This is all that should matter.

Of course, it is also true that when the accused is poor, he has not the resources to hire a lawyer of his choice. He usually is assigned a lawyer by the court. Because he is poor, he does not have money to ensure that he obtains all the evidence and all the expert testimony necessary to present a credible defence. When the accused is rich, he has all the resources to hire the best lawyers, and he has the money to challenge every piece of evidence presented by the prosecution.

Justice under the law is not true justice. It is judicial justice. It is not unheard of that a person who truly committed a crime has been acquitted because there was no sufficient evidence to convict him beyond reasonable doubt. It is not unheard of either that a person who has not committed a crime has been found guilty of having committed one. Justice often boils down to the impression made on the jury. It is the perception of the jury that matters whether or not a person will be found guilty or not guilty.

A jury consists of ordinary men and women who swear to hear evidence and evaluate it according to set rules and to determine if the evidence presented is enough to find the accused guilty. If any member of the jury has any mental reservation at all, then there can be no conviction. This is the rule of reasonable doubt. If any member of the jury has any doubt as to the probable guilt of the accused, then, the accused will have to be acquitted.

Justice is lofty not in the result but in the effort with which we ensure that it is carried out. Yes, occasionally, a guilty man may be acquitted and yes, an innocent man may be convicted. This does not mean that there is no justice. Justice cannot always be done, but justice must be served by going through the process of the justice system even if the end result does not suit everybody's sense of justice.

4.2.6 Focussing on Task B

Let "B" be Bersonal? OK, it does not exactly spell "personal" but it's close enough! The important point is to understand that you may attempt a different approach in the second writing task. But then again, nothing stops you from utilising the argumentative style in Task B.

Why so different?

Consider some of the criticisms aimed at young doctors: impressive "book knowledge" and technical ability but lacking skills in listening, communicating and empathising. Is it a fact that younger people are less empathetic because of a lack of experience? Can interpersonal skills - including empathy - be the focus of a section of a standardised exam? How does one evaluate empathy?

Ideas and imagination

They need to know whether you can imagine someone else's perspective. This does not mean that you need to write a creative story using the imagination of Isaac Asimov! It simply means that you have to be able to visualise and explain how other people may be feeling and experiencing life; thus the personal-interpersonal and social theme.

Introspection and Reasoning

The logical presentation of your views on the theme (i.e. your reasoning process) will still be part of the marking criteria in Task B. You can also demonstrate empathy using the discursive format. On the other hand, you may find that using pathos through personal reflection would be more effective in supporting your thesis.

A personal reflection is a narrative about a remarkable event in your life. It can be your own experience or one that involved a close friend or a family member. It must be recounted with enough details in order to help the readers understand where your perspectives are coming from. However, it should neither read like a confession nor a diary. Rather, it should serve as an example from which you can extract life-lessons that are germane to the theme.

Unlike a pure narrative or a creative non-fiction, you have to be explicit in your realisations, perceptions, and opinions. This personal example is your proof, taken from first-hand experience, to validate a point that you are trying to make. In addition, it should highlight a shift in perspectives or a fresh insight into a prevalent interpersonal-social problem such as bullying, domestic violence, discrimination and the likes.

UNDERSTANDING THE GAMSAT

Extending your personal realisations to a social issue exhibits another aspect of reasoning ability: the ability to be mentally resilient. When you can learn from an experience, take a personal truth and apply it to a novel situation, you are showing that you can continue to educate yourself outside formal teaching, adapt ideas and make them work under different circumstances.

The Personal and Social Relevance

When discussing the social issue part in your essay, it might help to imagine as if you are talking to a patient or a relative of a patient who is in a challenging condition. The person may be feeling frustrated, discriminated, or starting to lose self-esteem because of a debilitating disease. In this case, you would like to share your story as a possible source of inspiration.

The conversation can go something like "I (or my friend) once was. . . But I came to realise that . . . so then I decided to . . . and now I feel that (state a possible solution based on your personal triumph). . ." Of course this is just one strategy. An alternative would be to pick a quote from the given comments that easily pose a personal-social significance. This way, both themes can be interwoven in a single thread of discussion.

The organisation of the Task B essay can be summarised as follows:

Gold Standard Structure for Writing Test B

1. **Introduction:** the first paragraph should acquaint the reader with the topic. In addition, it should give the markers a glimpse of what to expect from the body of your text, which you can do by clearly stating your specific assertion and point of view. Make sure your introduction is written in an active tone, with strong verbs and powerful statements.

2. **The body:** the second paragraph (and sometimes a 3rd and/or 4th) should focus on one main idea that supports your assertions in the Introduction. Dissect that main idea into three distinct parts: the main assertion, a specific supporting example or examples, and a summary (each could be one paragraph depending on how much you can write effectively in the limited time).

3. **Conclusion:** the last paragraph summarises the main point(s), reasserts your view and ends the essay with impact. This will be the last thing markers will get from your essay, so make sure it ties everything together succinctly as well as creates a lasting impression in their mind.

==Remember to write your Task B with feeling==.

The following is a more detailed outline in writing a personal reflection:

Gold Standard Detailed Structure (Test B)

Paragraph 1: Begin with a thesis statement.

a. Paraphrase the comments. Explain what they mean to you in light of the overall theme.

b. State whether you agree or disagree with the main idea in the comments and why.

c. Briefly discuss one argument that supports your stance. This is the transitional sentence for you to introduce your narrative. Your personal experience of an event or a condition will be your main argument.

Paragraph 2: Begin the narrative.

a. This is your personal illustration thus it must be written in your own point of view (avoid the third person).

b. It must be a story of something that happened to you or to someone very close to you and which you experienced vicarious pain or joy, stress, discomfort or fear.

c. You must choose an event that is rich with emotion and one that is pivotal in your life.

Note: Sometimes, the narrative can take several paragraphs.

Paragraph 3: Reflect upon the narrative you just described.

a. You must say what you learned from the narrative or experience.

b. Describe how you felt, how you thought and what made you change your mind or your perspective.

c. There must be a 'before-and-after' description of your state of mind and state of heart.

Paragraph 4: Apply the reflection or life-lesson you learned.

a. Find a problem that is relevant to the problem you described in your narrative.

b. The problem must be something that affects a large segment of society.

c. Your life-lesson can be an insight you can share with those people who may be similarly situated; it could be a source of inspiration or a challenge for them.

Section II Practice Worksheet IV found in Section 4.11 corresponds to a Task B Template. You can use it as a guide when attempting your Task B essays. We have placed two sample responses to the quotations on parenting or parents' love. They were both written within the prescribed time limit. Consider attempting the 30-minute essay before reviewing the sample responses.

Writing Task B

Read the following statements and write a response to any one or more of the ideas presented.

Your essay will be evaluated on the value of your thoughts on the theme, logical organisation of content and effective articulation of your key points.

* * * * *

Comment 1

Parents are always more ambitious for their children than they are for themselves.

* * * * *

Comment 2

We never know the love of a parent till we become parents ourselves.

Henry Ward Beecher

* * * * *

Comment 3

Parents can only give good advice or put them on the right paths, but the final forming of a person's character lies in their own hands.

Anne Frank

* * * * *

Comment 4

Some mothers are kissing mothers and some are scolding mothers, but it is love just the same, and most mothers kiss and scold together.

Pearl S. Buck

* * * * *

Comment 5

A father's goodness is higher than the mountain, a mother's goodness deeper than the sea.

Japanese Proverb

Sample Response 1 (Reflective Essay)

Every time I saw my father, I saw disappointment in his eyes. And why should he not be disappointed? He spent for my education through grade school, high school, university and post graduate studies in law. I was a lawyer and I left my law practice to tend to my sick son. It was once said that "parents are always more ambitious for their children than they are for themselves." However, I believe that the way I live my life, raise my own family and define success is still up to me.

My son developed jaundice on the second day of his life because there was bile sludge in his bile duct. He needed surgery and after the successful surgery, he needed follow-up. I was at the peak of my career, but I made the difficult decision to concentrate on nursing my son back to health instead of going to court everyday and leaving my sick son in the care of strangers.

I was a full-time and hands-on kind of mother. I breastfed the baby, changed him, cleaned him, played with him and rocked him to sleep. I read to him, sang to him and talked to him. We were inseparable. I was with him to every doctor's appointment. I held him and comforted him through every inoculation and every blood test. This was militant mother's love – the kind that is untiring in promoting and ensuring the health and well-being of her child.

I did this 24/7. I wanted to go back to work when he was about a year old but I found myself pregnant with my second child. I thought to myself that it was unfair to mother my son militantly and then leave my daughter to be raised by strangers. I did it all over again. Instead of having one child to care for, I had two. I did it every day for years that it became second nature to think of my children first before thinking of myself.

My own mother told me that I was cruising for a major disappointment because I was pouring myself into my children. She said that if I poured my entire being into my children, imprinting into them my very person, I would exhaust myself and then there would be no strength left for me. My mother said that someday, these children I had loved so intensely will grow up and leave and then, where would I be? I'd be left empty with no sense of achievement that I can proudly share with my own family.

I did not say a word when my mother said that. I did not argue with her. It made me understand her – that is why my mother was always stand-offish. All the while I was growing up, I felt that she was keeping something back from me, pulling from me each time we could be close. I thought she didn't really like me. Now I know. She loved me, but she just couldn't pour herself into me because she was afraid I would leave her one day. The result was that I had gotten accustomed to turn to myself for comfort and affection because I did not get sufficient comfort, attention or affection from my mother. I grew up without her, and I learned to fend for myself without her. Now that she is old, she reaches out to me, she wants us to hang out but there is just no love or affection between us - there is just nothing there on which to build a meaningful relationship upon.

My mother may be right – now that my kids are grown up, they go to school on their own, they go out with friends more often, and I'm left on my own again. I feel like my world is shaking – I am beginning to feel orphaned and naked. My children were like leaves on my tree and flowers on my bush. When they leave, I would be purposeless and meaningless. My life would be without prettiness because I think that my children made my life pretty. I like having them around, and I think they like having me around, too. They tell me things they wouldn't tell others. They ask me things they do not dare ask others. When they leave my nest, my nest will be empty.

So what should I do then? I've already done it – I got myself a dog. Dogs cannot take the place of my children, but they do fill the space and the hours when my kids are away. The dogs are there so that I'd have something to keep me occupied while I wait for my kids to come home. They really can't stay away too long – they are sure they will get love and attention here from me. I realise that I didn't take care of my children because they were mine and I was their mother. I took care of my children because that is who I am – I am a person who derives pleasure and meaning from taking care of others. In taking care of them, I was effectively actualising myself.

Mothering was what I was meant to do, this was what I was meant to be – I am a mother. And a mother's job is to raise kids so strong that they can survive without her. My mother and I just went about raising our kids in different ways: I would like to think that we both raised kids so strong they can survive without us. The only difference is, my kids would rather not survive without me. I have made their lives pretty just as they made mine pretty. That is the only difference.

Sample Response 2 (Discursive Essay)

Parenting As a Social Responsibility

Would you starve your own daughter until she masters a very difficult lesson? This is what American lawyer, book author, and Yale Law School professor Amy Chua almost did to her younger daughter. In her book **Battle Hymn of the Tiger Mother**, Amy Chua confesses having a highly authoritarian parenting style. In one extreme situation, she did not allow her daughter, Lulu, to get up - not even for water or for bathroom breaks - until Lulu perfected playing a difficult piano piece. Professor Chua justifies her methods, claiming it is all about believing in your child more than they believe in themselves and making them realise their own potentials.

On the other hand, we've also heard of parents adopting a more positive and affectionate child-rearing style and advocates the same aspirations that Professor Chua hopes to achieve. Certainly, parents often have to use "carrot and stick" in order to instill discipline and values in a child. In any case, they are driven by one common reason: they love their children hence they will do whatever it takes to turn them into better and successful individuals. However, I do not agree that parenting should just be about developing your child's full potential and securing his or her bright future. Parenting should also be about raising children who will eventually become positive contributions to society.

Open communication and reasoning - explaining to a child the reasons why he or she is being pushed to the limits and at times punished - are quite important in developing individuals who are not merely focussed on self-improvement but also on the welfare and the rights of others. An example of this inductive approach is when a child - let's name him Andy - is found taking his classmate Ben's lunch without permission and worse, he does not own up to the misdemeanour. As his punishment, Andy is not allowed to watch TV and play video games for a month. But his parents also discuss crucial questions with him ranging from "How could have Ben possibly felt when he didn't have anything to eat during lunch?" to "How would your classmates and teachers feel now that they have someone in class whom they can no longer trust?"

Of course, the next time Andy feels like committing a similar misconduct, he would not only remember the punishment but also the uncomfortable thoughts and feelings attributed to the act: "I'd feel bad if someone did that to me. . . I don't want to lose their trust again. . . Our family does not take what's not ours." Hence Andy would discourage himself from misbehaving again. The benefits of inductive discipline for developing pro-social behaviour is further supported by a study conducted by Krevans and Gibbs in 1996. Their case study shows that parents who explain to their children the reasons and consequences of bad behaviour tend to develop empathy early in a child. These children also exhibit more self-control, moral reasoning, and consideration of how others feel.

The same approach can be employed when encouraging a child to excel in a skill. Instead of using pressure and threats, the parent draws from positive reinforcement and reasoning: "If you practiced real hard today, you'll be able to perfect your piano piece very shortly. We'll have time to go to the beach this weekend, and you'll still be all set for a superb performance next week! Everyone's happy." Or better yet, a socially responsible parent would be able to reinforce his or her teenager's decision to take up a health-related course that will help treat a disabled sibling and others with the same affliction.

Nonetheless, some child psychologists believe that moral reasoning may not always work with children who either have stronger and fearless temperament or too weak and fearful. Children who take on an adventurous outlook on life will take risks in repeating their offences. In this case, discipline may take more than explanations and simple punishment. Even emotional support may have to be in the form of firm rules and ultimatums. This is probably what drove Amy Chua to resort to extreme measures with her daughter, Lulu, who she described as a "real fireball".

Another danger of moralising and reasoning especially to a young child is when an act of punishment is not properly processed. Parents are by no means developmental experts and may use words and situations that are not age-appropriate. For example, a five-year-old girl caught taking her friend's favourite toy without permission may be made to think of the consequences of stealing. The concept of stealing may not even be fully clear at this age. This could result to confusion and unwarranted guilt on the part of the child.

Despite these contrary opinions on inductive parenting, open communication remains an effective tool in shaping socially and morally responsible children - and families. Even Amy Chua admits that her need to reach out to her daughter Lulu, who was rebelling at the time, served as the impetus to her (in)famous book. Showing the manuscript of her book to her husband and her daughters was cathartic to their family and saved their relationships. In the same manner, a parent who constantly talks and reasons with his or her child would know the most appropriate types of punishment and motivation to carry out. Hence, the argument against over-moralising would be more of a few exceptions than the rule.

In the end, it all boils down to a parent's sense of purpose. If one is to merely mould a self-actualised individual and overlook the social responsibility that comes with raising a child, then any parenting method would do as long as the results are achieved. On the other hand, if one is to inculcate moral and social sensibility in a child, then open communication and moral reasoning should be a significant component of a family. The hope is that, as a child grows to adulthood, and as the presence of an authority figure correspondingly fades, he or she will develop a sense of internal moral compass to reason his or her way through life's dilemmas rather than be on the lookout for any external promise of reward or threat of punishment.

Notes on Writing Task B Sample Response #2

The second essay reflects upon a personal issue that the writer feels strongly about. Using the third person (instead of the first person point of view) does not diminish the strong personal conviction of the writer that underlies each and every single idea expressed. While the essay is about child rearing, it cannot be overlooked that the author is actually formulating an opinion on child discipline based upon strongly-held personal beliefs which the author then measures up against the standards of psychological theories. It is implied that the author is actually reacting to the extreme form of child rearing that s/he not only heard about or read about, the author may actually be reacting to the insensitive and inattentive parenting that he or she witnesses all around.

The essay also works (despite its argumentative stance) because it highlights the social responsibility of parenting. That is to say, the author's ideas on how children should be raised is extrapolated to the way we, as a society, is equipping the next generation to learn discernment and circumspection in choosing how we behave and how we make decisions. This is (obliquely) a commentary on a social issue that confronts us: undisciplined children who grow up to be lawless adults; the lack of standards of behaviour that allow our children to conclude that they can do whatever they wish without thought of consequences.

Over all, this essay works because it is an educated opinion that is logically presented and organised. The control of language is superb even if there are a few grammatical errors. It has a clear message, and it conveys that message quite forcefully. It paints a good picture for the marker to take away after reading the essay. It shows a picture of us as a society, and it lays the accountability for our failure, as parents, to ensure reason and reasonableness in our children. The examples may not be gleaned from the writer's actual life experiences for it to be potent but because the examples are so commonplace, we see it every day; and therefore, readers can relate to the examples.

4.2.7 Timing

Timing skills should be developed during the early stages of your Section II preparation. Be careful not to get too engrossed in developing your great ideas that you might neglect containing those thoughts within a limited time. You need to be able to get used to writing two legibly handwritten and well-organised essays on two different themes within 60 minutes.

Getting used to writing within the time limit will teach you to include only the most pertinent and strongest arguments in your essays. Also, please note that several past candidates report being given full 60 minutes to complete the two writing tasks - that is, you can spend 20 minutes on Task A while 40 minutes on Task B.

Indeed, some students can generate ideas easier on issues involving socio-cultural concerns and can thus finish Task A in less than 30 minutes. Others can be quite persuasive using a narrative. Still, others are more efficient discussing a well-balanced presentation of pros and cons. You will learn which essay format or style will be the easiest for you to control if you have practiced writing in a timed setting way beforehand.

Speed Writing

Remember that GAMSAT is a paper-based exam, which means that your Section II responses will be written by hand. Even if you have a clear penmanship, there are still other factors that can affect its readability. Time pressure tends to bring about anxiety, causing you to constantly misspell and erase several words. This can make your paper look untidy and some parts difficult to read. If you are used to typing, writing fast by hand might be challenging as well and can even affect your thinking process.

It is therefore important that you practice writing by hand regularly within a maximum of 30 minutes per task. Just like any skill, timed writing can be done in small stages. The trick is to do it consistently.

At first, do not worry about whether or not you'll be able to come up with an excellent piece. Just get yourself used to thinking spontaneously and then wrapping up your main points within the limited time. To help keep your thoughts organised, use the practice worksheets found in the last section of this chapter.

Next, review your writing and identify your weaknesses. Analyse what could be the causes. Is it a lack of exposure to current news? Could it be because you are uncomfortable with the format? Perhaps, you have problems arranging your ideas. It might also help to have someone check if your handwriting is readable enough.

GAMSAT-Prep.com
THE GOLD STANDARD

Once you know what your weaknesses are, you can address them one at a time. Continue to practice writing essays on a regular basis but aim to improve at least one aspect for every attempt.

Finally, if you still have ample time for preparation, practice, practice, and practice to a point when you can almost tell how many minutes have elapsed as you get to Paragraph 1, to Paragraph 2, and so forth. **Most candidates arrive to sit the test having completed around 10-20 essays.** While this may sound significant, there is much to be gained by writing and rewriting up to fifty essays. By doing so, you will arrive with a much greater body of knowledge and a strong faith in your structures.

4.2.8 The Five Minute, Five Step Plan

Another important component of your Section II strategy, which is quite related to timing, is pre-planning. We know that while it is possible to write a structured, complete essay in 30 minutes, this requires practice for most students. This is because normally, an essay would be written over a considerable period of time. You would think about your essay, plan what you would write, actually write, correct and polish your essay, and perhaps rewrite sections.

However, a timed essay is not normal. It is a situation where your thoughts have to be ordered, structured and organised straight out of your head! You have to plan what you will write quickly and efficiently. This is what the Five Minute, Five Step Plan is all about. **The objective is for you to take 5 minutes to prepare and 5 steps to finish the essay.**

Step 1: Read the instructions and the stimulus material.

This may seem obvious, but you would be surprised by the number of students who misread or misinterpret what is expected of them. Carefully read the quotations in both Writing Task A and Writing Task B during the 5-minute reading time given at the start of this section.

Since you are not yet allowed to do any writing at this time, you can just mentally note keywords from the quotations. Then look at the relationships of each idea in the different comments. Actively ask yourself the following questions: How does this particular idea relate to the other ideas? Do they contradict or support each other? If they contradict each other, what is the debatable issue that must be addressed? If they all agree with each other, what is the unifying theme that ties them all together? Earlier, we mentioned having completed as many essays as possible. By doing so, you will increase your chances of being able to use material from one of your practice essays.

UNDERSTANDING THE GAMSAT

Consider the following quotations and create an essay in response to one or more of them.

Example of a quotation that could be chosen from stimulus material in Writing Task A:

The government is best that governs least.

Henry David Thoreau

Now, in your mind, you should be thinking of writing a comprehensive essay in which you accomplish the following objectives. Explain what you think the statement means. Describe a specific example in which the government's powers should be increased. Discuss the basis for increasing or decreasing the government's powers. The preceding outlines the structure of the 'classic' argumentative essay (section 4.2.5).

Step 2: Prewrite your Thesis (Task 1), Antithesis (Task 2) and Synthesis (Task 3).

Once the actual testing time starts, you should jot down notes in the margin of your test booklet or below the quotation (you will not be permitted "scrap" or "scratch" paper). Alternatively, a one-page notes section is provided in each booklet. You can write your rough outline for Task A on the notes page of the second booklet, and then for Task B on the first booklet. This way, you don't have to keep flipping the pages when you are composing your essay.

Generating ideas at this early stage will have the greatest impact on your final score.

Task 1: Usually, you will have to explain a statement which will not be simply factual or self-evident. For example, the statement, "The government is best which governs least," has to be explained and terms have to be defined. Make notes as the information comes to mind:

Ex.: Government: *-federal, state, provincial, municipal*

   -authority, power -a ruling body

   Governs: *- rules, delegates, guides*

   -creates laws

   -exerts control, authority

When it comes time to write (Step 4), you will formulate a statement which clearly addresses Task 1: "Explain what you think the statement means ." You should choose one clear definition from amongst the possibilities. You may also want to use an example to further illustrate the point of view you are presenting:

The ideal ruling body would strive to maintain, at a minimum, its exertion of authority over the population. Clearly, a government representing the people should not have the right to indiscriminately curb the freedom of an individual. The consequence would be a contradiction of democratic principles. Thus a government should avoid extending its powers; rather, government should use its authority prudently.

There are many different interpretations and examples which can be used to explain what the statement means. One possibility is to suggest that 'big' government produces excessive 'red tape' or bureaucracy which eventually may lead to higher taxes and a greater deficit. Also consider using a quotation about government (e.g., from John F. Kennedy).

Another possibility would be to mention that 'big' government leads to too much power, and "absolute power corrupts absolutely." There are an endless number of possibilities. The key is to choose one line of thinking and present it in a clear manner. {Note how the structure and length of the sentences vary in the example.}

Task 2: Follow a similar approach for tasks two and three. Write down any points you may want to include in your essay which contradict the statement even if you completely agree with it. You should be able to see the other side. If you cannot think of something to challenge the statement, try to think what someone who actively disagrees with the statement would say.

Ex.: i> *Rights of one person begins where another person's rights end: government ensures that happens.*

 ii> *National crisis*

 iii> *War/draft*

Choose one specific example and elaborate. Take (iii) as a case in point. The writer may use World War II as a specific example. The fact that the government increased its powers by legislating that certain members of the population must go to war (= draft) could be explored. The war prevented the Nazi government from becoming an even greater destructive force and its reign of terror ended. Thus the government expanded its powers for the greater good.

Task 3: For the third task, look back at the ideas you wrote down to address the first two tasks. You should then be able to reconcile the two opposing views. Write down what you think is the key component of your answer to the third task. Remember that you are not expected to solve all the problems in the world. Simply try to find the best way you know to solve the dilemma outlined by the first two tasks. There are no right or wrong answers for this assignment. What is being graded is your reasoning and your ability to express your thoughts.

Ex.: i> *When the survival of the community is endangered*

 ii> *Government should govern for the benefit of its citizens*

Prewriting the tasks is not like writing a formal outline. It is simply a way to structure your ideas in order to enable you to write a well-organised essay in 30 minutes. While prewriting might seem like a waste of time, it is the key to helping you complete all three tasks in the time allowed.

Step 3: Organise your notes

Once you have completed the three tasks, you will want to organise and clarify your ideas. This will allow you to review your ideas before you write and to see how they fit together. You may want to remove some ideas and reformulate others. At this stage, you will decide in which order you will address the three tasks (normally, however, you will keep the order as Tasks 1, 2, 3, respectively). Once you have done this, you will be ready to write the essay. At this point, you will have spent five or six minutes prewriting the tasks. In doing so, you will have created a structure for your essay which will make writing it much easier.

Step 4: Write

When you write, pace yourself. This will be much easier as your notes will provide a framework to work with in writing. You will want to ensure you have a few (about five) minutes to review your masterpiece! Make sure that your essay flows. Use transition words and phrases between your paragraphs. Pay attention to your spelling, punctuation and grammar. Be sure to vary the structure and length of the sentences in your text.

Do not assume that the reader can read your mind! Be explicit in your presentation. Providing a specific, well-illustrated example can impress the marker. And finally, be sure to not digress from the theme of your essay.

Step 5: Proofread

Reread your text. You want to spend your last five minutes proofreading your essay. Look for and correct mistakes and ensure you followed the plan you established as you prewrote the tasks. At this point you want to simply polish your essay.

4.3 Building Your Vocabulary

Clarity of expression makes a GAMSAT Section II essay an easy read. On the other hand, it also helps to make an impression on the marker by interweaving words that will add a "wow" factor in your writing. Of course, you don't use "big words" just for the sake of it. You have to make sure that they make sense within the sentence's context. Simply using one or two of these words in your essay will elevate it above many others.

One way to improve or strengthen your vocabulary skills is to keep a "beautiful words" notebook. You can build your list by writing down a new word in this notebook every time you find a term that you feel would make your sentences sound more elegant in an essay. The following list is meant to help get you started. Consider making flashcards or an mp3 with the words you like most to help with repetition.

Accoutrement - *(noun)* additional clothing or equipment; accessories

> The Freedom of Information Act is the perfect **accoutrement** to the Bill of Rights.

Affectation - *(noun)* a display of behaviour or attitude that is artificial or pretentious but meant to impress others. This is different from affection which is a feeling of liking or caring for another person

> *The daughter-in-law held her mother-in-law's hand and touched it to her cheek: clearly an **affectation** intending to convey fondness for the old lady who held the family's purse.*

Allegory - *(noun)* the representation of abstract ideas or principles by characters, figures, or events in narrative, dramatic, or pictorial form

> *The book, Animal Farm, is an **allegory** of communism and the pitfalls of having a common identity.*

Altruism - *(noun)* a selfless commitment to the service of others

> ***Altruism** is a rare gift, exemplified by the likes of Mother Teresa and Princess Diana.*

Aphorism - *(noun)* a brief statement containing a general truth or opinion; an adage

> *He is the master of Shakespearean **aphorisms**.*

Apocryphal - *(adjective)* of doubtful authority or authenticity but widely made out to be the truth

> *Historians are always faced with the challenge of distinguishing authentic happenings from **apocryphal** stories.*

Arcane - *(adjective)* understood by a select few who have the knowledge or interest; mysterious; concealed

> *Only real poets can speak the **arcane** language of poetry.*

UNDERSTANDING THE GAMSAT

Bellwether - *(noun)* someone who leads the flock; a person or entity at the forefront of a trend, profession, industry or any other endeavour; trendsetter

> Our biology professor is a **bellwether** of practical science.

Bifurcate - *(verb)* to divide into two separate branches; forked

> The end of the road **bifurcates**, leading you into two different directions.

Caveat - *(noun)* a warning or word of caution; specific limits

> As comprehensive and eloquent as this policy is, there is still one **caveat**: it fails to mention where jurisdiction resides.

Chicanery - *(noun)* the use of tricks to deceive someone (usually to extract money from them)

> **Chicanery** made him rich and so will be his downfall.

Circumlocution - *(noun)* an indirect way of conveying one's thoughts and ideas; excessive use of words to express a simple meaning

> Laws have become a series of **circumlocutions**, disconnecting the people from the government and marginalising the poorest of the poor.

Circumvent - *(verb)* to evade or avoid using strategic or deceptive means; to bypass or go around; to entrap

> Individuals who **circumvent** the law are regarded by society as deviants.

Conundrum - *(noun)* a serious problem with some degree of difficulty; a puzzle, riddle or question asked for the sake of amusement

> Through unity and cooperation, social institutions can combat this **conundrum**.

Conviviality - *(noun)* a quality marked by good cheer, liveliness and friendliness

> His **conviviality** and trustworthiness brought him to the heights of success.

Cupidity - *(noun)* overwhelming desire (to the point of greed); the excessive urge to possess or covetousness

> Human **cupidity** has been subject to much contention in the field of sociology.

Cynosure - *(noun)* the center of attention because of its beauty; a guide

> An uncompromising policy against corruption is the **cynosure** of the new government.

Demagogue - *(noun)* a leader who tries to stir up people by appealing to their emotions and prejudices for the purpose of gaining power

> Adolf Hitler was the greatest **demagogue** of all time as history itself certifies this claim.

Discombobulate - (verb) to upset, disconcert; to provoke feelings of confusion or frustration

> If you try to **discombobulate** me, I will stop talking to you for months.

Ebullient - (adjective) energetic, enthusiastic or in high spirits; in a boiling state

> His **ebullient** personality made a lot of people weary except me.

Eclectic - (adjective) adopting, made up of or combining elements from varying sources; acceptance of or adherence to more than one system of thought, belief, culture or practice

> My friend embraces an **eclectic** way of life, being a Buddhist, a Christian and a Muslim all at the same time.

Egalitarian - *(adjective)* an assertion and manifestation of or belief in the equality of all people especially in political and socio-economic matters; favouring equality in all aspects

> The French Revolution was a prime example of an uprising fueled by **egalitarian** sentiments.

Egregious - (adjective) outstandingly bad; notorious

> Such an **egregious** mistake should never be committed again.

UNDERSTANDING THE GAMSAT

Enfranchise - *(verb)* grant freedom to, as from slavery or servitude; to afford rights or privileges that were previously withheld

*This new system could **enfranchise** and empower women in the labour sector, who feel underrepresented and voiceless.*

Ephemeral - *(adjective)* a temporary condition, situation or state of being; short-lived

*The passing of Princess Diana shows us that no matter how brightly she shined, her glow was still **ephemeral**.*

Epistemology - *(noun)* a system, method or manner of learning; a theory on human knowledge and the process of learning

*From this **epistemology**, he arrived at the conclusion that knowledge and consciousness are distinct entities.*

Equanimity - *(noun)* exuding grace under pressure; composure even in the face of tension

*For the quick delivery of relief services, both public servants and victims must practice **equanimity**.*

Erudite - *(adjective)* characterised by extensive reading or knowledge; well instructed; highly educated or learned

*An **erudite** person like you should go to medical school.*

Excogitate - *(verb)* to devise a plan or think something through; to understand something by carefully studying it

*During the meeting, we **excogitated** the best solution to the problem at hand.*

Existential - *(adjective)* relating to or affirming existence; grounded on existence or the experiences of existence; empirical (can be apprehended by the five senses of man, thus, capable of being measured)

*Bruno Bettelheim believed that fairy tales that have been passed generation to generation are society's way of helping children deal with **existential** anxieties.*

Expurgate - *(verb)* to omit or modify parts considered indelicate or inappropriate

*Economic policies are thoroughly **expurgated** prior to publication.*

Facetious - *(adjective)* characterised by wit and pleasantry; no serious or literal meaning

*His **facetious** remarks entertained the crowd.*

Fait accompli - *(noun)* an accomplished and presumably irreversible deed or fact; a done deal

*For this bill to be made into law is **fait accompli**.*

Fatuous - *(adjective)* devoid of intelligence; mindless or foolish

*Use your head if you don't want to be a **fatuous** victim of love.*

Gasconade - *(noun)* excessive boasting; a boastful manner of talking

*You can actually tell the difference between a sincere memoir and one that's full of **gasconade**.*

Gerrymander - *(verb)* to divide unfairly and to one's advantage; to manipulate boundaries, as in voting districts, for self-serving reasons

*Politicians found guilty of **gerrymandering** will face legal charges and be made to answer to the court of law.*

Halcyon - *(adjective)* pertaining to peaceful, tranquil, undisturbed and happy

*The **halcyon** days are gone, replaced by war and strife.*

Hegemony - *(noun)* the dominance or leadership of one social group or nation over others; the pursuit of world domination through aggressive or expansionist acts

*Imposing one's political beliefs on other people is a manifestation of **hegemony**.*

Hubris - *(noun)* an excess of pride or self-confidence

> *He who falls prey to **hubris** shall fail to see the real meaning of life.*

Hyperbole - *(noun)* a deliberate exaggeration; a figure of speech characterised by extravagant expressions

> *To say that Helen of Troy's beauty can launch a thousand ships is nothing more than a **hyperbole**.*

Iconoclast - *(noun)* one who attacks and seeks to overthrow traditional or popular beliefs and ideas of institutions under the assumption of error or irrationality

> *During the Byzantine era, **iconoclasts** from the Eastern Orthodox faith destroyed religious statues and images that belonged to the Roman Catholic Church.*

Idiosyncratic - *(adjective)* an unusual way in which a particular person behaves or thinks; may also refer to an eccentric feature of something

> *Dishevelled and unruly hair is **idiosyncratic** of Albert Einstein as purple socks are idiosyncratic to my grandmother.*

Inchoate - *(adjective)* partially but not fully in existence or operation; underdeveloped or incomplete; still at the initial stages

> *According to the principles of International Law, unless you fully occupy a piece of land, merely discovering it will only give you an **inchoate** title.*

Incognito - *(can be used as a noun, an adjective or an adverb)* without revealing or concealing one's identity in order to avoid notice

> *The monarch of a 19th century superpower country traveled **incognito** to Australia.*

Irony - *(noun)* an amusing or comical situation that arises from the contradiction of things, especially when expectations are at odds with the resulting reality

> *Note: **Irony** is also used in debate and in cross-examination (Socratic irony: where a person who seems to be ignorant, asks questions of someone who appears to be*

smart only to expose that the "smart' person is anything but smart). It is also used in drama (When the sequence of events leads the audience to expect a particular ending but the ending does not conform to expectations, the ending is said to be one of dramatic irony).

It is **ironic** that the prankster slipped and fell as he was setting up a prank on someone else.

Jejune - *(adjective)* not of interest; not distinctive or remarkable in any way; insipid

The *jejune* lecture caused me to doze off.

Ken - *(noun)* understanding, perception or knowledge (of an idea or circumstance); to comprehend, recognise or discern

Math is a subject that has always been beyond my **ken**.

Lexicon - *(noun)* a stock of terms used in a particular profession, subject or style; a vocabulary list or a record, collection or inventory of words and terms

Adorbs and clickbait are now part of the global **lexicon**.

Magnanimous - *(adjective)* refers to a person's generous and kind nature; may also refer to a lofty and courageous spirit; suggests nobility of feeling and generosity of mind

Bill Gates was **magnanimous** in his contributions to charity.

Milieu - *(noun)* social or cultural environment; backdrop or setting

Our definition of marital union is often dictated by the standards of a particular **milieu**.

Moiety - *(noun)* one of two (approximately) equal parts; a part of something

Ethnic tribes comprise one **moiety** of the whole nation.

Myopic - *(adjective)* lack of discernment or long-range perspective in thinking or planning; inability to act with prudence or foresight; narrow-minded

Racists and chauvinists have a **myopic** mindset, which can be corrected through immersion in and constant exposure to a pluralist community.

Nefarious - *(adjective)* wicked in the extreme; promulgates injustice

*I knew he was plotting something **nefarious** when I saw him enter the warehouse.*

Nihilism - *(noun)* complete denial or outright rejection of all established authority, systems and institutions, be it political, economic or social; a preference for anarchy, revolution or absolute destruction

*The Holocaust was a clear manifestation of **nihilism**.*

Obviate - *(verb)* to prevent or eliminate by interception; to render unnecessary

*Studying will **obviate** the risk of getting a low score.*

Oligarchy - *(noun)* a political system governed by a few people, usually of significant wealth and influence; pertains to any other system (economic or social) or institution whereby power is concentrated in the hands of a select group of people

***Oligarchy** is the reason why 75% of our country's population continues to live below the poverty line.*

Ostentatious - *(adjective)* a display of wealth or knowledge that is meant to attract attention admiration or envy; also refers to a fondness for conspicuous and vainglorious and pretentious display

*A peacock, displaying his multicoloured tail feathers to attract a peahen, is not really being **ostentatious**; it assures the peahen that their offspring will be likely as strong and attractive as the peacock, thus ensuring the propagation of their species.*

Paragon - *(noun)* a perfect example of; a model of excellence

*This government is no longer a **paragon** of transparency and accountability.*

Parsimonious - *(adjective)* of or having a thrifty, frugal or stingy disposition

*Experiencing financial failure taught our family to be more **parsimonious**.*

Patrician - *(noun)* a highly educated person of refined upbringing, manners and taste; an aristocrat or someone from a noble or privileged lineage

*The upper echelons of society house individuals with a **patrician** background.*

Pecuniary - *(adjective)* relating to money or monetary transactions

*All **pecuniary** concerns must be directed to the finance officer.*

Pedantic - *(adjective)* learning in an attempt to impress others; bookish or excessively concerned with tiny details

*There's nothing **pedantic** about me joining the Ivy League Debaters Club.*

Pejorative - *(adjective)* has a disparaging, belittling or derogatory impact

*Not to be **pejorative** about it, but the lesson was simply uninteresting.*

Perfidy - *(noun)* intentional treachery or breaking off of trust; any treacherous or dishonest act

*Officials found guilty of **perfidy** should answer for their crimes.*

Pernicious - *(adjective)* results to harm or injury; deadly

*This **pernicious** beast must be tamed before he swallows us all.*

Perspicacious - *(adjective)* having a sharp mental perception; discerning

*Choosing the right candidate requires **perspicacious** judgement.*

Plenary - *(can be used as an adjective or a noun)* fully constituted or complete; a gathering characterised by the presence of all qualified members

*The **plenary** session of the Senate will not start until a quorum is formed.*

Pragmatism - *(noun)* a reasonable and logical way of doing things or thinking about problems that is based on dealing with specific situations instead of on ideals and theories

*Choosing to work from home as a blogger shows the **pragmatism** of a stay-at-home mom of three toddlers: she can earn money while keeping an eye on her children.*

Prevaricate - *(verb)* to create false truths or impressions with the intention to mislead or deceive; to deviate from the truth

*The proletariats believe that the bourgeoisie **prevaricate** their way to the top.*

Probity - *(noun)* honesty, uprightness; with integrity

*Citizens are encouraged to vote for political candidates with a proven reputation for **probity** and fairness.*

Proclivity - *(noun)* a natural inclination

*The dentist's receptionist has a **proclivity** for discussing trivial details.*

Proficuous - *(adjective)* useful, profitable, advantageous

*A **proficuous** turn of events propelled the economy to full recovery.*

Puerile - *(adjective)* displaying a lack of maturity or child-like characteristics; relating to children or youthfulness

*What a **puerile** way of looking at things.*

Pusillanimous - *(adjective)* lacking in courage; faint-hearted or cowardly

*A person with a **pusillanimous** nature will have a hard time in the military.*

Quotidian - *(adjective)* daily; ordinary; the usual; a common or mundane occurrence

*I don't understand why you're so excited when it's just a **quotidian** event.*

Rancor - *(noun)* consumed by bitterness or resentment for a long time

*The moment her sister asked for forgiveness, the **rancor** she felt all those years began to melt.*

Renege - *(verb)* to revoke a given promise or commitment

*Find another supplier if this one tries to **renege** or demand an unreasonable sum.*

GAMSAT-Prep.com
THE GOLD STANDARD

Res Ipsa Loquitur - *(noun)* a legal doctrine referring to situations where an injury was obviously caused by negligence; a legal jargon for "what you see is what you get"

> This accident is a case of **res ipsa loquitor**, seeing that there is not one warning device found anywhere in the vicinity.

Sangfroid - *(noun)* composure or coolness of mind, sometimes excessive, as shown in dangerous situations or under trying circumstances

> To commit a crime with **sangfroid** is far from normal.

Sanguine - *(adjective)* confidently optimistic or cheerful; relating to blood or the color red

> What a **sanguine** face this baby has.

Sardonic - *(adjective)* bitterly sarcastic; mocking or sneering

> I want to wipe that **sardonic** grin off his face.

Satire - *(noun)* humour derived from poking fun at social issues and human follies in general

> George Orwell's novel, Animal Farm, is a good example of a political **satire** as it exposes the folly of our notions of equality and sums it up in one phrase: "Everyone is created equal, but some are more equal than others."

Scintilla - *(noun)* a minute amount; an iota or trace

> Not even a **scintilla** of my fortune will go to that scheming relative.

Soliloquy - *(noun)* a speech you make or a long diatribe to yourself; a monologue

> She delivered a **soliloquy** in an empty auditorium just to make herself feel better.

Suffragist - *(noun)* an advocate of the extension of voting rights (especially to women); one who promotes or supports the idea that everyone has the right to vote

> Louisa May Alcott, the author of Little Women, was a famed **suffragist**.

Susurrus - *(noun)* whispering, humming or rustling sounds; soft murmurs or mutters

   The **susurrus** of leaves was like a lullaby that brought my baby to sleep.

Tautological - *(adjective)* unnecessary repetition of the same sense in different words; redundant use of words, statements or ideas to the point of vagueness

   This book often makes **tautological** conclusions.

Temperament - *(noun)* typical behaviour, condition or disposition

   Though he does not have a pleasant **temperament**, he still wins friends wherever he goes.

Touche - *(interjection)* an expression used to acknowledge a striking point or a clever remark made by another person in a discussion

   Touche! Your suggestion hit the nail on the head.

Ubiquitous - *(adjective)* universal, omnipresent or being everywhere; accepted by all

   His name became **ubiquitous** in the current news because of the atrocities exposed during his leadership.

Unctuous - *(adjective)* unpleasantly and excessively suave; insincere

   Even her charitable works were perceived to be **unctuous** by her disgruntled constituents.

Usufruct - *(noun)* the right or privilege to enjoy the use and advantages of a property owned by another, not including the destruction or misuse of its substance

   They may not have ownership rights but tenants have **usufruct** rights over their landlord's territory.

GAMSAT-Prep.com
THE GOLD STANDARD

● **Helpful Latin Expressions**

The Western world owes much to the classical language of Latin. Some expressions we use today are borrowed from Latin. Even the terms and concepts that serve as basis for our current systems of government, education, science and philosophy are derived from Latin. For this reason, although no one speaks this language nowadays, Latin lives on as part of English expressions. Here are some of them that might come handy when you write your Section II essays. You can choose to use one up to a maximum of two of these phrases in your essay:

A priori - *(adjective)* means something assumed or known even without experience; self-evident

> The analysis provided by the speaker mostly stems from **a priori** discernment of one's moral values.

Ad hoc - *(adjective)* means something that is set up only for this one instance, to address a singular and particular set of circumstances, problem or situation and not as something permanent

> The President formed an **ad hoc** committee to assess the rehabilitation needs of places affected by the supertyphoon Haiyan.

Ad infinitum - *(adverb)* means "endless"; to remember the meaning of this phrase, you only have to remember Buzz Lightyear as this is his catchphrase: "To infinity and beyond."

> The nagging wife made it a point to rehearse her husband's faults to his face **ad infinitum.**

Ad nauseum - *(expression)* signifies a boring and tedious repetition

> The doting mother extolled, **ad nauseam**, the virtues of her beloved son, to anyone who cared to listen.

Barba tenus sapientes - *(expression)* A man described as barba tenus sapientes is literally said to be "wise as far as his beard". In other words, he might look intelligent but he's actually far from it. This is just one of a number of phrases that show how the Romans associated beards with intelligence, alongside barba non facit philosophum, "a beard does not make a philosopher," and barba crescit caput nescit, meaning "the beard grows, but the head doesn't grow wiser."

> Robert doesn't shave off his beard; he thinks it makes him look **barba tenus sapientes**.

Bona fide - *(adjective)* means something genuine, honest, authentic and sincere; especially without any intention to deceive or beguile

*As per his client's wishes, and against the better judgment of the stockbroker, he made a **bona fide** offer to buy the shares of stock of Enron.*

Brutum fulmen - *(noun)* a harmless or empty threat; literally means "senseless thunderbolt"

*When a man who is swaying on his feet from drunkenness tells you he is going to beat you up, you can be sure it's just **brutus fulmen**.*

Carpe diem - *(expression)* literally means "to seize the day"; conveys the same meaning as "make hay while the sun shines" meaning, seize the opportunities that present themselves. In the movie Dead Poets' Society, the actor Robin Williams played the role of a professor in a prep school who urged his students to "carpe diem" - seize the day.

*My 70 year-old grandmother, wishing to tick-off items on her bucket list, went bungee jumping – the last thing she said before jumping off was **"Carpe diem!"***

Caveat emptor - *(noun)* a doctrine in both law and business that someone who wishes to buy anything must be aware of the conditions, circumstances and consequences of the purchase as the seller cannot be held responsible unless expressed in a warranty

*When buying a second-hand car, always look for the car's registration papers and insurance; check that the chassis and engine numbers which appear on the car match the numbers on the registration. After all, this is due diligence because of **caveat emptor**.*

Cogito ergo sum - *(expression or idea)* literally means **"I think, therefore, I am."**; the conclusion reached by the person who wonders whether he exists. In the work by Rene Descartes, the phrase was in French ("Je pense donc je suis."). This phrase became the basis for Western philosophy. For Rene Descartes, existence is self-awareness and self-awareness presumes existence.

Compos mentis - *(adjective)* literally means "of sound mind" ; this phrase usually appears in the negative "non compos mentis" which means "not of a sound mind"; this phrase is often used to describe people who are incompetent to stand trial, to act with legal effect in entering binding contracts

*The heirs of the 90-year old billionaire went to court asking that he be declared **"non compos mentis"** and therefore, put into their guardianship.*

GAMSAT-Prep.com
THE GOLD STANDARD

Coup de grace - *(noun)* means the final touch or decisive stroke; In art, it is the last brush-stroke to a masterpiece. In murder novels, it is the "last strike or the last stroke" meaning, the death blow.

> *The fencer lunges with a* **coup de grace** *- his foil hits the mark near the heart of his opponent. It was his winning move.*

Cui bono - *(expression)* literally means "Who benefits?"; a rhetorical Latin legal phrase used to imply that whoever appears to have the most to gain from a crime is probably the culprit. More generally, it is used in English to question the meaningfulness or advantages of carrying something out.

> *The police detective, all dressed up in the fashion of Sherlock Holmes, turned around most theatrically and said to the relatives of the victim:* **"Cui bono**? *He who has the most to gain from the crime probably had the strongest motive to commit it."*

De facto - *(noun)* In law and business, it means to exist as a fact even without legal sanction or legal right.

> *In Australia, when a man and a woman live together sharing domestic life, they are considered a* **de facto** *couple and are entitled to the same rights given to married couples.*

De jure - *(noun)* according to law; by legal right

> *Adultery is illegal,* **de jure**, *in many states, but the laws are never enforced.*

De novo - *(adverb)* used in English to mean "anew" or "afresh"

> *When one appeals a lower court decision, the appellate court usually reviews the evidence* **de novo**.

Dum spiro spero - *(expression or motto)* literally means, "While I breathe, I hope."; the English equivalent is "Hope springs eternal."

> *My grandmother, on a hospital bed after suffering a stroke, said to the doctor who told her that she might not be able to drive a car anymore:* **"Dum spiro spero."**

UNDERSTANDING THE GAMSAT

E pluribus unum - *(expression or motto)* literally means "out of many, one"

> The Latin phrase "**E pluribus unum**" appears on the seal of the United States as it is the official motto of the United States of America, signifying the federal system of government.

Errare humanum est - *(expression)* literally means "to err is human"; It means that it is expected for mortal men to make mistakes. This harks back to the Biblical story of the first man, Adam, and how he and his wife, Eve, fell into sin. The rest of humanity which was begotten of them, therefore inherited the tendency to err, to make mistakes and to sin. The entire phrase is: "Errare humanum est, et ignoscere divinum." (Translated: To err is human, and to forgive, divine.")

Félix cupla - *(noun)* literally a "happy fault"; an apparent mistake or disaster that actually ends up having surprisingly beneficial consequences

> Losing my job when I was laid off, although quite a stressful experience, turned out to be a **félix culpa** since I started a business, which is now quite profitable.

Imperium in emperio - *(noun)* meaning "an empire within an empire"; can be used literally to refer to a self-governing state confined within a larger one; or to a rebellious state fighting for independence from another; or, more figuratively, to a department or a group of workers in an organisation who, despite appearing to work for themselves, are still answerable to an even larger corporation.

> The IT Department at our office is an **imperium in imperio**: it is made up of techie geeks who work independently, often ignoring the office dress code and the designated office hours.

Je ne sais quoi - *(noun)* This is actually French phrase which literally means "I don't know what"; its English equivalent is 'a certain something'; refers to an innate quality of a person or thing that makes them attractive but which cannot be quantified, articulated, or put into words

> To be a supermodel, it is not enough to be merely tall or beautifully proportioned; one also needs to have a presence, a certain **je ne sais quoi**.

Mea culpa - *(expression)* literally means "the fault is mine"; it is the Latin equivalent of a plea of guilty in court; also a form of apology

> The witness exclaimed, "**Mea culpa!**" when the opposing lawyer showed her a discrepancy in her recollection of events.

Modus operandi - *(noun)* often used to describe a signature move or signature moves of criminals

> *Most internet scammers have the same* **modus operandi**: *they send you an email informing you that you have won several thousand dollars but in order to receive the entire amount, you are to deposit a certain smaller amount to "verify" your account and whereabouts.*

Non sequitur - *(noun)* an illogical conclusion; the opposite of "et sequitur" which means "and so on and so forth"; usually indicates that there is a logical gap between two propositions

> *Just because I agreed to go out on one date with you, it doesn't mean I love you or I want to marry you – that is* **non sequitur**.

Panem et circensēs - *(noun)* means "bread and circuses"; refers to the basic needs and desires - i.e., food and entertainment - to keep a person happy

> *In order to keep the Roman citizens from becoming an unruly mob, the emperors took it as their political duty to provide them with* **panem et circensēs** *to keep them quiet and compliant.*

Persona non grata - *(noun)* literally means "an unwelcome person"; the term is primarily used of diplomatic officials from other countries when they have committed crimes in a host country and are expelled from that host country

> *Even when he was accused of sexually harassing his personal assistant, the attaché could not be criminally charged but he was declared "***persona non grata***" and he left for his home country.*

Quid pro quo - *(noun)* literally means "this for that"; the original phrase signifies an exchange of things with equivalent value; the English equivalent is "tit for tat" signifying an equivalent retaliation;

> *The serial killer Hannibal Lester refused to answer the FBI agent's questions unless the FBI agent herself answers his questions regarding her personal life; he told her "***Quid pro quo***, Clarisse."*

Semper Fi - *(noun)* This is the motto of the US Marines which means "Always faithful" or "Always keep the faith". This motto comes with a twin "Marines leave no man behind." This signifies the camaraderie in arms of the Marines that in battle, at great risk to themselves, they will bring home the men with whom they fought side by side, be they dead or alive. It also signifies that Marines will always be faithful to their oath to uphold their nation's defense.

Sine qua non - *(noun)* something you cannot do without; in law, it is an absolute condition, that is, it is a condition that must be met before entering into a privilege or a right

> *When Sara's grandmother bequeathed to her one million dollars in her will, she made Sara's marriage a **sine qua non** to the inheritance.*

Status quo - *(noun)* In law, this phrase is used as "status quo ante" which means, the status or state of affairs prior to the present controversy; in everyday language, the term "status quo" means the actual state of affairs in the present. The best way to remember this phrase is by calling to mind the Disney movie High School Musical:

> *The popular girl, Sharpe Adams, was opposed to the basketball athletes and Math wizards joining the drama club and the musical so she sang, "stick to the **status quo**."*

Tempus fugit - *(expression)* literally means "time flies"; in English, the phrase "time flies when you're having fun" comes from the Latin phrase 'tempus fugit'.

Veni, vidi, vici - *(expression or motto)* This is what Julius Ceasar said when he reported to the Roman Senate after he conquered the Gauls (of France) "I came, I saw, I conquered."

Verbatim - *(can be used as adverb or adjective)* means "word for word"; a precise and exact quote of what someone said

> *The senator said to the reporter who was interviewing him: "You can quote me on that, in fact, quote me **verbatim**, why don't you?"*

Veto - *(can be used as noun or verb)* the political power to single-handedly stop or make void a law

> *The new immigration bill passed by a slim margin in Congress, but the President is likely to **veto** it.*

Vox populi - *(noun)* literally means "the voice of the people"; refers to public opinion

> *When elected viva voce by the Roman mob, this is what the elected official says when he accepts the elected position "**vox populi**, vox dei" which means, God has spoken through the people.*

GAMSAT-Prep.com
THE GOLD STANDARD

4.4 Practice Materials

It is great to know the structure, as previously described, for Task A and Task B. However, you must practice generating ideas and expressing yourself.

Practice Problems
• Brainstorm using famous quotes (Section 4.5)
• Generate thesis statements using sets of quotes (Section 4.6)
• ACER Automatic Scoring
• GS Essay Correction Service

Full-length Practice Tests
• GS
• ACER

If you want to find out how you would fare according to ACER's marking guide, ACER offers a paid automated essay scoring service. On the other hand, if you are very concerned about your performance and feel that you need personalised comments from an expert, you can find an essay correcting service available at GAMSAT-prep.com.

4.5 Advice on How to Generate Ideas

Many candidates struggle in generating their initial ideas for an essay. One possible root cause may be a difficulty in comprehending the idea expressed in a quotation. In most cases, you will simply not know enough about the topic. By writing a timed essay, and then revising it by doing research outside of exam conditions, you will grow your body of knowledge. This body of knowledge is what separates the very high achievers from the median in Section II.

As your knowledge builds, you may still experience issues attempting to piece together your arguments and evidence. One way to address this problem is by having a ready set of guide questions that you can actively ask yourself while you consider a given quotation. The following are some of these possible questions:

Main idea/Introduction:

1. What is the quotation talking about?
2. What is its main point?

Thesis/Body:

1. What is my immediate thought or reaction to the quotation?

UNDERSTANDING THE GAMSAT

2. What is the significant issue / first-hand experience that I can relate to my thesis?

3. Check for focus and relevance: How does it connect to the view reflected by the quotation?

Antithesis/Body:

1. What opinion or situation can I recall, based on knowledge or experience, that will counter my initial view in the thesis?

2. Check again for focus and relevance: How does it connect to the central idea presented in the quotation?

Synthesis/Conclusion:

1. How do I reconcile the two opposing views with my thesis?

2. How do I connect these views in my present socio-cultural or interpersonal context?

We have placed 50 quotations for you to work through. Half for Writing Task A and the other half for Writing Task B. Please consider re-reading Sections 4.2.5 and 4.2.6. Your aim is to quickly key in on the idea being presented and generate ideas in point form in less than 5 minutes. Frankly, your efficiency should increase in the last 10 essays in each section. Do not try to complete all the exercises in one sitting.

You can discuss the way you structured your essay with other students in our Forum.

4.5.1 Writing Task A Quotations

1. Let us never negotiate out of fear. But let us never fear to negotiate.

    John F. Kennedy

    Thesis _____
    Antithesis _____
    Synthesis _____

2. We live in a moment in history where change is so speeded up that we begin to see the present only when it is already disappearing.

    R.D. Laing

    Thesis _____
    Antithesis _____
    Synthesis _____

3. All diplomacy is a continuation of war by other means.

    Chou En-Lai

    Thesis _____
    Antithesis _____
    Synthesis _____

UNDERSTANDING THE GAMSAT 233

4. It is better that ten guilty persons escape than one innocent suffer.
William Blackstone

Thesis _____
Antithesis _____
Synthesis _____

5. Money is like the sixth sense without which you cannot make a complete use of the other five.
W. Somerset Maugham

Thesis _____
Antithesis _____
Synthesis _____

6. That man is richest whose pleasures are the cheapest.
Henry David Thoreau

Thesis _____
Antithesis _____
Synthesis _____

7. The technologies which have had the most profound effects on human life are usually simple.
Freeman Dyson

Thesis _____
Antithesis _____
Synthesis _____

8. The great growling engine of change - technology.
Alvin Toffler

Thesis _____
Antithesis _____
Synthesis _____

9. Ability is a poor man's wealth.
John Wooden

Thesis _____
Antithesis _____
Synthesis _____

10. The mother of revolution and crime is poverty.
Aristotle quotes

Thesis _____
Antithesis _____
Synthesis _____

11. It is better to be defeated on principle than to win on lies.
Arthur Calwell

Thesis _____
Antithesis _____
Synthesis _____

12. Those who make peaceful revolution impossible will make violent revolution inevitable.

    John F. Kennedy

    Thesis _____
    Antithesis _____
    Synthesis _____

13. Injustice anywhere is a threat to justice everywhere.

    Martin Luther King, Jr.

    Thesis _____
    Antithesis _____
    Synthesis _____

14. ...government of the people, by the people, for the people, shall not perish from the earth.

    Abraham Lincoln

    Thesis _____
    Antithesis _____
    Synthesis _____

15. In the long-run every Government is the exact symbol of its People, with their wisdom and unwisdom.

    Thomas Carlyle

    Thesis _____
    Antithesis _____
    Synthesis _____

16. The cost of liberty is less than the price of repression.

    W. E. B. Du Bois

    Thesis _____
    Antithesis _____
    Synthesis _____

17. I have to follow them, I am their leader.

    Alexandre-Auguste Ledru-Rollin

    Thesis _____
    Antithesis _____
    Synthesis _____

18. I would rather be exposed to the inconveniences attending too much liberty than those attending too small a degree of it.

    Thomas Jefferson

    Thesis _____
    Antithesis _____
    Synthesis _____

19. Those who expect to reap the blessings of freedom, must, like men, undergo the fatigues of supporting it.
Thomas Jefferson

Thesis _____
Antithesis _____
Synthesis _____

20. The only way to make sure people you agree with can speak is to support the rights of people you don't agree with.
Eleanor Holmes Norton

Thesis _____
Antithesis _____
Synthesis _____

21. I disapprove of what you say, but I will defend to the death your right to say it.
Voltaire

Thesis _____
Antithesis _____
Synthesis _____

22. He that would make his own liberty secure must guard even his enemy from oppression.
Thomas Paine

Thesis _____
Antithesis _____
Synthesis _____

23. War settles nothing.
Dwight D. Eisenhower

Thesis _____
Antithesis _____
Synthesis _____

24. You can't hold a man down without staying down with him.
Booker T. Washington

Thesis _____
Antithesis _____
Synthesis _____

25. Men prize the thing ungained, more than it is.
Shakespeare

Thesis _____
Antithesis _____
Synthesis _____

4.5.2 Writing Task B Quotations

1. It is amazing how complete the delusion that beauty is goodness.
   Leo Tolstoy
   Introduction _____
   Body _____
   Conclusion _____

2. Whether you think you can or think you can't - you are right.
   Henry Ford
   Introduction _____
   Body _____
   Conclusion _____

3. From the deepest desires often come the deadliest hate.
   Socrates
   Introduction _____
   Body _____
   Conclusion _____

4. The error of youth is to believe that intelligence is a substitute for experience, while the error of age is to believe that experience is a substitute for intelligence.
   Lyman Bryson
   Introduction _____
   Body _____
   Conclusion _____

5. Conform and be dull.
   James Frank Dobie
   Introduction _____
   Body _____
   Conclusion _____

6. You can stay young as long as you can learn, acquire new habits and suffer contradictions.
   Marie von Ebner-Eschenbach
   Introduction _____
   Body _____
   Conclusion _____

7. Hatred is the coward's revenge for being intimidated.
   George Bernard Shaw
   Introduction _____
   Body _____
   Conclusion _____

8. The young always have the same problem – how to rebel and conform at the same time. They have now solved this by defying their parents and copying one another.

Quentin Crisp

Introduction _____
Body _____
Conclusion _____

9. Youth is the best time to be rich, and the best time to be poor.

Euripides

Introduction _____
Body _____
Conclusion _____

10. Some people say they haven't yet found themselves. But the self is not something one finds; it is something one creates.

Thomas Szasz

Introduction _____
Body _____
Conclusion _____

11. My youth is escaping without giving me anything it owes me.

Ivy Compton-Burnett

Introduction _____
Body _____
Conclusion _____

12. You can't get rid of poverty by giving people money.

P.J. O'Rourke

Introduction _____
Body _____
Conclusion _____

13. Nobody can make you feel inferior without your consent.

Eleanor Roosevelt

Introduction _____
Body _____
Conclusion _____

14. Youth is something very new: twenty years ago no one mentioned it.

Coco Chanel

Introduction _____
Body _____
Conclusion _____

UNDERSTANDING THE GAMSAT

15. There are three things extremely hard: steel, a diamond, and to know one's self.

    Benjamin Franklin

    Introduction _____
    Body _____
    Conclusion _____

16. Comedy is the last refuge of the nonconformist mind.

    Edward Albee

    Introduction _____
    Body _____
    Conclusion _____

17. When she stopped conforming to the conventional picture of femininity she finally began to enjoy being a woman.

    Betty Naomi Friedan

    Introduction _____
    Body _____
    Conclusion _____

18. When you can't remember why you're hurt, that's when you're healed.

    Jane Fonda

    Introduction _____
    Body _____
    Conclusion _____

19. Laughter is the shortest distance between two people.

    Victor Borge

    Introduction _____
    Body _____
    Conclusion _____

20. In prison, those things withheld from and denied to the prisoner become precisely what he wants most of all.

    Eldridge Cleaver

    Introduction _____
    Body _____
    Conclusion _____

21. People travel to wonder at the height of mountains, at the huge waves of the sea, at the long courses of rivers, at the vast compass of the ocean, at the circular motion of the stars, and they pass themselves by without wondering.

    St. Augustine

    Introduction _____
    Body _____
    Conclusion _____

22. Ask the young. They know everything.

Joseph Joubert

Introduction _____
Body _____
Conclusion _____

23. A sense of humor is a major defense against minor troubles.

Mignon McLaughlin

Introduction _____
Body _____
Conclusion _____

24. If the misery of the poor be caused not by the laws of nature, but by our institutions, great is our sin.

Charles Darwin

Introduction _____
Body _____
Conclusion _____

25. They can't hurt you unless you let them.

Multiple attributions

Introduction _____
Body _____
Conclusion _____

4.6 Exercises for Developing a Logical Response

Other candidates may not have much of a problem understanding quotations. But they do find difficulty in identifying the central theme or issue of the different quotations. We have prepared 20 sets of 5 comments each as supplementary exercises - 10 for Writing Task A and the remaining 10 for Writing Task B.

You may want to review Section 4.2.1 before going through these exercises. You may also use the templates found in Section 4.11 as guides in developing your essays.

4.6.1 Writing Task A Exercises

Exercise 1:

Comment 1

Without censorship, things can get terribly confused in the public mind.

William Westmoreland

* * * * *

Comment 2

I don't believe in censorship, but I do believe that an artist has to take some moral responsibility for what he or she is putting out there.

Tom Petty

* * * * *

Comment 3

If you have to be careful because of oppression and censorship, this pressure produces diamonds.

Tatyana Tolstaya

* * * * *

Comment 4

The most dangerous untruths are truths moderately distorted.

Georg Christoph Lichtenberg

* * * * *

Comment 5

To forbid us anything is to make us have a mind for it.

Michel de Montaigne

Topic:_____
Socio-cultural Theme/Issue: _____
Thesis Statement:_____

Exercise 2:

Comment 1

Only when the last tree has died and the last river been poisoned and the last fish been caught will we realise we cannot eat money.

Indian Cree Proverb

* * * * *

Comment 2

Environmentally friendly cars will soon cease to be an option . . . they will become a necessity.

Fujio Cho

* * * * *

Comment 3

I would feel more optimistic about a bright future for man if he spent less time proving that he can outwit Nature and more time tasting her sweetness and respecting her seniority.

Elwyn Brooks White

* * * * *

Comment 4

Every human has a fundamental right to an environment of quality that permits a life of dignity and well-being.

* * * * *

Comment 5

After one look at this planet any visitor from outer space would say "I want to see the manager".

William S. Burroughs

Topic:_____
Socio-cultural Theme/Issue: _____
Thesis Statement:_____

Exercise 3:

Comment 1

My personal opinion (not speaking for IBM) is that DRM [Digital Rights Management] is stupid, because it can never be effective, and it takes away existing rights of the consumer.

David Safford

* * * * *

Comment 2

Digital files cannot be made uncopyable, any more than water can be made not wet.

Bruce Schneier

* * * * *

Comment 3

Trusted systems presume that the consumer is dishonest.

Mark J. Stefik

* * * * *

Comment 4

Hoaxes use weaknesses in human behavior to ensure they are replicated and distributed. In other words, hoaxes prey on the Human Operating System.

Stewart Kirkpatrick

* * * * *

Comment 5

It's baffling to me that the content industries don't look at the experience of the software industry in the 80's, when copy protection on software was widely tried, and just as widely rejected by consumers.

Tim O'Reilly

Topic:_____
Socio-cultural Theme/Issue: _____
Thesis Statement:_____

Exercise 4:

Comment 1

If the past cannot teach the present and the father cannot teach the son, then history need not have bothered to go on, and the world has wasted a great deal of time.

Russell Hoban

* * * * *

Comment 2

The best of my education has come from the public library . . . my tuition fee is a bus fare and once in a while, five cents a day for an overdue book. You don't need to know very much to start with, if you know the way to the public library.

Lesley Conger

* * * * *

Comment 3

He who opens a school door, closes a prison.

Victor Hugo

* * * * *

Comment 4

Education is an ornament in prosperity and a refuge in adversity.

Aristotle

* * * * *

Comment 5

Education... has produced a vast population able to read but unable to distinguish what is worth reading.

G. M. Trevelyan

Topic:_____
Socio-cultural Theme/Issue: _____
Thesis Statement:_____

Exercise 5:

Comment 1

Technology makes it possible for people to gain control over everything, except over technology.

John Tudor

* * * * *

Comment 2

Humanity is acquiring all the right technology for all the wrong reasons.

R. Buckminster Fuller

* * * * *

Comment 3

If it keeps up, man will atrophy all his limbs but the push-button finger.

Frank Lloyd Wright

* * * * *

Comment 4

The real danger is not that computers will begin to think like men, but that men will begin to think like computers.

Sydney J. Harris

* * * * *

Comment 5

It has become appallingly obvious that our technology has exceeded our humanity.

Albert Einstein

Topic:_____
Socio-cultural Theme/Issue: _____
Thesis Statement:_____

Exercise 6:

Comment 1

Government, even in its best state, is but a necessary evil; in its worst state, an intolerable one.

Thomas Paine

* * * * *

Comment 2

The worst thing in this world, next to anarchy, is government.

Henry Ward Beecher

* * * * *

Comment 3

Freedom is when the people can speak, democracy is when the government listens.

Alastair Farrugia

* * * * *

Comment 4

Good government is no substitute for self-government.

Mahatma Gandhi

* * * * *

Comment 5

Every civilised society needs a government that will protect the people's lives and rights to liberty and property.

Topic:_____
Socio-cultural Theme/Issue: _____
Thesis Statement:_____

Exercise 7:

Comment 1

> Globalization has changed us into a company that searches the world, not just to sell or to source, but to find intellectual capital – the world's best talents and greatest ideas.
>
> Jack Welch

* * * * *

Comment 2

> It has been said that arguing against globalization is like arguing against the laws of gravity.
>
> Kofi Annan

* * * * *

Comment 3

> Globalization means we have to re-examine some of our ideas, and look at ideas from other countries, from other cultures, and open ourselves to them.
>
> Herbie Hancock

* * * * *

Comment 4

> Globalization has created this interlocking fragility. At no time in the history of the universe has the cancellation of a Christmas order in New York meant layoffs in China.
>
> Nassim Nicholas Taleb

* * * * *

Comment 5

> Globalization by the way of McDonald's and KFC has captured the hearts, the minds, and from what I can see through the window, the growing bellies of the folks here.
>
> Raquel Cepeda

Topic:_____
Socio-cultural Theme/Issue: _____
Thesis Statement:_____

Exercise 8:

Comment 1

Capitalism is an organised system to guarantee that greed becomes the primary force of our economic system and allows the few at the top to get very wealthy and has the rest of us riding around thinking we can be that way, too.

Michael Moore

* * * * *

Comment 2

I am opposing a social order in which it is possible for one man who does absolutely nothing that is useful to amass a fortune of hundreds of millions of dollars, while millions of men and women who work all the days of their lives secure barely enough for a wretched existence.

Eugene V. Debs

* * * * *

Comment 3

Capitalism tries for a delicate balance: It attempts to work things out so that everyone gets just enough stuff to keep them from getting violent and trying to take other people's stuff.

George Carlin

* * * * *

Comment 4

Today's consumers are not opposed to companies making a profit; they want more empathic, enlightened corporations that seek a balance between profit and purpose.

* * * * *

Comment 5

You cannot help the poor by destroying the rich. . . You cannot lift the wage earner by pulling the wage payer down . . . You cannot help people permanently by doing for them, what they could and should do for themselves.

Abraham Lincoln

Topic:_____
Socio-cultural Theme/Issue: _____
Thesis Statement:_____

Exercise 9:

Comment 1

People demand freedom of speech as a compensation for the freedom of thought which they seldom use.

Soren Kierkegaard

* * * * *

Comment 2

Freedom of speech means freedom for those who you despise, and freedom to express the most despicable views.

Alan Dershowitz

* * * * *

Comment 3

The Internet's like one big bathroom wall with a lot of people who anonymously can say really mean things.

Zooey Deschanel

* * * * *

Comment 4

If liberty means anything at all, it means the right to tell people what they do not want to hear.

George Orwell

Comment 5

Freedom of speech does not protect you from the consequences of saying stupid shit.

Jim C. Hines

Topic:_____
Socio-cultural Theme/Issue: _____
Thesis Statement:_____

Exercise 10:

Comment 1

Helping those who have been struck by unforseeable misfortunes is fundamentally different from making dependency a way of life.

Thomas Sowell

* * * * *

Comment 2

Dependency is death to initiative, to risk-taking and opportunity. It's time to stop the spread of government dependency and fight it like the poison it is.

Mitt Romney

* * * * *

Comment 3

We must promote upward mobility, starting with solutions that speak to our broken education system, broken immigration policy, and broken safety net programs that foster dependency instead of helping people get back on their feet.

Paul Ryan

* * * * *

Comment 4

Once you go on welfare, it changes you. Even if you get off welfare, you never escape the stigma that you were a charity case.

Jeannette Walls

* * * * *

Comment 5

I do not believe that the power and duty of the General Government ought to be extended to the relief of individual suffering which is in no manner properly related to the public service or benefit.

Grover Cleveland

Topic:_____
Socio-cultural Theme/Issue: _____
Thesis Statement:_____

4.6.2 Writing Task B Exercises

Exercise 1:

Comment 1

    A man's growth is seen in the successive choirs of his friends.

                                                                   Ralph Waldo Emerson

                              * * * * *

Comment 2

    Friendship is a single soul dwelling in two bodies.

                                                                                  Aristotle

                              * * * * *

Comment 3

    I have friends in overalls whose friendship I would not swap for the favor of the kings of the world.

                                                                 Thomas Edison

                              * * * * *

Comment 4

    The bird a nest, the spider a web, man friendship.

                                                                  William Blake

                              * * * * *

Comment 5

    True friends stab you in the front.

                                                                    Oscar Wilde

Topic:_____
Personal/Social Issues: _____
Thesis Statement:_____

GAMSAT-Prep.com
THE GOLD STANDARD

Exercise 2:

Comment 1

In every man's heart there is a secret nerve that answers to the vibrations of beauty.

Christopher Morley

* * * * *

Comment 2

I see beauty as the grace point between what hurts and what heals, between the shadow of tragedy and the light of joy. I find beauty in my scars.

* * * * *

Comment 3

What makes the desert beautiful is that somewhere it hides a well..

The Little Prince, Antoine de Saint Exupery

* * * * *

Comment 4

When you have only two pennies left in the world, buy a loaf of bread with one, and a lily with the other.

Chinese Proverb

* * * * *

Comment 5

We ascribe beauty to that which is simple; which has no superfluous parts; which exactly answers its end; which stands related to all things; which is the mean of many extremes.

Ralph Waldo Emerson

Topic:_____
Personal/Social Issues: _____
Thesis Statement:_____

Exercise 3:

Comment 1

> Where love rules, there is no will to power; and where power predominates, there love is lacking. The one is the shadow of the other.
>
> Carl Jung

* * * * *

Comment 2

> Contrary to Pascal's saying, we don't love qualities, we love persons; sometimes by reason of their defects as well as of their qualities.
>
> Jacques Martain

* * * * *

Comment 3

> Love is like racing across the frozen tundra on a snowmobile which flips over, trapping you underneath. At night, the ice-weasels come.
>
> Tom Robbins

* * * * *

Comment 4

> If somebody says, "I love you", to me, I feel as though I had a pistol pointed at my head. What can anybody reply under such conditions but that which the pistol-holder requires? "I love you, too".
>
> Kurt Vonnegut, Jr.

* * * * *

Comment 5

> They do not love that do not show their love. The course of true love never did run smooth. Love is a familiar. Love is a devil. There is no evil angel but Love.
>
> William Shakespeare

Topic:_____
Personal/Social Issues: _____
Thesis Statement:_____

Exercise 4:

Comment 1

Experience is not what happens to you. It is what you do with what happens to you.

Aldous Huxley

* * * * *

Comment 2

It is not only for what we do that we are held responsible, but also for what we do not do.

Moliere

* * * * *

Comment 3

Experience is a hard teacher because she gives the test first, the lesson afterward.

Vernon Law

* * * * *

Comment 4

Life teaches none but those who study it.

V. O. Kliuchevsky

* * * * *

Comment 5

Experience is a great advantage. The problem is that when you get the experience, you're too damned old to do anything about it.

Jimmy Connors

Topic:_____
Personal/Social Issues: _____
Thesis Statement:_____

Exercise 5:

Comment 1

The road of excess leads to the palace of wisdom.

William Blake

* * * * *

Comment 2

One's first step in wisdom is to question everything - and one's last is to come to terms with everything.

Georg Christoph Lichtenberg

* * * * *

Comment 3

Wisdom begins at the end.

Daniel Webster

* * * * *

Comment 4

The wisest mind has something yet to learn.

George Santayana

* * * * *

Comment 5

He who devotes sixteen hours a day to hard study may become at sixty as wise as he thought himself at twenty.

Mary Wilson Little

Topic:_____
Personal/Social Issues: _____
Thesis Statement:_____

Exercise 6:

Comment 1

Heroes are ordinary people who make themselves extraordinary.

Gerard Way

* * * * *

Comment 2

Anyone who does anything to help a child in his life is a hero to me.

Fred Rogers

* * * * *

Comment 3

I would describe a hero as a person who has no fear of life, who can face life squarely.

Alexander Lowen

* * * * *

Comment 4

Those who say that we're in a time when there are no heroes, they just don't know where to look.

Ronald Reagan

* * * * *

Comment 5

The real hero is always a hero by mistake; he dreams of being an honest coward like everybody else.

Umberto Eco

Topic:_____
Personal/Social Issues: _____
Thesis Statement:_____

Exercise 7:

Comment 1

    Forgiveness is a virtue of the brave.

                                                   Indira Gandhi

* * * * *

Comment 2

    It is easier to forgive an enemy than to forgive a friend.

                                                   William Blake

* * * * *

Comment 3

    You can make up a quarrel, but it will always show where it was patched.

                                                 Edgar Watson Howe

* * * * *

Comment 4

    To err is human; to forgive, divine.

                                                 Alexander Pope

* * * * *

Comment 5

    There is no revenge so complete as forgiveness.

                                               Josh Billings

Topic:_____
Personal/Social Issues: _____
Thesis Statement:_____

Exercise 8:

Comment 1

The worst loneliness is not to be comfortable with yourself.

Mark Twain

* * * * *

Comment 2

Solitude is the profoundest fact of the human condition. Man is the only being who knows he is alone.

Octavio Paz

* * * * *

Comment 3

Loneliness is a barrier that prevents one from uniting with the inner self.

Carl Rogers

* * * * *

Comment 4

At the innermost core of all loneliness is a deep and powerful yearning for union with one's lost self.

Brendan Francis

* * * * *

Comment 5

To dare to live alone is the rarest courage; since there are many who had rather meet their bitterest enemy in the field, than their own hearts in their closet.

Charles Caleb Colton

Topic:_____
Personal/Social Issues: _____
Thesis Statement:_____

UNDERSTANDING THE GAMSAT

Exercise 9:

Comment 1

If you want creative workers, give them enough time to play.

John Cleese

* * * * *

Comment 2

There is a time for work and there is a time for play. Don't ever mix both.

* * * * *

Comment 3

This is the real secret of life - to be completely engaged with what you are doing in the here and now. And instead of calling it work, realise it is play.

Alan Wilson Watts

* * * * *

Comment 4

There is virtue in work and there is virtue in rest. Use both and overlook neither.

Alan Cohen

* * * * *

Comment 5

You can discover more about a person in an hour of play than in a year of conversation.

Plato

Topic:_____
Personal/Social Issues: _____
Thesis Statement:_____

Exercise 10:

Comment 1

    Attitude is a little thing that makes a big difference.

                                                     Winston Churchill

*****

Comment 2

    Excellence is not a skill. It is an attitude.

                                                         Ralph Marston

*****

Comment 3

    Our attitude towards others determines their attitude towards us.

                                                        Earl Nightingale

*****

Comment 4

    You cannot change what has already happened - but your attitude can.

*****

Comment 5

    Weakness of attitude becomes weakness of character.

                                                        Albert Einstein

Topic:_____
Personal/Social Issues: _____
Thesis Statement:_____

UNDERSTANDING THE GAMSAT

4.7 The Scoring Key

Your score in the Written Communication section will mostly be based on how you present your ideas. Although technical issues - like occasional grammar and spelling errors - essentially influence the quality of your writing, these are only assessed relative to the effectiveness of your general response. Your personal stand and attitude towards the subject matter will not be part of the assessment. The following are two primary criteria on which Section II is assessed: thought and content, and organisation and expression.

Thought and content refers to the substance of your ideas in response to a text. The GAMSAT gives emphasis on generative thinking, which is basically about generating values and innovative ideas in your writing within the thirty minutes per essay time limit. The way you effectively carry out your thoughts and feelings as responses to the task give weight to this criterion.

Organisation and expression is how you develop those fresh ideas in a logical and coherent manner. Control of language, i.e., grammar and fluency, is an inherent consideration in the assessment. However, your skills in this area will only be secondary to the overall content of your response.

Most papers are evaluated on common scoring descriptions. Although ACER has an automated Essay Correction Service, for the real GAMSAT, ==essays have been historically hand marked separately by three individuals, and adjudicated when necessary.== It is advisable that you ask someone to correct your essay to get a general idea. Have this person go through the following guide. Please be reminded that this is not endorsed by ACER and should only be considered as a guide to provide you with a general idea of the process.

Typical Essay Grade	Characteristics of a Paper	Estimated Conversion to a GAMSAT Score
6/6	Thought and content shows clear and coherent transitions of ideas. The writer stays focussed on the subject or issue. There is evidence of a logical build-up of arguments (i.e., normally just Task A but possibly Task B) or reflective discussion (i.e., Task B). Command of the language is excellent.	≥ 72

GAMSAT-Prep.com
THE GOLD STANDARD

Typical Essay Grade	Characteristics of a Paper	Estimated Conversion to a GAMSAT Score
5/6	Writing shows clarity of ideas with a certain extent of complexity. The argument stays focussed on the issue while main ideas are well-developed. Control of the language is strong.	65–71
4/6	The essay observes clarity of thought and some depth in ideas. There is also a development of major points and some focus. Control of the language is adequate.	58–64
3/6	There is evidence of some problems with integration and transition of ideas. Major ideas need to be organised and discussed clearly. Errors in grammar and mechanics are evident.	51–57
2/6	Thought and content are disorganised and unclear. There is a lack of logical organisation of main ideas. There are numerous errors in grammar, usage and structure.	44–50
1/6	The essay shows a lack of comprehension about the writing task. There is no development and organisation of ideas. Poor handling of the language prevents the reader from following the points of the writer.	≤ 43

In the next section (4.8), you will find a couple of corrected Section II essays and later, in section 4.9, we will present some excellent essays for your perusal. Also, we have placed dozens of Section II essays online that were corrected using the Gold Standard (GS) Essay Correction Service. You can access all these essays by logging in to your GAMSAT-prep.com Account and clicking on Lessons in the top menu. Of course, you can also leave comments at gamsat-prep.com/forum.

4.8 Sample Corrected Essays

In this section, you will find two response essays with corresponding comments. If you wish, use this as yet another exercise. Get a pen and some lined paper. Time yourself (30 minutes) and create an essay in response to the instructions below. Subsequently, compare your response to the graded essays that follow.

WRITING TASK A

Consider the following comments and develop a piece of writing in response to one or more of them.

Your writing will be judged on the quality of your response to the theme; how well you organise and present your point of view, and how effectively you express yourself. You will not be judged on the views or attitudes you express.

* * * * * *

"Laws made by common consent must not be trampled on by individuals."
George Washington

"The final test of civilization of a people is the respect they have for law."
Lewis F. Korns

"In matters of conscience, the law of the majority has no place."
Mahatma Gandhi

"In Republics, the great danger is that the majority may not sufficiently respect the rights of the minority."
James Madison

"All, too, will bear in mind this sacred principle, that though the will of the majority is in all cases to prevail, that will to be rightful must be reasonable; that the minority possess their equal rights, which equal law must protect, and to violate would be oppression."
Thomas Jefferson

SAMPLE ESSAY #1

A   A   A   A   A

The law of the majority Unimportant?

"In matters of concience the law of the majority has no place". For instance, a h.s. student, greatly feels peer pressure would choose not to smoke eventhough the majority of his peers feel that it is a desirable thing to do. According to the statement this student should make his choice based on what he believes not to be right, regardless of the general consoesnus of his peers.

There are some situations in which the law of majority is important in matters of conscience. For instance, a politician that believes in firearms can not make a law to force his constituents to carry guns, if they are horrible opposed to such weapons in the first place. Therefore the politician, in doing what he feels is right wouldn't be able to ignore the general consensus of the people of his province about firearms because his decision about such a law would affect them as well as him.

Certain circumstances would govern whether the law of majority is important or not in matters of conscience. If a person acts in such a way that he can live with, and it doesn't have adverse effects on other people who may

IF YOU NEED MORE SPACE, CONTINUE ON THE NEXT PAGE.

UNDERSTANDING THE GAMSAT

SAMPLE ESSAY #1

A   A   A   A   A

feel quite differently, then the law of majority is unimportant. If a person's conscience tells them to act in ways that hurt others, then the conscience of the majority must be taken into account. For instance, a Christian school teacher can't force her class that is majority Jewish to sing christmas songs because she believes it's the proper thing to do during the christmas holidays. That would antagonize the class, which would have been taken into consideration when she wanted to do what's right.

GAMSAT-Prep.com
THE GOLD STANDARD

Analysis of Sample Essay #1

Score
2/6   44–50

Task 1 – not really achieved. Although the statement was used in the first sentence, it was never really defined as a thesis nor otherwise defined. Encountering the typographical error "concience" instead of "conscience" or the mistake in spelling the quote in the beginning, seriously hurts the credibility of the writer. Peer evaluation or pressure is somewhat analogous to the making of laws by the majority, but quite loose as an association. For these reasons, clarity of thought and concrete examples to support a given thesis seem cloudy and unfocussed.

Task 2 – an antithesis is never really developed to the extent needed. While the politician example whom is juxtaposed in relation to a general consensus, could be developed, the idea of "forcing" people to carry weapons, seems an example, a bit absurd and reaching. The credibility of the writer is also questioned, when the use of "horrible" instead of the correct "horribly" (Para. 2, Line 2) is used adding to a general tone of inconsistency in care of grammar, and overall approach to the subject.

Task 3 – Because neither of the above tasks were completed with the necessary organisational and supportive devices and materials, providing a synthesis of arguments presented is impossible. A touchy feely context-based qualification in the surmounting to a "well, it all depends on the circumstance," is an intellectual and academic cop-out. The example of the Christian school teacher with Jewish students not forcing them to sing Christian songs, could be developed in more detail, if such an example is chosen.

Overall – some good ideas, but unfocussed, not organised to the extent needed. There seems to be some misunderstanding of the quote. The writer needs to reveal the Gandhi meaning that non-violent resistance to certain political repressions was not only necessary, but morally correct and in opposition to the laws of the majority. Hypothetical examples could be explored also: suppose that there was a law passed that said you could not protest or peaceably assemble to protest, or a law prohibiting you from enjoying "life, liberty, and the pursuit of happiness." In many ways, the subject of the essay concerns "personal liberty" vs. "collective responsibility" or "subjective reactions" to "legislative mandates or laws." This juxtaposition, or fulcrum needs to be explored and balanced to a larger degree.

Technical errors, spelling, and typographical errors deflated the essay – as previously noted. A stronger organisational pattern is needed, which follows a sequential and logical progression.

Evaluation (*see* Section 4.5): 2/6. This essay completely fails to address adequately one or more of the tasks. There may be recurring mechanical errors (i.e. spelling and grammar). Problems with analysis and organisation are typical (though organisation was fine in this instance).

2	These essays may show some problems with clarity or complexity of thought. The treatment of the writing assignment may show problems with integration or coherence. Major ideas may be underdeveloped. There may be numerous errors in mechanics, usage, or sentence structure.

UNDERSTANDING THE GAMSAT

SAMPLE ESSAY #2

A   A   A   A   A

My Rights Begin Where Yours End

In our democratic society, we have created many laws or rules gained through legislation. These rules are discussed, developed and enacted by elected officials who represent the majority of their constituents. However, the laws produced in this manner may be in conflict with a particular individual's beliefs or values. Thus the statement suggests that when such a conflict is evident, the individuals beliefs superceed the law, rendering the rules of the majority irrelevant. "In matters of conscience, the law of the majority has no place," spoken by a man of peace regarding a non violent struggle. However, there are those who have used such ideas for darker purposes...

For example, in 1996 many churches frequented by the African-American community were set ablaze by individuals – some of whom were members of racist movements. Both arson and such race-based acts are illegal in America. As in this case, the individuals who acted in defiance of the law of majority claimed they were abiding by their own beliefs and values. Thus they acted with a clear conscience destroying the lives and communities of innocent victims. Such a crime is immoral, unacceptable and – according to the rules of

IF YOU NEED MORE SPACE, CONTINUE ON THE NEXT PAGE.

A A A A A

the majority — illegal. Clearly, the law of majority must supercede the conscience of the perpetrators of such a crime.

The dividing line becomes clear. Life, liberty and the pursuit of happiness are the foundations of Constitution. The concept is both logical and moral. Our conscience should be our guide as we excercise our own freedom. However, since our neighbors and fellow Americans share the same rights, someone's conscience should never be used as a reason why someone's Constitutionally protected rights are stripped away. In conclusion, one's conscience should be one's guide but when it interferes with the rights of others, the law of majority becomes more important.

IF YOU NEED MORE SPACE, CONTINUE ON THE NEXT PAGE.

UNDERSTANDING THE GAMSAT

Analysis of Sample Essay #2

Score
5/6   65–71

Task 1 – A quick example could help buttress Task 1 in outlining the thesis matter, where subjective liberties are at odds with social, legislative, or governmental mandates. As noted in Essay #1, hypothetical examples could be used in supporting the thesis outline. Identifying the source of the quote as Gandhi, as a man of peace, helps further establish the credibility as a writer.

Task 2 – effective transition into an antithetical notion of when a sinister turn is taken between the dialectic of individual rights-beliefs and governmental mandates. Very good *specific* example and portrayal of the paradoxes of such a balance.

Task 3 – follows a logical progression, sequential with good analysis and reasoning. Good use of quotes in relation to a most relevant document concerning this juxtaposition: The Constitution (naturally, there are many effective international, national or regional examples depending on where you live or where you attend school).

Overall – good logical sequence, completion of tasks to an above average extent, clarity of focus, good development of ideas, clear and simple style of language.

The title did not necessarily - nor correctly - represent the outline of the ideas presented to the adequacy needed. The title is somewhat ambiguous and polysemantic, having several ways to interpret. Another minor observation – rules and laws are conflated to some extent, they could be differentiated more effectively, or simply omit the use of the word "rules".

Examples of some minor technical and typographical errors – "gained" in Paragraph (P) 1, Line (L) 2 is redundant, omit; P1, L9 – "supercede" not "superceed"; P3, L2 – insert "the" before "Constitution"; P3, L3 should be "These concepts are . . ."; P3, L4 doubled "our our"; P3, L9 – "constitutionally" – use lower case.

Evaluation (*see* Section 4.5): 5/6: All tasks are addressed by this essay. The treatment of the subject is substantial but not as thorough as for a 6 point essay. While some depth, structure and good vocabulary and sentence control are exhibited, this is at a lower level than for a 6 point essay.

> **5** These essays show clarity of thought, with some depth or complexity. The treatment of the rhetorical assignment is generally focussed and coherent. Major ideas are well developed. A strong control of language is evident.

GAMSAT-Prep.com
THE GOLD STANDARD

4.9 Frequently Asked Questions

Over the last 5 years, our Gold Standard GAMSAT Essay Correction Service has corrected thousands of student essays en route to improved GAMSAT Section II scores. From our experience, students tend to have similar concerns about essay writing for the GAMSAT.

How many quotes should I choose?

Your first 5 minutes of Section 2 is "reading time" and thus not counted as part of the overall time of 60 minutes for Section 2. This is your opportunity to read all 10 quotes and begin the process of brainstorming. For example, keeping the overall theme in mind, which quote or quotes generate(s) the best ideas?

There are students who have obtained exceptionally high scores exploring only 1 quote for their essay as there have been students who have explored 3 or more quotes. As long as you stick to the theme, the number of quotes that you choose should not be your focus. Compelling ideas which are well-illustrated must be the focus of your essay.

From our experience, an average science student without essay-writing experience tends to optimise their score by choosing 2 quotes in opposition for the argumentative essay (Writing Test A), and one quote - well explored - for the reflective essay (Writing Test B). Your personal experience and skills may lead you to a different path in order to optimise your score.

Ultimately, it all boils down to your experiences, writing skills and knowledge of the theme of the quotes.

Which quote should I choose?

Writing Test A: Consider the 3 tasks that we described as applied to the 5 quotes. Which generates the most clear, specific ideas? Can you mention dates with confidence? Can you mention names other than those provided alongside the quotes? Other specifics? Answering these questions will lead you naturally down the path to the ideal quote for you to optimise your score.

Writing Test B: Consider personal experiences/reflections to illustrate any of the 5 quotes. If that truly does not work, try the reverse (i.e. an argumentative approach). Consider the social implication for that point of view. Any quote, within the context of the overall theme, that generates the best ideas, should be pursued with vigour.

What do I do if I have strong argumentative ideas for Writing Test B?

Go with it! If your creative juices flow in a particular direction, you must go with the flow of ideas. The point of understanding the Gold Standard structure for Writing Tests A and B (sections 4.25 and 4.2.6) is that you keep in mind the objective. For example, even if you pursue an argumentative essay for Test B, consider the social implication and, most importantly, reflect on the personal meaning and related experience(s).

Accordingly, you can use a reflective or a personal narrative in response to Writing Test A. As discussed in Section 4.2.3, you may appeal to a reader's pathos in an argument. Besides, ACER does not impose any format for Section II. What they simply require is for you to generate a valuable response for the socio-cultural theme of Test A and the personal-social one in Test B. We've had past students who did well in Section II using the reflective approach for both tasks.

How personal is personal?

Your GAMSAT Writing Test B may include personal experiences that you are willing to share with, obviously, a stranger who is professional at marking essays (i.e. this is not your psychiatrist!!). In other words, this is unlikely to be the ideal venue to share experiences that you have never shared with anyone in your entire life.

On the other hand, "personal" must be sincere and must exemplify the point that you are trying to make. Being sincere and practicing your essay-writing skills optimise the chance that the reader buys into the experience that you are describing in your essay.

Examples of meaningful, personal expressions that, within context, seemed sincere: I wept, I felt, I failed, I was able to overcome my failure, I was hurt, I was the cause of his/her pain, I realised, I adapted, I was forced/compelled to reconsider, etc.

How many essays do top GAMSAT Section II students complete prior to the exam?

Top students complete 20-40 timed essays prior to the actual GAMSAT. Of course, students with natural charisma expressed by the pen or with a non-science background can get away with much less practice and still obtain a high Section II score.

How can I gauge my essay-writing progress?

We have placed our suggested scoring system in this book (section 4.7). You can have someone that you respect (a friend, family member, high school teacher or university professor), score some of your essays. ACER has a new automated GAMSAT Section II scoring service, which you can access by going to their website. Gold Standard has a personalised essay correction service, which you can access at GAMSAT-prep.com.

Is there anything useful to review for Section II the night before the exam?

Yes! Consider reviewing the answers you create for the Section II exercises in this book; the quotes, helpful words and Latin expressions from this book or from your personal notes; and review the notes you take from your practice exam experiences and/or from your exposure to the various resources we have previously described. In the end, well-explored ideas combined with 2-3 powerful words and/or expressions can produce tremendous results for GAMSAT Section II.

What is the ideal length of a GAMSAT essay?

Unless you can think fast and write as fast by hand at the same time, you really have time for only one and a half up to two pages. **The most important thing is to finish a well-organised essay with great ideas that is also easy to understand.**

What level of English skills would be required in Section II?

Part of the assessment is being able to put your ideas and emotions in words that are clear, appropriate and accurate. This means that your spelling skills must be decent enough that you can tell the difference between "eel and "ill" or "peach" and "pitch", for example.

You must also be able to construct complete sentences. Keep in mind that spoken English and written English have their own nuances. Colloquial terms and tone are highly discouraged. After all, you are applying for a graduate medicine program. It is only reasonable that you are expected to write formal, academic essays.

Another option is to enroll in a short-term writing class. You can inquire from your university's Student Services office to aid you in this area.

I have never been good at writing essays. My head goes blank every time I attempt to start writing. Do you have any suggestions?

You need to find out what could be causing the problem. Two common root causes are **exam anxiety** and **limited reading exposure**.

Sometimes, when you are too nervous trying to beat the limited time to write your essays, you end up with nothing essential - "your head goes blank". The solution is really very simple. Practice as often as you can. Just like any skills training, you have to keep practicing until you master the techniques.

If the problem is because you are always faced with unfamiliar topics and you have no idea on what to talk about, you need to read as much varied materials as you can - news, blogs, even scientific articles, and so on. But because you are preparing for the GAMSAT, an exam that requires you to write short essays, you might want to choose short articles from which to emulate good writing and concise arguments.

UNDERSTANDING THE GAMSAT

Is a title important?

A title is not required but if something original or engaging comes to mind after having planned your essay, then it could be of benefit.

How much time do I need to prepare for Section II?

Preparation time highly depends on your academic training and English writing skills. First, forming well-reasoned opinions for an on-the-spot topic can entail reading several sources prior to the test. Otherwise, you may be able to express agreement or disagreement on an idea, but you might find yourself inadequate to support your view with strong examples.

Even with candidates whose first language is English, expressing thoughts in a clear, logical manner may not be an easy task. You may feel like you have so many things to say within such a limited time. This entails discipline, and can take time to develop, in filtering only the most salient ideas that you will discuss in your essay.

Developing language skills and a writing style that suits you best can indeed take some time. The key is to determine your strengths and weaknesses months before the exam. Simulate a timed Section II test then do a post-test analysis. Most likely, you will then be able to know how much time and what kind of help you need.

GAMSAT-Prep.com
THE GOLD STANDARD

4.10 Common Grammatical Errors

Please do not read the following section unless either it is more than 6 weeks before the real exam or you have done some practice essays and you find that generating ideas and producing a well-structured essay is no longer challenging. At this point, improving details such as grammar and flexibility in the use of language can now become more interesting to explore as you aim to go from a very good score to an excellent score.

Some Basic Concepts

By definition, a sentence has the following properties:
- it contains a *subject*
- it contains a *verb*
- it expresses a *complete thought*

E.g., the sentence *"China prospers."* has a subject: "China"; a verb: "prospers"; and it conveys a complete thought or idea that makes sense.

Most sentences also have an *object* (receiver of the action); e.g., in the sentence "Mary baked a cake," the object is "a cake."

Run-on Sentences (fused sentences)

Incorrect usage	Correct usage	Explanation
He watched the movie ten times he really loved it.	He watched the movie ten times. He really loved it. He watched the movie ten times; he really loved it. He watched the movie ten times, for he really loved it. Since he really loved the movie, he watched it ten times.	Run-on sentences occur when two main clauses have no punctuation between them. Separate the two main ideas into separate complete sentences and punctuate each properly. Use a conjunction preceded by a comma to combine two ideas. Subordinate one of the main ideas into a clause.

Comma Faults (comma splices)

Incorrect usage	Correct usage	Explanations
He watched the movie ten times, he really loved it.	He watched the movie ten times, for he really loved it. He watched the movie ten times; he really loved it.	Comma faults occur when two main clauses are joined by only a comma. Use comma before a conjunction (*and, but, for, nor, or, so,* or *yet*) to join two complete thoughts (sentences). Use a semicolon to join two sentences. Omit the use of a conjunction, and start the second sentence in lowercase. Form two complete thoughts as separate sentences with the proper end marks. (See preceding example.) Join two thoughts by subordinating one of them. (See preceding example.)

Sentence Fragments

Incorrect usage	Correct usage	Explanation
Luke can read a book. And memorise it right after.	Luke can read a book and memorise it right after.	A sentence must have a subject and a verb.

Faulty Subordination

Incorrect usage	Correct usage	Explanation
I gazed out of the bus window, noticing a person getting mugged.	Gazing out of the bus window, I noticed a person getting mugged.	Place what you want to emphasise in the main clause, not the subordinate clause. Here the mugging should be emphasised and so should be in the main clause.

Errors in Subject-Verb Agreement

Rule: The verb should agree with the subject in terms of number (singular or plural) and person (first, second, or third).

Incorrect usage	Correct usage	Explanation
There is no glasses.	There are no glasses.	In this sentence, the subject is *glasses*, not there. *glasses* is plural; therefore, the verb should be plural (i.e. *are*).
She like diamonds.	She likes diamonds.	The subject *she* is in the second person, and is singular; therefore, the verb should also be in the second person, and be singular (i.e. *likes*).
Neither Emma nor Harry were there.	Neither Emma nor Harry was there.	In sentences where subjects are joined by *or* or *nor*, the verb agrees with the subject closer to it. In this example, "Harry" is the nearer subject. It is singular, so the verb should be also.
Neither Mary nor the others was there.	Neither Mary nor the others were there.	"Others" is the subject that is nearer to the verb. It is plural, so the verb should be also.
All of the team were there.	All of the team was there.	"Team" is singular, so the verb should be also.
All the players was present.	All the players were present.	"Players" is plural, so the verb should be also.
There are a variety of fruits.	There is a variety of fruits.	"Variety" is singular.
	There is a lot of birds here *or* there are a lot of birds here.	Both are correct. The first is correct since "lot" is singular. The second is correct because it is gaining acceptance through popular use.
Here is your shoes and tie.	Here are shoes and tie.	This sentence is in the inverted order, i.e., the subject/s come/s after the verb. When re-stated in the normal order, this sentence will be: *Your shoes and tie are here.* Subjects joined by *and* always take the plural form. Therefore, "shoes and tie" is plural, so the verb should be also.

Incorrect usage	Correct usage	Explanation
Fiona is one of the worst singers who has performed in this bar.	Fiona is one of the worst singers who have performed in this bar.	When relative pronouns *who*, *which*, or *that* are used as subjects of dependent adjective clauses, the verb of the adjective clause must agree in number with the antecedent of the pronoun. In this sentence, the antecedent of *who* is *singers*. "Singers" is plural, so the verb should be also (i.e. "have").
"I forget" or "I forgot".	I've forgotten.	Note that "I often forget" and "I forgot my umbrella yesterday" are correct.
Everybody are happy with the results.	Everybody is happy with the results.	Words like *everybody, everyone, everything, somebody, someone, each, either, nothing* and *anything* are examples of indefinite pronouns in singular form. Always remember that only the following are indefinite pronouns that are plural in form: *both, few, many, others,* and *several*. *All, any, more, most, none, some* may take singular or plural forms depending on the context of the sentence.
The queen, together with invited guests, face the media.	The queen, together with invited guests, faces the media.	The subject in this sentence is "queen". "Invited guests" is a noun of the intervening phrase that merely adds information about the subject. "Queen" is singular, so the verb should be also in its singular form, "faces".
Two-thirds of the project were assigned to me.	Two-thirds of the project was assigned to me.	When the subject is a fraction, the verb agrees with the noun in the of-phrase (i.e. "project").
The number of applicants remain unaccounted.	The number of applicants remains unaccounted.	*The number of* is always singular. *A number of* is always plural.

Errors in Noun-Pronoun Agreement

Rule: Pronouns should agree with their nouns in terms of number (singular or plural), person (first, second, or third), and gender (masculine or feminine).

Incorrect usage	Correct usage	Explanation
Did everyone remember their assignment?	Did everyone remember his assignment?	*Everyone* is singular, so the pronoun should be as well.
It was them who apologized.	It was they who apologized.	The nominative case (I, you, he, she, it, we, you, they, who) is used following some form of the verb *to be*.
If I were him, I would go.	If I were he, I would go.	As above.
It is me.	It is I.	As above.
Whom will succeed?	Who will succeed?	A simple rule-of-thumb is to use "who" when "he" would also make sense; and use "whom" when "him" would also make sense (e.g. "Him will succeed" does not sound right, while "he will succeed" does).
Who did you give it to?	Whom did you give it to?	As above. "You gave it to he" does not sound right, while "you gave it to him" does. Thus, use "whom".
It belongs to he and I.	It belongs to him and me.	The *objective* case of pronoun (i.e. me, you, him, her, it, us, you, them, whom) is used as the object of a preposition, such as "to".
Hugh fired he.	Hugh hired him.	The *objective* case of pronoun (i.e. me, you, him, her, it, us, you, them, whom) is used as the *object* of a verb.
He is as proficient as me.	He is as proficient as I.	Try stretching the sentence out: "He is as proficient as *I am proficient*, not "he is as proficient as *me am proficient*."
He was in the same class as us.	He was in the same class as we.	Try stretching the sentence out: "He was in the same class as *we were in*."
I trust Bob more than he.	I trust Bob more than him.	Try stretching the sentence out: "I trust Bob more than *I trust him*."
Now sing without me coaching you.	Now sing without my coaching you.	Use the *possessive* case of the pronoun (i.e. my, your, his, her, its, our, your, their, whose) in sentences like this.

Special Problems in Pronoun Agreement

Incorrect usage	Correct usage	Explanation
The movie was disappointing because *they* never made the plot seem realistic.	The *movie* was disappointing because *it* never made the plot seem realistic. The movie was disappointing because *the writers* never made the plot seem realistic.	Pronoun must agree with antecedents that are either clearly stated or understood. Otherwise, use a specific noun.
In 17th century England, *you* had to choose between following the Church or the King.	In 17th century England, *Puritans* had to choose between following the Church or the King.	Use *YOU* only when the reference is truly addressed to the reader.
Charles asked *William* about the state of his marriage. William tried to evade the topic, but confused about the situation, *he* tried to carry on a pleasant conversation.	*Charles* asked *William* about the state of his marriage. William tried to evade the topic, but confused about the situation, *Charles* tried to carry on a pleasant conversation.	Always use a pronoun close enough to its antecedent to avoid confusion.
I placed my passport in my bag, but I can't find *it*.	I placed my passport in my bag, but I can't find *my bag*.	Use pronouns to refer to an obvious antecedent.

Dangling Modifiers

Rule: Avoid dangling modifiers (i.e. adjectives or adverbs that do not refer to the noun or pronoun they are intended to refer to).

Incorrect usage	Correct usage	Explanation
While dialling the phone, the lights went out.	While *I was* dialling the phone, the lights went out.	The modifying phrase "while dialling the phone" does not refer to a particular noun or pronoun (i.e. it dangles).
After attending the mass, pizza was eaten.	After attending the mass, we ate pizza.	As above.

GAMSAT-Prep.com
THE GOLD STANDARD

Misplaced Modifiers

Incorrect usage	Correct usage	Explanation
Nina won almost 1 million euros.	Nina almost won 1 million euros.	The first sentence does not mean what it is intended to mean. The modifier "almost" is misplaced.
I only want you.	I want only you.	Same as above.

"Were" to be used in the Subjunctive Mood

Rule: Use *"were"* in the subjunctive mood, i.e. when expressing a wish, regret, or a condition that does not exist.

Incorrect usage	Correct usage	Explanation
If I was prettier, I would be famous.	If I were prettier, I would be famous.	This sentence is in the subjunctive mood.
Mum treats him as if he is a slave.	Mum treats him as if he were a slave.	As above.

That, Which, and Who

Incorrect usage	Correct usage	Explanation
This is the novel which he loved.	This is the novel that he loved.	When commas are not used, use "that".
This gown, that is designed by Monique, is expensive and elegant.	This gown, which is designed by Monique, is expensive and elegant.	When commas are used, use "which".
She is the person that designed the gown.	She is the person who designed the gown.	For persons, use "who". Do not use "who" for animals.
The President, which is an avid golfer, was on the course.	The President, who is an avid golfer, was on the course.	For persons, use "who", even when commas are used.

Note: Often the above pronouns can be omitted making a sentence more concise. Thus:

This is the novel he loved. ("That" is implied.) This gown, designed by Monique, is expensive and elegant. She designed the gown. The President, an avid golfer, was on the course.

Faulty Parallelism

Incorrect usage	Correct usage	Explanation
She likes to read, swim and shopping a lot.	She likes to read, swim and shop a lot. She likes to read, to swim and to shop a lot.	Similar ideas should be expressed in grammatically similar forms. (E.g., nouns with nouns, adjectives with adjectives, words with words, phrases with phrases)
The professor was asked to submit his report quick and accurately.	The professor was asked to submit his report quickly and accurately.	Similar ideas should be expressed in grammatically similar structures (i.e. same word order, consistent verb tenses).

Mixed Constructions

Incorrect usage	Correct usage	Explanation
Will asked Lizzie to marry him?	Will asked Lizzie to marry him?	Don't mix a statement with a question.
The reason is because I don't have a nanny.	The reason is that I don't have a nanny.	Don't mix two different sentence constructions.

Split Infinitives

Incorrect usage	Correct usage	Explanation
I need to mentally prepare.	I need to prepare mentally.	"To prepare" is an infinitive. Splitting infinitives with other words tends to be awkward.

Commas

Incorrect usage	Correct usage	Explanation
Uncle has money, wealth and power.	Uncle has money, wealth, and power.	Use a comma before the last item in a series to avoid any confusion.
The food was served late cold and smelly.	The food was served late, cold, and smelly.	Use commas to separate adjectives that could be joined with "and." You could say that "the food was served late and cold and smelly."
Jonas is a popular, varsity player.	Jonas is a popular varsity player.	Don't use commas to separate adjectives that could not be joined with "and." It would be ridiculous to say that " Jonas is a popular and varsity player."

GAMSAT-Prep.com
THE GOLD STANDARD

Incorrect usage	Correct usage	Explanation
You wait here, and I'll get your coat.	You wait here and I'll get your coat.	Don't use a comma to set off clauses that are short or have the same subject. However, always use a comma before "for", "so," and "yet" to avoid confusion.
The doctor gave detailed precise instructions to the nurse.	The doctor gave detailed, precise instructions to the nurse.	Use commas to separate adjectives of same or equal rank.
India has a rigid, social caste system.	India has a rigid social caste system.	Do not use commas to separate adjectives that must stay in a specific order.

Semicolons

Incorrect usage	Correct usage	Explanation
The car is old, however, it is in good condition.	The car is old; however, it is in good condition. The car is old; it is, however, in good condition.	Use a semicolon with a conjunctive adverb (e.g. nevertheless, however, otherwise, consequently, thus, therefore, meanwhile, moreover, furthermore).

Apostrophes

Correct usage	Explanation
Maggie Holmes' dog is lost. Maggie Holmes 's dog is lost.	Since there is disagreement on which is correct, both are acceptable.
The girl's doll fell in the mud. The girls' doll fell in the mud.	Common errors arise when apostrophes are misplaced in singular and plural nouns. In the first sentence, placing the apostrophe in between the noun and an *s* indicates a singular noun. In the second sentence, an apostrophe placed after a plural noun hints that the "doll" is commonly owned by at least two girls.

Troublesome Verbs

TRANSITIVE (followed by an object)	INTRANSITIVE (not followed by an object)
raise, raising, raised: The farmer is raising chickens.	**rise, rising, rose**: The moon is rising.
lay, laying, laid: I am laying the dress on the bed.	**lie, lying, lain**: I am lying on the bed.

"A" or "The"

Correct usage	Explanation
I dated **the** cheerleader back in college.	The definite article **the** is used when referring to a specific subject or member of a group. The speaker in the sentence could have been acquainted with many cheerleaders; but he was able to date only one particular cheerleader.
I dated **a** cheerleader back in college.	Use the indefinite article **a** to refer to a non-specific subject. The sentence implies that the speaker dated someone who could have been any member of a cheerleading group.

Proper Usage of *"The"*

• The Thames flow through Oxford and London. • The Gibson Desert is home to indigenous Australians. • Myths say that Santa Claus lives in the North Pole. • The equator is approximately 3,500 miles from the southernmost part of the United Kingdom. • The Chinese are hardworking people.	USE **the** when referring to • the proper names of rivers, oceans and seas; • deserts, forests, gulfs, and peninsulas • geographical areas • points on the globe • some countries like *the* Netherlands, *the* Dominican Republic, *the* Philippines, *the* United States • the people of a nation
Anna shops in Bond Street. Blue Lake attracts many tourists in Australia. St. Patrick's Island is a sanctuary for seabirds. Galtymore ranks 14th among Ireland's highest mountain peak. English is the main language used in the United Kingdom.	DO NOT USE **the** when referring to • street names • names of lakes except with a group of lakes • bays • most countries/territories but NOT cities, states or towns • names of mountains in general • names of continents • names of islands except with island chains • names of languages and nationalities

Verb or Participle

Not all verbs demonstrate an action. There are those that merely express a condition or an existence. These are called linking verbs. Words that describe (adjectives) or identify (another noun) should follow the linking verb.

Examples:

Incorrect Usage	Correct Usage
Nicole Kidman **sounds** sarcastically in the interview.	Nicole Kidman **sounds** sarcastic in the interview. The verb "sounds" expresses the state of emotions (sarcastic) of the subject (Nicole Kidman) at the time of the interview.
	Sir Edward Hallstrom **is** a philanthropist. The verb "is" connects the noun "philanthropist" to the subject "Sir Edward Hallstrom".

Participles are words that look like verbs but function in the sentence as nouns.

Example: **Exploring** Lake Argyle is one of the most wonderful outdoor adventures in Australia.
"Exploring" is a participle that functions as the noun-subject in the sentence and should not be confused with the main verb "is".

Common errors involving confusion between verbs and participles lead to **Sentence Fragments.**

Incorrect Usage	Correct Usage	Explanation
Dancing on her toes. The ballerina **was** superb.	**Dancing** on her toes, the ballerina **was** superb.	The main thought of the sentence is a description of the level of performance of the subject (ballerina) - "superb". The action word "dancing" merely adds information about what the subject (ballerina) does.

4.11 Section II Practice Worksheets

Section II Practice Worksheet I (Formulating the Thesis Statement)

Comment #	Repeated words	Ideas for or against the subject
1		
2		
3		
4		
5		
Topic:		
Theme or Issue:		
My Debatable Claim		

Section II Practice Worksheet I (Writing the Introduction)

This is where you express your interpretation of the comments' theme. You may state it as a direct statement or you may use a creative device.	
This is where you expound your ideas in relation to your initial statement by quoting or paraphrasing one or two of the given comments. Alternatively, you can continue discussing your narrative or metaphor.	
Your last sentence in the paragraph is your thesis statement. Make sure that it is clear, and it is debatable claim.	

Section II Practice Worksheet III (Task A Template)

Note: This template may also be used if you are more comfortable using an argumentative format for Writing Task B.

(Optional) Choose a title that summarises - in one short phrase - the overall idea of your essay.	
This is your introductory paragraph. Remember to include the following: - Aim to open with a catchy statement or anecdote - Express what the overall theme or one of the comments means to you - Include your debatable thesis statement in the last sentence of the paragraph (**Note:** Sometimes, if your introduction is too lengthy, you can discuss your thesis statement in the second paragraph.)	
In this paragraph, your aim is to explain and support your thesis statement. - Give one reason or argument in support of your thesis - Provide a concrete example or examples to support your argument - Explain how the examples relate to the argument	

This is where you present the strongest counterargument to your thesis. - Your counterargument should be related or parallel to the thesis' supporting example - Provide a clear illustration of your counter-argument's example.	
This is the paragraph where you show that your thesis' arguments are superior to the antithesis. Your aim here is to show that you have carefully considered all arguments for and against your idea and you have made up your mind to choose your arguments because it is better than the best opposition to it.	
This is your closing paragraph. - Summarise the main ideas discussed in the preceding paragraphs. - Tie up or reconcile conflicting ideas. - Propose your plan of action for the consideration of the reader - End with a memorable statement.	

Section II Practice Worksheet IV (Task B Template)

Note: This template may also be used if you are more comfortable using a personal piece for Writing Task A.

(Optional) Choose a title that summarises - in one short phrase - the overall idea of your essay.	
This is your introductory paragraph. Remember to explain: - what the comments mean to you. - why you agree or disagree with the comments idea. Briefly present your thesis statement towards the end of the paragraph.	
This is where you begin your personal narrative. It must be about an event that is pivotal in your life. It must also be relevant to the theme of the comments and/or your thesis.	

This is where you share your realisations from the personal narrative. Describe: - how you felt - how you thought and - what made you change your mind or point of view **There must be a 'before-and-after' description of your state of mind and state of heart.**	
This is where you state an application of your personal realisation. Cite a social problem that is relevant to your experience. How can your life-lesson serve as an inspiration to those who may be similarly situated? What new perspectives can you offer to the social problem that you cited?	

4.12 Samples of Excellent Essays

Writing Task A:

Comment 1

> Only when the last tree has died and the last river been poisoned and the last fish been caught will we realise we cannot eat money.
>
> Indian Cree Proverb

* * * * *

Comment 2

    Environmentally friendly cars will soon cease to be an option . . . they will become a necessity.

                                                                    Fujio Cho

* * * * *

Comment 3

    I would feel more optimistic about a bright future for man if he spent less time proving that he can outwit Nature and more time tasting her sweetness and respecting her seniority.

                                                          Elwyn Brooks White

* * * * *

Comment 4

    Every human has a fundamental right to an environment of quality that permits a life of dignity and well-being.

* * * * *

Comment 5

    After one look at this planet any visitor from outer space would say "I want to see the manager".

                                                         William S. Burroughs

THE AIR-CONDITIONED NIGHTMARE

    Such is the current global demand for energy that humanity now purportedly faces its greatest challenge: the growth of consumption while slowing and eventually reversing environmental impact. The issue surrounds developed society's inability to manage the exponential growth of consumption that has come with great affluence. In energy per capita, Australians consume 8 times the world average and a staggering 50 times the average of developing nations. Such figures are the premise of Toyota Chairman Fujio Cho's statement that, "Environmentally friendly cars will soon cease to be an option, they will become a necessity.' Cho's advocacy for efficiency is relevant in any age: why would any engineering-savvy civilisation opt for inefficient means of living when there are alternatives? Implicitly, Cho also warns of the impending end of the fossil fuel age and society's need to embrace what most would deem 'green' technology. While 'greener' technologies are the most promising technology for the long-term amelioration of our seemingly mutually exclusive aims of growing consumption and cleaning up the biosphere, it will be argued herein that in the medium-term, green technology is insufficient. Instead the solution to the current crisis entails words few would like to hear: the developed world needs to reduce its consumption.

Firstly, Cho's quote can be endorsed by a brief analysis of the energy requirements of the world, and the inherent inefficiencies in world energy use. When we talk of the world's energy needs, it is safe to reduce the discourse to that of the developed world due to its enormous proportion of world consumption (as detailed above). Developed nations consume most of the world's annual demand of 6×10^{20} joules of energy, and a significant amount is driven by desire rather than necessity. Ignoring the 75% of waste energy lost as heat in modern power plants, we will focus our discussion on the household and the individual. Many people continue to drive heavy vehicles with large capacity engines; build homes with minimum efficiency standards and live lifestyles that are unnecessarily energy intensive. For instance, most Australian and North American homes are built to the minimum standard utilising 2x4 inch framework while studies have shown that the price of a home built using 2x6 inch framework would only cost 5% more yet save 50% of the energy required for perpetual climate management. Cho's statement can be extrapolated from vehicles to – in this instance – houses and many other energy intensive aspects of life. For instance, studies have also shown that individuals will select an average air-conditioner temperature at a level low enough to trigger the desire for heating if the season were winter. On reflection of the current lifestyle of the affluent Westerner, it would appear that there is no perception of a necessity to restrict consumption and or become more efficient as Cho suggests.

Secondly, one becomes more sceptical of Cho's statement when his position and the state of fossil fuel capacity is considered critically. Despite the current schedule of communication, the world is not 'running out' of any of its resources if we consider this to mean the world will have no fossil fuels left in the medium term. Until the late nineteenth century, the primary fuel of the US remained wood (in China, this was the case until 1960) and it was not until the 1960's that the primary fuel of the great machine that is the USA became oil. The 20th century was very much the world's century of coal, not oil. The switch to oil as a primary fuel only came later due to easier access and efficiencies of energy generation. Today, the energy evolution continues and natural gas is becoming more popular due to the price of oil. Tomorrow, better extraction and refinement techniques –such as horizontal drilling - will see shale-gas/oil become a more economical alternative and this pattern will continue into the future: before the world runs out of any resource, it will become so expensive that demand for the resource on a global scale will reach zero. Cho is correct to say that cars and lifestyles in general need to become more efficient for the betterment of the environment, however his statement feels more like an endorsement of the current 'green' pandemic that many corporations have endorsed on the premise of positioning and selling their products.

The last two decades have witnessed an explosion in environmentally friendly products, institutions, government advisory bodies and even political parties such as the Greens. The purpose of the 'green' groundswell is noble: to prevent further destruction and pollution of the natural environment. Solutions such as solar, wind, geothermal and hydroelectric power are put forward by this movement in an attempt to unify growing consumption with environmental utopia. At the level of the household, these solutions are viable. For instance, much like water tanks, solar-powered households are able to consume electricity as desired as they have invested in technology that is future proofing their level of consumption. However, on a national scale this is not possible. On his Twitter account, scientist Dr. Karl Kruszelnicki recently endorsed plans for a 30-kilometre square solar farm in Africa's Sahara desert. The farm is the result of an energy think-tank and in theory is capable of supplying the world with a surplus of energy. In reality, there are no means of storing or transporting this amount of energy. The largest battery in the world can only store 1.3×10^{11} joules meaning virtually every citizen in the world would need one these batteries. Furthermore, there exist no global networks for energy distribution. The US estimates it would cost US$12 trillion to replace its own failing power grid habitually rated a D- in annual audits by civil engineers. Pragmatically, these considerations also apply to the hero electric product from Cho's Toyota corporation: the Prius. Toyota is not alone. GM also spent billions developing its Volt model and the Tesla was also developed by the US Tesla corporation at great cost. So far, sales of these vehicles have been much lower than forecast. Like much of the green movement's ideas, the products are more idealistic than functional. To date, there exists no network to publicly recharge such vehicles outside of the pioneering California state. More critically, the root resource of powering these vehicles remains fossil fuels. The same 25% efficiency steam-turbo generators that power our houses and pollute the atmosphere will be required to charge these electric cars. While all of these 'green' efforts are dignified and should remain in development, humanity should not be expecting them to become the primary source of energy for a long time – they remain in their infancy.

As the environmental programs of governments and private enterprise remain underdeveloped, the only solution for managing current environmental pressures and the emergence of developing nations is for the developed world to consume less. Efforts are already underway to mitigate consumption. While free-markets shoulder a significant portion of the responsibility for the destruction of the natural world, they are now effecting a redress. This can be seen in the pricing of emissions such as in Australia's move initially toward a carbon tax and now toward an emissions trading scheme. These policies are required as an interim measure to minimise the damage of fossil fuels while other technologies are developed. As in many areas of life, restrictions and parameters breed innovation and though many people will choose to ignore the increasing price of energy in the future, forced behaviour modification in the form of reduced consumption will be inevitable. It is an indictment on Western norms that we would prefer to work so hard to develop a host of new technologies rather than make what can only be defined as simple but effective modifications to mitigate our profligacy.

Writing Task B:

Comment 1

>Ambition makes you look pretty ugly.
>
>>Radiohead

* * * * *

Comment 2

>Ambition can creep as well as soar.
>
>>Edmund Burke

* * * * *

Comment 3

>Ambition has one heel nailed in well, though she stretch her fingers to touch the heavens.
>
>>Lao Tzu

* * * * *

Comment 4

>Ambition is pitiless. Any merit that it cannot use it finds despicable.
>
>>Eleanor Roosevelt

* * * * *

Comment 5

>All ambitions are lawful except those which climb upward on the miseries or credulities of mankind.
>
>>Joseph Conrad

WELL IS IT KNOWN THAT AMBITION CAN CREEP AS WELL AS SOAR

"Ambition makes you look pretty ugly", Thom Yorke wails in the song Paranoid Android by Radiohead. The lyric is perfectly demonstrative of the oxymoronic qualities of ambition: it can make one look pretty, yet also ugly. Edmund Burke was before Yorke's time, but he also expressed the dualistic notion of ambition when he stated it was capable of both 'creeping' and 'soaring'. So, what is the difference between virtuous and evil ambition? Some would say that ambition perpetrated to the resultant benefaction of humankind is virtuous, while 'that which climbs upwards on the miseries and credulities of mankind', to quote Joseph Conrad, is malignant. The following is an examination of ambition in the context of modern socioeconomics. Where ambition is given room for expression, the virtuosity of ambition is not black and white, it is an indiscrete continuum. Whether ambition is merited as benevolent or malevolent should be based on the effects it has on society, such as those experienced in the 2008 financial crisis.

Ambition can be used for evil as much as it can for good. When ambition takes on qualities extending beyond the general desire to succeed, undesirable traits such as egomania and indifference ensue. This was evidenced by the collapse of the entire world economic system in late 2008. The collapse was caused by a minute group of investment bankers from corporations such as Goldman Sachs and Lehman Brothers. These investment banks - like most companies - are run for the profit of their shareholders, and rightly so. However, sometime in the early-mid noughties, the investment banker's ambition bulged greedily, and grew excessively bold: they decided they would continue to make sub-prime mortgage loans to people they knew could never pay them back. The mortgages were then hastily packaged up, and sold as securities to everyday investors to absolve the banks of risk. The bankers heeded the insatiable Gordon Gecko mantra, "greed is good" and before anyone realised the gravity of the situation, the unfettered ambition of the Wall Street plutocrats had already caused devastation to the lives of millions.

The evils of hyper-ambition were on display at the US Congressional trials of investment oligarchs Richard Fuld and Lloyd Blankfein, both of whom have taken home a collective US $ 1 billion in bonuses in their time. The heads of the aforementioned banking firms admitted to selling - in their companies own words - 'shitty' deals to retirement investment funds, and then 'shorting' those deals, effectively betting that the investments would fail. Basically, the enterprise the banks operated was akin to taking your vehicle to a mechanic, the mechanic filling your car with cooking oil, taking your money and then betting with a third-party that your car will not last a week on the road - though on a huge scale. For any ambitious enterprise to be considered positive, it must pay dividends to both the pursuing individual or individuals, and society at large.

While the bankers rode ambition to its lowest form, another man demonstrated a great and benevolent form of ambition in the establishment of a not-for-profit organisation that directly attacked the injustices of the world; that man was Julian Assange, and his organisation is Wikileaks. Assange saw the injustices of the world - ironically some of which were actually caused by ambition - perpetrated by authority and was compelled to deliver a solution. Due to Assange's ambitious, and dangerous, quest to deliver justice and truth, the citizens of the world now have a conduit through which to expose injustice and malpractice. If it were not for Assange's deep desire and vision, the world would be a more opaque place.

So, if Assange's ambition was just as grand as that of the Wall Street bankers, what is the difference?

One may be inclined to disagree with the evils of the investment bankers; one could well argue that their actions were intensified by the continued deregulation of the money markets. One could argue further that the actions and ambition of Assange have placed more lives at risk than they have saved as vested information becomes public domain. Despite these arguments, it is quite clear that ambition, in the case of the bankers, was far more detrimental to society than any negative effects propagated by Wikileaks. This is the difference: the fact that the ambition of the bankers was almost purely self-serving at the expense of a huge portion of society. In what would seem contrary to the crimes, Assange is currently holed-up in an Ecuadorian embassy in London fleeing persecution from the USA while investment bankers have not faced a single conviction, and continue to enjoy their massive bonuses. While the virtue of ambition should be based on how it manifests itself in society, it seems in modern times the world has quite a perverted discretion when it comes to judging the ambitious. The world would be a much greater place if, like Assange, the ambitious gave more than they took.

Writing Task A:

Comment 1

> Education is what remains after one has forgotten what one has learned in school.
>
> Albert Einstein

* * * * *

Comment 2

> Education is an admirable thing, but it is well to remember from time to time that nothing worth knowing can be taught.
>
> Oscar Wilde

Comment 3

    We must remember that intelligence is not enough. Intelligence plus character - that is the goal of true education.

                                                    Martin Luther King, Jr.

* * * * *

Comment 4

    Educating the mind without educating the heart is no education at all.

                                                    Aristotle

* * * * *

Comment 5

    The aim of education should be to teach us rather how to think, than what to think.

                                                  Bill Beattie

KNOWLEDGE

    Wilde's statement seems to define education quite narrowly as a formal means of training within an academy. While Wilde admits that a formal education by teachers can teach one many things, most of them are without value when compared to the teachings one receives at the hands of experience. For the purpose of the following, we will use Wilde's definition, even though education is occasionally attributed to those with great intelligence who have never received formal training. On the matter of knowledge, as Wilde implies, experience is a greater contributor than formal education.

    Firstly, it is a non sequitur that those holding certification of an academy possess knowledge. Often, formal education only enables one to attain knowledge within a certain context. It follows that this knowledge attained within academic boundaries often fails to apply to the complexities of real issues; these issues require experience. A chief economist or foreign minister hold great executive powers not because they are well-educated; rather, because they are well-educated and heavily experienced. When this author departed university wielding an Honours degree in business, he quickly found that he would have to begin a new educational experience: how to apply his skills in a real business. This experience is common to many graduates leaving the comfort of university; they must teach themselves and be sunned at the furnace of life. This is the essence of Wilde's quote: nothing worth knowing can be learnt from another.

Secondly, it is no wonder society has no school or academy for equipping people with the many skills necessary for a happy and successful life; many of these skills are simply impossible to formally teach. For instance, one can study to be a doctor, a pilot, a builder or a dancer; however humanity is horribly uneducated when it comes to dealing with an instinct such as love, failure, personal tragedy or courage. All of these experiences or traits are developed as a result of one's personal vicarious contact with the world; they are impossible to teach in the classroom. Sporting aptitude and other physical aptitudes - such as musicianship - that many learn from birth are also impossible to learn via dictation. Testament to Wilde's statement is that his insight can be applied on many levels. While the skill of loving or overcoming failure cannot be taught, neither can the aptitude of acquiring such skills.

While a person's experience is unquestionably important, some would argue that the acquisition of knowledge can, and is attained directly from others. Many have learned a great deal from the professors of the world, however those purporting this argument would likely emphasise the more important knowledge learned from family and close confidantes. For example, one's parents may set a great example of how to build long-lasting relationships or how to persevere through hardship. On reflection of Wilde's quote, he would likely argue that through interaction with one's parents, one is receiving that lived, hands-on experience that is the premise for knowledge. For instance, when one's parents fight or divorce, a child may witness and learn a valuable lesson about relationships; however, the greatest and most important lesson impressed upon them are the new feelings and circumstances they face. Though the lesson was catalysed by their parents, the child is faced with his own vicarious learning experience that is a platform for further personal growth.

Certainly no formal means of education could ever teach one how to build or indeed manage a relationship; this can only be learnt in the midst of real life. Therefore, while education is necessary in helping one attain the specific knowledge in what is likely to be an economic vocation, it is exceedingly rare that it can teach one how to manage life's most arduous and testing of times. To be well equipped for these, one needs to have experienced and built a panoply of robust skills in the real world. Without doing so, one would be worryingly underequipped to face many of life's great challenges.

Writing Task B:

Comment 1

> The only way to get through life is to laugh your way through it.
>
> Marjorie Pay Hinckley

* * * * *

Comment 2

> There's no life without humour. It can make the wonderful moments of life truly glorious, and it can make tragic moments bearable.
>
> Rufus Wainwright

* * * * *

Comment 3

> Humour is the weapon of unarmed people: it helps people who are oppressed to smile at the situation that pains them.
>
> Simon Wiesenthal

* * * * *

Comment 4

> Every survival kit should include a sense of humor.

* * * * *

Comment 5

> If I had no sense of humor, I would long ago have committed suicide.
>
> Mahatma Gandhi

My brother died when he was only 6 years old. It was the 5th of August. He fell from a window as he was trying to 'fly'. His death was so sudden and so unexpected. We could not comprehend it and for the first few days, all we could do was shed tears. I shed tears when I was alone and when I caught my sister's eye. I could not keep myself from crying. The loss was so real, it brought on a hollow kind of feeling in my stomach, an emptiness that was gnawing at my insides.

At his funeral, my father was inconsolable. My Dad was a joker. He usually cracked jokes and teased us. For the first time in my life, I saw my father shed tears. My father was sobbing. My brothers, sister and I were all seated together during the service. My father was seated across from us. As we were listening to the eulogy, my father started crying – he was bawling like a child whose favourite toy got broken, a child who had skinned his knee and was crying for his mum. We stopped and stared at my Dad. Tears were still streaming down our faces but my father's sobs got our attention. We started laughing at the sight of my Dad's face: red and contorted with his sobs. He looked like a clown.

It was so out of place, the sound of our laughter at the funeral service. It was so contradictory, the sound of our laughter while my Dad was wracked with sobs. But we couldn't help it – my Dad's face looked so funny as he sobbed. We have never seen him cry before and we found it funny to see our Dad shedding tears like a child – like ourselves. Pretty soon, my Dad looked at us – wondering what we found so funny. We couldn't tell him – we all tried to contort our faces imitating the way he looked when he was crying and we all started laughing.

When we first learned that my brother had died, I wondered to myself if we would come out of that situation intact – if we would fall apart, if we would become bitter or deathly afraid. I wondered if any of us would get depressed or anxious. A death in the family – it alters the family. Grief alters people. When I started laughing at my brother's funeral, I had a fleeting thought that I was becoming unhinged. I was afraid that I was falling apart, but then, I also felt relief. I knew that we would be alright at some point in the future. I was crying now, but the fact that I could still see something funny and laugh at it could only mean that my brother's death had not unhinged me.

It was alright, I realised, to feel the hurt, to grieve and to mourn, to cry and shed tears – the death and loss of someone so dear is reason enough for all that. However, I also realised that the grief will someday lose its sharpness until it becomes a dull ache and then, a memory and a sigh. It will leave a mark on us but we had a choice as to how our grief will mark us. I realised that we could let the grief overwhelm and overshadow us, or else, we could let it motivate us to cherish each other more because life is so short and death is so sure. We could live our lives so afraid of death, or we could live our lives thankful for another day.

Every August 5th, I remember my brother. I remember his death, and the grief has become a dull ache. Every April 11th – my brother's birthday, I mark just how old he would have been. I sigh. The grief is still real but it has lost its power over me. My grief has been transformed by time. It is now mingled with hope. I realise that I too will die someday, and it doesn't seem as scary as it did years before. When I think of dying, I feel sad at the pain my death will inflict on those I love and those who love me and who will miss me. But with this sadness, there is also a hope that death will not be so uncertain – I can look forward to being with my brother.

I realise that I cannot control life or death, I cannot predict when death will come or how it will come. Death can come when we least expect it. Grief is intense and the loss is often unfathomable. However, the grief passes, too. Grief is a process that one must go through. Grief however, does not need to rob me of my joy forever. The ability to laugh in the midst of grief, even at the most trivial things - is a sign of hope that grief will pass and laughter will become more precious, more intense because it provides a counterpoint to the grief. When I can still laugh even in the midst of my grief, it only means that I am coping and doing my best to mend what death has broken inside me.

> If you give a sincere effort and really develop content for sections 4.5.1, 4.5.2, 4.6.1, 4.6.2 and 4.11, then in the days and hours leading up to the GAMSAT, reviewing that content will be one of your most valuable tools to optimize your Section II GAMSAT score. Good luck!

UNDERSTANDING THE GAMSAT

PROLOGUE TO GAMSAT SECTION 3

Common Root Words of Scientific Terms

The following is a list of root words, prefixes, and suffixes, which you may find helpful for GAMSAT Section 3 review, problems and/or tests. Of course, a prefix is a group of letters added to the beginning of a word; a suffix is added to the end of a word.

Prefixes

A
aden- gland
adip- fat
aero- air
agri- field; soil
alb- white
alg-/algia- pain
alto- high
ambi- both
ameb- change; alternation
amni- fetal membrane
amphi-; ampho- both
amyl- starch
ana- up; back; again
andro- man; masculine
anemo- wind
angi- blood vessel; duct
ante- before; ahead of time
anter- front
antho- flower
anthropo- man; human
aqu- water
archaeo- primitive; ancient
arteri- artery
arthr- joint; articulation
aster-; astr- ; astro- star
ather- fatty deposit
atmo- vapor
audi- hear

aur- ear
auto- self

B
bacter-/bactr- bacterium; stick; club
baro- weight
bath- depth; height
bene- well; good
bi- (Latin) two; twice
bi-/bio- (Greek) life; living
brachi- arm
brachy- short
brady- slow
branchi- fin
bronch- windpipe

C
calor- heat
capill- hair
capit- head
carcin- cancer
cardi-/cardio- heart
carn- meat; flesh
carp- fruit
carpal- wrist
cata- breakdown; downward
caud- tail
cente- pierce
centi- hundredth

centr- center
cephal- head
cerat- horn
cerebr- brain
cervic- neck
chel- claw
chem- dealing with chemicals
chir- hand
chlor- green
chondr- cartilage
chrom-/chromo- color
chron- time
circa-; circum- around; about
cirru- hairlike curls
co- with; together
cocc- seed; berry
coel- hollow
coll- glue
coni- cone
contra- against
corp- body
cort-/cortic- outer layer
cosmo- world; order; form
cotyl- cup
counter- against
crani- skull
cresc-/cret- begin to grow
crypt- hidden; covered

Prefixes

cumul- heaped
cuti- skin
cyt- cell; hollow container

D
dactyl- finger
deca- ten
deci- tenth
deliquesc- become fluid
demi- half
dendr- tree
dent- tooth
derm- skin
di-/dipl- (Latin) two; double
di-/dia- (Greek) through; across; apart
dia- (Latin) day
digit- finger; toe
din- terrible
dis- apart; out
dorm- sleep
dors- back
du-/duo- two
dynam- power
dys- bad; abnormal; difficult

E
ec- out of; away from
echin- spiny; prickly
eco- house
ecto- outside of
en-/endo-/ent- in; into; within
encephal- brain
enter- intestine; gut
entom- insects
epi- upon; above; over

erythro- red
eso- inward; within; inner

F
ferro- iron
fibr- fiber; thread
fiss- split
flor- flower
flu-; fluct-; flux flow
foli- leaf
fract- break

G
gastr- stomach
geo- land; earth
gloss- tongue
gluc-/glyc- sweet; sugar
glut- buttock
gnath- jaw
gymno- naked; bare
gyn- female
gyr- ring; circle; spiral

H
halo- salt
hapl- simple
hecto- hundred
hem- blood
hemi- half
hepar/hepat- liver
herb- grass; plants
hetero- different; other
hex- six
hibern- winter
hidr- sweat
hipp- horse
hist- tissue
holo- entire; whole
homo- (Latin) man; human
homo- (Greek) same; alike
hort- garden
hydr- water
hygr- moist; wet
hyper- above; beyond; over
hyph- weaving; web
hypno- sleep
hypo- below; under; less
hyster- womb; uterus

I
ichthy- fish
infra- below; beneath
inter- between
intra- within; inside
iso- equal; same

K
kel- tumor; swelling
kerat- horn
kilo- thousand
kine- move

L
lachry- tear
lact- milk
lat- side
leio- smooth
leuc-/leuk- white; bright; light
lign- wood
lin- line
lingu- tongue
lip- fat
lith-; -lite stone; petrifying

Prefixes

loc- place
lumin- light

M
macr- large
malac- soft
malle- hammer
mamm- breast
marg- border; edge
mast- breast
med- middle
meg- million; great
mela-/melan- black; dark
mes- middle; half; intermediate
met-/meta- between; along; after
micro- small; millionth
milli- thousandth
mis- wrong; incorrect
mito- thread
mole- mass
mono- one; single
mort- death
morph- shape; form
multi- many
mut- change
my- muscle
myc- fungus
mycel- threadlike
myria- many
moll- soft

N
nas- nose
necr- corpse; dead
nemat- thread
neo- new; recent
nephro- kidney

neur- nerve
noct-/nox- night
non- not
not- back
nuc- center

O
ob- against
ocul- eye
oct- eight
odont- tooth
olf- smell
oligo- few; little
omni- all
onc- mass; tumor
opthalm- eye
opt- eye
orb- circle; round; ring
ornith- bird
orth- straight; correct; right
oscu- mouth
oste- bone
oto- ear
ov-/ovi- egg
oxy- sharp; acid; oxygen

P
pachy - thick
paleo- old; ancient
palm- broad; flat
pan- all
par-/para- beside; near; equal
path- disease; suffering
pent- five
per- through
peri- around
permea- pass; go
phag- eat

pheno- show
phon- sound
photo- light
phren- mind; diaphragm
phyc- seaweed; algae
phyl- related group
physi- nature; natural qualities
phyt- plant
pino- drink
pinni- feather
plan- roaming; wandering
plasm- formed into
platy- flat
pleur- lung; rib; side
pneumo- lungs; air
poly- many; several
por- opening
port- carry
post- after; behind
pom- fruit
pre- before; ahead of time
prim- first
pro- forward; favoring; before
proto- first; primary
pseudo- false; deceptive
psych- mind
pter- having wings or fins
pulmo- lung
puls- drive; push
pyr- heat; fire

Q
quadr- four
quin- five

Prefixes

R
radi- ray
ren- kidney
ret- net; made like a net
rhe- flow
rhin- nose
rhiz- root
rhodo- rose
roto- wheel
rubr- red

S
sacchar- sugar
sapr- rotten
sarc- flesh
saur- lizard
schis-/schiz- split; divide
sci- know
scler- hard
semi- half; partly
sept- partition; seven
sex- six
sol- sun
solv- loosen; free
som-/somat- body
somn- sleep
son- sound
spec-/spic- look at
spir- breathe

stat- standing; staying
stell- stars
sten- narrow
stern- chest; breast
stom- mouth
strat- layer
stereo- solid;
   3-dimensional
strict- drawn tight
styl- pillar
sub- under; below
super-/sur- over; above;
   on top
sym-/syn- together

T
tachy- quick; swift
tarso- ankle
tax- arrange; put in order
tele- far off; distant
telo- end
terr- earth; land
tetr- four
thall- young shoot
toxico- poison
top- place
trache- windpipe
trans- across

tri- three
trich- hair
turb- whirl

U
ultra- beyond
uni- one
ur- urine

V
vas- vessel
vect- carry
ven-/vent- come
ventr- belly; underside
vig- strong
vit-/viv- life
volv- roll; wander

X
xanth- yellow
xero- dry
xyl- wood

Z
zo- animal
zyg- joined together
zym- yeast

Suffixes

A
-ap/-aph -touch
-ary/-arium -place for
   something
-ase -forms names of
   enzymes

B
-blast -sprout; germ;
   bud

C
-cell -chamber; small
   room

-chrome -color
-chym -juice
-cid/-cis -cut; kill; fall
-cul/-cule -small;
   diminutive
-cyst -sac; pouch;
   bladder

PROLOGUE TO GAMSAT SECTION 3

-cyte -cell; hollow container

D
-duct -lead

E
-elle -small
-emia -blood
-en -made of
-eous -nature of; like
-err -wander; go astray

F
-fer -bear; carry; produce
-fid -divided into
-flect/-flex -bend

G
-gam -marriage
-gene -origin; birth
-gest -carry; produce; bear
-glen -eyeball
-glob -ball; round
-gon -angle; corner

H
-hal/-hale -breathe; breath
-helminth -worm

I
-iac -person afflicted with disease
-iasis -disease; abnormal condition
-ism -a state or condition
-ist -person who deals with...
-itis -inflammation; disease

-ium -refers to a part of the body

K
-kary -cell nucleus

L
-less -without
-log -word; speech
-logist -one who studies...
-logy -study of...
-lys/-lyt/-lyst -decompose; split; dissolve

M
-mer -part
-meter/-metry measurement
-mot -move

N
-ner -moist; liquid
-node -knot
-nom/-nomy -ordered knowledge; law

O
-oid -form; appearance
-oma -abnormal condition; tumor
-orium/-ory -place for something
-osis -abnormal condition

P
-pathy -disease; suffering
-ped -foot
-ped -child
-phil -loving; fond of
-phone -sound

-phore; pher -bear; carry
-phyll -leaf
-phyte -plant
-plast -form
-pod -foot

R
-rrhage -burst forth
-rrhea -flow

S
-scop -look; device for seeing
-septic -infection; putrefaction
-sis -condition; state
-sperm -seed
-spher -ball; round
-spire -breathe
-spor -seed
-stasis -placed
-stome -mouth

T
-the/-thes -put
-thel -cover a surface
-therm -heat
-tom -cut; slice
-trop -turn; change
-troph -nourishment; one who feeds

U
-ul/-ule -diminutive; small
-ura -tail

V
-verge -turn; slant
-vor -devour; eat

Z
-zoa -animal

GAMSAT-Prep.com
THE GOLD STANDARD

The Natural Order to Learn Science

This textbook is arranged such that each section presumes that you have completed your review of the previous section.

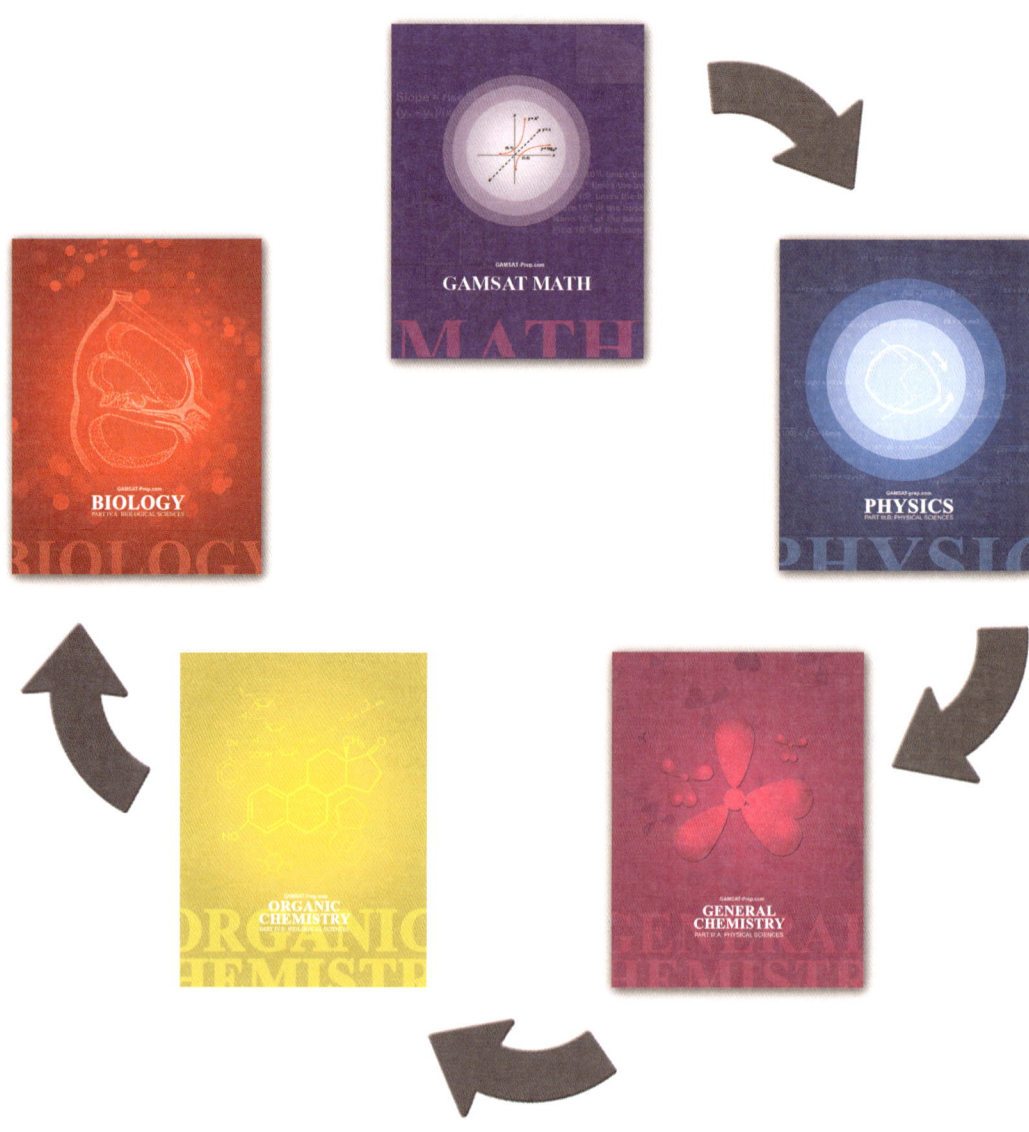

GAMSAT-Prep.com

GAMSAT MATH

NUMBERS AND OPERATIONS
Chapter 1

Memorize	Understand	Not Required
Properties of Real Numbers Order of Operations Rules on Zero Important Fraction-Decimal Conversions Properties of Exponents Common squares and cubes of integers	* Integer, Rational, and Real Numbers * Basic Operations and Definitions * Fractions, Mixed Numbers, Decimals and Percentages * Exponent Manipulations * Ratios and Proportions	* Advanced Level Math * Memorizing mathematical terms

GAMSAT-Prep.com

Introduction

There will never be a GAMSAT question where you would need to know mathematical terms in order to get the right answer (i.e. terms such as 'rational numbers' or 'integers' or 'associative laws', etc.). However, if we are to have an understanding of the math used in the GAMSAT then, for some students, we will need to start with the basics. If the math is too basic for you, either skim through until it gets to your level, or at least complete the practice questions at the end of the chapters to ensure that you are up to speed.

Additional Resources

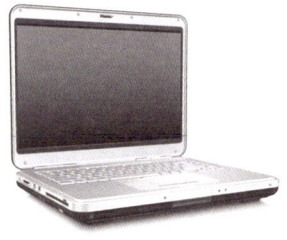

Free Online Forum

Special Guest

GAMSAT MATH   GM-03

GAMSAT-Prep.com
THE GOLD STANDARD

1.1 Integers, Rational Numbers, and the Number Line

1.1.1 Integers

Integers are whole numbers without any decimal or fractional portions. They can be any number from negative to positive infinity including zero.

> **EXAMPLES** −2, −1, 0, 1, 2, 3 etc.

1.1.2 Rational Numbers

Rational numbers are numbers that can be written as fractions of integers. "Rational" even contains the word "ratio" in it, so if you like, you can simply remember that these are ratio numbers.

EXAMPLES

$$\frac{1}{2}$$

$$-5 \left(-5 = \frac{-5}{1} \right)$$

$$1.875 \left(1.875 = \frac{15}{8} \right)$$

> **NOTE**
> Every integer is also a rational number, but not every rational number is an integer. You can write them as fractions simply by dividing by 1.

Make sure you are extra careful when ratios and fractions are involved because they are notorious for causing mistakes.

Irrational numbers are numbers that cannot be written as fractions of integers. Irrational numbers are normally numbers that have a decimal number that goes on forever with no repeating digits.

EXAMPLES

$\sqrt{2} = 1.4142135623730950...$

$Pi = \pi = 3.14159265358979...$

$e = 2.718281828459045...$

For GAMSAT math, it is expected that you have memorized pi to 3.14 and you will work faster during the exam if you recognize root 2 as 1.4 and root 3 as 1.7.

We will discuss the number *e* in context (natural logs) in Chapter 3.

1.1.3 Real Numbers and the Number Line

Real numbers are all numbers that can be represented on the number line. These include both rational and irrational numbers.

EXAMPLES

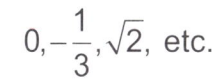
$0, -\frac{1}{3}, \sqrt{2}$, etc.

The **number line** is an infinite straight line on which every point corresponds to a real number. As you move up the line to the right, the numbers get larger, and down the line to the left, the numbers get smaller.

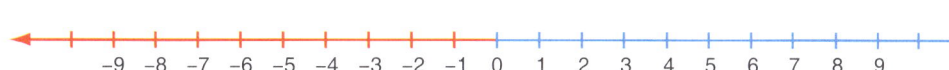

1.2 Basic Arithmetic

1.2.1 Basic Operations

An **operation** is a procedure that is applied to numbers. The fundamental operations of arithmetic are addition, subtraction, multiplication, and division.

A **sum** is the number obtained by adding numbers.

EXAMPLE

The sum of 7 and 2 is 9 since $2 + 7 = 9$.

A **difference** is the number obtained by subtracting numbers.

EXAMPLE

In the equation $7 - 2 = 5$, 5 is the difference of 7 and 2.

A **product** is the number obtained by multiplying numbers.

EXAMPLE

The product of 7 and 2 is 14 since $7 \times 2 = 14$.

A **quotient** is the number obtained by dividing numbers.

EXAMPLE

In the equation 8 ÷ 2 = 4, 4 is the quotient of 8 and 2.

> Unlike a sum or a product, difference and quotient can result in different numbers depending on the order of the numbers in the expression:
>
> 10 − 2 = 8 while 2 − 10 = −8
> 20 ÷ 5 = 4 while 5 ÷ 20 = 0.25

The sum and difference of positive numbers are obtained by simple addition and subtraction, respectively. The same is true when adding negative numbers, except that the sum takes on the negative sign.

EXAMPLES

(-3) + (-9) = -12

(-5) + (-12) + (-44) = -61

On the other hand, when adding two integers with unlike signs, you need to ignore the signs first, and then subtract the smaller number from the larger number. Then follow the sign of the larger number in the result.

EXAMPLES

(-6) + 5 = 6 − 5 = -1

7 + (-10) = 10 − 7 = - 3

When subtracting two numbers of unlike signs, start by changing the minus sign into its reciprocal, which is the plus sign. Next reverse the sign of the second number. This will make the signs of the two integers the same. Now follow the rules for adding integers with like signs.

EXAMPLES

(-6) − 5 = (-6) + (-5) = -11

7 − (-10) = 7 + 10 = 17

Multiplication and division of integers are governed by the same rules: If the numbers have like signs, the product or quotient is positive. If the numbers have unlike signs, the answer is negative.

EXAMPLES

$5 \times 6 = 30$
$-5 \times -3 = 15$
$81 \div 9 = 9$
$-20 \div -4 = 5$
$7 \times -4 = -28$
$-9 \times 6 = -54$
$-15 \div 3 = -5$
$16 \div -2 = -8$

An **expression** is a grouping of numbers and mathematical operations.

EXAMPLE

2 + (3 × 4) × 5 is a mathematical expression.

An **equation** is a mathematical sentence consisting of two expressions joined by an equals sign. When evaluated properly, the two expressions must be equivalent.

EXAMPLE

$2 \times (1+3) = \frac{16}{2}$ is an equation since the expressions on both sides of the equals sign are equivalent to 8.

> **NOTE**
>
> Whenever you see simple calculations in these chapters, take the time to make sure that you are able to make the presented calculations quickly and efficiently. We know that you have learnt all of these skills before, we just want to firmly rebuild your foundation for more complex, speed-driven, GAMSAT-level math.

1.2.1.1 Summary of Properties of Positive and Negative Integers

Positive + Positive = Positive

$5 + 4 = 9$

Negative + Negative = Negative

$(-6) + (-2) = -8$

Positive + Negative = Sign of the highest number and then subtract

$(-5) + 4 = -1$
$(-8) + 10 = 2$

Negative − Positive = Negative

$(-7) - 10 = -17$

Positive − Negative = Positive + Positive = Positive

$6 - (-4) = 6 + 4 = 10$

Negative − Negative = Negative + Positive = Sign of the highest number and then subtract

$(-8) - (-7) = (-8) + 7 = -1$

Negative × Negative = Positive

$(-2) \times (-5) = 10$

Positive/Positive = Positive

$8/2 = 4$

Negative × Positive = Negative

$(-9) \times 3 = -27$

Positive/Negative = Negative

$64/(-8) = -8$

1.2.2 Properties of the Real Numbers

Whenever you are working within the real numbers, these properties hold true. It isn't necessary to memorize the name of each property, but you must be able to apply them all.

Symmetric Property of Equality: The right and left hand sides of an equation are interchangeable, so if $a = b$, then $b = a$.

Transitive Property of Equality: If $a = b$ and $b = c$, then $a = c$. This means that if you have two numbers both equal to one other number, those two numbers are also equal.

Commutative Property of Addition: When adding numbers, switching the position of the numbers will not change the outcome, so $a + b = b + a$.

Associative Property of Addition: When adding more than two numbers, it doesn't matter what order you do the addition in, so $(a + b) + c = a + (b + c)$.

Commutative Property of Multiplication: When multiplying numbers, switching the position of the numbers will not change the outcome, so $a \times b = b \times a$.

Associative Property of Multiplication: When multiplying more than two numbers, it doesn't matter what order you do the multiplication in, so $(a \times b) \times c = a \times (b \times c)$.

Identity Property of Addition: When zero is added or subtracted to any number, the answer is the number itself, so $10b - 0 = 10b$.

Identity Property of Multiplication: When a number is multiplied or divided by 1, the answer is the number itself, so $6a \times 1 = 6a$.

Distributive Property of Multiplication: When multiplying a factor on a group of numbers that are being added or subtracted, the factor may be distributed by multiplying it by each number in the group, so $a(b - c) = ab - ac$.

> Subtraction and division do not follow associative laws.

1.2.3 Order of Operations

Knowing the order of operations is fundamental to evaluating numerical expressions. If you follow it properly, you will always come up with the correct answer! Here it is in list form, to be followed from the top down:

Parentheses
Exponents (including square roots)
Multiplication
Division
Addition
Subtraction

This forms the simple acronym **PEMDAS**, which is a great way to keep the operations straight. Alternatively, some people find it easier to remember the phrase "**P**lease **E**xcuse **M**y **D**ear **A**unt **S**ally."

If you don't like either of these techniques, feel free to come up with your own. It's important to have this down because, as simple as it may seem, being able to carry out the order of operations quickly is crucial.

Using PEMDAS, let's evaluate this expression composed only of integers.

$$2^2 + [(3 + 2) \times 2 - 9]$$

First, evaluate the expression contained in the inner set of parentheses.

$$= 2^2 + [(5) \times 2 - 9]$$

You can then choose to strictly follow the PEMDAS order by evaluating the exponent next. Alternately, you can perform the operations within the square brackets, working your way outward, for a more organized procedure as follows:

First, perform the multiplication.

$$= 2^2 + (10 - 9)$$

Then, perform the subtraction.

$$= 2^2 + 1$$

Now evaluate the exponent.

$$= 4 + 1$$

Finally, evaluate the remaining expression.

$$= 5$$

> **NOTE**
>
> - Multiplication and division have the same rank. It is generally recommended to do them in order from left to right as they appear in the expression, but you can also do them in whatever order that makes most sense to you.
> - The same goes for addition and subtraction. Execute them from left to right, or in the order that feels most comfortable.
> - When you encounter nested parentheses, evaluate the innermost ones first then work your way outward.

GAMSAT-Prep.com
THE GOLD STANDARD

1.3 Rules on Zero

1.3.1 Addition and Subtraction with Zero

Zero is a unique number, and it has special properties when it comes to operations.

Zero is known as the **additive identity** of the real numbers since whenever it is added to (or subtracted from) a number, that number does not change.

Let's examine a simple expression.

$$(3 + 2) - 4$$

We can add or subtract zero anywhere within the expression and the value will not change:

$$(3 - 0 + 2) - 4 + 0$$
$$= (3 + 2) - 4$$

The addition or subtraction of the two zeros has no effect whatsoever on the outcome.

1.3.2 Multiplication and Division with Zero

When adding zero in an expression, it is easy to come up with a practical picture of what the operation represents; you begin with a collection of things and add zero more things to them. When multiplying and dividing with zero, however, such a conceptualization is more difficult. The idea of using zero in this manner is far more abstract.

Fortunately, you don't need to wrestle with trying to picture what multiplication or division with zero looks like. You can simply remember these easy rules:

Multiplying by Zero: The result of multiplying any quantity by zero is *always* equal to zero.

Remember that by the commutative property of multiplication, $a \times b = b \times a$, so if we let $b = 0$, then we have $a \times 0 = 0 \times a$. This means that instead of trying to imagine multiplying a number by zero, you can reverse the thought and consider multiplying zero by a number instead. This second statement is more natural to visualize. You start with nothing, and then no matter how many times you duplicate that nothing, you still end up with nothing.

EXAMPLE

$3 \times 0 = 0$

$123.79 \times 0 = 0$

$\left[1.2 + \left(37 - \sqrt{5}\right) \times 2.331\right] \times 0$

In the last example, there is no need to go through the order of operations and evaluate the expression inside the parentheses. Because you can see immediately that the entire parenthetical expression is being multiplied by zero, you know that the end result will be zero.

Zero Divided by a Number: The result of dividing zero by any quantity is *always* equal to zero. As with multiplication by zero, if you start with nothing and then take a portion of that nothing, you still end up with nothing.

EXAMPLE

$0 \div 3 = 0$

$0 \div 123.79 = 0$

$0 \div \left[1.2 + \left(37 - \sqrt{5}\right) \times 2.331\right] = 0$

Just like with the multiplication by zero example, you do not need to evaluate the parenthetical expression in order to know that the solution is zero.

Dividing by Zero: Dividing any nonzero quantity by zero results in a solution that is not defined and is therefore undefined.

You should never have to deal with this case on the GAMSAT. If you end up with division by zero in a calculation, you have probably made a mistake. Similarly, you should never end up with zero divided by zero (an undefined quantity). If you do, you should go back and check your work.

1.4 Fractions, Decimals, and Percentages

1.4.1 Fractions

A **fraction** is the quotient of two numbers. It represents parts of a whole and may be seen as a proportion. The number on top is the *numerator*, and the one on the bottom is the *denominator*. Another way of understanding fractions is to consider one as the number of parts present (*numerator*) and the amount of parts it takes to make up a whole (*denominator*). These values can be divided by each other, and this fraction is the quotient.

EXAMPLE

$$\frac{2}{7}$$

In this fraction, 2 is the numerator and 7, the denominator.

Remember, all rational numbers (including integers) can be written as fractions.

1.4.2 Manipulating Fractions

A. Fraction Multiplication

To multiply fractions, simply multiply the numerators together (this will be the new numerator) and then multiply the denominators together (this will be the new denominator).

EXAMPLE

$$\frac{2}{3} \times \frac{4}{5}$$

Multiply the numerators and denominators separately.

$$= \frac{(2 \times 4)}{(3 \times 5)}$$

$$= \frac{8}{15}$$

B. Fraction Division

A **reciprocal** is the number obtained by switching the numerator with the denominator of a fraction. For example, the reciprocal of $\frac{2}{3}$ is $\frac{3}{2}$.

To divide a number by a fraction, multiply that number by the reciprocal of the fraction.

EXAMPLE

$$3 \div \frac{4}{3}$$

Switch the numerator and the denominator in the fraction and multiply. Remember that 3 is really 3 ÷ 1 so the new denominator would be the product of 1 × 4.

$$= \frac{3}{1} \times \frac{3}{4}$$

$$= \frac{9}{4}$$

C. Fraction Addition and Subtraction

With fractions, addition and subtraction are not so easy. You can only add or subtract fractions from each other if they have the same denominator. If they satisfy this condition, then to add or subtract, you do so with the numerators only and leave the denominator unchanged.

EXAMPLE

$$\frac{1}{5} + \frac{3}{5}$$

Both fractions have the same denominator, so add the numerators.

$$= \frac{1+3}{5}$$

$$= \frac{4}{5}$$

EXAMPLE

$$\frac{3}{5} - \frac{1}{5}$$

Both fractions have the same denominator, so subtract the numerators.

$$= \frac{3-1}{5}$$

$$= \frac{2}{5}$$

What if the denominators of two fractions you are adding or subtracting are not the same? In this case, you must find the Lowest Common Denominator (LCD), the smallest number that is divisible by both of the original denominators.

Ideally, you would like to find the smallest common denominator because smaller numbers in fractions are always easier to work with. But this is not always easy to do, and usually it isn't worth the extra time it will take to do the necessary calculation. The simplest way to find a common denominator is to multiply each fraction by a new fraction in which the numerator and denominator are both the same as the denominator of the other fraction.

EXAMPLE

$$\frac{2}{3} + \frac{2}{7}$$

Don't be confused by the fact that the numerators are the same. We still need to find a common denominator because the denominators are different.

$$= \left(\frac{2}{3} \times \frac{7}{7}\right) + \left(\frac{2}{7} \times \frac{3}{3}\right)$$

$$= \frac{14}{21} + \frac{6}{21}$$

Now that we have the same denominator, we can add the numerators.

$$= \frac{20}{21}$$

This method of finding common denominators utilizes the fact that any number multiplied by 1 is still the same number. The new fractions we introduce are always made of equivalent numerators and denominators, which make the fraction equal to 1, so the values of the original fractions do not change.

D. Comparing Fractions

Another method with which you should be familiar when manipulating fractions is comparing their values (i.e., which of the given fractions is greater than or lesser than the other) when they have different denominators. We will show you three ways to do this.

When you are confronted with only two fractions, finding their common denominator makes the task of evaluating the values easier.

1. Similar to the preceding discussion on adding or subtracting fractions that have different denominators, the fastest way to come up with a common denominator is to multiply both the numerator and denominator of each fraction by the other's denominator.

Let's say you are given the two fractions:

$$\frac{4}{5} \text{ and } \frac{3}{7}$$

Multiply the first fraction by 7 over 7 and the second fraction by 5 over 5. (The 7 comes from the fraction $\frac{3}{7}$ while 5 from $\frac{4}{5}$.)

$$\frac{4}{5} \times \frac{7}{7} = \frac{28}{35}$$

$$\frac{3}{7} \times \frac{5}{5} = \frac{15}{35}$$

With both fractions having 35 as the common denominator, you can now clearly see that 28 must be greater than 15. Therefore, $\frac{4}{5}$ is greater than $\frac{3}{7}$.

2. Another way to go about this is through cross-multiplication. Using the same fractions as examples, you first multiply the numerator of the first fraction by the denominator of the second fraction. The product will then serve as the new numerator of the first fraction.

$$\frac{4}{5} \searrow \frac{3}{7} \Rightarrow 4 \times 7 = 28$$

Next, multiply the denominators of the two fractions. The product will now serve as the new denominator of the first fraction.

$$\frac{4}{5} \rightarrow \frac{3}{7} \Rightarrow 5 \times 7 = 35$$

The resulting new fraction would be $\frac{28}{35}$.

Now, let's work on the second fraction. To get its new numerator, this time, multiply the numerator of the second fraction by the denominator of the first fraction. Then multiply the denominators of both fractions.

$$\frac{4}{5} \swarrow \frac{3}{7} \Rightarrow 3 \times 5 = 15$$

$$\frac{4}{5} \leftarrow \frac{3}{7} \Rightarrow 7 \times 5 = 35$$

The second fraction will now become $\frac{15}{35}$. Thus comparing the first and second fractions, we get the same result as we had in the first method.

Because $\frac{28}{35}$ is greater than $\frac{15}{35}$,

therefore $\frac{4}{5}$ is greater than $\frac{3}{7}$.

Both procedures follow the same basic principles and prove to be efficient when dealing with two given fractions. But what if you were given three or four fractions (since the GAMSAT is multiple choice, this will happen from time to time)?

3. A much simpler way is to convert each fraction to decimals, and then compare the decimals. All you have to do is divide the numerator of the fraction by its own denominator. With a little practice, you can actually train your brain to work fast with arithmetic.

Now let's say a third fraction is introduced to our previous examples: $\frac{4}{5}, \frac{3}{7}, \frac{9}{13}$. Working on the first fraction, simply divide 4 by 5; on the second fraction, 3 by 7; and on the last, 9 by 13 (you should try this yourself to ensure that you can perform these basic calculations quickly and correctly).

$\frac{4}{5} = 4 \div 5 = 0.8$

$\frac{3}{7} = 3 \div 7 = 0.43$

$\frac{9}{13} = 9 \div 13 = 0.69$

Comparing the three fractions in their decimal forms, 0.43 ($\frac{3}{7}$) is the smallest, 0.69 ($\frac{9}{13}$) is the next, and the largest is 0.8 ($\frac{4}{5}$).

> **NOTE**
>
> For the GAMSAT, decimals should be the recourse of last resort. When needed, try to complete calculations using fractions which will improve your speed.

E. Reduction and Cancelling

To make calculations easier, you should always avoid working with unnecessarily large numbers. To reduce fractions, you can cancel out any common factors in the numerator and denominator.

EXAMPLE

$$\frac{20}{28}$$

First, factor both the numerator and denominator.

$$= \frac{(4 \times 5)}{(4 \times 7)}$$

Since both have a factor of four, we can cancel.

$$= \frac{5}{7}$$

When multiplying fractions, it is possible to cross-cancel like factors before performing the operation. If there are any common factors between the numerator of the first fraction and the denominator of the second fraction, you can cancel them. Likewise, if there are common factors between the numerator of the second and the denominator of the first, cancel them as well.

EXAMPLE

$$\frac{5}{9} \times \frac{6}{25}$$

First, factor the numerators and denominators.

$$= \frac{5}{(3 \times 3)} \times \frac{(2 \times 3)}{(5 \times 5)}$$

Now, we see that we can cross-cancel 5s and 3s.

$$= \frac{1}{3} \times \frac{2}{5}$$

$$= \frac{2}{15}$$

F. Mixed Numbers

You may encounter numbers on the GAMSAT that have both an integer part and a fraction part. These are called mixed numbers.

EXAMPLE

$$3\frac{1}{2}$$

Mixed numbers should be thought of as addition between the integer and the fraction.

EXAMPLE

$$3\frac{1}{2} = 3 + \frac{1}{2}$$

Now in order to convert a mixed number back to a fraction, all you have to do is consider the integer to be the fraction of itself over 1 and perform fraction addition.

EXAMPLE

$$3\frac{1}{2}$$

$$= \frac{3}{1} + \frac{1}{2}$$

Obtain a common denominator.

$$= \left(\frac{3}{1}\right)\left(\frac{2}{2}\right) + \frac{1}{2}$$

$$= \frac{6}{2} + \frac{1}{2}$$

$$= \frac{7}{2}$$

To add or subtract mixed numbers, you can deal with the integer and fraction portions separately.

EXAMPLE

$$3\frac{1}{2} - 2\frac{1}{2}$$

$$= (3-2) + \left(\frac{1}{2} - \frac{1}{2}\right)$$

$$= 1$$

> **NOTE**
>
> To convert a mixed number to a fraction, keep the denominator of the fraction while multiplying the integer part of the mixed number by the denominator. Then add to the numerator of the mixed number.
>
> **EXAMPLE**
>
> $$6\frac{2}{5} = (6 \times 5) + \frac{2}{5} = 30 + \frac{2}{5} = \frac{32}{5}$$

1.4.3 Decimals and Percentages

There are two other ways to represent non-integer numbers that you will encounter on the GAMSAT: As decimals and as percentages.

A. Decimals

Decimal numbers can be recognized by the decimal point (a period) that they contain. Whatever digits are to the left of the decimal point represent a whole number, the integer portion of the number. The digits to the right of the decimal point are the decimal portion.

EXAMPLE

12.34

The integer portion of the number is 12, and .34 is the fractional portion.

The value of the decimal portion of a number operates on a place-value system just like the integer portion. The first digit to the right of the decimal point is the number of tenths (1/10 is one tenth), two digits over is the number of hundredths (1/100 is one hundredth), three digits over is the number of thousandths, then ten-thousandths, etc.

For example, in the decimal 0.56789:

- the 5 is in the tenths position;
- the 6 is in the hundredths position;
- the 7 is in the thousandths position;
- the 8 is in the ten thousandths position;
- the 9 is in the one hundred thousandths position.

Thus, to convert a decimal into a fraction, just drop the decimal point and divide by the power of ten of the last decimal digit. To convert a fraction to a decimal, simply perform the long division of the numerator divided by the denominator.

EXAMPLE

$$0.34 = \frac{34}{100}$$

B. Operations with Decimals

Addition and Subtraction: Adding and subtracting decimals is the same as with integers. The only difference is that you need to take care to line up the decimal point properly. Just like with integers, you should only add or subtract digits in the same place with each other.

EXAMPLE

Add 3.33 to 23.6.

$$\begin{array}{r} 23.60 \\ + 03.33 \end{array}$$

Notice how we have carried the decimal point down in the same place. Also, to illustrate the addition more clearly, we have added zeros to hold the empty places. Now perform the addition as if there were no decimal points.

$$\begin{array}{r} 23.60 \\ + 03.33 \\ \hline 26.93 \end{array}$$

Multiplication: You can multiply numbers with decimals just as you would with integers, but placing the decimal point in the solution is a little tricky. To decide where the decimal point goes, first count the number of significant digits after the decimal points in each of the numbers being multiplied. Add these numbers together to obtain the total number of decimal digits. Now, count that number of digits in from the right of the solution and place the decimal point in front of the number at which you end.

EXAMPLE

Multiply 3.03 by 1.2.

$$\begin{array}{r} 3.03 \\ \times\ 1.20 \end{array}$$

We have written in a zero as a placeholder at the end of the second number, but be careful not to include it in your decimal count. Only count up to the final nonzero digit in each number (the 0 in the first number counts because it comes before the 3). Thus our decimal digit count is 2 + 1 = 3, and we will place our decimal point in the solution 3 digits in from the right; but first, perform the multiplication while ignoring the decimal.

$$\begin{array}{r} 3.03 \\ \times\ 1.20 \\ \hline 606 \\ + 3030 \\ \hline 3636 \end{array}$$

Now, insert the decimal point to obtain the final solution.

$$= 3.636$$

When counting significant digits, remember to consider the following:

1. all zeros between nonzero digits

   EXAMPLE

   $0.45078 \rightarrow 5$ significant figures

2. all zeros in front of a nonzero number

   EXAMPLE

   $0.0056 \rightarrow 4$ significant figures

3. ignore all zeros after a nonzero digit

   EXAMPLE

   $0.2500 \rightarrow 2$ significant figures

Division: We can use our knowledge of the equivalence of fractions to change a decimal division problem into a more familiar integer division problem. Simply

> **NOTE**
>
> Unfortunately this last math rule is not so simple because in science labs, significant figures (= significant digits = sig figs) represent the accuracy of measurement. The good news is that if there were ever a question on the GAMSAT involving significant figures, they would clarify which rule to apply before asking questions.

multiply each number by the power of ten corresponding to the smallest significant digit out of the two decimal numbers being divided, and then, perform the division with the integers obtained.

This operation is acceptable because it amounts to multiplying a fraction by 1.

EXAMPLE

Divide 4.4 by 1.6

$$\frac{4.4}{1.6}$$

Since the smallest decimal digit in either number is in the tenth place, we multiply the top and bottom by 10.

$$= \frac{4.4}{1.6} \times \frac{10}{10}$$

$$= \frac{44}{16}$$

$$= \frac{11}{4}$$

If you like, you can convert this back to a decimal.

$$= 2.75$$

Rounding Decimals: Rounding decimals to the nearest place value is just like rounding an integer. Look at the digit one place further to the right of the place to which you are rounding. If that digit is 5 or greater, add 1 to the previous digit and drop all the subsequent digits. If it is 4 or less, leave the previous digit alone and simply drop the subsequent digits.

Consider the number 5.3618:

(a) Round to the nearest tenth.

$$= 5.4$$

Since the digit after the tenth place is a 6, we add 1 tenth and drop every digit after the tenth place.

(b) Round to the nearest hundredth.

$$= 5.36$$

Since the digit after the hundredth place is a 1, we do not change any digits. Just drop every digit after the hundredth place.

Fraction-Decimal Conversions to Know: Having these common conversions between fractions and decimals memorized will help you save valuable time on the test.

Fraction	Decimal
1/2	.5
1/3	~ .33
1/4	.25
1/5	.2
1/6	~ .167
1/8	.125
1/10	.1

C. Percentages

Percentages are used to describe fractions of other numbers. One percent (written 1%) simply means 1 hundredth. This is easy to remember since "percent" can literally be broken down into "per" and "cent", and we all know that one cent is a hundredth of a dollar.

We can use this conversion to hundredths when evaluating expressions containing percents of numbers, but a percentage has no real meaning until it is used to modify another value. For example, if you see 67% in a problem you should always ask "67% of what?"

EXAMPLE

What is 25% of 40?

$$= .25 \times 40$$
$$= 10$$

To find what percentage a certain part of a value is of the whole value, you can use what is known as the **percentage formula**:

Percent = (Part/Whole) × 100

EXAMPLE

What percentage of 50 is 23?

Percentage = (23/50) × 100
$$= (46/100) \times 100$$
$$= 46\%$$

1.5 Roots and Exponents

1.5.1 Properties of Exponents

To multiply exponential values with the same base, keep the base the same and add the exponents.

EXAMPLE

$$a^2 \times a^3 = a^{2+3} = a^5$$

To divide exponential values with the same base, keep the base the same and subtract the exponent of the denominator from the exponent of the numerator.

EXAMPLE

$$\frac{x^5}{x^3} = x^{5-3} = x^2$$

To multiply exponential values with different bases but the same exponent, keep the exponent the same and multiply the bases.

EXAMPLE

$$2^x \times 3^x = (2 \times 3)^x = 6^x$$

To divide exponential values with different bases but the same exponent, keep the exponent the same and divide the bases.

EXAMPLE

$$\frac{6^x}{2^x} = \left(\frac{6}{2}\right)^x = 3^x$$

To raise an exponential value to another power, keep the base the same and multiply the exponents.

EXAMPLE

$$(x^3)^4 = x^{(3 \times 4)} = x^{12}$$

Even though all of the preceding examples use only positive integer exponents, these properties hold true for all three of the types described in section 1.5.3.

1.5.2 Scientific Notation

Scientific notation, also called exponential notation, is a convenient method of writing very large (or very small) numbers. Instead of writing too many zeroes on either side of a decimal, you can express a number as a product of a power of ten and a number between 1 and 10. For example, the number 8,765,000,000 can be expressed as 8.765×10^9.

The first number 8.765 is called the coefficient. The second number should always have a base of ten with an exponent equal to the number of zeroes in the original numbers. Moving the decimal point to the left makes a positive exponent while moving to the right makes a negative exponent.

In multiplying numbers in scientific notation, the general rule is as follows:

$$(a \times 10^x)(b \times 10^y) = ab \times 10^{x+y}$$

EXAMPLE

To multiply 2.0×10^4 and 10×10^2

(i) Find the product of the coefficients first.

$2.0 \times 10 = 20$

(ii) Add the exponents.

$4 + 2 = 6$

(iii) Construct the result.

20×10^6

(iv) Make sure that the coefficient has only one digit to the left of the decimal point. This will also adjust the number of the exponent depending on the number of places moved.

2.0×10^7

Dividing numbers in scientific notation follows this general rule:

$$\frac{(a \times 10^x)}{(b \times 10^y)} = \frac{a}{b} \times 10^{x-y}$$

Going back to our preceding example, let's divide 2.0×10^4 and 10×10^2 this time:

(i) Divide the coefficients.

$2.0 \div 10 = 0.2$

(ii) Subtract the exponents.

$4 - 2 = 2$

(iii) Construct the result and adjust the values to their simplest forms.

$0.2 \times 10^2 = 2 \times 10 = 20$

In adding and subtracting numbers written in scientific notation, you need to ensure that all exponents are identical. You would need to adjust the decimal place of one of the numbers so that its exponent becomes equivalent to the other number.

EXAMPLE

Add 34.5×10^{-5} and 6.7×10^{-4}

(i) Choose the number that you want to adjust so that its exponent is equivalent to the other number. Let's pick 34.5 and change it into a number with 10^{-4} as its base-exponent term.

$3.45 \times 10^{-4} + 6.7 \times 10^{-4}$

(ii) Add the coefficients together:

$3.45 + 6.7 = 10.15$

(iii) The exponents are now the same, in this case 10^{-4}, so all you have to do is plug it in:

10.15×10^{-4}

(iv) Adjust the end result so that the coefficient is a number between 1 and 10:

1.015×10^{-3}

The same procedure basically applies to subtraction.

> **NOTE**
>
> Notice in the examples in this section, when you lower the power from the coefficient (i.e. by moving the decimal to the left), you must add to the exponent, and vice-versa.

1.5.3 Types of Exponents

Positive Integer Exponents: This is the type of exponent you will encounter most often. Raising a base number b to a positive integer exponent x is equivalent to making x copies of b and multiplying them together.

EXAMPLE

$2^4 = 2 \times 2 \times 2 \times 2 = 16$

Fractional Exponents: Fractional exponents are also known as roots. Let x be the fraction. To raise a base number b to the x power we make use of the fifth property of exponents in section 1.5.1.

We can write $b^{\frac{n}{d}}$ as $\left(b^{\frac{1}{d}}\right)^n$. The value $b^{\frac{1}{d}}$ is known as the d-th root of b. So the base b raised to the x power is the same as the d-th root of b raised to the n power.

EXAMPLE

$8^{\frac{2}{3}}$

$= \left(8^{\frac{1}{3}}\right)^2$

The expression inside the parentheses is the cube root of 8. Since $2 \times 2 \times 2 = 8$, the cube root of 8 is 2.

$= 2^2$
$= 4$

Consider the following: What is the cube root of 125, and separately, what is the cube root of -125? The number 5 multiplied by itself 3 times equals 125. Similarly, the number -5 multiplied by itself 3 times equals -125. Thus the answers are 5 and -5, respectively.

Negative Exponents: The value of a base raised to a negative power is equal to the reciprocal of the base, raised to a positive exponent of the same value. For any exponential value b^{-x}, b^{-x} is equivalent to $\dfrac{1}{(b^x)}$.

EXAMPLE

$$3^{-2}$$

Take the reciprocal and invert the sign of the exponent.

$$= \frac{1}{(3^2)}$$

$$= \frac{1}{(3 \times 3)}$$

$$= \frac{1}{9}$$

1.5.4 Zero and Exponents

Raising a Number to the Zero: Any number raised to the zero power is equal to 1.

We can see that this follows the rules of exponents (see section 1.5), because $a^0 = a^1 \times a^{-1} = a/a = 1$.

> **NOTE**
>
> The quantity 0^0 (read as zero to the zero power) is 1.

EXAMPLES

$$3^0 = 1$$
$$123.79^0 = 1$$
$$\left[1.2 + \left(37 - \sqrt{5}\right) \times 2.331\right]^0 = 1$$

As with multiplication and division, you should not waste time evaluating the parenthetical expression.

1.5.5 Summary of the Rules for Exponents

$$a^0 = 1 \qquad a^1 = a$$

$$a^n \, a^m = a^{n+m} \qquad a^n/a^m = a^{n-m}$$

$$(a^n)^m = a^{nm} \qquad a^{\frac{1}{n}} = \sqrt[n]{a}$$

1.5.6 Recognizing Number Patterns

==It is possible to save a lot of time during the real GAMSAT by avoiding unnecessary calculations by the recognition of certain patterns.== One helpful way to achieve this is by knowing at least the following relationships that are typically memorized in high school math class (see table below).

Test makers choose their numbers carefully. The moment you see 1.44 on the GAMSAT, there would be a high likelihood that taking the square root, which gives 1.2, would be required (because, of course, the square root of 144 is 12, the square root of 1.44 must be 1.2). Likewise, the square root of 1.7, being an approximation of 1.69, must be 1.3 (the square root of 169 being 13).

EXAMPLE 1

If you have not done your Physics review yet, don't worry, we will discuss simple harmonic motion later (SHM; PHY 7.2.3). Please try the following practice questions before looking at the worked solutions. For now, just focus on the math. If you have done your Physics review, in the small angle approximation, the motion of a simple pendulum is approximated by the following equation:

$$T = 2\pi \sqrt{\frac{\ell}{g}}$$

where T is the period of a mass attached to a pendulum of length ℓ with gravitational acceleration g.

x	1	2	3	4	5	6	7	8	9	10	11	12	13	14	15	20
x^2	1	4	9	16	25	36	49	64	81	100	121	144	169	196	225	400
x^3	1	8	27	64	125	-	-	-	-	1000	-	-	-	-	-	-

GAMSAT-Prep.com
THE GOLD STANDARD

Again, please ignore Physics for now. If the length of the pendulum increases by 70%, by what percentage will the period increase?

A. 30%
B. 40%
C. 50%
D. 70%

If the length increases by 70%, that is the same as saying 1.70(ℓ), 1.70 is similar to 1.69 and since we know that square root 1.69 is 1.3 (because 13 squared is 169), this means that the original square root of ℓ has increased by 30%.

$$T = 2\pi\sqrt{\frac{\ell}{g}}$$

$$T = 2\pi\sqrt{\frac{(1.69)\ell}{g}}$$

$$T = 1.30\left[2\pi\sqrt{\frac{\ell}{g}}\right]$$

Translation: the original equation is 1.30 times higher which means 30% greater. Answer: **A**.

EXAMPLE 2

If the pendulum is in an environment with 1/50th of Earth's gravity, what would be the change in the period?

A. It would be 15 times the original.
B. It would be 10 times the original.
C. It would be 7 times the original.
D. It would be 1/10th times the original.

$$T = 2\pi\sqrt{\frac{\ell}{g}}$$

By observing that gravity will change and a square root is imminent (as well as the fact that the answer choices are not very 'tight' or close together), let's estimate 50 as 49 which has a simple square root:

$$T = 2\pi\sqrt{\frac{\ell}{g/49}}$$

A denominator in a denominator is the same as a numerator (in other words, if you divide by a fraction, it is the same as multiplying by the inverse; see GM 1.4.2B):

$$T = 2\pi\sqrt{\frac{(49)\ell}{g}}$$

Of course, the square root of 49 is 7:

$$T = 7\left[2\pi\sqrt{\frac{\ell}{g}}\right]$$

Translation: the original equation is 7 times greater. Answer: **C**. Note that the actual square root of 50 is approximately 7.1 so our estimate is valid considering the answer choices.

> **NOTE**
>
> Try to complete all the chapter review warm-up exercises as quickly as possible and, of course, without the use of a calculator.

GAMSAT MATH

1.6 Ratio and Proportion

1.6.1 What is a Ratio?

A **ratio** is the relation between two numbers. There are multiple ways they can be written, but ratios can always be denoted as fractions.

These are all ways to represent the same ratio:

$$3 \text{ to } 4 = 3:4 = \frac{3}{4}$$

If a ratio is written out in words, the first quantity stated should generally be placed in the numerator of the equivalent fraction and the second quantity in the denominator. Just make sure you keep track of which value corresponds to which category.

1.6.2 Solving Proportions

A **proportion** is a statement of equality between two or more ratios.

Solving for an unknown variable is the most common type of proportion problem. If you have just a ratio on either side of an equation, you can rewrite the equation as the numerator of the first times the denominator of the second equal to the denominator of the first times the numerator of the second. This allows you to find the missing information more easily.

EXAMPLE

Solve for x in the following equation.

$$\frac{2}{3} = \frac{5}{x}$$

Cross multiply to eliminate fractions.

$$2 \times x = 3 \times 5$$
$$2x = 15$$
$$x = \frac{15}{2} = 7\frac{1}{2}$$

This means that the ratio 2 to 3 is equivalent to the ratio 5 to $7\frac{1}{2}$.

Unless it is stated, a proportion does not describe a specific number of things. It can only give you information about quantities in terms of other quantities. But if it is explicitly stated what one of the two quantities is, the other quantity can be determined using the proportion.

GOLD STANDARD WARM-UP EXERCISES

CHAPTER 1: Numbers and Operations

1. What is the approximate value of $0.125 + \sqrt{\frac{1}{9}}$?

   A. 0.40
   B. 0.46
   C. 0.50
   D. 0.45

2. 0.8 is to 0.9 as 80 is to:

   A. 9
   B. 100
   C. 8
   D. 90

3. If you invest in Bank A, you will receive 19% interest on the amount you invest. If you invest in Bank B, you will receive 21% interest. The maximum amount you can invest in Bank A is $6,430, and the maximum amount you can invest in Bank B is $5,897. How much more interest will you earn if you invest the maximum amount in Bank B than if you invest the maximum amount in Bank A?

   A. $16.67
   B. $16.30
   C. $101.27
   D. $111.93

4. Board C is 3/4 as long as Board B. Board B is 4/5 as long as Board A. What is the sum of the lengths of all three Boards if Board A is 100 m long?

   A. 255 m
   B. 225 m
   C. 240 m
   D. 235 m

5. The proportion of the yellow marbles in a jar of yellow and green jars is 7 out of 9. If there are 999 marbles in the jar, how many of these are yellow?

   A. 111
   B. 777
   C. 2
   D. 222

6. If 0.25 months is equal to one week, what fraction of a month is equal to one day?

   A. 1/7
   B. 4/7
   C. 1/30
   D. 1/28

GAMSAT MATH

7. Which of the following is 6.4% of 1,000?
   A. $64^{\frac{3}{4}}$
   B. $256^{\frac{3}{4}}$
   C. $\left(\frac{64}{100}\right)^2$
   D. 6.4 / 100

8. $2 + \left[71 - 8\left(\frac{6}{2}\right)^2\right]$ is what percent of $\sqrt{2500}$?
   A. 50%
   B. 1%
   C. 44%
   D. 2%

9. Which is the largest?
   A. 0.636
   B. 0.136
   C. 0.46
   D. 0.163

10. Determine the sum of 9, -5, and 6.
    A. 20
    B. – 20
    C. – 10
    D. 10

11. Determine the value of 1.5×10^7 divided by 3.0×10^4.
    A. 5.0×10^3
    B. 5.0×10^2
    C. 5.0×10^{-2}
    D. 0.5×10^{-3}

12. Try to complete the following calculation in under 30 seconds: Determine the value of .333 x .125. {Reminder: all calculations in this book should be performed without the use of a calculator.}
    A. 0.02
    B. 0.03
    C. 0.04
    D. 0.05

GS ANSWER KEY

CHAPTER 1

			Cross-Reference				Cross-Reference
1.	B	GM 1.2.3, 1.4.3		7.	B	GM 1.2.3, 1.4.3, 1.5.2
2.	D	GM 1.6.2		8.	D	GM 1.2.3, 1.4.3
3.	A	GM 1.4.3		9.	A	GM 1.4.3
4.	C	GM 1.4.2		10.	D	GM 1.2.1
5.	B	GM 1.6.2		11.	B	GM 1.5.2
6.	D	GM 1.6.1		12.	C	GM 1.4.3

* Worked solutions can be found at the end of the GAMSAT Math chapters. If something is still not clear, go to the forum at GAMSAT-prep.com.

GOLD NOTES

SCIENTIFIC MEASUREMENT
Chapter 2

Memorize

...ersions between units in the ... system (whenever applicable) ...its

Understand

* SI prefixes
* How to convert between units
* Dimensional analysis

Not Required

* Memorizing conversion factors between different systems of units.

GAMSAT-Prep.com

Introduction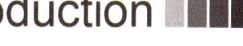

It is extremely important to know the SI system of measurement for the GAMSAT. The metric system is very much related to the SI system. The British system, though familiar, does not need to be memorized for the GAMSAT (related questions would only be asked if relevant conversion factors were provided).

Additional Resources

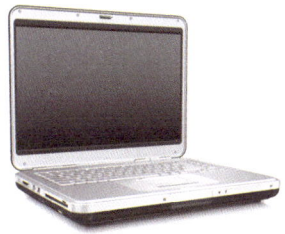

Free Online Forum

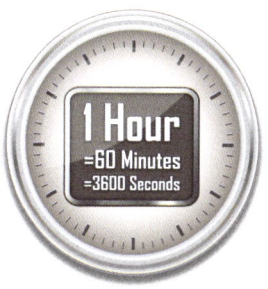

Special Guest

GAMSAT-Prep.com
THE GOLD STANDARD

2.1 Systems of Measurement

2.1.1 British Units (Imperial System of Measurement)

You are probably already familiar with several of these units of measurement, but we recommend reviewing them at least once.

A. Length: These units are used to describe things like the length of physical objects, the displacement of a physical object, the distance something has traveled or will travel, etc. Area and volume are also measured as the square and cube (respectively) of these units.

Inches	The *inch* is the smallest measurement of length in the British System.
Feet	There are 12 inches in every foot. 1 ft. = 12 in.
Yards	There are 3 feet in every yard. 1 yd. = 3 ft.
Miles	The *mile* is the largest unit of length in the British System. There are 5,280 feet in every mile. 1 mi. = 5,280 ft.

B. Time: These units describe the passage of time.

Seconds	The *second* is the smallest unit of time in the British System.
Minutes	There are 60 seconds in every minute. 1 min. = 60 s.
Hours	There are 60 minutes in every hour. 1 h. = 60 min.
Days	There are 24 hours in every day. 1 day = 24 h.
Years	The *year* is the largest unit of time in the British System. There are 365 days in every year. 1 yr. = 365 days

C. Mass/Weight: These terms are not technically the same and we will discuss the differences in Physics. The following units describe the amount of matter in an object.

Ounces	The *ounce* is the smallest unit of mass in the British System.
Pounds	There are 16 ounces in every pound. 1 lb. = 16 oz.
Tons	The *ton* is the largest unit of mass in the British System. There are 2,000 pounds in every ton. 1 ton = 2,000 lb.

2.1.2 Metric Units

Measuring with Powers of 10: Unlike the British System, the Metric System has only one unit for each category of measurement. In order to describe quantities that are much larger or much smaller than one of the base units, a prefix is chosen from a variety of options and added to the front of the unit. This changes the value of the unit by some power of 10, which is determined by what the prefix is. The following are the most common of these prefixes (with the representative symbols in brackets):

Milli (m)	One thousandth (10^{-3}) of the base unit
Centi (c)	One hundredth (10^{-2}) of the base unit
Deci (d)	One tenth (10^{-1}) of the base unit
Deca (da)	Ten (10^{1}) times the base unit
Kilo (k)	One thousand (10^{3}) times the base unit

There is a mnemonic that may be used to identify these prefixes:

King	Kilometer	Kilo
Henry	Hectometer	Hecto (h)
Died	Decameter	Deca
Unexpectedly	Unit Base	Unit
Drinking	Decimeter	Deci
Chocolate	Centimeter	Centi
Milk	Milimeter	Milli

As you go down, you divide by 10 and as you go up, you multiply by 10 in order to convert between the units.

EXAMPLE

How many meters is 1 kilometer?

$$1 \text{ km} = 1,000 \text{ m}$$

From general knowledge, we know that kilo means one thousand. This means there are 1,000 meters in a kilometer. But just in case you get confused, you can also use the clue from the mnemonic. Now we know that Kilo is three slots upward from the Unit base. Hence we multiply 3 times by 10: 10 x 10 x 10 = 1000.

An even less confusing way to figure out how to do the metric conversions quickly and accurately, is to use a metric conversion line. This is quite handy with any of the common units such as the *meter*, *liter*, and *grams*.

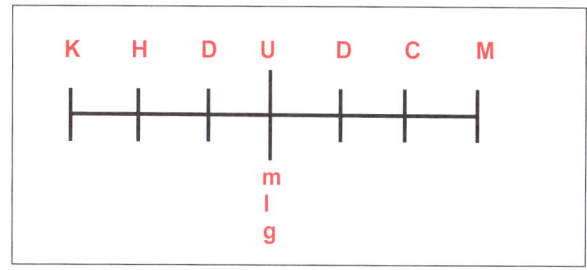

Figure GM 2.1: The Metric Conversion Line. The letters on top of the metric line stands for the "King Henry" mnemonic. On the other hand, the letters below the metric line - **m**, **l**, **g** – stand for the unit bases, **m**eter, **l**iter, or **g**ram, respectively.

To use this device, draw out the metric line as shown in Fig GM 2.1. From the centermost point **U**, the prefixes going to the left represent those that are larger than the base unit (kilo, hecto). These also correspond to the decimal places that you will be moving from the numerical value of the unit to be converted. Those going to the right are for the ones smaller than the unit (deci, centi, milli).

EXAMPLE

How much is 36 liters in milliliters?
Step 1: Place your pen on the given unit, in this case L (liter). Then count the number of places it takes you to reach the unit being asked in the problem (milliliter).

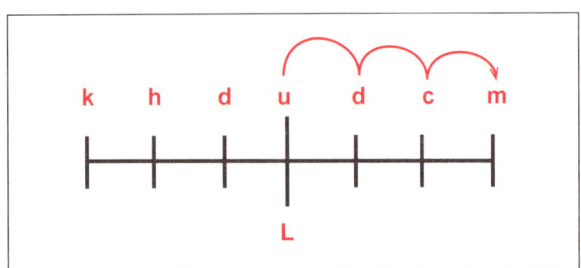

Fig GM 2.2: Converting liter to milliliter using the metric conversion line.

Step 2: Because it took you three places going to the right to move from the liter to the milliliter units, you also need to add three places from the decimal point of the number 36.0.

36 L = 36,000 ml

Now, let's try converting centimeter to kilometer: What is 6.3 cm in km?

1. Place your pen on the **c** (centi) point in the metric line.

2. Moving from **c** to **k** (kilo) takes five places going to the left. This also means moving five places from the decimal point of the number 6.3.
6.3 cm = .000063 km

Using this method definitely makes doing the metric conversions so much faster than the fraction method!

There are other prefixes that are often used scientifically:

Tera (T) 10^{12} times the base unit
Giga (G) 10^{9} times the base unit
Mega (M) 10^{6} times the base unit
Micro (μ) 10^{-6} of the base unit
Nano (n) 10^{-9} of the base unit
Pico (p) 10^{-12} of the base unit

A. Length: As with British length units, these are used to measure anything that has to do with length, displacement, distance, etc. Area and volume are also measured as the square and cube (respectively) of these units.

Meters	The *meter* is the basic unit of length in the Metric System.
Other Common Forms	millimeter, centimeter, kilometer

GM-36   SCIENTIFIC MEASUREMENT

GAMSAT MATH

B. Time: These are units that quantify the passage of time.

Seconds	Just as in the British System, the *second* is the basic unit of time in the Metric System. Minutes, hours, and the other British units are not technically part of the Metric System, but they are often used anyway in problems involving metric units.
Other Common Forms	millisecond

C. Mass: These are units that describe the amount of matter in an object.

Grams	The *gram* is the basic metric unit of mass.
Other Common Forms	milligram, kilogram

2.1.3 SI Units

SI units is the **International System of Units** (abbreviated **SI** from the French *Le Système International d'Unités*) and is a modern form of the metric system. SI units are used to standardize all the scientific calculations that are done anywhere in the world. Throughout this book, and during the real exam, you will see the application of base SI units and the units derived from the base SI units.

> **NOTE**
>
> Typically, because of Chemistry, students think that the liter (L) is an SI unit. It is not. The cubic meter is the SI unit for volume. It is important that you know that 1 L = 1000 cubic centimeters (= cc or mL) = 1 cubic decimeter.

Table 1: SI Base Units

Base quantity	Name	Symbol
	SI base unit	
length	meter	m
mass	kilogram	kg
time	second	s
electric current	ampere	A
thermodynamic temperature	kelvin	K
amount of substance	mole	mol

Table 2: Examples of SI Derived Units

	SI derived unit	
area	square meter	m^2
volume	cubic meter	m^3
speed, velocity	meter per second	m/s
acceleration	meter per second squared	m/s^2

Table 3: SI Derived Units with Special Names and Symbols

			SI base unit	
frequency	hertz	Hz	-	s^{-1}
force	newton	N	-	$m \cdot kg \cdot s^{-2}$
pressure, stress	pascal	Pa	N/m^2	$m^{-1} \cdot kg \cdot s^{-2}$
energy, work, quantity of heat	joule	J	$N \cdot m$	$m^2 \cdot kg \cdot s^{-2}$
power	watt	W	J/s	$m^2 \cdot kg \cdot s^{-3}$
electric charge, quantity of electricity	coulomb	C	-	$s \cdot A$
electric potential difference, electromotive force	volt	V	W/A	$m^2 \cdot kg \cdot s^{-3} \cdot A^{-1}$

> **NOTE**
>
> We will see all the units from these 3 tables in the Physics and Chemistry chapters.
>
> Do not try to memorize the last 2 columns in Table 3. However, if this is your second time reviewing this page, you should be able to derive all the units displayed in the last 2 columns of Table 3. In fact, the derivation of units through dimensional analysis is a regular type of GAMSAT question. You will be tested on this point with the online chapter review practice questions in Physics and Chemistry that are included with this textbook.

GAMSAT MATH

2.2. Mathematics of Conversions (Dimensional Analysis)

The Process: In order to convert a quantity from one type of unit to another type of unit, all you have to do is set up and execute multiplication between ratios. Each conversion from the preceding sections is actually a ratio.

Let's look at the conversion from feet to inches.

"There are 12 inches in 1 foot."

This can be rewritten as a ratio in two ways: "12 inches to 1 foot" or "1 foot to 12 inches."

$$= \frac{12 \text{ in}}{1 \text{ ft}} \text{ or } \frac{1 \text{ ft}}{12 \text{ in}}$$

When you are performing a conversion, you should treat the units like numbers. This means that when you have a fraction with a certain unit on top and the same unit on bottom, you can cancel out the units leaving just the numbers.

You can multiply a quantity by any of your memorized conversions, and its value will remain the same as long as all of the units, but one, cancel out.

EXAMPLE

Given that there are 2.54 cm in an inch, how many inches are there in 3 feet?

First, determine which conversion will help. Of course we have a conversion directly between feet and inches, so that is what we'll use and we'll ignore the distractor (cm).

Next, determine which of the two possible conversion ratios we should use. The goal is to be able to cancel out the original units (in this case, feet), so we want to use whichever ratio has the original units in the denominator (in this case, inches/feet).

$$3 \text{ ft} = 3 \text{ ft} \times \frac{12 \text{ in}}{1 \text{ ft}}$$

Now perform the unit cancellation.

$$= 3 \times \frac{12 \text{ in}}{1}$$
$$= 36 \text{ in}$$

In many instances, you will not have a direct conversion. All you have to do in such a case is multiply by a string of ratios instead of just one.

EXAMPLE

How many inches are there in 5.08 meters? {Try the conversion yourself before looking at the solution.}

We cannot convert meters directly into inches, but we can convert meters to centimeters and then centimeters into inches. We can set up both these conversions at the same time and evaluate.

$$5.08 \text{ m} = 5.08 \text{ m} \times \frac{100 \text{ cm}}{1 \text{ m}} \times \frac{1 \text{ in}}{2.54 \text{ cm}}$$

Next, cancel the units.

$$= 5.08 \times \frac{100}{1} \times \frac{1 \text{ in}}{2.54}$$

$$= \frac{508 \text{ in}}{2.54}$$

$$= 200 \text{ in}$$

> **NOTE**
>
> Make sure you check and see that all of your units cancel properly! A lot of unnecessary errors can be avoided simply by paying attention to the units. "Dimensional analysis" is the formal term given to these types of calculations that are solved while keeping an eye on the relations based on units. The solutions to many problems on the real GAMSAT are dependent on dimensional analysis.

GAMSAT MATH

GOLD STANDARD WARM-UP EXERCISES

CHAPTER 2: Scientific Measurement

1. How many millimeters are there in 75 meters?

   A. 750 mm
   B. 75 mm
   C. 7,500 mm
   D. 75,000 mm

2. Which of the following is the shortest distance?

   A. 10 m
   B. 1,000 mm
   C. 10 cm
   D. 0.1 km

3. A triathlon has three legs. The first leg is a 12 km run. The second leg is a 10 km swim. The third leg is a 15 km bike ride. How long is the total triathlon in meters?

   A. 37,000 m
   B. 3,700 m
   C. 1,000 m
   D. 37 m

4. If a paperclip has a mass of one gram and a staple has a mass of 0.05 g, how many staples have a mass equivalent to the mass of one paperclip?

   A. 10
   B. 100
   C. 20
   D. 25

5. Which of the following is the number of minutes equivalent to $17\frac{5}{6}$ hours?

   A. 1,080
   B. 1,056
   C. 1,050
   D. 1,070

6. The three children in a family weigh 67 lbs., 1 oz., 93 lbs., 2 oz., and 18 lbs., 5 oz. What is the total weight of all three children? {You may go back to section 2.1 to find an appropriate conversion factor.}

   A. 178.8 lbs.
   B. 178.5 lbs.
   C. 178.08 lbs.
   D. 179.8 lbs.

7. A lawyer charges clients $20.50 per hour to file paperwork, $55 per hour for time in court, and $30 per hour for consultations. How much will it cost for a 90-minute consultation, $\frac{8}{6}$ hours time filing paperwork, and 1 hour in court?

   A. $110.28
   B. $100.75
   C. $88.25
   D. $127.33

8. If a car moving at a constant speed travels 20 centimeters in 1 second, approximately how many feet will it travel in 25% of a minute? {You may go back to section 2.1 to find an appropriate conversion factor.}

   A. 10
   B. 15
   C. 12
   D. 9

9. The Dounreay Nuclear Power Station has been in operation for quite some time. Over the last six years, they have turned out a total of two megawatt-years of energy. Assuming that operations were continuous over a six year period at a constant rate, what was its power in watts (W)?

   A. 3.3×10^5 W
   B. 6.6×10^5 W
   C. 3.3×10^2 W
   D. 6.6×10^2 W

10. The dimension of a physical quantity can be expressed as a product of the basic physical dimensions of mass (M), length (L) and time (T). For example, the dimension of the physical quantity speed or velocity (meters/second = m/s) is length/time (L/T).

    Given that $F = at^{-1} + bt^2$ where F is the force and t is the time, then the dimensions of a and b must be, respectively (note: this is a challenging question but it is at the level of the real GAMSAT. You can look at the table in section 2.1 to guide you to the dimensions that should apply to the force F but that would not be given to you on the real exam. Don't worry if you could not do this problem. We will revisit this question type in our online Physics practice problems and in the practice exam at the back of the book.):

    A. LT^{-2}, T^{-2}
    B. T, T^{-2}
    C. LT^{-1}, T^{-2}
    D. MLT^{-1}, MLT^{-4}

GS ANSWER KEY

Chapter 2

Cross-Reference

1. D GM 2.2.2
2. C GM 2.1.2
3. A GM 2.2
4. C GM 2.1
5. D GM 2.2.2

Cross-Reference

6. B GM 2.2.2
7. D GM 2.1.1, 2.2
8. A GM 2.2.2; dimensional analysis
9. A PHY 5.7, dimensional analysis
10. D dimensional analysis

* Worked solutions can be found at the end of the GAMSAT Math chapters. If something is still not clear, go to the forum at GAMSAT-prep.com.

GOLD NOTES

ALGEBRA
Chapter 3

Memorize	Understand	Not Required

#1 Rule of Algebra
e-Intercept Form for linear
ations
es of logarithms
	* Basic equations and methods
	  of equation solving
	* Simplifying equations
	* Solving one or more linear equations
	* Manipulating logs and exponents
	* Graph analysis, slopes, area under curves
	* 2D (x, y) and 3D (x, y, z) graphs
		* Multiplying polynomials
		* Inequalities
		* Memorizing math expressions like
		  "Cartesian Coordinates"

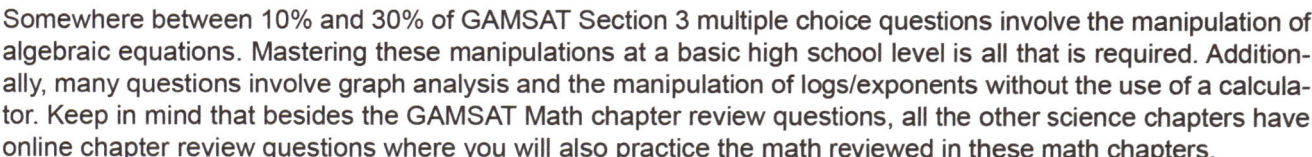

Introduction

Somewhere between 10% and 30% of GAMSAT Section 3 multiple choice questions involve the manipulation of algebraic equations. Mastering these manipulations at a basic high school level is all that is required. Additionally, many questions involve graph analysis and the manipulation of logs/exponents without the use of a calculator. Keep in mind that besides the GAMSAT Math chapter review questions, all the other science chapters have online chapter review questions where you will also practice the math reviewed in these math chapters.

Additional Resources

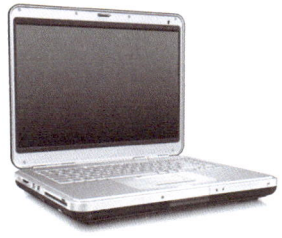

Free Online Forum

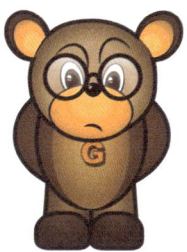

Special Guest

GAMSAT MATH GM-45

3.1 Equation Solving and Functions

3.1.1 Algebraic Equations

Before we jump into more complicated algebra, let's review the basics.

A. Terms

Variable: A variable is a symbol - usually in the form of a small letter - that represents a number. It can take on any range of values.

Most problems that are strictly algebraic in nature will provide you with an equation (or equations) containing one or more unknown variables. Based on the information given, the values of the variables will most likely be fixed. Your job is to solve for those values.

Constant: A constant is a fixed value. A constant can be a number on its own, or sometimes it is represented by a letter such as a, b, k, π, e, etc. In the chapters to come, you will discover that there are many constants in nature.

Polynomial: A polynomial is an expression (usually part of a function or an equation) that is composed of the sum or difference of some number of terms. Please note that some of the terms can be negative. The **order** of a polynomial is equal to the largest exponent to which a variable is raised in one of the terms.

EXAMPLE $3x^2 + x + 5$

This expression is a polynomial. The variable here is x, and the order of the polynomial is 2 because that is the largest exponent to which x is raised.

B. Preserving Equality

The #1 Rule of Algebra: Whatever you do to one side of an equation, you *must* do to the other side also!

The equals sign implies equality between two different expressions. When you are given an equation, the equality established must be considered to be always true for that problem (unless you are told otherwise). So if you change one side of the equation and you do not also change the other side in the same way, you fundamentally alter the terms of the equation. The equation will no longer be true.

EXAMPLE

Consider this equation:

$$2x + 3 = 5$$

The following manipulation violates the above rule:

$$(2x + 3) - 3 = 5$$

Here, we have subtracted three from one side but not the other, so the equality no longer holds.

This manipulation, however, does not violate the rule:

$$(2x + 3) - 3 = 5 - 3$$

Here, we have subtracted three from both sides, so the equality still holds true.

C. Solving Basic Equations

We can use the rule of algebra described in Part B to help solve algebraic equations for an unknown variable. Keep in mind that addition and subtraction,

> **NOTE**
>
> If two sides of an equation are equal, you can add or subtract the same amount to/from both sides, and they will still be equal.
>
> **EXAMPLE**
> $a = b$
> $a + c = b + c$
> $a - c = b - c$
>
> The same rule applies to multiplication and division.
>
> **EXAMPLE**
> $a = b$
> $ac = bc$
> $a \div c = b \div c$

along with multiplication and division, are inverse operations: They undo each other. First decide the operation that has been applied and then use the inverse operation to undo this (make sure to apply the operation to both sides of the equation). The idea is to isolate the variable on one side of the equation. Then, whatever is left on the other side of the equation is the value of the variable.

EXAMPLE

Solve: $2x + 3 = 5$

$2x + 3 - 3 = 5 - 3$
$2x = 2$

Subtracting 3, however, has not isolated the variable x. Hence, we need to continue undoing by dividing 2 on both sides.

$2x \div 2 = 2 \div 2$
$x = 1$

Here's a little more complicated equation for you to try: $2x + 2/3 = 3x - 2$

Objective: isolate the variable in order to provide a solution to the equation. When you have an equation with the variable on both sides, choose whichever you think will be easier to focus on. In this case, we will isolate x on the right. First, subtract $2x$ from both sides.

$$(2x + 2/3) - 2x = (3x - 2) - 2x$$

$$\Rightarrow 2/3 = x - 2$$

Next, add 2 to both sides to isolate *x*.

$$(2/3) + 2 = (x - 2) + 2$$
$$\Rightarrow 8/3 = x$$

3.1.2 Addition and Subtraction of Polynomials

When adding or subtracting polynomials, the general rules for exponents are applied and like terms are grouped together. You can think of it as similar to collecting the same things together.

EXAMPLE

$$4x^3y + 5z^2 + 5xy^4 + 3z^2$$

$$= 4x^3y + 5xy^4 + (5+3)z^2$$
$$= 4x^3y + 5xy^4 + 8z^2$$

By grouping the similar terms, seeing which terms may be added or subtracted becomes easier.

3.1.3 Simplifying Algebraic Expressions

Algebraic expressions can be factored or simplified using standard formulae:

$$a(b + c) = ab + ac$$
$$(a + b)(a - b) = a^2 - b^2$$
$$(a + b)(a + b) = (a + b)^2 = a^2 + 2ab + b^2$$
$$(a - b)(a - b) = (a - b)^2 = a^2 - 2ab + b^2$$
$$(a + b)(c + d) = ac + ad + bc + bd$$

3.2 Simplifying Equations

In order to make solving algebraic equations easy and quick, you should simplify terms whenever possible. The following are the most common and important ways of doing so.

3.2.1 Combining Terms

This is the most basic thing you can do to simplify an equation. If there are multiple terms being added or subtracted in your equation that contain the same variables, you can combine them.

EXAMPLE

Simplify the equation: $3x + 4xy - 2 = xy + 1$

Notice that there are two terms we can combine that contain xy and two terms we can combine that are just constants.

$(3x + 4xy - 2) - xy = (xy + 1) - xy$
$\Rightarrow 3x \quad 3xy - 2 = 1$

$(3x + 3xy - 2) + 2 = 1 + 2$
$\Rightarrow 3x + 3xy = 3$

$\Rightarrow \left(\dfrac{3x + 3xy}{3}\right) = \dfrac{3}{3}$

$\Rightarrow x + xy = 1$

Always make sure to look for like terms to combine when you are solving an algebra problem.

3.2.2 Variables in Denominators

When you are trying to manipulate an equation, having variables in the denominators of fractions can make things difficult. In order to get rid of such denominators entirely, simply multiply the entire equation by the quantity in the denominator. This will probably cause other terms to become more complicated, but you will no longer have the problem of a variable denominator.

EXAMPLE

Simplify the expression: $\dfrac{3}{2x} + 5x = 4$.

The problem denominator is $2x$, so we multiply both sides by $2x$.

$(\dfrac{3}{2x} + 5x)2x = (4)2x$

$\Rightarrow 3 + 10x^2 = 8x$

When there are different denominators containing variables, cross multiply the denominator to cancel out. Try the following example.

EXAMPLE

$\dfrac{5}{(x+3)} = \dfrac{2}{x} - \dfrac{1}{3x}$

Multiply 3x on both sides:

$$\frac{5}{(x+3)}(3x) = \frac{2}{x} - \frac{1}{3x}(3x)$$

$$\frac{15x}{(x+3)} = 6 - 1$$

Multiply (x+3) on both sides:

$$\frac{15x}{(x+3)}(x+3) = 5(x+3)$$

$$15x = 5x + 15$$

$$15x - 5x = 5x + 15 - 5x$$

$$10x = 15$$

$$x = \frac{15}{10} = \frac{3}{2}$$

3.2.3 Factoring

If every term of a polynomial is divisible by the same quantity, that quantity can be factored out. This means that we can express the polynomial as the product of that quantity times a new, smaller polynomial.

EXAMPLE

Factor the following expression:

$$2x^3 - 4x^2 + 4x$$

Every term in this polynomial is divisible by 2x, so we can factor it out of each term. The simplified expression, then, is

$$2x(x^2 - 2x + 2).$$

To verify that you have properly factored an expression, multiply out your solution. If you get back to where you started, you've done it correctly.

3.3 Linear Equations

3.3.1 Linearity

Linear equation is an equation between two (or three) variables that gives a straight line when plotted on a graph (GM 3.5.1). In a linear equation, there can neither be variables raised to exponents nor variables multiplied together.

GM-50   ALGEBRA

(a) $3x + 2y = z + 5$

This equation is linear.

(b) $3x^2 - 2xy = 1$

This equation is not linear. The terms $3x^2$ and $2xy$ cannot appear in a linear equation.

The reason such equations are called "linear" is that they can be represented on a Cartesian graph as a straight line. "Cartesian" is the basic coordinate system composed of an x axis and a y axis (and sometimes z axis as well) which we will review shortly.

3.3.2 Solving Linear Equations with Multiple Variables

In the previous sections we have only considered equations with single variables. In some cases though, GAMSAT problems will require you to deal with a second variable.

A. Isolating a Variable

When you have a single equation with two variables, you will not be able to solve for specific values. What you can do is solve for one variable in terms of the other. To do this, pick a variable to isolate on one side of the equation and move all other terms to the other side.

EXAMPLE

Solve the following for y: $4y - 3x = 2y + x - 6$.

Let's isolate y on the left side:

$(4y - 3x) + 3x - 2y = (2y + x - 6) + 3x - 2y$

$$\frac{(2y)}{2} = \frac{(4x - 6)}{2}$$

$$y = 2x - 3$$

Now we know the value of y, but only in relation to the value of x. If we are now given some value for x, we can simply plug it in to our solution and obtain y. For example, if $x = 1$ then $y = 2 - 3 = -1$.

B. Solving Systems of Equations

How do you know if you will be able to solve for specific values in an equation or not? The general rule is that if you have the same number of unique equations as variables (or more equations), you will be able find a specific value for every variable. So for the example in Part A, since we have two variables and only one equation, in order to solve for the variables, we would need one more unique equation.

In order for an equation to be unique, it must not be algebraically derived from another equation.

EXAMPLE

$$300 = 30x - 10y$$
$$30 = 3x - y$$

From the above example, the two equations describe the same line and therefore are not unique since they are scalar multiples of each other.

There are two strategies you should know for solving a system of equations:

I. **Substitution.** This strategy can be used every time, although, it will not always be the fastest way to come up with a solution. You begin with one equation and isolate a variable as in Part A. Next, wherever the isolated variable appears in the second equation, replace it with the expression this variable is equal to. This effectively eliminates that variable from the second equation.

If you only have two equations, all you need are two steps. Once you have followed the procedure above, you can solve for the second variable in the second equation and substitute that value back into the first equation to find the value of the first variable. If you have more than two variables and equations, you will need to continue this process of isolation and substitution until you reach the last equation.

EXAMPLE

Solve the following system of equations for x and y.

$$4y - 3x = 2y + x - 6$$
$$3x + y = 12$$

We have already isolated y in the first equation, so the first step is done. The new system is as follows:

$$y = 2x - 3$$
$$3x + y = 12$$

Next, we substitute $2x - 3$ for y in the second equation.

$$3x + (2x - 3) = 12$$
$$\Rightarrow 5x - 3 = 12$$
$$\Rightarrow 5x = 15$$
$$\Rightarrow x = 3$$

Now, we have a value for x, but we still need a value for y. Substitute 3 for x in the y-isolated equation.

$$y = 2(3) - 3$$
$$y = 3$$

So our solution to this system of equations is $x = 3$, $y = 3$.

II. **Equation Addition or Subtraction.** You will not always be able to apply this strategy, but in some cases, it will save you from having to do all of the time-consuming substitutions of Strategy I. The basic idea of equation addition or subtraction is exactly what you would expect: Addition or subtraction of equations directly to each other.

Say you have two equations, A and B. Because both sides of any equation are by definition equal, you can add, say, the left side of equation A to the left side of equation B and the right side of equation A to the right side of equation B without changing anything. In performing this addition, you are doing the same thing to both sides of equation B.

The purpose of performing such an addition is to try and get a variable to cancel out completely. If you can accomplish this, you can solve for the other variable easily (assuming you only have two variables, of course). Before adding the equations together, you can manipulate either of them however you like (as long as you maintain equality) in order to set up the cancellation of a variable.

If the only way to cancel out a variable is by subtracting the equation, this may be done as well.

EXAMPLE

Use equation addition or subtraction to solve the following for x and y.

$$2x - 2y = 1$$
$$4x + 5y = 11$$

If we multiply the first equation by two, we will have $4x$ present in each equation. Then if we subtract, the $4x$ in each equation will cancel.

$$4x - 4y = 2$$
$$-(4x + 5y = 11)$$
$$\overline{0x - 9y = -9}$$
$$\Rightarrow y = 1$$

Now, we can substitute this value of y into whichever equation looks simpler to solve for x (either one will work though).

$$2x - 2(1) = 1$$
$$\Rightarrow 2x = 3$$
$$\Rightarrow x = \frac{3}{2}$$

So our solution to this system of equations is $y = 1$, $x = \frac{3}{2}$.

> **NOTE**
>
> A 'classic' GAMSAT-style question requires an understanding of Strategy II to solve Hess' Law problems (CHM 8.3).

3.4 Graphing Linear Functions

3.4.1 Linear Equations and Functions

Every linear equation can be rewritten as a linear function. To do so, simply isolate one of the variables as in GM 3.1.1C. This variable is now a function of the variables on the other side of the equation.

EXAMPLE

Rewrite the equation $3y - 2x = 6$ as a function of x.

$$3y - 2x = 6$$
$$\Rightarrow 3y = 2x + 6$$
$$\Rightarrow y = \frac{2}{3}x + 2$$

Now that we have isolated y, it is actually a function of x. For every input of x, we get a unique output of y. If you like, you can rewrite y as $f(x)$.

$$f(x) = \frac{2}{3}x + 2$$

3.4.2 Cartesian Coordinates in 2D

The Cartesian coordinate system is the most commonly used system for graphing. A Cartesian graph in two dimensions has two axes: The x-axis is the horizontal one, and the y-axis is the vertical one. The independent variable is always along the x-axis and the dependent variable is along the y-axis. The independent variable is controlled and the output depends on the independent variable.

The further right you go on the x-axis, the larger the numbers get; and on the y-axis, the numbers get larger the further up you go. A point on the graph is specified as an ordered pair of an x value and a y value like this: (x, y). This point exists x units from the origin (the point $(0, 0)$ where the axes cross) along the x-axis, and y units from the origin along the y-axis.

EXAMPLE

Find the point $(3, -1)$ on the Cartesian graph shown.

To plot this point, simply count three units to the right along the x-axis and one unit down along the y-axis.

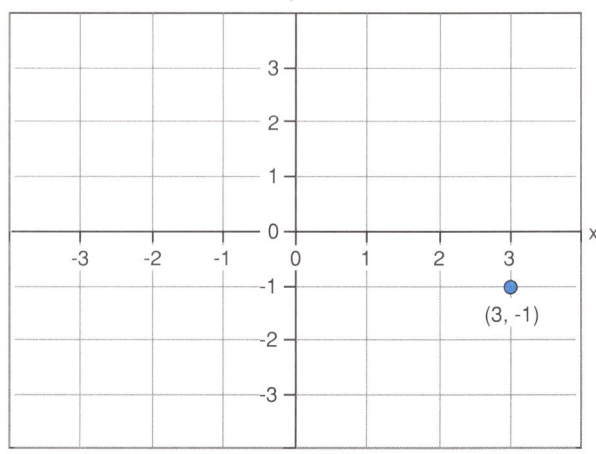

GM-54   ALGEBRA

3.4.3 Graphing Linear Equations

In order to graph a straight line in Cartesian coordinates, all you need to know is two points. Every set of two points has only one unique line that passes through both of them.

To find two points from a linear equation, simply choose two values to plug in for one of the variables. It is best to pick values that will make your calculations easier, such as 0 and 1. Plugging in each of these values, we can solve for y and obtain two points.

EXAMPLE

Graph the line defined by $2x + y = 3$.

First, let's plug in $x = 0$ and $x = 1$ to find two points on the line.

$$2(0) + y = 3$$
$$\Rightarrow y = 3$$
$$2(1) + y = 3$$
$$\Rightarrow y = 1$$

Now, we have two points: (0, 3) and (1, 1). To graph the line, all we have to do is plot these points on a graph and draw a straight line between them.

3.4.4 Slope-Intercept Form

There are two pieces of information that are very useful in the graphing of a linear equation: The slope of the line and its y-intercept.

Slope refers to the steepness of a line. It is the ratio (slope = rise/run) of the number of units along the y-axis to the number of units along the x-axis between two points.

EXAMPLE

$y = 5x + 3$ and $y = 5x + 10$

These two equations would be parallel to each other since both slopes (m) = 5.

$$y = 3x + 6 \text{ and } y = -\frac{1}{3x} + 3$$

These two equations are perpendicular. The line of the first equation has a positive slope and the perpendicular line has a decreasing slope and therefore both slopes have opposite signs. In fact, the general rule is that when slopes are negative reciprocals of each other, the 2 lines in question must be perpendicular to each other.

The *y*-**intercept** of a line is the *y*-coordinate of the point at which the line crosses the *y*-axis. The value of *x* where the line intersects, is always zero and its coordinates will be (0, *y*).

One of the standard forms of a linear equation is the slope-intercept form, from which the slope and the *y*-intercept of the line are immediately obvious. This form resembles $y = mx + b$. Here *m* and *b* are constants such that *m* is the slope of the line and *b* is the *y*-intercept.

EXAMPLE

Rewrite the following equation in slope-intercept form: $2y + 5x = 8$.

$$\Rightarrow 2y = -5x + 8$$
$$\Rightarrow y = -\frac{5}{2}x + 4$$

This is now in slope-intercept form. In this case, the slope *m* is $-\frac{5}{2}$ and the *y*-intercept is 4.

Slope-intercept form is also useful for constructing the equation of a line from other information. If you are given the slope and the intercept, obviously you can simply plug them in to $y = mx + b$ to get the equation. It is also very simple to obtain the slope and intercept if you know two points on the line, (x_1, y_1) and (x_2, y_2). The slope can be obtained directly from this information:

$$\text{Slope} = \text{rise/run} = (y_2 - y_1)/(x_2 - x_1)$$

Once the slope *m* is obtained, you only need to solve for *b*. To do so, plug in one of the points as well as *m* into the slope-intercept equation. You can then solve for *b*.

EXAMPLE

Find the equation for the line passing through (1, 1) and (2, 3).

First, determine the slope.

$$m = \frac{(3-1)}{(2-1)} = 2$$

Now plug *m* and a point into the slope-intercept equation to find *b*.

$$y = mx + b$$
$$\Rightarrow 1 = 2(1) + b$$
$$\Rightarrow -1 = b$$

Plugging in all of this information, we now have a complete equation.

$$y = 2x - 1$$

GAMSAT MATH

3.5 Basic Graphs

3.5.1 The Graph of a Linear Equation

Given any two points (x_1, y_1) and (x_2, y_2) on the line, we have:

$$y_1 = ax_1 + b$$

and

$$y_2 = ax_2 + b.$$

Subtracting the upper equation from the lower one and dividing through by $x_2 - x_1$ gives the value of the slope,

$$\boxed{\begin{array}{l} a = (y_2 - y_1)/(x_2 - x_1) \\ = \Delta y/\Delta x = \text{rise/run} \end{array}}$$

Lines that have positive slopes, slant "up hill" (as viewed from left to right), like the graph on this page. Lines that have negative slopes, slant "down hill" (as viewed from left to right). Lines that are horizontal have no slope (= a slope of zero; see PHY 1.4.1).

> **NOTE**
>
> Often on the real GAMSAT, you will need to either calculate the slope of a line or the area under a graph or line, or both.

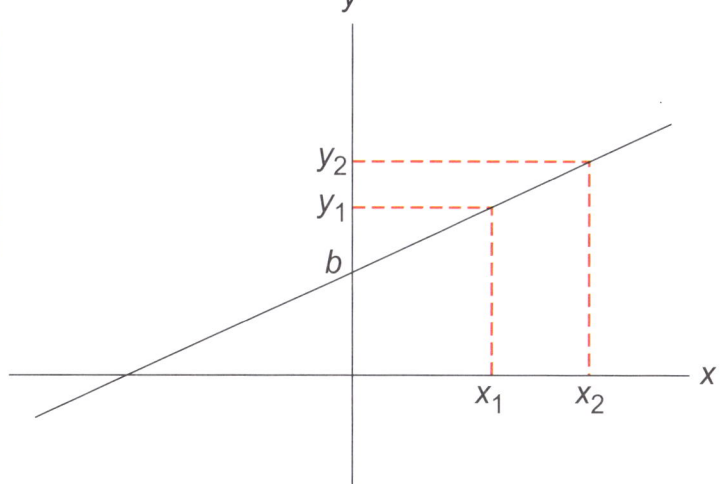

> **NOTE**
>
> Don't get attached to variables in equations. Only focus on the meaning of the equation. Among and within different textbooks and exams, different variables may be used in the same equations (*a* or *m* for slope; S or d or x for displacement, and many others). Some exam questions are designed to catch students who try to memorize without understanding equations.

3.5.2 Reciprocal Curve

For any real number x, there exists a unique real number called the multiplicative inverse or *reciprocal* of x denoted $1/x$ or x^{-1} such that $x(1/x) = 1$. The graph of the reciprocal $1/x$ for any x is:

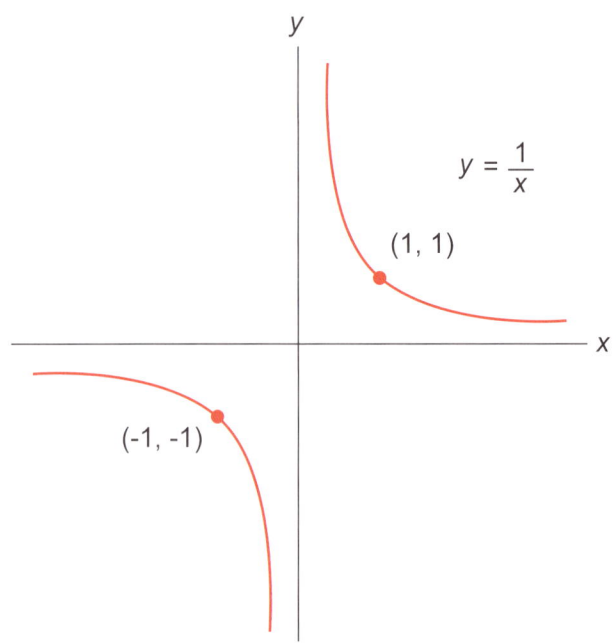

3.5.3 Miscellaneous Graphs

There are classic curves which are represented or approximated in the science text as follows: Sigmoidal curve (CHM 6.9.1, BIO 7.5.1), sinusoidal curve (GM 5.2.3, PHY 7.1), and hyperbolic curves (CHM 9.7 Fig III.A.9.3, BIO 1.1.2). Another type of graph that you will certainly see during the real GAMSAT is where one or both axes are logarithmic (so called semi-log and log-log graphs, respectively; CHM 4.3.3, CHM 6.9.1/2).

If you were to plot a set of experimental data, often one can draw a line or curve which can "best fit" the data. The preceding defines a *regression* line or curve (GM 6.3.1). One purpose of the regression graph is to predict what would likely occur outside of the experimental data.

3.5.4 Tangential Slope and Area under a Curve

During the real GAMSAT, you will very likely need to calculate a slope based on a curve (i.e. the slope of the straight line must just glance the curve at a specific point = *tangential*), and you will likely have to calculate the area under a curve (depending on the presentation, you would estimate the answer by either counting boxes below the graph or by multiplying some part of the x axis by some part of the y axis; the question could be in Physics, Chemistry or Biology).

As long as you pay attention to the units (dimensional analysis), then you do not have to memorize these common facts: velocity is the slope of a displacement vs. time graph (PHY 1.3); acceleration is the slope and displacement is the area under the curve of a velocity vs. time graph (PHY 1.4.1); the change in momentum (= impulse) is the area under a force vs. time graph (PHY 4.3); work is the area under the force vs. displacement graph (PHY 7.2.1).

Do not worry about the physics for now. Just focus on the math. Let's examine a velocity vs. time graph of a bullet fired from a gun. The y axis is velocity which is in the SI units of meters/second (m/s). The x axis is time in the SI units of seconds (s).

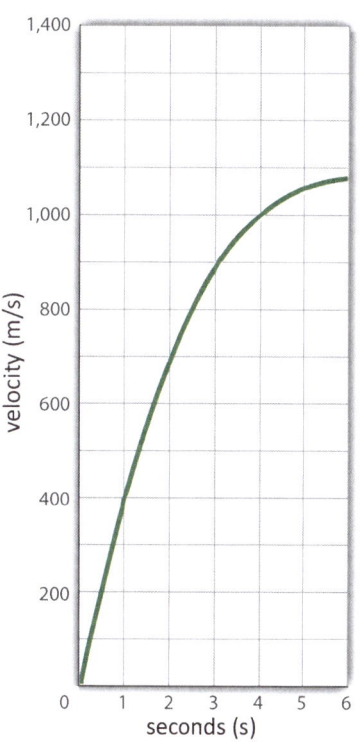

Here are 2 questions that you can try to work out before looking at the solutions:

(1) Given that acceleration is in units of m/s^2, calculate the instantaneous acceleration at time = 3 seconds.

(2) Given that displacement is in the units of meters (m), calculate the displacement of the bullet in the first 2 seconds of being fired.

GAMSAT-Prep.com
THE GOLD STANDARD

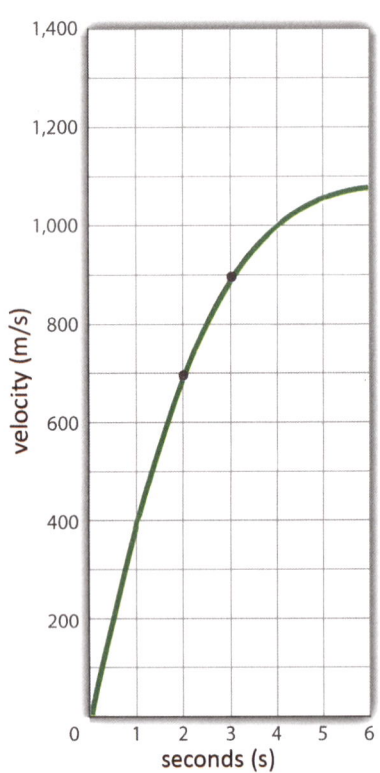 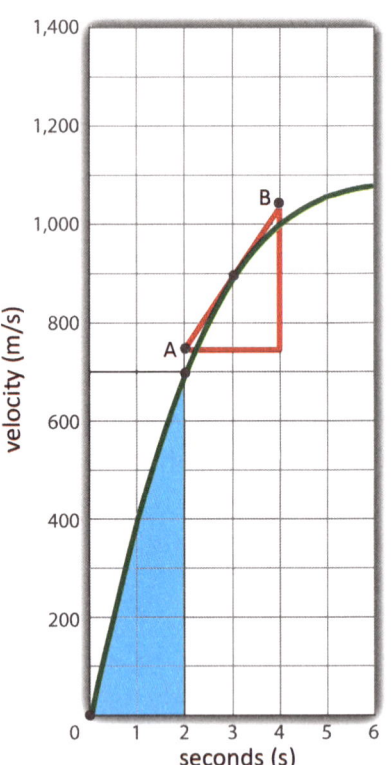

Hints if required:

(1) Hint: try to calculate the slope of a straight line off the curve at 3 seconds. Why does the slope solve the problem? Take a look at the units. A slope is the change of y divided by the change of x. In terms of units, this would make m/s/s = m/s^2 = acceleration.

(2) Hint: determine the area of the curve below that segment of the graph (i.e. the first 2 seconds). One way to do so is to calculate the area of one box and then estimate how many boxes are below the curve. Why the area? Again, the units: the area of a square or rectangle is one side times the other side. For a graph, it is x times y. So here is what happens to the units: m/s x s = m = meters which is displacement.

GM-60   ALGEBRA

GAMSAT MATH

ANSWERS

(1) To calculate the slope at a point, the line that you draw needs to be tangential to the curve as described previously (see the preceding graphs). The line can be as long or as short as you want (basically, you choose the length to make the calculation as easy as possible).

We chose a change in x (i.e. from points A to B as seen from the x axis) which is easy to calculate = 2 seconds (i.e. 4 − 2 = 2). The change in y (i.e. from points A to B as seen from the y axis) is also easy = 300 m/s (1050 − 750 = 300). The slope is the change in y divided by the change in x so: (300 m/s)/(2 s) = 150 m/s^2.

Notice that point A in the graph is our point (x_1, y_1) and point B is (x_2, y_2); see GM 3.5.1. While sitting the GAMSAT, you may need to assess a slope by laying down a pen or pencil on the exam paper followed by a reasonable estimate of the data points.

(2) As explained in the "hint", we are trying to calculate the area under the curve in the first 2 seconds. If you put your pen in the line (0, 0) to (2, 700), you will notice that your pen approximates the green line (do not use a ruler because they are not permitted during the GAMSAT!).

In other words, if we were to imagine a rectangle that includes the points (0, 0) to (2, 700), then the area under the curve seems to be about ½ that value. Because a rectangle is simply one side times the other, we can multiply 2 seconds x 700 m/s = 1400 meters. The area below the green graph is about ½ that or 700 meters, which is thus the displacement.

Of course, it depends on the multiple choice answers. Careful observation will show you that the area under the curve is slightly more than 700 m.

An alternative way to calculate the area in blue would be to calculate the area of one single small box from the graph: 100 m/s times 1 s = 100 meters. If you carefully count the boxes in the blue shaded area (which you can see better from the graph on the left), you will be able to count about 7 complete boxes (i.e. approx. 700 m; of course, sometimes you need to add 2 incomplete boxes to make one full box).

Yet another alternative may have been the first choice of those with a science background: estimate the area in blue as a triangle (which we will discuss in GM 4.2.2) which is 1/2(base)(height) = 1/2(2)(700) = 700 m.

3.6 Cartesian Coordinates in 3D

The GAMSAT will sometimes present 3D (3 dimensional) graphs to see if you are capable of a basic analysis.

Consider the following illustration of a 3D Cartesian coordinate system. Notice the origin O and the 3 axis lines X, Y and Z, oriented as shown by the arrows. The tick marks on the axes are one length unit apart. Look carefully at the black dot. What coordinate (x, y, z) would you give to identify the position of that dot? The black dot represents a point with coordinates x = 2, y = 3, and z = 4, or (2,3,4).

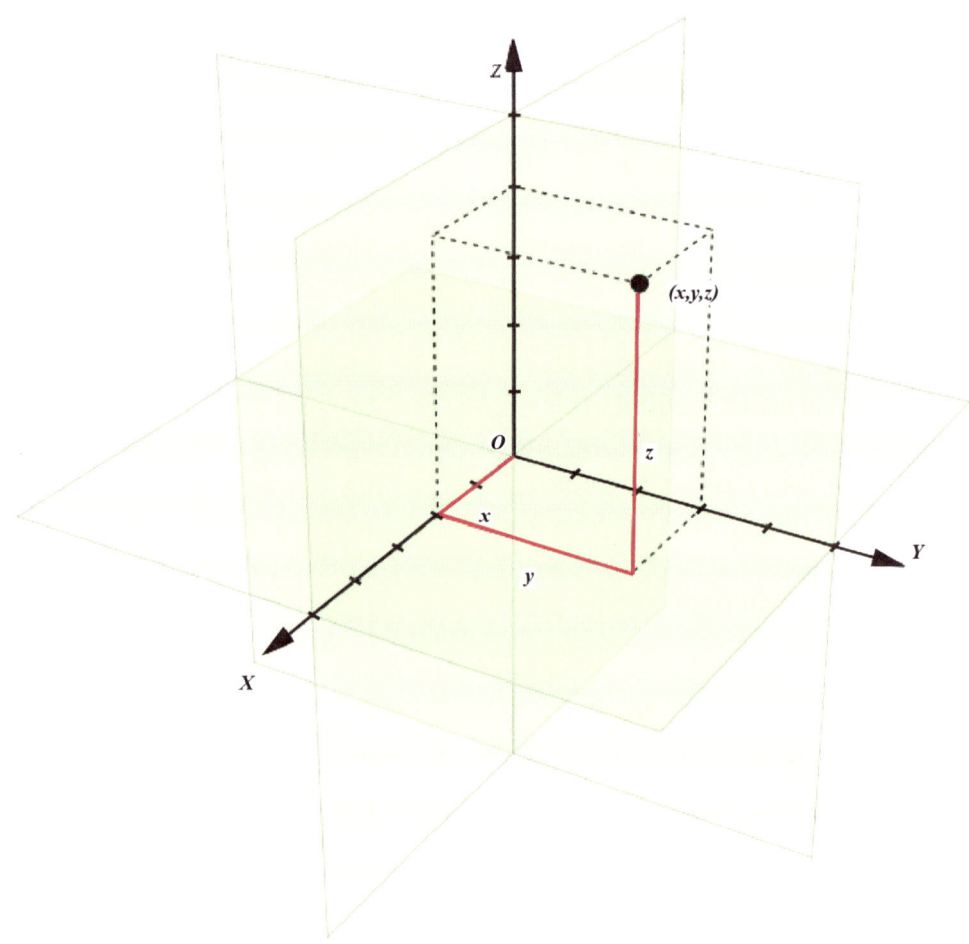

Figure IV.3.1: Three dimensional Cartesian coordinate system. (Stolfi)

GAMSAT MATH

EXAMPLE

We will be looking at phase diagrams in General Chemistry Chapter 4. For now, we'll ignore the chemistry and just focus on graph analysis. So as an exercise to read 3D graphs, comment on the relative magnitudes of temperature and pressure for the SOLID (only) portion of the curve in Figure IV.3.2.

First, you must see the graph as a 3 dimensional object. This particular graph looks like a wooden block with parts of 4 sides gouged out, as well as part of the middle. The 3 arrows in the graph indicate increasing magnitudes in the directions of the arrows. Notice that the pressure for solids could be either high or low. However, the specific volume is always relatively low as is the temperature in the region where the graph shows only solid (of course, it makes sense that something that is solid takes up less volume than the gaseous state; also, because of our experience with water - for example, ice and steam - we expect solids to be at low temperatures and gas to be at high temperatures with liquid somewhere in between).

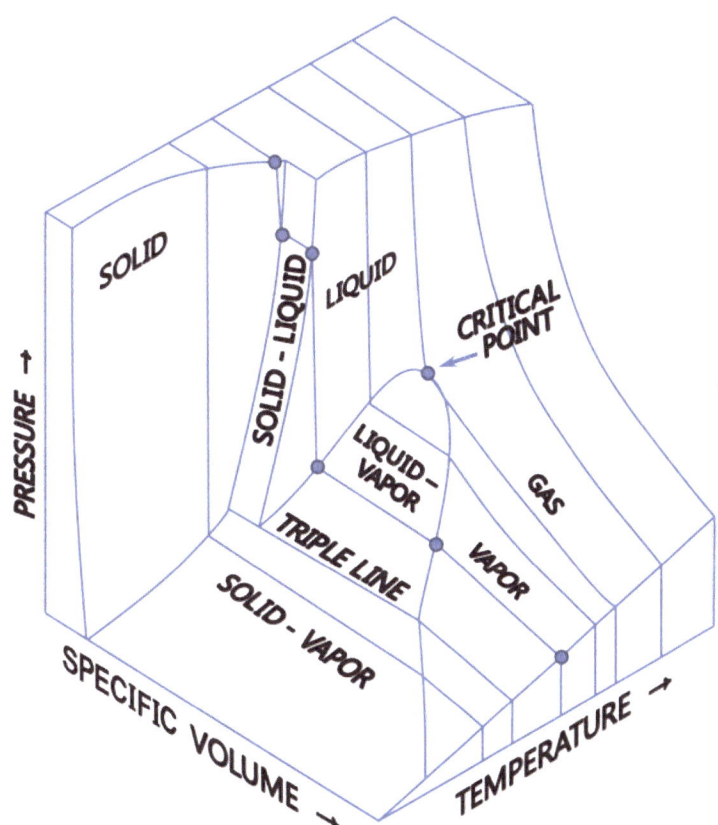

Figure IV.3.2: Pressure-volume-temperature diagram for a pure substance. (Lee/Padleckas)

In conclusion, the relative magnitude of the temperature for the SOLID (only) portion of the curve is low while the pressure can range from high to low.

EXAMPLE

In Figure IV.3.2, which of the following can be relatively high at the solid-vapor equilibrium: pressure, temperature or specific volume?

Notice the pressure is always low at the solid-vapor equilibrium (i.e. the part of the graph that says SOLID-VAPOR near the bottom). Temperature also seems to be relatively low at the SOLID-VAPOR part of the graph. However, the volume can be either high or low and thus the volume would be the correct answer.

Just as an aside, the line on the surface called a **triple line** is where solid, liquid and vapor can all coexist in equilibrium.

> **NOTE**
>
> When you start to complete GS Biology chapter review questions and practice tests online, you will find more questions based on 3D diagrams and log curves.

3.7 Logarithms

3.7.1 Log Rules and Logarithmic Scales

The rules of logarithms are also discussed in context of Acids and Bases in General Chemistry (CHM 6.5.1). These basic log rules also apply to the "natural logarithm" which is the logarithm to the base e, where "e" is an irrational constant approximately equal to 2.71... (GM 1.1.2). The natural logarithm is usually written as $\ln x$ or $\log_e x$.

In general, the power of logarithms is to reduce wide-ranging numbers to quantities with a far smaller range. For example, the graphs commonly seen in this text, including the preceding 2-dimensional graphs, are drawn to a unit or *arithmetic scale*. In other words, each unit on the x and y axes represents exactly *one* unit. This scale can be adjusted to accommodate rapidly changing curves. For example, in a unit scale the numbers 1 ($= 10^0$), 10 ($= 10^1$), 100 ($= 10^2$), and 1000 ($= 10^3$), are all far apart with varying intervals. Using a logarithmic scale, the sparse values suddenly become separated by one unit: $\log 10^0 = 0$, $\log 10^1 = 1$, $\log 10^2 = 2$, $\log 10^3 = 3$, and so on.

In practice, logarithmic scales are often used to convert a rapidly changing curve

GAMSAT MATH

(e.g. an exponential curve) to a straight line. It is called a *semi-log* scale when either the x axis *or* the y axis is logarithmic. It is called a *log-log* scale when both the x axis *and* the y axis are logarithmic. Note: if not specified otherwise, when you just see "log" with no base, then it is considered to be the "common log" which means log base 10.

Here are the rules you must know:

1) $\log_a a = 1$
2) $\log_a M^k = k \log_a M$
3) $\log_a(MN) = \log_a M + \log_a N$
4) $\log_a(M/N) = \log_a M - \log_a N$
5) $10^{\log_{10} M} = M$
6) $\log_a(1) = 0$, given "a" is greater than zero.

EXAMPLE

Given:

$$pH = -\log_{10}[H^+]$$

Let us calculate the pH of 0.001 H^+ (for now, ignore the chemistry, focus only on the math):

$[H^+] = 0.001$
$-\log[H^+] = -\log(0.001)$
$\quad pH = -\log(10^{-3})$
$\quad pH = 3 \log 10 \quad$ (rule #2)
$\quad pH = 3 \quad\quad\quad$ (rule #1, a = 10)

EXAMPLE

What is log (1 000 000)?
log (1 000 000) = log 10^6 = 6

EXAMPLE

What is log (1/100)?
log (1/100) = log 10^{-2} = -2

EXAMPLE

Given that ln2 = 0.69, what is $\ln 2e^3$?

Try to solve the problem while keeping in mind: (1) ln is the natural logarithm, meaning that it is log to the base e; (2) our 3rd rule of logarithms permits you separate factors.

$\ln 2e^3 = \ln 2 + \ln e^3 = 0.69 + 3 = 3.69$

Notice that if you have the base of the log and the base of the number with the exponent the same, then the answer is simply the exponent. Thus

$\text{Log}(1000) = \log 10^3 = \ln e^3 = 3$

NOTE

GAMSAT log problems come in the form of pH, pKa, pKb, rate law, Nernst equation, semi-log graphs, log-log graphs, decibels/sound intensity (PHY 8.3), Gibbs free energy (CHM 9.10), just to name a few! The relevant equations are usually provided. In other words, the 'science' reduces to a basic math problem.

GAMSAT-Prep.com
THE GOLD STANDARD

EXAMPLE

Approximate log(200).

Because the number 200 is between 100 and 1000 (but clearly closer to 100), and since log(100) = 2 and log(1000) = 3, log(200) must be a number between 2 and 3 but closer to the number 2. Such an approximation is sufficient for a multiple choice exam. {Incidentally, log(200) happens to be approximately 2.3.}

> **NOTE**
>
> The common log and the natural log (ln) are common features of the GAMSAT.

3.8 Exponential and Logarithmic Curves

The exponential and logarithmic functions are *inverse functions*. That is, their graphs can be reflected about the $y = x$ line which you can see in Figure IV.3.3.

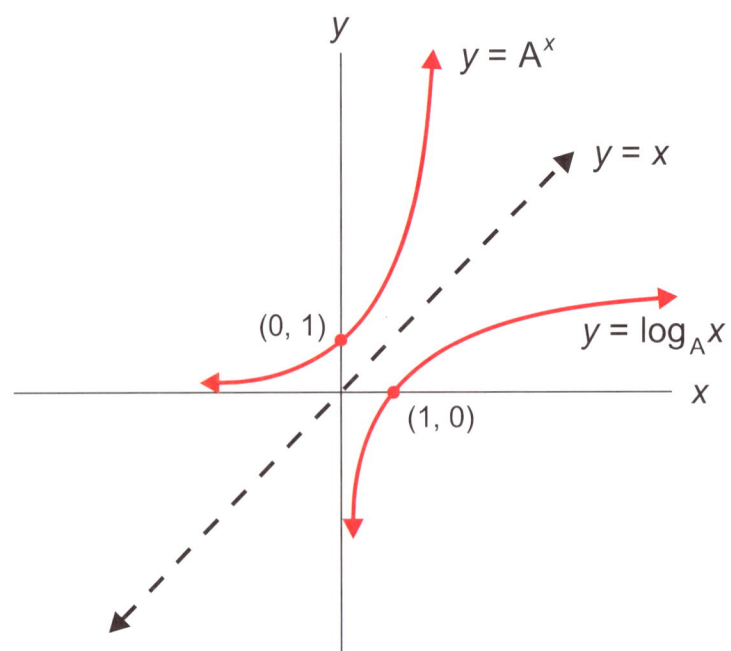

Figure IV.3.3: Exponential and Logarithmic Graphs. $A > 0$, $A \neq 1$. Notice that when a positive number is raised to the power of 1, then the result is 0 [i.e. the point (0, 1); see also GM 1.5.4, 1.5.5 for rules of exponents]. Also note that log(1) = ln (1) = 0 [i.e. the point (1, 0) on the generic logarithmic curve].

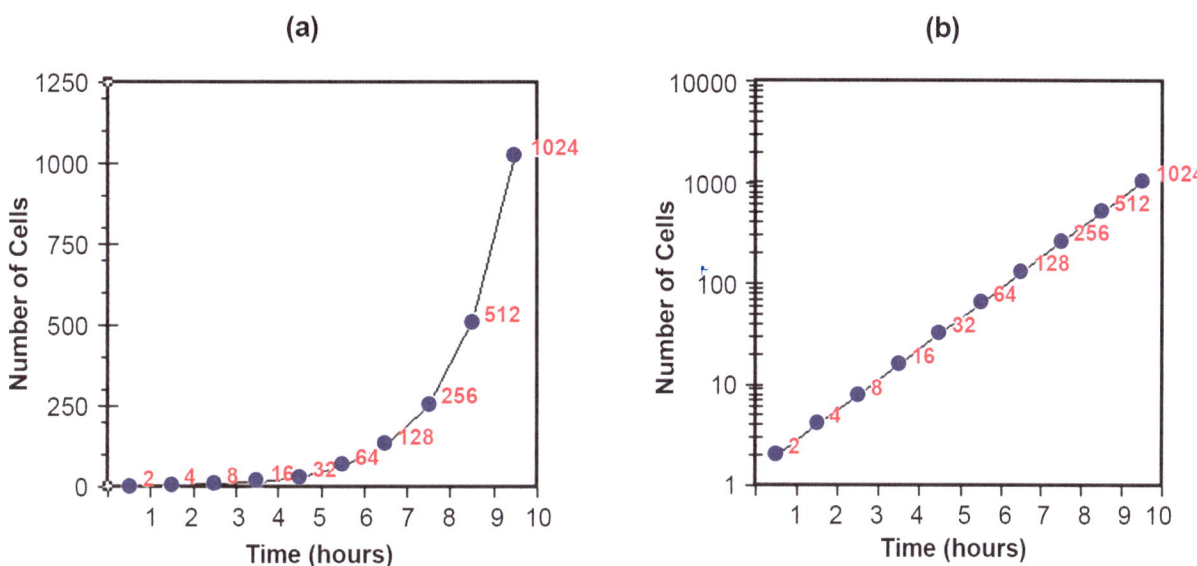

Figure IV.3.4: Growth curves of cells dividing mitotically. (a) An exponential curve with a linear scale for the x and y axis. (b) A logarithmic scale on the y axis converts the data rising exponentially into a linear graph. This is referred to as a semi-log graph or semi-log plot. Notice that it is observation or analysis that leads to the conclusion as to what type of graph is being assessed as neither graph is labelled "exponential" nor "logarithm" anywhere.

Let's revisit one of the key reasons for using logarithms: when the data points vary from low numbers to very high numbers, sometimes a log helps to better demonstrate all the data points on one graph. Consider Figure IV.3.4: two growth curves that both represent the same data of bacteria doubling over time ($2^n = 2, 2^2, 2^3, 2^4, 2^5, 2^6, 2^7, 2^8, 2^9, 2^{10}$ which is 1024; BIO 2.2).

Notice that in the first graph, the y axis increases in a linear fashion: the difference between each major marking is 250 cells and it starts at zero. The problem however is that the first 4 or 5 points on the exponential curve are not really distinguishable. They are all such small relative numbers making the first ½ of the curve quite flat before it increases rapidly. It is that rapid rise that we recognize visually as an exponential increase (even though, of course, it is the entire curve which is exponential, being 2 to the power of n).

On the other hand, the second graph uses a logarithmic scale on the y axis (i.e. each number is 10 times the preceding number and equally spaced; the 4th number does not represent 4 times some number, rather, it represents 10 to the power of 4 times which is 10 000 times larger); suddenly the exponential curve is converted to a manageable, more clear, linear relationship where small and large

GAMSAT-Prep.com
THE GOLD STANDARD

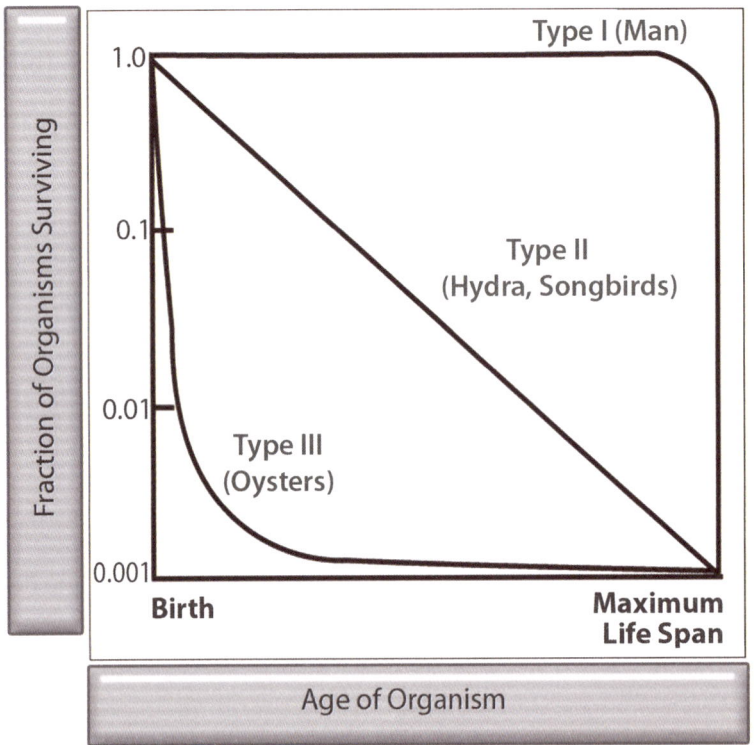

Figure IV.3.5: Type I, II and III survivorship curves scaled to a maximum life span for each species.

data points are easily visible on one graph. Notice that if you took the log of the 5 numbers along the y axis, you would get the quite regular result of 0, 1, 2, 3 and 4 (recall that log 10000 = log10^4 = 4). Incidentally, because the x axis increases in a linear fashion, the preceding is a semi-log graph.

Thus a graph that has a scale that is logarithmic on one axis but is linear on the other axis is semi-log. The term for the graph is unimportant for the GAMSAT but recognizing that you are dealing with such a graph is often critical to answering the questions properly. We will now explore another semi-log graph (Figure IV.3.5) and we will work through some log-log graphs online (Biology chapter review questions).

Spend a few moments considering Figure IV.3.5.

QUESTION 1

Based on the diagram provided, is it true that approximately ½ of songbirds would be expected to survive ½ of their maximum lifespan?

QUESTION 2

One perspective regarding the biological success of a species would be to equate success with the absolute number of individual organisms belonging to the species in question. Given this perspective, if oysters, songbirds and humans are all equally successful, based on the diagram, which of the three likely produces the least number of organisms (i.e. the least number of offspring per organism)?

EXPLANATION 1

NO! Not even close!! First, let's get a sense of the scales. We must assume that the x axis is linear because no other information is provided. However, the y axis is clearly logarithmic. It looks like it is regular (in a linear sense) but when you look at the numbers, they are increasing logarithmically. Each marking on the y axis is 10 times the previous marking. After 3 markings, 1000 times or 10^3. If you take the log of the 4 numbers on the y axis, you would get the very regular numbers of -3, -2, -1 and 0.

Now let's look at ½ of the maximum life span (so ½ of the length of the x axis). When you look at the Type II line at that point (signifying songbirds and hydra; it's not important that you know what hydra means) and look across to the y axis, you get a point ½ way between 0.01 and 0.1. Even if we imagine the higher of the 2 numbers, 0.1, that is only 1/10th of the surviving organisms (0.1 = 1/10 = 10%). And because the lower number is 1/100th (= 1%) of the surviving organisms, the actual result is between the two which is far lower than ½ of surviving organisms (i.e. 50%). This is a common question type that can appear in any of the GAMSAT science subtopics. If you do not understand the scale, you will get the wrong answer.

EXPLANATION 2

Presumably, for the next generation to exist, the current generation must survive long enough to reproduce. The survivorship curve with the most extreme change between birth and a presumed age of reproductive ability would be the Type III survivorship curve. Let's see what we can infer from the shapes of that curve.

Most individuals in populations with Type III survivorship must produce many

> **NOTE**
>
> Notice that neither Figure IV.3.4 nor Figure IV.3.5 had a clear origin of (0, 0). This fact was not important here but sometimes questions are designed to test whether you observed that the origin was other than (0, 0) and that you took it into account when necessary. We will see some questions like that in Biology.

thousands of individuals, most of whom, according to the diagram, die right away. Once this initial period is over, survivorship is relatively constant. Examples of this would likely include fish, seeds, marine larvae, and of course oysters. Relatively little effort or parental care is likely invested in each individual.

Type I survivorship includes humans, likely, we could reason, in developed countries. As a result of environment and the resources invested in each individual, there is a high survivorship throughout the life cycle. Most individuals, according to the graph, die of old age. If Type III must produce a lot of individuals to survive the 'die off' and still be successful, then Type I requires relatively few offspring to be successful because the survivorship is better than the other two groups. Thus the answer is: humans.

GOLD STANDARD WARM-UP EXERCISES
CHAPTER 3: Algebra

1. If $y = \dfrac{12}{4x^3 - 6x + 5}$, then if $x = 2$ then y equals:

   A. 12/17
   B. 12/49
   C. 12/9
   D. 12/25

2. $13xy^2z$ is to $39y$ as $9xyz^6$ is to:

   A. $3z^5$
   B. $27z$
   C. $9y$
   D. $27z^5$

3. At what point do the lines $y = 2x - 1$ and $6x - 5y = -3$ intersect?

   A. (2, 3)
   B. (0.5, 0)
   C. (−1, −3)
   D. (−0.5, −2)

4. Loubha has a total of $.85. If she has two less dimes than nickels, how many dimes and nickels does she have?

   A. 5 nickels, 7 dimes
   B. 6 nickels, 4 dimes
   C. 4 nickels, 2 dimes
   D. 7 nickels, 5 dimes

5. If $2.5 \times 10^3 (3 \times 10^x) = 0.075$, then x equals:

   A. −3
   B. −5
   C. 0
   D. −4

6. A plank of wood is leaning against the left side of a house with vertical walls. Both are on level ground. If the plank touches the ground 7 feet away from the base of the house, and touches the house at a point 5 feet above the ground, at what slope is the plank lying?

   A. −5/7
   B. 7/5
   C. −7/5
   D. 5/7

7. If $n + n = k + k + k$ and $n + k = 5$, then $n = ?$

   A. 9
   B. 6
   C. 5
   D. 3

8. Let $x = 4$ and $y = 8$. Evaluate the expression: $((y^{-2/3})^{1/2}) / (x^{-1/2})$.

   A. 8
   B. 4
   C. 1
   D. 1/2

9. Evaluate the expression: $\log_6(24) + \log_6(9)$.

  A. 3
  B. 2
  C. 1
  D. 1/2

10. Solve for x: $\log_{10}(70) = x + \log_{10}(7)$.

  A. 0
  B. 1
  C. 2
  D. 3

11. Simplify the expression: $x(\log_b(y)) + y(\log_b(y))$.

  A. $\log_b(y^{x-y})$
  B. $\log_b(y^{x+y})$
  C. $\log_b(y^{xy})$
  D. $\log_b(xy^{xy})$

12. Evaluate the expression: $\ln(e^3)\log_3(27) + \ln(1)\ln(e)$.

  A. e
  B. 3
  C. 6
  D. 9

13. Which equation matches the graph below?

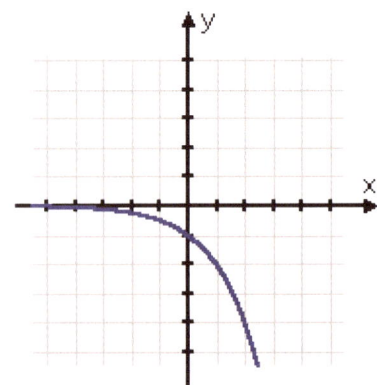

  A. $y = 2^x - 1$
  B. $y = -(2^x) + 1$
  C. $y = 2^x$
  D. $y = -(2^x)$

14. Which equation matches the graph below?

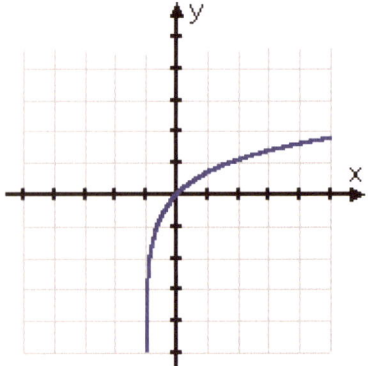

  A. $y = \ln(x)$
  B. $y = -\ln(x - 1)$
  C. $y = -\ln(x + 1)$
  D. $y = \ln(x + 1)$

15. pH is measured on a logarithmic scale given by the equation pH = $-\log_{10}(H)$. Given that H is positive but less than 1, as H decreases, the slope of the graph of pH vs H:

   A. decreases.
   B. increases.
   C. remains constant.
   D. sometimes decreases, sometimes increases.

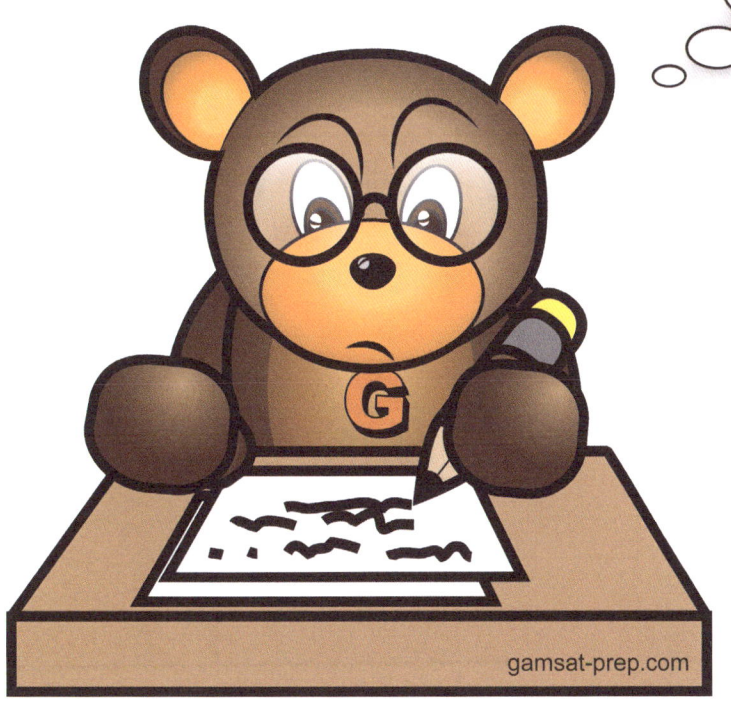

GS ANSWER KEY
CHAPTER 3

		Cross-Reference				Cross-Reference
1.	D	GM 3.1.4	9.	A	GM 3.7	
2.	D	GM 3.3.2, 3.3.3	10.	B	GM 3.7	
3.	A	GM 3.4.2A, 3.4.2B	11.	B	GM 1.5, 3.7	
4.	D	GM 3.4.2B	12.	D	GM 1.5, 3.7	
5.	B	GM 3.3.1	13.	D	GM 3.7, 3.8	
6.	D	GM 3.5.4	14.	D	GM 3.7, 3.8	
7.	D	GM 3.3.1, 3.4.2A, 3.4.2B	15.	B	GM 3.7, 3.8	
8.	C	GM 1.5				

* Worked solutions can be found at the end of the GAMSAT Math chapters. If something is still not clear, go to the forum at GAMSAT-prep.com.

GOLD NOTES

GOLD NOTES

GEOMETRY
Chapter 4

Memorize	Understand	Not Required
Pythagorean Theorem Perimeter, Area, and Volume Formulas Properties of Triangles	* Points in Cartesian Coordinates * Parallel and Perpendicular Lines * Similar Polygons * Types of Triangles and Angles * Problems with Figures and Solids	* Vertices, cones, volumes of complex solids

GAMSAT-Prep.com

Introduction

Geometry is a very visual branch of mathematics dealing with lines and shapes and relations in space, so drawing and labeling pictures can be extremely helpful when you are confronted with certain GAMSAT physics problems. But don't forget about algebra! More often than not, these problems are simply algebraic equations in disguise.

Additional Resources

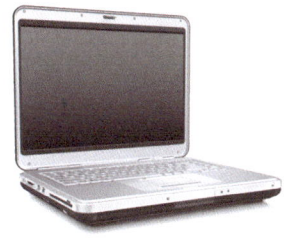

Free Online Forum

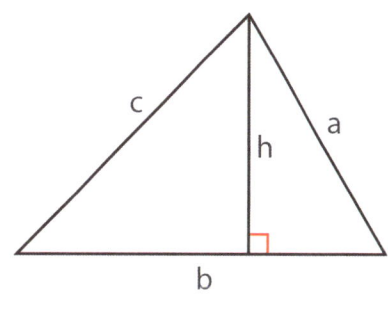

Special Guest

4.1 Points, Lines and Angles

4.1.1 Points and Distance

Knowing your way around the Cartesian coordinate systems begins with understanding the relationships between simple points. As discussed in section 3.5, points on a graph are represented as an ordered pair of an *x* and *y* coordinate, (*x*, *y*).

A. Addition and Subtraction of Points

To add or subtract two points, simply add or subtract the two *x* values to obtain the new *x* value and add or subtract the two *y* values to obtain the new *y* value.

EXAMPLE

Add the points (2, 3) and (1, -5).

(2, 3) + (1, -5)
= (2 + 1, 3 – 5)
= (3, -2)

Graphically, addition of points is easy to visualize. All you are doing when you add two points is treating the first point as the new origin. You then plot the second point in terms of this new origin to find the sum of the two points.

You can add more than two points in the same way. Just add all of the *x* values together, and then add all of the *y* values together.

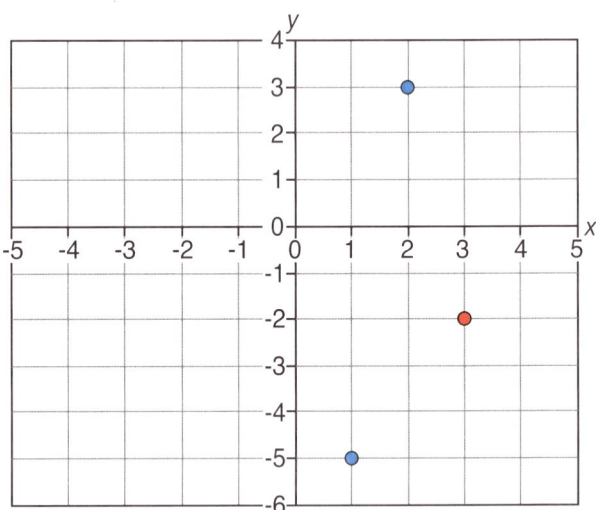

B. Distance between Points

Finding the distance between two points requires the use of the Pythagorean Theorem. This theorem is probably the most important tool you have for solving geometric problems.

Pythagorean Theorem: $x^2 + y^2 = z^2$

This theorem describes the relationship between the lengths of the sides of a right triangle. The lengths *x* and *y* correspond to the two legs of the triangle adjacent to the right angle, and the length *z* corresponds to the hypotenuse of the triangle.

In order to find the distance between two points (x_1, y_1) and (x_2, y_2), consider there to be a line segment connecting them. This line segment (with length z equivalent to the distance between the points) can be thought of as the hypotenuse of a right triangle. The other two sides extend from the points: One is parallel to the x-axis; the other, to the y-axis (with lengths x and y, respectively).

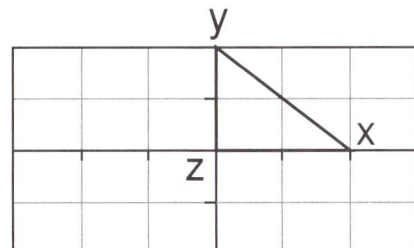

To find the distance between the two points, simply apply the Pythagorean Theorem.

$x = (x_2 - x_1)$
$y = (y_2 - y_1)$
$z = \sqrt{(x^2 + y^2)}$

Plugging in the point coordinates will yield z, the distance between the two points.

EXAMPLE

Find the distance between the points (5, 0) and (2, -4).

$x = (2 - 5) = -3$
$y = (-4 - 0) = -4$
$z = \sqrt{(-3^2 + -4^2)}$
$= \sqrt{(9+16)} = \sqrt{25} = 5$

So the distance between the points is $z = 5$.

4.1.2 Line Segments

A. Segmentation Problems

These problems are a kind of geometry-algebra hybrid. You are given a line segment that has been subdivided into smaller segments, and some information is provided. You are then asked to deduce some of the missing information.

In a segmentation problem, some of the information you are given may be geometric, and some may be algebraic. There is not, however, a clear algebraic equation to solve. You will need to logically determine the steps needed to reach a solution.

EXAMPLE

The line segment QT of length $4x + 6$ is shown in the figure that follows. Point S is the midpoint of QT and segment RS has length x – 1. What is the length of line segment QR?

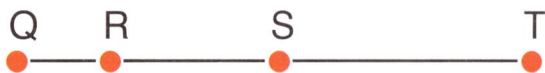

First, determine what information you know. The length of QT and RS are given. Also, since we have a midpoint for QT, the length of QS and ST are simply half of the length of QT.

Now, determine an algebraic relationship regarding the length of QR, which is what we are looking for. We can see that the length of QR is simply QS with the RS segment removed.

$$QR = QS - RS$$

Plugging in our information, we get the following:

$$QR = \frac{(4x+6)}{2} - (x-1)$$
$$= 2x + 3 - x + 1$$
$$= x + 4$$

Before you start working out a solution, it can be extremely helpful to list the information you are given. This will help you understand and organize the problem, both in your own mind and on the page.

B. Segments in the Plane

In segmentation problems, you only have to deal with one dimension. However, line segments can also turn up in problems dealing with a two dimensional Cartesian graph.

To determine the length of a line segment in a plane, simply find the distance between its endpoints using the Pythagorean Theorem (see section 4.1.1).

Any line segment in a plane corresponds to a single linear equation. This can be determined as in chapter 3 from any two points on the line segment. Knowing this linear equation can help you find other points on the line segment.

4.1.3 Angles

An **angle** is formed by the intersection of two lines.

In problems that are not trigonometric, angles are almost always measured in degrees. A full circle makes 360°.

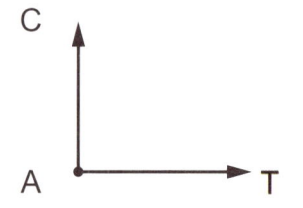

A **right angle** is an angle that is exactly 90°.

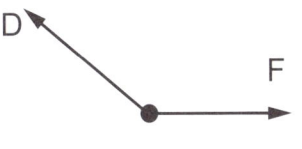

An **obtuse angle** is an angle that is greater than 90°.

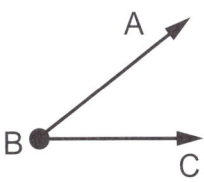

An **acute angle** is an angle that is less than 90°.

A **straight angle** is an angle that is exactly 180°.

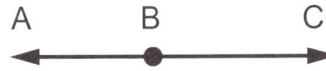

A **vertical angle** is the angle opposite of each other that is formed by two intersecting lines. The two angles across from each other are equal in measure. The following example shows that angles 1 and 3 are vertical angles and equal to each other. Same are angles 2 and 4. At the same time, adjacent vertical angles 1 and 4 or 2 and 3 are also supplementary angles and will form 180°.

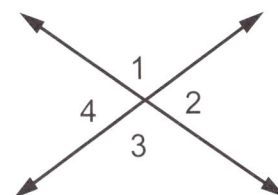

Complementary angles are two angles that add up to 90°. The example that follows shows that angles A and B add up to 90°.

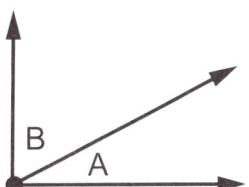

Supplementary angles are two angles that add up to 180°. This example shows that angles A and B add up to 180°.

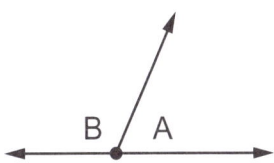

A. Angles and Lines in the Plane

If two lines are **parallel**, they have the same slope. Such lines will never intersect, and so they will never form angles with one another.

If two lines are **perpendicular**, their intersection forms only 90° angles. If the slope of a given line is a/b, then the slope of any perpendicular line is $-b/a$.

EXAMPLE

Consider the line defined by $y = 2x + 3$.

(a) Give the equation for a parallel line:

$$y = 2x + 2.$$

Any line that still has a slope of 2 will suffice. So, in slope-intercept form, any line of the form $y = 2x + a$ will be a parallel line.

GAMSAT MATH   GM-81

(b) Give the equation for the perpendicular line that intersects the given line at the *y*-axis.

In this case, there is only one solution since the line can only intersect the *y*-axis once. The solution will be a line with the same *y*-intercept (which is 3) and the negative reciprocal slope (which is -½): rule from GM 3.4.4.

$$y = -\frac{1}{2}x + 3$$

The standard kind of angle-line problem deals with a setup of two parallel lines that are cut by a transversal, like the one in the following diagram (this type of geometry may present in Physics Chapter 11: Light and Geometric Optics).

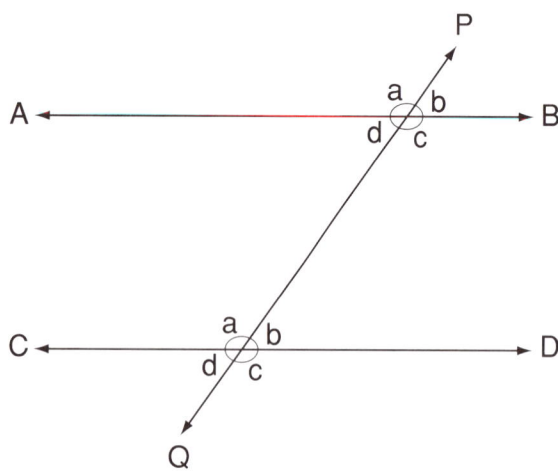

The trick with these problems is to realize that there are only ever two values for the angles.

First, think of the two areas of intersection as exact duplicates of each other.

The upper left angles are equivalent, as are the upper right, the lower left, and the lower right. Using just this information, you automatically know the value of the twin of any angle that is given to you.

Also, angles that are opposite each other are equivalent. So the lower left angle is the same as the upper right and vice versa.

The other fact you can use to determine unknown angles is that the angle along a straight line is 180°. When you are given an angle *a*, you can find supplement *b* by subtracting 180° - *a*.

EXAMPLE

In the figure that follows, if angle *a* is 35°, what is the value of angle *b*?

Angle *b* is the twin of the supplement of *a*, so *b* is equal to 180° - *a*.

$$b = 180° - 35° = 145°$$

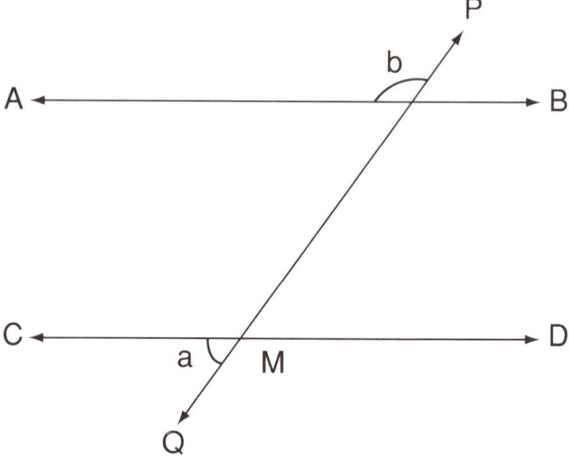

B. Properties of Parallel Line Angles

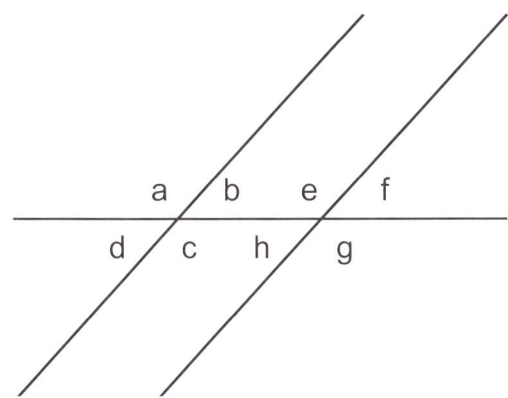

When two parallel lines are cut by a transversal line:

1. both pairs of acute angles as well as obtuse angles are equal: *a = e, b = f, d = h, c = g*.
2. alternate interior angles are equal in measure as well: *c = e, b = h*.

C. Interior Angles of a Polygon

Sometimes you may be dealing with a shape that you are not familiar with and that you do not know the total of all interior angles. A polygon is a flat (i.e. plane) figure with at least three straight sides and angles. If the polygon has *x* sides, the sum, S, is the total of all interior angles for that polygon. For a polygon with *x* sides, the sum may be calculated by the following formula:

$$S = (x - 2)(180°)$$

EXAMPLE

A triangle has 3 sides, therefore,

$S = (3 - 2) \times 180°$
$S = 180°$

A rectangle has 4 sides,

$S = (4 - 2) \times 180°$
$S = 360°$.

Given the total angles for a polygon, you can determine each interior angle of a polygon by dividing the sum of the polygon by the number of sides.

EXAMPLE

A rectangle has a sum of 360°. Given that x = 4, 360° ÷ 4 = 90°. Therefore, each angle in a rectangle is 90°.

> **NOTE**
>
> Though not common, these question types are usually related to projectile motion, inclined planes and optics which will be explored in Physics.

4.2 2D Figures

Make sure you know how to find the area, perimeter, side lengths, and angles of all the figures in this section. There are all kinds of ways to combine different shapes into the same problem; but if you can deal with them all individually, you'll be able to break down any problem thrown your way!

4.2.1 Rectangles and Squares

A **rectangle** is a figure with four straight sides and four right angles. In rectangles, opposite sides always have the same length, as do the two diagonals that can be drawn from corner to corner.

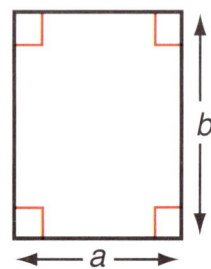

Perimeter: The perimeter of a rectangle is equal to the sum of its sides.

Perimeter = $a + b + a + b = 2a + 2b$

Area: The area of a rectangle is equal to the product of its length and width.

Area = Length × Width = $a \times b$

A **square** is a rectangle with all four sides of the same length, so $a = b$.

The perimeter of a square is

$P = a + a + a + a = 4a$.

The area of a square is

$A = a \times a = a^2$.

4.2.2 Types of Triangles

While there are a wide variety of types of triangles, every one shares these properties:

(i) The sum of the interior angles of a triangle is always equal to 180°. In the following figure, a, b, and c are interior angles.

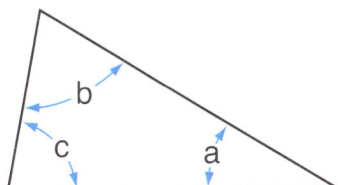

$3x - 10 = 25 + x + 15$
$2x = 10 + 25 + 15$
$2x = 50$
$x = 25$

(ii) The sum of the exterior angles of a triangle is always equal to 360°. The following figure shows *d, e,* and *f* to be exterior angles.

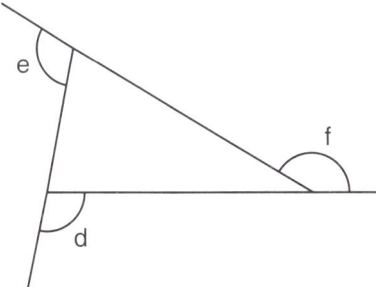

(iv) The perimeter of a triangle is equal to the sum of its sides.

(v) The area of a triangle is always half the product of the base and the height.

$$\text{Area} = \frac{1}{2} \text{Base} \times \text{Height}$$

You can pick any side of the triangle to function as the base, and the height will be the line perpendicular to that side that runs between it and the opposite vertex (i.e. highest point).

(iii) The value of an exterior angle is equal to the sum of the opposite two interior angles.

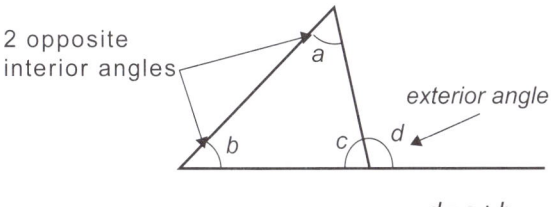

$d = a + b$

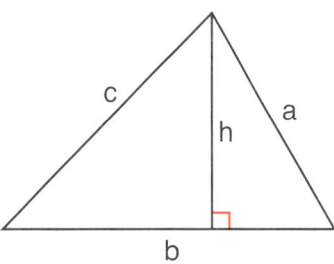

EXAMPLE

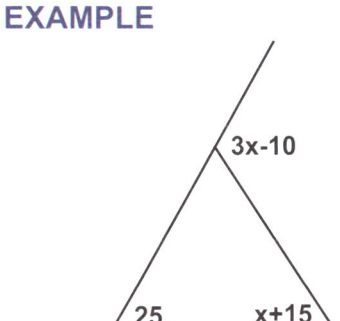

NOTE

If you ever see a triangular shaped graph during the GAMSAT, check the units of one axis multiplied by the other. If the units match the answer choices of any of the questions then you are likely 1/2 way to getting the correct answer without even having read the question yet! As an example, see the 2nd question and the 2nd graph (blue shaded area) in GM 3.5.4.

GAMSAT MATH   GM-85

A. Right Triangles

A **right triangle** is a triangle that contains a right angle. The other two angles in a right triangle add up to 90°.

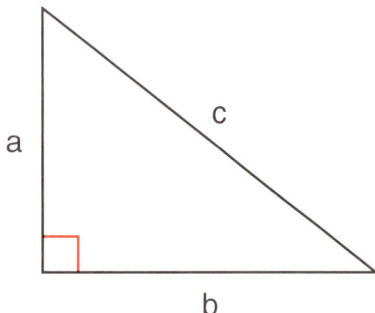

The two short legs of a right triangle (the legs that come together to form the right angle) and the hypotenuse (the side opposite the right angle) are related by the Pythagorean Theorem:

$$a^2 + b^2 = c^2$$

To find a missing side of the triangle, plug the values you have into the Pythagorean Theorem and solve algebraically.

The two legs of a right triangle are its base and height. So to find the area, compute as shown.

> **NOTE**
>
> The area of a triangle, the Pythagorean Theorem and its special ratios appear regularly on the real GAMSAT.

$$\text{Area} = \frac{1}{2}(a \times b)$$

Special Cases: There are a few cases of right triangles you should know. First, the ratios of side lengths 3:4:5 and 5:12:13 are often used. Identifying that a triangle corresponds to one of these cases can save you precious time since you will not have to solve the Pythagorean Theorem.

There are also two special ratios of interior angles for right triangles: 30°-60°-90° and 45°-45°-90°. The sides of a 30°-60°-90° triangle have the ratio $1:\sqrt{3}:2$ and the sides of a 45°-45°-90° triangle have the ratio $1:1:\sqrt{2}$.

B. Isosceles Triangles

An **isosceles triangle** is a triangle that has two equal sides. The angles that sit opposite the equal sides are also equal.

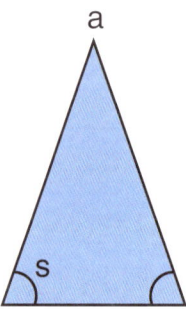

For an isosceles triangle, use the odd side as the base and draw the height line to the odd vertex. This line will bisect the side, so it is simple to determine the height using the Pythagorean Theorem on one of the new right triangles formed.

GAMSAT MATH

> **NOTE**
>
> **Pythagorean Theorem**
>
> Knowing any two sides of a right triangle lets you find the third side by using the Pythagorean formula: $a^2 + b^2 = c^2$.
>
> 3-4-5 triangle: if a right triangle has two legs with a ratio of 3:4, or a leg to a hypotenuse ratio of either 3:5 or 4:5, then it is a 3-4-5 triangle.
>
> 5-12-13 triangle: if a right triangle has two legs with a ratio of 5:12, or a leg to a hypotenuse ratio of either 5:13 or 12:13, then it is a 5-12-13 triangle.
>
> 45°-45°-90° triangle: if a right triangle has two angles that are both 45°, then the ratio of the three legs is $1:1:\sqrt{2}$.
>
> 30°-60°-90° triangle: if a right triangle has two angles of 30° and 60°, then the ratio of the three legs is $1:\sqrt{3}:2$.
>
> Confirm for yourself that the ratio of sides in the 4 preceding triangles actually fulfill the Pythagorean Theorem.

C. Equilateral Triangles

An **equilateral triangle** is a triangle with all three sides equal. All three interior angles are also equal, so they are all 60°.

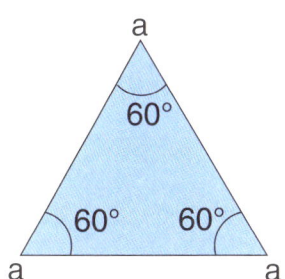

Drawing a height line from any vertex will divide the triangle into two 30°-60°-90° triangles, so you can easily solve for the area.

D. Scalene Triangles

A **scalene triangle** is any triangle that has no equal sides and no equal angles. To find the value for the height of this kind of triangle requires the use of trigonometric functions (see Chapter 5).

E. Similar Triangles

Two triangles are **similar** if they have the same values for interior angles. This means that ratios of corresponding sides will be equal. Similar triangles are triangles with the same shape that are scaled to different sizes.

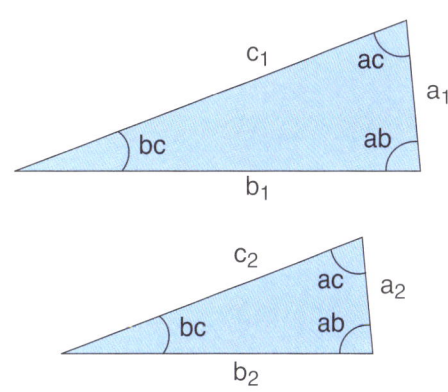

GAMSAT MATH   GM-87

To solve for values in a triangle from information given about a similar triangle, you will need to use ratios. The ratios of corresponding sides are always equal, for example $\frac{a_1}{a_2} = \frac{b_1}{b_2}$. Also, the ratio of two sides in the same triangle is equal to the corresponding ratio in the similar triangle, for example $\frac{a_1}{b_1} = \frac{a_2}{b_2}$.

4.2.3 Circles

A **circle** is a figure in which every point is the same distance from the center. This distance from the center to the edge is known as the **radius** (*r*). The length of any straight line drawn from a point on the circle, through the center, and out to another point on the circle is known as the **diameter** (*d*). The diameter is twice the radius.

$$d = 2 \times r \quad \text{or} \quad r = \frac{1}{2}d$$

There are no angles in a circle.

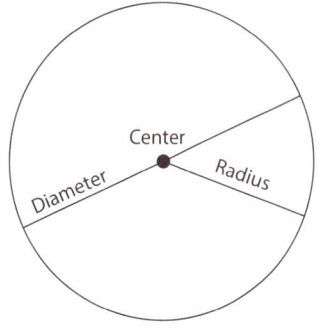

Circumference: The circumference of a circle is the total distance around a circle. It is equal to pi times the diameter.

$$\text{Circumference} = \pi \times d = 2\pi \times r$$

Area: The area of a circle is equal to pi times the square of the radius.

$$\text{Area} = \pi \times r^2 = \frac{1}{4}\pi \times d^2$$

Length: Length of an arc is defined as a piece of circumference formed by an angle of *n* degrees measured as the arc's central angle in a circle of radius *r*.

$$L = \frac{n°}{360°} \times 2\pi r$$

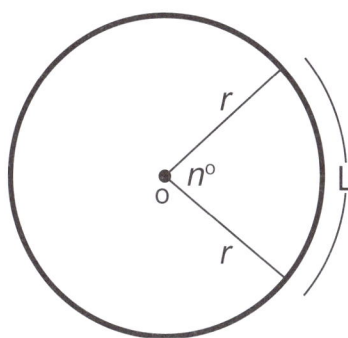

$$\text{Area (sector)} = \frac{1}{2}r^2\theta \quad \text{(in radians)}$$

$$\text{Area (sector)} = \frac{n^\circ}{360^\circ} \times \pi r^2 \quad \text{(in degrees)}$$

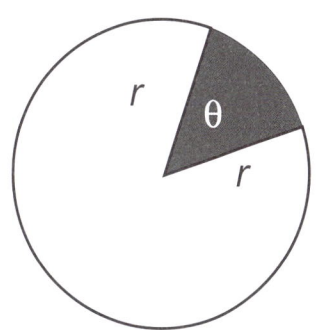

Area of a sector: The area of a sector is a portion of the circle formed by an angle of n degree measured as the sector's central angle in a circle of radius r.

4.2.4 Trapezoids and Parallelograms

A. Trapezoids

A **trapezoid** is a four-sided figure with one pair of parallel sides and one pair of non-parallel sides.

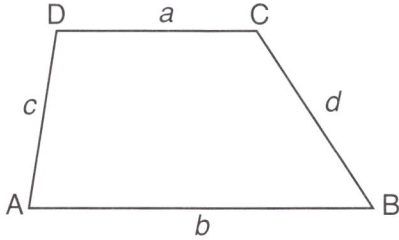

Usually the easiest way to solve trapezoid problems is to drop vertical lines down from the vertices on the smaller of the two parallel lines. This splits the figure into two right triangles on the ends and a rectangle in the middle. Then, to find information about the trapezoid, you can solve for the information (side length, area, angles, etc.) of these other shapes.

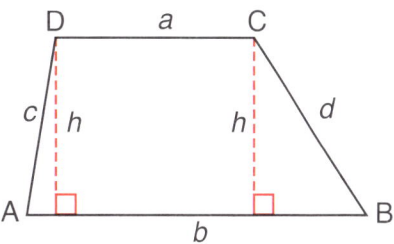

1. The area of a trapezoid is calculated as

$$\frac{a+b}{2}h$$

GAMSAT MATH   GM-89

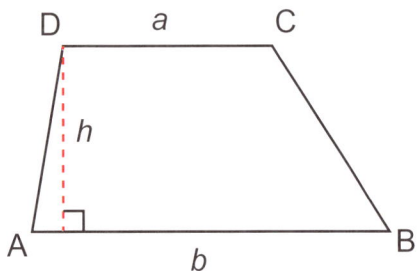

2. The upper and lower base angles are supplementary angles (i.e., they add up to 180°).

Angle A + Angle D = 180°
Angle B + Angle C = 180°

> **NOTE**
>
> "Really, will the GAMSAT ever specifically ask for the area of a trapezoid?" No! But they may occasionally present a graph that is shaped like a trapezoid and the question requires you to calculate the area under the graph or 'curve' (i.e. the area of the trapezoid).

Sometimes it can be useful to draw a line from vertex to vertex and construct a triangle that way, but this usually only makes sense if the resulting triangle is special (i.e. isosceles).

Isosceles Trapezoids: Just like isosceles triangles, **isosceles trapezoids** are trapezoids with two equal sides. The sides that are equal are the parallel sides that form angles with the base of the trapezoid. Similarly, if the left and right sides are of the same lengths, these angles are the same as well.

In this isosceles trapezoid, ABCE means that Angle A = Angle D, Angle B = Angle C, and Diagonal AC = Diagonal BD.

The perimeter = a + b + 2c

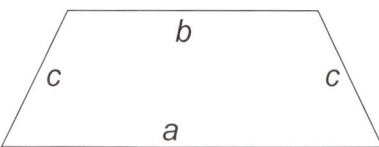

B. Parallelograms

A **parallelogram** is a quadrilateral that has two sets of parallel sides. A square, for example, is a special kind of parallelogram, as is a rhombus (which has four sides of equal length but, unlike a square, has two different pairs of angle values).

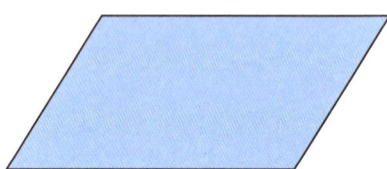

Area: The area of a parallelogram is simply the base times the height.

Area = (Base) × (Height)

The height of a parallelogram can be found by dropping a vertical from a vertex to the opposite side and evaluating the resulting right triangle.

The sum of all the angles in a parallelogram is 360°. Opposite angles are equivalent, and adjacent angles add up to 180°.

4.3 3D Solids

In three dimensions, it doesn't always make sense to talk about perimeters. Shapes with defined edges (such as boxes and pyramids) still have them, but rounded shapes (such as spheres) do not. Instead, we are generally concerned with the values of surface area and volume.

4.3.1 Boxes

Boxes are the three-dimensional extension of rectangles. Every angle in a box is 90°, and every box has six rectangular faces, twelve edges, and eight vertices. Opposite (and parallel) faces are always of the same length, height, and width, as are opposite (and parallel) edges. None of the equations in these sections (4.3.1, 4.3.2, 4.3.3) should be memorized. Hopefully, most of the equations will make sense to you in some way.

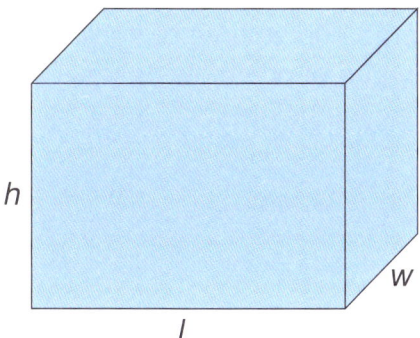

Perimeter: The perimeter of a box is the sum of its edges. There are, however, only three different lengths and four edges corresponding to each one. So to find the perimeter, we can simply take the sum of four times each the width, length, and height.

$$\text{Perimeter} = 4l + 4w + 4h = 4(l + w + h)$$

Surface Area: The surface area of a box is the sum of the area of each of its faces. Since there is one duplicate of each unique face, we only need to find three products, double them, and add them together.

$$\text{Surface Area} = 2lw + 2wh + 2lh$$
$$= 2(lw + wh + lh)$$

Volume: Calculating the volume of a box can be visualized as taking the surface of any of its rectangular faces and dragging it through space, like you were blowing a box-shaped bubble. So you start with the product of a width times a height, and then you multiply that by a length.

$$\text{Volume} = l \times w \times h$$

4.3.2 Spheres

The definition of a sphere is basically identical to that of a circle, except that it is applied in three dimensions rather than two: It is a collection of points in three dimensions that are all of the same distance from a particular center point. Again, we call this distance the radius, and twice the radius is the diameter. A sphere has no vertices or edges, so it has no circumference.

Surface Area:

$$\text{Surface Area} = 4\pi \times r^2$$

Volume:

$$\text{Volume} = (4/3)\pi \times r^3$$

4.3.3 Cylinders

Spheres may be the 3D equivalent of circles, but if you start with a circle and extend it into the third dimension, you obtain the tube shape known as a cylinder. Cylinders have two parallel circular faces, and their edges are connected by a smooth, edgeless surface.

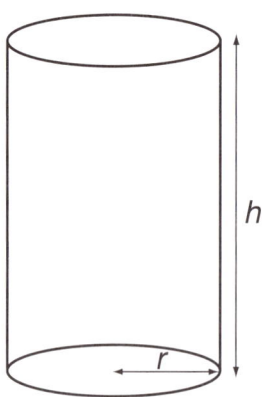

Surface Area: The surface area of a cylinder is composed of three parts: The two circular faces and the connecting portion. To find the total area of a cylinder, add the areas of these two parts. We already know how to calculate area for circles; and for the connecting surface, all we need to do is extend the circumference of one of the circles into three dimensions. So, multiply the circumference by the height of the cylinder.

$$\text{Surface Area} = 2(\pi \times r^2) + (2\pi \times r) \times h$$

Volume: The volume of a cylinder is equal to the area of one of its bases (circle) multiplied by the height.

$$\text{Volume} = (\pi \times r^2) \times h$$

NOTE

Notice that a cylinder approximates a pipe (Physics) or a small part of a blood vessel (Biology).

GAMSAT MATH

GOLD STANDARD WARM-UP EXERCISES
CHAPTER 4: Geometry

1. The area of a circle is 144π. What is its circumference?
   A. 6π
   B. 24π
   C. 72π
   D. 12π

2. The points (2,-3) and (2,5) are the endpoints of a diameter of a circle. What is the radius of the circle?
   A. 64
   B. 4π
   C. 8
   D. 4

3. A and B are similar 45°-45°-90° triangles. If B has an area of 12 square meters, and A has three times the area of B, what is the length of A's hypotenuse?
   A. $\sqrt{72}$ m
   B. 36 m
   C. 72 m
   D. 12 m

4. Leslie drives from Highway 1 to the parallel Highway 2 using the road that crosses them, as in the given figure below. Leslie misses the turn onto Highway 1 at point Q and drives 2 km further, to point P. Driving in a straight line from point P to get back to Highway 1, how much further will Leslie travel?

   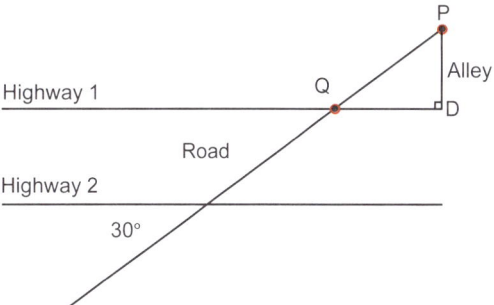

   A. 1/2 km
   B. $\sqrt{3}$ km
   C. 1 km
   D. 2 km

5. A circle is inscribed in a square with a diagonal of length 5. What is the area of the circle?
   A. $\frac{25}{8}\pi$
   B. $\frac{25}{2}\pi$
   C. $\frac{25}{16}\pi$
   D. $\frac{25}{4}\pi$

6. A circle is drawn inside a larger circle so that they have the same center. If the smaller circle has 25% the area of the larger circle, which of the following is the ratio of the radius of the small circle to that of the larger circle?

   A. $\dfrac{1}{8}$

   B. $\dfrac{3}{4}$

   C. $\dfrac{1}{4}$

   D. $\dfrac{1}{2}$

7. A circle passes through the point (0,0) and the point (10,0). Which of the following could NOT be a third point on the circle?

   A (1, -3)
   B (2, 4)
   C (7, 4)
   D (5, 0)

8. Consider a box with length l, width w and height h, if the thickness of the cardboard is t, how much space is inside this cardboard box?

   A. l x w x h
   B. (l - t) x (w - t) x (h - t)
   C. (l + t) x (w + t) x (h + t)
   D. (l - 2t) x (w - 2t) x (h - 2t)

GS ANSWER KEY

Chapter 4

Cross-Reference

1. B GM 4.2, 4.2.3
2. D GM 4.2, 4.2.3
3. D GM 4.2, 4.2.2
4. C GM 4.1, 4.1.3

Cross-Reference

5. A GM 4.2, 4.2.1, 4.2.3
6. D GM 4.2, 4.2.3
7. D GM 4.1, 4.1.1, 4.2.3
8. D GM 4.3.1; deduce

* Worked solutions can be found at the end of the GAMSAT Math chapters. If something is still not clear, go to the forum at GAMSAT-prep.com.

GOLD NOTES

TRIGONOMETRY
Chapter 5

Memorize	Understand	Not Required
Formulas for Sine, Cosine, and Tangent Important Values of Sine and Cosine	* Graphing Sine, Cosine, and Tangent * The Unit Circle * Degrees vs. Radians * Inverse Trigonometric Functions	* Memorizing the unit circle

GAMSAT-Prep.com

Introduction

Trigonometry is the most conceptually advanced branch of mathematics with which you will need to be familiar for the GAMSAT test. But don't let that scare you. Basically, everything in this section boils down to right triangles, and after Chapter 5, you'd be a triangle pro!

Additional Resources

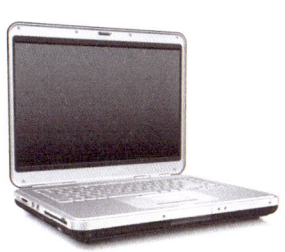

Free Online Forum

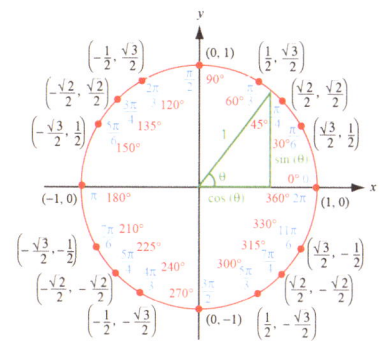

Special Guest

GAMSAT MATH GM-97

GAMSAT-Prep.com
THE GOLD STANDARD

5.1 Basic Trigonometric Functions

The trigonometric functions describe the relationship between the angles and sides of right triangles. The angle in question is generally denoted by θ, the Greek letter theta, but you will never see the right angle used as θ.

We call the leg connecting to the corner of θ: the *adjacent side* ("b" in the diagram); and the leg that does not touch: the *opposite side* ("a" in the diagram). The edge across from the right angle is called the *hypotenuse* ("c" in the diagram).

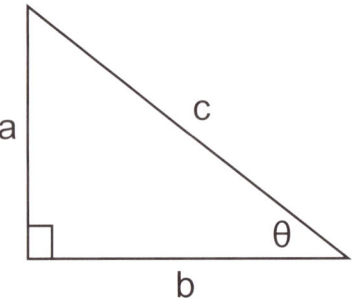

5.1.1 Sine

A lot of people like to use the mnemonic device "SOH-CAH-TOA" to remember how to evaluate the three basic trigonometric functions: Sine, cosine, and tangent. The first three letters, "SOH," refer to the first letter of each word in the following equation.

$$\text{Sine} = \frac{\text{Opposite}}{\text{Hypotenuse}}$$

Sine of an angle θ is written sin(θ). So to calculate this value, simply divide the length of the opposite side by the length of the hypotenuse.

EXAMPLE

What is sin(θ) in the following triangle?

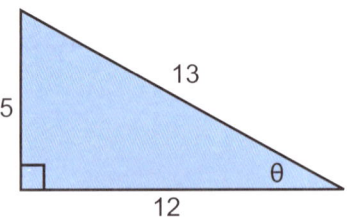

The opposite side has length 5, and the hypotenuse has length 13, so

$$\sin(\theta) = \frac{5}{13}$$

5.1.2 Cosine

The second set of three letters in SOH-CAH-TOA refers to the equation for the cosine of an angle.

$$\text{Cosine} = \frac{\text{Adjacent}}{\text{Hypotenuse}}$$

The abbreviation for the cosine of an angle is $\cos(\theta)$.

EXAMPLE

In the 5–12–13 triangle in Section 5.1.1, what is $\cos(\theta)$?

Dividing the adjacent side by the hypotenuse, we obtain the following solution:

$$\cos(\theta) = \frac{12}{13}$$

5.1.3 Tangent

The final three letters in SOH-CAH-TOA refer to the equation for finding the tangent of an angle.

$$\text{Tangent} = \frac{\text{Opposite}}{\text{Adjacent}}$$

You can also find the tangent of an angle if you know the value for sine and cosine. Notice that the hypotenuse cancels out if you divide sine and cosine.

$$\text{Tangent} = \frac{\text{Sine}}{\text{Cosine}}$$

You can also manipulate this equation to express sine or cosine in terms of the tangent.

EXAMPLE

In the 5–12–13 triangle in Section 5.1.1, what is $\tan(\theta)$?

Dividing the opposite side by the adjacent side, we obtain:

$$\tan(\theta) = \frac{5}{12}$$

5.1.4 Secant, Cosecant, and Cotangent

These three functions are far less commonly used than sine, cosine, and tangent, but you should still be familiar with them. They are not very hard to remember because they are just the reciprocals of the main three functions.

$$\text{Cosecant} = \frac{1}{\text{Sine}}$$

$$= \frac{\text{Hypotenuse}}{\text{Opposite}}$$

$$\text{Secant} = \frac{1}{\text{Cosine}}$$

$$= \frac{\text{Hypotenuse}}{\text{Adjacent}}$$

$$\text{Cotangent} = \frac{1}{\text{Tangent}}$$

$$= \frac{\text{Adjacent}}{\text{Opposite}}$$

The abbreviations for these functions are sec, csc, and cot, respectively. Unlike sine, cosine and tangent, you do not need to memorize these unusual functions.

5.2 The Unit Circle

5.2.1 Trig Functions on a Circle

As you can see from the equations in Section 5.1, the trigonometric functions are ratios of side lengths. This means that every angle has a value for each of the functions that *does not* depend on the scale of the triangle.

In Section 5.1 we looked at examples with a 5–12–13 triangle. Our solutions were as follows:

$$\sin(\theta) = \frac{5}{13}$$

$$\cos(\theta) = \frac{12}{13}$$

$$\tan(\theta) = \frac{5}{12}$$

Let's compare these results with the trigonometric functions for the similar triangle 10, 24, 26, which clearly has longer sides but the same angle θ:

GAMSAT MATH

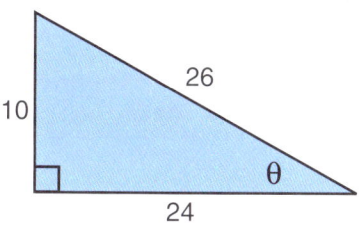

$$\sin(\theta) = \frac{10}{26} = \frac{5}{13}$$

$$\cos(\theta) = \frac{24}{26} = \frac{12}{13}$$

$$\tan(\theta) = \frac{10}{24} = \frac{5}{12}$$

As you can see, the trigonometric values for the angle remain the same.

Also, the absolute value of sine and cosine is never greater than 1 for any angle. This makes perfect sense because the hypotenuse of a triangle is always its longest side, and for sine and cosine, the hypotenuse is in the denominator.

If we plot the graph of sine and cosine for θ from 0° to 360° in Cartesian Coordinates with $x = \cos(\theta)$ and $y = \sin(\theta)$, we

obtain a circle of radius 1. This is known as the **unit circle**, as shown in the succeeding picture. The angle formed at the vertex of the x-axis is equal to θ.

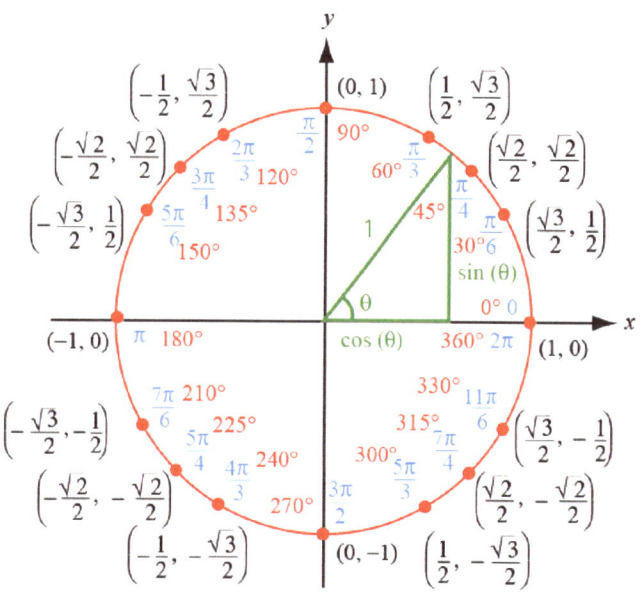

When simply dealing with right triangle figures, we never use negative numbers because negative length does not make sense. With the unit circle, though, legs of the triangle can be in negative space on the Cartesian plane. This can result in negative values for sine and cosine. You do not need to memorize the results of the unit circle.

5.2.2 Degrees and Radians

Up until this point, we have measured angles using degrees. When dealing with trigonometric functions, however, it is often more convenient to use the unit-less measurement of **radians**. There are 2π radians in 360°, so one trip around the unit circle is an increase in θ by 2π radians.

GAMSAT-Prep.com
THE GOLD STANDARD

2π radians = 360°

This translates to 1 radian = $\frac{360}{2\pi}$, but you will usually be working with radians in multiples of π, so it is not necessary to memorize this.

Here is a list of important angles (in degrees and radians) and their sine and cosine values that are helpful to know from the unit circle:

Degrees	Radians	Sine	Cosine
0°	0	0	1
30°	$\frac{\pi}{6}$	$\frac{1}{2}$	$\frac{\sqrt{3}}{2}$
45°	$\frac{\pi}{4}$	$\frac{1}{\sqrt{2}}$	$\frac{1}{\sqrt{2}}$
60°	$\frac{\pi}{3}$	$\frac{\sqrt{3}}{2}$	$\frac{1}{2}$
90°	$\frac{\pi}{2}$	1	0

Note that $\frac{1}{\sqrt{2}}$ is the same as $\frac{\sqrt{2}}{2}$.

These major angles repeat for each quadrant of the unit circle, but the signs of the sine and cosine values change. Moving counterclockwise around the circle and beginning with the upper right, the quadrants are labeled I, II, III, and IV.

Quadrant	Sine	Cosine
I	+	+
II	+	−
III	−	−
IV	−	+

NOTE

How many degrees are there in $\frac{3(\pi)}{4}$ radians?

Because 2π radians = 360°, this makes 1(π) radian = 180°.

Solution:

1π radian = 180°

$\frac{3\pi}{4} = \frac{3\pi}{4} \times \frac{180°}{\pi}$

= 135°

How many radians are there in 270°?

Solution:

1π radian = 180°

$270° \times \frac{\pi}{180°} = \frac{3\pi}{2}$

GM-102 TRIGONOMETRY

5.2.3 Graphing Trig Functions

Looking at the unit circle, it is very apparent that the trigonometric functions are **periodic**. This means that they continue to repeat the same cycle infinitely. After you go once around the circle, a full 360°, you end up right back at the beginning and begin to cycle through again.

A. Sine

As you can see from the table in 5.2.2, the sine function increases for the first 90°. For the next 90° it decreases while staying positive, then it continues to decrease into the negatives, and finally for the last 90°, it increases from −1 back to 0. From this information, we can picture the general shape of the graph, and we know that the period of the function is a full 360° or 2π radians.

The graph itself looks like this:

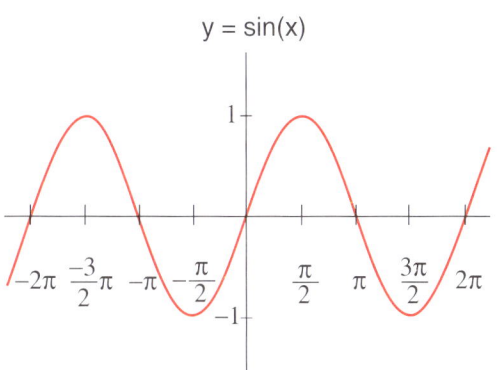

As you can see in the graph, the sine function reaches a maximum at $\frac{\pi}{2} + 2\pi \times n$, has an x-intercept at $\pi \times n$, and a minimum at $\frac{3\pi}{2} + 2\pi \times n$ where n is any integer.

B. Cosine

The cosine function is identical to the sine function, except that it is shifted along the x-axis by half a period. So rather than starting at 0 and increasing, it starts at one and decreases. The period is still 2π radians.

The graph looks like this:

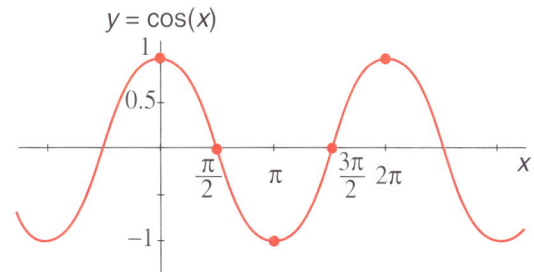

Just like with the sine function, you can see where the maxima, minima, and intercepts of the cosine function are from the graph. It reaches a maximum at $2\pi \times n$, an x-intercept at $\frac{\pi}{2} + \pi \times n$, and a minimum at $2\pi \times n + \pi \times n$ where n is any integer.

GAMSAT MATH GM-103

C. Tangent

The graph of the tangent function differs from sine and cosine graphs in a few important ways. First of all, the tangent function repeats itself every π radian instead of every 2π. So it is π-periodic rather than 2π-periodic. Also, it has vertical **asymptotes**, vertical lines that the function approaches but never crosses, at $(n)\left(\frac{\pi}{2}\right)$ for every odd integer *n*. The value of the tangent goes infinity as it approaches an asymptote from left to right; and negative infinity as it approaches from right to left.

> **NOTE**
> We will see the application of sine curves when we discuss Wave Characteristics and Periodic Motion in Physics Chapter 7.

Remember, the tangent function is the ratio of the sine function to the cosine function, so the asymptotes occur when the cosine of an angle is equal to zero, where cos(x) = 0, because division by zero is undefined. 0/0 is never possible for the tangent function, so it is irrelevant.

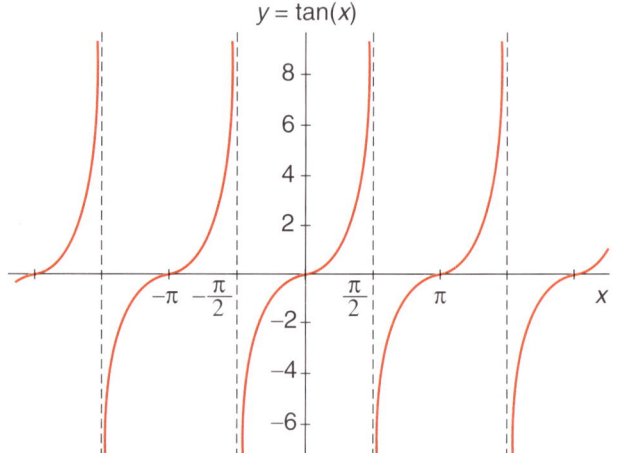

5.3 Trigonometric Problems

5.3.1 Inverse Trig Functions

We have discussed the formulas for finding the value of trigonometric functions for different angles, but how can you find the value of an angle if all you know is the value of one of the functions? This is where the inverse trigonometric functions come into play.

The **inverse** of a trigonometric function takes an input value *x* and outputs an angle. The value of the inverse trigonometric function of x is equal to the angle. To represent an inverse function, we write −1 in superscript like we would an exponent. But remember, this is not actually an exponent.

Inverse sine is represented as sin^{-1} and it is defined as such:

$$\sin(\sin^{-1}(x)) = x$$

So, $\sin(\theta) = x$ and $\sin^{-1}(x) = \theta$.

Now that we have inverse functions in our toolbox, we can begin to solve algebraic problems that contain trigonometric functions.

Solve the following equation for x.

$$\pi - \tan 2x = \left(\frac{4}{3}\right)\pi$$

$$\Rightarrow -\tan 2x = \left(\frac{1}{3}\right)\pi$$

$$\Rightarrow \tan 2x = \frac{-\pi}{3}$$

$$\Rightarrow 2x = \tan^{-1}\left(\frac{-\pi}{3}\right)$$

We did not list values for tangent in the tables in Section 5.2.2, but we can use the sine and cosine values to find them. Remember that tan = sin/cos. We can use the values for $\frac{\pi}{3}$ in quadrant IV:

$$\Rightarrow 2x = \frac{-\left(\frac{\sqrt{3}}{2}\right)}{\frac{1}{2}}$$

$$\Rightarrow 2x = -\sqrt{3}$$

$$\Rightarrow x = -\frac{\sqrt{3}}{2}$$

GOLD STANDARD WARM-UP EXERCISES

CHAPTER 5: Trigonometry

> **NOTE**
>
> All these questions are "open book" practice questions. Please feel free to find information in this chapter to help you solve these problems. This type of practice helps to improve your deductive reasoning. Of course, please do not use a calculator.

1. What percentage of the unit circle is represented by the angle $8\pi/5$?
   A. 1.6%
   B. 80%
   C. 0.25%
   D. 160%

2. Which of the following is the value of $-\cos(\pi/2)$?
   A. 0
   B. −1
   C. 1
   D. $1/\sqrt{2}$

3. The tangent of one of the acute angles in a right triangle is 3/2. If the leg opposite this angle has a length of 12, what is the length of the hypotenuse?
   A. 8
   B. $6\sqrt{13}$
   C. $4\sqrt{13}$
   D. 18

4. Given that the sine of an acute angle is equal to the cosine of its complement, and vice versa, the value of $\cos(\pi/6)$ equals the value of which of the following? (note: for complementary angles, see GM 4.1.3)

   A. $\sin(\pi/2)$
   B. $\sin(\pi/4)$
   C. $\sin(\pi/6)$
   D. $\sin(\pi/3)$

GS ANSWER KEY

Chapter 5

Cross-Reference

1. B GM 5.2, 5.2.1
2. A GM 5.5

Cross-Reference

3. C GM 5.1, 5.1.3, 5.3, 5.3.3
4. D GM 4.1.3, 5.2, 5.2.3

* Worked solutions can be found at the end of the GAMSAT Math chapters. If something is still not clear, go to the forum at GAMSAT-prep.com.

GOLD NOTES

PROBABILITY AND STATISTICS
Chapter 6

Memorize	Understand	Not Required
Formula for Average Formula for Probability	* Determining Probabilities * Combining Probabilities of Multiple Events * Mode, Median, Variance, Standard Deviation and its Corresponding Graph * Correlation Coefficient * Regression lines ("lines of best fit")	* Permutations and combinations * Formulae for standard deviation and variance

GAMSAT-Prep.com

Introduction

Probability and statistics are relatively minor subjects for the GAMSAT. This section will help you keep things straight such as when to multiply and when to add probabilities – simple questions that can often be the most confusing probabilities.

Additional Resources

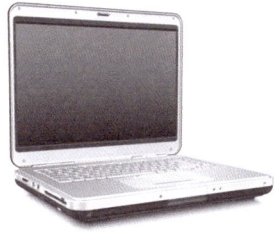

Free Online Forum

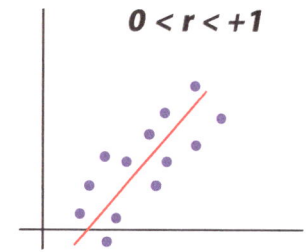

Special Guest

GAMSAT MATH GM-109

GAMSAT-Prep.com
THE GOLD STANDARD

6.1 Probability

6.1.1 What is Probability?

Probability is a measure of the likelihood that something will happen.

In mathematics, probability is represented as a ratio of two numbers. The second number - the denominator - corresponds to the total number of possible outcomes the situation can have. The first number - the numerator - corresponds to the number of ways the particular outcome in question can occur.

$$\text{Probability} = \frac{\text{(number of ways the outcome can occur)}}{\text{(number of possible outcomes)}}$$

Let's look at a simple example.

Let's consider the flipping of a coin. Of course, we know that there are only two possible outcomes of a coin flip, heads or tails. So the total number of outcomes is 2, which will be our denominator.

Say we want to find the probability that a flipped coin will be heads. There is only one way this outcome can come about, so the numerator will be 1. Therefore, the probability of flipping heads is 1 in 2:

$$\text{Probability of Heads} = \frac{1}{2}$$

It is important to note that the quantity in the numerator of a probability ratio is a subset of the quantity in the denominator. The number of ways an outcome can occur is always less than or equal to the total number of outcomes. This means that a probability will never be more than 1, since 1 would mean the outcome is the *only* possibility. Also, the sum of the probabilities of all possible outcomes will always be 1.

Let's look at a slightly more complicated example.

Say you have a typical six-sided die with the sides labeled 1 through 6. If you roll the die once, what is the probability that the number will not be divisible by 3?

Let's begin by finding the total number of outcomes. Be careful here. The only outcomes we wish to determine the probability of are rolls of numbers divisible by 3, but the total number of possible outcomes is not affected by this restriction. There are still 6 in total, one for each number it is possible to roll.

Now we want to know how many ways out of these 6 we can roll a number that is not divisible by 3. Well, the only two numbers that are divisible by 3 that are possibilities are 3 and 6. So 1, 2, 4, and 5 are not. This means that there are 4 ways for the outcome to occur.

$$\text{Probability} = \frac{4}{6}$$

Reducing fractions is usually fine when working with probability; just know that if you do, the numerator and denominator will not necessarily correspond to the number of possibilities anymore.

$$\text{Probability} = \frac{2}{3}$$

The simplest way to complicate a probability problem is to allow for multiple correct outcomes. To find the total probability, simply add the individual probabilities for each correct outcome. For the above example, the total probability is actually the sum of the probabilities of rolling 1, 2, 4, and 5.

6.1.2 Combining Probabilities

What if you are asked to find the probability that multiple events will occur?

The solution to such a problem will still be a ratio in which the numbers represent the same quantities as before. The new difficulty is figuring out how many different outcome possibilities there are. Luckily, there is an easy way to calculate this. All you have to do is find the probability of each individual event and then multiply them together.

Why does this work? Think about it this way: For each possible outcome of the first event, there is still every possible outcome for the second. So the total number of possibilities will be the number of outcomes in the first times the number of outcomes in the second.

EXAMPLE

Let's go back to the flipping coin! If you flip it twice, what is the probability that the first flip will turn up heads and the second tails?

When dealing with multiple events, always focus on one event at a time before combining. So start with the first flip. We know that the probability it will be heads is ½. Now for the second flip, the probability it will be tails is also ½.

Now to find the probability that both of the events will occur, we multiply the individual probabilities:

$$\text{Probability} = \frac{1}{2} \times \frac{1}{2}$$
$$= \frac{1}{4}$$

Let's look at another coin flip example.

EXAMPLE

If you flip a coin twice, what is the probability that it will come up heads exactly one time?

This question seems almost identical to the previous example, but be careful! The difference is that the phrasing of this question does not specify particular outcomes for the individual events.

Let's solve this in two ways:

(i) Let's combine both events into one. To find the total number of possible outcomes, multiply the totals of each event, so there are 2 × 2 = 4 possibilities. Now count the number of ways we can flip heads once. Well, we could have heads on the first flip and tails on the second, so that is 1, or we could have tails then heads, so that is 2. Therefore, the probability of flipping heads exactly once is 2 to 4.

$$\text{Probability} = \frac{2}{4}$$

(ii) Now let's treat the events separately. Ask yourself: What are the odds that an outcome of the first event will be compatible with flipping heads once? The answer is $\frac{2}{2}$ since we can still achieve the overall desired outcome with the second flip no matter what the first flip is.

Now what are the odds that an outcome of the second event will be compatible with flipping heads once? Since you already have a first flip determined, there is only one outcome for the second flip that will give the desired result. If the first flip was heads we need a tails flip, and if the first flip was tails we need a heads flip. So the odds for the second flip are ½.

$$\text{Probability} = \frac{2}{2} \times \frac{1}{2}$$
$$= \frac{2}{4}$$

There are all kinds of confusing ways probability problems can be written. You have to be extra careful to break them down and determine exactly what is being asked because the test writers love to try and trick you. Double and triple-check that you have the setup right for probability problems because it is so easy to accidentally overlook something.

> **NOTE**
>
> When you want to know the probability of event A or B, the probabilities must be added. If you want to know the probability of events A and B, the probabilities must be multiplied.

6.2 Statistics

6.2.1 Averages

When given a collection of numbers, the **average** is the sum of the numbers divided by the total number of numbers.

$$\text{Average} = \frac{(\text{sum of numbers})}{(\text{number of numbers})}$$

EXAMPLE

What is the average of the set {4, 7, 6, 7}?

Add up the numbers and, since there are 4 of them, divide by 4.

$$\begin{aligned}\text{Average} &= \frac{(4+7+6+7)}{4} \\ &= \frac{24}{4} \\ &= 6\end{aligned}$$

The average may or may not actually appear in the set of numbers, but it is a common way to think of the typical value for the set.

6.2.2 Mode, Median, Mean

Here are a few other statistics terms you should know:

The **mode** of a set of values is the number that appears the most times. Mode can be bimodal or multimodal. Simply stated, bimodal means that two numbers are repeated the most while multimodal indicates two or more numbers are repeated the most.

The **median** of a set of values is the number that appears exactly in the center of the distribution. This means there are an equal number of values greater than and less than the median.

Arithmetic mean is just another name for the average of a set of numbers. The terms are interchangeable.

EXAMPLE

Find the mode, median, and mean of the following set: {3, 5, 11, 3, 8}.

Let's begin with the mode. All we need to do is see which value or values repeat the most times. In this case, the only one that repeats is 3.

$$\text{Mode} = 3$$

To find the median we always need to first arrange the set in numerical order.

$$\{3, 3, 5, 8, 11\}$$

Now the median is whichever number lies in the exact center.

$$\text{Median} = 5$$

Since the mean is the same as the average, we add the values and divide by 5.

$$\text{Mean} = \frac{(3 + 3 + 5 + 8 + 11)}{5}$$
$$= \frac{30}{5}$$
$$= 6$$

NOTE

If a set has an even number of values, there will be no value exactly in the center. In this case, the median is the average of the two values that straddle the center.

Example

Given: 3, 4, 5, 6, 6, 8, 9, 10, 10, 12

The median is the average of the two middle data: $\frac{(6+8)}{2} = 7$

6.3 More Tools for Probability and Statistics

6.3.1 The Correlation Coefficient

The correlation coefficient r indicates whether two sets of data are associated or *correlated*. The value of r ranges from -1.0 to 1.0. The larger the absolute value of r, the stronger the association. Given two sets of data X and Y, a positive value for r indicates that as X increases, Y increases. A negative value for r indicates that as X increases, Y decreases.

GAMSAT MATH

Imagine that the weight (X) and height (Y) of everyone in the entire country was determined. There would be a strong positive correlation between a person's weight and their height. In general, as weight increases, height increases (*in a population*). However, the correlation would not be perfect (i.e. r < 1.0). After all, there would be some people who are very tall but very thin, and others who would be very short but overweight. We might find that $r = 0.7$. This would suggest there is a strong positive association between weight and height, but it is not a perfect association.

If two sets of data are correlated, does that mean that one *causes* the other? Not necessarily; simply because weight and height are correlated does not mean that if you gained weight you will necessarily gain height! Thus association does not imply causality.

Note that a correlation greater than 0.8 is generally described as strong, whereas a correlation that is less than 0.5 is generally described as weak. However, the interpretation and use of these values can vary based upon the "type" of data being examined. For example, a study based on chemical or biological data may require a stronger correlation than a study using social science data. You will regularly see regression lines with well correlated data in ACER's practice materials and during the real GAMSAT.

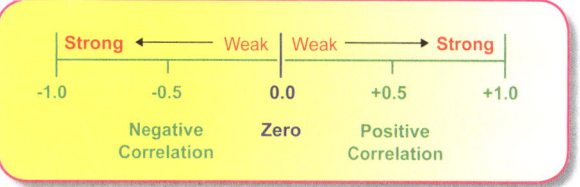

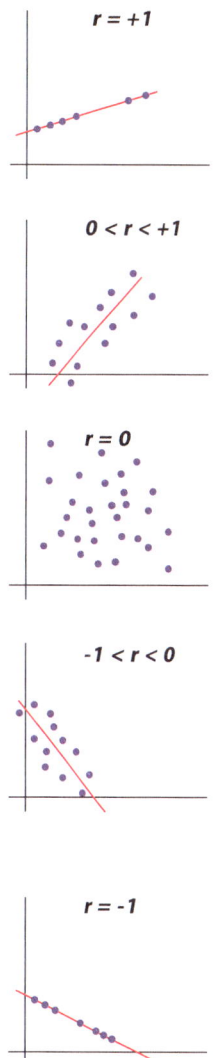

Varying values of the correlation coefficient (r) based on data plotted for two variables (= scatter diagrams). In red is the line of "best fit" (= *regression line*).

6.3.2 The Standard Deviation

When given a set of data, it is often useful to know the average value, *the mean*, and the *range* of values. As previously discussed, the mean is simply the sum of the data values divided by the number of data values. The range is the numerical difference between the largest value and the smallest value.

Another useful measurement is the *standard deviation*. The standard deviation indicates the dispersion of values around the mean. Given a bell-shaped distribution of data (i.e., the height and weight of a population, the GPA of undergraduate students, etc.), each standard deviation (SD) includes a given percentage of data. For example, the mean +/– 1 SD includes approximately 68% of the data values, the mean +/– 2 SD includes 95% of the data values, and the mean +/– 3 SD includes 99.7% of the data values.

For example, imagine that you read that the mean GPA required for admission to Belcurve University's Dental School is 3.5 with a standard deviation of 0.2 (SD = 0.2). Thus approximately 68% of the students admitted have a GPA of 3.5 +/– 0.2, which means between 3.3 and 3.7. We can also conclude that approximately 95% of the students admitted have a GPA of 3.5 +/– 2(0.2), which means between 3.1 and 3.9. Therefore the standard deviation becomes a useful measure of the dispersion of values around the mean 3.5.

> **NOTE**
>
> To see a Normal Curve displaying GAMSAT score results, go to www.GAMSAT-prep.com/GAMSAT-scores.

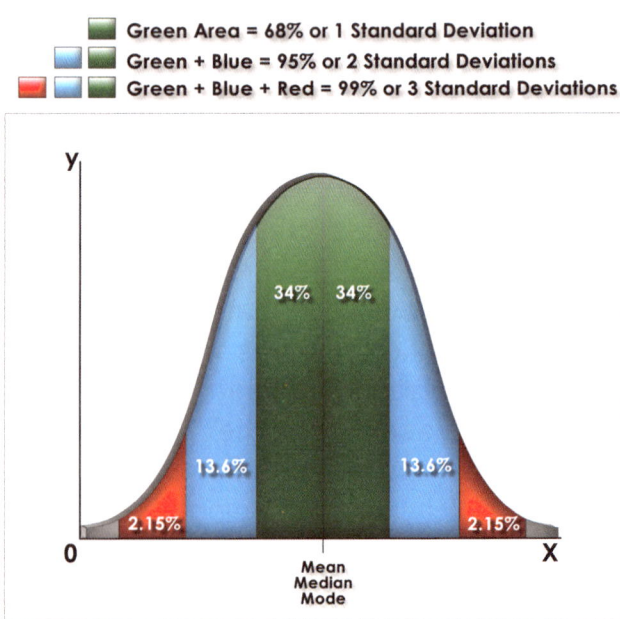

Figure 6.1: The Normal Curve (also referred to as: the Normal Distribution Curve).

6.3.3 Variance

Variance is another measure of how far a set of numbers is spread out or, in other words, how far numbers are from the mean. Thus variance is calculated as the average of the squared differences from the mean.

There are three steps to calculate the variance:

1. Determine the mean (the simple average of all the numbers)
2. For each number: subtract the mean and square the result (the squared difference)
3. Determine the average of those squared differences

The variance is also defined as the square of the standard deviation. Thus unlike standard deviation, the variance has units that are the square of the units of the variable itself.

For example, a variable measured in meters will have a variance measured in meters squared.

You are unlikely to need to calculate the standard deviation nor the variance. But having a basic understanding of these statistical measures can help when reading passages or analysing graphs during the GAMSAT.

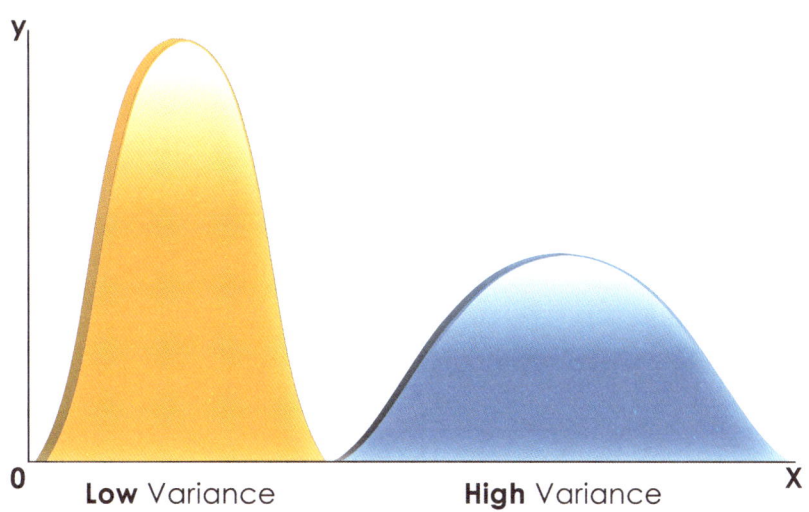

Figure 6.2: Variance.

6.3.4 Simple Probability Revisited

Let's apply a formula to simple probability. If a phenomenon or experiment has n equally likely outcomes, s of which are called successes, then the probability P of success is given by $P = \dfrac{s}{n}$.

EXAMPLE

- if "heads" in a coin toss is considered a success, then
$$P(\text{success}) = \frac{1}{2};$$

- if a card is drawn from a deck and diamonds are considered successes, then
$$P(\text{success}) = \frac{13}{52}.$$ It follows that $P(\text{success}) = 1 - P(\text{failure})$.

NOTE

Any of the 4 GAMSAT sciences may require the use of simple probability but it must often presents itself in Genetics (Biology Chapter 15).

GAMSAT MATH

GOLD STANDARD WARM-UP EXERCISES

CHAPTER 6: Probability and Statistics

1. A jar contains 4 red marbles and 6 blue marbles. What is the probability that a marble chosen at random will be red?
   A. 4/6
   B. 4/10
   C. 2/6
   D. 6/10

2. A box contains 6 yellow balls and 4 green balls. Two balls are chosen at random without replacement. What is the probability that the first ball is yellow and the second ball is green?
   A. 5/12
   B. 1/10
   C. 6/25
   D. 4/15

3. An English teacher wants to prepare a class reading list that includes 1 philosophy book, 1 work of historical fiction, and 1 biography. She has 3 philosophy books, 2 works of historical fiction, and 4 biographies to choose from. How many different combinations of books can she put together for her list?
   A. 32
   B. 288
   C. 9
   D. 24

4. An in-state medical training survey shows that the distribution of the residents' annual income is a bell curve. 2,516 residents are within one standard deviation of the average annual income. How many residents were in the survey's sample?
   A. 3,700
   B. 2,648
   C. 2,524
   D. 2,523

5. The average time it takes 3 students to complete a test is 35 minutes. If 1 student takes 41 minutes to complete the test and another takes 37 minutes, how many minutes does the third student take to complete the test?
   A. 4
   B. 38
   C. 27
   D. 39

6. A small library receives a shipment of gray books, blue books, black books, and brown books. If the librarian decides to shelve all the books of one color on Monday, all of the books of another color on Tuesday, and the rest of the books on Wednesday, in how many different ways can the book shelving be completed?

- **A.** 3
- **B.** 4
- **C.** 8
- **D.** 12

7. When you roll a die, what is the probability to first get a 3 and then a 1 or a 2?

- **A.** 1/6
- **B.** 1/8
- **C.** 1/32
- **D.** 1/18

GS ANSWER KEY

CHAPTER 6

Cross-Reference

1. B GM 6.1.1
2. D GM 6.1, 6.1.2
3. D GM 6.3, 6.3.5
4. A GM 6.3.2

Cross-Reference

5. C GM 6.2, 6.2.1
6. D GM 6.3.5
7. D GM 6.1, 6.1.2

* Worked solutions can be found at the end of the GAMSAT Math chapters. If something is still not clear, go to the forum at GAMSAT-prep.com.

GOLD NOTES

Chapter Review Solutions
GAMSAT Math

Chapter Review Solutions — Chapter 1

Question 1   B
See: GM 1.2.3, 1.4.3

According to the rules of order of operations, we work with the square root first: $0.125 + \sqrt{\frac{1}{9}} = 0.125 + \frac{1}{3}$. Since the answers are in decimal form, this problem is easiest to solve if all values are in decimal form. From the list of fraction-to-decimal conversions, $\frac{1}{3} \approx 0.33$, and so, $0.125 + \frac{1}{3} \approx 0.125 + 0.33 = 0.455$. All of the answers have only two decimal places, so we must round this answer off to the hundredths decimal place. The digit in the thousandths decimal place is a 5, and so the digit in the hundredths decimal place increases by 1 to become 6. 0.455 therefore rounds off to 0.46.

Quick Solution:

$$0.125 + \sqrt{\frac{1}{9}} = 0.125 + \frac{1}{3} \approx 0.125 + 0.333$$

$$= 0.458 \approx 0.46.$$

Question 2   D
See: GM 1.6.2

This is a proportion problem, so there will be two equivalent ratios. We construct the first ratio as $\frac{0.8}{0.9}$ and the second as $\frac{80}{x}$. If we set them equal, we get $\frac{0.8}{0.9} = \frac{80}{x}$, and cross-multiplication gives us $0.8x = (0.9)(80)$, or $0.8x = 72$. Therefore, $x = \frac{72}{0.8} = 90$.

Quick Solution: 80 differs from 0.8 by a factor of 100. This means that the answer must be related to 0.9 by the same factor: $x = 100(0.9) = 90$

Question 3   A
See: GM 1.4.3

The interest earned by investing $5,897 in Bank B is 21% of $5,897, or $(0.21)($5,897) = 1238.37. The interest earned by investing $6,430 in Bank A is 19% of $6,430, or $(0.19)($6,430) = 1221.70. Subtracting the smaller from the larger, we get $1238.37 − $1221.70 = $16.67.

Though you won't be asked about interest for the GAMSAT, the words will be different but the math will be the same. Also, you must be quick and precise with your calculations.

Question 4   C
See: GM 1.4.2

We must work backwards to find the lengths of boards B and C. Board B is 4/5 as long as Board A, which is $\frac{4}{5}(100\text{m}) = 80\text{m}$. Board C is 3/4 as long as this, which is $\frac{3}{4}(80\text{m}) = 60\text{m}$. To find the sum of these lengths, we add the three values: 100m + 80m + 60m = 240m.

Question 5   B
See: GM 1.6.2

This is a proportion problem in which the following are given: The proportion of the yellow marbles in the jar of yellow and green marbles is 7 out of 9. This makes the ratio of the number of yellow marbles to green marbles 7:2. The total number of marbles is 999. Therefore, the number of yellow marbles = (7/9) × 999 = 777 marbles.

Question 6   D
See: GM 1.6.1

This is a ratio problem involving different units. The given ratio is 0.25 months per week. We need to re-write this as a fraction: 0.25 months per week $= \frac{25}{100}$ months/week $= \frac{1}{4}$ months/week. This ratio tells us that there are four weeks in one month. We can express the number of months corresponding to one day using an intermediate relationship. There are 7 days in one week, which we can express with the ratio $\frac{1}{7}$ weeks/day. To express the number of months per day, we must multiply the first ratio by the second: $(\frac{1}{4}$ months/week$)(\frac{1}{7}$ weeks/day$) = \frac{1}{28}$ months/day. Notice that the weeks units cancel so that the only units left are months and days. If we had used a ratio expressing the number of days per week (the reciprocal of weeks per day), $\frac{7}{1}$ days/week, this cancellation would not occur and the final answer would not have the correct units of months per day.

Quick Solution: To convert a ratio that expresses a relationship between months and weeks to one that expresses a relationship between months and days, multiply it by a ratio that expresses a relationship between weeks and days:

$$(\tfrac{1}{4} \text{ months/week})(\tfrac{1}{7} \text{ weeks/day}) = \tfrac{1}{28} \text{ months/day}.$$

CHAPTER REVIEW SOLUTIONS — CHAPTER 1

Question 7   B
See: GM 1.2.3, 1.4.3, 1.5.2
The first step in this problem is to find the value of 6.4% of 1,000. We convert the percentage to a decimal (0.064) and multiply by one thousand: 0.064(1,000) = 64. Next, we find which of the answer choices is equal to this value. Choice A is obviously incorrect because 64 taken to any power besides 1 does not equal 64. The order of operations tells us that we must perform the calculation inside the parentheses first in choice C, which is a decimal (0.64). Squaring this value does not give us 64. Choice D begins with a small number (6.4) and divides it by a much larger number, so we know that the answer will be even smaller, and therefore not equal to 64. The correct choice is B. To check this, note that $256^{3/4} = (256^{1/4})^3 = (4)^3$ (because $4 \times 4 \times 4 \times 4 = 256$) and $(4)^3 = 64$.

Question 8   D
See: GM 1.2.3, 1.4.3
First, simplify the expressions according to the rules of the order of operations:

$$2 + \left[71 - 8\left(\frac{6}{2}\right)^2\right] = 2 + (71 - 8(3)^2)$$
$$= 2 + (71 - 8(9))$$
$$= 2 + (71 - 72)$$
$$= 2 + (-1) = 1$$

and $\sqrt{2500} = 50$. So, we need to find the percentage of 50 that is constituted by 1. Using the formula

Percent = Part/Whole × 100

$$\frac{1}{50} \times 100 = 0.02 \times 100 = 2,$$

we see that the answer is 2%.

Question 9   A
See: GM 1.4.3
The tenths decimal place is the largest occupied in each number. Comparing the digits in this decimal place, it is clear that the .6 in .636 is the largest.

Question 10   D
See: GM 1.2.1
Following the rule of adding like and unlike signs:

= 9 + −5 + 6
= 4 + 6
= 10

Question 11   B
See: GM 1.5.2
Dividing the coefficients 1.5 and 3.0 gives an answer of 0.5. Then the correct exponent value is determined by subtracting the exponents involved, which are 7 and 4. The final answer in scientific notation is $0.5 \times 10^3 = 5.0 \times 10^2$

Question 12   C
See: GM 1.4.3
It is usually easier to calculate using fractions than decimals. You should instantly recognize .333 as 1/3 and .125 as 1/8 (GM 1.4.3).

1/3 x 1/8 = 1/24 which is approximately 1/25 = 4/100 = 0.04.

You may be surprised at how often the test makers for the GAMSAT choose numbers to give you the option to work faster with fractions.

CHAPTER REVIEW SOLUTIONS — CHAPTER 2

Question 1   D
See: GM 2.2.2
Construct a ratio comparing millimeters to meters using the definition of the prefix "milli." Remember that we want to convert from meters to millimeters, so the denominator of the fraction we use for this ratio must contain the units of meters:

$\frac{1000\,mm}{1\,m}$. Now multiply this ratio and the given value:

$$75\,m\left(\frac{1000\,mm}{1\,m}\right) = 75,000\,mm.$$

Question 2   C
See: GM 2.1.2
Start with any of the choices and compare it to the rest:

0.1km = 100m > 10 m

0.1 km > 10 m

10 cm < 10 m

1000mm = 1m > 10 cm

Chapter Review Solutions

Question 3   A
See: GM 2.2
The total length of the triathlon is 12 km + 10 km + 15 km = 37 km. Express the ratio of kilometers to meters as a fraction, with kilometers in the denominator to cancel the units of 37 km:

$\frac{1000 \text{ m}}{1 \text{ km}}$. Now multiply: $37 \text{ km} \left(\frac{1000 \text{ m}}{1 \text{ km}} \right) = 37{,}000 \text{ m}$.

Question 4   C
See: GM 2.1
Construct an equation that expresses an unknown number of staples, times the weight of each, equals the weight of one paper-clip:

$$0.05x = 1$$
$$x = \frac{1}{0.05} = 20$$

Question 5   D
See: GM 2.2.2
Convert the mixed number to an improper fraction (which you should be able to 'do in your head' because 17 times 6 can be broken down to 10 times 6 = 60 PLUS 7 times 6 = 42 so SUBTOTAL = 102 PLUS 5 for a TOTAL = 107):

$$17\frac{5}{6} = \frac{107}{6}$$

Convert using the fact that 60 minutes equals 1 hour (notice that the number 6 cancels so the problem is reduced to 107 times 10 = 1070):

$$\left(\frac{107}{6} \text{ hours} \right) \left(\frac{60 \text{ minute}}{1 \text{ hour}} \right) = 1070 \text{ minutes}$$

Question 6   B
See: GM 2.2.2
Add like units:

$$67 \text{ lbs.} + 93 \text{ lbs.} + 18 \text{ lbs.} = 178 \text{ lbs.}$$
$$1 \text{ oz.} + 2 \text{ oz.} + 5 \text{ oz.} = 8 \text{ oz.}$$

Convert to pounds the part of the total weight that is in ounces and add to the rest of the weight:

$$(8 \text{ oz.}) \left(\frac{1 \text{ lbs.}}{16 \text{ oz.}} \right) = 0.5 \text{ lbs.}$$
$$178 \text{ lbs.} + 0.5 \text{ lbs.} = 178.5 \text{ lbs.}$$

Question 7   D
See: GM 2.1.1, 2.2
Given that the charges are:

$20.50 per hour to file paper,
$55 per hour for time in court,
$30 per hour for consultations,

a 90-minute consultation = $30 + $15 = $45.
8/6 hours = 80 minutes time filing paper work = $20.50 + $6.83 = $27.33

Since 20 minutes = $6.83

1 hour in court = $55

Total charges = $45 + $27.33 + $55 = $127.33

Notice that the first and third charge add to $100 making the calculation trivial.

Question 8   A
See: GM 2.2.2; dimensional analysis
Multiply by all ratios necessary to convert centimeters to feet (via inches) and seconds to minutes, and divide by 4 to calculate the speed for only 25% of a minute:

$$(20 \text{ cm/sec.}) \left(\frac{1}{2.54} \text{ in./cm} \right)$$
$$\left(\frac{1}{12} \text{ ft./in.} \right) (60 \text{ sec./min.}) \left(\frac{1}{4} \right) \approx 10 \text{ ft./min.}$$

Question 9   A
See: PHY 5.7, dimensional analysis
This problem is strictly a matter of dimensional analysis.
In the SI system, "mega" means 10^6
1 Megawatt = 10^3 kW = 10^6 W
Therefore, power in watts = (Total number of watt-years)/(Number of years)
Notice that the equation is constructed to allow "years" to cancel (i.e. it is in the numerator and in the denominator).
2 x 10^6 watt-years/6 years = 0.33 x 10^6 W = 3.3 x 10^5 W

Question 10   D
See: dimensional analysis
We will explore force in Physics. Force is in units called 'newtons' which is mass times acceleration, thus a newton is equivalent to a kg(m/s^2) [see section 2.1] and since kg is M (mass), m is L (length) and s is T (time), we get that the force is dimensionally equivalent to ML/T^2. Now the terms added on the right side of the equation must also be dimensionally equal to ML/T^2. Let's first solve for 'a' (note: most of the steps that we will show are really mental manipulations but we'll show the steps in case you are not used to it):

$ML/T^2 = at^{-1} = aT^{-1} = a/T$

To isolate 'a', multiply through by T:

$$(T)ML/T^2 = (T)a/T$$

Cancel T:

$$ML/T = a = MLT^{-1}$$

Now we solve for 'b':

$$ML/T^2 = bt^2 = bT^2$$

To isolate 'b', divide both sides by T^2:

$$ML/T^2/T^2 = ML/T^4 = b$$

Chapter Review Solutions

Question 1   D
See: GM 3.1.4
Substitute 2 for x in the function:

$$y = \frac{12}{4(2)^3 - 6(2) + 5}$$
$$= \frac{12}{4(8) - 12 + 5}$$
$$= \frac{12}{32 - 12 + 5} = \frac{12}{25}$$

Question 2   D
See: GM 3.3.2, 3.3.3
Create a ratio with the first two values and simplify:

$$\frac{13xy^2z}{39y} = \frac{xyz}{3}$$

The unknown ratio must also be equal to this value. Let k represent the variable and cross-multiply:

$$\frac{9xyz^6}{k} = \frac{xyz}{3}$$
$$3(9xyz^6) = (xyz)k$$
$$\frac{27xyz^6}{xyz} = k$$
$$27z^5 = k$$

Question 3   A
See: GM 3.4.2A, 3.4.2B
Substitute the first equation into the second, replacing y:

$$6x - 5y = -3$$
$$6x - 5(2x - 1) = -3$$
$$6x - 10x + 5 = -3$$
$$-4x + 5 = -3$$
$$-4x = -8$$
$$x = 2$$

Substitute this value back into either equation to find y:

$$y = 2x - 1$$
$$y = 2(2) - 1$$
$$y = 3$$

Question 4   D
See: GM 3.4.2B
We will need to write equations that correspond to the sentences. Let d represent the number of dimes, and n represent the number of nickels. Since there are two less dimes than nickels,

$$d = n - 2.$$

The amount of money a group of coins is worth is equal to the value of the coins times the number of coins. The total value of Loubha's nickels is $\$0.05n$ and the total value of her dimes is $\$0.10d$. These add up to all of the money she has:

$$\$0.05n + \$0.10d = \$0.85.$$

Substitute the first equation into the second for n:

$$\$0.05n + \$0.10(n - 2) = \$0.85$$
$$\$0.05n + \$0.10n - \$0.20 = \$0.85$$
$$\$0.15n = \$0.85 + \$0.20$$
$$\$0.15n = \$1.05$$

$$n = \$1.05 / \$0.15$$
$$n = 7$$

There are 7 nickels. We can plug this into either of the two original equations, but the first is easiest to use:

$$d = n - 2$$
$$d = 7 - 2$$
$$d = 5$$

NOTE: In this particular problem, the fastest way is to just try the different answers until one fits the requirements. We have shown the work in case it was a different question type then you would still know the approach.

CHAPTER REVIEW SOLUTIONS   CHAPTER 3

Question 5   B
See: GM 3.3.1
Simplify the expression:

$$(2.5 \times 10^3)(3 \times 10^x) = 0.075$$
$$(2.5 \times 3)(10^3 \times 10^x) = 0.075$$
$$(7.5)(10^{3+x}) = 0.075$$

Divide both sides of the equation 7.5, or simply note that 0.075 is one–hundredth $(\frac{1}{100}) = 10^{-2}$ of 7.5:

$$10^{3+x} = 10^{-2}$$
$$3 + x = -2$$
$$x = -5$$

Question 6   D
See: GM 3.5.4
If we think of the plank as a straight line in a coordinate system, we can use the points at which its ends are located to find its slope. The origin can be anywhere we choose, and the base of the house's left wall is a good choice. This point of the house must be located at (0, 0), and so the base of the plank, 7 feet to the left, is located at (−7, 0). The point at which the plank touches the left wall is 5 feet above the origin, at (0, 5). The slope of the plank is therefore

$$m = \frac{0-5}{-7-0} = \frac{-5}{-7} = \frac{5}{7}$$

Question 7   D
See: GM 3.3.1, 3.4.2A, 3.4.2B
It is given that $2n = 3k$, which implies that $\frac{2}{3}n = k$. $n + k = 5$ can therefore be rewritten:

$$n + \frac{2}{3}n = 5$$
$$\frac{5}{3}n = 5$$
$$n = 3$$

Question 8   C
See: GM 1.5
First combine the exponents where possible, and rearrange so they are all positive:

$$((y^{-2/3})^{1/2}) / (x^{-1/2})$$
$$= (y^{-1/3}) / (x^{-1/2})$$
$$= (x^{1/2}) / (y^{1/3})$$

Now plug in x=4 and y=8. Notice that $4=2^2$ and $8=2^3$.

$$= (4^{1/2}) / (8^{1/3})$$
$$= (2^{(2)1/2}) / (2^{(3)1/3})$$
$$= 2^1/2^1$$
$$= 1.$$

Question 9   A
See: GM 3.7
When adding logarithms of the same base, combine them by multiplying the numbers in parentheses. In this case:

$$\log_6(24) + \log_6(9)$$
$$= \log_6(24*9)$$
$$= \log_6(216)$$
$$= \log_6(6^3)$$

Now remember, a logarithm is an exponent. The question it poses is, "the base raised to what power is equal to the number in the parentheses?" So 6 raised to what power is equal to 6^3? The answer is, of course, 3.

Question 10   B
See: GM 3.7
First isolate the x terms on one side and all other terms on the other side of the equation.

$$\log_{10}(70) = x + \log_{10}(7)$$
$$\log_{10}(70) - \log_{10}(7) = x$$

Now combine the logarithms. When subtracting logarithms of the same base, combine them by dividing the numbers in parentheses.

$$\log_{10}(70/7) = x$$
$$\log_{10}(10) = x$$
$$1 = x.$$

Question 11   B
See: GM 1.5, 3.7
A coefficient multiplied by a logarithm can by brought inside the parentheses as an exponent.

$$x(\log_b(y)) + y(\log_b(y))$$
$$= \log_b(y^x) + \log_b(y^y)$$
$$= \log_b(y^x y^y)$$
$$= \log_b(y^{x+y}).$$

Question 12   D
See: GM 1.5, 3.7
The natural log has base e. Note that a logarithm of 1, no matter what the base, is equal to 0. And a log of its own base is equal to 1. So:

$$\ln(e^3)\log_3(27) + \ln(1)\ln(e)$$

Chapter Review Solutions — Chapter 3

$= \ln(e^3)\log_3(27) + 0*1$

$= 3\log_3(27)$

$= 3(3)$

$= 9$.

Question 13   D

See: GM 3.5, 3.7, 3.8

There are some useful pieces of information to notice that will help you answer this problem.

- What is the x and/or y intercept, if there is one?
- Where is the vertical asymptote? [Note: an 'asymptote' refers to a line that keeps approaching a given curve but does not meet the curve at any finite distance (GM 5.2.3C).] And does the curve approach positive or negative infinity?

In this case there is no x intercept, but the y intercept is at the point (0, -1). Plugging $x = 0$ into the given equations we can rule out all options except $y = -(2^x)$, so that is the solution.

Question 14   D

See: GM 3.7, 3.8

There are some useful pieces of information to notice that will help you answer this type of problem.

- What is the x and/or y intercept, if there is one?
- Where is the vertical asymptote? And does the curve approach positive or negative infinity?

The x and y intercept of this graph are the same, at (0, 0). Plugging in $y = 0$ to the given equations we can eliminate all but $y = \ln(x+1)$ and $y = -\ln(x+1)$. Next find the vertical asymptote.

It appears to be located at $x = -1$, and the curve approaches negative infinity. When x is small, $-\ln(x+1)$ is positive, so it cannot be the solution. Thus the graph represents $y = \ln(x+1)$.

Question 15   B

See: GM 3.7, 3.8

You can think of pH and H as corresponding to y and x respectively. So the graph you are considering is $y = -\log_{10}(x)$, the logarithm graph reflected about the x-axis. So the slopes along the curve are the opposite of the positive logarithm graph. Therefore when we decrease the value of x (moving right to left along the axis) the slope increases. If you are unsure of your solution, plug in test points to check. To see a positive log graph: GM 3.8.

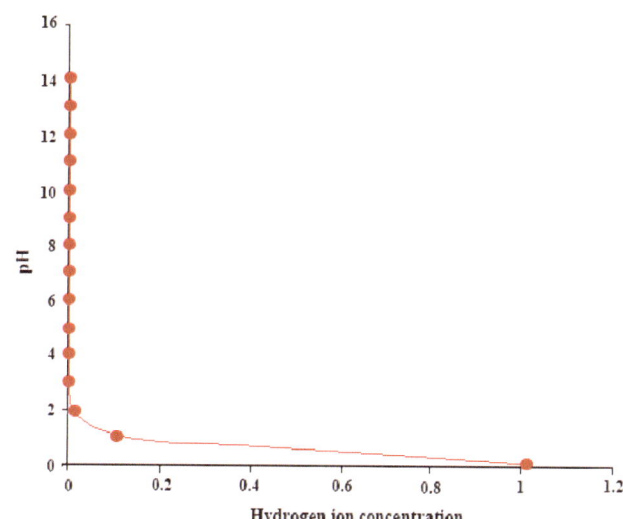

Chapter Review Solutions — Chapter 4

Question 1   B

See: GM 4.2, 4.2.3

Using the given information to write an equation, we have:

$$\pi r^2 = 144\pi$$

We need the value of the radius to find the circumference, so we solve for r:

$$r^2 = \frac{144\pi}{\pi}$$

$$r = \sqrt{144}$$

$$r = 12$$

The formula for the circumference of a circle gives us:

$$2\pi r = 2\pi(12) = 24\pi$$

Question 2   D

See: GM 4.2, 4.2.3

The length of the radius is half of the length of the diameter, which is $d = \sqrt{(2-2)^2 + (-3-5)^2} = \sqrt{0 + 64} = 8$ units long. The radius is therefore equal to 4.

Question 3   D

See: GM 4.2, 4.2.2

Triangle A has an area of $\frac{bh}{2} = 3(12m^2) = 36m^2$ which means that its base times its height is equal to 72 square feet. The base and height of all 45°–45°–90° triangles are the same, so (b × h)/2 = (b × b)/2 = 36. Solving for b gives us $b = \sqrt{72}$. Using the Pythagorean Theorem, we can solve for the hypotenuse. $h^2 = (\sqrt{72})^2 + (\sqrt{72})^2 = 144$, therefore $h = \sqrt{144} = 12$.

Question 4   C
See: GM 4.1, 4.1.3

The angle PQD has a measure equal to that of the given angle, 30 degrees, because the highways are parallel and the road forms a transversal across them. The hypotenuse of the right triangle PQD is 2 km long, and the alley, which forms the leg of the triangle that is opposite angle PQD, has a length of

$$(2 \text{ km}) \sin(30°) = 1 \text{ km}$$

Don't worry if you did not know or remember how to solve a problem with the sine function. As long as you understand the set up for the solution, that's fine for now. We will discuss trigonometric functions in the next GAMSAT Math chapter and again in Physics Chapter 1.

Question 5   A
See: GM 4.2, 4.2.1, 4.2.3

The relationship between the length of a side s and the length of the diagonal d of a square is (i.e. because the diagonal cuts the square into 45-45-90 triangles and remembering the ratio of that triangle's sides):

$$d = s\sqrt{2}$$

The length of a side of the given square is therefore

$$s = \frac{d}{\sqrt{2}} = \frac{5}{\sqrt{2}}$$

This is always the length of the diagonal of the inscribed circle, which has a radius of length $\frac{5}{\sqrt{2}} \div 2 = \frac{5}{2\sqrt{2}}$. The area of the circle is therefore

$$\pi\left(\frac{5}{2\sqrt{2}}\right)^2 = \frac{25\pi}{8}$$

Question 6   D
See: GM 4.2, 4.2.3

Represent the areas of the large and small circle by πr_L^2 and πr_S^2, respectively. 25% is equivalent to $\frac{1}{4}$, so

$$\pi r_S^2 = \frac{1}{4}(\pi r_L^2)$$

$$r_S^2 = \frac{1}{4} r_L^2$$

$$\sqrt{r_S^2} = \sqrt{\frac{1}{4} r_L^2}$$

$$r_S = \frac{1}{2} r_L$$

and the ratio of the radii is $\frac{r_S}{r_L} = \frac{\frac{1}{2} r_L}{r_L} = \frac{1}{2}$.

Question 7   D
See: GM 4.1, 4.1.1, 4.2.3

(0, 0), (10, 0), and any given point except (5, 0) can be connected by an arc, which can form part of a circle. (0, 0), (10, 0), and (5, 0) can only be connected by a line, which can never form part of a circle.

Question 8   D
See: GM 4.3.1; deduce

Because it is cube-like, we need to multiply 3 different sides together in order to get the volume. Consider that if you were to just multiply the 3 sides together, you would get a volume which includes the actual cardboard (i.e. calculating the volume that way would get a result which is somewhat greater than the actual volume INSIDE the box). However, if we were to examine the length for example, the space available inside the box would be less than the length of the box because of the thickness at BOTH ends.

Thus the inside measurements are reduced by the thickness of each side:

- The inside length will be l-2t
- The inside width will be w-2t
- The inside height will be h-2t

Thus the space (volume) inside the box = (l - 2t) x (w - 2t) x (h - 2t)

This style of reasoning including the development of an equation (during the exam!) that you have never seen before is a common though infrequent part of the real GAMSAT.

Note: Answer choice A is a reasonable approximation but answer choice D is the best answer among the choice provided. Part of the challenge of multiple choice exams is getting in the habit of identifying the best among options.

Chapter Review Solutions — Chapter 5

Question 1 B
See: GM 5.2, 5.2.1
A circle covers a total of 2π radians, and

$$\frac{\frac{8\pi}{5}}{2\pi} = \frac{4}{5}$$

which is equivalent to 80%.

Question 2 A
See: GM 5.5

$$-\cos\left(\frac{\pi}{2}\right) = \cos\left(\frac{\pi}{2}\right) = 0$$

Question 3 C
See: GM 5.1, 5.1.3, 5.3, 5.3.3
In a right triangle, the tangent of an angle represents the ratio of sides $\frac{opposite}{adjacent}$, so the given values form the proportion $\frac{3}{2} = \frac{12}{x}$, where x is the side adjacent the angle in question.
Cross-multiplication gives us $3x = 24$, or $x = 8$, and we can find the length of the hypotenuse using the Pythagorean Theorem:

$$12^2 + 8^2 = c^2$$
$$144 + 64 = c^2$$
$$\sqrt{208} = c$$
$$\sqrt{4 \times 4 \times 13} = c$$
$$4\sqrt{13} = c$$

Question 4 D
See: GM 4.1.3, 5.2, 5.2.3
The cosine of an angle is equal to the sine of its complement. $\frac{\pi}{6}$, or $\left(\frac{\pi}{6}\right)\left(\frac{180°}{\pi}\right) = 30°$, is the complement of $\frac{\pi}{3} = 60°$.

Chapter Review Solutions — Chapter 6

Question 1 B
See: GM 6.1.1
There are four red marbles, and a total of 4 red + 6 blue = 10 marbles, so the probability is $\frac{4}{10}$.

Question 2 D
See: GM 6.1, 6.1.2
With a total of 10 balls and 6 yellow balls, the probability that the first ball is yellow is $\frac{6}{10} = \frac{3}{5}$. After the first ball is chosen, there are 9 left, of which 4 are green. The probability of choosing a green ball at this point is therefore $\frac{4}{9}$. The total probability is

$$\left(\frac{3}{5}\right)\left(\frac{4}{9}\right) = \frac{4}{15}$$

Question 3 D
See: GM 6.3, 6.3.5
Multiply all possible choices: $3 \times 2 \times 4 = 24$

Question 4 A
See: GM 6.3.2
The 2516 residents represent 68% of the total number of residents x:

$$2516 = 0.68x$$
$$3700 = x$$

Question 5 C
See: GM 6.2, 6.2.1
If the third student takes x minutes to complete the test:

$$\frac{41 + 37 + x}{3} = 35$$
$$78 + x = 105$$
$$x = 27$$

Question 6 D
See: GM 6.3.5
There are 4 different book colors, so there are 4 different choices for books to shelve on Monday. There are only 3 choices on Tuesday. On Wednesday, the rest of the books will be shelved, so there is only 1 choice. This gives a total of $4 \times 3 \times 1 = 12$ different ways to shelve the books.

Question 7 D
See: GM 6.1, 6.1.2
A die has a total of 6 possible sides. There is only one side that displays a 3, so the probability of rolling a 3 is $\frac{1}{6}$. Similarly, the probability of rolling any other number is also $\frac{1}{6}$. The probability of rolling a 1 or a 2 is the sum of their individual probabilities: $\frac{1}{6} + \frac{1}{6} = \frac{1}{3}$. Because this probability is independent of the probability of first rolling a 3, we multiply the results to get the total probability: $\left(\frac{1}{6}\right)\left(\frac{1}{3}\right) = \frac{1}{18}$.

GAMSAT-prep.com
PHYSICS
PART III.B: PHYSICAL SCIENCES

IMPORTANT: Before doing your science survey for the GAMSAT, be sure you have read the Preface, Introduction and Part II, Chapter 2. The beginning of each science chapter provides guidelines as to what you should Memorize, Understand and what is Not Required. These are guides to get you a top score without getting lost in the details. Our guides have been determined from an analysis of all ACER materials plus student surveys. Additionally, the original owner of this book gets a full year access to many online features described in the Preface and Introduction including an online Forum where each chapter can be discussed.

TRANSLATIONAL MOTION
Chapter 1

Memorize	Understand	Not Required*
onometric functions: definitions hagorean theorem ne: displacement, velocity, eleration ations: acceleration, kinematics	* Scalar vs. vector * Add, subtract, resolve vectors * Determine common values of functions * Conversion of the angle to other units * Displacement, velocity, acceleration (avg. and instant.) including graphs	* Advanced level college info * Any derivatives with or without vectors * Complex vector systems

GAMSAT-Prep.com

Introduction

Translational motion is the movement of an object (or particle) through space without turning (rotation). Displacement, velocity and acceleration are key vectors — specified by magnitude and direction — often used to describe translational motion. Being able to manipulate and resolve vectors is critical for problem solving in GAMSAT Physics.

Whether science or non-science background: (1) please complete the GAMSAT Math chapters prior to starting Physics; (2) key in on information underlined, in italics, in red boxes or highlighted in yellow; (3) go to your online access account and consider: watching videos, printing our GAMSAT Physics Equation List or making your own, and irrespective of your initial comfort level, try some online practice questions because they will begin with the basics and then work up to challenge you.

Additional Resources

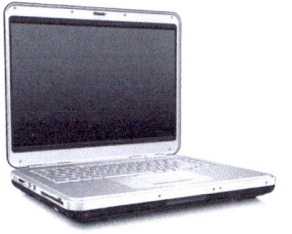   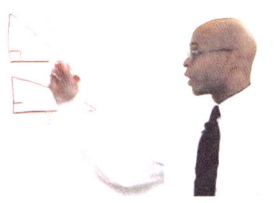   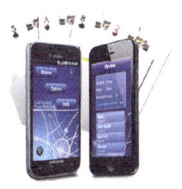   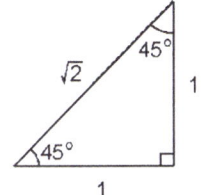

Free Online Q&A + Forum   Video: Online or DVD   Flashcards   Special Guest

THE PHYSICAL SCIENCES   PHY-03

---

* The real GAMSAT may have advanced level information presented (ie. in a passage) but previous knowledge of said information is not required to answer the questions that would follow. Practice ACER and GS practice GAMSATs can help you clarify this point.

1.1 Scalars and Vectors

Scalars, such as speed, have magnitude only and are specified by a number with a unit (55 miles/hour). Scalars obey the rules of ordinary algebra. *Vectors*, like velocity, have both magnitude **and** direction (100 km/hour, west). Vectors are represented by arrows where: i) the length of the arrow indicates the magnitude of the vector, and ii) the arrowhead indicates the direction of the vector. Vectors obey the special rules of vector algebra. Thus vectors can be moved in space but their orientation must be kept the same.

Addition of Vectors: Two vectors **a** and **b** can be added geometrically by drawing them to a common scale and placing them head to tail. The vector connecting the tail of **a** to the head of **b** is the sum or resultant vector **r**.

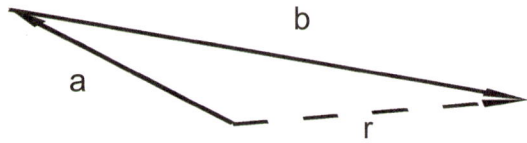

Figure III.B.1.1: The vector sum a + b = r.

Subtraction of Vectors: To subtract the vector **b** from **a**, reverse the direction of **b** then add to **a**.

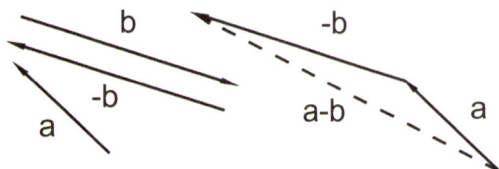

Figure III.B.1.2: The vector difference a - b = a + (-b).

Resolution of Vectors: Perpendicular projections of a vector can be made on a coordinate axis. Thus the vector **a** can be *resolved* into its x-component (a_x) and its y-component (a_y).

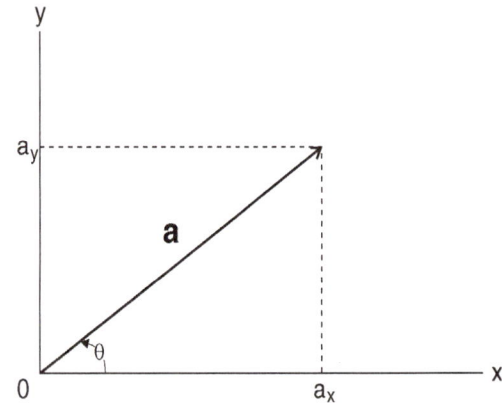

Figure III.B.1.3: The resolution of a vector into its scalar components in a coordinate system.

Analytically, the resolution of vector **a** is as follows:

$$a_x = \mathbf{a} \cos \theta \quad \text{and} \quad a_y = \mathbf{a} \sin \theta$$

Conversely, given the components, we can reconstruct vector **a**:

$$\mathbf{a} = \sqrt{a_x^2 + a_y^2} \quad \text{and} \quad \tan \theta = a_y / a_x$$

We will now foreshadow the scalar and vector quantities that we will be exploring over the 12 Physics chapters. You may already have a sense as to the logic of the classification but, if not, after you have completed Physics, please return to this section to confirm.

PHY-04 TRANSLATIONAL MOTION

Examples of Scalar Quantities	Examples of Vector Quantities
distance, speed, time, temperature, mass, area, volume, energy, entropy, electric charge	displacement, velocity, acceleration, force, momentum, gravitational field, electrical field

1.1.1 Trigonometric Functions

The power in trigonometric functions lies in their ability to relate an angle to the ratio of scalar components or *sides* of a triangle. These functions may be defined as follows:

$$\sin \theta = opp/hyp = y/r$$

$$\cos \theta = adj/hyp = x/r$$

[*opp* = the length of the side *opposite* angle θ, *adj* = the length of the side *adjacent* to angle θ, *hyp* = the length of the *hypotenuse*]

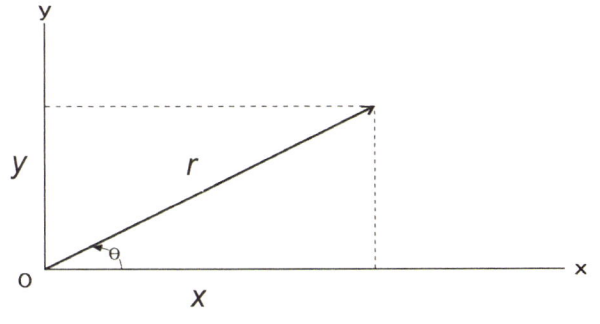

Thus sine (*r*sin θ) gives the y-component and cosine (*r*cos θ) gives the x-component of vector r. The tangent function (*tan* θ) and two important trigonometric identities relate sine and cosine:

$$\tan \theta = \sin \theta / \cos \theta = opp/adj = y/x$$

$$\sin^2 \theta + \cos^2 \theta = 1$$

and

$$\sin 2\theta = 2 \sin \theta \cos \theta$$

Other functions of very little importance for GAMSAT physics include: cotangent (*cot* θ = x/y), secant (*sec* θ = r/x) and cosecant (*csc* θ = r/y).

The Pythagorean Theorem relates the sides of the right angle triangle according to the following:

$$r^2 = x^2 + y^2.$$

THE PHYSICAL SCIENCES   PHY-05

1.1.2 Common Values of Trigonometric Functions

There are special angles which produce standard values of the trigonometric functions. These values should be memorized. Several of the values are derived from the following triangles:

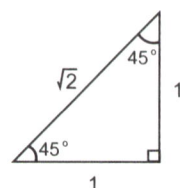 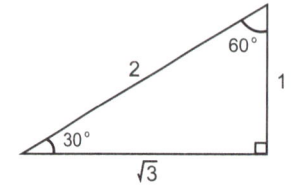

θ	sin θ	cos θ	tan θ
0°	0	1	0
30°	1/2	√3/2	1/√3
45°	1/√2	1/√2	1
60°	√3/2	1/2	√3
90°	1	0	∞
180°	0	-1	0

Table III.B.1.1:
Common values of trigonometric functions. The angle θ may be given in radians (R) where $2\pi^R$ = 360°= 1 revolution. Recall √3 ≈1.7, √2 ≈ 1.4.

Note that 1° = 60 arcminutes, 1 arcminute = 60 arcseconds. These conversions do not need to be memorized because they would be given on the exam if needed.

Each trigonometric function (i.e. sine) contains an inverse function (i.e. $\sin^{-1}$), where if sin θ = x, θ = $\sin^{-1}$ x. Thus cos 60° = 1/2, and 60° = $\cos^{-1}$ (1/2). Some texts denote the inverse function with "arc" as a prefix. Thus arcsec (2) = $\sec^{-1}$ (2).

1.2 Distance and Displacement

Distance is the amount of separation between two points in space. It has a magnitude but no direction. It is a scalar quantity and is always positive.

Displacement of an object between two points is the difference between the final position and the initial position of the object in a given referential system. Thus, a displacement has an origin, a direction and a magnitude. It is a vector.

The sign of the coordinates of the vector displacement depends on the system under study and the chosen referential system. The sign will be positive (+) if the system is moving towards the positive axis of the referential system and negative (-) if not.

The units of distance and displacement are expressed in length units such as *feet (ft), meters (m), miles* and *kilometers (km)*. The International System of Units (SI), the standard for the GAMSAT and science in general, uses the meter for length (see GM 2.1.3).

1.3 Speed and Velocity

Speed is the rate of change of distance with respect to time. It is a scalar quantity, it has a magnitude but no direction, like distance, and it is always positive.

Velocity is the rate of change of displacement with respect to time. It is a vector, and like the displacement, it has a direction and a magnitude. Its value depends on the position of the object. The sign of the coordinates of the vector velocity is the same as that of the displacement.

The instantaneous velocity of a system at a given time is the slope of the graph of the displacement of that system vs. time at that time. The magnitude of the velocity decreases if the vector velocity and the vector acceleration have opposite directions.

The units of speed and velocity are expressed in length divided by time such as *feet/sec., meters/sec. (m/s)* and *miles/hour.*

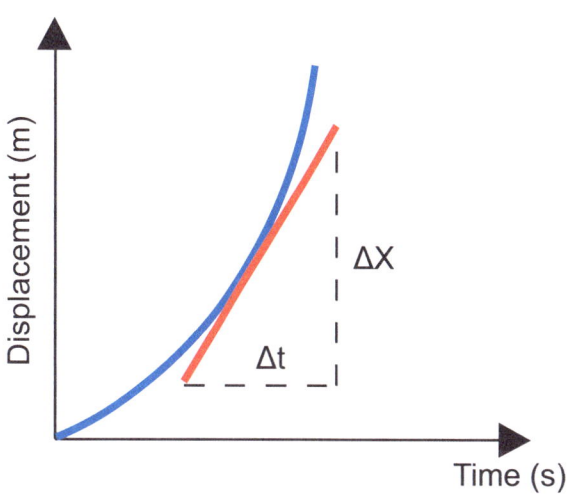

Figure III.B.1.4: Displacement vs. time. Please note that the capital letter X denotes displacement as opposed to referring to the x-axis (small letter x) which is time.

Dimensional Analysis: remember from High School math that a slope is "rise over run" meaning it is the change in the y-axis divided by the change in the x-axis (GM 3.5, 3.5.4). This means when we pay attention to the units, we get, for example, m/s which is velocity in SI units.

1.4 Acceleration

Acceleration (a) is the rate of change of the velocity (v) with respect to time (t):

$$a = v/t$$

Like the velocity, it is a vector and it has a direction and a magnitude.

The sign of the vector acceleration depends on the net force applied to the system and the chosen referential system. The units of acceleration are expressed as velocity divided by time such as meters/sec^2 (m/s^2; SI units). The term for negative acceleration is deceleration.

1.4.1 Average and Instantaneous Acceleration

The average acceleration av between two instants t and t' = t + Δt, measures the result of the increase in the speed divided by the time difference,

$$a_v = \frac{v' - v}{\Delta t}$$

The instantaneous acceleration can be determined either by calculating the **slope** (*see Appendix A.3.1*) of a velocity vs. time graph at any time, or by taking the limit when Δt approaches zero of the preceding expression.

$$a_v = \lim_{\Delta t \to 0} \frac{v' - v}{\Delta t}$$

Math involving "limits" does not exist on the GAMSAT. So let's discuss what this definition is describing in informal terms. The limit is the value of the change in velocity over the change in time as the time approaches 0. It's like saying that the change in velocity is happening in an instant. This allows us to talk about the acceleration in that incredibly fast moment: the instantaneous acceleration which can be determined graphically.

Consider the following events illustrated in the graph (Fig. III.B.1.4): your car starts at rest (0 velocity and time = 0); you steadily accelerate out of the parking lot (the change in velocity increases over time = acceleration); you are driving down the street at constant velocity (change in velocity = 0 and thus acceleration is 0 divided by the change in time which means: a = 0); you see a cat dart across the street safely which made you slow down temporarily (change in velocity is negative thus negative acceleration which, by definition, is deceleration); you now enter the on-ramp for the highway so your velocity is now increasing at a faster and faster rate (increasing acceleration). You can examine the instantaneous acceleration at any one point (or instant) during the period that your acceleration is increasing.

==To determine the displacement (*not* distance), take the area under the graph or curve.== To calculate area: a rectangle is base (b) times height (h); a triangle is ½b × h; and for a curve, they can use graph paper and expect you would count the boxes under the curve to estimate the area.

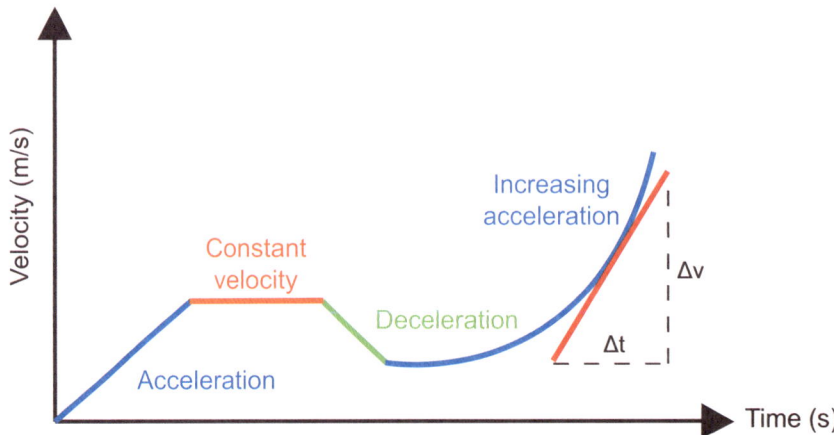

Figure III.B.1.4: Velocity vs. time. Note that at constant velocity, the slope and thus the acceleration are both equal to zero.

1.5 Uniformly Accelerated Motion

The magnitude and direction of the acceleration of a system are solely determined by the exterior forces acting upon the system. If the magnitude of these forces is constant, the magnitude of the acceleration will be constant and the resulting motion is a *uniformly accelerated motion*. The initial displacement, the velocity and the accelera-tion at any given time contribute to the over-all displacement of the system:

$x = x_0$ – displacement due to the initial displacement x_0.

$x = v_0 t$ – displacement due to the initial velocity v_0 at time t.

$x = \frac{1}{2}at^2$ – displacement due to the acceleration at time t.

The total displacement of the uniformly-accelerated motion is given by the following formula:

$$x = x_0 + v_0 t + \tfrac{1}{2}at^2$$

The translational motion is the motion of the center of gravity of a system through space, illustrated by the above equation.

1.6 Equations of Kinematics

Kinematics is the study of objects in motion with respect to space and time. There are three related equations which must be memorized. The first is above (PHY 1.5), the others are:

$$v = v_0 + at \quad \text{and}$$
$$v^2 = v_0^2 + 2ax$$

where v is the final velocity; we will put these equations to use in PHY 2.6.

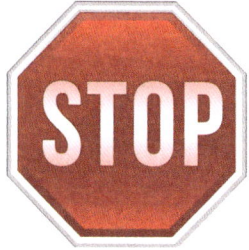

Reminder: Chapter review questions are available online for the original owner of this textbook. Doing practice questions will help clarify concepts and ensure that you study in a targeted way. First, register at gamsat-prep.com, then login and click on GAMSAT Textbook Owners in the right column so you can use your Online Access Card to have access to the Lessons section.

No science background? Consider watching the relevant videos at gamsat-prep.com and you have support at gamsat-prep.com/forum. Don't forget to check the Index at the beginning of this book to see which chapters are HIGH, MEDIUM and LOW relative importance for the GAMSAT.

Your online access continues for one full year from your online registration.

GOLD NOTES

FORCE, MOTION, AND GRAVITATION
Chapter 2

Memorize	Understand	Not Required*
with units: weight, mass n's laws, Law of Gravitation ion for uniformly accelerated motion	* Mass, weight, center of gravity * Newton's laws * Law of Gravitation, free fall motion * Projectile motion equations and calculations	* Advanced level college info * Memorizing values for K,G

GAMSAT-Prep.com

Introduction

Force is a vector (often a push or pull) that can cause a mass to change velocity thus motion. Forces can be due to gravity, magnetism or anything that causes a mass to accelerate. Nuclear forces (strong) are far greater than electrostatic forces (opposite charges attract), which in turn are far greater than gravitational forces (one of the weakest forces in nature).

Additional Resources

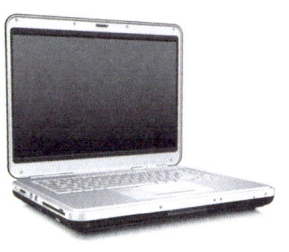 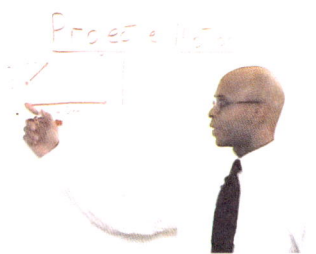 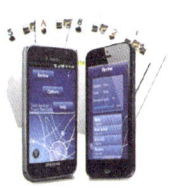 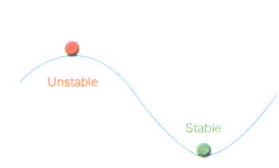

ree Online Q&A + Forum   Video: Online or DVD   Flashcards   Special Guest

THE PHYSICAL SCIENCES   PHY-11

* The real GAMSAT may have advanced level information presented (ie. in a passage) but previous knowledge of said information is not required to answer the questions that would follow. Practice ACER and GS practice GAMSATs can help you clarify this point.

2.1 Mass, Center of Mass, Weight

The mass (m) of an object is its measure of inertia. It is the measure of the capacity of that object to remain motionless or to move with a constant velocity if the sum of the forces acting upon it is zero. This definition of inertia is derived from Newton's First Law.

The *center of mass* of an object is a point whose motion can be described like the motion of a particle through space. The center of mass of an object always has the simplest motion of all the points of that object.

The center of gravity (COG) is also the center of mass seen as the center of application of all the gravitational forces acting on the object. For example, for a uniform plank hanging horizontally, the COG is at half the length of the plank.

The COG can be determined experimentally by suspending an object by a string at different points and noting that the direction of the string passes through the COG.

The intersection of the projected lines in the different suspensions is the COG.

An object is in *stable equilibrium* if the COG is as low as possible and any change in orientation will lead to an elevation of the COG. An object is in *unstable equilibrium* if the COG is high relative to the support point or surface and any change in orientation will lead to a lowering of the COG.

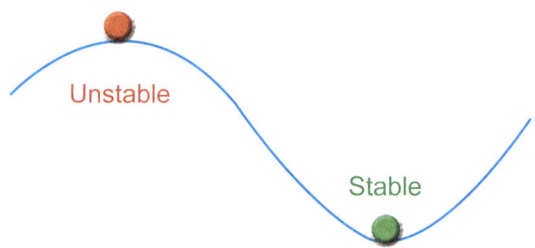

The *weight* is a force (i.e. newtons, pounds). It is a vector unlike the *mass* which is a scalar (i.e. kilograms, slugs). The weight is proportional to the mass. It is the product of the mass by the vector gravitational acceleration g.

$$W = m \times g$$

2.2 Newton's Second Law

Newton's Second Law, also called the fundamental dynamic relation, states that the sum of all the exterior forces acting upon the center of mass of a system is equal to the product of the mass of the system by the acceleration of its center of mass.

Therefore, if there is a net force, the object must accelerate. It is a vectorial equality which asserts that <u>a net force against an object *must* result in acceleration</u>:

$$\Sigma F = m \times a$$

It is important to note that for a system in complex motion, Newton's Second Law can only determine the acceleration of the center of mass. It does not give any indication about the motion of the other parts of the system.

Whereas, for a system in translational motion, Newton's Second Law gives the acceleration of the system.

In your daily life, you would already have the sense that objects with a greater mass (m) require a greater force (F) to get it to move with increasing speed (a). If you maintain a net force on an object, it will not only move, it must accelerate. We will be exploring more consequences of Newton's Second Law both in this and later chapters.

2.3 Newton's Third Law

For every action there is an equal and opposite reaction. If one object exerts a force, F, on a second object, the second object exerts a force, F', on the first object. F and F' have opposite direction but the same magnitude.

One conclusion would be that forces are found in pairs. Consider the time you sit in a chair. Your body exerts a force downward (mg) and that chair needs to exert an equal force upward (the normal force N) or the chair will collapse. There is symmetry. Acting forces encounter other forces in the opposite direction. Consider shooting a cannonball. When the explosion fires the cannonball through the air, the cannon is pushed backward. The force pushing the ball out is equal to the force pushing the cannon back, but the effect on the cannon is less noticeable because it has a much larger mass and it may be restrained. Similarly, a gun experiences a "kick" backwards when a bullet is fired forward.

2.4 The Law of Gravitation

The Law of Gravitation states that there is a force of attraction existing between any two bodies of masses m_1 and m_2. The force is proportional to the product of the masses and inversely proportional to the square of the distance between them.

$$F = K_G(m_1 m_2 / r^2)$$

r is the distance between the bodies; K_G is the universal constant of gravitation, and its value depends on the units being used.

2.5 Free Fall Motion

The free fall motion of an object is the upward or downward vertical motion of that object with reference to the earth.

The motion is always uniformly accelerated with the acceleration g: vertical, directed towards the center of the earth and the magnitude is considered constant during the free fall motion.

Also, during the free fall motion, the air resistance is considered negligible. The equation of the motion can easily be derived from Newton's Second Law.

$$\Sigma F = ma$$

Where ΣF represents all the forces acting on the object, m is the mass of the object and a is the acceleration of the center of mass of the object. Hence, a can be replaced by g since $a = g$ by definition. In the free fall motion, the only force acting on the object is the gravitational force, which gives the following equality:

$$K_G m_{object} \frac{M_{earth}}{r^2_{earth}} = m_{object}\, g$$

dividing both sides by m_{object} we get:

$$g = K_G \frac{M_{earth}}{r^2_{earth}}$$

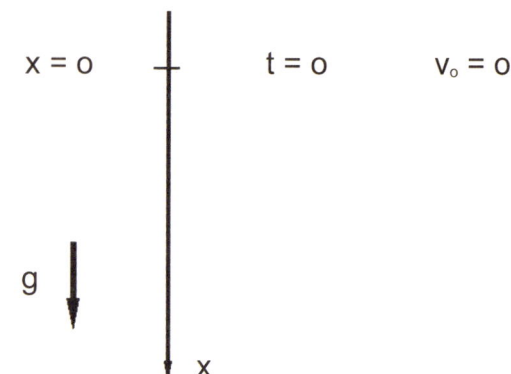

Figure III.B.2.1: Free fall motion.

The values of g are: 32 ft/s^2 (Imperial units), 980 cm/s^2 (CGS units), or 9.8 m/s^2 (**SI** units). The equation for uniformly accelerated motion is applicable by replacing a by g:

$$x = x_0 + v_0 t + 1/2\, gt^2$$

$$v = gt$$

$$a = g$$

Before doing any calculation, the reference point and a positive direction must be chosen. In the free fall of an actual object, the value of g is modified by the buoyancy of air and resistance of air. This results in a *drag force* which depends on the location on earth, shape and size of the object, and the velocity of the object (as free fall velocity increases, the drag force increases). When the drag force reaches the force of gravity, the object reaches a final velocity called the terminal velocity and continues to fall at that velocity.

2.6 Projectile Motion

The projectile motion is the motion of any object fired or launched at some angle α from the horizontal. The motion defines a parabola (see Figure III.B.2.2) in the plane O-x-y that contains the initial (*original*) vector velocity v_o.

The motion can be decomposed into two distinct motions: a vertical component, affected by g, and a horizontal component, independent of g.

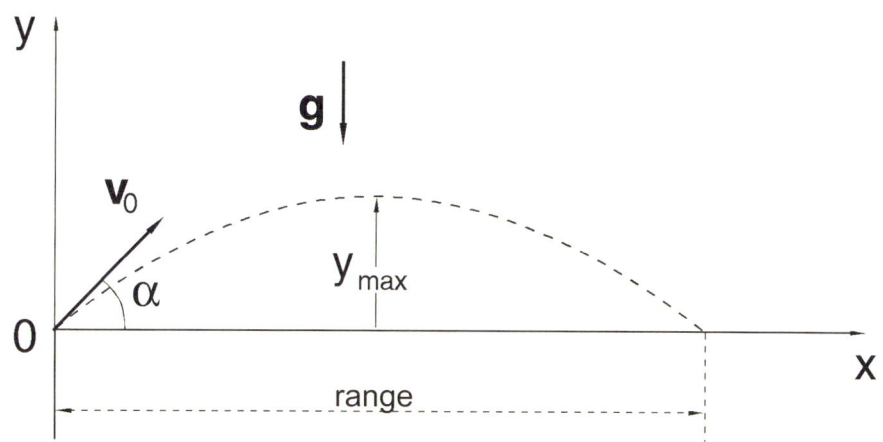

Figure III.B.2.2: Projectile motion.

Vertical component (free fall)
- initial speed : $V_{oy} = V_o \sin α$
- displacement at time t: $y = V_{oy}t + 1/2 gt^2$
- speed at any time t: $V_y = V_{oy} + gt$

Horizontal component (linear with constant speed)
- initial speed : $V_{ox} = V_o \cos α$
- displacement at any time t: $x = V_{ox}t$
- speed at any time t: $V_x = V_{ox}$ (speed is constant)

Initial velocity

- magnitude: $|V_o| = \sqrt{V_{ox}^2 + V_{oy}^2}$

- direction: *alpha*: $\tan α = V_{oy} / V_{ox}$

- important points to consider:
1) Neglecting air resistance, there is no acceleration in the horizontal direction: V_x is constant.
2) V_y is zero at Y_{max}, then $V_y = 0 = V_{oy} + gt_{up}$ or $-V_{oy} = gt_{up}$ can be solved for t.

3) Also, by eliminating the variables y and t in the equations, we can get the following equality :
$$x = \frac{V_o^2 \sin 2α}{g}$$

The horizontal distance from the origin to where the object strikes the ground (= *the range*) is maximum for a given V_o when $\sin 2α = 1$, hence for $2α = (π/2)^R$ => $α = (π/4)^R$ or $α = 45$ degrees.

2.6.1 Projectile Motion Problem (Imperial units)

In the Rugby World Cup, a player kicks the ball at an angle of 30° from the horizontal with an initial speed of 75 ft/s. Assume that the ball moves in a vertical plane and that air resistance is negligible.

(a) Find the time at which the ball reaches the highest point of its trajectory.
{key: height refers to the y-component; we can define *gravity* as a negative vector since it is directed downwards}

V_y is zero at Y_{max} (= the highest point), thus:

$V_y = 0$, $V_o = 75$ ft/s, $\alpha = 30°$, $g = -32$ ft/s²

$V_y = V_o \sin \alpha + g t_{up}$

Isolate t_{up}:

$$t_{up} = \frac{V_y - V_o \sin \alpha}{g} = \frac{-75(\sin 30°)}{-32}$$

$= 1.2$ seconds

(b) How high does the ball go?

$Y_{max} = V_o (\sin \alpha) t_{up} + 1/2 g t_{up}^2$

$Y_{max} = 75(\sin 30°)1.2 + 1/2(-32)(1.2)^2 = 22$ feet

(c) How long is the ball in the air and what is its range?
{key: time is the same for x- and y-components, range = x-component}

Once the ball strikes the ground its vertical displacement y = 0, thus:

$y = 0 = V_o (\sin \alpha) t + 1/2 g t^2$

Divide through by t then isolate:

$t = 2V_o (\sin \alpha)/g = 2.4$ seconds.

Since $t = 2t_{up}$, we can conclude that the time required for the ball to go up to Y_{max} is the same as the time required to come back down: 1.2 seconds in either direction.

The range $x = V_o (\cos \alpha) t$

$x = 75(\cos 30°)2.4 \approx 150$ feet

or

$x \approx 150$ ft (1 yd/ 3 ft) = 50 yards

{Had the player kicked the ball at 45° from the horizontal he would have maximized his range. He should be benched for not having done his physics!}

(d) *What is the velocity of the ball as it strikes the ground?*

{*key: velocity* is the resultant vector of V_x and V_y - the final velocities in the *x* and *y* directions}

$V_x = V_o \cos \alpha = 75(\cos 30°) = 65$ ft/s

$V_y = V_o \sin \alpha + gt$

$= 75(\sin 30°) + (-32)(2.4) = -39$ ft/s

$V = \sqrt{V_x^2 + V_y^2} = \sqrt{(65)^2 + (-39)^2}$

$= \sqrt{(13 \times 5)^2 + (13 \times -3)^2}$

$V = 13\sqrt{(5)^2 + (-3)^2} = 13\sqrt{34}$

To estimate $\sqrt{34}$ we must first recognize that the answer must be at least 5 ($5^2 = 25$) but closer to 6 ($6^2 = 36$). Try squaring 5.7, 5.8, 5.9. Squaring 5.8 is the closest estimate (= *33.6*), thus

$V = 13(5.8) = 75$ ft/s.

Please note:
- With no air resistance and a symmetric problem (the ball is launched and returns to the same vertical point), the initial and final speeds are the same (75 ft/s).
- Usually ACER will use SI units in GAMSAT problems, but many problems are solved using dimensional analysis, with or without SI units.
- Please be sure you can do all the preceding calculations efficiently. To learn more about SI units, *see* GM 2.1.3.

Go online to GAMSAT-prep.com for free chapter review Q&A and forum.

GOLD NOTES

PARTICLE DYNAMICS
Chapter 3

Memorize	Understand	Not Required*
Centripetal force and acceleration Circumference and area of a circle	* Equations: f_{max}, μ * Static vs. kinetic friction * Resolving vectors, calculate for incline plane * Uniform circular motion * Solve pulley system, free body diagram	* Advanced level college info * Memorizing values of μ

GAMSAT-Prep.com

Introduction

Particle dynamics is concerned with the physics of motion. Among other topics, particle dynamics includes Newton's laws, frictional forces, and problems dealing with incline planes, uniform circular motion and pulley systems.

Additional Resources

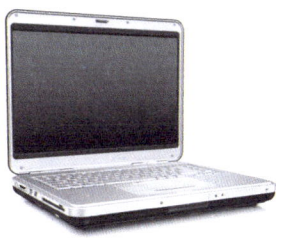

Free Online Q&A + Forum

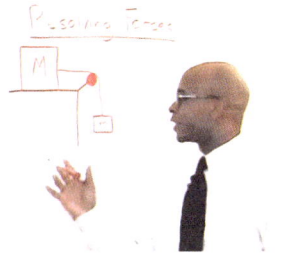

Video: Online or DVD

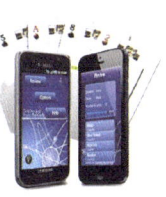

Flashcards

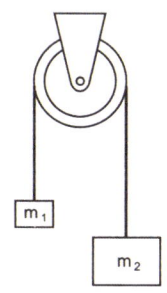

Special Guest

THE PHYSICAL SCIENCES PHY-19

* The real GAMSAT may have advanced level information presented (ie. in a passage) but previous knowledge of said information is not required to answer the questions that would follow. Practice ACER and GS practice GAMSATs can help you clarify this point.

3.1 Overview

For the GAMSAT, particle dynamics is concerned with the physics of motion. Among other topics, particle dynamics includes Newton's laws, frictional forces, and problems dealing with incline planes, uniform circular motion and pulley systems.

3.2 Frictional Forces

Frictional forces are nonconservative (mechanical energy is not conserved) and are caused by molecular adhesion between tangential surfaces but are independent of the area of contact of the surfaces. Frictional forces always oppose the motion. The maximal frictional force has the following expression: $f_{max} = \mu N$, where μ is the coefficient of friction and N is the normal force to the surface on which the object rests, it is the reaction of that surface against the weight of the object. Thus N always acts perpendicular to the surface.

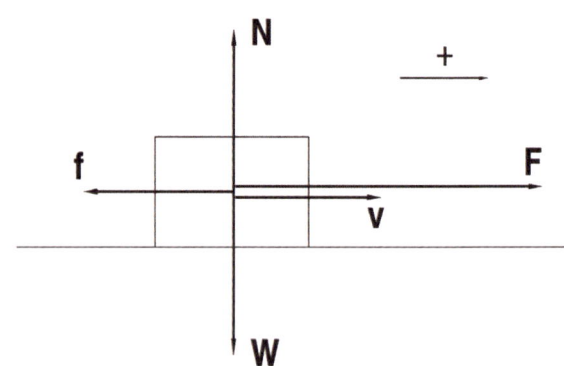

Figure III.B.3.1: Frictional force f and force normal N.

Static friction is when the object is not moving, and it must be overcome for motion to begin. The coefficient of static friction μ_s is given as:

$$\mu_s = \tan \alpha$$

where α is the angle at which the object first begins to move on an inclined plane as the angle is increased from 0 degrees to α degrees (see Figure III.B.3.2). There is also a coefficient of kinetic friction, μ_k, which exists when surfaces are in motion; $\mu_k < \mu_s$ always.

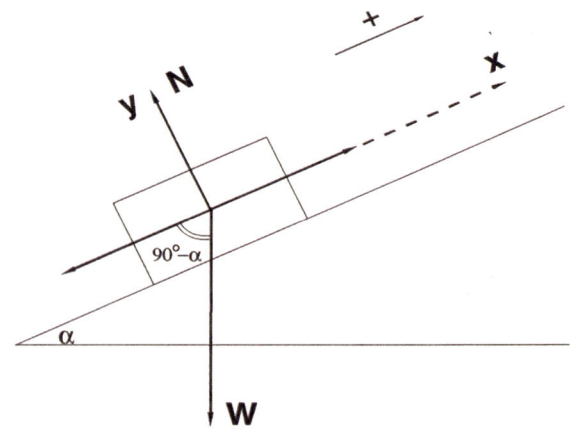

Figure III.B.3.2:
Analysis of motion on an incline. To understand the relationship of the angles in the diagram, see Geometry GM 4.1.3.

The weight (W) due to gravity (g) may be sufficient to cause motion if friction is overcome. The reference axes are usually chosen as shown such that one (the x) is along the surface of the incline.

Note that W is directed downward and N is directed upward but *perpendicular* to the surface of the incline (i.e. in the positive y direction).

3.2.1 Incline Plane Problem with Friction (SI units)

A 50 kilogram block is on an incline of 45°. The coefficient of sliding (= *kinetic*) friction between the block and the plane is 0.10.

Determine the acceleration of the block. {key: motion is along the plane, so only the x-components of the force is relevant to the acceleration}

Begin with Newton's Second Law:

$$F = m \times a$$

thus

$$F_x = f_k - W\sin\alpha = \mu_k N - W\sin\alpha = m \times a$$

The force normal (N) can be determined by summing the forces in the y direction where the acceleration is zero:

$$F_y = N - W\cos\alpha = m \times a = 0$$

Therefore,

$$N = W\cos\alpha$$

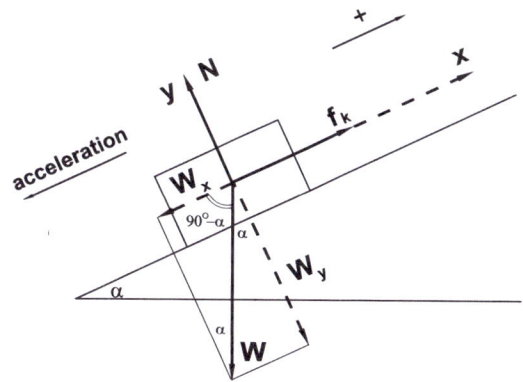

Figure III.B.3.3: Resolving the weight W into its x-component (W sinα) and its y-component (W cosα).

Solving for a and combining our first and last equations we get (*recall:* $W = mg$):

$$a = (\mu_k W\cos\alpha - W\sin\alpha)/m$$
$$= mg(\mu_k\cos\alpha - \sin\alpha)/m = g(\mu_k\cos\alpha - \sin\alpha)$$

Substituting the values:

$$a = 9.8 \text{ m/s}^2(0.10\cos45° - \sin45°) = -6.2 \text{ m/s}^2$$

- Thus the block accelerates at 6.2 m/s² *down* the plane. Also note that the *mass* of the block is irrelevant.

THE PHYSICAL SCIENCES

3.3 Uniform Circular Motion

In Chapter 1 we saw that acceleration is due to a change in velocity (PHY 1.4). For a particle moving in a circle at constant speed (= *uniform circular motion*), the velocity vector changes continuously in <u>direction</u> but the <u>magnitude</u> remains the same.

The velocity is always tangent to the circle and since it is always changing (i.e. *direction*) it creates an acceleration directed radially inward called the *centripetal* acceleration (a_c). The magnitude of the acceleration a_c is given by v^2/r where r is the radius of the circle.

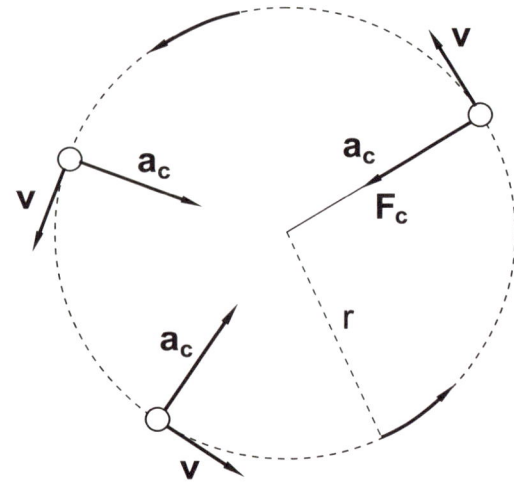

Figure III.B.3.4: Uniform Circular Motion.

Every accelerated particle must have a force acting on it according to Newton's Second Law. Thus we can calculate the *centripetal* force,

$$F_c = ma_c = mv^2/r.$$

The centripetal force can be produced in many ways: a taut string which is holding a ball at the end that is spinning in a circle; a radially directed frictional force like when a car drives around a curve on an unbanked road; a contact force exerted by another body like driving around a curve on a banked road or like the wall of an amusement park rotor.

Any particle moving in a circle with *non-uniform* speed will experience both centripetal *and* tangential forces and accelerations. {Reminder: the circumference of a circle is $2\pi r$ and the area is πr^2}

3.4 Pulley Systems

Consider two unequal masses connected by a string which passes over a frictionless, massless pulley (see Figure III.B.3.5). Let us determine the following parameters: i) the tension T in the string which is a force and ii) the acceleration of the masses given that m_2 is greater than m_1.

Always begin by drawing vector or *free-body* diagrams of a problem. The position of each mass will lie at the origin O of their respective axes. Now we assign positivity or negativity to the directions of motion. We can arbitrarily define the upward direction as positive. Thus if the acceleration of m_1 is a then the acceleration of m_2 must be $-a$.

Using Newton's Second Law we can derive the equation of motion for m_1:

$$F = T - m_1 g = m_1 a$$

and for m_2:

$$F = T - m_2 g = -m_2 a$$

Subtracting one equation from the other eliminates T then we can solve for a:

$$a = \frac{m_2 - m_1}{m_2 + m_1} g$$

Solve for a using the equations of motion, equate the formulas, then we can solve for T:

$$T = \frac{2 m_1 m_2}{m_1 + m_2} g$$

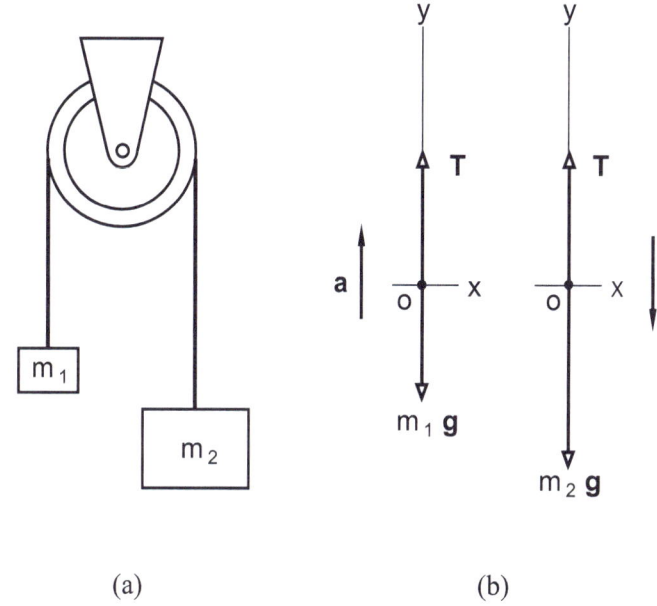

Figure III.B.3.5: A Pulley System. (a) Two unequal masses suspended by a string from a pulley (= Atwood's machine). (b) Free-body diagrams for m_1 and m_2.

Let us solve the problem using Imperial units where m_2 is 3.0 slugs ($W_2 = m_2 g = 96$ pounds - lb) and m_1 is 1.0 slug ($W_1 = m_1 g = 32$ lb):

$$a = \frac{3.0 - 1.0}{3.0 + 1.0} g = g/2 = 16 \text{ ft/s}^2$$

and

$$T = \frac{2 (1.0)(3.0)}{1.0 + 3.0} (32) = 48 \text{ lb}.$$

- Note that T is always between the weight of mass m_1 and that of m_2. The reason is that T must exceed $m_1 g$ to give m_1 an upward acceleration, and $m_2 g$ must exceed T to give m_2 a downward acceleration.

Go online to GAMSAT-prep.com for free chapter review Q&A and forum.

GOLD NOTES

EQUILIBRIUM
Chapter 4

Memorize	Understand	Not Required*
finitions and equations to solve que problems wton's First Law, inertia uations for momentum, impulse	* Solve torque, collision problems * Choosing an appropriate pivot point * Create vector diagrams * Elastic vs. inelastic vs. conservation of E. * Solve momentum problem, significant figures	* Advanced level college info * Complex torque or collision problems * Torque as a function of time * Machine torque

GAMSAT-Prep.com

Introduction

Equilibrium exists when a mass is at rest or moves with constant velocity. Translational (straight line) and rotational (turning) equilibria can be resolved using linear forces, torque forces, Newton's first law and inertia. Momentum is a vector that can be used to solve problems involving elastic (bouncy) or inelastic (sticky) collisions.

Additional Resources

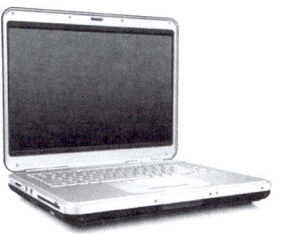

ee Online Q&A + Forum

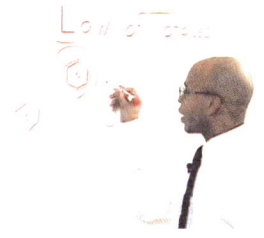

Video: Online or DVD

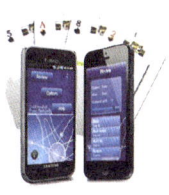

Flashcards

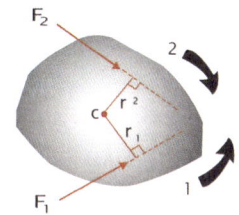

Special Guest

* The real GAMSAT may have advanced level information presented (ie. in a passage) but previous knowledge of said information is not required to answer the questions that would follow. Practice ACER and GS practice GAMSATs can help you clarify this point.

4.1 Translational, Rotational and Complex Motion

When a force acts upon an object, the object will undergo translational, rotational or complex (translational and rotational) motion.

Rotational motion of an object about an axis is the rotation of that object around that axis caused by perpendicular forces to that axis. The effective force causing rotation about an axis is the torque (L).

The torque is like a *turning force*. Consider a hinged door. If you were to apply a force F at the pivot point (*the hinge*), the door would not turn (L=0). If you apply the *same* force further and further from the pivot point, the turning force multiplies and the acceleration of the door increases. Thus the torque can be defined as the force applied multiplied by the perpendicular distance from the pivot point (= *lever or moment arm = r*).

$$L = (\text{force}) \times (\text{lever arm})$$

Thus according to Figure III.B.4.1:

$$L_1 = F_1 \times r_1 = \text{counterclockwise torque (1)} = \text{positive}$$

and

$$L_2 = F_2 \times r_2 = \text{clockwise torque (2)} = \text{negative.}$$

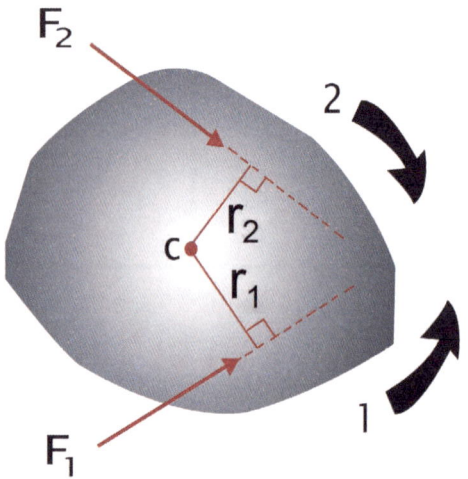

Figure III.B.4.1: Rotational Motion.

Positivity and negativity are arbitrary designations of the two opposite directions of motion. To determine the direction of rotation caused by the torque, imagine the direction the object would rotate if the force is pushing its moment arm at right angles. The net torques acting upon an object is obtained by summing the counterclockwise (+) and the clockwise (−) torques. An object is at equilibrium when the net forces and the net torques acting upon the object is zero. Thus, the object is either motionless or moving at a constant velocity due to its internal inertia.

The conditions of equilibrium are:

For translational equilibrium:

$$\Sigma F_x = 0 \text{ and } \Sigma F_y = 0$$

For rotational equilibrium:

$$\Sigma L = 0$$

In terms of translational equilibrium, the meaning of the equations can be summarized as: all upward forces equal all downward forces (y axis), all forces to the left equal all forces to the right (x axis), all forces towards you equals all forces away from you (z axis, $\sum F_z = 0$; the latter is possible, but not likely to be found as a GAMSAT question).

In terms of rotational equilibrium, if the torques sum to zero about one point in an object, they will sum to zero about any point in the object. If the point chosen as reference (= *pivot point or fulcrum*) includes the line of action of one of the forces, that force need not be included in calculating torques.

4.1.1 Torque Problem (SI units)

A 70 kg person sits 50 cm from the edge of a non-uniform plank which weighs 100 N and is 2.0 m long (*see Figure III.B.4.2*). The weight supported by point B is 250 N. Find the center of gravity (COG) of the plank.

{key: draw a vector diagram then choose an unknown value as the pivot point i.e. point A; see section 2.1 for a definition of COG}

(a)   (b)

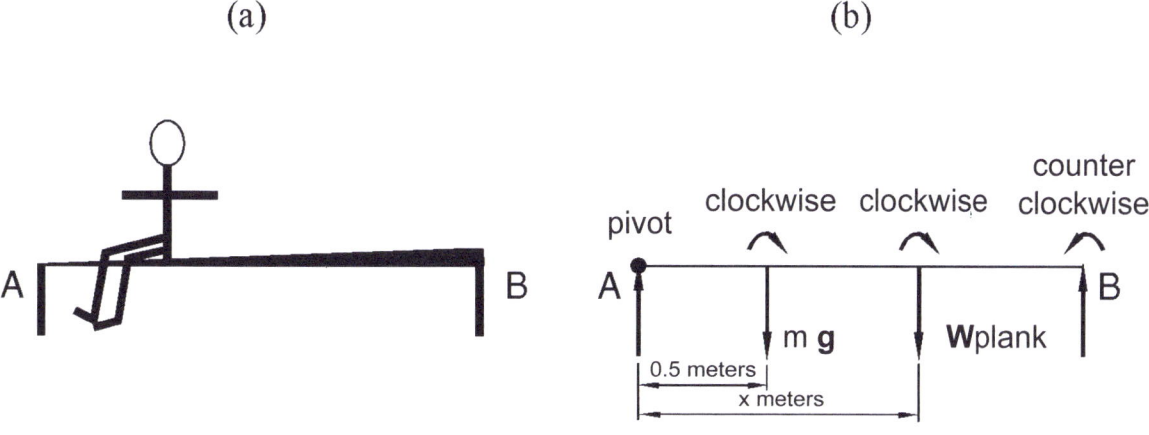

Figure III.B.4.2: Torque Problem.
(a) A person sitting on a non-uniform bench which is composed of a plank with two supports A and B. (b) Vector diagram with point A as the reference point. The torque force at point A is zero since its distance from itself is zero.

GAMSAT-Prep.com
THE GOLD STANDARD

The counterclockwise torque (CCW) is given by the force at point *B* multiplied by its distance from the reference point *A*:

$$CCW = F_B r_B = 250(2.0) = 500 \text{ Nm}$$

The clockwise torques (CW) are given by the force exerted by the person (= the weight *mg*) multiplied by the distance from the pivot point ($r = 50$ cm $= 0.5$ m) *and* the force exerted by the plank (= the weight) multiplied by the distance from the pivot point where the weight of the plank acts (= COG):

$$CW = mgr + W(COG)$$
$$= 70(10)0.5 + 100(COG)$$
$$= 350 + 100(COG)$$

Gravity was estimated as 10 m/s². Now we have:

$$\Sigma L = CCW - CW = 500 - 350 - 100(COG) = 0$$

Isolate COG

$$COG = 150/100 = 1.5 \text{ m from point } A.$$

- Note that had the plank been uniform its COG would be at its center which is 1.0 m from either end.

- Had the problem requested the weight supported at point *A*, it would be easy to determine since $\Sigma F_y = 0$. If we define upward forces as positive, we get:

$$\Sigma F_y = F_A + F_B - mg - W_{plank} = 0$$

Isolate F_A

$$F_A = 70(10) + 100 - 250 = 550 \text{ N}.$$

4.2 Newton's First Law

<u>Newton's First Law</u> states that objects in motion or at rest tend to remain as such unless acted upon by an outside force. That is, objects have inertia (resistance to motion). For translational motion, the mass (*m*) is a measure of inertia.

For rotational motion, a quantity derived from the mass called the moment of inertia (*I*) is the measure of inertia. In general $I = \Sigma mr^2$ where r is the distance from the axis of rotation. However, the exact formulation depends on the structure of the object.

PHY-28 EQUILIBRIUM

4.3 Momentum

The momentum (*M*) is a vector quantity. The momentum of an object is the product of its mass and its velocity.

$$M = m v$$

Linear momentum is a measure of the tendency of an object to maintain motion in a straight line. The greater the momentum (*M*), the greater the tendency of the object to remain moving along a straight line in the same direction. The momentum (*M*) is also a measure of the force needed to stop or change the direction of the object.

The impulse *I* is a measure of the change of the momentum of an object. It is the product of the force applied by the time during which the force was applied to change the momentum.

$$I = F \Delta t = \Delta M$$

where *F* is the acting force and Δt is the elapsed time during which the force was acting. The momentum is also conserved just like energy. The total linear momentum of a system is constant when the resultant external force acting on the system is zero.

4.4 Collisions

During motion, objects can collide. There are two kinds of collisions: *elastic* and *inelastic*. During an elastic collision (objects rebound off each other), there is a conservation of momentum and conservation of kinetic energy. Whereas, during an inelastic collision (objects stick together), there is conservation of momentum but not conservation of kinetic energy. Kinetic energy is lost as heat or sound, so total energy is conserved.

Examples of elastic collisions include 2 rubber balls colliding, particle collisions in ideal gases, and the slingshot type gravitational interactions between satellites and planets popularized in science fiction movies. Examples of inelastic collisions include 2 cars colliding at high speed becoming stuck together and a ballistic pendulum which can be a huge chunk of wood used to measure the speed of a moving object (i.e. bullet) which becomes completely embedded in the wood. If, however, the bullet were to emerge from the wood block, then it would be an elastic collision since the objects did not stick together.

Imagine two spheres with masses m_1 and m_2 and the velocity components before the collision v_{1i} and v_{2i} and after the collision v_{1f} and v_{2f}. If the momentum and the velocity are in the same directions, and we define that direction as positive, from the conservation of momentum we obtain:

$$m_1 v_{1i} + m_2 v_{2i} = m_1 v_{1f} + m_2 v_{2f} .$$

If the directions are not the same then each momentum must be resolved into x- and y-components as necessary.

- In the explosion of an object at rest, the total momentum of all the fragments must sum to zero because of the conservation of momentum and because the original momentum was zero.

- If one object collides with a second identical object that is at rest, there is a total trans-fer of kinetic energy, that is the first object comes to rest and the second object moves off with the momentum of the first one.

4.4.1 Collision Problem (CGS units)

A bullet of mass 10 g and a speed of 5.0×10^4 cm/s strikes a 700 g wooden block at rest on a very smooth surface. The bullet emerges with its speed reduced to 3.5×10^4 cm/s.

Find the resulting speed of the block. {CGS uses centimeters, grams, and seconds as units; the CGS unit of force is a dyne}.

Let m_1 = the mass of the bullet (10 g), v_{1i} = the speed of the bullet before the collision (5.0×10^4 cm/s), m_2 = the mass of the wooden block (700 g), v_{2i} = the speed of the block before the collision (0 cm/s), v_{1f} = the speed of the bullet after the collision (3.5×10^4 cm/s), and v_{2f} = the speed of the block after the collision (unknown), now we have:

$$m_1v_{1i} + m_2v_{2i} = m_1v_{1f} + m_2v_{2f}$$

Solving for v_{2f}

$$v_{2f} = (m_1v_{1i} - m_1v_{1f})/m_2$$
$$= (5.0 \times 10^5 - 3.5 \times 10^5)/(700)$$
$$= 2.1 \times 10^2 \text{ cm/s}.$$

- Note: the least precise figures that we are given in the problem contain at least two digits or <u>significant figures</u>. Thus our answer can not be more precise than two significant figures. The exponent 10^x is not considered when counting significant figures unless you are *told* that the measurement was more precise than is evident {For more on significant figures see GM 1.4.3, 1.5.2 and PHY 8.5.1}.

- Note: Sometimes, during the exam, you will want to convert to SI units (i.e. meters, kilograms, etc.; GM 2.1-2-3); however, depending on the answer choices and the nature of the equation or any constants, it may be faster to avoid any conversions. Experience with practice questions will enable you to decide efficiently.

Go online to GAMSAT-prep.com for free chapter review Q&A and forum.

NOTES

GOLD NOTES

WORK AND ENERGY
Chapter 5

Memorize	Understand	Not Required*
equation, units: work ons and units: potential energy ons and units: kinetic energy, power	* Path independence of work done in a g field * Work-Energy Theorem * Conservation of E.; conservative forces * Solving Conservation of E. problems	* Advanced level college info

GAMSAT-Prep.com

Introduction

Work and energy are used to describe how bodies or masses interact with the environment or other bodies or masses. Conservation of energy, work and power describe the forms of energy and the changes between these forms.

Additional Resources

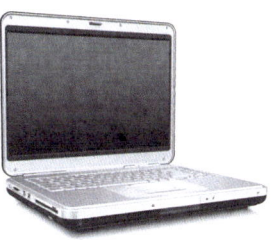

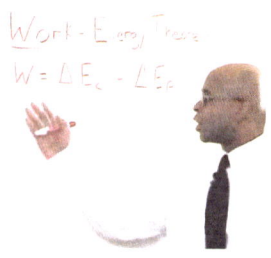

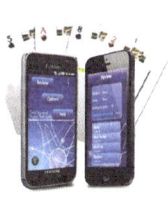

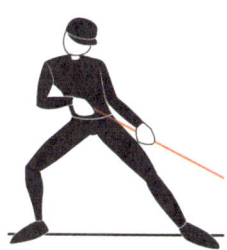

ee Online Q&A + Forum

Video: Online or DVD

Flashcards

Special Guest

* The real GAMSAT may have advanced level information presented (ie. in a passage) but previous knowledge of said information is not required to answer the questions that would follow. Practice ACER and GS practice GAMSATs can help you clarify this point.

5.1 Work

The work of a force *F* on an object is the product of the force by the distance travelled by the object where the force is in the direction of the displacement.

• *Units*: both work and energy are measured in joules where 1 *joule (J)* = 1 N × 1 m. {Imperial units: the *foot-pound*, CGS units: the *dyne-centimeter* or *erg*}

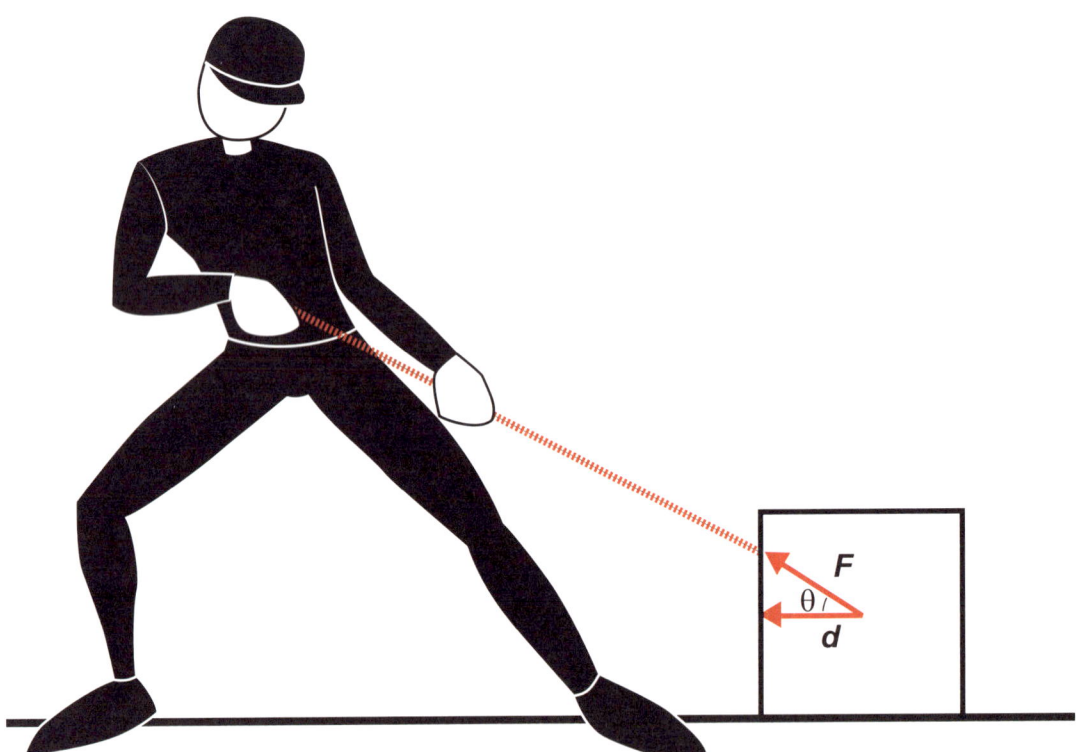

Figure III.B.5.1: Work. The displacement depends on the final and initial positions of the object. The angle θ is necessary to determine the component of a constant force F in the same direction of the displacement. Note that if F acts perpendicular to the displacement then the work $W = F\,d\,cos(90°) = 0$.

5.2 Energy

We usually speak of mechanical, electrical, chemical, potential, kinetic, sound, atomic and nuclear energy, to name a few. In fact, these different kinds of energy are different forms or manifestations of the same energy. Energy is a scalar. It is defined as a physical quantity capable of producing work.

5.3 Kinetic Energy

1) Definition of kinetic energy

Kinetic energy (E_k) is the energy of motion which can produce work. It is proportional to the mass of the object and its velocity:

$$E_k = 1/2\ mv^2.$$

2) The Work-Energy Theorem

A net force is the sum of interior and exterior forces acting upon the system. The variation of the kinetic energy of a system is equal to the work of the net force applied to the system:

$$W \text{ (of the resultant force)} = \Delta E_k.$$

Consequently, if the speed of a particle is constant, $\Delta E_k = 0$, then the work done by the resultant force must be zero. For example, in uniform circular motion the speed of the particle remains constant thus the centripetal force does no work on the particle. A force at right angles to the direction of motion merely changes the direction of the velocity but not its magnitude.

5.4 Potential Energy

Potential energy (E_p) is referred to as potential because it is accumulated by the system that contained it. It varies with the configuration of the system, i.e., when distances between particles of the system vary, the interactions between these particles vary. The variation of the potential energy is equal to the work performed by the interior forces caused by the interaction between the particles of the system. The following are examples of potential energy:

a) potential energy (= electric potential = E_p) derived from the Coulomb force (r is the distance between point charges q_1 and q_2, PHY 9.1.4):

$$E_p = k\ q_1 q_2 / r$$

b) potential energy derived from the universal attraction force (r is the distance between the COG of masses m_1 and m_2):

$$E_p = G\ m_1 m_2 / r$$

c) potential energy derived from the gravitational force (h is the height):

$$E_p = mgh$$

d) potential energy derived from the elastic force (i.e. a compressed spring):

$$E_p = kx^2/2.$$

{k = the spring constant, x = displacement, cf. PHY 7.2.1}

5.5 Conservation of Energy

a) *Definition*

The mechanical energy (E_T) of a system is equal to the sum of its kinetic energy and its potential energy:

$$E_T = E_k + E_p.$$

b) *Theorem of mechanical energy*

The variation of the mechanical energy of a system is equal to the work of exterior forces acting on the system.

c) *Consequence*

An isolated system, i.e., which is not being acted upon by any exterior force, keeps a constant mechanical energy. The kinetic energy and the potential energy may vary separately but their sum remains constant. This makes conservation of energy a very simple way to solve many different types of physics problems.

5.5.1 Conservation of Energy Problem (SI units)

A 6.8×10^3 kg frictionless roller coaster car starts at rest 30 meters above ground level. Determine the speed of the car at (a) 20 m above ground level; (b) at ground level.

$$E_T = E_k + E_p = 1/2 mv^2 + mgh$$

Initially $v = 0$ since the car starts at rest, $h = 30$ m, and the constant $g \approx 10$ m/s², thus

$$E_T = 0 + m(10)(30) = 300m \text{ joules.}$$

Situation (a) where $h = 20$ m:

$$E_T = 300m = 1/2 mv^2 + mgh$$

m cancels, multiply through by 2, solve for v:

$$v = \sqrt{2(300) - 2(10)20} = \sqrt{2(100)}$$
$$= \sqrt{2(10)} = 14 \text{ m/s}$$

Situation (b) at ground level $h = 0$:

$$E_T = 300m = 1/2 mv^2 + 0$$

m cancels, multiply through by 2, solve for v:

$$v = \sqrt{600} = \sqrt{6(100)} = 10\sqrt{6} = 24 \text{ m/s}$$

- Note: the mass of the roller coaster is irrelevant!
- Note: you must be able to quickly estimate square roots (PHY 1.1.2, 2.6.1).

5.6 Conservative Forces

The three definitions of a conservative force are: i) after a round trip the kinetic energy of a particle on which a force acts must return to its initial value; ii) after a round trip the work done on a particle by a force must be zero; iii) the work done by the force on a particle depends on the initial and final positions of the particle and not on the path taken.

Examples: Friction disobeys all three of the preceding criteria thus it is a non-conservative force. The force $F_s = -kx$ (Hooke's Law, PHY 7.2.1) of an ideal spring on a frictionless surface is a conservative force. Gravity is a conservative force. If you throw a ball vertically upward, it will return with the same kinetic energy it had when it left your hand (*neglect air resistance*).

5.7 Power

The power P applied during the work W performed by a force F is equal to the work divided by the time necessary to do the work. In other words, power is the rate of doing work:

$$P = \Delta W / \Delta t.$$

- The SI unit for power is the *watt* (W) which equals one *joule per second* (J/s).

- Power can also be expressed as the product of a force on an object and the object's velocity: $P = Fv.$

Go online to GAMSAT-prep.com for free chapter review Q&A and forum.

GOLD NOTES

FLUIDS AND SOLIDS
Chapter 6

Memorize	Understand	Not Required*
uation: density nsity of water uations for pressure, ssure change	* Buoyancy force, SG and height immersed * Streamline, turbulent flow; continuity/ Bernouilli's equation * Fluid viscosity, Archimedes' principle, surface tension; vapor press., atmospheric press. * Elastic properties of solids; effect of temperature	* Advanced level college info * Memorizing all the equations for solids * Memorizing equations: Continuity, hydrostatic pressure, Bernouilli's

GAMSAT-Prep.com

Introduction

A fluid is a substance that flows (*deforms*) under shear stress. This includes all gases and liquids. It is important to understand the properties without movement (hydrostatic pressure, Archimedes' principle) and with movement (continuity, Bernoulli's). On the other hand, a solid *resists* being deformed or submitting to changes in volume. A basic understanding of this *elastic* property of solids is required.

Additional Resources

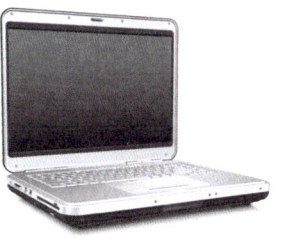

Free Online Q&A + Forum

Video: Online or DVD

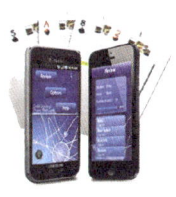

Flashcards

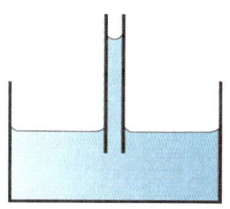

Special Guest

THE PHYSICAL SCIENCES PHY-39

* The real GAMSAT may have advanced level information presented (ie. in a passage) but previous knowledge of said information is not required to answer the questions that would follow. Practice ACER and GS practice GAMSATs can help you clarify this point.

6.1 Fluids

6.1.1 Density, Specific Gravity

The *density* of an object is defined as the ratio of its mass to its volume.

$$\text{density} = \text{mass} / \text{volume}$$

This definition holds for solids, fluids and gases. From the definition, it is easy to see that solids are more dense than liquids which are in turn more dense than gases. This is true because for a given mass, the average distance between molecules of a given substance is bigger in the liquid state than in the solid state. Put simply, the substance occupies a bigger volume in the liquid state than in the solid state and a much bigger volume in gaseous state than in the liquid state.

At a given temperature, the *specific gravity* (SG) is defined as:

$$SG = \frac{\text{density of a substance}}{\text{density of water}}$$

The density of water is about 1 g/ml (= 1 g/cm^3 = 10^3 kg/m^3) over most common temperatures. So in most instances the specific gravity of a substance is the same as its density.

Note that the dimension of density is mass per unit volume, whereas the specific gravity is dimensionless. Density is one of the key properties of fluids (liquids or gases) and the other is pressure.

6.1.2 Hydrostatic Pressure, Buoyancy, Archimedes' Principle

Pressure (P) is defined as the force (F) per unit area (A):

$$P = F/A.$$

The force F is the normal (*perpendicular*) force to the area. The SI unit for pressure is the *pascal* (1 Pa = 1 N/m^2). Other units are: 1.00 atm = 1.01 × 10^5 Pa = 1.01 bar = 760 mmHg = 760 torr = 14.7 lb/in^2.

Pressure is also formulated as potential energy per unit volume as follows:

$$P = \frac{F}{A} = \frac{mg}{A} = \frac{(mg/A)}{(h/h)} = \frac{mgh}{V} = \rho g h$$

ρ = density and h = depth below surface; if the depth is changing we can write:

$$\Delta P = \rho g \Delta h.$$

We will now examine 6 key rules of incompressible fluids (liquids) that are not moving (*statics*).

1) In a fluid confined by solid boundaries, pressure acts perpendicular to the boundary – it is a <u>normal force</u>, sometimes called a *surface force*.

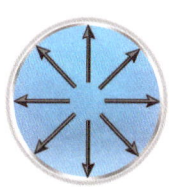
pipe or tube

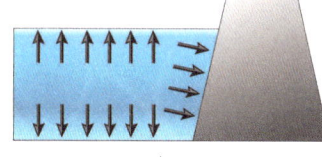
dam

2) At any particular depth, the pressure of the fluid is the same in all directions.

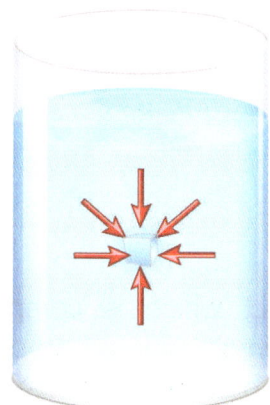

3) The fluid or *hydrostatic pressure* depends on the density and the depth of the fluid. So it is easy to calculate the change in pressure in an open container, swimming pool, the ocean, etc.:

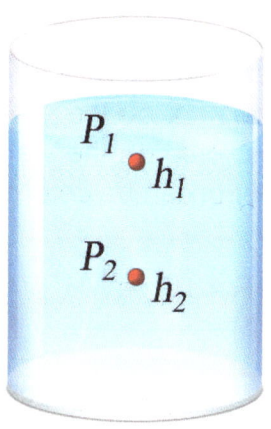

P_1 = atmospheric pressure
h_1 = surface = a depth of 0
$P_2 - P_1 = \Delta P$
$h_2 - h_1 = \Delta h$

$\Delta P = \rho g \Delta h$

Vertical plane surfaces

We can now combine rules 1, 2 and 3 about fluids to examine a special case which is that of a vertical plane surface like a vertical wall that is underwater.

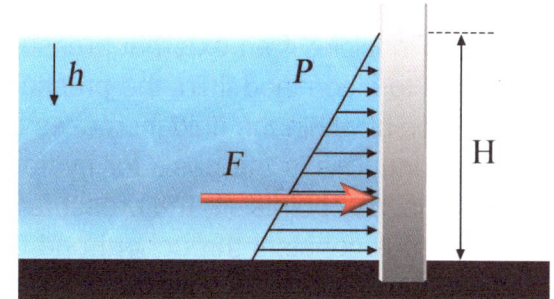

Of course pressure varies linearly with depth because $\Delta P = \rho g \Delta h$.

GAMSAT-Prep.com
THE GOLD STANDARD

If the height of the vertical rectangular wall is H and the width W, with the help of calculus (which is *not* on the GAMSAT!), the equation for the force on the wall, or vertical plane, at any depth can be determined to be:

$$F = 1/2 \, \rho g W H^2$$

4) The size or shape of a container does not influence the pressure (= *hydrostatic paradox*). Note that the pressure is the same at the bottom of all 3 containers because the height h and fluid density are the same.

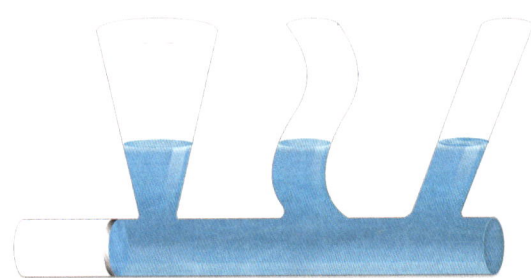

Hydraulic systems, like the brakes in a car, can multiply the force applied. For example, if a 50 N force is applied by the left piston in the diagram and if the right piston has an area five times greater, then the force out at F_2 is 250 N (thus the force vector F_2 is 5 times longer).

$$F_2 = A_2(F_1/A_1) = 5A_1(F_1/A_1) = 5(F_1)$$

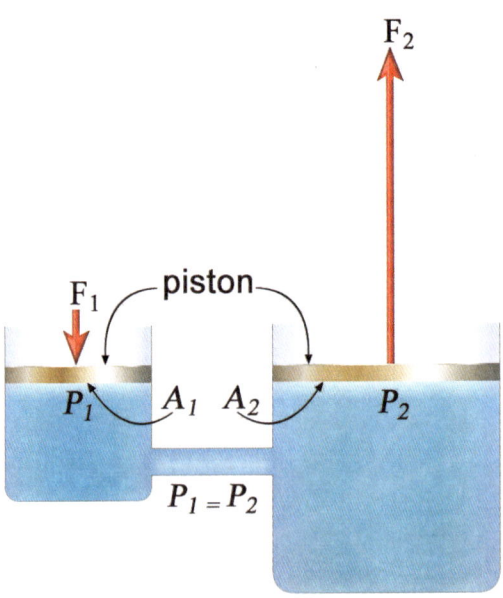

5) Pascal's Principle: If an external pressure is applied to a confined fluid, the pressure at every point within the fluid increases by that amount. This is the basis for hydraulic systems. Key points: (1) the pressure of the system is constant throughout and (2) by definition, P = F/A, so we get:

$$F_1/A_1 = F_2/A_2$$

6) An object which is completely or partially submerged in a fluid experiences an upward force equal to the weight of the fluid displaced (*Archimedes' principle*).

This buoyant force F_b is :

$$F_b = V\rho g = mg$$

PHY-42 FLUIDS AND SOLIDS

where ρ is the density of the fluid displaced. An object that floats must displace at most its own weight.

Archimedes' principle can be used to calculate specific gravity. And in turn, specific gravity is equivalent to the fraction of the height of a buoyant object below the surface of the fluid. Thus if SG = 0.90, then 90% of the height of the object would be immersed in water. Therefore, less dense objects float.

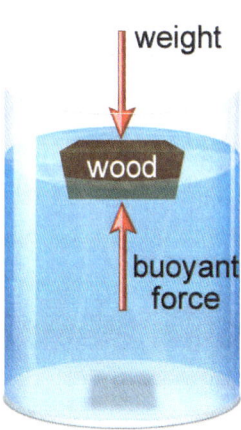

6.1.2.1 Atmospheric Pressure

Atmospheric pressure is the force per unit area exerted against a surface by the weight of the air above that surface. If the number of air molecules above a surface increases, there are more molecules to exert a force on that surface and thus, the pressure increases. On the other hand, a reduction in the number of air molecules above a surface will result in a decrease in pressure. Atmospheric pressure is measured with a "barometer", which is why atmospheric pressure is also referred to as *barometric* pressure.

Atmospheric pressure is often measured with a mercury (Hg) barometer, and a height of approximately 760 millimeters (30 in) of mercury represents atmospheric pressure at sea level (760 mmHg).

Unit	Definition or Relationship
SI Unit: 1 pascal (Pa)	1 kg m^{-1} s^{-2} = 1 N/m^2
1 bar	1 x 10^5 Pa
1 atmosphere (atm)	101,325 Pa = 101.3 kPa
1 torr	1 / 760 atm
760 mmHg	1 atm
14.7 pounds per sq. in. (psi)	1 atm

Units of Pressure

GAMSAT-Prep.com
THE GOLD STANDARD

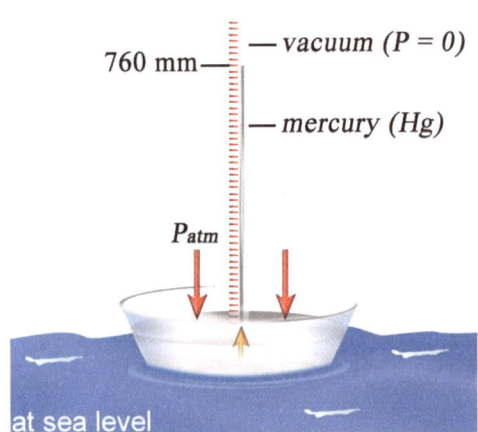

When the altitude or elevation increases, we get closer to "outer space" so there is less overlying atmospheric mass from gases, so that pressure decreases with increasing elevation.

Figure III.B.6.0: Atmospheric pressure decreases with elevation. Mount Everest is about 8,800 meters (m) and a 747 can cruise at an altitude of 10,000 m but requires increased cabin pressure to prevent passengers from having altitude sickness and low oxygen (hypoxia).

6.1.2.2 Gauge Pressure

When you measure the pressure in your tires, you are measuring the pressure difference between the tires and atmospheric pressure, which is the *gauge* (or *gage*) pressure.

Absolute pressure is the pressure of a fluid relative to the pressure in a vacuum. The absolute pressure is then the sum of the gauge pressure, which is what you measure, and the atmospheric pressure.

$$P_{abs} = P_{atm} + P_{gauge}$$

Pressure can be measured in devices in which one or more columns of a liquid (i.e. mercury or water) are used to determine the pressure difference between two points (i.e. U-tube manometer, inclined-tube manometer). Of course, electronic instruments for measurement are used more frequently.

PHY-44 FLUIDS AND SOLIDS

6.1.3 Fluids in Motion, Continuity Equation, Bernoulli's Equation

Fluids in motion are described by two equations, the continuity equation and Bernoulli's equation. Fluids are assumed to have <u>streamline</u> (= *laminar*) flow which means that the motion of every particle in the fluid follows the same path as the particle that preceded it. <u>Turbulent</u> flow occurs when that definition cannot be applied, resulting in molecular collisions, irregularly shaped whirlpools, energy is then dissipated and frictional drag is increased. The rate (R) of streamline flow is given by:

$$R = \text{(volume past a point)}/\text{time} = Avt/t = Av$$

volume = (cross-sectional area) (length) = (A) (vt) = Avt

length = distance = (velocity) (time) = vt

cross-sectional area of a tube = ==area of a circle== = πr^2 where π can be estimated as 3.14 and *r* is the radius of the circle.

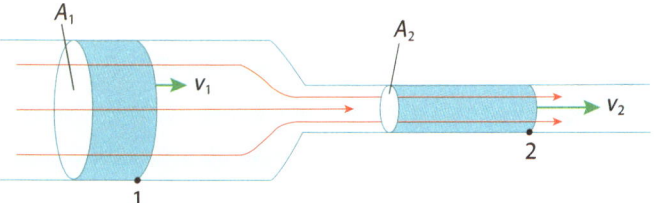

Figure III.B.6.0.1 Application of the continuity equation. When a tube narrows, the same volume occupies a greater length. For the same volume to pass points 1 and 2 in a given time, the speed must be greater at point 2.

- The equation can also be written as the **continuity equation**:

$$A_1v_1 = A_2v_2 = \text{constant}$$

where subscripts 1 and 2 refer to different points in the line of flow. The continuity equation can be used for an incompressible fluid flowing in an enclosed tube. For a compressible fluid:

$$\rho_1 A_1 v_1 = \rho_2 A_2 v_2 = \text{constant}$$

- **Bernoulli's equation** is an application of the law of conservation of energy and is:

$$P + \rho g h + 1/2\, \rho v^2 = \text{constant}$$

It follows:

$$P_1 + \rho g h_1 + 1/2\, \rho v_1^2 = P_2 + \rho g h_2 + 1/2\, \rho v_2^2$$

where subscripts 1 and 2 refer to different points in the flow.

A commonly encountered consequence of Bernoulli's equation is that where the height is relatively constant and the velocity of a fluid is high, the pressure is low, and vice versa.

{Various applications of the preceding equations will be explored in GS-1, the first practice test!}

6.1.4 Fluid Viscosity and Determining Turbulence

Viscosity is analogous to friction between moving solids. It may, therefore be viewed as the resistance to flow of layers of fluid (as in streamline or laminar flow) past each other. This also means that viscosity, as in friction, results in dissipation of mechanical energy. As one layer flows over another, its motion is transmitted to the second layer and causes this layer to be set in motion. Since a mass m of the second layer is set in motion and some of the energy of the first layer is lost, there is a transfer of momentum between the layers.

The greater the transfer of this momentum from one layer to another, the more energy that is lost and the slower the layers move.

The viscosity (η) is the measure of the efficiency of transfer of this momentum. Therefore the higher the viscosity coefficient, the greater the transfer of momentum and loss of mechanical energy, and thus loss of velocity. The reverse situation holds for a low viscosity coefficient.

Consequently, a high viscosity coefficient substance flows slowly (e.g. molasses), and a low viscosity coefficient substance flows relatively fast (e.g. water or, especially helium). Note that the transfer of momentum to adjacent layers is in essence, the exertion of a force upon these layers to set them in motion.

Whether flow is streamline or turbulent depends on a combination of factors already discussed. A convenient measure is Reynolds Number (R):

$$R = vd\rho / \eta$$

v = velocity of flow
d = diameter of the tube
ρ = density of the fluid
η = viscosity coefficient

In general, if R < 2000 the flow is streamline; if R > 2000 the flow is turbulent. Note that as v, d or ρ increases or η decreases, the flow becomes more turbulent.

6.1.5 Surface Tension

Molecules of a liquid exert attractive forces toward each other (cohesive forces), and exert attractive forces toward the surface they touch (adhesive forces). If a liquid is in a gravity free space without a surface, it will form a sphere (smallest area relative to volume).

If the liquid is lining an object, the liquid surface will contract (due to cohesive forces) to the lowest possible surface area. The forces between the molecules on this surface will create a membrane-like effect. Due to the contraction, a potential energy (PE) will present in the surface.

This PE is directly proportional to the surface area (A). An exact relation is formed as follows:

$$PE = \gamma A$$

γ = surface tension = PE/A = joules/m²

An alternative formulation for the surface tension (γ) is:

$$\gamma = F/l$$

F = force of contraction of surface
l = length along surface

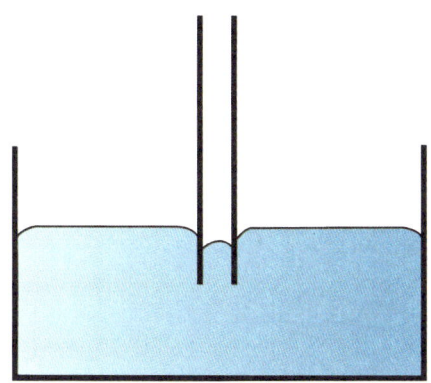

(a) cohesive > adhesive

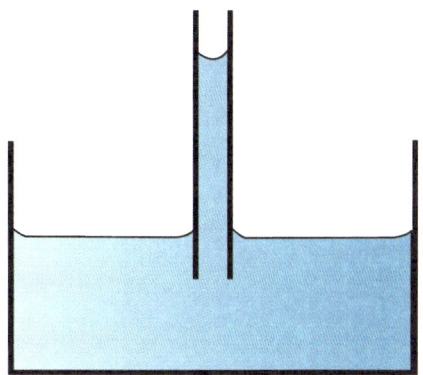

(b) adhesive > cohesive

Figure III.B.6.1: Effects of adhesive and cohesive forces. The distance the liquid rises or falls in the tube is directly proportional to the surface tension γ and inversely proportional to the liquid density and radius of the tube. Examples of 2 liquids consistent with the illustrations include: (a) mercury; (b) water.

Because of the contraction, a small object which would ordinarily sink in the liquid may float on the surface membrane. For example, a small insect like a "water strider."

The liquid will rise or fall on a wall or in a capillary tube if the adhesive forces are greater than cohesive or vice versa (see Figure III.B.6.1).

6.2 Solids

6.2.1 Elastic Properties of Solids

When a force acts on a solid, the solid is deformed. If the solid returns to its original shape, the solid is elastic. The effect of a force depends on the area over which it acts. Stress is defined as the ratio of the force to the area over which it acts. Strain is defined as the relative change in dimensions or shape of the object caused by the stress. This is embodied in the definition of the modulus of elasticity (ME) as:

$$ME = \frac{stress}{strain}$$

Some different types of stresses are tensile stress (equal and opposite forces directed away from each other), compressive stress (equal and opposite forces directed towards each other), and shearing stress (equal and opposite forces which do not have the same line of action). There are two commonly used moduli of elasticity:

1) Young's Modulus (Y) for compressive or tensile stress:

$$Y = \frac{longitudinal\ stress}{longitudinal\ strain}$$

$$Y = \frac{(F/A)}{(\Delta l/l)} = \frac{F \times l}{A \Delta l}$$

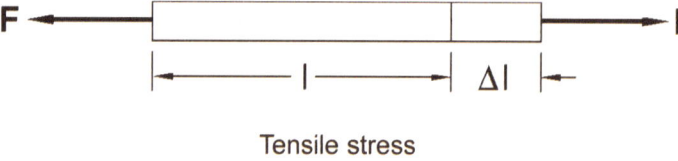

Tensile stress

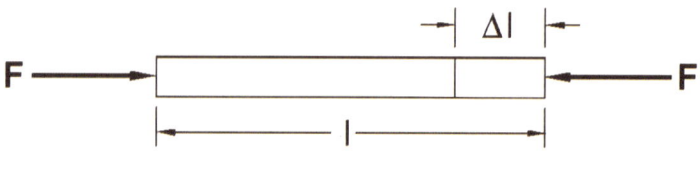

Compressive stress

Figure III.B.6.2: Compressive and Tensile Stress.

2) Shear modulus (S) or the modulus of rigidity is:

S = shearing stress / shearing strain

$$S = (F/A) / \tan \phi$$

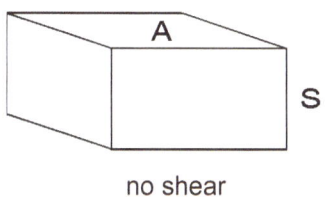
no shear

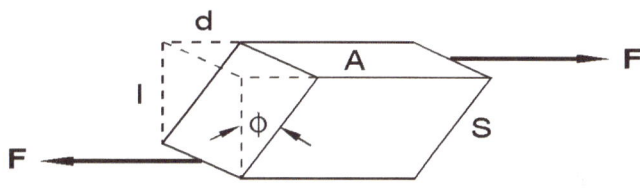

Figure III.B.6.3: Shear Stress. A is the area tangential to the force F.

6.3 The Effect of Temperature on Solids and Liquids

When substances gain or lose heat they usually undergo expansion or contraction.

Expansion or contraction can be by linear dimension, by area or by volume.

Table III.B.6.1: Substance thermal expansion.

Type	Final	Original	Change caused by heat
(1) Linear	L $L = L_0 + \alpha \Delta T L_0$ $L = L_0(1 + \alpha \Delta T)$ α = coefficient of linear thermal expansion ΔT = change in temperature	L_0	$\alpha \Delta T L_0$
(2) Area	A $A = A_0 + \gamma \Delta T A_0$ $A = A_0(1 + \gamma \Delta T)$ γ = coefficient of area thermal expansion = 2α	A_0	$\gamma \Delta T A_0$
(3) Volume	V $V = V_0 + \beta \Delta T V_0$ $V = V_0(1 + \beta \Delta T)$ β = coefficient of volume thermal expansion = 3α	V_0	$\beta \Delta T V_0$

Go online to GAMSAT-prep.com for free chapter review Q&A and forum.

GOLD NOTES

WAVE CHARACTERISTICS AND PERIODIC MOTION
Chapter 7

Memorize	Understand	Not Required*
avelength, frequency, velocity, e ntensity, constructive/destructive ice, beat freq. : relating velocity to frequency, th : Hooke's Law, work (periodic motion)	* SHM, transverse vs. longitudinal waves, phase * Resonance, nodes, antinodes, pipes (standing waves) * Harmonics, overtones * Periodic motion: force, accel., vel., diplace., period * The simple pendulum, theory and calculations	* Advanced level college info * Memorizing displacement/elementary vibration equations * Memorizing equation for harmonics, simple pendulum

Introduction

Wave characteristics and periodic motion describe the motion of systems that vibrate. Topics include transverse and longitudinal waves, interference, resonance, Hooke's law and simple harmonic motion (SHM). Some basic equations must be memorized but for most of the material, you must seek a comfortable understanding.

Additional Resources

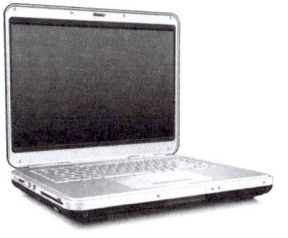

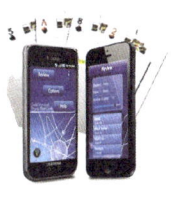

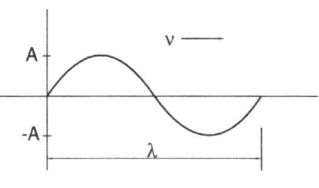

ree Online Q&A + Forum   Video: Online or DVD   Flashcards   Special Guest

THE PHYSICAL SCIENCES   PHY-51

* The real GAMSAT may have advanced level information presented (ie. in a passage) but previous knowledge of said information is not required to answer the questions that would follow. Practice ACER and GS practice GAMSATs can help you clarify this point.

7.1 Wave Characteristics

7.1.1 Transverse and Longitudinal Motion

A wave is a disturbance in a medium such that each particle in the medium vibrates about an equilibrium point in a simple harmonic (*periodic*) motion. If the direction of vibration is perpendicular to the direction of propagation of the wave, it is called a transverse wave (e.g. light or an oscillating string under tension).

If the direction of vibration is in the same direction as the propagation of the wave, it is called a longitudinal wave (e.g. sound). Longitudinal waves are characterized by condensations (regions of crowding of particles) and rarefactions (regions where particles are far apart) along the wave in the medium.

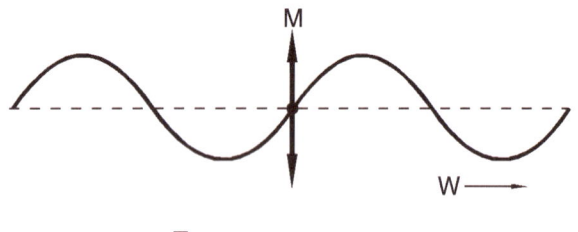

Transverse wave

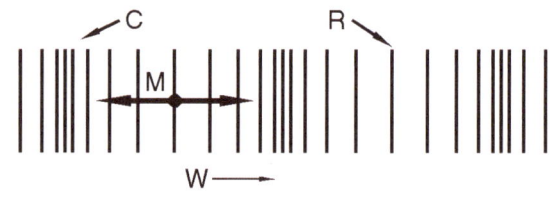

Longitudinal wave

Figure III.B.7.1: Transverse and longitudinal waves. W = wave propagation, R = rarefaction, C = condensation, M = motion of particle.

7.1.2 Wavelength, Frequency, Velocity, Amplitude, Intensity

The wavelength (λ) is the distance from crest to crest (or valley to valley) of a transverse wave. It may also be defined as the distance between two particles with the same displacement and direction of displacement. In a longitudinal wave, the wavelength is the distance from one rarefaction (or condensation) to another. The *amplitude* (A) is the maximum displacement of a particle in one direction from its equilibrium point. The *intensity* (I) of a wave is the square of the amplitude.

Frequency (f) is the number of cycles per unit time (per second = s^{-1} = hertz = Hz = SI unit). Period (T) is the duration of one cycle, it is the inverse of the frequency. *The velocity* (v) of a wave is the velocity of the propagation of the disturbance that forms the wave through the medium.

The velocity is inversely proportional to the inertia of the medium. The velocity can be calculated according to the following important equation:

$$v = \lambda f$$

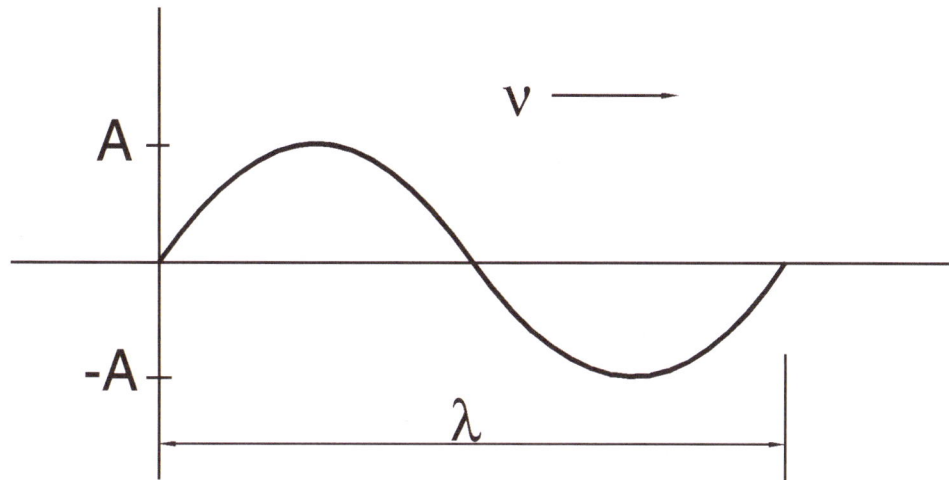

Figure III.B.7.2: Characteristics of waves.

7.1.3 Superposition of Waves, Phase, Interference, Addition

The superposition principle states that the effect of two or more waves on the displacement of a particle is independent. The final displacement of the particle is the resultant effect of all the waves added algebraically, thus the amplitude may increase or decrease. The *phase* of a particle under vibration is its displacement at the time of origin (t=0). The displacement can be calculated as follows:

$$x = A\sin(\omega t + \varphi)$$

where x is the displacement, A is the amplitude, ω is the angular velocity, t is the time, and φ is the phase.

Interference is the summation of the displacements of different waves in a medium. Certain criteria must first be established:

- *synchrony sources*: vibrations emitted by synchrony sources have the same phase.
- *coherent vibrations*: the phases of the vibrations are related, this means that the duration of the light impressions on the retina is much longer than the duration of a wave train between two emissions.
- *parallel vibrations*: the displacements of parallel vibrations keep parallel directions in space.

• *interference conditions*: two or more vibrations can interfere only when the are coherent, parallel and have the same period.

• *beat frequency*: the difference in frequency of two waves creates a new frequency (*see* Beats, PHY 8.4).

Given an elementary vibration $S_i = A_i \sin(w_t + \varphi_i)$ the composition of n vibrations that interfere is given by:

$S_1 + S_2 + S_3 + ... + S_n = a_1\sin(wt+\varphi_1) + a_2\sin(wt+\varphi_2) + ... + a_n\sin(wt+\varphi_n) = A\sin(wt+\Phi)$

where A is the resultant amplitude and Φ the resultant phase. Constructive interference (*see Figure III.B.7.4*) is when the waves add to a larger resultant wave than either original. This occurs maximally when the phase difference φ is a whole wavelength λ which corresponds to multiples of π.

This occurs at $\varphi = 0$, 2π, 4π, etc. Since $\varphi = 2\pi\Delta L/\lambda$, where ΔL equals the difference in path to a point of two waves of equal wavelength, these waves interfere constructively when $\Delta L = 0$, λ, 2λ, 3λ, *etc.* See Figure III.B.7.3 for the definition of ΔL.

Destructive interference (*see Figure III.B.7.5*) is when the waves add to a smaller resultant wave than either original wave. This occurs maximally when $\varphi = \pi$, 3π, 5π, *etc.*, which are multiples of one-half of a wavelength where $180° = \pi$ which corresponds to ½λ. This occurs when $\Delta L = \lambda/2$, $3\lambda/2$, $5\lambda/2$, etc.

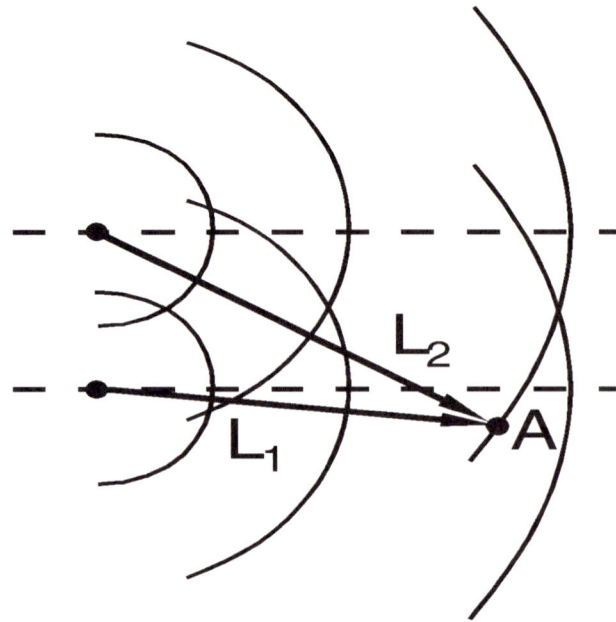

Figure III.B.7.3: Schematic for ΔL.
L_1 and L_2 are distances from the origins of the waves to point A. Thus $\Delta L = |L_2 - L_1|$ (absolute value).

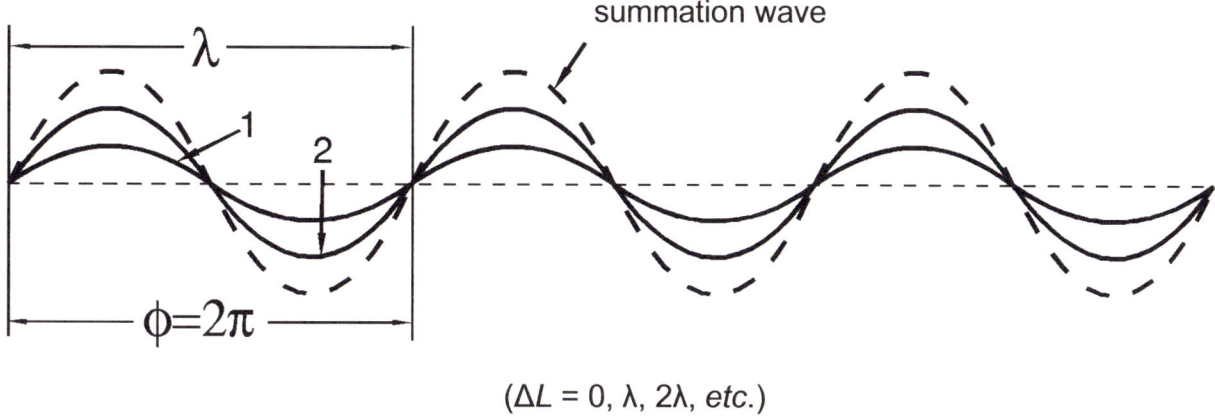

($\Delta L = 0, \lambda, 2\lambda, etc.$)

Figure III.B.7.4: Maximal constructive interference. Waves (1) and (2) begin at the points shown, have the same λ but different amplitudes. The summation wave is maximal (i.e. highest amplitude but same wavelength) since ΔL = λ *in this example.*

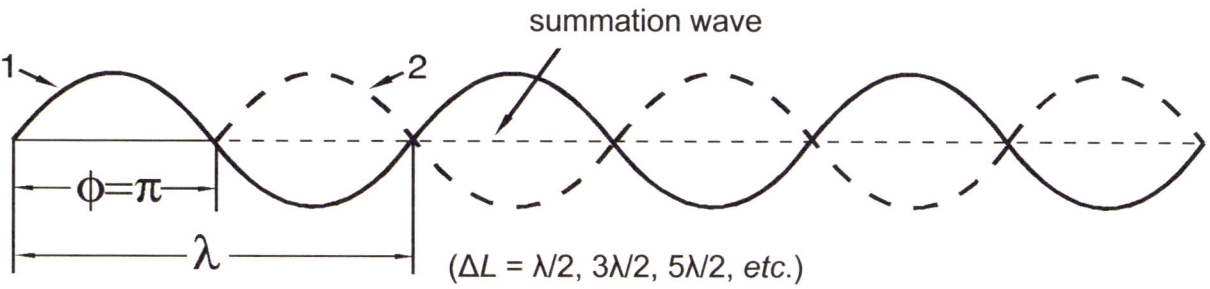

($\Delta L = \lambda/2, 3\lambda/2, 5\lambda/2, etc.$)

Figure III.B.7.5: Maximal destructive interference.

GAMSAT-Prep.com
THE GOLD STANDARD

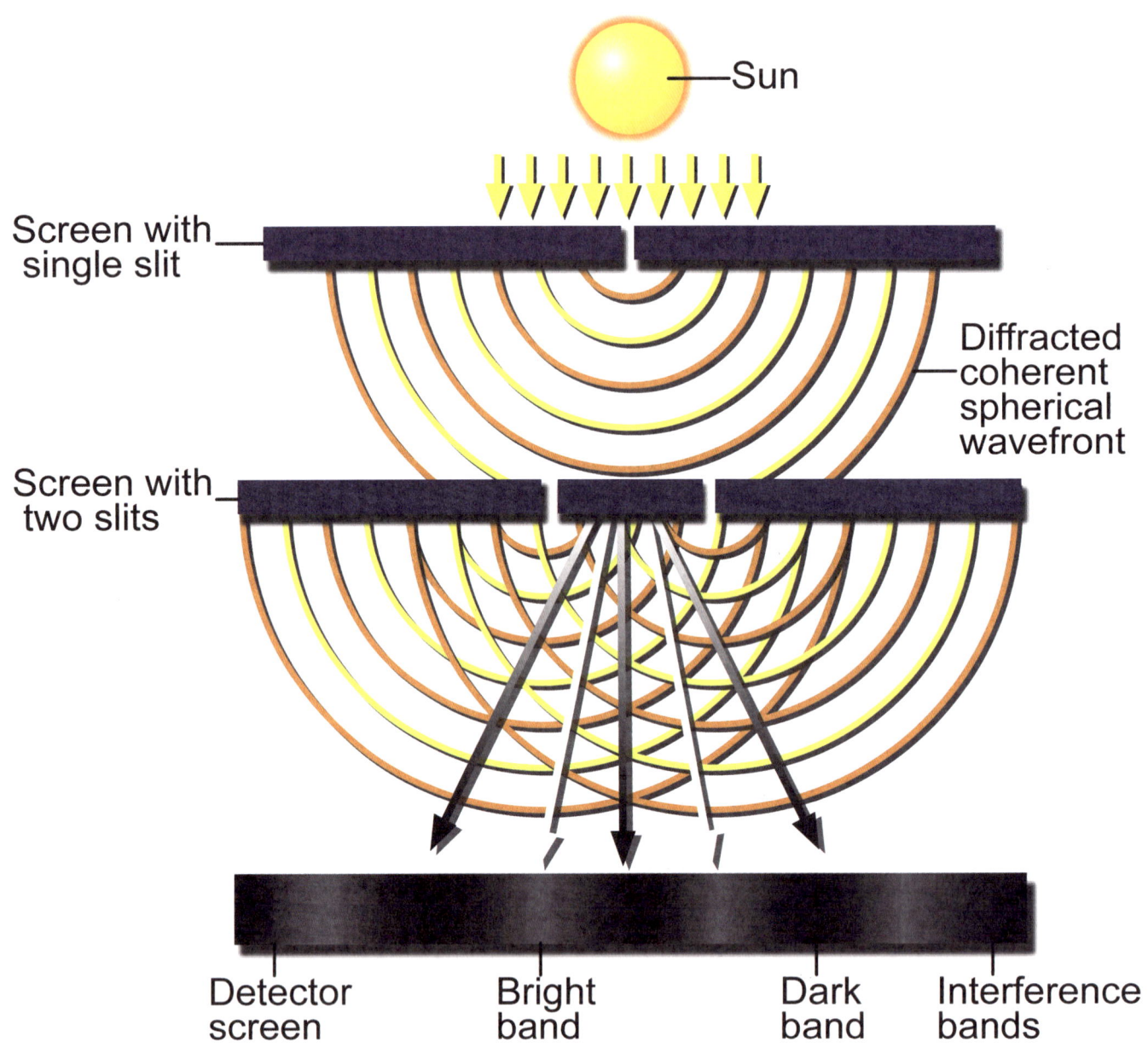

Figure III.B.7.5.1: Thomas Young's Double Slit Experiment Young's experiment demonstrates both the wave and particle natures of light. A coherent light source illuminates a thin plate with two parallel slits cut in it, and the light passing through the slits strikes a screen behind them. The wave nature of light causes the light waves passing through both slits to interfere, creating an interference pattern of bright and dark bands on the screen. However, at the screen, the light is always found to be absorbed as though it were made of discrete particles (photons). The double slit experiment can also be performed (using different apparatus) with particles of matter such as electrons with the same results. Again, this provides an additional circumstance demonstrating particle-wave duality. Diffraction is the apparent bending of a wave around a small obstacle. We see diffracted light waves through each of the slits above.

7.1.4 Resonance

Forced vibrations occur when a series of waves impinge upon an object and cause it to vibrate. Natural frequencies are the intrinsic frequencies of vibration of a system. If the forced vibration causes the object to vibrate at one of its natural frequencies, the body will vibrate at maximal amplitude. This phenomenon is called *resonance*. Since energy and power are proportional to the amplitude squared, they also are at their maximum.

7.1.5 Standing Waves, Pipes and Strings

Standing waves result when waves are reflected off a stationary object back into the oncoming waves of the medium and superposition results. *Nodes* are points where there is no particle displacement, which are similar to points of maximal destructive interference.

Nodes occur at fixed end points (points that cannot vibrate). Antinodes are points that undergo maximal displacements and are similar to points of maximal constructive interference. Antinodes occur at open or free end points (*see Figure III.B.7.6*).

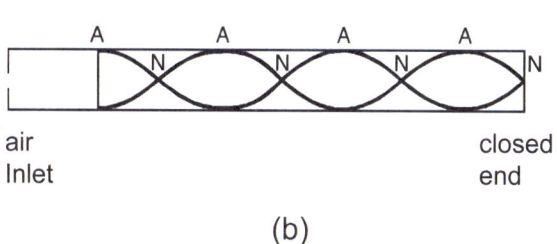

Figure III.B.7.6: Standing waves.
(a) <u>String</u>: Standing waves produced by an experimenter wiggling a string or rubber tube at point X towards a fixed point Y at the correct frequency. (b) <u>Pipe</u>: Standing wave produced in a pipe with a closed end point i.e. in a closed organ pipe where sound originates in a vibrating air column (A = antinode and N = node).

7.1.6 Harmonics

Consider a violin. A string is fixed at both ends and is bowed, transverse vibrations travel along the string; these disturbances are reflected at both ends producing a standing wave. The vibrations of the string give rise to longitudinal vibrations in the air which transmits the sound to our ears.

A string of length *l*, fixed at both ends, can resonate at frequencies *f* given by:

$$f_n = nv/(2l)$$

where the velocity *v* is the same for all frequencies and the number of antinodes $n = 1, 2, 3, ...$

The lowest frequency, $f_1 = v/(2l)$, is the *fundamental* frequency, and the others are called *overtones*. The fundamental is the first *harmonic*, the second harmonic $2f_1$ is the first overtone, the third harmonic $3f_1$ is the second overtone, etc. Overtones whose frequencies are integral multiples of the fundamental are called *harmonic series*.

7.2 Periodic Motion

7.2.1 Hooke's Law

The particles that are undergoing displacement when a wave passes through a medium undergo motion called simple harmonic motion (SHM) and are acted upon by a force described by Hooke's Law. SHM is caused by an inconstant force (called a *restoring force*) and as a result has an inconstant acceleration. The force is proportional to the displacement (*distance from the equilibrium point*) but opposite in direction,

$$F = -kx \text{ (Hooke's Law)}$$

where *k* = the spring constant, *x* = displacement from the equilibrium. The work *W* can be determined according to $W = \frac{1}{2}kx^2$.

Notice that the equation for the work done by the spring is identical to the potential energy of a spring (PHY 5.4). This is because when an external force stretches the spring, this work is stored in the force field, which is said to be stored as potential energy. If the external force is removed, the force field acts on the body to perform the work as it moves the body back to the initial position, reducing the stretch of the spring. For example, an archer applies human force over a distance (= work; PHY 5.1) to pull an arrow back in the bow, elastic potential energy is now stored in the stretched bow, when the arrow leaves the bow, the potential energy turns into kinetic energy.

Examples of objects that have elastic potential energy include stretched or compressed elastic bands, springs, bungee cords, shock absorbers (cars, trucks, bicycles), trampolines, etc.

The work done in compressing or stretching a spring can be determined by taking the area under a Force vs. Displacement graph for the spring.

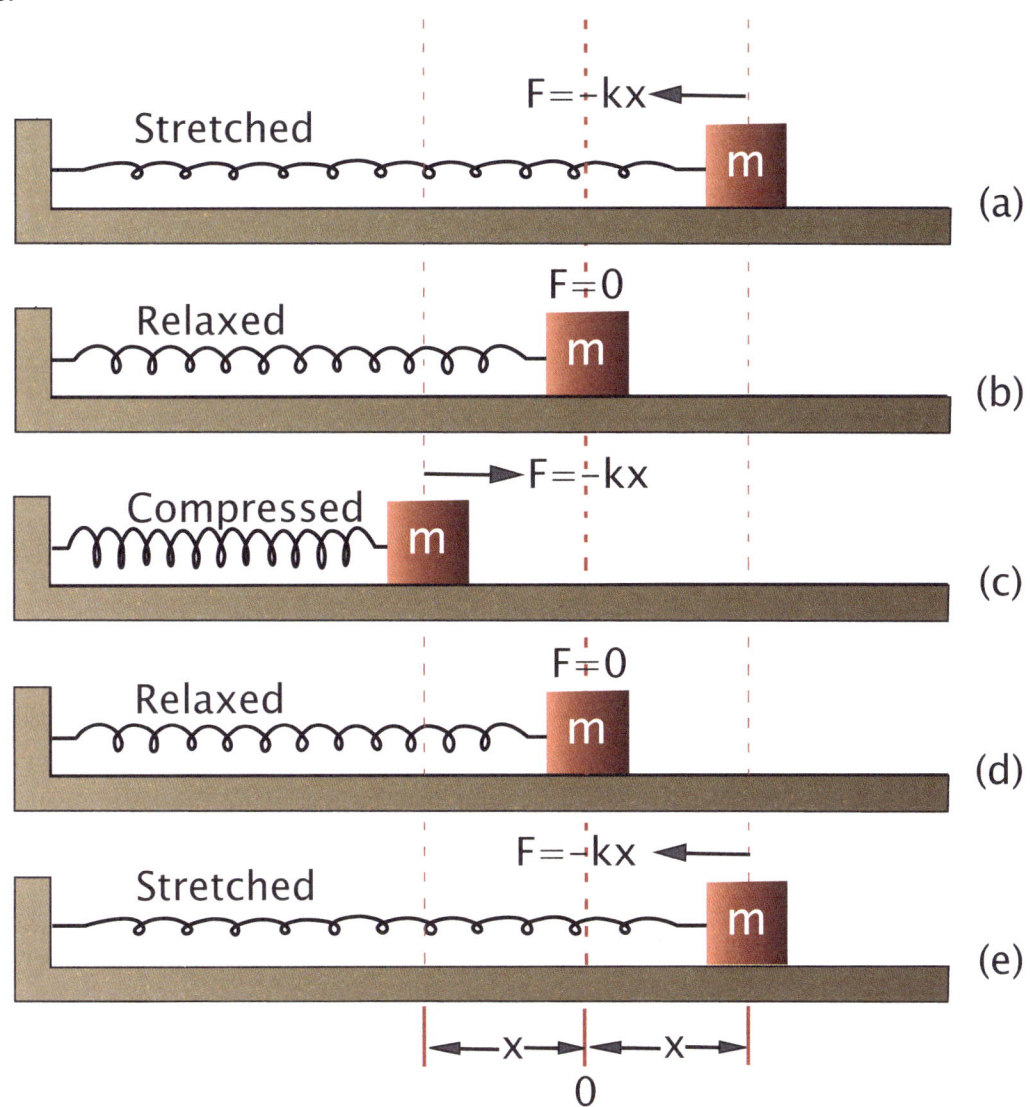

Figure III.B.7.7: Simple harmonic motion.
A block of mass m exhibiting SHM. The force F exerted by the spring on the block is shown in each case. Notice that the restoring force F is always pointing in the opposite direction to the direction of the displacement x. Because these two vectors are always opposite to each other, there is a negative sign built into the equation $F = -kx$.

7.2.2 Features of SHM and Hooke's Law

1) Force and acceleration are always in the same direction.
2) Force and acceleration are always in the opposite direction of the displacement (*this is why there is a negative sign in the equation for force*).
3) Force and acceleration have their maximal value at +A and -A; they are zero at the equilibrium point (*the amplitude A equals the maximum displacement x*).
4) Velocity direction has no constant relation to displacement and acceleration.
5) Velocity is maximum at equilibrium and zero at A and -A.
6) The period T can be calculated from the mass m of an oscillating particle:

$$T = 2\pi\sqrt{m/k}$$

where k is the spring constant. The frequency *f* is simply 1/*T*.

7.2.3 SHM Problem: The Simple Pendulum

A simple pendulum consists of a point mass m suspended by a light inextensible cord of length l. When pulled to one side of its equilibrium position, the pendulum swings under the influence of gravity producing a periodic, oscillatory motion (= SHM). Given that the angle θ with the vertical is small, thus $\sin\theta \approx \theta$, determine the general equation for the period T.

The tangential component of mg is the restoring force since it returns the mass to its equilibrium position. Thus the restoring force is:

$$F = -mg\sin\theta.$$

Recall $\sin\theta \approx \theta$, $x = l\theta$, and for SHM $F = -kx$:

$$F = -mg\theta = -mgx/l = -(mg/l)x = -kx.$$

Hence $mg/l = k$, thus the equation for the period T becomes:

$$T = 2\pi\sqrt{\frac{m}{k}} = 2\pi\sqrt{\frac{m}{mg/l}} = 2\pi\sqrt{\frac{l}{g}}$$

The equation for the period in the simple pendulum is therefore independent of the mass of the particle.

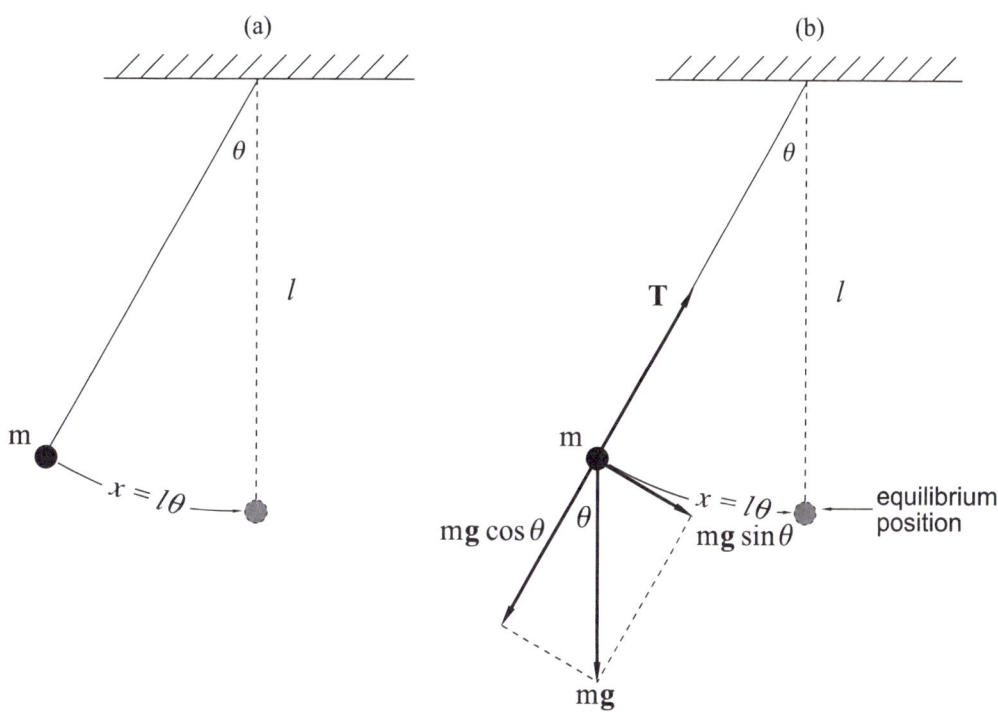

Figure III.B.7.8: The Simple Pendulum.
(a) The problem as it could be presented; the displacement x along the section of the circle (arc) is $l\theta$. (b) The vector components that should be drawn to solve the problem. The forces acting on a simple pendulum are the tension **T** in the string and the weight mg of the mass. The magnitude of the radial component of mg is mgcosθ and the tangential component is mgsinθ.

A rough approximation of SHM would be a grandfather clock or a child on a swing. However, note that the *length l* in the equation of a simple pendulum refers to the length of the cord to the bob's or child's center of gravity (COG; PHY 2.1). For some common manipulations involving the equation for the period of a simple pendulum, *see* GM 1.5.6.

What do physicists enjoy doing the most at football games?
The 'wave'   :)

Go online to GAMSAT-prep.com for free chapter review Q&A and forum.

GOLD NOTES

SOUND
Chapter 8

Memorize	Understand	Not Required*
ory vs. physical correspondence earing	* Relative velocity of sound in solids, liquids and gases * The relation of intensity to P, area, f, amplitude * Calculation of the intensity level * Rules of logarithms * Doppler effect and calculations	* Advanced level college info *Memorizing specific frequencies, speed of sound, dB's

GAMSAT-Prep.com

Introduction

Sound waves are longitudinal waves which can only be transmitted in a material, elastic medium. Speed, intensity, resonance (Chapter 7) and the Doppler effect help to describe the behavior of sound in different media. If the equations for sound intensity or the Doppler effect are required for the GAMSAT, they will be provided.

Additional Resources

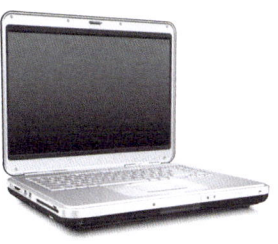

ree Online Q&A + Forum

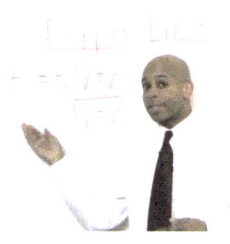

Video: Online or DVD

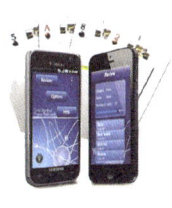

Flashcards

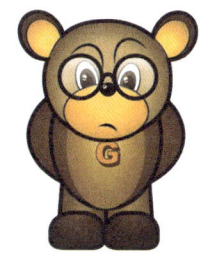

Special Guest

THE PHYSICAL SCIENCES PHY-63

* The real GAMSAT may have advanced level information presented (ie. in a passage) but previous knowledge of said information is not required to answer the questions that would follow. Practice ACER and GS practice GAMSATs can help you clarify this point.

8.1 Production of Sound

Sound is a longitudinal mechanical wave which travels through an elastic medium. Sound is thus produced by vibrating matter. There is no sound in a *vacuum* because it contains no matter.

Compressions (condensations) are regions where particles of matter are close together; they are also high pressure regions. Rarefactions are regions where particles are sparse, they are low pressure regions of sound waves (PHY 7.1.1).

8.2 Relative Velocity of Sound in Solids, Liquids, and Gases

The velocity of sound is proportional to the square root of the elastic restoring force and inversely proportional to the square root of the inertia of the particles (e.g., density is a measure of inertia). Thus as a rule, the velocity of sound is higher in liquids as compared to gases, and highest in solids.

Furthermore, an increase in temperature increases the velocity of sound; conversely, a decrease in temperature decreases the velocity of sound in that medium.

8.3 Intensity, Pitch

Hearing is subjective but its characteristics are closely tied to physical characteristics of sound.

The quality depends on the number and relative intensity of the overtones of the waveform. Frequency, and therefore pitch are perceived by the ear from 20 to 20,000 Hz (hertz = cycles/second = s^{-1}). Frequencies below 20 Hz are called infrasonic. Frequencies above 20,000 Hz are called ultrasonic.

Sensory	Physical
loudness	intensity
pitch	frequency
quality	waveform

Table III.B.8.1:
Sensory and physical correspondence of hearing.

Sound intensity (I) is the rate of energy (power) propagation through space:

$I = $ (power/area) which is proportional to $(f^2 A^2)$

where f = frequency, A = amplitude.

The loudness varies with the frequency. The ears are most sensitive (hears sounds of lowest intensity) at approximately 2,000 to 4,000 Hz. I_o is taken to be 10^{-12} watts/cm², is barely audible and is assigned a value of 0 dB (zero *decibels*). Then intensity level (I) of a sound wave in dB is,

$$dB = 10 \log_{10}(I/I_o)$$

where dB = the sound level, I = the intensity at a given level, I_o = the threshold intensity. {To calculate a change in the sound level or volume ΔV in units of dB, given two values for sound intensity, the given equation can be modified thus: $\Delta V = 10\log(I_{new}/I_{old})$}

Examples of some values of dB's are: whisper (20), normal conversation (60), subway car (100), pain threshold (120), and jet engine (160). Continual exposure to sound greater than 90 dB can lead to hearing impairment.

8.3.1 Calculation of the Intensity Level

What is the loudness or intensity level of Mr. Yell Alot's voice when he generates a sound wave ten million times as intense as I_o?

$I = (10,000,000) \quad I_o = (10^7) I_o$

Thus
$$dB = 10 \log_{10} (10^7 I_o/I_o)$$
$$= 10 \log_{10} 10^7$$
$$= 70 \log_{10} 10 = 70$$

{See chemistry section 6.5.1 for rules of logarithms. Question types involving logs including acids-bases (CHM Chapter 6) and rate law (CHM Chapter 9) are common amongst ACER's GAMSAT materials.}

8.4 Beats

When sound of different frequencies are heard together, they interfere. Constructive interference results in beats. The number of beats per second is the absolute value of the difference of the frequencies ($|f_1 - f_2|$).

Hence, the new frequency heard includes the original frequencies and the absolute difference between them.

8.5 Doppler Effect

The Doppler effect is the effect upon the observed frequency caused by the relative motion of the observer (o) and the source (s). If the distance is decreasing between them, there is a shift to higher frequencies and shorter wavelengths (to higher pitch for sound and toward blue-violet for light, PHY 8.3 and 9.2.4). If the distance is increasing between them, there is a shift to longer wavelengths and lower frequencies (to lower pitch for sound and toward red for light). The summary equation of the above in terms of frequency (f) is:

$$f_o = f_s(V \pm v_o)/(V \pm v_s)$$

V = speed of the wave, v = speed of the observer (o) or the source (s).

Choose the sign such that the frequency varies consistently with the relative motion of the source and the observer. In other words, when the distance between the source and observer is *decreasing* use $+v_o$ and $-v_s$; if the distance is *increasing* use $-v_o$ and $+v_s$.

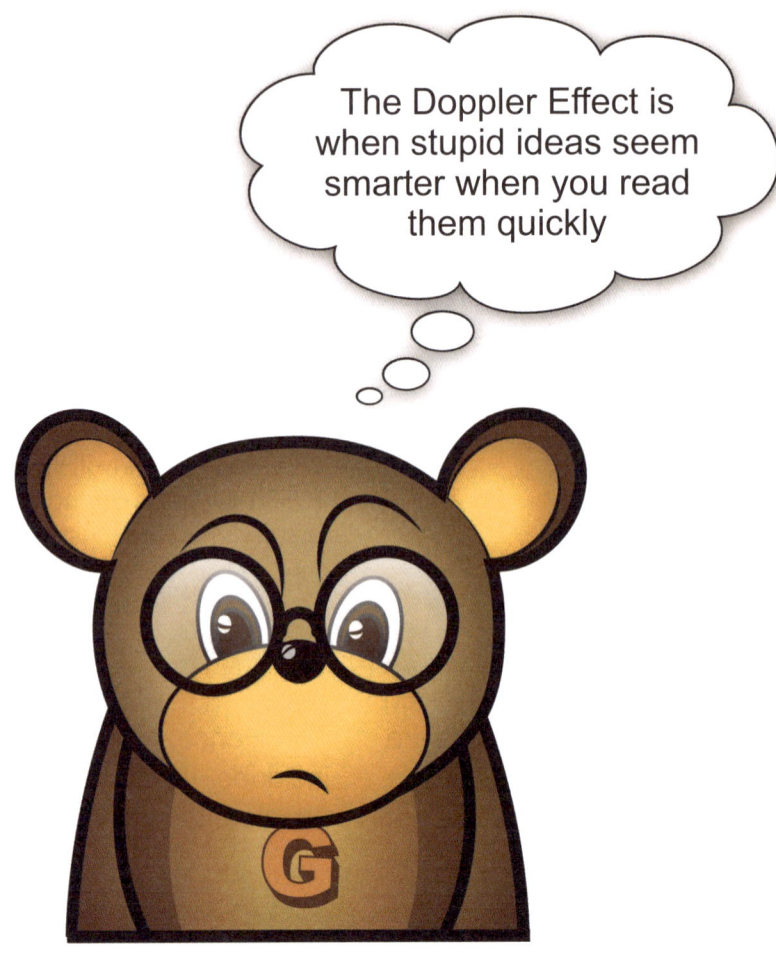

8.5.1 Doppler Effect Problem (SI units)

A car drives towards a bus stop with its car stereo playing opera. The opera singer sings the note middle C (= 262 Hz) loudly; however, the people waiting at the bus stop hear C sharp (= 277 Hz). Given that the speed of sound V in air is 331 m/s, how fast is the car moving?

{Remember the sign convention: since the distance between the source (the car) and the observer (people at the bus stop) is <u>decreasing</u> we use $+v_o$ and $-v_s$}

- the car (the *source* of the frequency) f_s = 262 Hz, v_s = unknown.

- the bus stop (where the *observers* are stationary) f_o = 277 Hz, v_o = 0 m/s.

$$f_o = f_s(V + v_o)/(V - v_s)$$

Thus

$$V - v_s = f_s(V + v_o)/f_o$$

Hence

$$v_s = -f_s(V + v_o)/f_o + V$$

Substitute

$$v_s = -262(331 + 0)/277 + 331 = 17.9 \text{ m/s.}$$

- Note that the answer contains three significant figures.

Go online to GAMSAT-prep.com for free chapter review Q&A and forum.

GOLD NOTES

ELECTROSTATICS AND ELECTROMAGNETISM
Chapter 9

Memorize	Understand	Not Required*
s: for charge Q, Coulomb's law, eld s: potential energy, absolute potential relating energy, planck's constant,	* Conservation of charge, use of Coulomb's law * Graphs/theory: electric field/potential lines, mag. induction * Potential difference, electric dipoles, mag. induction * Laplace's law, the right hand rule, magnetic field * Direction of F in magn. field; electromagnetism	* Advanced level college info * Memorizing coulomb's, permittivity or planck's constants * Memorizing equation with permittivity constant or dF * Calculus, derivatives, integrals, speed of light

GAMSAT-Prep.com

Introduction

Electrostatics (statics = usu. at rest) refers to the science of stationary or slowly moving charges. Such charges can interact and behave in ways described by charge, electric force, electric field and potential difference. When a charge is in motion, it creates a magnetic field. Electromagnetism describes the relationship between electricity (moving electrical charge) and magnetism. The electromagnetic spectrum includes light and X-rays.

Additional Resources

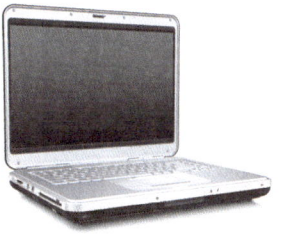

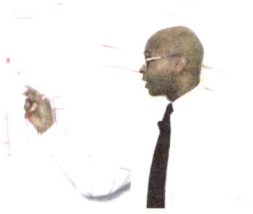

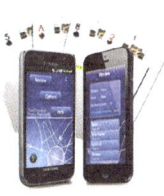

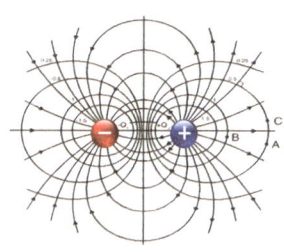

ree Online Q&A + Forum   Video: Online or DVD   Flashcards   Special Guest

THE PHYSICAL SCIENCES   PHY-69

* The real GAMSAT may have advanced level information presented (ie. in a passage) but previous knowledge of said information is not required to answer the questions that would follow. Practice ACER and GS practice GAMSATs can help you clarify this point.

GAMSAT-Prep.com
THE GOLD STANDARD

9.1 Electrostatics

9.1.1 Charge, Conductors, Insulators

By friction of matter we create between substances repulsive or attractive electric forces. These forces are due to two kinds of electric charges, distinguished by positive (+) and negative (−) signs. Each has a charge of 1.6×10^{-19} coulombs (= C = an SI derived unit; GM 2.1.3, Table 3) but differ in sign. The electron is the negative charge carrier, and the proton is the positive charge carrier. Substances with an excess of electrons have a net negative charge. Substances with a deficiency of electrons have a net positive charge. The total amount of charge Q of matter depends on the number of particles n and the charge e on each particle, thus $Q = ne$.

The conservation of charge states that a net charge cannot be created but that charge can be transferred from one object to another. One way of charging substances is by rubbing them (i.e., by contact).

For example, glass rubbed on fur becomes positive and rubber rubbed on fur becomes negative. Objects can also be charged by induction which occurs when one charged object is brought near to another uncharged object causing a charge redistribution in the latter to give net charge regions. Conductors transmit charge readily. Insulators resist the flow of charge.

9.1.2 Coulomb's Law, Electric Force

Charges exert forces upon each other. Like charges repel each other and unlike charges attract. For any two charges q_1 and q_2 the force F is given by Coulomb's Law:

$$F = k \frac{q_1 q_2}{r^2} = \frac{1}{4\pi\varepsilon_0}\left(\frac{q_1 q_2}{r^2}\right)$$

where k = coulomb's constant = 9.0×10^9 N-m²/C², ε_0 = permittivity constant = 8.85×10^{-12} C²/N-m², and r = the distance between the charges. Note that the relationship of force and distance follows an inverse square law. Thus if the distance r is doubled [$(2r)^2 = 4r^2$], the new force is quartered ($F_{new} = F/4$). {cf. Law of Gravity: PHY 2.4}

9.1.3 Electric Field, Electric Field Lines

A charge generates an electric field (E) in the space around it. Fields (force fields) are vectors. A field is generated by an object and it is that region of space around the object that will exert a force on a second object brought into that field. The field exists independently of that second object and is not altered by its presence. The force exerted on the second object depends upon that object and the field. The electric field E is given by:

$$E = F/q = k\, Q/r^2$$

where E and F are vectors, Q = the charge generating the field, and q = the charge placed in the field.

Charges exert forces upon each other through fields. The direction of a field is the direction <u>a positive charge would move if placed in it</u>. *Electric field lines* are imaginary lines which are in the same direction as E at that point. The direction is away from positive charges and toward negative charges, or put another way, the electric field is directed toward the decreasing potentials.

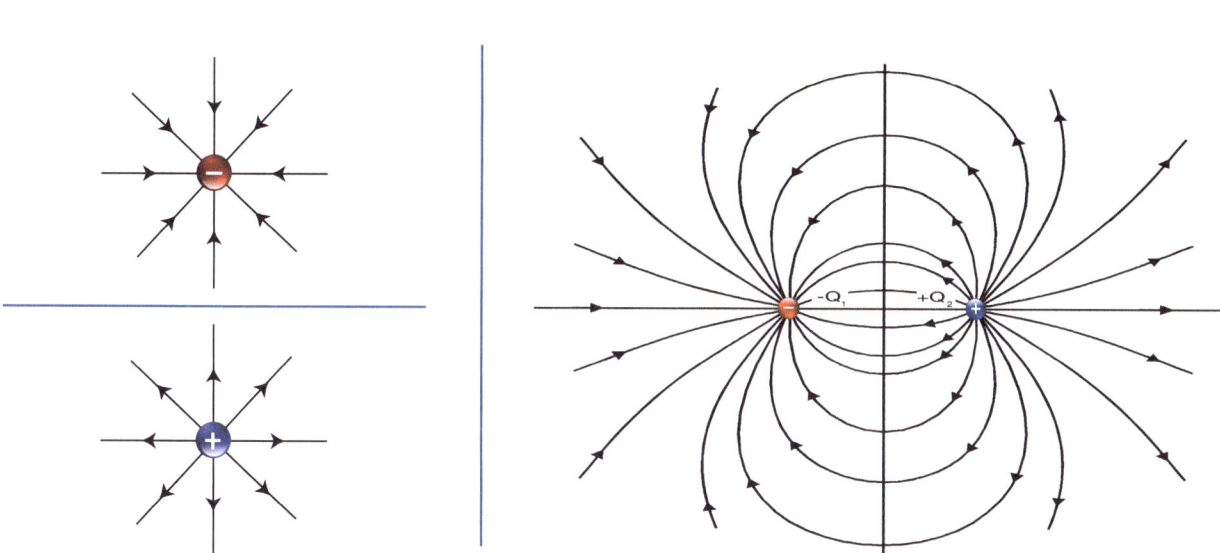

Figure III.B.9.1: Electric field lines. The electric field is generated by the charges $-Q_1$ and $+Q_2$. The arrowheads show the direction of the electric field.

If an electric potential is applied between two plates in a vacuum, and an electron is introduced, the electron will experience an attractive force to the positive plate (see Figure III.B.9.2).

The force will cause the electron to accelerate towards the positive plate in a straight line. It suffers no collisions because the area between the plates is *in vacuo*. This effect is used in thermoionic valves.

If the electron is given some motion, and the electric field is applied perpendicular to the motion, interesting things happen (see Figure III.B.9.3). For example, a beam of electrons is emitted from a device called an electron gun. These electrons are moving in the x direction.

As the electrons pass between the plates they are accelerated in the y direction, as explained before, but their velocity in the x direction is unaltered. The electron beam is thus deflected as shown.

By varying the potential applied to the plates, the angle of deflection can be controlled. This effect is the basis of the cathode ray oscilloscope.

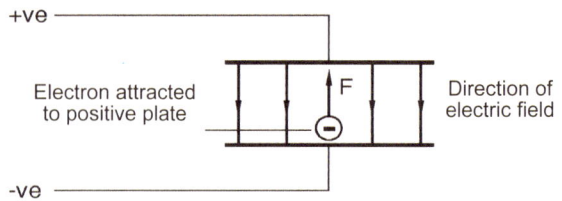

Figure III.B.9.2:
Electric field between parallel plates.

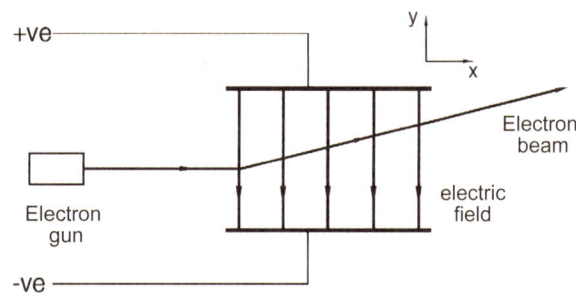

Figure III.B.9.3:
Electrostatic deflection of an electron beam.

9.1.4 Potential Energy, Absolute Potential

The *potential energy* (E_p) of a charged object in a field equals the work done on that object to bring it from infinity to a distance (r) from the charge setting up the electric field,

$$E_p = \text{work} = Fr = (qE)r = kQq/r$$

where Q = the charge setting up field, and q = the charge brought in to a distance r.

When a +q moves against E, its E_p increases. When a -q moves against the electric field E, its E_p decreases. If two positive or negative charges were brought together, work would have to be done to the system (and E_p would increase), and vice versa for charges of opposite charges.

The *absolute potential* (V) is a scalar, and it is defined at each distance (r) from a charge (Q) generating an electric field. It represents the negative of the work per unit charge in bringing a +q from infinity to r:

• $V = E_p/q = kQ/r$ in volts where 1 volt = 1 joule/coulomb.

• $V = Ed$ for a parallel plate capacitor where d = distance between the plates (PHY 10.4).

PHY-72   ELECTROSTATICS AND ELECTROMAGNETISM

9.1.5 Equipotential Lines, Potential Difference, Electric Dipoles

Equipotential lines are lines (and surfaces) of equal V and are *perpendicular* to electric field lines. Work can only be done when moving between surfaces of unequal V and is, therefore, independent of the path taken. No work is done when a charge (q) is moved along an equal potential (*equipotential*) surface (or line), because the component of force is zero along it. Potential (V) is defined in terms of positive charges such that V is positive when due to a +Q and negative when due a −Q. Potential (V) is added algebraically at a point (because it is a scalar).

See Figure III.B.9.4:

1) V_1, V_2 are two potentials perpendicular to the electric field E and the force F;
2) $V_2 - V_1$ is the potential difference (PD);
3) charge (q) moved from A ($V_1 = 0.5$) to B ($V_2 = 1$) has work (W) done on it:

$$W = q(V_2 - V_1) = q(PD)$$

4) charge (q) moved from A to C has no work done on it because this is along an equipotential surface (V = 0.5) and the non-zero component of force (F) is perpendicular to it;
5) the lines of F are along the lines of E.

The *potential difference* (PD) is the difference in V between two points, or it is the work per unit positive charge done by electric forces moving a small test charge from the point of higher potential to the point of lower potential:

$$PD = V_a - V_b = volts = work/charge$$

$$work = q(V_a - V_b) = q(PD).$$

An *electric dipole* consists of two charges separated by some finite distance (d). Usually the charges are equal and opposite. The laws of forces, fields, etc., apply to dipoles. A dipole is characterized by its *dipole moment* which is the product of the charge (q) and d.

Dipoles tend to line up with the electric field (Fig. III.B.9.5). Motion of dipoles against an electric field requires energy as discussed above.

If you consider a single isolated point charge and the circular equipotential line produced, in 3 D, it is a sphere where each point on the surface of the sphere has the same potential because it is the same distance from the charge. This imaginary 3 D shape is called a *gaussian* surface.

dipole moment = *(charge)(distance) = qd*

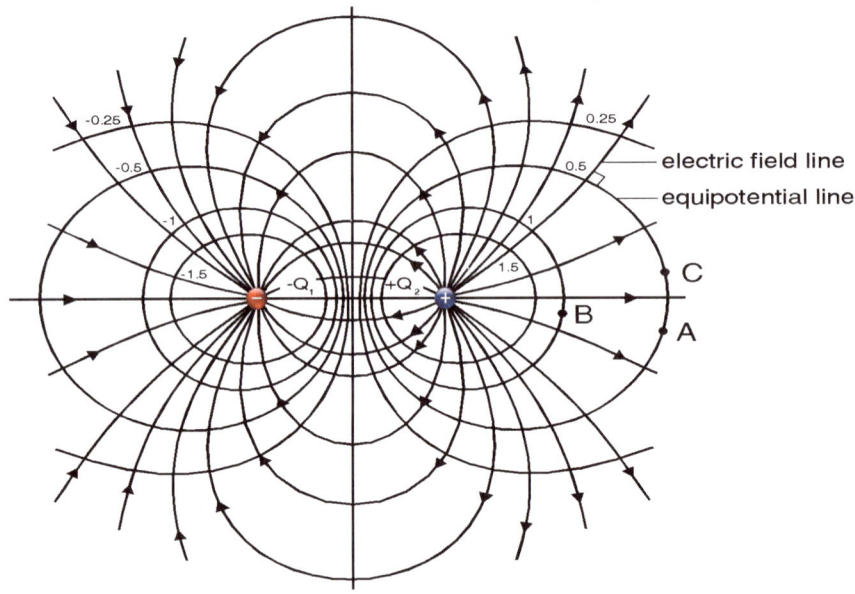

Figure III.B.9.4: Equipotential lines.
The circle-like curves around each charge $-Q_1$ and $+Q_2$ are the equipotential lines corresponding to each charge. The numbers represent the electric potential value (i.e. in millivolts) of the respective equipotential lines. Note the electric field lines as in Figure III.B.9.1.

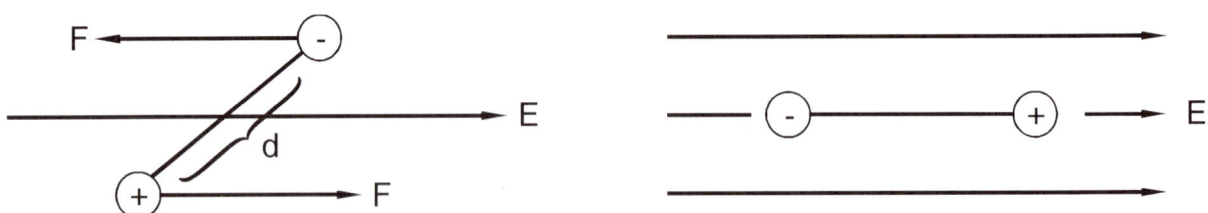

Dipole with equal and opposite charges

Alignment of dipole with E

Figure III.B.9.5: Dipole and electric field.
E = electric field, *F* = forces exerted by *E* on the dipole

9.2 Electromagnetism

9.2.1 Notion of Electromagnetic Induction

Coulomb's Law in electrostatics gives the nature of the forces acting upon electric charges at rest, but when the charges are moving, new forces appear.

They are not of the same nature as the electrostatic forces and they act differently on the electric charges. They are called electromagnetic forces.

9.2.2 Magnetic Induction Vector

Experiments have shown that two straight conductors (e.g. copper wires) traversed by electric currents of intensities I and I' in the same direction are acted upon by an attractive force proportional to the product of the intensities and inversely proportional to the distance between the two conductors. It can be demonstrated that when the electric current in one of the conductors disappears, the force also disappears.

Therefore, the force is due to the motion of the electric charges in both conductors.

We decompose the phenomenon by introducing a new physical quantity: the magnetic induction vector B, also created by magnets.

The SI unit for B is the tesla where 1 T = 1 N/(A·m) = 10^4 gauss.

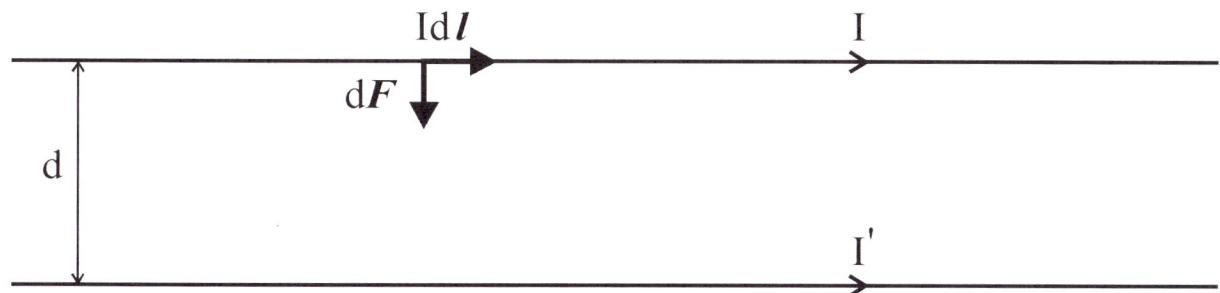

Figure III.B.9.6: Magnetic induction.
Two conductors a distance d apart; the current element Idl and the perpendicular force dF associated with the magnetic induction vector B are both shown. Vector B, which is not shown, has a direction perpendicular to both Idl and dF, pointing out of the page.

Thus, two effects have been shown by the preceding experiment:

1) a moving charge produces a magnetic induction.

2) a magnetic induction exerts a force on any nearby moving charge.

9.2.3 Laplace's Law

A test particle with charge dq moving at a velocity v in a magnetic induction field B is acted upon by a force dF given by the following formula:

$$dF = dq\, v \times B = dq\, v(B \sin \alpha)$$

where α is the angle formed by the direction of v with that of B (= the cross product).

The force dF is perpendicular to the magnetic induction vector and also to the displacement velocity vector of the charge (see Figure III.B.9.6).

When many charges are in motion so as to produce an electric current of intensity $I = dq/dt$ the force acting upon an elemental length of conductor dl traversed by that electric current is:

$$dF = I\, dl \times B = I\, dl(B \sin \alpha)$$

where α is the angle formed by the direction of the current element of conductor with that of B (= the cross product).

In order to determine the direction of a cross (= *vector*) product we can use the right-hand rule. If $c = a \times b$ then the right hand is held so that the curled fingers follow the rotation of *a* to *b*, the extended right thumb will point in the direction of *c* (dF in the preceding example). {Student's trick: "Grab the Wire!" Examine Fig. III.B.9.6. Turn the book around such that with your right hand open and thumb extended, the fingers point in the direction of dF and your thumb points in the direction Idl. As you begin to grab the wire, the initial direction of the tips of your fingers move perpendicular to both dF and Idl. Now the tips of your fingers make a circular motion around the wire. Those fingers have just described the direction of the magnetic induction vector B!}

9.2.4 Electromagnetic Spectrum, Radio, Infrared, X Rays

An electromagnetic field is described as having at every point of the field, two perpendicular vectors: *the electric field* vector E and the magnetic induction field vector B.

Radar (= *radio detection* and ranging) is an example of a radio wave.

Visible light can be broken down into colors remembered by the mnemonic (*from highest to lowest wavelength*), Roy G. BIV: Red, Orange, Yellow, Green, Blue, Indigo, Violet.

The separation of white light into these colors can occur as a result of refraction through a prism (PHY 11.4) or through water (i.e. mist or rain resulting in a rainbow).

Planck developed the relation between energy (E) and the frequency f of the electromagnetic radiation,

$$E = hf$$

where h = planck's constant. Thus high frequency or short wave length corresponds to high energy and vice versa.

The speed of light (= electromagnetic radiation), given by c, can be measured from the wavelength λ and the frequency f of an electromagnetic wave in a vacuum (= in vacuo = no pressure/no particles approximated by outer space). Recall that v = λf (PHY 7.1.2), and so we have the special case for the speed of light,

$$c = \lambda f$$

The result is the constant $c = 3 \times 10^8$ m/s which, if required to answer a question during the GAMSAT, would be given in the passage or question stem. The speed at which light propagates through transparent materials, such as glass, water or air, is less than c, given by the refractive index n of the material (n = c/v; PHY 9.2.4). The change in c in different materials (refraction) is responsible for the colors of a rainbow.

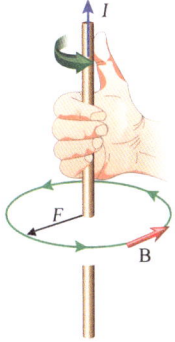

Figure III.B.9.6b: Right-hand rule.

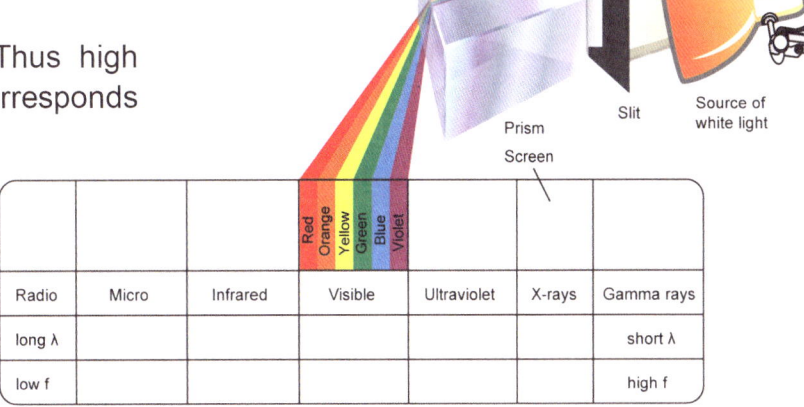

Figure III.B.9.7: The complete electromagnetic spectrum.

Go online to GAMSAT-prep.com for free chapter review Q&A and forum.

THE PHYSICAL SCIENCES PHY-77

GOLD NOTES

ELECTRIC CIRCUITS
Chapter 10

Memorize	Understand	Not Required*
tion/equation/units: current, resistance aw, resistors in series/parallel tance, capacitors in series/parallel ff's laws	* Battery, emf, voltage, terminal potential * Internal resistance of the battery, resistivity * Ohm's law, resistors in series/parallel * Parallel plate capacitor, series, parallel * Conductivity, power in circuits, Kirchoff's laws * Capacitor discharge curve (exponential decay)	* Advanced level college info * Complex/discrete/digital circuits * Transistors, FPGAs, microprocessors * Memorizing equations for rms voltage/current

GAMSAT-Prep.com

Introduction

Electric circuits are closed paths which includes electronic components (i.e. resistors, capacitors, power supplies) through which a current can flow. There are 3 basic laws that govern the flow of current in an electrical circuit: Ohm's law and Kirchoff's first and second laws.

Additional Resources

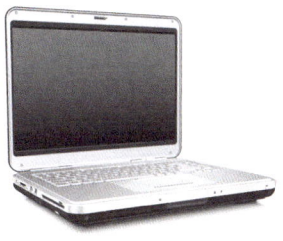

Free Online Q&A + Forum

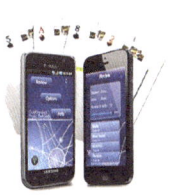

Video: Online or DVD

Flashcards

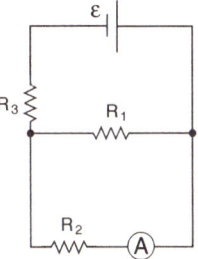

Special Guest

THE PHYSICAL SCIENCES

* The real GAMSAT may have advanced level information presented (ie. in a passage) but previous knowledge of said information is not required to answer the questions that would follow. Practice ACER and GS practice GAMSATs can help you clarify this point.

10.1 Current

The current (*I*) is the amount of charge (*Q*) that flows past a point in a given amount of time (*t*),

$$I = Q/t = amperes = coulombs/sec.$$

Current is caused by the movement of electrons between two points of significant potential difference of an electric circuit. Free electrons will accelerate towards the positive connection. As they move they will collide with atoms in the substance, losing energy which we observe as heat. The net effect is a drift of electrons at a roughly constant speed towards the positive connection. The motion of electrons is an *electric current*. As electrons are removed by the electric potential source at the positive connection, electrons are being injected at the negative connection. The potential can be considered as a form of *electron pump*.

This model explains many observed effects.

If the magnitude of the electric potential is increased, the electrons will accelerate faster and their mean velocity will be higher, i.e., the current is increased. The collisions between electrons and atoms transfer energy to the atoms. The collisions manifest themselves as heat. This effect is known as *Joule heating*. Materials such as these are termed ohmic conductors, since they obey the well-known Ohm's Law:

$$V = IR$$

where *V* is the voltage, *I* is the current, and *R* is the resistance.

The potential difference is maintained by a voltage source (emf). The direction of current is taken as the direction of positive charge movement, by convention. It is represented on a circuit diagram by arrows. Ammeters are used to measure the flow of current and are symbolized as in Figure III.B.10.1.

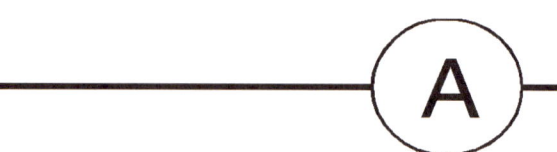

Figure III.B.10.1: Symbol of an ammeter.

10.2 Resistance, Resistivity, Series and Parallel Circuits

Resistance (R) is the measure of opposition to the flow of electrons in a substance. Resistivity (ρ) is an inherent property of a substance. It varies with temperature. For example, the resistivity of metals increases with increasing temperature.

Resistance is directly proportional to resistivity and length l but inversely proportional to the cross-sectional area A.

$$R = \rho l / A$$

Resistance increases with temperature because the thermal motion of molecules increases with temperature and results in more collisions between electrons which impede their flow.

The units of resistance are ohms, symbolized by Ω (omega). From Ohm's Law, 1 ohm = 1 volt/ampere.

When a positive current flows across a resistor, there is a voltage decrease and an energy loss:

$$\text{energy loss} = Vq = VIt = joules$$

$$\boxed{\text{power loss } (P) = VIt/t = VI = watts}$$

$$watts = volts \times amperes = joules/sec.$$

The energy loss may be used to perform work. These relations hold for power (P),

$$P = VI = (IR)(I) = I^2R = V(V/R) = V^2/R.$$

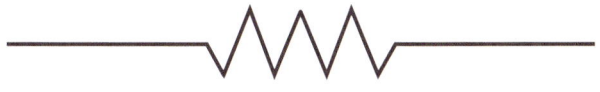
constant (normal) resistance
"classic" image of resistor

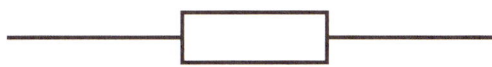
"modern" image of resistor

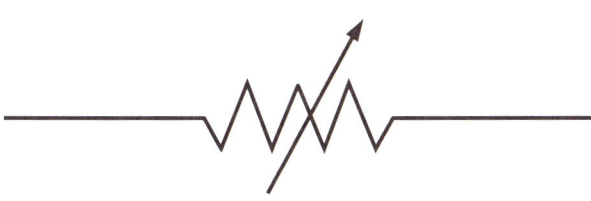
variable resistance (rheostat)

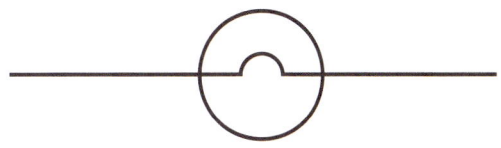
incandescent light bulb
treated like resistor

Figure III.B.10.2: Representations of resistors. Note that the filament inside of a light bulb (= *incandescent lamp* or *globe*) is a resistor. Because it resists the flow of current, it becomes hot and glows providing light. This is why a light bulb in a circuit is treated exactly like a resistor. The brightness of a light bulb depends on how much power it loses (= *dissipates*; P = VI).

THE PHYSICAL SCIENCES PHY-81

Circuit elements are either in series or in parallel. Two components are in series when they have only one point in common; that is, the current travelling from one of them back to the emf source must pass through the other. In a complete series circuit, or for individual series loops of a larger mixed circuit, the current (I) is the same over each component and the total voltage drop in the circuit elements (resistors, capacitors, inductors, internal resistance of emf sources, etc.) is equal to the sum V_t of all the emf sources. The value of the equivalent resistance R_{eq} in a series circuit is:

$$R_{eq} = R_1 + R_2 + R_3 + \ldots$$

Two components are in parallel when they are connected to two common points in the circuit; that is, the current travelling from one such element back to the emf source need not pass through the second element because there is an alternate path.

In a parallel circuit, the total current is the sum of currents for each path and the voltage is the same for all paths in parallel. The equivalent resistance in a parallel circuit is:

$$1/R_{eq} = 1/R_1 + 1/R_2 + 1/R_3 + \ldots$$

10.2.1 Resistance Problem in Series and Parallel

Determine the equivalent resistance between points *A* and *B* in Figure III.B.10.3.

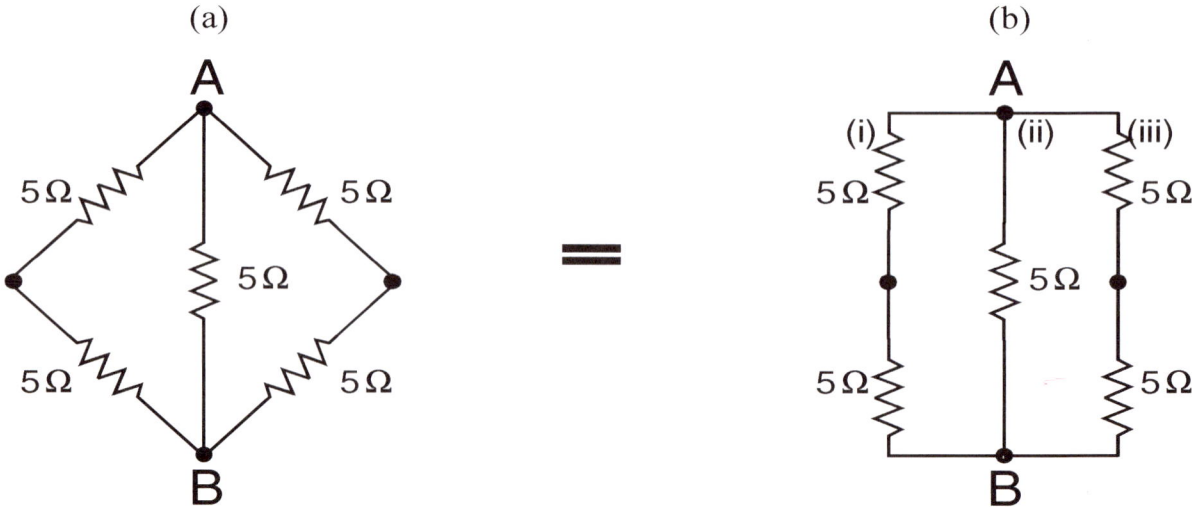

Figure III.B.10.3: Equivalent resistance.
(a) The problem as it could be presented; (b) the way you should interpret the problem.

- Wire (i) has two resistors in a row (*in series*): $R_{(i)} = 5 + 5 = 10\ \Omega$

- Wire (ii) has only one resistor: $R_{(ii)} = 5\ \Omega$

- Wire (iii) has two resistors in series: $R_{(iii)} = 5 + 5 = 10\ \Omega$

Between A and B we have three resistor systems in parallel: (i), (ii) and (iii), thus

$$1/R_{eq} = 1/R_{(i)} + 1/R_{(ii)} + 1/R_{(iii)}$$
$$= 1/10 + 1/5 + 1/10 = 4/10$$

multiply through by $10R_{eq}$ to get: $10 = 4R_{eq}$

thus $R_{eq} = 10/4 = 2.5\ \Omega$.

10.3 Batteries, Electromotive Force, Voltage, Internal Resistance

An *electromotive force (emf)* source maintains between its terminal points, a constant potential difference. The emf source replaces energy lost by moving electrons. Sources of emf are batteries (conversion of chemical energy to electrical energy) and generators (conversion of mechanical energy to electrical energy).

The source of emf does work on each charge to raise it from a lower potential to a higher potential.

Then as the charge flows around the circuit (naturally from higher to lower potential) it loses energy which is replaced by the emf source again.

energy supplied = energy lost

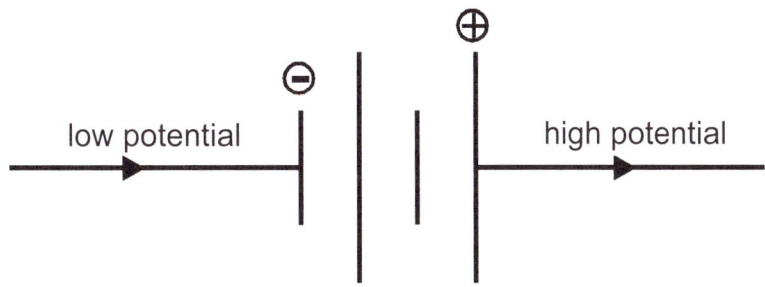

Figure III.B.10.4: Symbol of an emf source. Arrows show the normal direction of current.

Energy is lost whenever a charge (as current) passes through a resistor. The units of emf are volts. The actual voltage delivered to a circuit is not equal to the value of the source. This is reduced by an internal voltage lost which represents the voltage loss by the *internal resistance (r)* of the source itself. The net voltage is called the terminal voltage or *terminal potential V_t*.

Figure III.B.10.5: Simplified symbol of an emf source.

$V_t = V - Ir = IR_t$

I, R_t = totals for the circuit; V = maximal voltage output of the emf source.

When two emf sources are connected in opposition, (positive pole to positive pole) the charge loses energy when passing in the second emf source.

Therefore, if there is more than one emf source in a circuit, the total emf is the sum of the individual emf sources not in opposition reduced by the sum of individual sources in opposition in a given direction.

10.3.1 Kirchoff's Laws and a Multiloop Circuit Problem

Given that the emf of the battery $\varepsilon = 12$ volts and the resistors $R_1 = 12\ \Omega$, $R_2 = 4.0\ \Omega$, and $R_3 = 6.0\ \Omega$, determine the reading in the ammeter (*see* Figure III.B.10.6).

Ignore the internal resistance of the battery.

{*The ammeter will read the current which flows through it which is i_2*}

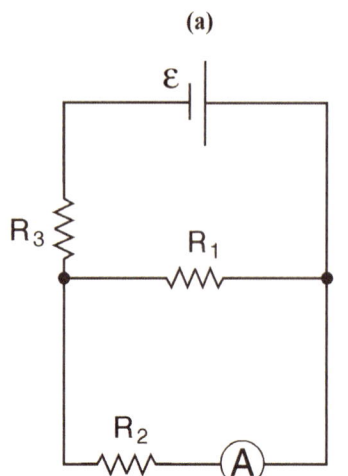
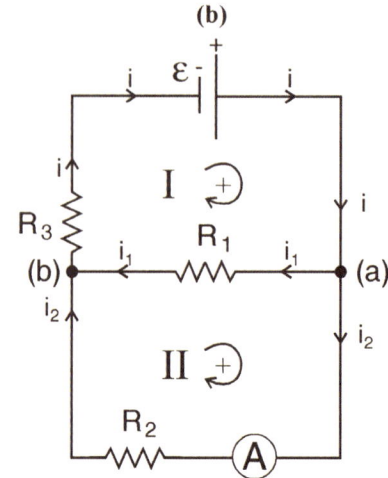

Figure III.B.10.6: A multiloop circuit.
(**a**) The problem as it could be presented; (**b**) the way you should label the diagram. Note that the current emanates from the positive terminal and is the same current i which returns to the emf source.

Kirchoff's Law I (*the junctional theorem*): when different currents arrive at a point (= *junction*, as in points (*a*) and (*b*) in the labelled diagram) the sum of current equals zero.

We can arbitrarily define all current *arriving* at the junction as positive and all current *leaving* as negative.

Kirchoff's Law I	$\Sigma i = 0$ at a junction

Thus at junction (a) $i - i_1 - i_2 = 0$

And for junction (b) $i_1 + i_2 - i = 0$

Both (a) and (b) reduce to equation (c):

$$i = i_1 + i_2$$

Kirchoff's Law II (*the loop theorem*): the sum of voltage changes in one continous loop of a circuit is zero. A single loop circuit is simple since the current is the same in all parts of the loop hence the loop theorem is applied only once.

In a multiloop circuit (loops *I* and *II* in the labelled diagram), there is more than one loop thus the current in general will not be the same in all parts of any given loop. We can arbitrarily define all voltage changes around the loop in the *clockwise* direction as positive and in the *counterclockwise* direction as negative.

Thus if by moving in the clockwise direction we can move from the battery's negative terminal (*low potential*) to its positive terminal (*high potential*), the value of the emf ε is negative.

Kirchoff's Law II	$\Sigma \Delta V = 0$ in a loop

Thus in loop *I* (*recall: V=IR*)

$$i_1 R_1 + i R_3 - \varepsilon = 0$$

And in loop II

$$i_2 R_2 - i_1 R_1 = 0$$

We now have simultaneous equations. There are three unknowns (i, i_1, i_2) and three equations (c, loop *I*, and loop *II*). We need only solve for the current i_2 which runs through the ammeter.

Substitute (c) into loop I

$$i_1 R_1 + (i_1 + i_2) R_3 - \varepsilon = 0$$

Thus

$$i_1 R_1 + i_1 R_3 + i_2 R_3 - \varepsilon = 0$$

Substitute i_1 from loop *II* where $i_1 = i_2 R_2 / R_1$, hence

$$i_2 R_2 + i_2 R_2 R_3 / R_1 + i_2 R_3 = \varepsilon$$

Begin isolating i_2

$$i_2 (R_2 + R_2 R_3 / R_1 + R_3) = \varepsilon$$

Isolate i_2

$$i_2 = \varepsilon (R_2 + R_2 R_3 / R_1 + R_3)^{-1}$$

Substitute

$$i_2 = 12[4 + (4)(6)/(12) + 6]^{-1} = 12/12 = 1.0 \text{ ampere.}$$

10.4 Capacitors and Dielectrics

Capacitors can store and separate charge. Capacitors can be filled with dielectrics which are materials which can increase capacitance. The capacitance (C) is an inherent property of a conductor and is formulated as:

C = charge/electric potential = Q/V = farad = coulomb/volt

The capacitance is the number of coulombs that must be transferred to a conductor to raise its potential by one volt.

The amount of charge that can be stored depends on the shape, size, surroundings and type of the conductor.

The higher the dielectric strength (i.e., the electric field strength at which a substance ceases to be an insulator and becomes a conductor) of the medium, the greater the capacitance of the conductor.

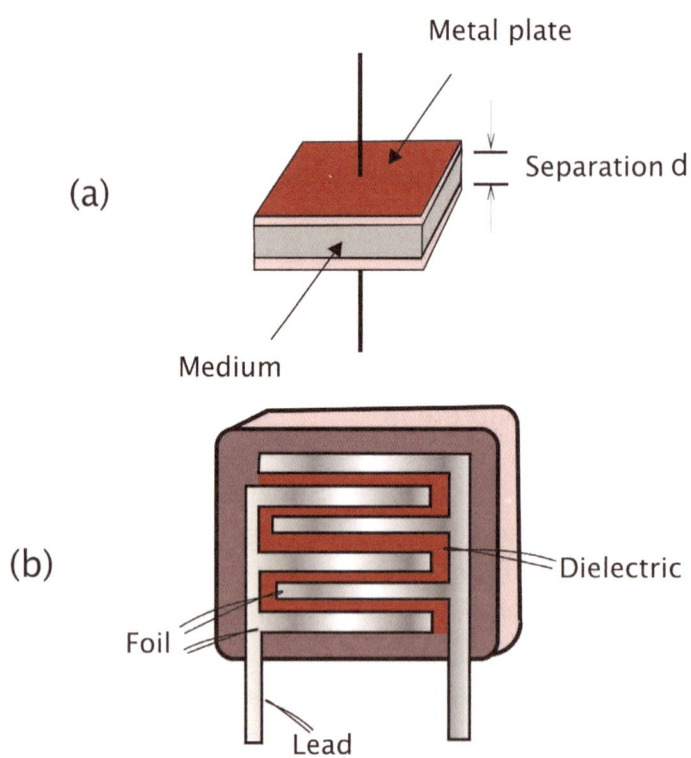

Figure III.B.10.7: (a) Parallel plate capacitor; (b) Ceramic capacitor.

A capacitor is made of two or more conductors with opposite but equal charges placed near each other.

A common example is the parallel plate capacitor. The important formulas for capacitors are:

1) $C = Q/V$ where V = the potential between the plates
2) $V = Ed$ where E = electric field strength, and d = distance between the plates
3) C is directly proportional to the surface area A of the plates and inversely proportional to the distance between the plates

$$C = \varepsilon_o A/d$$

for air as a medium between the plates. If the capacitor contains a dielectric, the above equation would by multiplied by the factor κ (= *dielectric constant*) whose value depends on the dielectric being used.

4) The equivalent capacitance C_{eq} for capacitors arranged in series and in parallel is:

Series: $1/C_{eq} = 1/C_1 + 1/C_2 + 1/C_3 \ldots$

Parallel: $C_{eq} = C_1 + C_2 + C_3 \ldots$

The dielectric substances set up an opposing electric field to that of the capacitor which decreases the net electric field and allows the capacitance of the capacitor to increase ($C = Q/Ed$). The molecules of the dielectric are dipoles which line up in the electric field.

{cf. Fig. III.B.9.5 from PHY 9.1.4 and Fig. III.B.10.8 in this section}

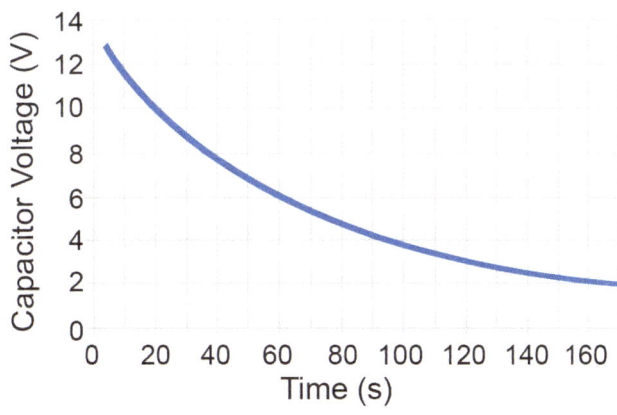

Figure III.B.10.7.1: Capacitor discharge curve. A capacitor is first charged by connecting it to a power supply. In this example, the capacitor is charged up to 14 volts. When the capacitor discharges through a resistor, the charge drains rapidly at first then decreases gradually. This pattern of decrease can be described as *exponential decay* and can be found in many areas of science (examples: first and second order reactions in General Chemistry, CHM 9.2; radioactive decay in Physics, PHY 12.4).

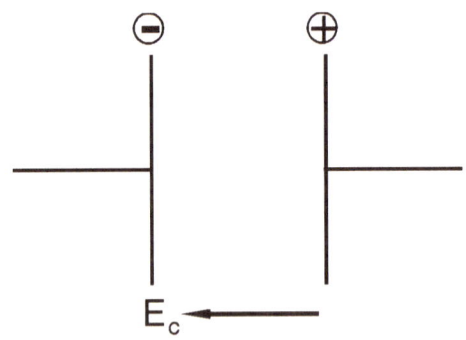
without dielectric

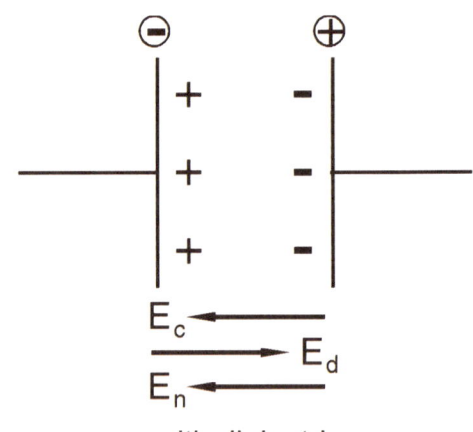
with dielectric

Figure III.B.10.8: Capacitors and dielectrics. Note that the capacitor is symbolized by two parallel lines of equal length. The electric fields: E_c generated by the capacitor, E_d generated by the dielectric, and E_n is the resultant electric field.

The energy associated with each charged capacitor is:

Potential Energy $(PE) = W = (1/2V)(Q) = 1/2QV$

also and

$W = 1/2(CV)(V) = 1/2CV^2$

$W = 1/2Q(Q/C) = 1/2Q^2/C$.

10.5 Root-Mean-Square Current and Voltage

DC (*direct current*) circuits contain a continuous current. Thus calculating power output is quite simple using $P = I^2R = IV$. However, AC (*alternating current*) circuits pulsate; consequently, we must discuss the average power output P_{av} where

$P_{av} = (I_{rms})^2 R = (I_{rms})(V_{rms})$

which is true for a purely resistive load where the root-mean-square (*rms*) values are determined from their maximal (*max*) values:

$I_{rms} = I_{max}/\sqrt{2}$ and $V_{rms} = V_{max}/\sqrt{2}$.

Thus by introducing the *rms* quantities the equations for DC and AC circuits have the same forms. AC circuit voltmeters and ammeters have their scales adjusted to read the *rms* values.

Go online to GAMSAT-prep.com for free chapter review Q&A and forum.

NOTES

GOLD NOTES

LIGHT AND GEOMETRICAL OPTICS
Chapter 11

Memorize

quations: PHY 11.3, 11.4, 11.5
ules for drawing ray diagrams

Understand

* Rules/equations: reflection, refraction, Snell's law
* Dispersion, total internal reflection
* Mirrors, lenses, real/virtual images
* Ray diagrams
* Lens strength, aberration

Not Required*

* Advanced level college info
* Memorization of constants

GAMSAT-Prep.com

Introduction

Geometrical optics describes the propagation of light in terms of "rays." Rays are then bent at the interface of 2 rather different substances (i.e. air and glass) thus the ray may curve. A basic understanding of the equations and the geometry of light rays is necessary for solving problems in geometrical optics. Discrete questions regarding total internal reflection are frequent. Usually for the real GAMSAT, they will provide you with the optics equations to solve problems when needed. However, sometimes knowing the equation will give you an edge for "theoretical" questions and this is why we recommend that many optics equations be memorized.

Additional Resources

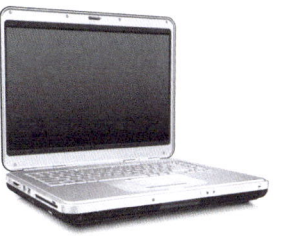

ree Online Q&A + Forum

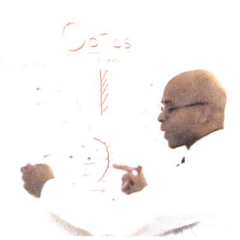

Video: Online or DVD

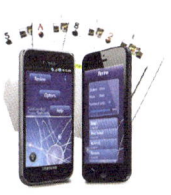

Flashcards

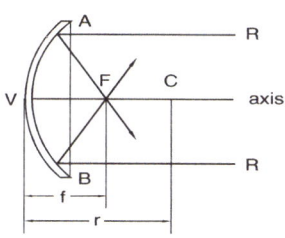

Special Guest

THE PHYSICAL SCIENCES   PHY-91

* The real GAMSAT may have advanced level information presented (ie. in a passage) but previous knowledge of said information is not required to answer the questions that would follow. Practice ACER and GS practice GAMSATs can help you clarify this point.

11.1 Visual Spectrum, Color

Geometrical optics is a first approximation of physical optics, which by its wavy nature, is part of the electromagnetic wave theory. The theory of light has a dualistic aspect:

- *particulate*: referring to a packet of energy called a photon when one wants, for example, to explain the photoelectric effect.

- *wavy*: when one wants to explain, for example, light interference and diffraction. Diffraction occurs when waves of light bend at the interface between two different media.

The optics domain of the electromagnetic wave theory corresponds to the following range of wavelengths of the electromagnetic spectrum (expressed in microns $1\mu = 10^{-6} m$):

$$0.4\mu < \lambda < 0.8\mu$$

or

$$0.4\mu < visible < 0.8\mu.$$

See PHY 9.2.4 for the colors in the visual spectrum. See PHY 9.2.4, 11.4 and 12.3 for the speed of light in a vacuum.

11.2 Polarization

An electromagnetic field is described as having at every point of the field two perpendicular vectors: *the electric field vector E and the magnetic induction field vector B.*

The electromagnetic wave front is polarized in a straight line when *E* and *B* are fixed at all times. Thus polarized light is light that has waves in only one plane.

11.3 Reflection, Mirrors

Reflection is the process by which light rays (= *imaginary lines drawn perpendicular to the advancing wave fronts*) bounce back into a medium from a surface with another medium (*versus being refracted or absorbed*). The ray that arrives is the *incident* ray while the ray that bounces back is the *reflected* ray. The laws of reflection are:

1) the angle of incidence (I) equals the angle of reflection (R) at the normal (N, the line perpendicular to the surface)
2) the I, R, N all lie in the same plane.

After a ray strikes a mirror or a lens it forms an image. A virtual image has no light rays passing through it and cannot be projected upon a screen.

A real image has light rays passing through it and can be projected upon a screen.

Mirrors have a plane surface, like an ordinary household mirror, or a non-plane surface. For a plane mirror, all incident light is reflected in parallel off the mirror and therefore all images seen are virtual, erect, left-right reversed and appear to be just as far (perpendicular distance) behind the mirror as the object is in front of the mirror.

In other words, the object (o) and the image (i) distances have the same magnitudes but have opposite directions ($i = -o$).

Spherical mirrors are non-plane mirrors which may have the reflecting surface convex (*diverges light*) or concave (*converges light*). Note the images formed by a converging mirror (concave) are like those for a converging lens (convex); and diverging mirrors (convex) and a diverging lens (concave) also form similar images. The terminology for spherical mirrors is :

r = radius of curvature
C = center of curvature
F = focal point

V = vertex (center of the mirror itself)
axis = line through C and V
f = focal length (distance from F to V)

i = image distance (distance from V to image along the axis)
o = object distance (distance from V to object along the axis)
AB = linear aperture (cord connecting the ends of the mirror; the larger the aperture, the better the resolution).

As a rule, capital letters refer to a point (*or position*) and small case letters refer to a distance.

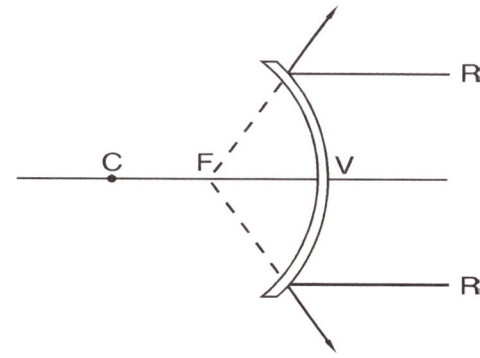

Concave (converging)   Convex (diverging)

Figure III.B.11.1: Reflection by spherical mirrors. R = the light rays.

With concave (spherical) mirrors the incident light is converged toward the axis. The path of light rays is as follows:

1)
if o < f, then the image is virtual and erect;
if o > f, then the image is real and inverted;
if o = f, then no image is formed;
2)
if o < r, then the image is enlarged in size;
if o > r, then the image is reduced in size;
if o = r, then the image is the same.

The relations are similar to those for a converging lens (convex). With convex (spherical) mirrors, the incident light is diverged from the axis after reflection. It is the backward extension (dotted lines in the diagram) that may pass through the focal point F. The path of light rays are as follows:

1) Incident rays parallel to the axis have backward extension of their reflections through F (see Figure III.B.11.1);
2) incident rays along a radius (that would pass C if extended) reflect back along themselves;
3) incident rays that pass through F (if extended) reflect parallel to the axis.

The image formed for a convex mirror is always virtual, erect and smaller than the object. The mirror equation and the derivations from it allow the above relations between object and image to be calculated instead of memorized. The equation is valid for convex and concave mirrors:

$$1/i + 1/o = 1/f$$

$$f = r/2$$

$$M = \text{magnification} = -i/o.$$

Convention:
• for i and o, *positive* values mean real, negative values mean virtual;
• for r and f, *positive* values mean converging, negative values mean diverging;
• for M, a *positive* value means erect, negative is inverted;
• for M > 1 the image is enlarged, M < 1 the image is diminished.

11.4 Refraction, Dispersion, Refractive Index, Snell's Law

Refraction is the bending of light as it passes from one transparent medium to another and is caused by the different speeds of light in the two media.

If θ_1 is taken as the angle (to the normal) of the incident light and θ_2 is the angle (to the normal) of the refracted light, where 1 and 2 represent the two different media, the following relations hold (Snell's Law):

where v = velocity and λ = wavelength.

$$\boxed{\frac{\sin \theta_1}{\sin \theta_2} = \frac{v_1}{v_2} = \frac{n_2}{n_1} = \frac{\lambda_1}{\lambda_2}}$$

$$\boxed{n = \frac{\text{speed of light in vacuum}}{\text{speed of light in medium}} = \frac{c}{v}}$$

$c = 3 \times 10^8$ m/sec or 181,000 mi/sec
$n = 1.0$ for air, $n = 1.33$ for H_2O
$n = 1.5$ for glass (at $\lambda = 589$ nm)
n = the refractive index which is a property of the medium
n_1 = refractive index of medium 1
n_2 = refractive index of medium 2
N = normal line to the surface
S = surface line, represents the separation between the two media (= interface = boundary)
I = incident light (= ray = beam)
R = refracted light (= ray = beam)

The speed at which light propagates through transparent materials, such as glass, water or air, is less than c, as you can tell from index of refractions above.

The angle θ is smaller (closer to the normal, e.g. θ_1) in the more optically dense (higher n) medium.

Also the smaller wavelength of the incident light (i.e. toward the violet end), the closer θ_2 is to the normal (i.e. it is smaller than θ_1).

This means longer wavelengths travel faster in a medium than shorter wavelengths (i.e. longer wavelengths are more subject to refraction).

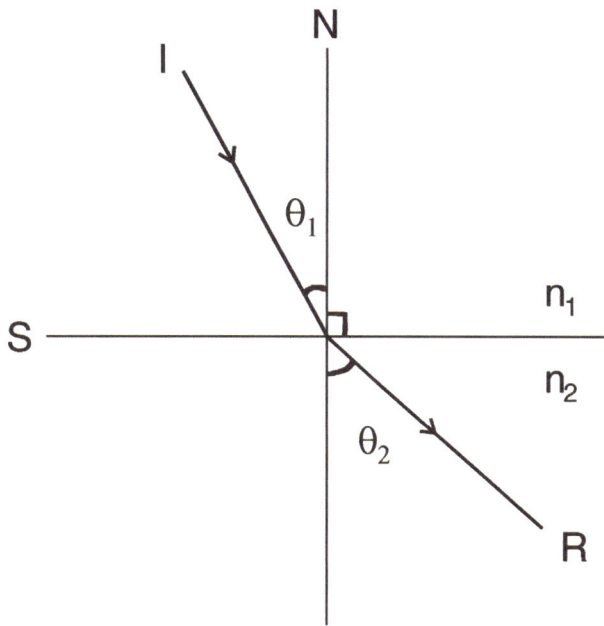

Figure III.B.11.2: Refraction.

This leads to *dispersion* which is the separation of white light (= *all colors together*) into individual colors by this differential refraction. For example, a prism disperses white light. See PHY 9.2.4.

The laws of refraction are:

1) The incident ray, the refracted ray and the normal ray all lie in the same plane.
2) The path of the ray (incident and refracted parts) is reversible.

When light passes from a more optically dense (higher n) medium into a less optically dense medium, there exists an angle of incidence such that the angle of refraction θ_2 is 90°.

This special angle of incidence is called the critical angle θ_c.

This is because when the angle of incidence is less then θ_c refraction occurs. If the angle of incidence is equal to θ_c, then neither refraction nor reflection occur.

And if $\theta_1 > \theta_c$, then total internal reflection (*ray is reflected back into the more optically dense medium*) occurs. The θ_c is found from Snell's Law:

$n_1 \sin\theta_c = n_2 \sin\theta_2$

and $\theta_2 = 90° \Rightarrow \sin\theta_2 = 1$

giving $n_1 \sin\theta_c = n_2 \times 1$

finally $\sin\theta_c = n_2/n_1$

where $n_2 < n_1$.

When looking at an object under water from above the surface, the object appears closer than it actually is. This is due to refraction. In general:

apparent depth/actual depth = n_2/n_1

where n_2 = the medium of the observer, and n_1 = the medium of the object.

11.5 Thin Lens, Diopters

A lens is a transparent material which refracts light. Converging lenses refract toward the axis, and diverging lenses refract the light away from the axis.

A converging lens is wider at the middle than at the ends, and the diverging lens is thinner at the middle than at the ends.

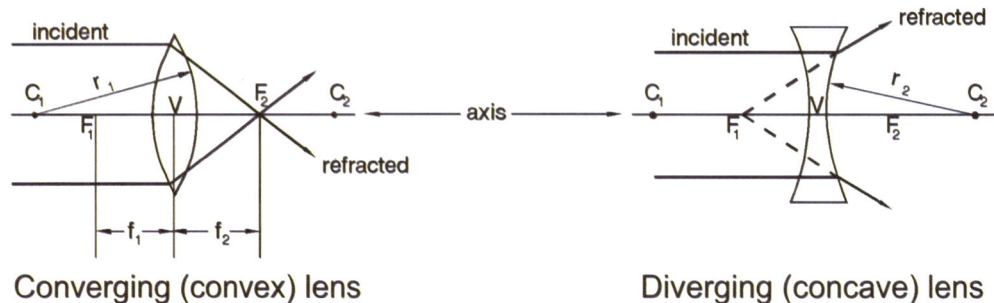

Converging (convex) lens　　　　Diverging (concave) lens

Figure III.B.11.3: Refraction by spherical lenses; *r* = the radius of curvature.

If the surface is convex, r is positive (e.g., r_1). If the surface is concave, r is negative (e.g., r_2).
Subscript 1 refers to the incident side, 2 refers to the refracted side.

C = center of curvature, F = focal point
V = the optical center of the lens or <u>v</u>ertex
axis = line through C and V

f = focal length is the distance between V and F
i = image distance (from V to the image)
o = object distance (from V to the object).

The path rays through a lens are:

1) incident rays parallel to the axis refract through F_2 of the converging lens, and appear to come from F_1 of a diverging lens (backward extensions of the refracted ray, see dotted line on diverging diagram);

2) an incident ray through F_1 of a converging lens or through F_2 of a diverging lens (if extended) are refracted parallel to the axis;

3) incident rays through V are not deviated (refracted).

For a converging lens (e.g., convex) the image formed depends on the object distance relative to the focal length (f). The relations (note similarity with a converging mirror) are:

1) if $o < f_1$, then image is virtual and erect;
   if $o > f_1$, the image is real and inverted;
   if $o = f_1$, then no image is formed;

2) if $o < 2f_1$, then the image is enlarged is size;
   if $o > 2f_1$, then the image is reduced in size;
   if $o = 2f_1$, then the image is the same.
   remember $2f_1 = r$.

For a diverging lens (e.g., concave), the image is always virtual, erect and reduced in size as for a diverging mirror.

The above relations can be calculated rather than memorized by use of the lens equation (similar to the mirror equation) and derivations from it,

1) $1/o + 1/i = 1/f$ (lens equation, same as mirror equation)

2) $D = 1/f = (n-1)(1/r_1 - 1/r_2)$, (lens maker's equation, n = index of refraction)

A <u>magnifying glass</u> (or "hand lens") is a convex lens that is used to produce a magnified image of an object. The lens is usually mounted in a frame with a handle. You can determine from the preceding rules that, in order to have an image that is erect (upright) and magnified for easier viewing, the object distance must be less than the focal length of the convex lens.

THE PHYSICAL SCIENCES

3) diopters (D) = 1/f where f is in meters, measures the refractive *power* of the lens; the larger the diopters, the stronger the lens. The diopters has a positive value for a converging lens and a negative value for a diverging lens.

To get the refractive power (D) of lenses in series just add the diopters which can then be converted into focal length:

$$D_T = D_1 + D_2 = 1/f_T \ (T = total).$$

4) Note that you can add only inverses of focal lengths :

$$1/f_T = 1/f_1 + 1/f_2 \ . \ . \ .$$

5) M = Magnification = $-i/o$ = $M_1 M_2$ for lenses in series.

Convention:
- for i and o, positive values mean real, negative values mean virtual;
- for r and f, positive values mean converging, negative values mean diverging;
- for M, a positive value means erect, negative is inverted.

The lens equation holds only for thin lenses (the thickness is small relative to other dimensions). For combination of lenses not in contact with each other, the image is found for the first lens (nearer the object) and then this image is used as the object of the second lens to find the image formed by it.

It should be noted that since concave lenses are concave on both sides they are sometimes called *biconcave*. Likewise, convex lenses may be called *biconvex*.

11.5.1 Lens Aberrations

In practice, the images formed by various refracting surfaces, as described in the previous section, fall short of theoretical perfection. Imperfections of image formation are due to several mechanisms or *aberrations*.

For example a nick or cut in a convex lens might create a microscopic area of concavity. Thus the light ray which strikes the aberration diverges instead of converging. Therefore the image will be less sharp or clear as the number or sizes of the aberrations increase.

Go online to GAMSAT-prep.com for free chapter review Q&A and forum.

GOLD NOTES

ATOMIC AND NUCLEAR STRUCTURE
Chapter 12

Memorize (Optional)	Understand	Not Required*
n relating energy and mass; half-life eta, gamma particles n for maximum number of electrons l n relating energy to frequency n for the total energy of the electrons om	* Basic atomic structure, amu * Fission, fusion; the Bohr model of the atom * Problem solving for half-life * Quantized energy levels for electrons * Fluorescence	* Advanced level college info * Memorizing mass: neutrons/protons/electrons * Memorizing constants, conversions

GAMSAT-Prep.com

Introduction

Atomic structure can be summarized as a nucleus orbited by electrons in different energy levels. Transition of electrons between energy levels and nuclear structure (i.e. protons, neutrons) are important characteristics of the atom. There is very little in this chapter that MUST be memorized for the GAMSAT. However, following our recommendations will give you an edge for many question types on this topic.

Additional Resources

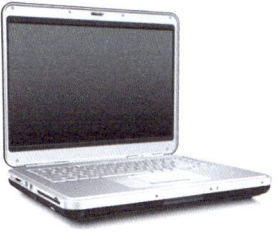

ree Online Q&A + Forum

Video: Online or DVD

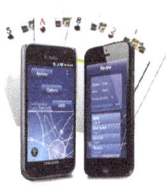

Flashcards

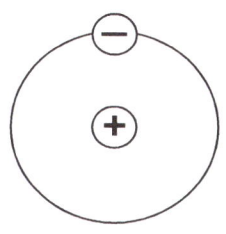

Special Guest

THE PHYSICAL SCIENCES PHY-101

* The real GAMSAT may have advanced level information presented (ie. in a passage) but previous knowledge of said information is not required to answer the questions that would follow. Practice ACER and GS practice GAMSATs can help you clarify this point.

12.1 Protons, Neutrons, Electrons

Only recently, with high resolution electron microscopes, have large atoms been visualized. However, for years their existence and properties have been inferred by experiments. Experimental work on gas discharge effects suggested that an atom is not a single entity but is itself composed of smaller particles. These were termed <u>elementary particles</u>. A more encompassing expression would be "subatomic" particles.

The atom appears as a small solar system with a heavy nucleus composed of positive particles and neutral particles: *protons and neutrons*. Around this nucleus, there are clouds of negatively charged particles, called *electrons*. The mass of a neutron is slightly more than that of a proton (both ≈ 1.7×10^{-24} g); the mass of the electron is considerably less (9.1×10^{-28} g).

Since an atom is electrically neutral, the negative charge carried by the electrons must be equal in magnitude (but opposite in sign) to the positive charge carried by the protons.

Experiments with electrostatic charges have shown that opposite charges attract (and like charges repel), so it can be considered that <u>electrostatic forces</u> hold an atom together. The difference between various atoms is therefore determined by their *composition*.

A hydrogen atom consists of one proton and one electron; a helium atom of two protons, two neutrons and two electrons. They are shown in diagram form in Figure III.B.12.1.

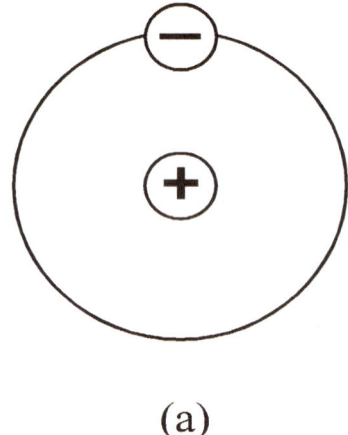
(a)

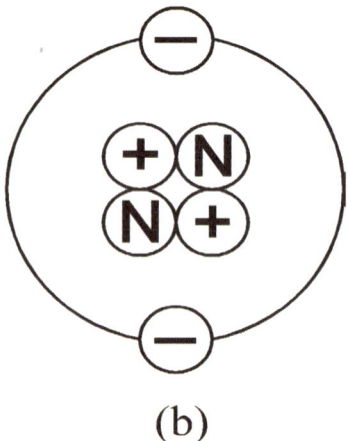
(b)

Figure III.B.12.1: Atomic structure simplified: (a) hydrogen atom; (b) helium atom.

12.2 Isotopes, Atomic Number, Atomic Weight

A proton has a mass of 1 a.m.u. (*atomic mass unit*) and a charge of +1, whereas, a neutron has a mass of 1 a.m.u. and no charge. The *atomic number* (*AN*) of an atom is the number of protons in the nucleus. In an atom of neutral charge, the atomic number (AN) is also equal to the number of electrons.

The atomic number is conventionally represented by the letter "Z". Each of the chemical elements has a unique number of protons which is identified by its own atomic number "Z". As an example, for the hydrogen H element, $Z = 1$ and for Na, $Z = 11$.

An *element* is a group of atoms with the same AN. *Isotopes* are elements which have the same atomic number (Z) but different number of neutrons and hence a different mass number (MN). As an example, the three carbon isotopes differ only in the number of neutrons and therefore have the same number of protons and electrons but differ in mass and are usually represented as follows: C-12, C-13 and C-14 or more specifically as follows: $^{12}_{6}C$, $^{13}_{6}C$ and $^{14}_{6}C$. It is therefore the number of protons that distinguishes elements from each other. The *weighted average* follows the natural abundance of the various isotopic compositions of an element.

The *mass number* (*MN*) of an atom is the number of protons and neutrons in an atom. The *atomic weight* (*AW*) is the weighted average of all naturally occurring isotopes of an element.

For example: Silicon is known to exist naturally as a mixture of three isotopes (Si-28, Si-29 and Si-30). The relative amount of each of the three different silicon isotopes is found to be 92.2297% with a mass of 27.97693, 4.6832% with a mass of 28.97649 and the remaining 3.0872% with a mass of 29.97377. The atomic weight of silicon is then determined as the weighted average of each of the isotopes as follows:

$$\begin{aligned} \text{Si mass} &= (27.97693 \times 0.922297) \\ &+ (28.97649 \times 0.046832) \\ &+ (29.97377 \times 0.030872) \\ &= 28.0854 \text{ g/mol.} \end{aligned}$$

It is also important to note that as the number of <u>protons</u> distinguishes *elements* from each other, it is their <u>electronic configuration</u> (CHM 2.1, 2.2, 2.3) that determines their *reactivity*.

The mass of a nucleus is always smaller than the combined mass of its constituent protons and neutrons. The difference in mass is converted to energy (E) which holds protons and neutrons together within the nuclear core.

Let's consider the number of protons and neutrons in two commonly discussed isotopes: carbon and hydrogen. Carbon C-12, C-13 and C-14 are isotopes with 12, 13 and 14 MN, respectively. The atomic number of carbon is 6 (this can be seen on a periodic table, CHM 2.4.1), which means that every carbon atom has 6 protons, so that the number of neutrons of these isotopes must be 6, 7 and 8, respectively. Likewise, hydrogen (AN = 1 = 1 proton) has 3 isotopes: H-1 (0 neutrons), H-2 (= deuterium, D; 1 neutron); and H-3 (= tritium, T; 2 neutrons).

12.3 Nuclear Forces, Nuclear Binding Energy, Stability, Radioactivity

Coulomb repulsive force (between protons) in the nuclei are overcome by nuclear forces. The nuclear force is a non-electrical type of force that binds nuclei together and is equal for protons and neutrons. The nuclear binding energy (E_b) is a result of the relation between energy and mass changes associated with nuclear reactions,

$$\Delta E = \Delta mc^2$$

in ergs in the CGS system, i.e. m = grams and c = cm/sec; ΔE = energy released or absorbed; Δm = mass lost or gained, respectively; c = velocity of light = 3.0×10^{10} cm/sec.

Conversions:
1 gram = 9×10^{20} ergs
1 a.m.u. = 931.4 MeV (Mev = 10^6 electron volts)
1 a.m.u. = 1/12 the mass of $_6C^{12}$.

The preceding equation is a statement of the law of conservation of mass and energy. The value of E_b depends upon the mass number (MN) as follows, (see Figure III.A.11.2):

The peak E_b/MN is at MN = 60. Also, E_b/MN is relatively constant after MN = 20. <u>Fission</u> is when a nucleus splits into smaller nuclei. <u>Fusion</u> is when smaller nuclei combine to form a larger nucleus. Energy is released from a nuclear reaction when nuclei with MN >> 60 undergo fission or nuclei with MN << 60 undergo fusion. Both fusion and fission release energy because the mass difference between the initial and the final nuclear states is converted into energy.

Not all combinations of protons are stable. The most stable nuclei are those with an even number of protons and an even number of neutrons. The least stable nuclei are those with an odd number of protons and an odd number of neutrons. Also, as the atomic number (AN) increases, there are more neutrons (N) needed for the nuclei to be stable.

According to the *Baryon number conservation*, the total number of protons and neutrons remains the same in a nuclear reaction even with the inter-conversions occurring between protons and neutrons.

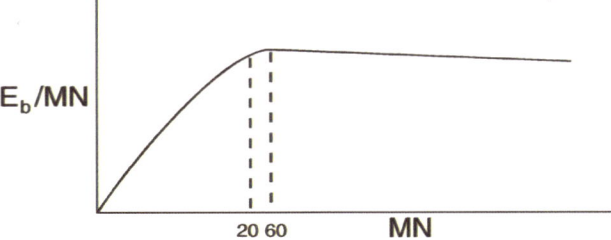

Figure III.A.11.2: Binding Energy per Nucleus. E_b/MN = binding energy per nucleus; this is the energy released by the formation of a nucleus.

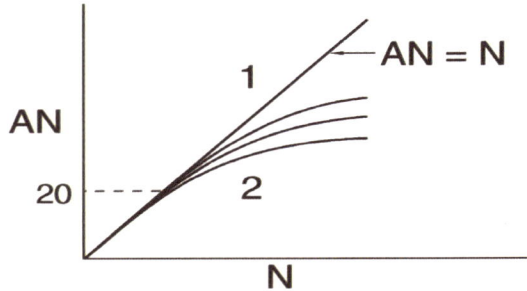

Figure III.A.11.3: Stability of Atoms. AN = atomic number and N = number of neutrons.

Up to AN = 20 (Calcium) the number of protons is equal to the number of neutrons, after this there are more neutrons. If an atom is in region #1 in Figure III.A.11.3, it has too many protons or too few neutrons and must decrease its protons or increase its neutrons to become stable. The reverse is true for region #2. All nuclei after AN = 84 (Polonium) are unstable.

Unstable nuclei become stable by fission to smaller nuclei or by absorption or emission of small particles. Spontaneous fission is rare. Spontaneous radioactivity (emission of particles) is common. The common particles are:

(1) alpha (α) particle = $_2He^4$ (helium nucleus);

(2) beta (β) particle = $_{-1}e^0$ (an electron);

(3) a positron $_{+1}e^0$ (same mass as an electron but opposite charge);

(4) gamma (γ) ray = no mass and no charge, just electromagnetic energy;

(5) orbital electron capture - nucleus takes electrons from K shell and converts a proton to a neutron. If there is a flux of particles such as neutrons ($_0n^1$), the nucleus can absorb these also.

> A neutron walks into a bar and asks the bartender: "How much for a beer?" The bartender answers: "For you, no charge." :)

12.4 Nuclear Reaction, Radioactive Decay, Half-Life

Nuclear reactions are reactions in which changes in nuclear composition occur. An example of a nuclear reaction which involves uranium and hydrogen:

$$_{92}U^{238} + _1H^2 \rightarrow _{93}Np^{238} + 2_0n^1$$

for $_{92}U^{238}$: 238 = mass number, 92 = atomic number. The sum of the lower (or higher) numbers on one side of the equation equals the sum of the lower (or higher) numbers on the other side of the equation. Another way of writing the preceding reaction is:

$_{92}U^{238}(_1H^2, 2_0n^1)_{93}Np^{238}$. {# neutrons (i.e. $_{92}U^{238}$) = superscript (238) – subscript (92) = 146}

Radioactive decay is a naturally occurring spontaneous process in which the atomic nucleus of an unstable atom loses energy by the emission of ionizing particles. Such unstable nuclei are known to spontaneously decompose and emit minute atomic sections to essentially gain some stability. The radioactive decay fragments are categorized into alpha, beta and gamma-ray decays. The radioactive decay can result in a nuclear change (*transmutation*) in which the parent and daughter nuclei are of different elements. For example, a C-14 atom may undergo an alpha decay and emit radiation and as a result, transform into a N-14 daughter nucleus. It is also possible that radioactive decay does not result in transmutation but only decreases the energy of the parent nucleus. As an example, a Ni-28 atom undergoing a gamma decay will emit radiation and then transform to a lower energy Ni-28 nucleus. The following is a brief description of the three known types of radioactive decay.

(1) **Alpha (α) decay:** Alpha decay is a type of radioactive decay in which an atomic nucleus emits an alpha particle. An alpha particle is composed of two protons and two neutrons which is identical to a helium-4 nucleus. An alpha particle is the most massive of all radioactive particles. Because of its relatively large mass, alpha particles tend to have the most potential to interact with other atoms and/or molecules and ionize them as well as lose energy. As such, these particles have the lowest penetrating power. If an atomic nucleus of an element undergoes alpha decay, this leads to a transmutation of that element into another element as shown below for the transmutation of Uranium-238 to Thorium-234:

$$^{238}_{92}U \rightarrow {}^{234}_{90}Th + {}^{4}_{2}He^{2+}$$
$$^{238}U \rightarrow {}^{234}Th + \alpha$$

(2) **Beta (β) decay:** Beta decay is a type of decay in which an unstable nucleus emits an electron or a positron. A positron is the antiparticle of an electron and has the same mass as an electron but opposite in charge. The electron from a beta decay forms when a neutron of an unstable nuclei changes into a proton and in the process, an electron is then emitted. The electron in this case is referred to as a beta minus particle or β⁻. In beta decays producing positron emissions, it is referred to as beta plus or β⁺. For an atomic nucleus undergoing beta decay, the process leads to the transmutation of that element into another as shown for the transmutation of Cesium-137 for beta minus and Na-22 for beta plus emissions:

$$^{137}_{55}Cs \rightarrow {}^{137}_{56}Ba + \beta^-$$
$$^{22}_{11}Na \rightarrow {}^{22}_{10}Ne + \beta^+$$

(3) **Gamma (γ) decay:** Gamma decay is different from the other two types of decays. Gamma decay emits a form of electromagnetic radiation. Gamma rays are high energy photons known to penetrate matter very well and are symbolized by the Greek letter gamma (γ). A source of gamma decay could be a case in which an excited daughter nucleus - following an alpha or beta decay - lowers its energy state further by gamma-ray emission without a change in mass number or atomic number. The following is an example:

$$^{60}Co \rightarrow {}^{60}Ni^* + \beta^-$$

Co-60 decays to an excited Ni*-60 via beta decay and subsequently, the excited Ni*-60 drops to ground state and emits gamma (γ) rays as follows:

$$^{60}Ni^* \rightarrow {}^{60}Ni + \gamma$$

To summarize, a gamma ray has no charge and no mass since it is a form of electromagnetic radiation. As shown, gamma rays are usually emitted in conjunction with other radiation emissions.

Spontaneous radioactive decay is a first order process. This means that the rate of decay is *directly* proportional to the amount of material present:

$$\Delta m/\Delta t = \text{rate of decay}$$

where Δm = change in mass, Δt = change in time.

The preceding relation is equalized by adding a proportionality constant called the decay constant (k) as follows,

$$\Delta m/\Delta t = -km.$$

The minus sign indicates that the mass is decreasing. Also, $k = -(\Delta m/m)/\Delta t$ = fraction of the mass that decays with time.

The *half-life* ($T_{1/2}$) of a radioactive atom is the time required for one half of it to disintegrate. The half-life is related to k as follows,

$$T_{1/2} = 0.693/k.$$

If the number of half-lifes n are known we can calculate the percentage of a pure radioactive sample left after undergoing decay since the fraction remaining $= (1/2)^n$.

For example, given a pure radioactive substance X with $T_{1/2}$ = 9 years, calculating the percentage of substance X after 27 years is quite simple,

$$27 = 3 \times 9 = 3\ T_{1/2}$$

Thus

$$n = 3,\ (1/2)^n = (1/2)^3 = 1/8 \text{ or } 13\%.$$

After 27 years of disintegration, 13% of pure substance X remains. {Similarly, note that *doubling time* is given by $(2)^n$; see BIO 2.2}

Table III.A.11.1: Modes of Radioactive Decay

Decay Mode	Participating particles	Change in (A, Z)	Daughter Nucleus
Alpha decay	α	A = –4, Z = –2	(A – 4, Z – 2)
Beta decay	β⁻	A = 0, Z = +1	(A, Z + 1)
Gamma decay	γ	A = 0, Z = 0	(A, Z)
Positron emission	β⁺	A = 0, Z = –1	(A, Z – 1)

GAMSAT-Prep.com
THE GOLD STANDARD

12.5 Quantized Energy Levels For Electrons, Emission Spectrum

Work by Bohr and others in the early part of the last century demonstrated that the electron orbits are arranged in shells, and that each shell has a defined maximum number of electrons it can contain.

For example, the first shell can contain two electrons, the second eight electrons (see CHM 2.1, 2.2). The maximum number of electrons in each shell is given by:

$$N_{electrons} = 2n^2$$

$N_{electrons}$ designates the number of electrons in shell n.

The state of each electron is determined by the four quantum numbers:

- principal quantum number n determines the number of shells, possible values are: 1 (K), 2 (L), 3 (M), etc...
- angular momentum quantum number l, determines the subshell, possible values are: 0 (s), 1 (p), 2 (d), 3 (f), n-1, etc...
- magnetic momentum quantum number m_l, possible values are: ±l, ... , 0
- spin quantum number m_s, determines the direction of rotation of the electron, possible values are: ±1/2.

Chemical reactions and electrical effects are all concerned with the behavior of electrons in the outer shell of any particular atom. If a shell is full, for example, the atom is unlikely to react with any other atom and

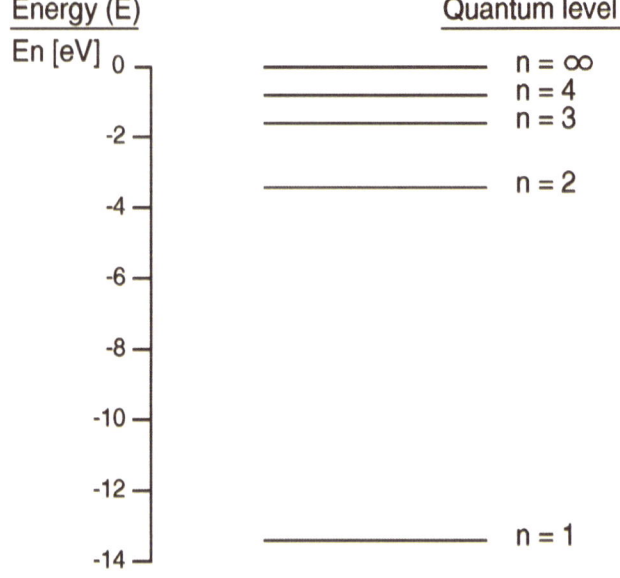

Figure III.A.11.4: Energy levels. The energy E_n in each shell n is measured in electron volts.

is, in fact, one of the noble (inert) gases such as helium.

The energy that an electron contains is not continuous over the entire range of possible energy. Rather, electrons in a atom may contain only discrete energies as they occupy certain orbits or shells. Electrons of each atom are restricted to these discrete energy levels. These levels have an energy below zero.

This means energy is released when an electron moves from infinity into these energy levels.

If there is one electron in an atom, its ground state is n = 1, the lowest energy level available. Any other energy level, n = 2, n = 3, etc., is considered an excited state for that electron. The difference in energy (E) between the levels gives the absorbed (or emitted) energy when an electron moves to a higher orbit (or lower orbit, respectively) and therefore, the frequency (f) of light necessary to cause excitation.

$$E_2 - E_1 = hf$$

where E_1 = energy level one, E_2 = energy level two, h = planck's constant, and f = the frequency of light absorbed or emitted.

Therefore, if light is passed through a substance (e.g., gas), certain wavelengths will be absorbed, which correspond to the energy needed for the electron transition. An *absorption* spectrum will result that has dark lines against a light background. Multiple lines result because there are possible transitions from all quantum levels occupied by electrons to any unoccupied levels.

An *emission* spectrum results when an electron is excited to a higher level by another particle or by an electric discharge, for example. Then, as the electron falls from the excited state to lower states, light is emitted that has a wavelength (which is related to frequency) corresponding to the energy difference between the levels since: $E_1 - E_2 = hf$.

The resulting spectrum will have light lines against a dark background. The absorption and emission spectrums should have the same number of lines but often will not. This is because in the absorption spectrum, there is a rapid radiation of the absorbed light in all directions, and transitions are generally from the ground state initially.

These factors result in fewer lines in the absorption than in the emission spectrum.

The total energy of the electrons in an atom, where KE is the kinetic energy, can be given by:

$$E_{total} = E_{emission} \text{ (or } E_{ionization}) + KE$$

12.6 Fluorescence

Fluorescence is an emission process that occurs after light absorption excites electrons to higher electronic and vibrational levels. The electrons spontaneously lose excited vibrational energy to the electronic states. There are certain molecular types that possess this property, e.g., some amino acids (tryptophan).

The fluorescence process is as follows:
- **step 1** - absorption of light;
- **step 2** - spontaneous deactivation of vibrational levels to zero vibrational level for electronic state;
- **step 3** - fluorescence with light emission (longer wavelength than absorption).

Figure III.B.12.5 shows diagrammatically the steps described above. Step 2 which is not shown in the figure is the intermediate step between light absorption and light emission. See BIO 1.5.1 for fluorescence as applied to microscopy.

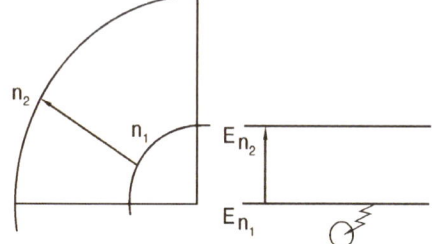
Step 1: light absorption

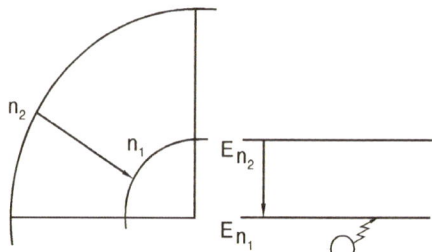
Step 3: light emission

Figure III.B.12.5: The fluorescence process. Represented is an atom with shells n_1, n_2 and their respective energy levels E_n.

NOTES

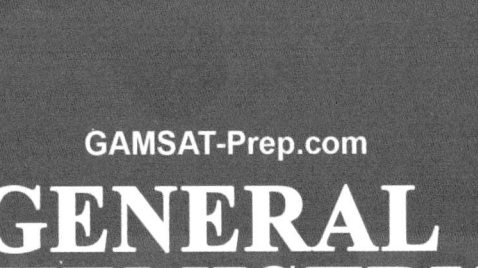

GAMSAT-Prep.com
GENERAL CHEMISTRY
PART III.A: PHYSICAL SCIENCES

IMPORTANT: Before doing your science survey for the GAMSAT, be sure you have read the Preface, Introduction and Part II, Chapter 2. The beginning of each science chapter provides guidelines as to what you should Memorize, Understand and what is Not Required. These are guides to get you a top score without getting lost in the details. Our guides have been determined from an analysis of all ACER materials plus student surveys. Additionally, the original owner of this book gets a full year access to many online features described in the Preface and Introduction including an online Forum where each chapter can be discussed.

STOICHIOMETRY

Chapter 1

Memorize	Understand	Not Required*
ine: molecular weight ine: empirical/molecular formula es for oxidation numbers	* Composition by % mass * Mole concept, limiting reactants * Avogadro's number * Calculate theoretical yield * Basic types of reactions * Calculation of ox. numbers	* Advanced level college info * Balancing complex equations * Stoichiometric coefficients in competing reactions

GAMSAT-Prep.com

Introduction

Matter can be described as the substance that makes up all observable physical objects. Chemistry is the study of the composition, structure, properties and change of matter. This includes atoms (Physics Chapter 12) and molecules. The latter is characterized by chemical bonds formed between atoms to create chemical compounds. Stoichiometry is simply the math behind the chemistry involving products and reactants. The math is quite simple, in part, because of the law of conservation of mass that states that the mass of a closed system will remain constant throughout a chemical reaction.

Additional Resources

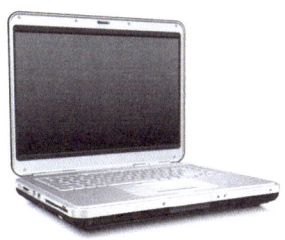

Free Online Q&A + Forum

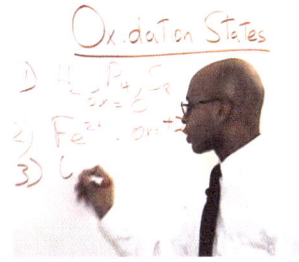

Video: Online or DVD

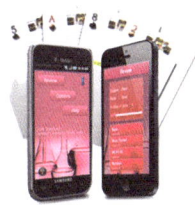

Flashcards

THE PHYSICAL SCIENCES   CHM-03

* The real GAMSAT may have advanced level information presented (ie. in a passage) but previous knowledge of said information is not required to answer the questions that would follow. Practice ACER and GS practice GAMSATs can help you clarify this point.

1.1 Generalities

Most substances known to us are mixtures of pure compounds. Air, for instance, contains the pure compounds nitrogen (~78%), oxygen (~21%), water vapor and many other gases (~1%). The compositional ratio of air or any other mixture may vary from one location to another. Each pure compound is made up of molecules which are composed of smaller units: the *atoms*. Atoms combine in very specific ratios to form molecules. A molecule is the smallest unit of a compound presenting the properties of that compound. During a chemical reaction molecules break down into individual atoms which then recombine to form new compounds. Stoichiometry establishes relationships between the above-mentioned specific ratios for individual molecules (or moles) or for molecules involved in a given chemical reaction.

1.2 Empirical Formula vs. Molecular Formula

The molecules of oxygen (O_2) are made up of two atoms of the same element. Water molecules on the other hand are composed of two different elements: hydrogen and oxygen in the specific ratio 2:1. Note that water is not a mixture of hydrogen and oxygen since this ratio is specific and does not vary with the location or the experimental conditions. The *empirical formula* of a pure compound is the simplest whole number ratio between the numbers of atoms of the different elements making up the compound. For instance, the empirical formula of water is H_2O (2:1 ratio) while the empirical formula of hydrogen peroxide is HO (1:1 ratio). The *molecular formula* of a given molecule states the exact number of the different atoms that make up this molecule. The empirical formula of water is identical to its molecular formula, i.e. H_2O; however, the molecular formula of hydrogen peroxide, H_2O_2, is different from its empirical formula (both correspond to a 1:1 ratio).

1.3 Mole - Atomic and Molecular Weights

Because of the small size of atoms and molecules chemists have to consider collections of a large number of these particles to bring chemical problems to our macroscopic scale. Collections of tens or dozens of atoms are still too small to achieve this practical purpose. For various reasons the number 6.02×10^{23} (Avogadro's number:N_A) was chosen. It is the number of atoms in 12 grams of the most abundant *isotope* of carbon (isotopes are elements which are identical chemically since the number of protons are the same; their masses differ slightly since the number of neutrons differ). A mole of atoms or molecules (or in fact any particles in general) contains an Avogadro number of these particles. The weight in grams of a mole of atoms of a given element is the gram-atomic weight, GAW, of that element (sometimes weight is measured in atomic mass units - see PHY 12.2, 12.3). Along the same lines, the weight in grams of a mole of molecules of a given compound is its gram-molecular weight, GMW. Here are some equations relating these concepts in a way that will help you solve some of the stoichiometry problems:

For an element:
$$\text{moles} = \frac{\text{weight of sample in grams}}{\text{GAW}}$$

For a compound:
$$\text{moles} = \frac{\text{weight of sample in grams}}{\text{GMW}}$$

The GAW of a given element is not to be confused with the mass of a single atom of this element. For instance the mass of a single atom of carbon-12 (GAW = 12 g) is $12/N_A = 1.993 \times 10^{-23}$ grams. Atomic weights are dimensionless numbers based on carbon-12 as the reference standard isotope and are defined as follows:

$$\frac{\text{mass of an atom of X}}{\text{mass of an atom of Y}} = \frac{\text{atomic weight of element X}}{\text{atomic weight of element Y}}$$

Clearly if the reference element Y is chosen to be carbon-12 (which is the case in standard periodic tables) the GAW of any element X is numerically equal to its atomic weight. In the table of atomic weights, all the elements then have values in which are relative to the carbon-12 isotope. The molecular weight of a given molecule is equal to the sum of the atomic weights of the atoms that make up the molecule. For example, the molecular weight of H_2O is equal to 18.0 amu/molecule (H = 1.008 and O = 16.00). The molar weight (or molar mass) of H_2O is numerically equal to the molecular weight (18.0) however, the units are in grams/mol as the molar weight is based on a mole amount of substance. Thus, molecular weight and molar weight are numerically equivalent however, molecular weight is the weight (amu) per molecule and molar weight is based on the weight (grams) per mole (1 mol = 6.02×10^{23} molecules).

1.4 Composition of a Compound by Percent Mass

The percentage composition of a compound is the percent of the total mass of a given element in that compound. For instance, the chemical analysis of a 100 g sample of pure vitamin C demontrates that there are 40.9 g of carbon, 4.58 g of hydrogen and 54.5 g of oxygen. The percentage composition of pure vitamin C is:

%C = 40.9; %H = 4.58; %O = 54.5

The composition of a compound by percent mass is closely related to its empirical formula. For instance, in the case of vitamin

C, the determination of the number of moles of atoms of C, H or O in a 100 g of vitamin C is rather straightforward:

moles of atoms of C in a 100 g of vitamin C = 40.9/12.0 = 3.41

moles of atoms of H in a 100 g of vitamin C = 4.58/1.01 = 4.53

moles of atoms of O in a 100 g of vitamin C = 54.5/16.0 = 3.41

[GAW can be determined from the periodic table in Chapter 2]

To deduce the smallest ratio between the numbers above, one follows the simple procedure:

(i) divide each one of the previously obtained numbers of moles by the smallest one of them (3.41 in our case):

for C: 3.41 mol/3.41 mol = 1.00
for H: 4.53 mol/3.41 mol = 1.33
for O: 3.41 mol/3.41 mol = 1.00

(ii) multiply the numbers obtained in the previous step by a small number to obtain a whole number ratio. In our case we need to multiply by 3 (in most cases this factor is between 1 and 5) so that:

for C: 1.00 × 3 = 3
for H: 1.33 × 3 = 4 and
for O: 1.00 × 3 = 3

Therefore, in this example, the simplest whole number ratio is 3C:4H:3O and we conclude that the empirical formula for vitamin C is: $C_3H_4O_3$.

In the previous example, instead of giving the composition of vitamin C by percent weight we could have provided the raw chemical analysis data and asked for the determination of that composition.

For instance, this data would be that the burning of a 4.00 mg sample of pure vitamin C yields 6.00 mg of CO_2 and 1.632 mg of H_2O. Since there are 12.0 g of carbon in 44.0 g of CO_2 the number of milligrams of carbon in 6.00 mg of CO_2 (which corresponds to the number of mg of carbon in 4.00 mg of vitamin C) is simply:

6.00 mg × (12.0 g C/44.0 g CO_2) = 1.636 mg of C in 6.00 mg of CO_2 or 4.00 mg of vitamin C for further clarification.

To convert this number into a percent mass is then trivial (GM 1.4.3). Similarly, the percent mass of hydrogen is obtained from the previous data and bearing in mind that there are 2.02 g of hydrogen (and not 1.01 g) in 18.0 g of water.

Incidentally, "burning" means <u>combustion</u> (CHM 1.5.1, ORG 3.2.1) which takes place in the presence of excess oxygen and results in the production of heat (exothermic), the conversion of the chemical species (new products), and light can be produced (glowing or a flame).

> The real GAMSAT does not usually provide a periodic table so the atomic weights (amu) will be given when required. Also, since calculators are not permitted, you should practice performing all calculations that you see in this textbook.

GENERAL CHEMISTRY

1.5 Description of Reactions by Chemical Equations

The convention for writing chemical equations is as follows: compounds which initially combine or react in a chemical reaction are called *reactants*; they are always written on the left-hand side of the chemical equation. The compounds which are produced during the same process are referred to as the *products* of the chemical reaction; they always appear on the right-hand side of the chemical equation. In the chemical equation:

$$2\ BiCl_3 + 3\ H_2O \rightarrow Bi_2O_3 + 6\ HCl$$

the coefficients represent the relative number of moles of reactants that combine to form the corresponding relative number of moles of products: they are the stoichiometric coefficients of the balanced chemical equation. The law of conservation of mass requires that the number of atoms of a given element remains constant during the process of a chemical reaction.

Balancing a chemical equation is putting this general principle into practice. Chemical equations must be balanced so that there are equal numbers of atoms of each element on both sides of the equation. Many equations are balanced by trial and error however, caution must be practiced when balancing a chemical equation. It is always easier to balance elements that appear only in one compound on each side of the equation; therefore, as a general rule, always balance those elements first and then deal with those which appear in more than one compound last. Thus, a general suggestive procedure for balancing equations would be as follows: (1) count and compare the atoms on both sides of the chemical equation, (2) balance each element one at a time by placing whole number coefficients in front of the formulas resulting in the same number of atoms of each element on each side of the equation. Remember that a coefficient in front of a formula multiplies every atom in the formula (i.e., $2BiCl_3 = 2Bi + 6Cl$). It is best to leave pure elements or metals until the end. Therefore, balance the carbon atoms in both the reactant and product side first. (3) Balance hydrogens in both the reactant and products; and (4) finally, check if all elements are balanced with the smallest possible set of whole number coefficients.

Given the preceding chemical reaction, if H_2O is present in excessive quantity, then $BiCl_3$ would be considered the **limiting reactant.** In other words, since the amount of $BiCl_3$ is relatively small, it is the $BiCl_3$ which determines how much product will be formed. Thus if you were given 316 grams of $BiCl_3$ in *excess* H_2O and you needed to determine the quantity of HCl produced (theoretical yield), you would proceed as follows:

▶ Determine the number of moles of $BiCl_3$ (see CHM 1.3) given Bi = 209 g/mol and Cl = 35.5 g/mol, thus $BiCl_3$ = (1 × 209) + (3 × 35.5) = 315.5 or approximately 316 g/mol:

moles $BiCl_3$ = (316 g)/(316 g/mol)
= 1.0 mole of $BiCl_3$.

▶ From the stoichiometric coefficients of the balanced equation:

- 2 moles of $BiCl_3$: 6 moles of HCl; therefore, 1 mole of $BiCl_3$: 3 moles of HCl
- Given H = 1.00 g/mol, thus HCl = 36.5 g/mol, we get:

3 moles × 36.5 g/mol = 110 g of HCl (approx.).

Please note: The theoretical yield is the calculated amount of product that can be predicted from a balanced chemical reaction and is seldom obtained in the laboratory. The actual yield is the actual amount of product produced and recovered in the laboratory. The Percentage yield = Actual yield/Theoretical Yield × 100%.

1.5.1 Categories of Chemical Reactions

Throughout the chapters in General Chemistry we will explore many different types of chemicals and some of their associated reactions. The various chemical reactions may be classified generally as either a redox type (see section 1.6) or as a non-redox type reaction. The following chart represents an overview of the chemical reaction classifications (categories) followed by a brief description of each of the reaction categories. Follow the chart like a story that you should revisit but do not memorize.

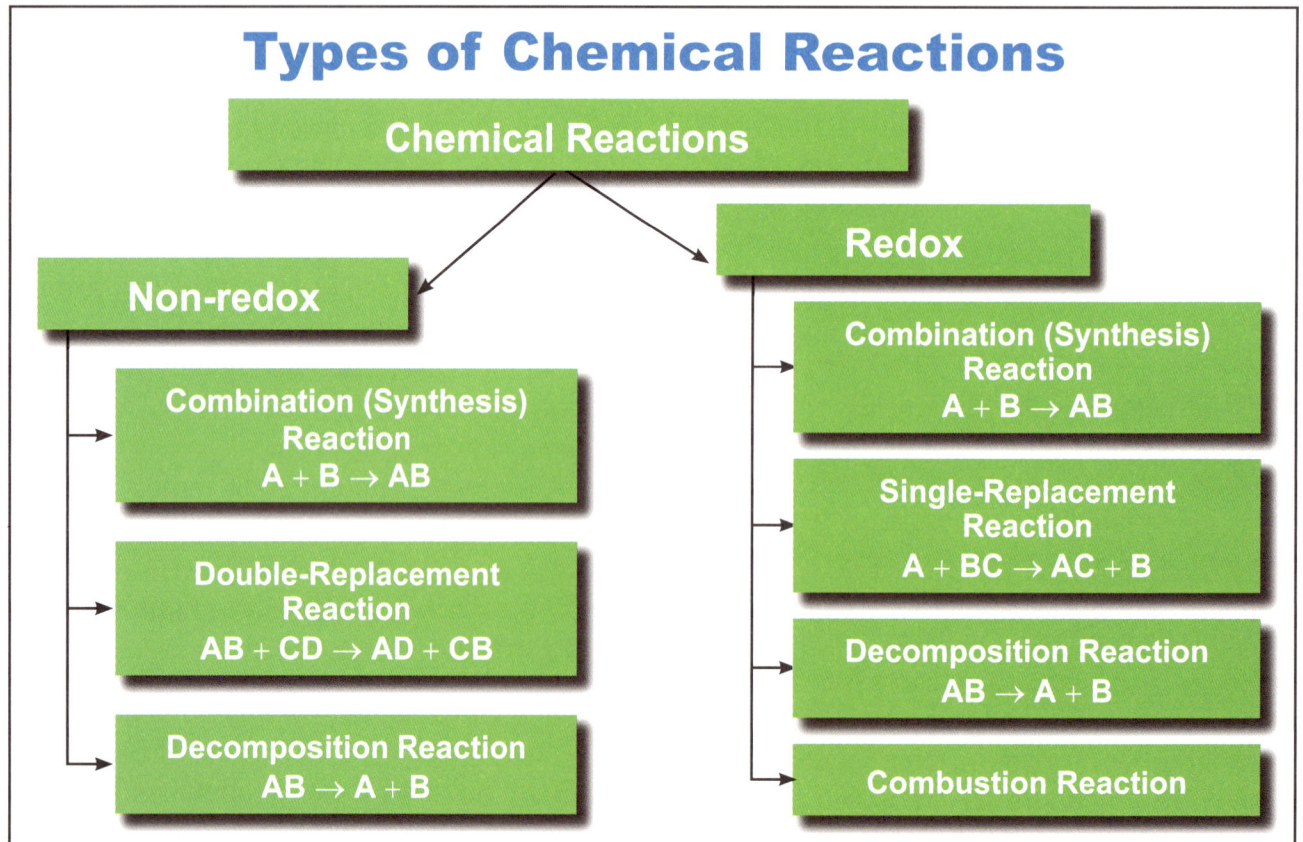

CHM-08 STOICHIOMETRY

GENERAL CHEMISTRY

Non-redox

Combination (Synthesis) Reaction

General equation: A + B → AB

Example: $SO_2(g) + H_2O(l) \rightarrow H_2SO_3(aq)$

Double-Replacement Reaction (or Metathesis Reaction)

(a) Precipitation Type

General equation: AB + CD → AD + CB

Example: $CaCl_2(aq) + Na_2CO_3(aq)$
$\rightarrow CaCO_3(s) + 2NaCl(aq)$

(b) Acid-Base Neutralization Type

General equation: HA + BOH → H$_2$O + BA
(HA = any H$^+$ acid & BOH = any OH$^-$ Base)

Example:
$2HCl(l) + Ba(OH)_2(aq) \rightarrow H_2O(l) + BaCl_2(aq)$

(c) Gas Evolution Type Reaction

General equation: HA + B → H$_2$O + BA
(HA = H$^+$ acid & B = special base salt NaHCO$_3$)

Example: $HCl(aq) + NaHCO_3(aq)$
$\rightarrow H_2CO_3(aq)^* + NaCl(aq)$
$\rightarrow H_2O(l) + CO_2(g) + NaCl(aq)$
(*H$_2$CO$_3$ is carbonic acid, the "fizz" in sodas, which degrades to CO$_2$(g) and H$_2$O(l))

Decomposition Reaction (CHM 4.3.1)

General equation: AB → A + B

Example: $H_2CO_3(aq) \rightarrow H_2O(l) + CO_2(g)$

Redox

Combination (Synthesis) Reaction

General equation: A + B → AB

Example: $SO_3(g) + H_2O(l) \rightarrow H_2SO_4(aq)$

Single-Replacement Reaction

General equation: A + BC → AC + B

Example:
$Zn(s) + CuSO_4(aq) \rightarrow Cu(s) + ZnSO_4(aq)$

Decomposition Reaction

General equation: AB → A + B

Example: $2NaCl(s) \rightarrow 2Na(l) + Cl_2(g)$
(electrolysis reaction)

Combustion Reaction

Example: $CH_4(g) + 2O_2(g) \rightarrow CO_2(g) + 2H_2O(g)$

Note that compounds in the preceding chart are identified as solid (s), liquid (l), gas (g) or solubilized in water which is an aqueous (aq) solution.

Combination (or synthesis) and decomposition type reactions are classified as both redox and non-redox reactions. Single replacement and combustion type reactions are classified as only redox type reactions; as the oxidation state of at least one atom species changes through electron transfer (oxidation/reduction) on either side of the chemical equation.

GAMSAT-Prep.com
THE GOLD STANDARD

The double-replacement type reactions are basically known as precipitation (or solid forming) type reactions or acid-base (neutralization) type reactions. A double replacement type reaction involves ions (CHM 5.2) which exchange partners and may or may not form precipitates depending on the water solubility of the products formed (CHM 5.3). In acid-base (neutralization) type reactions, the usual products formed are both water and a salt (CHM 6.7). Certain acid-base type reactions however are known to form gas products otherwise known as "Gas Evolution type reactions" due to the instability of an intermediate salt product formed as a result of the acid-base reaction (see preceding chart).

When replacement reactions occur, often there are ions known as "spectator ions" that do not undergo any changes and remain ionized in aqueous solutions (cf. ORG 1.6). These ions can be left out of the end equation known as a "net ionic equation" because it does away with the spectator ions that are not consequential to the reaction. Net ionic equations are used to show the actual chemical reaction that occurs during a single or double-replacement type reaction. Thus, it is essential to recognize and familiarize oneself to the various categories of reactions to enable one to further understand chemical reactivity.

1.6 Oxidation Numbers, Redox Reactions, Oxidizing vs. Reducing Agents

A special class of reactions known as *redox* reactions are better balanced using the concept of oxidation state. In a redox reaction, oxidation and reduction must occur simultaneously. Oxidation is defined as either an increase in oxidation number or a loss of one or more electrons and reduction is defined as a decrease in oxidation number or a gain of one or more electrons. This section deals with these reactions in which electrons are transferred from one atom (or a group of atoms) to another.

First of all, it is very important to understand the difference between the ionic charge and the oxidation state of an element. For this let us consider the two compounds sodium chloride (NaCl) and water (H_2O). NaCl is made up of the charged species or ions: Na^+ and Cl^-. During the formation of this ionic compound, one electron is transferred from the Na atom to the Cl atom. It is possible to verify this fact experimentally and determine that the charge of sodium in NaCl is indeed $+1$ and that the one for chlorine is -1. The elements in the periodic table tend to lose (oxidation) or gain (reduction) electrons to different extents. Therefore, even in non-ionic compounds electrons are always transferred, to different degrees, from one atom to another during the formation of a molecule of the compound. The actual partial charges that result from these partial transfers of electrons can also be determined experimentally. The oxidation state is not equal to such partial charges. It is rather an artificial concept that is used to perform some kind of "electron bookkeeping."

In a molecule like H₂O, since oxygen tends to attract electrons more than hydrogen, one can predict that the electrons that allow bonding to occur between hydrogen and oxygen will be displaced towards the oxygen atom. For the sake of "electron bookkeeping" we assign these electrons to the oxygen atom. The charge that the oxygen atom would have in this artificial process would be –2: this defines the oxidation state of oxygen in the H₂O molecule. In the same line of reasoning one defines the oxidation state of hydrogen in the water molecule as +1. The actual partial charges of hydrogen and oxygen are in fact smaller; but, as we will see later, the concept of oxidation state is very useful in stoichiometry.

Here are the general rules one needs to follow to assign oxidation numbers (or oxidation states) to different elements in different compounds:

1. In elementary substances, the oxidation number of an uncombined element regardless of whether it is monatomic (1 atom), diatomic (2 atoms) or polyatomic (multiple atoms), is zero. This is, for instance, the case for N in N_2 or Na in sodium element, O in O_2, or S in S_8.

2. In monatomic ions the oxidation number of the element that make up this ion is equal to the charge of the ion. This is the case for Na in Na⁺ (+1) or Cl in Cl⁻ (–1) or Fe in Fe³⁺ (+3). Clearly, monatomic ions are the only species for which atomic charges and oxidation numbers coincide.

3. In a neutral molecule the sum of the oxidation numbers of all the elements that make up the molecule is zero. In a polyatomic ion (e.g. SO_4^{2-}) the sum of the oxidation numbers of the elements that make up this ion is equal to the charge of the ion.

4. Some useful oxidation numbers to memorize:

For H: +1, except in metal hydrides (general formula XH where X is from the first two columns of the periodic table; CHM 2.4.1) where it is equal to –1.

For O: –2 in most compounds. In peroxides (e.g. in H_2O_2) the oxidation number for O is –1, it is +2 in OF_2 and –1/2 in superoxides (e.g. potassium superoxide: KO_2 which contains the O_2^- ion as opposed to the O^{2-} ion).

For alkali metals (first column in the periodic table): +1.

For alkaline earth metals (second column): +2.

Aluminium always has an oxidation number of +3 in all its compounds. (i.e. chlorides $AlCl_3$, nitrites $Al(NO_2)_3$, etc.)

The oxidation number of each Group VIIA element is –1; however, when it is combined with an element of higher electronegativity, the oxidation number is +1. For example, the oxidation number of Cl is –1 in HCl and the oxidation number of Cl is +1 in HClO.

An element is said to have been *reduced* during a reaction if its oxidation number decreased during this reaction, it is said to have been oxidized if its *oxidation* number increased. A simple example is:

$$Zn(s) + CuSO_4(aq) \longrightarrow ZnSO_4(aq) + Cu(s)$$

Oxid.#: Zn(s) = 0, CuSO₄(aq) = +2
Oxid.#: ZnSO₄(aq) = +2, Cu(s) = 0

During this reaction Cu is reduced (oxidation number decreases from +2 to 0) while Zn is oxidized (oxidation number increases from 0 to +2). Since, in a sense, Cu is reduced by Zn, Zn can be referred to as the reducing agent. Similarly, Cu is the oxidizing agent.

In chapters to come, we will discuss redox titrations (CHM 6.10) and more redox reactions in electrochemistry (CHM 10.1). Many of the redox agents in the table below will be explored in the chapters on Organic Chemistry.

Common Redox Agents	
Reducing Agents	**Oxidizing Agents**
* Lithium aluminium hydride (LiAlH₄) * Sodium borohydride (NaBH₄) * Metals * Ferrous ion (Fe²⁺)	* Iodine (I₂) and other halogens * Permanganate (MnO₄) salts * Peroxide compounds (i.e. H₂O₂) * Ozone (O₃); osmium tetroxide (OsO₄) * Nitric acid (HNO₃); nitrous oxide (N₂O)

How many moles are in guacamole?
Avocado's number.   :)

GOLD NOTES

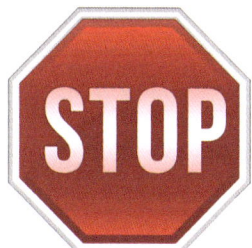

Reminder: Chapter review questions are available online for the original owner of this textbook. Doing practice questions will help clarify concepts and ensure that you study in a targeted way. First, register at gamsat-prep.com, then login and click on GAMSAT Textbook Owners in the right column so you can use your Online Access Card to have access to the Lessons section.

No science background? Consider watching the relevant videos at gamsat-prep.com and you have support at gamsat-prep.com/forum. Don't forget to check the Index at the beginning of this book to see which chapters are **HIGH**, **MEDIUM** and **LOW** relative importance for the GAMSAT.

Your online access continues for one full year from your online registration.

GOLD NOTES

ELECTRONIC STRUCTURE AND THE PERIODIC TABLE
Chapter 2

Memorize	Understand	Not Required*
• initions of quantum numbers • pes of s, p orbitals • er for filling atomic orbitals • location of the first 20 elements he periodic table	* Conventional notation, Pauli, Hund's * Box diagrams, IP, electronegativity * Valence, EA * Variation in shells, atomic size * Trends in the periodic table	* Advanced level college info * Memorizing Schroedinger's equation * IUPAC's systematic element names (gen. chem.)

GAMSAT-Prep.com

Introduction

The periodic table of the elements provides data and abbreviations for the names of elements in a tabular layout. The purpose of the table is to illustrate recurring (periodic) trends and to classify and compare the different types of chemical behavior. To do so, we must first better understand the atom. The periodic table is not usually provided in the real GAMSAT but you are still responsible for knowing the trends and relative locations of the most common atoms.

Additional Resources

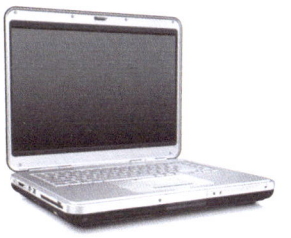　　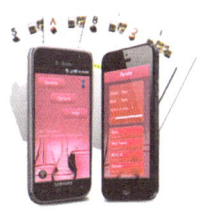　　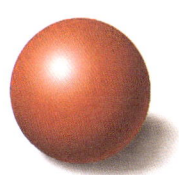

Free Online Q&A + Forum　　Video: Online or DVD　　Flashcards　　Special Guest

THE PHYSICAL SCIENCES   CHM-15

* The real GAMSAT may have advanced level information presented (ie. in a passage) but previous knowledge of said information is not required to answer the questions that would follow. Practice ACER and GS practice GAMSATs can help you clarify this point.

2.1 Electronic Structure of an Atom

The modern view of the structure of atoms is based on a series of discoveries and complicated theories that were put forth at the turn of the twentieth century. The atom represents the smallest unit of a chemical element. It is composed of subatomic particles: protons, neutrons and electrons. At the center of the atom is the nucleus composed of protons and neutrons surrounded by electrons forming an electron cloud.

The protons and neutrons have nearly identical masses of approximately 1 amu whereas electrons, by contrast, have an almost negligible mass. Protons and electrons both have electrical charges equal in magnitude but opposite in sign. Protons consist of a single positive (+1) charge, electrons consist of a single negative charge (–1) and neutrons have no charge (Physics Chapter 12).

Atoms have equal numbers of protons and electrons unless ionization occurs in which ions are formed. Ions are defined as atoms with either a positive charge (cation) due to loss of one or more valence electrons or negative charge (anion) as a result of a gain in electron(s). An atom's valence electrons are electrons furthest from the nucleus and are responsible for an element's chemical properties and are instrumental in chemical bonding (See CHM 2.2 and 2.3 and Chapter 3).

Atoms of a given element all have an equal number of protons however, may vary in the number of neutrons. Atoms that differ only by neutron number are known as isotopes. Isotopes have the same atomic number but differ in atomic mass due to the differences in their neutron numbers. As they have the same atomic number, isotopes therefore exhibit the same chemical properties.

In the following paragraphs, we will only present the main ideas behind the findings that shaped our understanding of atomic structure. The first important idea is that electrons (as well as any subatomic particles) are in fact waves as well as particles; this concept is often referred to in textbooks as the "dual nature of matter".

Contrary to classical mechanics, in this modern view of matter information on particles is not derived from the knowledge of their position and momentum at a given time but by the knowledge of the wave function (mathematical expression of the above-mentioned wave) and their energy. Mathematically, such information can be derived, in principle, by solving the master equation of quantum mechanics known as the Schrödinger equation. Moreover, the mathematical derivation of atomic orbitals and respective energies comes from solving the equation which includes the total energy profiles for the electrons as well as the wave function describing the wavelike nature of the electrons. Thus, the various solutions to the Schrödinger equation describes the atomic orbitals as complicated wave functions which may alternatively be graphically represented (See Figure III.A.2.1 and Figure III.A.2.2).

In the case of the hydrogen atom, this equation can be solved exactly. It yields the possible states of energy in which the electron can be found within the hydrogen atom and the wave functions associated with these states. The square of the wave function associated with a given state of energy gives the probability to find the electron, which is in that same state of energy, at any given point in space at any given time. These wave functions as well as their geometrical representations are referred to as the *atomic orbitals*. We shall explain further below the significance of these geometrical representations.

Atoms of any element tend to exist toward a minimal energy level (= ground state) unless subjected to an external environmental change. Even for a hydrogen atom there is a large number of possible states in which its single electron can be found (when it is subjected to different external perturbations). A labeling of these states is necessary. This is done using the quantum numbers. Hence, any orbital may be completely described by four quantum numbers; n, l, m_l and m_s. The position and energy of an electron and each of the orbitals are therefore described by its quantum number or energy state. The four quantum numbers are thus described as follows:

(i) n: *the principal quantum number*. This number takes the integer values 1, 2, 3, 4, 5… The higher the value of n the higher the energy of the state labelled by this n. This number defines the atomic shells K (n = 1), L (n = 2), M (n = 3) etc… or the size of an orbital.

(ii) l: *the angular momentum quantum number*. It defines the shape of the atomic orbital in a way which we will discuss further below. For a given electronic state of energy defined by n, l takes all possible integer values between 0 and n – 1. For instance for a state with n = 0 there is only one possible shape of orbital, it is defined by l = 0. For a state defined by n = 3 there are 3 possible orbital shapes with l = 0, 1 and 2.

All orbitals with l = 0 are called "s"-shaped, all with l = 1 are "p"-shaped, those with l = 2 or 3 are "d" or "f"-shaped orbitals respectively. The important shapes to remember are: i) s = spherical, and ii) p = 2 lobes or "dumbbell" (*see the following diagrams*). For values of l larger than 3, which occur with an n greater or equal to 4, the corresponding

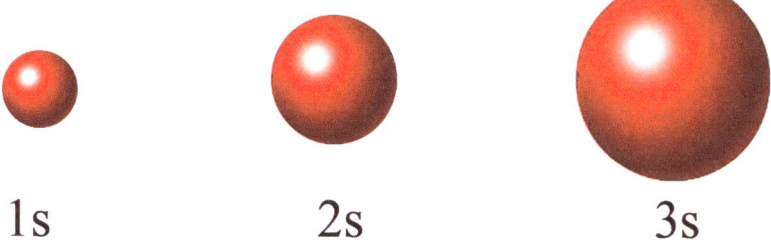

1s   2s   3s

Figure III.A.2.1: Atomic orbitals where l = 0. Notice that the orbitals do not reveal the precise location (position) or momentum of the fast moving electron at any point in time (Heisenberg's Uncertainty Principle). Instead, we are left with a 90% chance of finding the electron somewhere within the shapes described as orbitals.

THE PHYSICAL SCIENCES   CHM-17

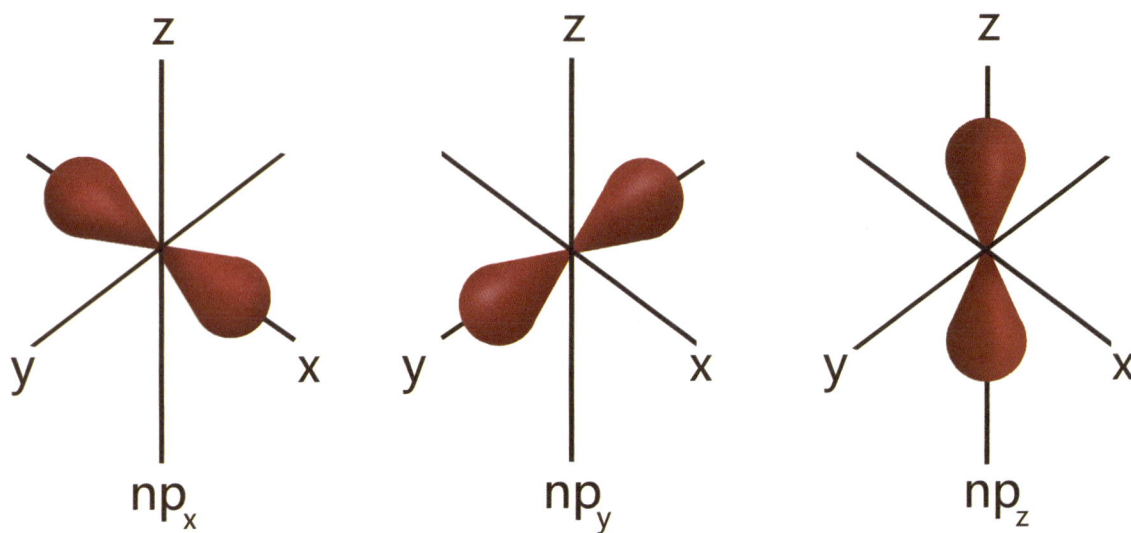

Figure III.A.2.2: Atomic orbitals where $l = 1$.

series of atomic orbitals follows the alphabetical order h, i, j, etc...

(iii) m_l: *the magnetic quantum number.* It defines the orientation of the orbital of a given shape. For a given value of l (given shape), m_l can take any of the $2l + 1$ integer values between $-l$ and $+l$. For instance for a state with $n = 3$ and $l = 1$ (3p orbital in notation explained in the previous paragraph) there are three possible values for m_l: -1, 0 and 1. These 3 orbitals are oriented along x, y or the z axis of a coordinate system with its origin on the nucleus of the atom: they are denoted as $3p_x$, $3p_y$ and $3p_z$. Figure III.A.2.2 shows the representation of an orbital corresponding to an electron in a state ns, np_x, np_y, and np_z. These are the 3D volumes where there is 90% chance to find an electron which is in a state ns, np_x, np_y, or np_z, respectively. This type of diagram constitutes the most common geometrical representation of the atomic orbitals (besides looking at the diagrams, consider watching one of the videos if you are having trouble visualizing these facts).

(iv) m_s: *the spin quantum number.* This number takes the values $+1/2$ or $-1/2$ for the electron. Some textbooks present the intuitive, albeit wrong, explanation that the spin angular momentum arises from the spinning of the electron around itself, the opposite signs for the spin quantum number would correspond to the two opposite rotational directions. We do have to resort to such an intuitive presentation because the spin angular moment has, in fact, no classical equivalent and, as a result, the physics behind the correct approach is too complex to be dealt with in introductory courses.

GENERAL CHEMISTRY

2.2 Conventional Notation for Electronic Structure

As described in the previous section, the state of an electron in an atom is completely defined by a set of four quantum numbers (n, *l*, m_l, m_s). If two electrons in an atom share the same n, *l* and m_l numbers their m_s have to be of opposite signs: this is known as the Pauli's exclusion principle which states that no two electrons in an atom can have the same four quantum numbers. This principle along with a rule known as Hund's rule which states that electrons fill orbital's singly first until all orbitals of the same energy are filled, constitutes the basis for the procedure that one needs to follow to assign the possible (n, *l*, m_l, m_s) quantum states to the electrons of a polyelectronic atom. Orbitals are "filled" in sequence, according to an example shown below. When filling a set of orbitals with the same n and *l* (e.g. the three 2p orbitals: $2p_x$, $2p_y$ and $2p_z$ which differ by their m_l's) electrons are assigned to orbitals with different m_l's first with parallel spins (same sign for their m_s), until each orbital of the given group is filled with one electron, then, electrons are paired in the same orbital with antiparallel spins (opposite signs for m_s). This procedure is illustrated in an example which follows. The electronic configuration which results from orbitals filled in accordance with the previous set of rules corresponds to the atom being in its lowest overall state of energy. This state of lowest energy is referred to as the ground state of the atom.

> **Note:** There are 2 periodic tables at the end of this chapter which you may want to consult from time to time.

The restrictions related to the previous set of rules lead to the fact that only a certain number of electrons is allowed for each quantum number:

for a given n (given shell): the maximum number of electrons allowed is $2n^2$. The greater the value of n, the greater the energy level of the shell.

for a given *l* (s, p, d, f…): this number is $4l + 2$.

for a given m_l (given orbital orientation): a maximum of 2 electrons is allowed.

There is a **conventional notation** for the electronic structure of an atom:

(i) orbitals are listed in the order they are filled (See Figure III.A.2.3)

(ii) generally, in this conventional notation, no distinction is made between electrons in states defined by the same n and l but which do not share the same m_l.

For instance the ground state electronic configuration of oxygen is written as:

$$1s^2\ 2s^2\ 2p^4$$

When writing the electronic configuration of a polyelectronic atom orbitals are filled (with electrons denoted as the superscripts of the configurations) in order of increasing energy: 1s 2s 2p 3s 3p 4s 3d … according to the following figure:

GAMSAT-Prep.com
THE GOLD STANDARD

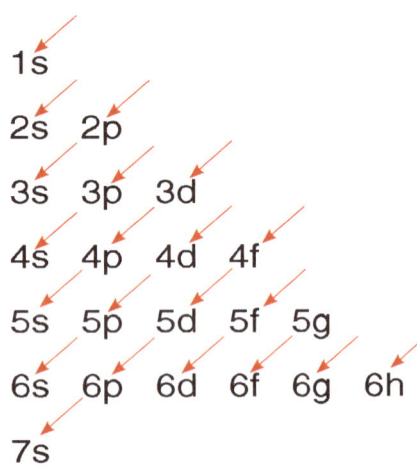

follow the direction of successive arrows moving from top to bottom

Figure III.A.2.3: The order for filling atomic orbitals.

Thus, the electronic configuration or the pattern of orbital filling of an atom generally abides by the following rules or principles:

1. Always fill the lowest energy (or ground state) orbitals first (Aufbau principle)

2. No two electrons in a single atom can have the same four quantum numbers; if n, l, and m_l are the same, m_s must be different such that the electrons have opposite spins. (Pauli exclusion principle) and

3. Degenerate orbitals of the subshell are each occupied singly with electrons of parallel spin before double occupation of the orbitals occurs (Hund's rule).

An alternative way to write the aforementioned electronic configuration is based on the avoidance in writing out the inner core electrons. Moreover, this is an abbreviation of the previous longer configuration or otherwise known as a short hand electronic configuration. Here, the core electrons are represented by a prior noble gas elemental symbol within brackets. As an example, calcium may be written in its expanded form or more commonly as a short hand notation represented as [Ar]4s^2 shown with the prior noble gas symbol for argon [Ar] written within brackets.

Another illustrative notation is also often used. In this alternate notation orbitals are represented by boxes (hence the referring to this representation as "box diagrams"). Orbitals with the same l are grouped together and electrons are represented by vertical ascending or descending arrows (for the two opposite signs of m_s).

For instance for the series H, He, Li, Be, B, C we have the following electronic configurations:

H: 1s^1 box diagram: [↑]
He: 1s^2 box diagram: [↑↓] and not [↑↑]
(rejected by Pauli's exclusion principle)
Li: 1s^2 2s^1
    [↑↓]   [↑]
Be: 1s^2 2s^2
    [↑↓]   [↑↓]
B: 1s^2 2s^2 2p^1
   [↑↓]   [↑↓]   [↑ | |]
C: 1s^2 2s^2 2p^2
   [↑↓]   [↑↓]   [↑ | ↑ |]

(to satisfy Hund's rule of maximum spin)

To satisfy Hund's rule the next electron is put into a separate 2p "box". The 4th 2p

CHM-20   ELECTRONIC STRUCTURE AND THE PERIODIC TABLE

electron (for oxygen) is then put into the first box with an opposite spin.

O: [↑↓]   [↑↓]   [↑↓|↑|↑]
    1s²   2s²   2p⁴

Within a given subshell l, orbitals are filled in such a way to maximize the number of half-filled orbitals with parallel spins. An unpaired electron generates a magnetic field due to its spin. Consequently, when a material is composed of atoms with unpaired electrons, it is said to be *paramagnetic* as it will be attracted to an applied external magnetic field (i.e. Li, Na, Cs). Alternatively, when the material's atoms have paired electrons, it is weakly repelled by an external magnetic field and it is said to be *diamagnetic* (i.e. Cu, molecular carbon, H_2, H_2O). Non-chemists simply call diamagnetic materials "not magnetic". The strongest form of magnetism is a permanent feature of materials like Fe, Ni and their alloys and is said to be *ferromagnetic* (i.e. a fridge magnet).

For the main group elements, the valence electrons of an atom are those that are involved in chemical bonding and are in the outermost principal energy level or shell. For example, for Group IA and Group IIA elements, only electrons from the s subshell are valence electrons. For Group IIIA through Group VIIIA elements, electrons from s and p subshell are valence electrons. Under certain circumstances, elements from Group IIIA through Group VIIA may accept electrons into its d subshell, leading to more than 8 valence electrons.

Finally, as previously mentioned, we should point out that electrons can be promoted to higher unoccupied (or partially occupied) orbitals when the atom is subjected to some external perturbation which inputs energy into the atom. The resulting electronic configuration is then called an excited state configuration (this concept was explored in PHY 12.5, 12.6).

2.3 Elements, Chemical Properties and The Periodic Table

Since most chemical properties of the atom are related to their outermost electrons (valence electrons), it is the orbital occupation of these electrons which is most relevant in the complete electronic configuration. The periodic table (there is one at the end of this chapter with a summary of trends) can be used to derive such information in the following way:

(i) the row or period number gives the "n" of the valence electrons of any given element of the period.

(ii) the first two columns or groups and helium (He) are referred to as the "s" block. The valence electrons of elements in these groups are "s" electrons.

(iii) groups 3A to 8A (13th to 18th columns) are the "p" group. Elements belonging to these groups have their ground state electronic configurations ending with "p" electrons.

(iv) Elements in groups 3B to 2B (columns 3 to 12) are called transition elements. Their electronic configurations end with $ns^2(n-1)d^x$ where n is the period number and x = 1 for column 3, 2 for column 4, 3 for column 5, etc… Note that these elements sometimes have unexpected or unusual valence shell electronic configurations.

This set of rules should make the writing of the ground-state valence shell electronic configuration very easy. For instance: Sc being an element of the "d" group on the 4th period should have a ground-state valence shell electronic configuration of the form: $4s^2 3d^x$. Since it belongs to group 3B (column 3) x = 1; therefore, the actual configuration is simply: $4s^2 3d^1$. However, half-filled (i.e. Cr) and filled (i.e. Cu, Ag, Au) d orbitals have remarkable stability. This stability behavior is essentially related to the closely spaced 3d and 4s energy levels with the stability associated with a half-filled (as in Cr) or completely filled (as in Cu) sublevel. Hence, this stability makes for unusual configurations (i.e. by the rules Cr = $4s^2 3d^4$, but in reality Cr = $4s^1 3d^5$ creating a half-filled d orbital). It can be noted that Cr therefore has an electronic configuration of $[Ar]4s^1 3d^5$, although four d electrons would be expected to be seen instead of five. This is because one electron from a s subshell jumps into the d orbital, giving the atom a half filled d subshell. As for Cu, it would have an electronic configuration of $[Ar]4s^2 3d^9$ by the rules. However, the Cu d shell is just one electron away from stability, and therefore, one electron from the s shell jumps into the d shell to convert it into $[Ar]4s^1 3d^{10}$.

==Some metal ions form colored solutions due to the transition energies of the d-electrons.==

A number of physical and chemical properties of the elements are periodic, i.e. they vary in a regular fashion with atomic numbers. We will define some of these properties and explain their trends:

(A) Ionization Energy

(i) The ionization energy (IE) is defined as the energy required to remove an electron from a gaseous atom or ion. The first ionization energy or potential (1st IE or IP) is the energy required to remove one of the outermost valence electrons from an atom in its gaseous state. The ionization potential increases from left to right within a period and decreases from the top to the bottom of a group or column of the periodic chart. The 1st IP drops sharply when we move from the last element of a period (inert gas) to the first element of the next period. These are general trends, elements located after an element with a half-filled shell, for instance, have a lower 1st IP than expected by these trends.

(ii) The second ionization is the energy or potential (2nd IE or IP) required to remove a second valence electron from the ion to form a divalent ion: the previous trends can be used if one remembers the relationship between 1st and 2nd ionization processes of an atom of element X:

$$X + energy \rightarrow X^+ + 1e^-$$
$$1^{st}\text{ ionization of X}$$
$$X^+ + energy \rightarrow X^{2+} + 1e^-$$
$$2^{nd}\text{ ionization of X}$$

The second ionization process of X can be viewed as the 1st ionization of X^+. With this in mind it is very easy to predict trends of 2nd IP's. For instance, let us compare the 2nd IP's of the elements Na and Al. This is equivalent to comparing the 1st IP's of Na^+ and Al^+. These, in turn, have the same valence shell electronic configurations as Ne and Mg, respectively. Applying the previous general principles on Ne and Mg we arrive at the following conclusions:

- the 1st IP of Ne is greater than the 1st IP of Mg
- the 1st IP of Na^+ is therefore expected to be greater than the 1st IP of Al^+
- the latter statement is equivalent to the final conclusion that the 2nd IP of Na is greater than the 2nd IP of Al.

(B) Electron Affinity

(iii) Electron affinity (EA) is the energy change that accompanies the following process for an atom of element X:

$$X(gas) + 1e^- \rightarrow X^-(gas)$$

This property measures the ability of an atom to accept an electron. The stronger the attraction of a nucleus for electrons, the greater the electron affinity (EA) will be. The electron affinity becomes more negative for non-metals than metals. Thus, halogen atoms (F, Cl, Br…) have a very negative EA because they have a great tendency to form negative ions. On the other hand, alkaline earth metals which tend to form positive rather than negative ions have very large positive EA's. The overall tendency is that EA's become more negative as we move from left to right across a period, they are more negative (less positive) for non-metals than for metals and they do not change considerably within a group or column.

(C) Atomic Radii

(iv) The atomic radius generally decreases from left to right across a period since the effective nuclear charge increases as the number of protons within an atom increases. The effective nuclear charge is the net charge experienced by the valence electrons as a result of the nucleus (ie, protons) and core electrons. Additionally, the atomic radius increases when we move down a group due to the shielding effect of the additional core electrons and the presence of another electron shell.

(D) Electronegativity

(v) Electronegativity is a parameter that measures the ability of an atom, when engaged in a molecular bond, to pull or repel the bond electrons. This parameter is determined from the 1st IE and the EA of a given atom. Electronegativity follows the same general trends as the 1st IE. The greater the electronegativity of an atom, the greater its attraction for bonding electrons. In general, electronegativity is inversely related to atomic size. Moreover, the larger the atom, the less the ability for it to attract electrons to itself in chemical bonding.

In conclusion, as one moves to the right across a row in the periodic table, the atomic radii decreases, the ionization energy (IE) increases and the electronegativity increases. As one moves down along a column within the periodic table, the atomic radii increases, the ionization energy (IE) decreases and electronegativity decreases.

2.3.1 Bond Strength

When there is a big difference in electronegativity between two atoms sharing a covalent bond then the bond is generally weaker as compared to two atoms with little electronegativity difference. This is because in the latter case, the bond is shared more equally and is thus more stable.

Bond strength is inversely proportional to bond length. Thus, all things being equal, a stronger bond would be shorter. Bonds and bond strength is further discussed in ORG 1.3-1.5.1.

2.4 Metals, Nonmetals and Metalloids

The elements of the periodic table belong in three basic categories: metals, nonmetals and metalloids (or semimetals).

Metals – high melting points and densities characterize metals. They are excellent conductors of heat and electricity due to their valence electrons being able to move freely. This fact also accounts for the major characteristic properties of metals: large atomic radius, low ionization energy, high electron affinities and low electronegativity. Groups IA and IIA are the most reactive of all metal species.

Of course, metals tend to be shiny and solid (with the exception of mercury, Hg, a liquid at STP). They are also *ductile* (they can be drawn into thin wires) and *malleable* (they can be easily hammered into very thin sheets).

Nonmetals – Nonmetals have high ionization energies and electronegativities. As opposed to metals, they do not conduct heat or electricity. They tend to gain electrons easily contrarily to metals that readily lose electrons when forming bonds.

GENERAL CHEMISTRY

Metalloids – The metalloids share properties with both metals and nonmetals. Their densities, boiling points and melting points do not follow any specific trends and are very unpredictable. Ionization energy and electronegativity values vary and can be found in between those of metals and nonmetals. Examples of metalloids are boron, silicon, germanium, arsenic, antimony and tellurium.

Table III A.2.1

Metals	Nonmetals	Metalloids
General characteristics of metals, nonmetals and metalloids		
• Hard and Shiny	• Gases or dull, brittle solids	• Appearence will vary
• 3 or less valence electrons	• 5 or more valence electrons	• 3 to 7 valence electrons
• Form + ions by losing e−	• Form − ions by gaining e−	• Form + and/or − ions
• Good conductors of heat and electricity	• Poor conductors of heat and electricity	• Conduct better than nonmetals but not as well as metals

*These are general characteristics. There are exceptions beyond the scope of the exam.

2.4.1 The Chemistry of Groups

Alkali metals – The alkali metals are found in Group IA and are different than other metals in that they only have one loosely bound electron in their outermost shell. This gives them the largest ionic radius of all the elements in their respective periods. They are also highly reactive (especially with halogens) due to their low ionization energies and low electronegativity and the relative ease with which they lose their valence electron.

Alkaline Earth metals – The alkaline earth metals are found in Group IIA and also tend to lose electrons quite readily. They have two electrons in their outer shell and experience a stronger effective nuclear charge than alkali metals. This gives them a smaller atomic radius as well as low electronegativity values.

Halogens – The halogens are found in Group VIIA and are highly reactive nonmetals with seven valence electrons in their outer shell. This gives them extremely high electronegativity values and makes them reactive towards alkali metals and alkaline earth metals that seek to donate electrons to form a complete octet. Some halogens are gaseous at Standard Temperature and Pressure (STP; CHM 4.1.1) (F_2 and Cl_2) while others are liquid (Br_2) or solid (I_2).

Noble gases – The noble gases, also called the inert gases, are found in Group VIII and are characterized by being a mostly non-reactive species due to their complete valence shell. This energetically favorable configuration of electrons gives them high ionization energies, low boiling points and no real electronegativities. They are all gaseous at room temperature.

Transition Elements – The transition elements are found in Groups IB to VIIIB and are characterized by high melting points and boiling points. Their key chemical characteristic is their ability to exist in a variety of different oxidation states. For the transition elements, the 4s shell gets filled prior to the 3d shell according to the Aufbau rule. However, electrons are lost from the 4s shell before the 3d shell. Thus, as the d electrons are held only loosely, this contributes to the high electrical conductivity and malleability of transition elements. This is because transition elements can lose electrons from both their s and d orbitals of their valence shell; the d electrons are held more loosely than the s electrons. They display low ionization energies and high electrical conductivities.

PERIODIC TABLE OF THE ELEMENTS

1 H 1.008																	2 He 4.003
3 Li 6.941	4 Be 9.012											5 B 10.81	6 C 12.011	7 N 14.007	8 O 15.999	9 F 18.998	10 Ne 20.179
11 Na 22.990	12 Mg 24.305											13 Al 26.982	14 Si 28.086	15 P 30.974	16 S 32.06	17 Cl 35.453	18 Ar 39.948
19 K 39.098	20 Ca 40.08	21 Sc 44.956	22 Ti 47.90	23 V 50.942	24 Cr 51.996	25 Mn 54.938	26 Fe 55.847	27 Co 58.933	28 Ni 58.70	29 Cu 63.546	30 Zn 65.38	31 Ga 69.72	32 Ge 72.59	33 As 74.922	34 Se 78.96	35 Br 79.904	36 Kr 83.80
37 Rb 85.468	38 Sr 87.62	39 Y 88.906	40 Zr 91.22	41 Nb 92.906	42 Mo 95.94	43 Tc (98)	44 Ru 101.07	45 Rh 102.906	46 Pd 106.4	47 Ag 107.868	48 Cd 112.41	49 In 114.82	50 Sn 118.69	51 Sb 121.75	52 Te 127.60	53 I 126.905	54 Xe 131.30
55 Cs 132.905	56 Ba 137.33	57 *La 138.906	72 Hf 178.49	73 Ta 180.948	74 W 183.85	75 Re 186.207	76 Os 190.2	77 Ir 192.22	78 Pt 195.09	79 Au 196.967	80 Hg 200.59	81 Tl 204.37	82 Pb 207.2	83 Bi 208.980	84 Po (209)	85 At (210)	86 Rn (222)
87 Fr (223)	88 Ra 226.025	89 **Ac 227.028	104 Unq (261)	105 Unp (262)	106 Unh (263)												

*	58 Ce 140.12	59 Pr 140.908	60 Nd 144.24	61 Pm (145)	62 Sm 150.4	63 Eu 151.96	64 Gd 157.25	65 Tb 158.925	66 Dy 162.50	67 Ho 164.930	68 Er 167.26	69 Tm 168.934	70 Yb 173.04	71 Lu 174.967
**	90 Th 232.038	91 Pa 231.036	92 U 238.029	93 Np 237.048	94 Pu (244)	95 Am (243)	96 Cm (247)	97 Bk (247)	98 Cf (251)	99 Es (254)	100 Fm (257)	101 Md (258)	102 No (259)	103 Lr (260)

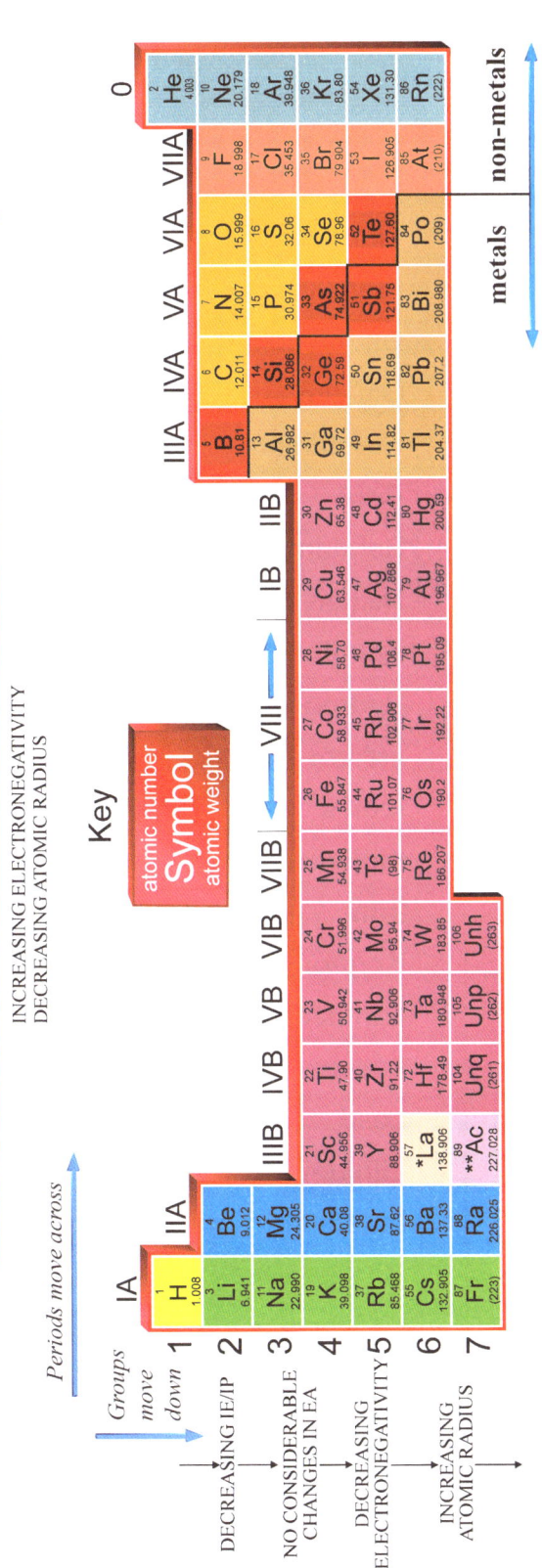
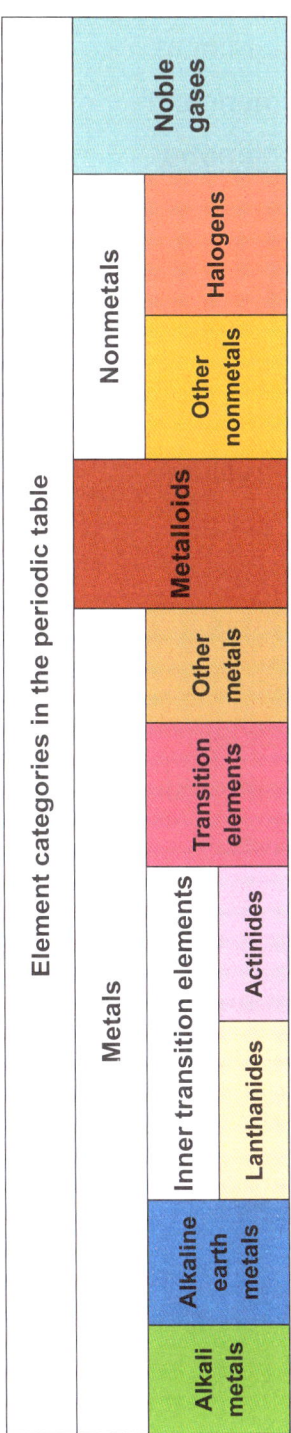

GAMSAT-Prep.com
THE GOLD STANDARD

Element	Symbol	Atomic Number
Actinium	Ac	89
Aluminum	Al	13
Americium	Am	95
Antimony	Sb	51
Argon	Ar	18
Arsenic	As	33
Astatine	At	85
Barium	Ba	56
Berkelium	Bk	97
Beryllium	Be	4
Bismuth	Bi	83
Boron	B	5
Bromine	Br	35
Cadmium	Cd	48
Calcium	Ca	20
Californium	Cf	98
Carbon	C	6
Cerium	Ce	58
Cesium	Cs	55
Chlorine	Cl	17
Chromium	Cr	24
Cobalt	Co	27
Copper	Cu	29
Curium	Cm	96
Dysprosium	Dy	66
Einsteinium	Es	99
Erbium	Er	68

Element	Symbol	Atomic Number
Europium	Eu	63
Fermium	Fm	100
Fluorine	F	9
Francium	Fr	87
Gadolinium	Gd	64
Gallium	Ga	31
Germanium	Ge	32
Gold	Au	79
Hafnium	Hf	72
Helium	He	2
Holmium	Ho	67
Hydrogen	H	1
Indium	In	49
Iodine	I	53
Iridium	Ir	77
Iron	Fe	26
Krypton	Kr	36
Lanthanum	La	57
Lawrencium	Lr	103
Lead	Pb	82
Lithium	Li	3
Lutetium	Lu	71
Magnesium	Mg	12
Manganese	Mn	25
Mendelevium	Md	101
Mercury	Hg	80
Molybdenum	Mo	42

ELECTRONIC STRUCTURE AND THE PERIODIC TABLE

GENERAL CHEMISTRY

Element	Symbol	Atomic Number
Neodymium	Nd	60
Neon	Ne	10
Neptunium	Np	93
Nickel	Ni	28
Niobium	Nb	41
Nitrogen	N	7
Nobelium	No	102
Osmium	Os	76
Oxygen	O	8
Palladium	Pd	46
Phosphorous	P	15
Platinum	Pt	78
Plutonium	Pu	94
Polonium	Po	84
Potassium	K	19
Praseodymium	Pr	59
Promethium	Pm	61
Protactinium	Pa	91
Radium	Ra	88
Radon	Rn	86
Rhenium	Re	75
Rhodium	Rh	45
Rubidium	Rb	37
Ruthenium	Ru	44
Samarium	Sm	62
Scandium	Sc	21

Element	Symbol	Atomic Number
Selenium	Se	34
Silicon	Si	14
Silver	Ag	47
Sodium	Na	11
Strontium	Sr	38
Sulfur	S	16
Tantalum	Ta	73
Technetium	Tc	43
Tellurium	Te	52
Terbium	Tb	65
Thallium	Tl	81
Thorium	Th	90
Thulium	Tm	69
Tin	Sn	50
Titanium	Ti	22
Tungsten	W	74
(Unnilhexium)	(Unh)	106
(Unnilpentium)	(Unp)	105
(Unnilquadium)	(Unq)	104
Uranium	U	92
Vanadium	V	23
Xenon	Xe	54
Ytterbium	Yb	70
Yttrium	Y	39
Zinc	Zn	30
Zirconium	Zr	40

Go online to GAMSAT-prep.com for free chapter review Q&A and forum.

GOLD NOTES

BONDING

Chapter 3

Memorize	Understand	Not Required*
hybrid orbitals, shapes Define Lewis: structure, acid, base Define: octet rule, formal charge	* Ionic, covalent bonds * VSEPR, Resonance * Dipole, covalent polar bonds * Trends in the periodic table	* Advanced level college info * Details of VSEPR * Memorizing hybrids with d, f * Memorizing dipole moment equation

GAMSAT-Prep.com

Introduction

Attractive interactions between atoms and molecules involve a physical process called chemical bonding. In general, strong chemical bonding is associated with the sharing or transfer of electrons between atoms. Molecules, crystals and diatomic gases are held together by chemical bonds which makes up most of the matter around us.

Additional Resources

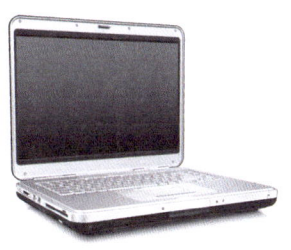   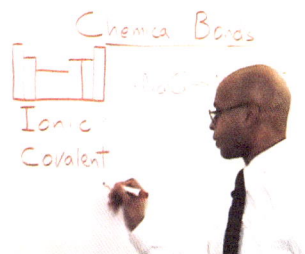   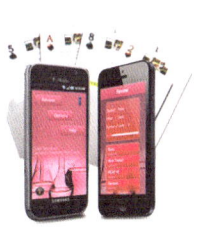   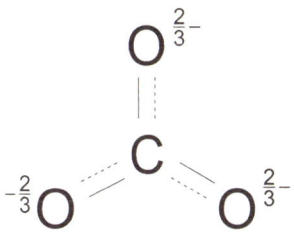

Free Online Q&A + Forum   Video: Online or DVD   Flashcards   Special Guest

THE PHYSICAL SCIENCES   CHM-31

* The real GAMSAT may have advanced level information presented (ie. in a passage) but previous knowledge of said information is not required to answer the questions that would follow. Practice ACER and GS practice GAMSATs can help you clarify this point.

GAMSAT-Prep.com
THE GOLD STANDARD

3.1 Generalities

Chemical bonds can form between atoms of the same element or between atoms of different elements. Chemical bonds are classified into three groups: ionic, covalent and metallic.

To summarize, if the electronegativity values of two atoms are:

- significantly different...
  - Ionic bonds are formed.
- similar...
  - Metallic bonds form between two metal atoms.
  - Covalent bonds form between two nonmetal atoms (or between metal and nonmetal atoms).
    - Non-polar covalent bonds form when the electronegativity values are very similar.
    - Polar covalent bonds form when the electronegativity values are somewhat further apart.

We will also see in this chapter that many bonds are formed according to the octet rule, which states that an atom tends to form bonds with other atoms until the bonding atoms obtain a stable electron configuration of eight valence electrons in their outermost shells, similar to that of Group VIIIA (noble gas) elements. There are certain exceptions to the octet rule such as, hydrogen forming bonds with two valence electrons; beryllium, which can bond to attain four valence electrons; boron, which can bond to attain six; and elements such as phosphorus and sulfur, which can incorporate d orbital electrons to attain more than eight valence electrons.

3.1.1 The Ionic Bond

Ionic bonds form when there is a complete transfer of one or more electrons between a metal and a nonmetal atom. When an element X with a low ionization potential is combined with an element Y with a large negative electron affinity, one or more electrons are transferred from the atoms of X to the atoms of Y. This leads to the formation of cations X^{n+} and anions Y^{m-}. These ions of opposite charges are then attracted to each other through electrostatic forces which then aggregate to form large stable spatial arrangements of ions: crystalline solids. The bonds that hold these ions together are called ionic bonds.

There exists a large difference in electronegativity between ionically bonded atoms. Electronegativity is defined as the ability of an atom to attract electrons towards its nucleus in bonding and each atomic element is assigned a numerical electronegativity value with a greatest value of 4.0 assigned to the most electronegative element, fluorine. Ionic compounds are known to have high melting and boiling points and high electrical conductivity. In our general example, note that to maintain electrical neutrality the empirical formula of this ionic compound has to be of the general form: $X_m Y_n$ (the total positive charge: $n \times m$ is equal to the total negative charge: $m \times n$ in a unit formula).

For instance, since aluminium tends to form the cation Al^{3+} and oxygen the anion O^{2-} the empirical formula for aluminium oxide is Al_2O_3. Thus, the empirical or simplest formula is written for each of the formula units (Al_2O_3) which are part of a larger crystalline solid. The actual ionic solid lattice formed however, consists of a large and equal number of ions packed together in a manner to allow maximal attraction of all the oppositely charged ions.

H	2.1												
Li	1.0	Be	1.5	B	2.0	C	2.5	N	3.0	O	3.5	F	4.0
Na	0.9	Mg	1.2	Al	1.5	Si	1.8	P	2.1	S	2.5	Cl	3.0
K	0.8	Ca	1.0	Ga	1.6	Ge	1.8	As	2.0	Se	2.4	Br	2.8
Rb	0.8	Sr	1.0	In	1.7	Sn	1.8	Sb	1.9	Te	2.1	I	2.5
Cs	0.7	Ba	0.9	Tl	1.8	Pb	1.9	Bi	1.9	Po	2.0	At	2.2

Table III.A.3.0: Pauling's values for the electronegativity of some important elements. Note that elements in the upper right hand corner of the periodic table have high electronegativities and those in the bottom left hand corner of the table have low electronegativities (CHM 2.3, 2.4.1). Note that Pauling's electronegativity is dimensionless since it measures electron attracting ability on a relative scale. Of course, the numbers do not need to be memorized but understanding the trends is very important for both GAMSAT General and Organic Chemistry.

3.2 The Covalent Bond

Atoms are held together in non-ionic molecules by covalent bonds. In this type of bonding two valence electrons are shared between two atoms. Two atoms sharing one, two or three electron pairs form single, double or triple covalent bonds, respectively. As the number of shared electron pairs increases, the two atoms are pulled closer together, leading to a decrease in bond length and a simultaneous increase in bond strength. As opposed to ionic bonds, atoms in covalent bonds have similar electronegativity. Ionic and covalent bonding are thus considered as the two extremes in bonding types. Covalent bonding is further categorized into the following subclasses; non-polar, polar and coordinate types of covalent bonding.

Non-polar covalent bonding occurs when two bonding atoms have either equal or similar electronegativities or a calculated electronegativity difference of less than 0.4.

Polar covalent bonding occurs when there is a small difference in electronegativity between atoms in the range of approximately 0.4 up to 2.0. When the difference in electronegativity is greater than 2.0, ionic bonding is then known to occur between two atoms. The more electronegative atom will attract the bonding electrons to a larger extent. As a result, the more electronegative atom acquires a partial negative charge and the less electronegative atom acquires a partial positive charge.

Coordinate covalent bonding occurs when the shared electron pair comes from the lone pair of electrons of one of the atoms in the bonding component. Typically coordinate bonds form between Lewis acids (electron acceptors) and Lewis bases (electron donors) as shown below.

$$A^+ + {}^-B \rightarrow A\text{—}B$$

Lewis Acid (Electron Acceptor) + Lewis Base (Electron Donor) → coordinate covalent bond

Al^{3+} (Lewis Acid) + H–Ö–H (Lewis Base) ⇌ $[Al(H_2O)_6]$

A <u>Lewis structure</u> is a representation of covalent bonding in which shared electrons are shown either as lines or as pairs of dots between two atoms. For instance, let us consider the H_2O molecule. The valence shell electronic configurations of the atoms that constitute this molecule are:

O: $2s^2 2p^4$
H: $1s^1$

Since hydrogen has only one electron to share with oxygen there is only one possible covalent bond that can be formed between the oxygen atom and each of the hydrogen atoms. Four of the valence electrons of the oxygen atom do not participate in this covalent bonding, these are called <u>non-bonding electrons or lone pairs</u>. The Lewis structure of the water molecule is:

H:Ö:H or H-Ö-H

Lewis formulated the following general rule known as the <u>octet rule</u> concerning these representations: atoms tend to form covalent bonds until they are surrounded by 8 electrons (with few exceptions such as for hydrogen which can be surrounded by a maximum of only 2 electrons; see CHM 3.1). To satisfy this rule (and if there is a sufficient number of valence electrons), two atoms may share more than one pair of electrons thus forming more than one covalent bond at a time. In such instances the bond between these atoms is referred to as a double or a triple bond depending on whether there are two or three pairs of shared electrons, respectively.

Some molecules cannot fully be described by a single Lewis structure. For instance, for the carbonate ion: CO_3^{2-}, the octet rule is satisfied for the central carbon atom if one of the C…O bonds is double (see the following diagrams). While this leads us to thinking that the three C…O bonds are not equivalent, every piece of experimental evidence concerning this molecule shows that the three bonds are in fact the same (same length, same polarity, etc…). This suggests that in such instances a molecule cannot be described fully by a single Lewis structure. However, a molecule may in fact be represented by two or more valid Lewis structures. Indeed, since there is no particular reason to choose one oxygen atom over another we can write three equivalent Lewis structures for the carbonate ion. These three structures are called <u>resonance structures represented with a double-headed arrow between each resonance structure.</u> The carbonate ion (CO_3^{2-}) actually exists as a hybrid of the three equivalent structures. It is the full set of resonance structures that describe such a molecule. In this picture, the C...O bonds are neither double nor single, they are intermediate and have both a single and a double bonded character (see the following diagrams).

CO_3^{2-}

$$\left[\begin{array}{c}:\ddot{O}-C=\ddot{O}\\|\\:\ddot{O}:\end{array}\right]^{2-} \leftrightarrow \left[\begin{array}{c}\ddot{O}=C-\ddot{O}:\\|\\:\ddot{O}:\end{array}\right]^{2-} \leftrightarrow \left[\begin{array}{c}:\ddot{O}-C-\ddot{O}:\\||\\:\ddot{O}:\end{array}\right]^{2-}$$

The actual structure of the carbonate ion is therefore one which is intermediate between the three resonance structures and is known as a resonance hybrid as shown:

$$\begin{array}{c} O^{\frac{2}{3}-}\\ \vdots\\ C\\ \diagup \quad \diagdown\\ ^{-\frac{2}{3}}O \qquad\qquad O^{\frac{2}{3}-} \end{array}$$

In many molecular structures, all of the respective resonance structures contribute equally to the hybridized representation. However, for some, resonance structures may not all contribute equally. Moreover, the more stable the resonance structure, the more contribution of that structure to the true hybrid structure based on formal charges.

Thus, based on their stabilities, non-equivalent resonance structures may contribute differently to the true overall hybridized structure representation of a molecule.

It is often interesting to compare the number of valence electrons that an atom possesses when it is isolated and when it is engaged in a covalent bond within a given molecule. This is often quantitatively described by the concept of <u>formal charge</u>.

Generally, a formal charge is a calculated conjured charge assigned to each individual atom within a Lewis structure allowing one to distinguish amongst various possible Lewis structures. The formal charge on any individual atom is calculated based on the difference between the atom's actual number of valence electrons and the number of electrons the atom possesses as part of a Lewis structure.

Moreover, the number of electrons attributed to an atom within a Lewis structure (covalently bonded) is not necessarily the same as the number of valence electrons that would be isolated within that free atom, and the difference is thus referred to as the "formal charge" of that atom. This concept is defined as follows:

Formal charge (of atom X) = Total number of valence electrons in a free atom (V) − [(total number of nonbonding electrons

(N) + ½ total number of bonding electrons (B) in a Lewis structure)].

Where, V is the number of valence electrons of the atom in isolation (atom in ground state); N is the number of non-bonding valence electrons on this atom in the molecule; and B is the total number of bonding electrons shared in covalent bonds with other atoms in the molecule (see structure of CO_3^{2-} in the previous illustrations).

Let us apply this definition to the two previous examples: H_2O and CO_3^{2-}. This process is fairly straightforward in the case of the water molecule:

total # of valence e⁻'s in free O:	6
– total # of non-bonding e⁻'s on O in H_2O:	4
– 1/2 (total # of bonding e⁻'s) on O in H_2O:	2
Formal charge of O in H_2O = 0	

In the case of the CO_3^{2-} ion, it is not as obvious. If we consider one of the three equivalent resonance forms, that of the oxygen with a double bond to carbon we have:

total # of valence e⁻'s in free O:	6
- total # of non-bonding e⁻'s on O in the ion:	4
- 1/2 (total # of bonding e⁻) on O in the ion:	2
Formal charge of O of C=O in the ion = 0	

Similarly, the calculation of the formal charge for one of the two singly bonded oxygen's of C–O in the same ion leads to the following: $6 - 6 - 1/2(2) = -1$. Considering that CO_3^{2-} is represented by three resonance forms, the actual formal charge of the oxygen atom is $1/3 (-1 -1 + 0) = -2/3$. This value formally reflects the idea that the oxygen atoms are equivalent and that any one of them has a –1 charge in 2 out of three of the resonance forms of this ion. Here are some simple rules to remember about formal charges:

(i) For neutral molecules, the formal charges of all the atoms should add up to zero.

(ii) For an ion, the sum of the formal charges must equal the ion's charge.

The following rules should help you select a plausible Lewis structure:

(i) If you can write more than one Lewis structure for a given neutral molecule; the most plausible one is the one in which the formal charges of the individual atoms are zero.

(ii) Lewis structures with the smallest formal charges on each individual atom are more plausible than the ones that involve large formal charges.

(iii) Out of a range of possible Lewis structures for a given molecule, the most plausible ones are the ones in which negative formal charges are found on the most electronegative atoms and positive charges on the most electropositive ones.

In addition to these rules, remember that some elements have a tendency to form molecules that do not satisfy the octet rule:

GENERAL CHEMISTRY

(i) When sulfur is the central atom in a molecule or a polyatomic ion, it almost invariably does not fulfill the octet rule.

(ii) The number of electrons around S in these compounds is usually 12 (e.g. SF_6, SO_4^{2-}). This situation (expanded octets) also occurs in other elements in and beyond the third period.

(iii) Molecules that have an element from the 3A group (B, Al, etc…) as their central atom do not generally obey the octet rule. In these molecules there are less than 8 electrons around the central atom (e.g. AlI_3 and BF_3).

(iv) Some molecules with an odd number of electrons can clearly not obey the octet rule (e.g. NO and NO_2).

3.3 Partial Ionic Character

Except for homonuclear molecules (molecules made of atoms of the same element, e.g. H_2, O_3, etc…), bonding electrons are not equally shared by the bonded atoms. Thus a diatomic (= *two atoms*) compound like Cl_2 shares its bonding electrons equally; whereas, a binary (= *two different elements*) compound like CaO (calcium oxide) or NaCl (sodium chloride) does not. Indeed, for the great majority of molecules, one of the two atoms between which the covalent bond occurs is necessarily more electronegative than the other. This atom will attract the bonding electrons to a larger extent (see CHM 3.2). Although this phenomenon does not lead to the formation of two separate ionic species, it does result in a molecule in which there are partial charges on these particular atoms: the corresponding covalent bond is said to possess partial ionic character. This polar bond will also have a dipole moment given by:

$$D = q \cdot d$$

where q is the absolute value of the partial charge on the most electronegative or the most electropositive bonded atom and d is the distance between these two atoms. To obtain the total dipole moment of a molecule one must add the individual dipole moment vectors present on each one of its bonds. Since this is a vector addition (see ORG 1.5), the overall result may be zero even if the individual dipole moment vectors are very large.

Non-polar bonds are generally stronger than polar covalent and ionic bonds, with ionic bonds being the weakest. However, in compounds with ionic bonding, there is generally a large number of bonds between molecules and this makes the compound as a whole very strong. For instance, although the ionic bonds in one compound are weaker than the non-polar covalent bonds in another compound, the ionic compound's melting point will be higher than the melting point of the covalent compound. Polar covalent bonds have a partially ionic character, and thus the bond strength is usually intermediate between that of ionic and that of non-polar covalent bonds. The strength of bonds generally decreases with increasing ionic character.

3.4 Lewis Acids and Lewis Bases

The Lewis model of acids and bases focuses on the transfer of an electron pair. Generally, a Lewis acid is defined as any substance that may accept an electron pair to form a covalent bond, while a Lewis base, is defined as any substance that donates an electron pair to form a respective covalent bond. Hence, as per the Lewis definition of an acid or base, a substance need not contain a hydrogen as defined by either Arrhenius or Bronsted-Lowry to be an acid, nor is a hydroxyl group (OH⁻) needed to be a base (see CHM 6.1). A Lewis acid therefore generally has an empty electronic orbital that can accept an electron pair whereas a Lewis base will contain a full electronic orbital or lone pair of electrons ready to be donated.

In CHM 3.2, we pointed out some exceptions to the Lewis' octet rule. Among these were molecules that had a deficiency of electrons around the central atom as described previously (e.g. BF_3). When such a molecule is put into contact with a molecule with lone pairs (e.g. NH_3) a reaction occurs. Such a reaction can be interpreted as a donation of a pair of electrons from the second type of molecule (Lewis base) to the first type of molecule (Lewis acid), or alternately by an acceptance of a pair of electrons by the first type of molecule. Thus, as previously shown, molecules such as BF_3 are referred to as <u>Lewis acids</u> while molecules such as NH_3 are known as <u>Lewis bases</u>. Thus some examples of Lewis acids are: BF_3, H^+, Cu^{2+}, and Cr^{3+} and Lewis bases are: NH_3, OH^-, and H_2O. {l**E**wis **A**cids: **E**lectron pair **A**cceptors}.

The Lewis acid BF_3 and the Lewis base NH_3. Notice that the green arrows follow the flow of electron pairs.

GENERAL CHEMISTRY

3.5 Valence Shell Electronic Pair Repulsions (VSEPR Models)

One of the shortcomings of Lewis structures is that they cannot be used to predict molecular geometries. In this context a model known as the <u>valence-shell electronic pair repulsion or VSEPR model</u> is very useful. In this model, the geometrical arrangement of atoms or groups of atoms bound to a central atom A is determined by the number of pairs of valence electrons around A. VSEPR procedure is based on the principle that these electronic pairs around the central atom are arranged in such a way that the repulsions between them are minimized. The general VSEPR procedure starts with the determination of the number of electronic pairs around A:

$$\begin{array}{l} \text{\# of valence electrons in a free atom of A} \\ + \text{ \# of sigma (or single) bonds involving A} \\ - \text{ \# of pi (or double) bonds involving A} \\ \hline = \text{(total \# of electrons around A)} \end{array}$$

The division of this total number by 2 yields the total number of electron pairs around A. Note the following important points:

(i) A single bond counts for 1 sigma bond, a double bond for 1 sigma bond and 1 pi bond and a triple bond for 1 sigma and two pi bonds.

(ii) The general calculation that we have presented is performed for the purposes of VSEPR modeling; its result can be quite different from the one obtained in the corresponding Lewis structure.

(iii) For all practical purposes, one always assigns a double bond (i.e. 1 sigma bond and one pi bond) to a terminal oxygen (an oxygen which is not a central atom and is not attached to any other atom besides the central atom).

(iv) A terminal halogen is always assigned a single bond.

Once the number of pairs around the central atom is determined, the next step is to use Figure III.A.3.1 to predict the geometrical arrangement of these pairs around the central atom.

The next step is to consider the previous arrangement of the electronic pairs and place the atoms or groups of atoms that are attached to the central atom in accordance with such an arrangement. The pairs of electrons which are not involved in the bonding between these atoms and the central atom are known as lone pairs. If we subtract the number of lone pairs from the total number of pairs of electrons, we readily obtain the number of bonding electron pairs. It is the number of bonding electron pairs which ultimately determines the molecular geometry in the VSEPR model according to Table III.A.3.1.

On the other hand, as for the *electronic geometrical arrangement* of a molecule, one is also to consider the free lone pair(s) of electrons. Consequently, a simple molecule such as SO_2 (see Table III.A.3.1) will have a trigonal planar electronic geometry with a bent molecular geometry with the respective differences in geometrical arrangement based solely on the lone pair of the central sulfur atom. ==Thus, the electron and molecular geometry of a molecule may be different.== (Note: electron geometry is based on the geometrical arrangement of electron pairs around a central atom, whereas, molecular geometry is based on the geometrical arrangement of the atoms surrounding a central atom). Let us consider three examples: CH_4, H_2O and CO_2.

1 – CH_4:

# of valence electrons on C:	4
+ # of sigma bonds:	+ 4
– # of pi bonds:	– 0
	= 8/2 = 4 pairs

According to Figure III.A.3.1 CH_4 corresponds to a tetrahedral arrangement. Each of these four pairs of electrons corresponds to a H atom bonded each to the central atom of carbon. Therefore, all 4 pairs of electrons are bonding pairs with a tetrahedral molecular and electronic geometry, respectively (due to a lack in lone pairs).

2 – H_2O:

# of valence electrons on O:	6
+ # of sigma bonds on the central O:	+ 2
– # of pi bonds on the central O:	– 0
	= 8/2 = 4 pairs

For the H_2O geometry, it also corresponds to a tetrahedral arrangement (i.e. 4 pairs). However, due to lone pairs surrounding each of the oxygen atoms, the molecular geometry is of a bent geometrical shape with a tetrahedral electronic geometrical configuration.

3 – CO_2:

# of valence electrons on C:	4
+ # of sigma bonds for terminal O's:	+ 2
– # of pi bonds for terminal O's:	– 2
	= 4/2 = 2 pairs

This total number of pairs corresponds to a linear arrangement. Since both of these electron pairs are used to connect the central C atom to the terminal O's there are no lone pairs left on C. Therefore, the number of bonding pairs is also 2 and both the molecular and electronic geometries are also linear.

Here are some additional rules when applying the VSEPR model:

(i) When dealing with a cation (<u>positive</u> ion) <u>subtract</u> the charge of the ion from the total number of electrons.

(ii) When dealing with an anion (<u>negative</u> ion) <u>add</u> the charge of the ion to the total number of electrons.

(iii) A lone pair repels another lone pair or a bonding pair very strongly. This causes some deformation in bond angles. For instance, the H–O–H angle is smaller than 109.5°.

GENERAL CHEMISTRY

Table III.A.3.1: Geometry of simple molecules in which the central atom A has one or more lone pairs of electrons (= e⁻).

Total number of e⁻ pairs	Number of lone pairs	Number of bonding pairs	Electron Geometry, Arrangement of e⁻ pairs	Molecular Geometry (Hybridization State)	Examples
3	1	2	Trigonal planar	Bent (sp^2)	SO_2
4	1	3	Tetrahedral	Trigonal pyramidal (sp^3)	NH_3
4	2	2	Tetrahedral	Bent (sp^3)	H_2O
5	1	4	Trigonal bipyramidal	Seesaw (sp^3d)	SF_4
5	2	3	Trigonal bipyramidal	T-shaped (sp^3d)	ClF_3

Note: dotted lines only represent the overall molecular shape and not molecular bonds. In brackets under "Molecular Geometry" is the hybridization, to be discussed in ORG 1.2.

THE PHYSICAL SCIENCES CHM-41

(iv) The previous rule also holds for a double bond. Note that in one of our previous examples (CO₂), the angle is still 180° since there are two double bonds and no lone pairs. Indeed, in this geometry, the strong repulsions between the two double bonds are symmetrical.

(v) The VSEPR model can be applied to polyatomic molecules. The procedure is the same as above except that one can only determine the arrangements of groups of atoms around one given central atom at a time. For instance, you could apply the VSEPR model to determine the geometrical arrangements of atoms around C or around O in methanol (CH₃OH). In the first case the molecule is treated as CH₃ – X (where –X is –OH) and in the second it is treated as HO–Y (where –Y is –CH₃). The

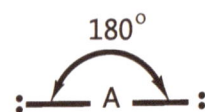

linear arrangement of 2 electron pairs around central atom A

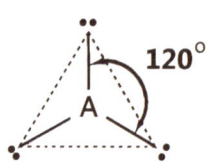

trigonal planar arrangement of 3 electron pairs around central atom A

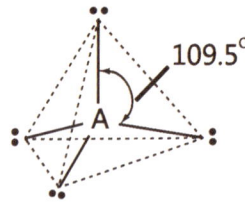

tetrahedral arrangement of 4 electron pairs around central atom A

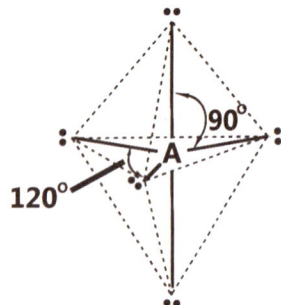

trigonal bipyramidal arrangement of 5 electron pairs around central atom A

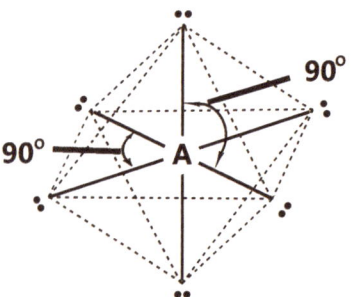

octahedral arrangement of 6 electron pairs around central atom A

Figure III.A.3.1: Molecular arrangement of electron pairs around a central atom A. Dotted lines only represent the overall molecular shape and not molecular bonds.

geometrical arrangement is tetrahedral in the first case which gives HCX or HCH angles close to 109°. The second case corresponds to a bent arrangement (with two lone pairs on the oxygen) and gives an HOY angle close to 109° as well. This also corresponds to a tetrahedral arrangement, however only two of these pairs are bonding pairs (connecting the H atoms to the central oxygen atom); therefore, the actual geometry according to Table III.A.3.1 is bent or V-shape geometry.

Go online to GAMSAT-prep.com for free chapter review Q&A and forum.

GOLD NOTES

PHASES AND PHASE EQUILIBRIA
Chapter 4

Memorize	Understand	Not Required*
ne: temp. (C, K), gas P and weight ne: STP, ideal gas, deviation ne: H bonds, dipole forces	* Kinetic molecular theory of gases * Maxwell distribution plot, H bonds, dipole F. * Deviation from ideal gas behavior * Equations: ideal gas/Charles'/Boyle's * Partial Press., mole fraction, Dalton's * Intermolecular forces, phase change/diagrams	* Advanced level college info * Memorizing Van der Waals' equation * Memorizing the gas constant R * Memorizing values: triple point of H_2O

GAMSAT-Prep.com

Introduction

A phase, or state of matter, is a uniform, distinct and usually separable region of material. For example, for a glass of water: the ice cubes are one phase (solid), the water is a second phase (liquid), and the humid air over the water is the third phase (gas = vapor). The temperature and pressure at which all 3 phases of a substance can coexist is called the triple point.

Additional Resources

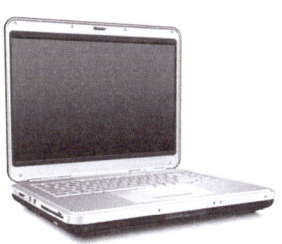

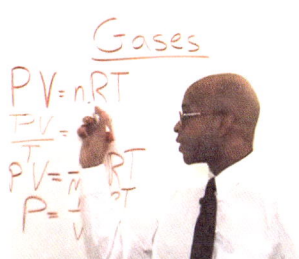

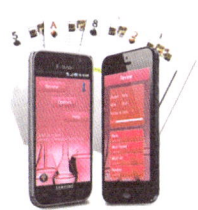

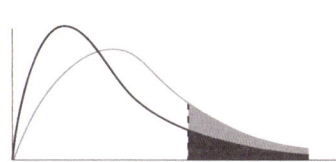

Free Online Q&A + Forum   Video: Online or DVD   Flashcards   Special Guest

THE PHYSICAL SCIENCES CHM-45

* The real GAMSAT may have advanced level information presented (ie. in a passage) but previous knowledge of said information is not required to answer the questions that would follow. Practice ACER and GS practice GAMSATs can help you clarify this point.

Elements and compounds exist in one of three states: <u>the gaseous state, the liquid state or the solid state</u>.

4.1 The Gas Phase

A substance in the gaseous state has neither fixed volume nor fixed shape: it spreads itself <u>uniformly</u> throughout any container in which it is placed.

4.1.1 Standard Temperature and Pressure, Standard Molar Volume

Any given gas can be described in terms of four fundamental properties: mass, volume, temperature and pressure. To simplify comparisons, the volume of a gas is normally reported at 0°C (273.15 K) and 1.00 atm (101.33 kPa = 760 mmHg = 760 torr); these conditions are known as the <u>standard temperature and pressure (STP)</u>. {Note: the SI unit of pressure is the pascal (Pa) and the old-fashioned Imperial unit is the pound per square inch because pressure is defined as force per unit area}

> The volume occupied by one mole of any gas at STP is referred to as the <u>standard molar volume</u> and is equal to 22.4 L.

4.1.2 Kinetic Molecular Theory of Gases (A Model for Gases)

The <u>kinetic molecular theory of gases</u> describes the particulate behavior of matter in the gaseous state. A gas that fits this theory exactly is called an <u>ideal gas</u>. The essential points of the theory are as follows:

1. Gases are composed of <u>extremely small</u> particles (either molecules or atoms depending on the gas) separated by distances that are relatively large in comparison with the diameters of the particles.

2. Particles of gas are in <u>constant motion,</u> except when they collide with one another.

3. Particles of an <u>ideal gas</u> exert no attractive or repulsive force on one another.

4. The collisions experienced by gas particles do not, on the average, slow them down; rather, they cause a <u>change</u> in the direction in which the particles are moving. If one particle loses energy as a result of a collision, the energy is gained by the particle with which it collides. <u>Collisions</u> of the particles of an ideal gas with the walls of the container <u>result in no loss of energy.</u>

5. The average kinetic energy of the particles (KE = 1/2 mv²) increases in direct proportion to the temperature of the gas (KE = 3/2 kT) when the temperature is measured on an absolute scale (i.e. the Kelvin scale) and k is a constant (the Boltzmann constant). The typical speed of a gas particle is directly proportional to the square root of the absolute temperature.

The plot of the distribution of collision energies of gases is similar to that of liquids. However, molecules in liquids require a minimum escape kinetic energy in order to enter the vapor phase (see Figure III.A.4.1 in CHM 4.1.2).

The properties of gases can be explained in terms of the kinetic molecular theory of ideal gases.

Experimentally, we can measure four properties of a gas:

1. The weight of the gas, from which we can calculate the number (N) of molecules or atoms of the gas present;

2. The pressure (P), exerted by the gas on the walls of the container in which this gas is placed (N.B.: a vacuum is completely devoid of particles and thus has *no* pressure);

3. The volume (V), occupied by the gas;

4. The temperature (T) of the gas.

In fact, if we know any three of these properties, we can calculate the fourth. So the minimum number of these properties required to fully describe the state of an ideal gas is three.

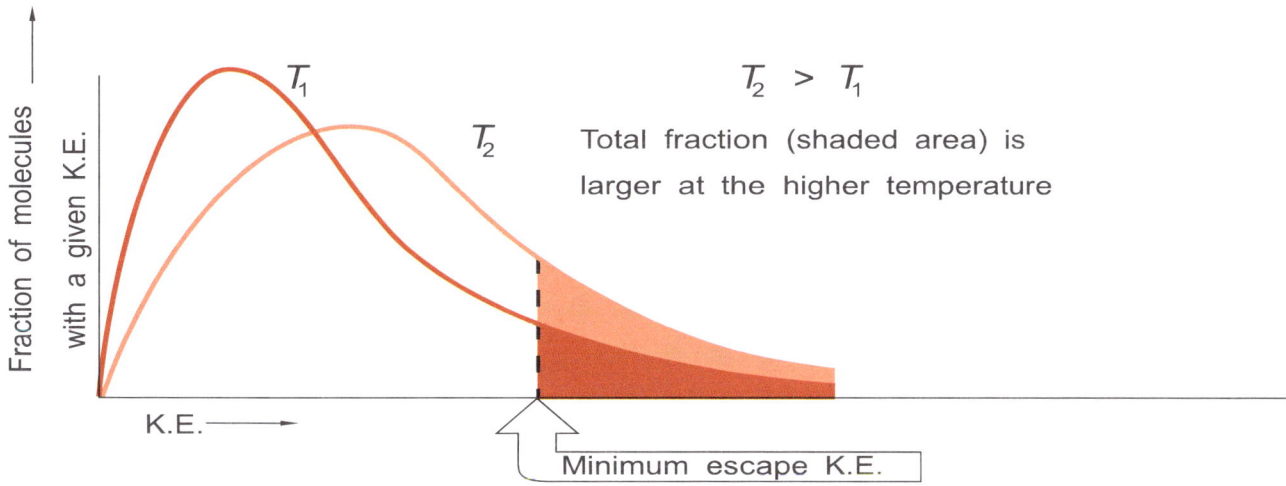

Figure III.A.4.1: The Maxwell Distribution Plot. At a higher temperature T₂, the curve peak is flattened, which means that gas particles within the sample are travelling at a wider range of velocities. Additionally, the larger shaded area at a temperature T₂ means that a greater proportion of molecules will possess the minimum escaping kinetic energy (KE) required to evaporate.

4.1.3 Graham's Law (Diffusion and Effusion of Gases)

Graham's law describes the mean (average) free path of any typical gas particle taken per unit volume. The process taken by such gas particles is known as *diffusion* and its related process *effusion* which are defined as follows:

Diffusion is the flow of gas particles spreading out evenly through random motion. Gas particles diffuse from regions of high concentration to regions of low concentration. The rate at which a gas diffuses is inversely proportional to the square root of its molar mass. The ratio of the diffusion rates of two different gases is inversely proportional to the square root of their respective molar masses. $Rate_1/Rate_2$ and M_1/M_2 represents diffusion rates of gases 1 and 2 and the molar mass of gases 1 and 2. Lighter particles diffuse quicker than heavier particles.

Effusion is the movement of a gas through a small hole or pore into another gaseous region or into a vacuum. If the hole is large enough, the process may be considered diffusion instead of effusion. The rates at which two gases effuse are inversely proportional to the square root of their molar masses, the same as that for diffusion:

$$\frac{Rate_1}{Rate_2} = \sqrt{\frac{M_2}{M_1}}$$

4.1.4 Charles' Law

The volume (V) of a gas is directly proportional to the absolute temperature (expressed in Kelvins) when P and N are kept constant.

$$V = \text{Constant} \times T \quad \text{or} \quad V_1/V_2 = T_1/T_2$$

NOTE: For Charles' Law and all subsequent laws, the subscripts 1 and 2 refer to both initial and final values of all variables for the gas in question.

4.1.5 Boyle's Law

The volume (V) of a fixed weight of gas held at constant temperature (T) varies inversely with the pressure (P).

$$V = \text{Constant} \times 1/P \quad \text{or} \quad P_1V_1 = P_2V_2$$

GENERAL CHEMISTRY

4.1.6 Avogadro's Law

The volume (V) of a gas at constant temperature and pressure is directly proportional to the number of particles or moles (n) of the gas present.

$$V/n = \text{Constant} \quad \text{or} \quad V_1/n_1 = V_2/n_2$$

4.1.7 Combined Gas Law

For a given constant mass of any gas the product of its pressure and volume divided by its Kelvin temperature is equal to a constant (k). Therefore, by using the combined gas law, one may calculate any of the three variables of a gas exposed to two separate conditions as follows:

This relationship depicts how a change in pressure, volume, and/or temperature of any gas (at constant mass) will be affected as a function of the other quantities (P_2, V_2 or T_2).

$$\frac{P_1V_1}{T_1} = k = \frac{P_2V_2}{T_2} \quad \text{(at constant mass)}$$

4.1.8 Ideal Gas Law

The combination of Boyle's law, Charles' law and Avogadro's law yields the "ideal gas law":

$$PV = nRT$$

where R is the <u>universal gas constant</u> and n is the number of moles of gas particles.

R = 0.0821 L-atm/K-mole
= 8.31 kPa-dm³/K-mole

A typical ideal gas problem is as follows: an ideal gas at 27 °C and 380 torr occupies a volume of 492 cm³. What is the number of moles of gas?

THE PHYSICAL SCIENCES CHM-49

GAMSAT-Prep.com
THE GOLD STANDARD

Ideal Gas Law problems often amount to mere exercises of unit conversions. The easiest way to do them is to convert the units of the values given to the units of the R gas constant.

$$P = 380 \text{ torr} = \frac{380 \text{ torr}}{(760 \text{ torr/atm})} = 0.500 \text{ atm}$$

$$T = 27\,°C = 273 + 27\,°C = 300 \text{ K}$$

$$V = 492 \text{ cm}^3 = 492 \text{ cm}^3 \times (1 \text{ liter}/1000 \text{ cm}^3)$$
$$= 0.492 \text{ liter}$$

$$PV = nRT$$

$$n = PV/RT$$

$$n = \frac{(0.500 \text{ atm} \times 0.492 \text{ L})}{(0.0821 \text{ L-atm/K-mole} \times 300 \text{ K})}$$

$$n = 0.0100 \text{ mole}$$

Also note that the ideal gas law could be used in the following alternate ways (Mwt = molecular weight):

(i) since n = (mass m of gas sample)/(Mwt M of the gas)

$$PV = (m/M)RT$$

(ii) since m/V is the density (d) of the gas:

$$P = \frac{dRT}{M}$$

4.1.9 Partial Pressure and Dalton's Law

In a mixture of unreactive gases, each gas distributes evenly throughout the container. All particles exert the same pressure on the walls of the container with equal force. If we consider a mixture of gases occupying a total volume (V) at a temperature (T) the term partial pressure is used to refer to the pressure exerted by one component of the gas mixture if it were occupying the entire volume (V) at the temperature (T).

Dalton's law states that the total pressure observed for a mixture of gases is equal to the sum of the pressures that each individual component would exert were it alone in the container.

$$P_T = P_1 + P_2 + \ldots + P_i$$

where P_T is the total pressure and P_i is the partial pressure of any component (i).

The mole fraction (X_i) of any one gas present in a mixture is defined as follows:

$$X_i = n_i/n_{(total)}$$

where n_i = moles of that gas present in the mixture and $n_{(total)}$ = sum of the moles of all gases present in the mixture (see CHM 5.3.1).

CHM-50   PHASES AND PHASE EQUILIBRIA

GENERAL CHEMISTRY

Of course, the sum of all mole fractions in a mixture must equal one:

$$\Sigma X_i = 1$$

The partial pressure (P_i) of a component of a gas mixture is equal to:

$$P_i = X_i P_T$$

The ideal gas law applies to any component of the mixture:

$$P_i V = n_i RT$$

4.1.10 Deviation of Real Gas Behavior from the Ideal Gas Law

The particles of an ideal gas have zero volume and no intermolecular forces. It obeys the ideal gas law. Its particles behave as though they were moving points exerting no attraction on one another and occupying no space. Real gases deviate from ideal gas behavior particularly when the gas particles are forced into close proximity under high pressure and low temperature, as follows:

1. They do not obey $PV = nRT$. We can calculate n, P, V and T for a real gas on the assumption that it behaves like an ideal gas but the calculated values will not agree with the observed values.

2. Their particles are subject to intermolecular forces (i.e. forces of attraction between different molecules like Van der Waal forces; CHM 4.2) which are themselves independent of temperature. But the deviations they cause are more pronounced at low temperatures because they are less effectively opposed by the slower motion of particles at lower temperatures. Similarly, an increase in pressure at constant temperature will crowd the particles closer together and reduce the average distance between them. This will increase the attractive force between the particles and the stronger these forces, the more the behavior of the real gas will deviate from that of an ideal gas. Thus, a real gas will act less like an ideal gas at higher pressures than at lower pressures. {Mnemonic: an ideal Plow and Thigh = an ideal gas exists when **Pressure** is **low** and **Temperature** is **high**}

3. The particles (i.e. molecules or atoms) occupy space. When a real gas is subjected to high pressures at ordinary temperatures, the fraction of the total volume occupied by the particles increases. At moderately high pressure, gas particles are pushed closer together and intermolecular attraction causes the gas to have a smaller volume than would be predicted by the ideal gas law. At extremely high pressure, gas particles are pushed even closer in such a way that the distance between them are becoming insignificant

THE PHYSICAL SCIENCES CHM-51

compared to the size of the particles, therefore causing the gas to take up a smaller volume than would be predicted by the ideal gas law. Under these conditions, the real gas deviates appreciably from ideal gas behavior.

4. Their size and mass also affect the speed at which they move. At constant temperature, the kinetic energy (KE = 1/2 mv^2) of all particles – light or heavy – is nearly the same. This means that the heavier particles must be moving more slowly than the lighter ones and that the attractive forces between the heavier particles must be exercising a greater influence on their behavior. The greater speed of light particles, however, tends to counteract the attractive forces between them, thus producing a slight deviation from ideal gas behavior. Thus, a heavier particle (molecule or atom) will deviate more widely from ideal gas behavior than a lighter particle. At low temperature, the average velocity of gas particles decreases and the intermolecular attraction becomes increasingly significant, causing the gas to have a smaller volume than would be predicted by the ideal gas law. {The preceding is given by Graham's law, where the rate of movement of a gas (*diffusion* or streaming through a fine hole – *effusion*) is inversely proportional to the square root of the molecular weight of the gas (see CHM 4.1.3)}

4.2 Liquid Phase (Intra- and Intermolecular Forces)

Liquids have the ability to mix with one another and with other phases to form solutions. The degree to which two liquids can mix is called their miscibility. Liquids have definite volume, but no definite shape. As we will discuss, molecules of liquids can be attracted to each other (*cohesion*) as they can be attracted to their surroundings (*adhesion*). The most striking properties of a liquid are its viscosity and surface tension (see CHM 4.2.1, PHY 6.1.5). Liquids also distinguish themselves from gases in that they are relatively incompressible. The molecules of a liquid are also subject to forces strong enough to hold them together. These forces are intermolecular and they are weak attractive forces that is, they are effective over short distances only. Molecules like methane (CH_4) are non-polar and so they are held together by weak intermolecular forces also known as Van der Waal forces (these include forces that are dipole-dipole, dipole-induced dipole and London forces). Whereas, molecules like water have much stronger intermolecular attractive forces because of the hydrogen bonding amongst the molecules. Hence, the most important forces are:

1. Dipole-dipole forces which depend on the orientation as well as on the distance between the molecules; they are inversely proportional to the fourth power of the distance. In addition to the forces between permanent dipoles, a dipolar

molecule induces in a neighboring molecule an electron distribution that results in another attractive force, the <u>dipole-induced dipole force</u>, which is inversely proportional to the seventh power of the distance and which is relatively independent of orientation.

2. <u>London forces</u> (or Dispersive forces) are attractive forces acting between nonpolar molecules. They are due to the unsymmetrical instantaneous electron distribution which induces a dipole in neighboring molecules with a resultant attractive force. This instantaneous unsymmetrical distribution of electrons causes rapid polarization of the electrons and formation of short-lived dipoles. These dipoles then interact with neighboring molecules, inducing the formation of more dipoles. Dispersion forces are thus responsible for the liquefaction of noble gases to form liquids at low temperatures (and high pressures).

3. <u>Hydrogen bonds</u> occur whenever hydrogen is covalently bonded to an atom such as O, N or F that attract electrons strongly. Because of the differences in electronegativity between H and O or N or F, the electrons that constitute the covalent bond are closer to the O, N or F nucleus than

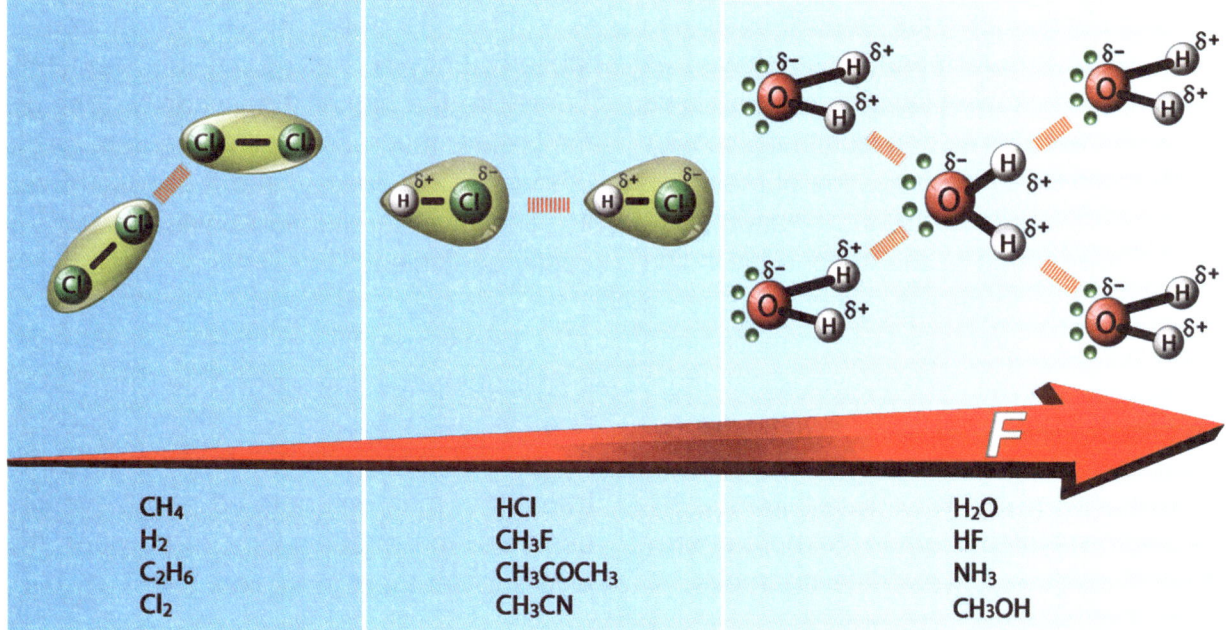

Table III.A.4.1: Van Der Waal's forces (weak) and hydrogen bonding (strong). London forces between Cl_2 molecules, dipole-dipole forces between HCl molecules and H-bonding between H_2O molecules. Note that a partial negative charge on an atom is indicated by δ^- (delta negative), while a partial positive charge is indicated by δ^+ (delta positive). Notice that one H_2O molecule can potentially form 4 H-bonds with surrounding molecules which is highly efficient. The preceding is one key reason that the boiling point of water is higher than that of ammonia, hydrogen fluoride or methanol.

to the H nucleus leaving the latter relatively unshielded. The unshielded proton is strongly attracted to the O, N or F atoms of neighboring molecules since these form the negative end of a strong dipole.

The slightly positive charge of the hydrogen atom will then be strongly attracted to the more electronegative atoms of nearby molecules. These forces are weaker than intramolecular bonds, but are much stronger than the other two types of intermolecular forces. Hydrogen bonding is a special case of dipole-dipole interaction. Hydrogen bonds are characterized by unusually strong interactions and high boiling points due to the vast amount of energy required (relative to other intermolecular forces) to break the hydrogen bonds. {Though the H-bonding atoms are often remembered by the mnemonic "Hydrogen is FON!", sulfur is also known to H-bond though far weaker than the more electronegative FON atoms.}

4.2.1 Viscosity

Viscosity is analogous to friction between moving solids. It may, therefore be viewed as the resistance to flow of layers of fluid or liquid past each other. This also means that viscosity, as in friction, results in dissipation of mechanical energy. As one layer flows over another, its motion is transmitted to the second layer and causes this layer to be set in motion. Since a mass m of the second layer is set in motion and some of the energy of the first layer is lost, there is a transfer of momentum between the layers.

The greater the transfer of this momentum from one layer to another, the more energy that is lost and the slower the layers move.

The viscosity (η) is the measure of the efficiency of transfer of this momentum. Therefore the higher the viscosity coefficient, the greater the transfer of momentum and loss of mechanical energy, and thus loss of velocity. The reverse situation holds for a low viscosity coefficient.

Consequently, a high viscosity coefficient substance flows slowly (e.g. molasses), and a low viscosity coefficient substance flows relatively fast (e.g. water). Note that the transfer of momentum to adjacent layers is in essence, the exertion of a force upon these layers to set them in motion.

GENERAL CHEMISTRY

4.3 Solid Phase

Solids have definite volume and shape and are incompressible under pressure. Intermolecular forces between molecules of molecular solids and electrostatic (i.e. coulombic or "opposite charges attract") interactive forces between ions of ionic solids are strong enough to hold them into a relatively rigid structure. A solid may be crystalline (ordered) or amorphous (disordered). A crystalline solid, such as table salt (NaCl) has a structure with an ordered geometric shape. Its atoms are arranged geometrically with a repeating pattern. It has a specific melting point. An amorphous solid, such as glass, has a molecular structure with no specific shape. It melts over a wide range of temperatures since the molecules require different amounts of energies to break bonds between them.

4.4 Phase Equilibria (Solids, Liquids and Gases)

4.4.1 Phase Changes

Elements and compounds can undergo transitions between the solid, liquid and gaseous states. They can exist in different phases and undergo phase changes which need not involve chemical reactions. Phase changes are reversible with an equilibrium existing between each of the phases. A phase is a homogeneous, physically distinct and mechanically separable part of a system. Each phase is separated from other phases by a physical boundary.

A few examples:

1. Ice/liquid water/water vapor (3 phases)

2. Any number of gases mix in all proportions and therefore constitute just one phase.

3. The system $CaCO_3(s) \rightarrow CaO(s) + CO_2(g)$ (2 phases, i.e. 2 solids: $CaCO_3$ and CaO and a gas: CO_2)

4. A saturated salt solution (3 phases: solution, undissolved salt, vapor)

An example of phase change is the vaporization of water into its vapor state. A system is considered homogeneous when it is uniform throughout its volume so that its properties are the same in all parts. This does not imply a single molecular species: a solution of sodium chloride is homogeneous provided its concentration is the same throughout.

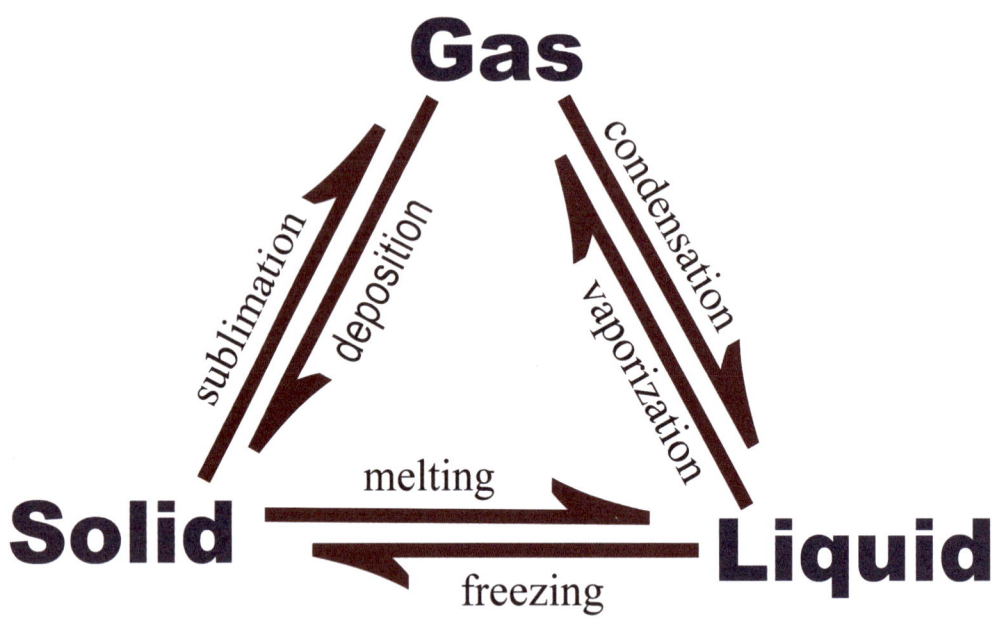

Figure III.A.4.2: Phase Changes

4.4.2 Freezing Point, Melting Point, Boiling Point

The conversion of a liquid to a gas is called <u>vaporization</u>. We can increase the rate of vaporization of a liquid by (i) increasing the temperature (ii) reducing the pressure, or (iii) both. Molecules escape from a liquid because, even though their average kinetic energy is constant, not all of them move at the same speed (see Figure III.A.4.1). A fast moving molecule can break away from the attraction of the others and pass into the vapor state. When a tight lid is placed on a vessel containing a liquid, the vapor molecules cannot escape and some revert back to the liquid state. The number of molecules leaving the liquid at any given time equals the number of molecules returning. Equilibrium is reached and the number of molecules in the fixed volume above the liquid remains constant. These molecules exert a constant pressure at a fixed temperature which is called the vapor pressure of the liquid. The vapor pressure is the partial pressure exerted by the gas molecules over the liquid formed by evaporation, when it is in equilibrium with the gas phase condensing back into the liquid phase. The vapor pressure of any liquid is dependent on the intermolecular forces that are present within the liquid and the temperature. Weak intermolecular forces result in volatile substances whereas strong intermolecular forces result in nonvolatile substances.

Boiling and evaporation are similar processes but they differ as follows: the vapor from a boiling liquid escapes with sufficient pressure to push back any other gas present,

GENERAL CHEMISTRY

rather than diffusing through it. Vapor pressure increases as the temperature increases, as more molecules have sufficient energy to break the attraction between each other to escape into the gas phase. The boiling point is therefore the temperature at which the vapor pressure of the liquid equals to the opposing external pressure. Under a lower pressure, the boiling point is reached at a lower temperature. Increased intermolecular interactions (i.e. H_2O see CHM 4.2, alcohol see ORG 6.1, etc.) will decrease the vapor pressure thus raising the boiling point. Other factors being equal, as a molecule becomes heavier (increasing molecular weight), it becomes more difficult to push the molecule into the atmosphere thus the boiling point increases (i.e. alkanes see ORG 3.1.1).

The freezing point of a liquid is the temperature at which the vapor pressure of the solid equals the vapor pressure of the liquid. Increases in the prevailing atmospheric pressure decreases the melting point and increases the boiling point.

When a solid is heated, the kinetic energy of the components increases steadily. Finally, the kinetic energy becomes great enough to overcome the forces holding the components together and the solid changes to a liquid. For pure crystalline solids, there is a fixed temperature at which this transition from solid to liquid occurs. This temperature is called the melting point. Pure solids melt completely at one temperature. Impure solids begin to melt at one temperature but become completely liquid at a higher temperature.

4.4.3 Phase Diagrams

Figure III.A.4.3 shows the temperature of ice as heat is added. Temperature increases linearly with heat until the melting point is reached. At this point, the heat energy added does not change the temperature. Instead, it is used to break intermolecular bonds and convert ice into water. There is a mixture of both ice and water at the melting point. After all of the complete conversion of ice into water, the temperature rises again linearly with heat addition. At the boiling point, the heat added does not change the temperature because the energy is again used to break the intermolecular bonds. After complete conversion of water into gas, the temperature will rise linearly again with heat addition.

Thus, during a phase change, there is no change in temperature. The energy that is added into the system is being used to weaken/break intermolecular forces; in other words, there is an increase in the potential energy of molecules rather than an increase in the average kinetic energy of molecules. The amount of energy to change one mole of substance from solid to liquid or from liquid to gas is called the molar *heat of fusion* and the molar *heat of vaporization* (CHM 8.7) Each

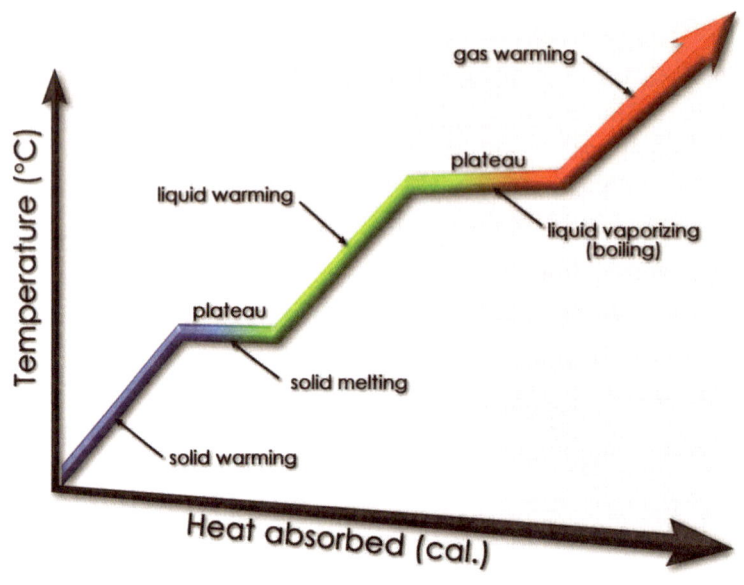

Figure III.A.4.3 Heating curve for H_2O

phase has its own specific heat. Enthalpy of vaporization is greater than that of fusion because more energy is required to break intermolecular bonds (from liquid phase to gas phase) than just to weaken intermolecular bonds (from solid phase to liquid phase).

The temperatures at which phase transitions occur are functions of the pressure of the system. The behavior of a given substance over a wide range of temperature and pressure can be summarized in a phase diagram, such as the one shown for the water system (Fig.III.A.4.4). The diagram is divided into three areas labeled **solid** (ice), **liquid** (water) and **vapor** in each of which only one phase exists. In these areas, P and T can be independently varied without a second phase appearing. These areas are bounded by curves AC, AD and AB. Line AB represents sublimation/deposition (sublimation curve). Line AC represents evaporation/condensation (vaporization curve) and Line AD represents melting/freezing (fusion curve). At triple point A, all three phases are known to coexist. At any point on these curves, two phases are in equilibrium. Thus on AC, at a given T, the saturated vapor pressure of water has a fixed value. The boiling point of water (N) can be found on this curve, 100 °C at 760 mmHg pressure. The curve only extends as far as C, the critical point, where the vapor and liquid are indistinguishable. In general, the gas phase is found at high temperature and low pressure; the solid phase is found at low temperatures and high pressure; and the liquid phase is found at high temperatures and high pressure. The temperature at which a substance boils when the pressure is 1 atm is called the normal boiling point.

GENERAL CHEMISTRY

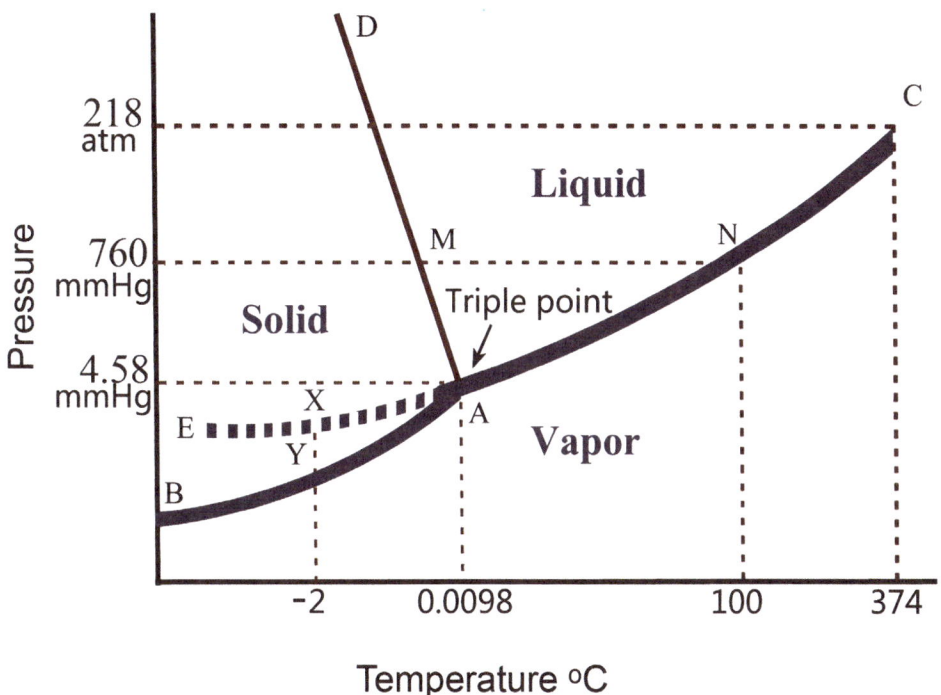

Figure III.A.4.4: Phase diagram for H₂O.

The extension of the curve CA to E represents the metastable equilibrium (*meta* = beyond) between supercooled water and its vapor. If the temperature is slightly raised at point X, a little of the liquid will vaporize until a new equilibrium is established at that higher temperature. Curve AB is the vapor pressure curve for ice. Its equilibria are of lower energy than those of AE and thus more stable.

The slope of line AD shows that an increase in P will lower the melting point of ice. This property is almost unique to water. Because of the negative slope of line AD, an isothermal increase in pressure will compress the solid (ice) into liquid (water). Thus H₂O is unique in that its liquid form is denser than its solid form. The high density of liquid water is due mainly to the cohesive nature of the hydrogen-bonded network of water molecules (see Table III.A.4.1 in CHM 4.2).

Most substances *increase* their melting points with increased pressure. Thus the line AD slants to the right for almost all substances. Point M represents the true melting point of ice, 0.0023 °C at 760 mmHg of pressure. (The 0 °C standard refers to the freezing point of water saturated with air at 760 mmHg). At point A, solid, liquid and vapor are in equilibrium. At this one temperature, ice and water have the same fixed vapor pressure. This is the triple point, 0.0098 °C at 4.58 mmHg pressure.

Go online to GAMSAT-prep.com for free chapter review Q&A and forum.

GOLD NOTES

SOLUTION CHEMISTRY

Chapter 5

Memorize	Understand	Not Required*
ine saturated, supersaturated, volatile nmon anions and cations in solution ts of concentration ine electrolytes with examples	* Colligative properties, Raoult's law * Phase diagram change due to coll. properties * Bp elevation, fp depression * Osmotic press, equation * Solubility product, common-ion effect * Solubility rules	* Advanced level college info * % solubility of glucose in water

GAMSAT-Prep.com

Introduction

A solution is a homogeneous mixture composed of two or more substances. For example, a solute (salt) dissolved in a solvent (water) making a solution (salt water). Solutions can involve gases in liquids (i.e. oxygen in water) or even solids in solids (i.e. alloys). Two substances are immiscible if they can't mix to make a solution. Solutions can be distinguished from non-homogeneous mixtures like colloids and suspensions.

Additional Resources

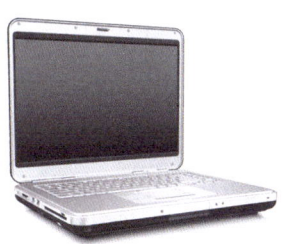   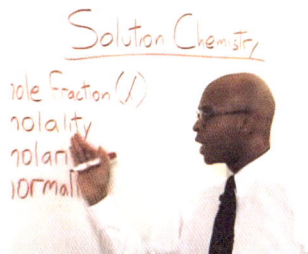   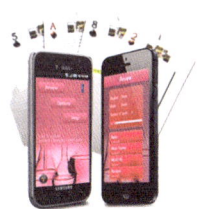   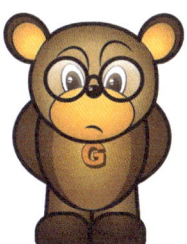

Free Online Q&A + Forum   Video: Online or DVD   Flashcards   Special Guest

THE PHYSICAL SCIENCES   CHM-61

The real GAMSAT may have advanced level information presented (ie. in a passage) but previous knowledge of said information is not required to answer the questions that would follow. Practice ACER and GS practice GAMSATs can help you clarify this point.

5.1 Solutions and Colligative Properties

Water (H₂O) is a universal solvent known as a pure substance or a one component system. Pure substances are often mixed together to form solutions. A solution is a sample of matter that is homogeneous but, unlike a pure substance, the composition of a solution can vary within relatively wide limits. Ethanol (= ethyl alcohol = "alcohol"; ORG 6.1) and water are each pure substances and each have a fixed composition, C_2H_5OH and H_2O, but mixtures of the two can vary continuously in composition from almost 100% ethanol to almost 100% water. Solutions of sucrose in water, however, are limited to a maximum percentage of sucrose - the solubility - which is 67% at 20°C, thus the solution is saturated. If the solution is heated, a higher concentration of sucrose can be achieved (i.e. 70%). Slowly cooling down to 20°C creates a supersaturated solution which may precipitate with any perturbation.

Intermolecular forces (see CHM 4.2) amongst various other parameters may either promote or may prevent the formation of a solution. The formation of solutions primarily involves the breaking of intermolecular forces between solutes and between solvents and the subsequent reformation of new intermolecular interactions amongst the solute and solvent. The initial step in solution formation (i.e. breakage of intermolecular forces amongst the solutes and solvent separately) is endothermic and the second step (i.e. reformation of intermolecular interactions between solute-solvent) is exothermic. If an overall reaction in solution formation is exothermic, the new intermolecular bonds between solute and solvent are more stable and a solution is formed. {Note: "endothermic" - absorbs heat, "exothermic" - releases heat; "enthalpy" is a measure of the total energy; see CHM chapters 7 and 8 for details}

In the energetic requirements of solution formation, the formation of a solution may result in either an increase or a decrease in the enthalpy of solution dependant on the magnitude of interactions between the solute and solvent. Hence, energy changes do occur when a solution forms (i.e exothermic or endothermic). An increase in enthalpy, a positive heat of solution, results in more energy in a system i.e. less stable and weaker bonds. Whereas a decrease in enthalpy, a negative heat of solution, results in less energy in a system i.e. more stable and stronger bonds and thus the respective drive to the formation of a solution.

Lastly, the formation of a solution always results in an increase in entropy or disorder due to the insidious tendency for energy to disperse.

Generally the component of a solution that is stable in the same phase as the solution is called the solvent. If two components of a solution are in the same phase, the component present in the larger amount is called the solvent and the other is called the solute. Many properties of solutions are dependent only on the relative number of molecules (or ions) of the solute and of the solvent. Properties that depend **only** on the number of particles present and not the kind of particles are called colligative properties. For all

GENERAL CHEMISTRY

colligative properties, a factor known as the Van't Hoff factor (*i*) is essentially required and defined as, the ratio of moles of particles or ions in a solution to the moles of all undissociated formula units (or molecules) within a solution. The factor (*i*) is therefore incorporated as a multiple of all the colligative properties equations, respectively (see below). Thus, for non-ionic solutions, the factor (*i*) is essentially equal to 1 as the particles are undissociated such as for sugar solutions. However, for ionic solutions, the factor (*i*) is dependent on the number of ions dissociated in solution (i.e., NaCl = 2, $CaCl_2$ = 3, etc.). Hence, the most important colligative properties can be found in the following sections.

5.1.1 Vapor-Pressure Lowering (Raoult's Law)

The vapor pressure of the components of an ideal solution behaves as follows:

$$p_i = X_i (p_i)_{pure}$$

where p_i = vapor pressure of component *i* in equilibrium with the solution
$(p_i)_{pure}$ = vapor pressure of pure component *i* at the same T
X_i = mole fraction of component *i* in the liquid.

Thus the vapor pressure of any component of a mixture is lowered by the presence of the other components. Experimentally, it can be observed that when dissolving a solute which cannot evaporate (= *nonvolatile*) into a solvent, the vapor pressure of the resulting solution is lower than that of the pure solvent. The extent to which the vapor pressure is lowered is determined by the mole fraction of the solvent in solution ($X_{solvent}$):

$$P = P°X_{solvent}$$

where P = vapor pressure of solution
$P°$ = vapor pressure of pure solvent (at the same temperature as P).

When rearranged this way, the vapor pressure of a solution is quantified by Raoult's law which states that the lowering of the vapor pressure of the solvent is proportional to the mole fraction of solvent and independent of the chemical nature of the solute.

Hence, to show by how much a solution's vapor pressure is lowered by a solute, we can therefore define the vapor pressure lowering (ΔP) by the following equation; $\Delta P = X_{solute} P°_{solvent}$. Where, $\Delta P = P°_{solvent} - P_{solution}$ and rearranging the differences between the solvent and solution vapor pressures and substituting the solvent mole fraction ($X_{solvent}$) with the solute mole fraction as $X_{solvent} = 1 - X_{solute}$, results in Raoult's law which indicates that the lowering of the vapor pressure is directly proportional to the solute mole fraction as stated previously.

THE PHYSICAL SCIENCES

5.1.2 Boiling-Point Elevation and Freezing-Point Depression

When the vapor-pressure curve of a dilute solution and the vapor-pressure curve of the pure solvent are plotted on a phase diagram (see Figure III.A.5.1), it can be seen that a vapor pressure lowering of a solution occurs at all temperatures and that the freezing point and boiling point of a solution must therefore be different from those of the pure liquid.

The freezing point of a pure solvent (water) is lowered or depressed with the addition of another substance; meaning that a solution (solvent + solute) has a lower freezing point than a pure solvent, and this phenomenon is called a "freezing point depression". Alternatively, the boiling point of a pure solvent (water) is elevated when another substance is added; meaning that a solution

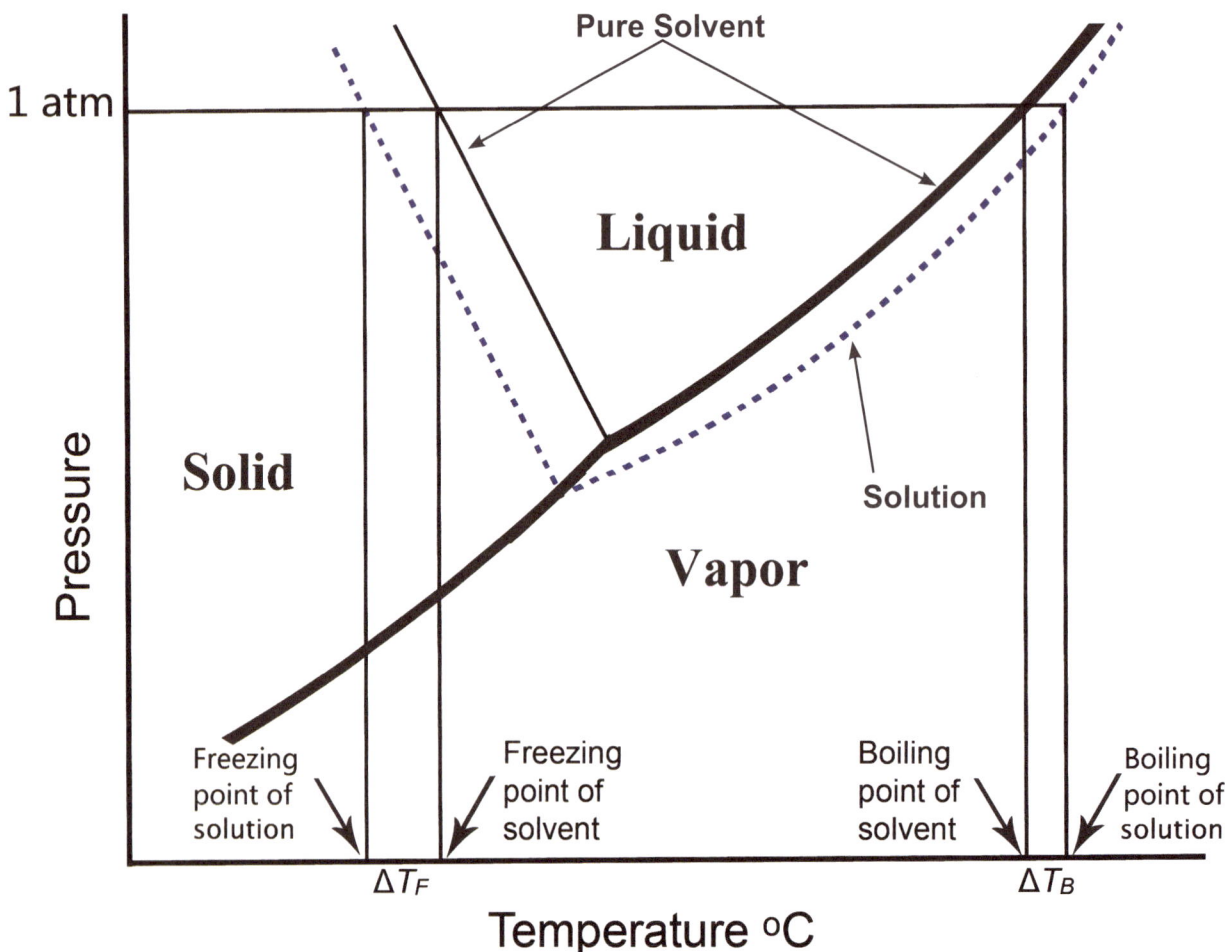

Figure III.A.5.1: Phase diagram of water demonstrating the effect of the addition of a solute.

has a higher boiling point than a pure solvent, and this phenomenon is called "boiling point elevation". The boiling point is therefore higher for the solution than for the pure liquid and the freezing point is lower for the solution than for the pure liquid. Since the decrease in vapor pressure is proportional to the mole fraction (see CHM 5.3.1) of solute, the boiling point elevation (ΔT_B) is also proportional to the mole fraction of solute and:

$$\Delta T_B = i\, K_B'\, X_B = i\, K_B\, m$$

where K_B' = boiling point elevation constant for the solvent
X_B = mole fraction of solute
m = molality (moles solute per kilogram of solvent; CHM 5.3.1)
i = Van't Hoff factor

K_B is related to K_B' through a change of units.

Similarly, for the freezing point depression (ΔT_F):

$$\Delta T_F = i\, K_F'\, X_B = i\, K_F\, m$$

where K_F' = freezing point depression constant for the solvent.

If K_F or K_B is known, it is then possible to determine the molality of a dilute solution simply by measuring the freezing point or the boiling point. These constants can be determined by measuring the freezing point and boiling point of a solution of known molality. If the mass concentration of a solute (in kg solute per kg of solvent) is known and the molality is determined from the freezing point of the solution, the mass of 1 mole of solute can be calculated.

It is important to recall that for a strong electrolyte solution such as NaCl which dissociates to positive and negative ions, the right hand side of the equation is multiplied by the Van't Hoff factor (*i*) equal to the number of ionic species generated per mole of solute. For NaCl n = 2 but for $MgCl_2$ n = 3. {Remember: colligative properties depend on the **number** of particles present}

5.1.3 Osmotic Pressure

The osmotic pressure (Π) of a solution describes the equilibrium distribution of solvent across semipermeable membranes separated by two compartments. When a solvent and solution are separated by a membrane permeable only to molecules of solvent (a semipermeable membrane), the solvent spontaneously migrates into the solution. The semipermeable membrane allows the solvent to pass but not the solute. Since pure solute cannot pass through the semipermeable membrane into the pure solvent side to equalize the concentrations, the pure solvent begins to then move into the solution side containing the solute. As it does so, the solution level rises and the pressure increases. Eventually a balance is achieved and the increased pressure difference on the solution side is the osmotic pressure. The solvent therefore migrates into the solution across the membrane until a sufficient hydrostatic pressure develops to prevent further migration of solvent. The pressure required to prevent migration of the solvent is therefore the osmotic pressure of the solution and is equal to:

$$\Pi = iMRT$$

where R = gas constant per mole
T = temperature in degrees K and
M = concentration of solute (mole/liter)
i = Van't Hoff factor

Note: molarity (M) is used in the osmotic pressure formulation in place of molality as is used for the other respective colligative properties as molarity is temperature dependent and molality is not temperature dependent.

Osmosis and osmotic pressure are also discussed in the context of biology in the following sections: BIO 1.1.1 and 7.5.2.

5.2 Ions in Solution

An important area of solution chemistry involves aqueous solutions. Water has a particular property that causes many substances to split apart into charged species, that is, to dissociate and form ions. Ions that are positively charged are called cations and negatively charged ions are called anions. {Mnemonic: anions are negative ions} As a rule, highly charged species (i.e. AlPO$_4$, Al^{3+}/PO$_4^{3-}$) have a greater force of attraction thus are much less soluble in water than species with little charge (i.e. NaCl, Na$^+$/Cl$^-$). The word "aqueous" simply means containing or dissolved in water. All the following ions can form in water.

Common Anions					
F$^-$	Fluoride	OH$^-$	Hydroxide	ClO$^-$	Hypochlorite
Cl$^-$	Chloride	NO$_3^-$	Nitrate	ClO$_2^-$	Chlorite
Br$^-$	Bromide	NO$_2^-$	Nitrite	ClO$_3^-$	Chlorate
I$^-$	Iodide	CO$_3^{2-}$	Carbonate	ClO$_4^-$	Perchlorate
O^{2-}	Oxide	SO$_4^{2-}$	Sulfate	SO$_3^{2-}$	Sulfite
S^{2-}	Sulfide	PO$_4^{3-}$	Phosphate	CN$^-$	Cyanide
N^{3-}	Nitride	CH$_3$CO$_2^-$	Acetate	MnO$_4^-$	Permanganate

GENERAL CHEMISTRY

Common Cations				
Na^+	Sodium	H^+	Hydrogen
Li^+	Lithium	Ca^{2+}	Calcium
K^+	Potassium	Mg^{2+}	Magnesium
NH_4^+	Ammonium	Fe^{2+}	Iron (II)
H_3O^+	Hydronium	Fe^{3+}	Iron (III)

Table III.A.5.1: Common Anions and Cations.

As opposed to Organic Chemistry, the GAMSAT does not normally ask Inorganic Chemistry nomenclature (= *naming*) questions but it may be useful to have some background regarding the International Union of Pure and Applied Chemistry (IUPAC) standard suffixes: (1) Single atom anions are named with an *-ide* suffix (i.e. fluoride); (2) Oxyanions (*polyatomic* or "many atom" anions containing oxygen) are named with *-ite* or *-ate*, for a lesser or greater quantity of oxygen. For example, NO_2^- is nitrite, while NO_3^- is nitrate. The hypo- and per- prefixes can also indicate less oxygen and more oxygen, respectively (see hypochlorite and perchlorate among the Common Anions in Table III.A.5.1). (3) -ium is a very common ending of atoms in the periodic table (CHM 2.3) and it is also common among cations; (4) Compounds with cations: The name of the compound is simply the cation's name (usually the same as the element's), followed by the anion. For example, NaCl is *sodium chloride* and Ca_3N_2 is *calcium nitride*.

5.3 Solubility

The solubility of any substance is generally defined as the amount of the substance (solute) known to dissolve into a particular amount of solvent at a given temperature. The solubility of a solute into a solvent is dependent on the entropy change of solubilization as well as the types of intermolecular forces involved (see CHM 4.2 and 5.1). Solvation or dissolution is the process of interaction between solute and solvent molecules. This process occurs when the intermolecular forces between solute and solvent are stronger than those between solute particles themselves. Generally, ionic and polar solutes are soluble in polar solvents and nonpolar solutes are soluble in nonpolar solvents. Consequently, the expression "like dissolves like" is often used for predicting solubility.

In the following section, the definitions of the various solution concentration units are given with examples.

GAMSAT-Prep.com
THE GOLD STANDARD

5.3.1 Units of Concentration

In the sections to follow, where possible, please try to complete the calculations as quickly as possible prior to looking at the solutions (i.e. apply dimensional analysis; GM 2.2).

There are a number of ways in which solution concentrations may be expressed.

Molarity (*M*): A one-molar solution is defined as one mole of substance in each liter of solution: M = moles of solute/liter of solution (solution = solute + solvent).

For example: If 55.0g of $CaCl_2$ is mixed with water to make 500.0 ml (0.5 L) of solution, what is the molarity (*M*) of the solution?

55.0g of $CaCl_2$ = 55.0 g/110.0 g/mol
= 0.500 mol of $CaCl_2$

Therefore, the Molarity = 0.500 mol $CaCl_2$/0.5L = 1.00 mol $CaCl_2$/L solution

Normality (*N*): A one-normal solution contains one equivalent per liter. An equivalent is a mole multiplied by the number of reacting units for each molecule or atom; the equivalent weight is the formula weight divided by the number of reacting units.

\# of Equiv. = mass (in g)/eq. wt. (in g/equiv.)
= Normality (in equiv./liter)
× Volume (in liters)

For example, sulfuric acid, H_2SO_4, has two reacting units of protons, that is, there are two equivalents of protons in each mole. Thus:

eq. wt. = 98.08 g/mole/2 equiv./mole
= 49.04 g/equiv.

and the normality of a sulfuric acid solution is twice its molarity. Generally speaking:

$$N = n\,M$$

where *N* is the normality,
M the molarity,
n the number of equivalents per unit formula.

Thus for 1.2 M H_2SO_4:

1.2 moles/L × 2 eq/mole = 2.4 eq/L = 2.4 N.

Molality (*m*): A one-molal solution contains one mole/1000g of solvent.

m = moles of solute/kg of solvent.

For example: If 20.0g of NaOH is mixed into 500.0g (0.50 kg) of water, what is the molality of the solution?

20.0g of NaOH = 20.0 g/40.0 g/mol
= 0.500 mol of NaOH

Therefore, the Molality = 0.500 mol NaOH/0.50 kg water = 1.0 mol NaOH/kg water

Molal concentrations are not temperature-dependent as molar and normal concentrations are (since the solvent volume is temperature-dependent).

GENERAL CHEMISTRY

Density (ρ): Mass per unit volume at the specified temperature, usually g/ml or g/cm³ at 20°C.

Osmole (*Osm*): The number of moles of particles (molecules or ions) that contribute to the osmotic pressure of a solution.

Osmolarity: A one-osmolar solution is defined as one osmole in each liter of solution. Osmolarity is measured in osmoles/liter of solution (Osm/L).

For example, a 0.001 *M* solution of sodium chloride has an osmolarity of 0.002 Osm/L (twice the molarity), because each NaCl molecule ionizes in water to form two ions (Na^+ and Cl^-) that both contribute to the osmotic pressure.

Osmolality: A one-osmolal solution is defined as one osmole in each kilogram of solution. Osmolality is measured in osmoles/kilogram of solution (Osm/kg).

For example, the osmolality of a 0.01 molal solution of Na_2SO_4 is 0.03 Osm/kg because each molecule of Na_2SO_4 ionizes in water to give three ions (2 Na^+ and 1 SO_4^{2-}) that contribute to the osmotic pressure.

Mole Fraction: Is expressed as a mole ratio as the amount of solute (in moles) divided by the total amount of solvent and solute (in moles).

For example: If 110.0g of $CaCl_2$ is mixed with 72.0g water, what are the mole fractions of the two components?

72.0g of H_2O = 72.0g/18.0 g/mol
= 4 mol H_2O

110.0g of $CaCl_2$ = 110.0g/110 g/mol
= 1 mol $CaCl_2$

Total mol = 4 mol H_2O + 1 mol $CaCl_2$
= 5 mol (H_2O and $CaCl_2$)

Therefore,
X($CaCl_2$) = 1mol $CaCl_2$/5 mol $CaCl_2$ + H_2O = 0.2
and
X(water) = 4 mol H_2O/5 mol H_2O + $CaCl_2$ = 0.8

Dilution: When solvent is added to a solution containing a certain concentration of solute it becomes diluted to produce a solution of a lower solute concentration. The equation representing this is:

$$M_i V_i = M_f V_f$$

Where M = molarity and
V = volume with the initial (*i*) and final (*f*) concentrations being measured.

For example: How many ml of a 10.0 mol/L NaOH solution is needed to prepare 500 ml of a 2.00 mol/L NaOH solution?

Given: $M_i V_i = M_f V_f$, where M_i = 10.0 mol/L, M_f = 2.00 mol/L and V_f = 500 ml. Therefore, rearranging the equation gives $V_i = M_f \times V_f / M_i$ and so V_i = (2.00 mol/L)(0.5 L)/(10.0 moL) = 100 mL.

THE PHYSICAL SCIENCES   CHM-69

5.3.2 Solubility Product Constant, the Equilibrium Expression

Any solute that dissolves in water to give a solution that contains ions, and thus can conduct electricity, is an *electrolyte*. The solid (s) that dissociates into separate ions surrounded by water is hydrated, thus the ions are aqueous (*aq*).

If dissociation is extensive and irreversible, we have a strong electrolyte:

$$NaCl\ (s) \rightarrow Na^+\ (aq) + Cl^-\ (aq)$$

If dissociation is incomplete and reversible, we have a weak electrolyte:

$$CH_3COOH\ (aq) \rightleftharpoons CH_3COO^-\ (aq) + H^+\ (aq)$$

If dissociation does not occur, we have a nonelectrolyte:

$C_6H_{12}O_6$ (aq) or glucose sugar does NOT dissociate.

Strong electrolytes: salts (NaCl), strong acids (HCl), strong bases (NaOH).

Weak electrolytes: weak acids (CH_3COOH), weak bases (NH_3), complexes ($Fe[CN]_6$), tap water, certain soluble organic compounds, highly charged species (CHM 5.2; $AlPO_4$, $BaSO_4$, exception: AgCl as it is a precipitate in aqueous solutions).

Nonelectrolytes: deionized water, soluble organic compounds (sugars).

The solubility of a solute substance is the maximum amount of solute that can be dissolved in an appropriate solvent at a particular temperature. It can be expressed in units of concentration such as molarity, molality and so on (see CHM 5.3.1). When a maximum amount of solute has been dissolved, the solution is in equilibrium and is said to be saturated. As temperature increases, the solubility of most salts generally increases. However, it is the opposite for gases, as the solubility of gases is known to generally decrease as temperature increases.

When substances have limited solubility and their solubility is exceeded, the ions of the dissolved portion exist in equilibrium with the solid material. When a compound is referred to as insoluble, it is not completely insoluble, but is slightly soluble.

For example, if solid AgCl is added to water, a small portion will dissolve:

$$AgCl\ (s) \rightleftharpoons Ag^+\ (aq) + Cl^-\ (aq)$$

The precipitate will have a definite solubility (i.e. a definite amount in g/liter) or molar solubility (in moles/ liter) that will dissolve at a given temperature.

An overall equilibrium constant can be written for the preceding equilibrium, called the solubility product, K_{sp}, given by the following

GENERAL CHEMISTRY

equilibrium expression:

$$K_{sp} = [Ag^+][Cl^-]$$

The preceding relationship holds regardless of the presence of any undissociated intermediate. In general, each concentration must be raised to the power of that ion's coefficient in the dissolving equation (in our example = 1). A different example would be Ag_2S which would have the following solubility product expression: $K_{sp} = [Ag^+]^2[S^{2-}]$. The calculation of molar solubility s in mol/L for AgCl would simply be: $K_{sp} = [s][s] = s^2$. On the other hand, the expression for Ag_2S would become: $K_{sp} = [2s]^2[s] = 4s^3$.

Knowing K_{sp} at a specified temperature, the molar solubility of compounds can be calculated under various conditions. The amount of slightly soluble salt that dissolves does not depend on the amount of the solid in equilibrium with the solution, as long as there is enough to saturate the solution. Rather, it depends on the volume of solvent. {Note: a low K_{sp} value means little product therefore low solubility and vice-versa}.

The following are examples of problems on solubility product constant and solubility calculations given one or the other.

Another example: The molar solubility of $PbCl_2$ in an aqueous solution is 0.0159 M. What is the K_{sp} for $PbCl_2$?

$$PbCl_2(s) \rightleftharpoons Pb^{2+}(aq) + 2Cl^-(aq)$$
$$K_{sp} = [Pb^{2+}][Cl^-]^2$$

For every mol of $PbCl_2$ that dissociates, one mol of Pb^{2+} and two mol of Cl^- are produced. Since the molar solubility is 0.0159M, $[Pb^{2+}]$ = 0.0159M and $[Cl^-]$ = 0.0159 × 2 = 0.0318M

Therefore,
$$K_{sp} = [0.0159][0.0318]^2 = 1.61 \times 10^{-5}$$

Another example: What are the concentrations of each of the ions in a saturated solution of Ag_2CrO_4 given that solubility product constant K_{sp} is 1.1×10^{-12}?

$$Ag_2CrO_4(s) \rightleftharpoons 2Ag^+(aq) + CrO_4^{2-}(aq)$$
$$K_{sp} = [Ag^+]^2[CrO_4^{2-}]$$

For every Ag_2CrO_4 that dissociates, two mol of Ag^+ ion and one mol of CrO_4^{2-} ion are produced.

Let x = concentration of CrO_4^{2-}, then 2x = concentration of Ag^+

Therefore,
$$K_{sp} = [2x]^2[x]$$
$$1.1 \times 10^{-12} = [2x]^2[x]$$
solving for x gives; x = 6.50×10^{-5} M

so,
$$[Ag^+] = 1.3 \times 10^{-4} \text{ M and}$$
$$[CrO_4^{2-}] = 6.5 \times 10^{-5} \text{ M}$$

"If you're not part of the solution, you're part of the precipitate!"   :)

5.3.3 Common-ion Effect on Solubility

If there is an excess of one ion over the other, the concentration of the other is suppressed. This is called the common ion effect. The solubility of the precipitate is decreased and the concentration can still be calculated from the K_{sp}.

For example, Cl^- ion can be precipitated out of a solution of AgCl by adding a slight excess of $AgNO_3$. If a stoichiometric amount of $AgNO_3$ is added, $[Ag^+] = [Cl^-]$. If excess $AgNO_3$ is added, $[Ag^+] > [Cl^-]$ but K_{sp} remains constant. Therefore, $[Cl^-]$ decreases if $[Ag^+]$ is increased. Because the K_{sp} product always holds, precipitation will not take place unless the product of $[Ag^+]$ and $[Cl^-]$ exceeds the K_{sp}. If the product is just equal to K_{sp}, all the Ag^+ and Cl^- ions would remain in solution. Thus, the solubility of an ionic compound in solution containing a common ion is decreased in comparison to the same compound's solubility in water. As another example, the solubility of CaF_2 in water at 25°C would be much larger in comparison to the solubility of the same CaF_2 compound in a solution containing a common ion such as NaF. This decrease in solubility of CaF_2 in a solution containing NaF would be due to the common fluoride (F^-) ion effect on the solubility of CaF_2.

5.3.4 Solubility Product Constant (K_{sp}) vs. Reaction Quotient (Q_{sp})

Solubility product constants are used to describe saturated solutions of ionic compounds of relatively low solubility. A saturated solution is in a state of dynamic equilibrium described by the equilibrium constant (K_{sp}).

$$M_xA_y(s) \leftrightarrow x\ M^{y+}(aq) + y\ A^{x-}(aq)$$

The solubility product constant $K_{sp} = [M^{y+}]^x [A^{x-}]^y$ in a solution at equilibrium (saturated solution). Note that "M" is meant to symbolize the metal and "A" represents the anion.

A reaction quotient is defined by the same formula: $Q_{sp} = [M^{y+}]^x [A^{x-}]^y$ in a solution at any point, not just equilibrium.

K_{sp} therefore represents the ion product at equilibrium while Q_{sp} represents the ion product at any point, not just at equilibrium; and in fact, equilibrium is just a special case of the reaction coefficient as we will see below:

If $Q_{sp} < K_{sp}$, the solution is unsaturated and no precipitate will form.

If $Q_{sp} = K_{sp}$, the solution is saturated and at equilibrium.

If $Q_{sp} > K_{sp}$, the solution is supersaturated and unstable. A solid salt will precipitate until ion product once again equals to K_{sp}.

5.3.5 Solubility Rules

The chemistry of aqueous solutions is such that solubility rules can be established:

1. All salts of alkali metals are soluble.
2. All salts of the ammonium ion are soluble.
3. All chlorides, bromides and iodides are water soluble, with the exception of Ag^+, Pb^{2+}, and Hg_2^{2+}.
4. All salts of the sulfate ion (SO_4^{2-}) are water soluble with the exception of Ca^{2+}, Sr^{2+}, Ba^{2+}, and Pb^{2+}.
5. All metal oxides are insoluble with the exception of the alkali metals and CaO, SrO and BaO.
6. All hydroxides are insoluble with the exception of the alkali metals and Ca^{2+}, Sr^{2+}, Ba^{2+}.
7. All carbonates (CO_3^{2-}), phosphates (PO_4^{3-}), sulfides (S^{2-}) and sulfites (SO_3^{2-}) are insoluble, with the exception of the alkali metals and ammonium.

> We do not suggest that you memorize the solubility rules. The rules should, however, confirm what you have been seeing regarding the common substances that have been presented in this chapter like sodium chloride, calcium chloride, sodium sulfate, sodium hydroxide, silver chloride, strong vs. weak electrolytes, etc. It is expected that you are familiar with the solubility of the common substances and, if reminded of the rules during an exam (or practice), that you can apply those rules to more unfamiliar substances.

Dear GAMSAT Chemistry, If I understand correctly, alcohol is *a solution?*

Go online to GAMSAT-prep.com for free chapter review Q&A and forum.

GOLD NOTES

ACIDS AND BASES
Chapter 6

Memorize	Understand	Not Required*
e: Bronsted acid, base, pH ples of strong/weak acids/bases STP, neutral H₂O pH, conjugate ase, zwitterions tions: K_a, K_b, pK_a, pK_b, K_w, pH, pOH alence point, indicator, rules of ithms	* Calculation of K_a, K_b, pK_a, pK_b, K_w, pH, pOH * Calculations involving strong/weak acids/bases * Salts of weak acids/bases, buffers; indicators * Acid-Base titration/curve, redox titration	* Advanced level college info * Specific values for K_a and/or K_b * Memorizing Henderson-Hasselback equation

GAMSAT-Prep.com

Introduction

Acids are compounds that, when dissolved in water, give a solution with a hydrogen ion concentration greater than that of pure water. Acids turn litmus paper (an indicator) red. Examples include acetic acid (in vinegar) and sulfuric acid (in car batteries). Bases may have [H⁺] less than pure water and turns litmus blue. Examples include sodium hydroxide (= lye, caustic soda) and ammonia (used in many cleaning products).

Additional Resources

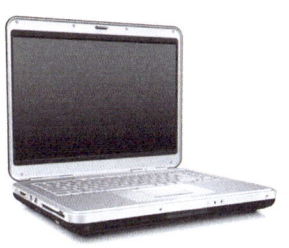   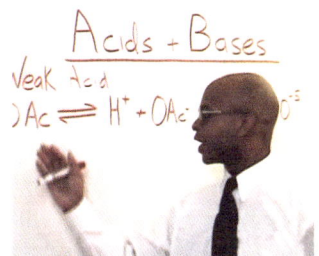   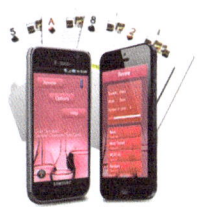

Free Online Q&A + Forum   Video: Online or DVD   Flashcards   Special Guest

THE PHYSICAL SCIENCES   CHM-75

* The real GAMSAT may have advanced level information presented (ie. in a passage) but previous knowledge of said information is not required to answer the questions that would follow. Practice ACER and GS practice GAMSATs can help you clarify this point.

GAMSAT-Prep.com
THE GOLD STANDARD

6.1 Acids

A useful definition is given by Bronsted and Lowry: an acid is a proton (i.e. hydrogen ion) donor (cf. Lewis acids and bases, see CHM 3.4). A substance such as HF is an acid because it can donate a proton to a substance capable of accepting it. In aqueous solution, water is always available as a proton acceptor, so that the ionization of an acid, HA, can be written as:

$$HA + H_2O \rightleftharpoons H_3O^+ + A^-$$

or:

$$HA \rightleftharpoons H^+ + A^-$$

The equilibrium constant is:

$$K_a = [H^+][A^-]/[HA]$$

Examples of ionization of acids are:

$HCl \rightleftharpoons H^+ + Cl^-$ $K_a = $ infinity
$HF \rightleftharpoons H^+ + F^-$ $K_a = 6.7 \times 10^{-4}$
$HCN \rightleftharpoons H^+ + CN^-$ $K_a = 7.2 \times 10^{-10}$

Acids are generally divided into two categories known as binary acids and oxyacids. The first category is that of acids composed of hydrogen and a nonmetal such as chlorine (HCl). For the halogen containing binary acids, the acid strength increases as a function of the halogen size. Moreover, as the halogen size increases, its bond length increases while its bond strength decreases and as such, its acidity increases. Thus, the acidity of HI > HBr > HCl > HF.

The second category of acids form from oxyanions (anions containing a nonmetal and oxygen such as the hydroxide or nitrate ions, see CHM 5.2) are known as the oxyacids. The oxyacids contain a hydrogen atom covalently bonded to an oxygen atom which is bonded to another central atom X (H-O-X-etc). The more oxygen atoms that are bounded to the central atom, the more acidic the oxyacids. Some examples of oxyacids are listed in Table III.A.6.1.

Note: a diprotic acid (two protons, i.e. H_2SO_4) would have K_a values for each of its two ionizable protons: K_{a1} for the first and K_{a2} for the second. Diprotic or any polyprotic acids are known to ionize in successive steps in which each of the steps contain their own dissociation or ionization acid constant, K_a. The first ionization constant (K_{a1}) is typically much larger than the subsequent ionization constants ($K_{a1} > K_{a2} > K_{a3}$, etc...).

Table III.A.6.1: Examples of acids that dissociate (CHM 5.2) completely (strong) and only partially (weak).

STRONG	WEAK	STRONG	WEAK
Perchloric $HClO_4$ Chloric $HClO_3$ Nitric HNO_3 Hydrochloric HCl	Hydrocyanic HCN Hypochlorous HClO Nitrous HNO_2 Hydrofluoric HF	Sulfuric H_2SO_4 Hydrobromic HBr Hydriodic HI Hydronium Ion H_3O^+	Sulfurous H_2SO_3 Hydrogen Sulfide H_2S Phosphoric H_3PO_4 Benzoic, Acetic and other Carboxylic acids

GENERAL CHEMISTRY

6.2 Bases

A base is defined as a <u>proton acceptor</u>. In aqueous solution, water is always available to donate a proton to a base, so the ionization of a base B, can be written as:

$$B + H_2O \rightleftharpoons HB^+ + OH^-$$

The equilibrium constant is:

$$K_b = [HB^+][OH^-]/[B]$$

Examples of ionization of bases are:

$$CN^- + H_2O \rightleftharpoons HCN + OH^- \quad K_b = 1.4 \times 10^{-5}$$
$$NH_3 + H_2O \rightleftharpoons NH_4^+ + OH^- \quad K_b = 1.8 \times 10^{-5}$$
$$F^- + H_2O \rightleftharpoons HF + OH^- \quad K_b = 1.5 \times 10^{-11}$$

Strong bases include any hydroxide of the group 1A metals. The most common weak bases are ammonia and any organic amine.

6.3 Conjugate Acid-Base Pairs

The <u>strength</u> of an acid or base is related to the extent that the dissociation proceeds to the right, or to the magnitude of K_a or K_b; the larger the dissociation constant, the stronger the acid or the base. From the preceding K_a values, we see that HCl is the strongest acid (almost 100% ionized), followed by HF and HCN. From the K_b's given, NH_3 is the strongest base listed, followed by CN^- and F^-. Clearly, when an acid ionizes, it produces a base. The acid, HA, and the base produced when it ionizes, A^-, are called a <u>conjugate acid-base</u> pair, so that the couples HF/F^- and HCN/CN^- are conjugate acids and bases.

Thus, an acid that has donated a proton becomes a conjugate base and a base that has accepted a proton becomes a conjugate acid of that base. For example, HCO_3^-/CO_3^{2-} are a conjugate acid/base pair, wherein HCO_3^- is the acid and CO_3^{2-} is the conjugate base. Both dissociate partially in water and reach equilibrium.

A strong acid (HCl) has a weak conjugate base (Cl^-) and a strong base (NaOH) has a weak conjugate acid (OH^-). Whereas, a weak acid (CH_3COOH) has a strong conjugate base (CH_3COO^-) and a weak base (NH_3) has a related strong conjugate acid (NH_4^+).

Another example of conjugate acid-base pairs is amino acids. Amino acids bear at least 2 ionizable weak acid groups, a carboxyl (–COOH) and an amino ($-NH_3^+$) which act as follows:

$$R-COOH \rightleftharpoons R-COO^- + H^+$$
$$R-NH_3^+ \rightleftharpoons R-NH_2 + H^+$$

R–COO⁻ and R–NH₂ are the conjugate bases (i.e. proton acceptors) of the corresponding acids. The carboxyl group is thousands of times more acidic than the amino group. Thus in blood plasma (pH ≈ 7.4) the predominant forms are the carboxylate anions (R–COO⁻) and the protonated amino group (R–NH₃⁺). This form is called a *zwitterion* as demonstrated by the amino acid alanine at a pH near 7:

$$CH_3\text{-}CH\text{-}COO^-$$
$$|$$
$$NH_3^+$$

Alanine

The zwitterion bears no net charge.

6.4 Water Dissociation

Water itself can ionize:

$$H_2O + H_2O \rightleftharpoons H_3O^+ + OH^-$$

or:

$$H_2O \rightleftharpoons H^+ + OH^-$$

At STP, $K_w = [H^+][OH^-] = 1.0 \times 10^{-14}$ = ion product constant for water. It increases with temperature and in a neutral solution, $[H^+] = [OH^-] = 10^{-7}$ M. Note that $[H_2O]$ is not included in the equilibrium expression because it is a pure liquid and it is a large constant ($[H_2O]$ is incorporated in K_w).

6.5 The pH Scale

The pH of a solution is a convenient way of expressing the concentration of hydrogen ions $[H^+]$ in solution, to avoid the use of large negative powers of 10. It is defined as:

$$pH = -\log_{10}[H^+]$$

Thus, the pH of a neutral solution of pure water where $[H^+] = 10^{-7}$ is 7.

A similar definition is used for the hydroxyl ion concentration:

$$pOH = -\log_{10}[OH^-]$$

Since, $K_w = [H^+][OH^-]$

And so, $1.0 \times 10^{-14} = [H^+][OH^-]$

And taking the –log of both sides gives $-\log[1.0 \times 10^{-14}] = -\log[H^+][OH^-]$

So, $14.0 = -\log[H^+] + -\log[OH^-]$

Therefore, $14.0 = pH + pOH$

Finally, at 25°C, pH + pOH = 14.0

A pH of 7 is neutral. Values of pH that are greater than 7 are alkaline (basic) and values that are lower are acidic. The pH can be measured precisely with a pH meter (quantitative) or globally with an indicator which will have a different color over different pH ranges (qualitative). For example, *litmus paper* (very common) becomes blue in basic solutions and red in acidic solutions; whereas, *phenolphthalein* is colorless in acid and pink in base.

We will see in CHM 6.9 that a weak acid or base can serve as a visual (qualitative) indicator of a pH range. Usually, only a small quantity (i.e. drops) of the indicator is added to the solution as to minimize the risk of any side reactions.

6.5.1 Properties of Logarithms

Many GAMSAT problems every year rely on a basic understanding of logarithms (GM 3.7, 3.8) for one or more of: pH problems, reaction rates (CHM 9.5), Gibbs Free Energy (CHM 9.10), the Nernst equation (CHM 10.3), and decibels/sound (PHY 8.3). Here are the rules you must know:

1) $\log_a a = 1$
2) $\log_a M^k = k \log_a M$
3) $\log_a(MN) = \log_a M + \log_a N$
4) $\log_a(M/N) = \log_a M - \log_a N$
5) $10^{\log_{10} M} = M$

For example, let us calculate the pH of 0.001 M HCl. Since HCl is a strong acid, it will completely dissociate into H^+ and Cl^-, thus:

$[H^+] = 0.001$
$-\log[H^+] = -\log(0.001)$
pH $= -\log(10^{-3})$
pH $= 3 \log 10$ (rule #2)
pH $= 3$ (rule #1, a = 10)

Reminder: We worked out the shape of the graph for pH vs. hydrogen ion concentration in GM chapter 3, review question 15.

6.6 Weak Acids and Bases

Weak acids (HA) and bases (B) partially dissociate in aqueous solutions reaching equilibrium following their dissociation. The following is the generic reaction of any weak acid (HA) dissociation in an aqueous solution.

$$HA + H_2O \rightleftharpoons A^- + H_3O^+$$

Now let us begin by taking a closer look at the development of the acid and base equilibrium constants. Like all equilibrium, acid/base dissociation will have a particular equilibrium constant (K_a or K_b) which will determine the extent of the dissociation (CHM 6.3). Thus, from the preceding equation for any generic acid (HA), the acid dissociation constant $K = [H_3O^+][A^-]/[H_2O][HA]$.

Very little water actually reacts and thus the concentration of water during the reaction is constant and can therefore be excluded from the expression for K. Therefore, this gives rise to the acid dissociation constant known as K_a.

Where, $K_a = K[H_2O] = [H_3O^+][A^-]/[HA]$

Likewise for a weak base dissociation in equilibrium,

$$B + H_2O \rightleftharpoons OH^- + BH^+$$

This gives rise to the base dissociation constant known as K_b.

Where, $K_b = K[H_2O] = [OH^-][BH^+]/[B]$

Weak acids and bases are only <u>partially ionized</u>. The ionization constant can be used to calculate the amount ionized, and from this, the pH.

Since weak acids are not completely dissociated, one needs to find the $[H^+]$ from the acid dissociation and then use a method known in most textbooks as the "ICE method". ICE is an acronym used in which, I = Initial acid $[H^+]$ concentration, C = Change in acid $[H^+]$ concentration and E = acid $[H^+]$ concentration at equilibrium. Thus, the acid concentration $[H^+]$ also represented as (x) at equilibrium is then used to calculate the pH. NOTE: the equilibrium concentration x is usually very small as the acid (or base) is weak and partially dissociated (or ionized). The following is an example of the application of the ICE method in solving for the $[H^+] = x$ at equilibrium and subsequently determining the pH of a weak acid solution.

Example: Calculate the pH and pOH of a 10^{-2} M solution of acetic acid (HOAc). K_a of acetic acid at 25°C = 1.75×10^{-5}.

$$HOAc \rightleftharpoons H^+ + OAc^-$$

The concentrations are:

	[HOAc]	[H⁺]	[OAc⁻]
Initial	10^{-2}	0	0
Change	–x	+x	+x
Equilibrium	10^{-2} –x	x	x

$K_a = [H^+][OAc^-]/[HOAc] = 1.75 \times 10^{-5}$
$\quad = (x)(x)/(10^{-2} - x)$

The solution is a quadratic equation which may be simplified if <u>less than 5%</u> of the acid is ionized by neglecting x compared to the concentration (10^{-2} M in this case). We then have:

$$x^2/10^{-2} = 1.75 \times 10^{-5}$$
$$x = 4.18 \times 10^{-4} = [H^+]$$

And $\quad$ pH = –log (4.18×10^{-4}) = 3.38
$\quad\quad$ pOH = 14.00 – 3.38 = 10.62

To confirm the 5% criterion one needs to calculate as follows: $(4.18 \times 10^{-4})/(1.00 \times 10^{-2}) \times 100 = 4.18\%$ which is less than 5% and therefore justifies the usage of the 5% criterion.

Similar calculations hold for weak bases. Note that all the preceding can be estimated without a calculator once you know the squares of all numbers between 1 and 15. The root of 1.69 (a fair estimate of 1.75) is thus 1.3 (also see CHM 6.6.1 to see how to estimate an answer without a calculator).

GENERAL CHEMISTRY

6.6.1 Determining pH with the Quadratic Formula

If you need to calculate pH on the GAMSAT, it is very unlikely that you would need to use the quadratic equation; however, you are expected to be familiar with the different ways to calculate pH and that is why it is presented here.

The solutions of the quadratic equation

$$ax^2 + bx + c = 0$$

are given by the formula (QR 4.6, 4.6.2)

$$x = [-b \pm (b^2 - 4ac)^{1/2}]/2a$$

The problem in CHM 6.6 can be reduced to

$$K_a = (x)(x)/(10^{-2} - x) = 1.75 \times 10^{-5}$$

or

$$x^2 + (1.75 \times 10^{-5})X + (-1.75 \times 10^{-7}) = 0$$

Using the quadratic equation where $a = 1$, $b = 1.75 \times 10^{-5}$ and $c = -1.75 \times 10^{-7}$, and doing the appropriate multiplications we get:

$$X = [-1.75 \times 10^{-5} \pm (3.06 \times 10^{-10} + 7.0 \times 10^{-7})^{1/2}]/2$$

Thus $x = [-1.75 \times 10^{-5} \pm (7.00 \times 10^{-7})^{1/2}]/2$
$= [-1.75 \times 10^{-5} \pm 8.37 \times 10^{-4}]/2$

Hence the two possible solutions are

$$X = [-1.75 \times 10^{-5} - 8.37 \times 10^{-4}]/2 = -4.27 \times 10^{-4}$$

Or

$$X = = [-1.75 \times 10^{-5} + 8.37 \times 10^{-4}]/2$$
$$= 4.10 \times 10^{-4}$$

The first solution is a negative number which is physically impossible for [H⁺], therefore pH = $-\log(4.10 \times 10^{-4}) = 3.39$

Our estimate in CHM 6.6 (pH = 3.38) was valid as it is less than 1% different from the more precise calculation using the quadratic formula.

Given a multiple choice question with the following choices: 2.5, 3.4, 4.3 and 6.8 – the answer can be easily deduced.

$$-\log(4.10 \times 10^{-4}) = -\log 4.10 - \log 10^{-4}$$
$$= 4 - \log 4.10$$

however

$$0 = \log 10^0 = \log 1 < \log 4.10 << \log 10 = 1$$

Thus a number slightly greater than 0 but significantly less than 1 is substracted from 4. The answer could only be 3.4.

6.7 Salts of Weak Acids and Bases

A *salt* is an ionic compound in which the anion is not OH^- or O^{2-} and the cation is not H^+.

Acids and bases react with each other, forming a salt and water in a reaction known as <u>neutralization reaction</u>. Salts are compounds composed of both a cation and anion (i.e. Na_2SO_4). As salts contain both a cation and anion, salts may therefore form acidic, basic or neutral solutions when dissolved into water. Hence, a salt can react with water to give back an acid or base in a reaction known as <u>salt hydrolysis</u> and thus affect the solution's pH. Moreover, a salt composed of an anion from a weak acid (CH_3COO^-) and a cation from a strong base (Na^+) dissociates and reacts in water to give rise to OH^- ions (a basic solution). Whereas, a salt composed of an anion from a strong acid (Cl^-) and a cation from a weak base (NH_4^+) dissociates and reacts in water to give rise to H^+ (an acidic solution).

Examples:

NaClO dissociates in water:

$$ClO^- + H_2O \rightleftharpoons HClO + OH^- \text{ (Basic)}$$

NH_4NO_3 dissociates in water:

$$NH_4^+ + H_2O \rightleftharpoons H_3O^+ + NH_3 \text{ (Acidic)}$$

The salt of a weak acid is a <u>Bronsted base</u>, which will accept protons. For example,

$$Na^+ OAc^- + H_2O \rightleftharpoons HOAc + Na^+ OH^-$$

The HOAc here is undissociated and therefore does not contribute to the pH. Because it hydrolyzes, sodium acetate is a weak base (the conjugate base of acetic acid). The ionization constant is equal to the basicity constant of the salt. ==The weaker the conjugate acid, the stronger the conjugate base,== that is, the more strongly the salt will combine with a proton.

$$K_H = K_b = [HOAc][OH^-]/[OAc^-]$$

K_H is the <u>hydrolysis constant</u> of the salt. The product of K_a of any weak acid and K_b of its conjugate base is always equal to K_w.

$$K_a \times K_b = K_w$$

For any salt of a weak acid, HA, that ionizes in water:

$$A^- + H_2O \rightleftharpoons HA + OH^-$$
$$[HA][OH^-]/[A^-] = K_w/K_a.$$

The pH of such a salt is calculated in the same manner as for any other weak base.

Similar equations are derived for the salts of weak bases. They hydrolyze in water as follows:

$$BH^+ + H_2O \rightleftharpoons B + H_3O^+$$

B is undissociated and does not contribute to the pH.

$$K_H = K_a = [B][H_3O^+]/[BH^+]$$

And

$$[B][H_3O^+]/[BH^+] = K_w/K_b.$$

In conclusion, there are four types of salts formed based on the reacting acid and base strengths as follows:

(1) Strong acid + strong base:

$HCl(aq) + NaOH(aq) \rightleftharpoons NaCl(aq) + H_2O(l)$

Salts in which the cation and anion are both conjugates of a strong base and a strong acid form neutral solutions.

(2) Strong acid + weak base:

$HCl(aq) + NH_3(aq) \rightleftharpoons NH_4Cl(aq)$

Salts that are formed based on a strong acid reacting with a weak base form acidic solutions.

(3) Weak acid + strong base:

$HOAc(aq) + NaOH(aq) \rightleftharpoons NaOAc(aq) + H_2O(l)$
(note: HOAc = acetic acid = CH_3COOH)

A salt in which the cation is the counterion of a strong base and the anion is the conjugate base of a weak acid results in the formation of basic solutions.

(4) Weak acid + weak base:

$HOAc(aq) + NH_3(aq) \rightleftharpoons NH_4OAc(aq)$

A salt in which the cation is a conjugate acid of a weak base and the anion is the anion of a weak acid will form a solution in which the pH will be dependent on the relative strengths of the acid and base.

> Note: Using the rules of logarithms (GM 3.7; CHM 6.5.1), we can change
> $K_a K_b = K_w$ to $-\log(K_a K_b) = -\log K_w$
> which is the same as
> $(-\log K_a) + (-\log K_b) = -\log K_w$.
> Thus $pK_a + pK_b = pK_w$.

6.8 Buffers

A <u>buffer</u> is defined as a solution that resists change in pH when a small amount of an acid or base is added or when a solution is diluted. A buffer solution consists of a <u>mixture of a weak acid and its salt or of a weak base and its salt</u>.

For example, consider the acetic acid-acetate buffer. The acid equilibrium that governs this system is:

$HOAc \rightleftharpoons H^+ + OAc^-$

Along with the acid equilibrium component of the buffer solution as shown above, the buffer solution must also contain a significant amount of the conjugate base of the acid as a salt. The following equation depicts the conjugate base salt dissociation of the acetic acid-acetate buffer solution:

$$NaOAc \rightarrow Na^+ + OAc^-$$

Thus, the buffer is made up of two components (1) a weak acid (HOAc) and (2) the conjugate base of the weak acid as a salt (NaAOc) so that both components are part of the buffer system in apt concentrations to make for a fully functional buffer.

When a small amount of NaOH base is added to the acetic acid/acetate buffer solution, the OH^- ions from the base will react with the free H^+ ions present in the buffer solution from the acetic acid dissociation. This will shift the equilibrium of the buffer toward the right which means more dissociation of the acid (HOAc). Thus, an increase in $[OH^-]$ from the addition of base to the buffer solution does not change pH significantly due to the reaction of the basic OH^- ions with the free protons (H^+) in solution.

The resistance to pH change is also noted with the addition of an acid (H^+) to the acetic acid/acetate buffer solution. The addition of acidic H^+ from the acid will react with the acetate ions (HOAc$^-$) from the salt dissociation of the buffer and this will also allow for the buffering capacity of the solution. Thus, due to the presence of both a weak acid and a conjugate base from the salt (or common ion), the buffer solution thus is known to maintain a pH within a certain range known as the buffering capacity.

Buffers must contain a significant amount of both a weak acid or weak base and its conjugate salts. A strong acid or strong base would not have any buffering capacity or effect within a buffer system as the dissociation would be irreversible and so the buffer capacity would not be present. In addition, a weak acid or base in itself would also not be able to work as a buffer system regardless of the fact that there is the presence of their conjugates as the concentrations of the conjugate acid or base from the weak acids or bases would not be sufficient to neutralize the addition of acids (H^+) or bases (OH^-). Thus, buffers require the addition of a conjugate acid or base as a salt to the weak acid or base component so to increase the salt concentration of the buffer solution.

If we were to add acetate ions into the system (i.e. from the salt), the H^+ ion concentration is no longer equal to the acetate ion concentration. The hydrogen ion concentration is:

$$[H^+] = K_a ([HOAc]/[OAc^-])$$

Taking the negative logarithm of each side, where $-\log K_a = pK_a$, yields:

$$pH = pK_a - \log ([HOAc]/[OAc^-])$$

or

$$pH = pK_a + \log([OAc^-]/[HOAc])$$

This equation is referred to as the Henderson-Hasselbach equation. It is useful for calculating the pH of a weak acid solution containing its salt. A general form can be written for a weak acid, HA, that dissociates into its salt, A⁻ and H⁺:

$$HA \rightleftharpoons H^+ + A^-$$

$$pH = pK_a + \log([salt]/[acid])$$

The <u>buffering capacity</u> of the solution is determined by the concentrations of HA and A⁻. The higher their concentrations, the more acid or base the solution can tolerate. The buffering capacity is also governed by the ratios of HA to A⁻. It is maximum when the ratio is equal to 1, i.e. when pH = pK_a.

Similar calculations can be made for mixtures of a weak base and its salt:

$$B + H_2O \rightleftharpoons BH^+ + OH^-$$

And

$$pOH = pK_b + \log([salt]/[base])$$

Many biological reactions of interest occur between pH 6 and 8. One useful series of buffers is that of phosphate buffers. By choosing appropriate mixtures of $H_3PO_4/H_2PO_4^-$, $H_2PO_4^-/HPO_4^{2-}$ or HPO_4^{2-}/PO_4^{3-}, buffer solutions covering a wide pH range can be prepared. Another useful clinical buffer is the one prepared from tris(hydroxymethyl) aminomethane and its conjugate acid, abbreviated Tris buffer.

Amphoteric Species: Some substances such as water can act as either an acid or a base (i.e. a dual property). These types of substances are known as amphoteric substances. Water behaves as an acid when reacted with a base (OH⁻) and alternatively, water behaves as a base when reacted with an acid (H⁺). Many metal oxides and hydroxides are also known to be amphoteric substances. Furthermore, molecules that contain both acidic and basic groups such as amino acids are considered to be amphoteric in nature as well (ORG 12.1.2). The following are examples of the amphoteric nature of HCO_3^- reacting with an acid and a base and water (H_2O) reacting with an acid and base.

In acids: $HCO_3^- + H_3O^+ \rightarrow H_2CO_3 + H_2O$
In bases: $HCO_3^- + OH^- \rightarrow CO_3^{2-} + H_2O$
In acids: $H_2O + HCl \rightarrow H_3O^+ + Cl^-$
In bases: $H_2O + NH_3 \rightarrow NH_4^+ + OH^-$

6.9 Acid-base Titrations

The purpose of a titration is usually the determination of concentration of a given sample of acid or base (<u>the analyte</u>) which is reacted with an equivalent amount of a strong base or acid of known concentration (<u>the titrant</u>). The end point or equivalence point is reached when a stoichiometric amount of titrant has been added. This end point is usually detected with the use of an <u>indicator</u> which changes color when this point is reached. Note: the end point is not exactly the same as the equivalence point. The equivalence point is where a reaction is theoretically complete whereas an end point is where a physical change in solution such as a color change is determined by indicators.

Regardless, the volume difference between an end point and an equivalence point can usually be ignored.

The end point is determined precisely by measuring the pH at different points of the titration. The curve pH = f(V) where V is the volume of titrant added is called a <u>titration curve</u>. While a strong acid/strong base titration will have an equivalence point at a neutralization pH of 7, the equivalence point of other titrations do not necessarily occur at pH 7. In fact, a weak acid/strong base titration will result in an equivalence point of a pH > 7 and a strong acid/weak base titration results in an equivalence point of a pH < 7. The differential pH effects at the relative equivalence points are due to the conjugate acids and/or bases formed. An indicator for an acid-base titration is a weak acid or base.

==The weak acid and its conjugate base should have two different colors in solution.== Most indicators require a <u>pH transition range</u> during the titration of about two pH units. An indicator is chosen so that its pK_a is close to the pH of the equivalence point.

6.9.1 Strong Acid versus Strong Base

In the case of a strong acid versus a strong base, both the titrant and the analyte are completely ionized. For example, the titration of hydrochloric acid with sodium hydroxide:

$H^+ + Cl^- + Na^+ + OH^- \rightarrow H_2O + Na^+ + Cl^-$

The H^+ and OH^- combine to form H_2O and the other ions remain unchanged, so the net result is the conversion of the HCl to a neutral solution of NaCl. A typical strong-acid-strong base titration curve is shown in Fig. III.A.6.1 (case where the titrant is a base).

If the analyte is an acid, the pH is initially acidic and increases very slowly. When the equivalent volume is reached the pH sharply increases. Midway between this transition jump is the equivalence point. In the case of strong acid-strong base titration the equivalence point corresponds to a neutral pH (because the salt formed does not react with water). If more titrant is added the pH increases and corresponds to the pH of a solution of gradually increasing concentration of the titrant base. This curve is simply reversed if the titrant is an acid.

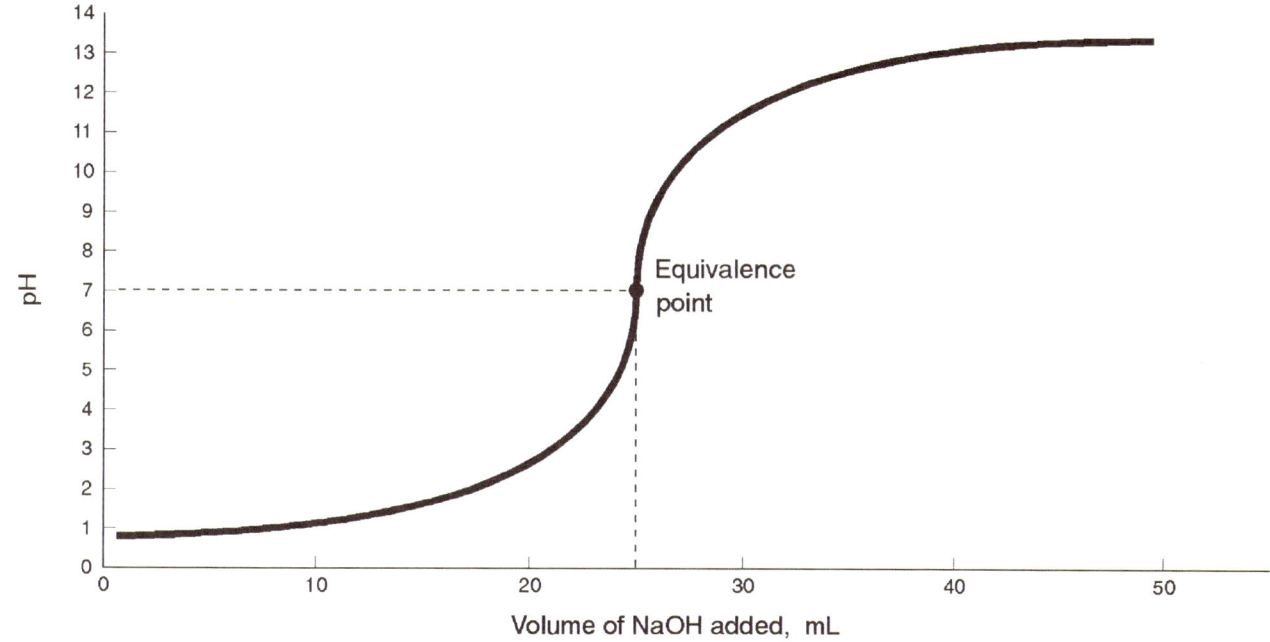

Figure III.A.6.1: The titration curve for a strong acid-strong base is a relatively smooth S-shaped curve with a very steep inclination close to the equivalence point. A small addition in titrant volume near the equivalence point will result in a large change in pH.

6.9.2 Weak Acid versus Strong Base

The titration of acetic acid with sodium hydroxide involves the following reaction:

$$HOAc + Na^+ + OH^- \rightarrow H_2O + Na^+ + OAc^-$$

The acetic acid is only a few percent ionized. It is neutralized to water and an equivalent amount of the salt, sodium acetate. Before the titration is started, the pH is calculated as described for weak acids. As soon as the titration is started, some of the HOAc is converted to NaOAc and a buffer system is set up. As the titration proceeds, the pH slowly increases as the ratio [OAc⁻]/[HOAc] changes. Halfway towards the equivalence point, [OAC⁻] = [HOAC] and the pH is equal to pK_a. At the equivalence point, we have a solution of NaOAc. Since it hydrolyzes, the pH at the equivalence point will be alkaline. The pH will depend on the concentration of NaOAc. The greater the concentration, the higher the pH. As excess NaOH is added, the ionization of the base, OAc⁻, is suppressed and the pH is determined only by the concentration of excess OH⁻. Therefore, the titration curve beyond the equivalence point follows that for the titration of a strong acid. The typical titration curve in this case is illustrated in Figure III.A.6.2.

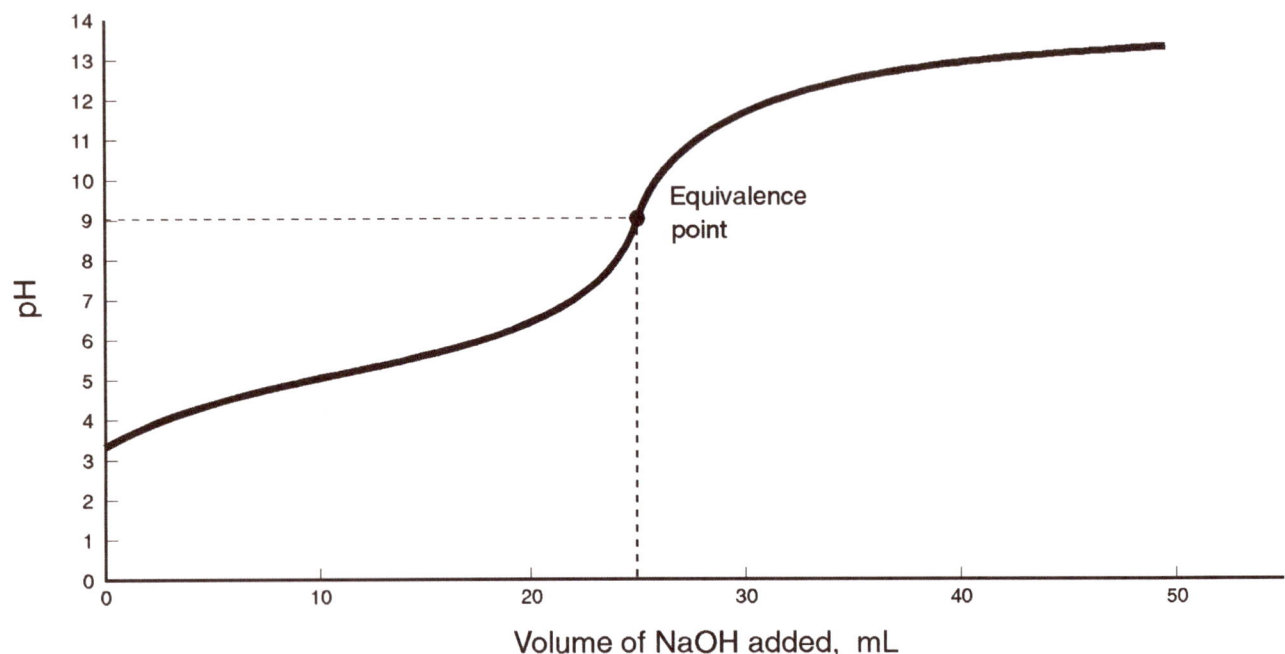

Figure III.A.6.2: The titration curve for a weak acid-strong base or alternatively a strong acid-weak base is somewhat irregular. The pH at the start of the titration prior to base addition is greater than that of a strong acid as the acid is a weak acid. The inclination close to the equivalence point is less significant due to the buffering effect of the solution prior to the equivalence point. A small addition in titrant volume near the equivalence point will therefore result in a small change in pH.

6.9.3 Weak Base versus Strong Acid

The titration of a weak base with a strong acid is analogous to the previous case except that the pH is initially basic and gradually decreases as the acid is added (curve in preceding diagram is reversed). Consider ammonia titrated with hydrochloric acid:

$$NH_3 + H^+ + Cl^- \rightarrow NH_4^+ + Cl^-$$

At the beginning, we have NH_3 and the pH is calculated as for weak bases. As soon as some acid is added, some of the NH_3 is converted to NH_4^+ and we are in the buffer region. At the midpoint of the titration, $[NH_4^+]$ = $[NH_3]$ and the pH is equal to $(14 - pK_b)$. At the equivalence point, we have a solution of NH_4Cl, a weak acid which hydrolyzes to give an acid solution. Again, the pH will depend on concentration: the greater the concentration, the lower the pH. Beyond the equivalence point, the free H^+ suppresses the ionization and the pH is determined by the concentration of H^+ added in excess. Therefore, the titration curve beyond the

CHM-88   ACIDS AND BASES

equivalence point will be similar to that of the titration of a strong base. {The midpoint of the titration is the equivalence point of the titration curve}

6.10 Redox Titrations

Redox titrations are based on a redox reaction or reduction-oxidation type reaction between an analyte (or sample) and a titrant. More specifically, redox titrations involve the reaction between an oxidizing agent, which accepts one or more electrons, and a reducing agent, which reduces the other substance by donating one or more electrons (CHM 1.6).

The most useful oxidizing agent for titrations is potassium permanganate - $KMnO_4$. Solutions of this salt are colorful since they contain the purple MnO_4^- ion. On the other hand, the more reduced form, Mn^{++}, is nearly colorless. So here is how this redox titration works: $KMnO_4$ is added to a reaction mixture with a reducing agent (i.e. Fe^{++}). MnO_4^- is quickly reduced to Mn^{++} so the color fades immediately. This will continue until there is no more reducing agent in the mixture. When the last bit of reducing agent has been oxidized (i.e. all the Fe^{++} is converted to Fe^{+3}), the next drop of $KMnO_4$ will make the solution colorful since the MnO_4^- will have nothing with which to react. Thus if the amount of reducing agent was unknown, it can be calculated using stoichiometry guided by the amount of potassium permanganate used in the reaction.

There are more questions on acids-bases in ACER's GAMSAT practice materials than any other General Chemistry subject. Though this fact does not guarantee what could be emphasized on any 1 new exam, it does underline the relative importance of this chapter.

Go online to GAMSAT-prep.com for free chapter review Q&A and forum.

GOLD NOTES

THERMODYNAMICS

Chapter 7

Memorize	Understand	Not Required*
Define: state function Conversion: thermal to mechanical E.	* System vs. surroundings * Law of conservation of energy * Heat transfer * Conduction, convection, radiation	* Advanced level college info * Memorizing: conversion between temperature scales or thermal units * Memorizing: 1st Law of Thermodynamics

GAMSAT-Prep.com

Introduction

Thermodynamics, in chemistry, refers to the relationship of heat with chemical reactions or with the physical state. Thermodynamic processes can be analyzed by studying energy and topics we will review in the next chapter including entropy, volume, temperature and pressure.

Additional Resources

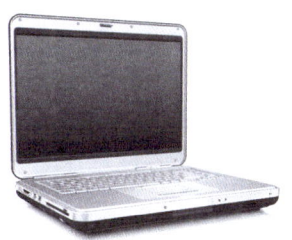   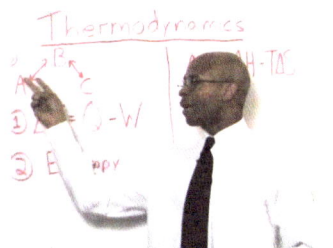   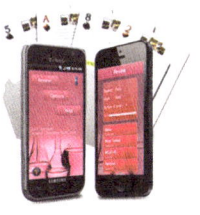   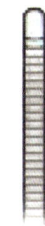

Free Online Q&A + Forum   Video: Online or DVD   Flashcards   Special Guest

THE PHYSICAL SCIENCES CHM-91

* The real GAMSAT may have advanced level information presented (ie. in a passage) but previous knowledge of said information is not required to answer the questions that would follow. Practice ACER and GS practice GAMSATs can help you clarify this point.

7.1 Generalities

Thermodynamics deals with fundamental questions concerning energy transfers. One difficulty you will have to overcome is the terminology used. For instance, remember that heat and temperature have more specific meanings than the ones attributed to them in every day life.

A thermodynamic transformation can be as simple as a gas leaking out of a tank or a piece of metal melting at high temperature or as complicated as the synthesis of proteins by a biological cell. To solve some problems in thermodynamics we need to define a "system" and its "surroundings." The system is simply the object experiencing the thermodynamic transformation. The gas would be considered as the system in the first example of transformations. Once the system is defined any part of the universe in direct contact with the system is considered as its surroundings. For instance, if the piece of metal is melted in a high temperature oven: the system is the piece of metal and the oven constitutes its surroundings.

In other instances, the limit between the system and its surroundings is more arbitrary, for example if one considers the energy exchanges when an ice cube melts in a thermos bottle filled with orange juice; the inside walls of the thermos bottle could be considered as part of "the system" or as part of the surroundings. In the first case one would carry out all calculations as though the entire system (ice cube + orange juice + inside walls) is isolated from its surroundings (rest of the universe) and all the energy exchanges take place within the system. In the second case the system (ice cube + orange juice) is not isolated from the surroundings (walls) unless we consider that the heat exchanges with the walls are negligible. There is also no need to include any other part of the universe in the latter case since all exchanges take place within the system or between the system and the inside walls of the thermos bottle.

Some systems may exchange both matter and energy with the surroundings. This is called an "open system". Alternatively, some systems may exchange energy only but not matter with the surroundings. This is called a "closed system". Finally, some systems do not exchange matter or energy with their surroundings. This is called an "isolated system". An isolated system therefore does not interact with its surroundings in any way.

7.2 The First Law of Thermodynamics

Heat, internal energy and work are the first concepts introduced in thermodynamics. Heat is thermal energy (a dynamic property defined during a transformation only), it is not to be confused with temperature (a static property defined for each state of the system). Internal energy is basically the average total mechanical energy (kinetic + potential) of the particles that make up the system. The first law of thermodynamics is often expressed as follows: when a system absorbs an amount of heat Q from the surroundings and does a quantity of work W on the same surroundings its internal energy changes by the amount:

$$\Delta E = Q - W$$

This law is basically the law of conservation of energy for an isolated system. Indeed, it states that if a system does not exchange any energy with its surroundings, its internal energy should not vary. If on the other hand a system does exchange energy with its surroundings, its internal energy should change by an amount corresponding to the energy it takes in from the surroundings.

The sign convention related to the previous mathematical expression of the first law of thermodynamics is:

- heat absorbed by the system: $Q > 0$
- heat released by the system: $Q < 0$
- work done by the system on its surroundings: $W > 0$
- work done by the surroundings on the system: $W < 0$

Caution: Some textbooks prefer a different sign convention: any energy (Q or W) flowing from the system to the surroundings (lost by the system) is negative and any energy flowing from the surroundings to the system (gained by the system) is positive. Within such a sign convention the first law is expressed as:

$$\Delta E = Q + W$$

i.e. the negative sign in the previous equation is incorporated in W.

7.3 Equivalence of Mechanical, Chemical and Thermal Energy Units

The previous equation does more than express mathematically the law of conservation of energy, it establishes a relationship between thermal energy and mechanical energy. Historically thermal energy was always expressed in calories (abbreviated as cal.) defined as the amount of thermal energy required to raise the temperature of 1 g of water by 1 degree Celcius. The standard unit used for mechanical work is the "Joule" (J). This unit eventually became the standard unit for any form of energy. The conversion factor between the two units is:

$$1 \text{ cal} = 4.184 \text{ J}$$

Chemists often refer to the amount of energies exchanged between the system and its surroundings to the mole, i.e., quantities of energy are expressed in J/mol or cal/mol. To obtain the energy per particle (atom or molecule), you should divide the energy expressed in J or cal by Avogadro's number.

GAMSAT-Prep.com
THE GOLD STANDARD

7.4 Temperature Scales

There are three temperature scales in use in science textbooks: the Celsius scale, the absolute temperature or Kelvin scale, and the Farenheit scale. In the Celsius scale the freezing point and the boiling point of water are arbitrarily defined as 0 °C and 100 °C, respectively. The scale is then divided into equal 1/100th intervals to define the degree Celsius or centigrade (from latin centi = 100). The absolute temperature or Kelvin scale is derived from the centigrade scale, i.e., an interval of 1 degree Celsius is equal to an interval of 1 degree Kelvin. The difference between the two scales is in their definitions of the zero point:

$$0 \text{ K} = -273.13 \text{ °C}.$$

Theoretically, this temperature can be approached but never achieved, it corresponds to the point where all motion is frozen and matter is destroyed. The Farenheit scale used in English speaking countries has the disadvantage of not being divided into 100 degrees between its two reference points: the freezing point of water is 32 °F and its boiling point is 212 °F. To convert Farenheit degrees into Celsius degrees you have to perform the following transformation:

$$(X \text{ °F} - 32) \times 5/9 = Y \text{ °C}$$

or

$$\text{°F} = 9/5 \text{ °C} + 32.$$

7.5 Heat Transfer

There are three ways in which heat can be transferred between the system and its surroundings:

(a) heat transfer by conduction

(b) heat transfer by convection

(c) heat transfer by radiation

In the first case (a) there is an intimate contact between the system and its surroundings and heat propagates through the entire system from the heated part to the unheated parts. A good example is the heating of a metal rod on a flame. Heat is initially transmitted directly from the flame to one end of the rod through the contact between the metal and the flame. When carrying out such an experiment you would notice at some point that the part of the rod which is not in direct contact with the flame becomes hot as well (please do not attempt!).

In the second case (b), heat is transferred to the entire system by the circulation of a hot liquid or a gas through it. The difference between this mode of transfer and the previous one, is that the entire system or a major part of it is heated up directly by the surroundings and not by propagation of the thermal energy from the parts of the system which are in direct contact with the heating source and the parts which are not.

In the third case (c) there is no contact between the heating source and the system. Heat is transported by radiation. The perfect example is the microwave oven where the water inside the food is heated by the microwave source. Most heat transfers are carried out by at least two of the above processes at the same time.

Note that when a metal is heated it expands at a rate which is proportional to the change in temperature it experiences. {For a definition of the coefficient of expansion, see PHY 6.3.}

7.6 State Functions

As previously mentioned, the first law of thermodynamics introduces three fundamental energy functions, i.e., the internal energy E, heat Q, and work W. Let us consider a transformation that takes the system from an initial state (I) to a final state (F) (which can differ by a number of variables such as temperature, pressure and volume). The change in the internal energy during this transformation depends only on the properties of the initial state (I) and the final state (F). In other words, suppose that to go from (I) to (F) the system is first subjected to an intermediate transformation that temporarily takes it from state (I) to an intermediate state (Int.) and then to another transformation that brings it from (Int.) to (F), the change in internal energy between the initial state (I) and the final state (F) are independent of the properties of the intermediate state (Int.). The internal energy is said to be a path-independent function or a state function. This is not the case for W and Q. In fact, this is quite conceivable since the amount of W or Q can be imposed by the external operator who subjects the system to a given transformation from (I) to (F). For instance, Q can be fixed at zero if the operator uses an appropriate thermal insulator between the system and its surroundings. In which case the change in the internal energy is due entirely to the work w ($\Delta E = -w$). It is easy to understand that the same result [transformation from (I) to (F)] could be achieved by supplying a small quantity of heat q while letting the system do more work W on the surroundings so that q – W is equal to –w. In which case we have:

	Work	Heat	Change in internal energy
1st transf.	w	0	–w
2nd transf.	$W = w + q$	q	–w

and yet in both cases the system is going from (I) to (F).

W and Q are not state functions. They depend on the path taken to go from (I) to (F). If you remember the exact definition of the internal energy you will understand that a system changes its internal energy to respond to an input of Q and W. In other words, contrary to Q and W, the internal energy cannot be directly imposed on the system.

The fact that the internal energy is a state function can be used in three other equivalent ways:

(i) If the changes in the internal energy during the intermediate transformation are known, they can be used to calculate the change for the entire process from (I) to (F): the latter is equal to the sum of the changes in the internal energy for all the intermediate steps.

(ii) If the change in the internal energy to go from a state (I) to a state (F) is $E_{I \to F}$ the change in the internal energy for an opposite transformation that would take the system from (F) to (I) is:

$$\Delta E_{F \to I} = -\Delta E_{I \to F}$$

(iii) If we start from (I) and go back to (I) through a series of intermediate transformations the change in the internal energy for the entire process is zero.

<u>W can be determined experimentally by calculating the area under a pressure-volume curve</u>. The mathematical relation is presented in CHM 8.1.

GOLD NOTES

GOLD NOTES

ENTHALPY AND THERMOCHEMISTRY
Chapter 8

Memorize	Understand	Not Required*
Define: endo/exothermic	* Area under curve: PV diagram * Equations for enthalpy, Hess's law, free E. * Calculation: Hess, calorimetry, Bond diss. E. * 2nd law of thermodynamics * Entropy, free E. and spontaneity	* Advanced level college info * Memorizing constants for latent heats * Memorizing equations

GAMSAT-Prep.com

Introduction

Thermochemistry is the study of energy absorbed or released in chemical reactions or in any physical transformation (i.e. phase change like melting and boiling). Thermochemistry for the GAMSAT includes understanding and/or calculating quantities such as enthalpy, heat capacity, heat of combustion, heat of formation, and free energy.

Additional Resources

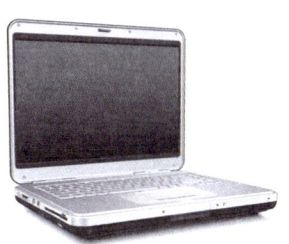

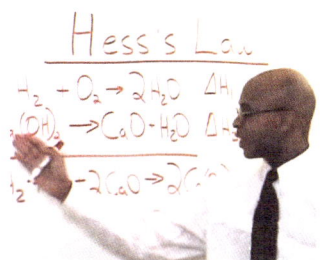

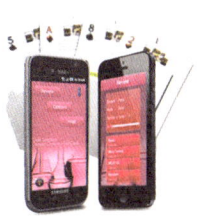

$\Delta G = \Delta H - T \Delta S$

Free Online Q&A + Forum   Video: Online or DVD   Flashcards   Special Guest

THE PHYSICAL SCIENCES CHM-99

* The real GAMSAT may have advanced level information presented (ie. in a passage) but previous knowledge of said information is not required to answer the questions that would follow. Practice ACER and GS practice GAMSATs can help you clarify this point.

8.1 Enthalpy as a Measure of Heat

The application of the general laws of thermodynamics to chemistry lead to some simplifications and adaptations because of the specificities of the problems that are dealt with in this field. For instance, in chemistry it is critical, if only for safety reasons, to know in advance what amounts of heat are going to be generated or absorbed during a reaction. In contrast, chemists are generally not interested in generating mechanical work and carry out most of their chemical reactions at constant pressure. For these reasons, although internal energy is a fundamental function its use is not very adequate in thermochemistry. Instead, chemists prefer to use another function derived from the internal energy: the enthalpy (H). This function is mathematically defined as:

$$\Delta H = \Delta E + P \times (\Delta V)$$

where P and V are respectively the pressure and the volume of the system. Hence, the enthalpy change (ΔH) of any system is the sum of the change in its internal energy (ΔE) and the product of its pressure (P) and volume change (ΔV). As the three components, internal energy, pressure and volume are all state functions, the enthalpy (H) or enthalpy change (ΔH) of a system is therefore also a state function. Thus, enthalpy change depends only on the enthalpies of the initial and final states (ΔH) and not on the path and therefore it is an example of a state function itself. The enthalpy change of a reaction is defined by the following equation $\Delta H = H_{final} - H_{initial}$; where ΔH is the enthalpy change, H_{final} is the enthalpy of the products of a reaction, and $H_{initial}$ is the enthalpy of the reactants of a reaction. A positive enthalpy change ($+\Delta H$) would indicate the flow of heat into a system as a reaction occurs and is called an "endothermic reaction". A cold pack added over an arm swelling would provide for a good example of an endothermic reaction. A negative enthalpy change ($-\Delta H$) would be called an "exothermic reaction" which essentially gives heat energy off from a system into its surroundings. A bunsen burner flame (= a small adjustable gas burner used in chem. labs) would be an appropriate example of an exothermic reaction.

You may wonder about the use of artificially introducing another energy function when internal energy is well defined and directly related to kinetic and potential energy of the particles that make up the system. To answer this legitimate question you need to consider the case of the majority of the chemical reactions where P is constant and where the only type of work that can possibly be done by the system is of a mechanical nature. In this case, since a change in internal energy (ΔE) occurring during a chemical reaction is basically a measure of all the systems energy as heat and work (Q + W) exchange with the system's surroundings, therefore, $\Delta E = Q + W$ and since, $W = -P\Delta V$, then, the change in enthalpy during a chemical reaction reduces to: $\Delta H = \Delta E + P \times V = (Q + W) + P \times V = Q + W - W = Q$ In other words, the change in enthalpy during a chemical reaction reduces to:

$$\Delta H = \Delta E + P \times V = (Q + W) + P \times V = Q$$

In other words, the change of enthalpy is a direct measure of the heat that evolves or is absorbed during a reaction carried out at constant pressure.

GENERAL CHEMISTRY

8.1.1 The Standard Enthalpy of Formation or Standard Heat of Formation ($\Delta H_f°$):

The standard enthalpy of formation, $\Delta H_f°$, is defined as the change of enthalpy that would occur when one mole of a substance is formed from its constituent elements in a standard state reaction. All elements in their standard states (oxygen gas, solid carbon as graphite, etc., at 1 atm and 25°C) have a standard enthalpy of formation of zero, as there is no change involved in their formation. The calculated standard enthalpy of various compounds can then be used to find the standard enthalpy of a reaction. For example, the standard enthalpy of formation for methane (CH_4) gas at 25°C would be the enthalpy of the following reaction:

$$C(s, graphite) + 2H_2(g) \rightarrow CH_4(g),$$

where $\Delta H_f° = -74.6$ KJ/mol. Thus, the chemical equation for the enthalpy of formation of any compound is always written with respect to the formation of 1 mole of the studied compound.

The standard enthalpy change for a reaction denoted as $\Delta H°_{rxn}$, is the change of enthalpy that would occur if one mole of matter is transformed by a chemical reaction with all reactants and products under standard state. It can be expressed as follows:

$$\Delta H°_{rxn} = (\text{sum of } n_f \Delta H°_f \text{ of products})$$
$$- (\text{sum of } n_r \Delta H°_f \text{ of reactants}),$$

where n_r represents the stoichiometric coefficients of the reactants and n_f the stoichiometric coefficients of the products. The $\Delta H°_f$ represents the standard enthalpies of formation.

8.2 Heat of Reaction: Basic Principles

As discussed, a reaction during which heat is released is said to be *exothermic* (ΔH is negative). If a reaction requires the supply of a certain amount of heat it is *endothermic* (ΔH is positive).

Besides the basic principle behind the introduction of enthalpy there is a more fundamental advantage for the use of this function in thermochemistry: it is a state function. This is a very practical property. For instance, consider two chemical reactions related in the following way:

reaction 1:   A + B → C
reaction 2:   C → D

If these two reactions are carried out consecutively they lead to the same result as the following reaction:

overall reaction: A + B → D

THE PHYSICAL SCIENCES   CHM-101

Because H is a state function we can apply the same arguments here as the ones we previously used for E. The initial state (I) corresponding to A + B, the intermediate state (Int.) to C, and the final state (F) to the final product D. If we know the changes in the enthalpy of the system for reactions 1 and 2, the change in the enthalpy during the overall reaction is:

$$\Delta H_{OVERALL} = \Delta H_1 + \Delta H_2$$

This is known as Hess's law. Remember that Hess's law is a simple application of the fact that H is a state function.

Thus, since the enthalpy change of a reaction is dependant only on the initial and final states, and not on the pathway that a reaction may follow, the sum of all the reaction step enthalpy changes must therefore be equivalent to the overall reaction enthalpy change (ΔH). The enthalpy change for a reaction can then be calculated without any direct measurement by using previously determined enthalpies of formation values for each reaction step of an overall equation. Consequently, if the overall enthalpy change is determined to be negative ($\Delta H_{net} < 0$), the reaction is exothermic and is most likely to be of a spontaneous type of reaction and a positive ΔH value would correspond to an endothermic reaction. Thus, Hess's law claims that enthalpy changes are additive and thus the ΔH for any single reaction can be calculated from the difference between the heat of formation of the products and the heat of formation of the reactants as follows:

$$\Delta H°_{reaction} = \Sigma \Delta H°_{f\ (products)} - \Sigma \Delta H°_{f\ (reactants)}$$

where the ° superscript indicates standard state values.

8.3 Hess's Law

Hess's law can be applied in several equivalent ways which we will illustrate with several examples:

Example: assume that we know the following enthalpy changes:

$2H_2(g) + O_2(g) \rightarrow 2H_2O(l)$
$\Delta H_1 = -136.6$ kcal : R1

$Ca(OH)_2(s) \rightarrow CaO(s) + H_2O(l)$
$\Delta H_2 = 15.3$ kcal : R2

$2CaO(s) \rightarrow 2\ Ca(s) + O_2(g)$
$\Delta H_3 = +303.6$ kcal : R3

and are asked to compute the enthalpy change for the following reaction:

$Ca(s) + H_2(g) + O_2(g) \rightarrow Ca(OH)_2(s)$: R

It is easy to see that reaction (R) can be obtained by the combination of reactions (R_1), (R_2) and (R_3) in the following way:

$-\ 1/2\ (R3):\quad Ca(s) + 1/2\ O_2(g) \rightarrow CaO(s)$
$+\ 1/2\ (R1):\quad H_2(g) + 1/2\ O_2(g) \rightarrow H_2O(l)$
$-\quad\ \ (R2):\quad CaO(s) + H_2O(l) \rightarrow Ca(OH)_2(s)$
$\overline{}$
$\quad\quad\quad\quad\ \ Ca(s) + H_2(g) + O_2(g) \rightarrow Ca(OH)_2(s)$

As we previously explained, since H is a state function the enthalpy change for (R) will be given by:

$$\Delta H = -1/2\Delta H_3 + 1/2\Delta H_1 - \Delta H_2$$

Example: assume that we have the following enthalpy changes as shown below:

R1: B_2O_3 (s) + $3H_2O$ (g) → $3O_2$ (g) + B_2H_6 (g)
(ΔH_1 = 2035 kJ/mol)

R2: H_2O (l) → H_2O (g)   (ΔH_2 = 44 kJ/mol)

R3: H_2 (g) + $(1/2)O_2$ (g) → H_2O (l)
(ΔH_3 = −286 kJ/mol)

R4: 2B (s) + $3H_2$ (g) → B_2H_6 (g)
(ΔH_4 = 36 kJ/mol)

and are then asked to find the enthalpy change or ΔH_f of the following reaction (R):

R: 2B (s) + $(3/2)O_2$ (g) → B_2O_3 (s)   (ΔH_f = ?)

After the required multiplication and rearrangements of all step equations (and their respective enthalpy changes), the result is as follows:

(−1) × (R1) B_2H_6 (g) + $3O_2$ (g)
→ B_2O_3 (s) + $3H_2O$ (g)
(ΔH_1 = −2035 kJ/mol)

(−3) × (R2) $3H_2O$ (g) → $3H_2O$ (l)
(ΔH_2 = -132 kJ/mol)

(−3) × (R3) $3H_2O$ (l) → $3H_2$ (g) + $(3/2)O_2$ (g)
(ΔH_3 = 858 kJ/mol)

(+1) × (R4) 2B (s) + $3H_2$ (g) → B_2H_6 (g)
(ΔH_4 = 36 kJ/mol)

adding the equations while canceling out all common terms, we finally obtain:

2B (s) + $(3/2)O_2$ (g) → B_2O_3 (s)
(ΔH_f = −1273 kJ/mol)

As noted in the initial example, it is shown that the enthalpy change (ΔH_f) for the final reaction is given by the following:

$$\Delta H_f = (-1)\Delta H_1 + (-3)\Delta H_2 + (-3)\Delta H_3 + (1)\Delta H_4$$

There are no general rules that would allow you to determine which reaction to use first and by what factor it needs to be multiplied. It is important to proceed systematically and follow some simple ground rules:

(i) For instance, you could start by writing the overall reaction that you want to obtain through a series of reaction additions.

(ii) Number all your reactions.

(iii) Keep in mind as you go along that the reactants of the overall reaction should always appear on the left-hand side and that the products should always appear on the right-hand side.

(iv) Circle or underline the first reactant of the overall reaction. Find a reaction in your list that involves this reactant (as a reactant or a product). Use that reaction first and write it in such a way that this reactant appears on the left-hand side with the appropriate stoichiometric coefficient (i.e., if this reactant appears as a product of a reaction on your list you should reverse the reaction).

(v) Suppose that in (iv) you had to use the second reaction on your list and that you had to reverse and multiply this reaction by a factor of 3 to satisfy the preceding rule. In your addition, next to this reaction or on top of the arrow write $-3 \times \Delta H_2$.

(vi) Repeat the process for the other reactants and products of the overall reaction until your addition yields the overall reaction. As you continue this process, make sure to cross out the compounds that appear on the right and left-hand sides at the same time.

8.4 Standard Enthalpies

Hess's law has a very practical use in chemistry. Indeed, the enthalpy change for a given chemical reaction can be computed from simple combinations of known enthalpy changes of other reactions. Because enthalpy changes depend on the conditions under which reactions are carried out it is important to define standard conditions:

(i) Standard pressure: 1 atmosphere pressure (approx. = 1 bar).

(ii) Standard temperature for the purposes of the calculation of the standard enthalpy change: generally 25 °C. The convention is that if the temperature of the standard state is not mentioned then it is assumed to be 25 °C, the standard temperature needs to be specified in all other instances.

(iii) Standard physical state of an element: it is defined as the "natural" physical state of an element under the above standard pressure and temperature. For instance, the standard physical state of water under the standard temperature and pressure of 1 atm and 25 °C is the liquid state. Under the same conditions oxygen is a gas.

Naturally, the standard enthalpy change (notation: $\Delta H°$) for a given reaction is defined as the enthalpy change that accompanies the reaction when it is carried out under standard pressure and temperature with all reactants and products in their standard physical state.

Note that the standard temperature defined here is <u>different from the standard temperature for an ideal gas</u> which is: 0 °C.

8.5 Enthalpies of Formation

The enthalpy of formation of a given compound is defined as the enthalpy change that accompanies the formation of the compound from its constituting elements. For instance, the enthalpy of formation of water is the $\Delta H_f°$ for the following reaction:

$$H_2 + 1/2\ O_2 \rightarrow H_2O$$

To be more specific the standard enthalpy of formation of water $\Delta H_f°$ is the enthalpy change during the reaction:

$$H_2(g) + 1/2 O_2(g) \xrightarrow[\text{1 atm}]{25°C} H_2O(l)$$

where the reactants are in their natural physical state under standard temperature and pressure.

Note that according to these definitions, several of the reactions considered in the previous sections were in fact examples of reactions of formation. For instance, in section 8.3 on Hess's law, reaction (R1) is the reaction of formation of two moles of water, if reversed reaction (R3) would be the reaction of formation of two moles of CaO and the overall reaction (R) is the reaction of formation of 1 mole Ca(OH)$_2$. Also note that although one could use the reverse of reaction (R2) to form Ca(OH)$_2$, this reaction, even reversed, is not the reaction of formation of Ca(OH)$_2$. The reason is that the constitutive elements of this molecule are: calcium (Ca), hydrogen (H$_2$) and oxygen (O$_2$) and not CaO and H$_2$O. Enthalpies of formation are also referred to as heats of formation. As previously explained, if the reaction of formation is carried out at constant pressure, the change in the enthalpy represents the amount of heat released or absorbed during the reaction.

8.6 Bond Dissociation Energies and Heats of Formation

The bond dissociation energy, also known as the bond dissociation enthalpy, is a measure of bond strength within a particular molecule defined as a standard enthalpy change in the *homolytic* cleavage (= 2 free radicals formed; CHM 9.4) of any studied chemical bond. An example of bond dissociation energies would be the successive homolytic cleavage of each of the C-H bonds of methane (CH$_4$) to give, CH$_3$• + •H, CH$_2$• + •H, CH• + •H and finally C• + •H. The bond dissociation energies for each of the homolytic CH bond cleavage of methane are determined to be as follows: 435 KJ/mol, 444 KJ/mol, 444 KJ/mol and 339 KJ/mol, respectively. The average of these four individual bond dissociation energies is known as the bond energy of the CH bond and is 414 KJ/mol. Thus, with the exception of all diatomic molecules where only one chemical bond is involved so that bond energy and bond dissociation energy are in this case equivalent, the bond dissociation energy is not exactly the same as bond energy. Bond energy is more appropriately defined as the energy required to sever 1 mole of a chemical bond in a gas and not necessarily the measure of a chemical bond strength within a particular molecule. Bond energy is therefore a measure of bond strength. Moreover as just described, bond energy may be considered as an average energy calculated from the sum of bond dissociation energies of all bonds within a particular compound. Bond energies are always positive values as it always takes energy to break bonds apart.

The difficulty in defining bond dissociation energies in polyatomic molecules is that the amounts of energy required to break a given bond (say an O–H bond) in two different polyatomic molecules (H_2O and CH_3OH, for instance) are different. Bond dissociation energies in polyatomic molecules are approximated to an average value for molecules of the same nature. Within the framework of this commonly made approximation we can calculate the <u>enthalpy change of any reaction</u> using the *sum* of bond energies of the reactants and the products in the following way:

$$\Delta H°_{(reaction)} = \Sigma BE_{(reactants)} - \Sigma BE_{(products)}$$

where BE stands for bond energies.

Standard enthalpy changes of chemical reactions can also be computed using enthalpies of formation in the following way:

$$\Delta H°_{(reaction)} = \Sigma \Delta H_{(bonds\ broken)} + \Sigma \Delta H_{(bonds\ formed)}$$
$$= \Sigma BE_{(reactants)} - \Sigma BE_{(products)}$$

Note how this equation is similar but not identical to the one making use of bond energies. This comes from the fact that a bond energy is defined as the energy required to <u>break</u> (and not to form) a given bond. Also note that the standard enthalpy of formation of a mole of any **element** is zero.

8.7 Calorimetry

Measurements of changes of temperature within a reaction mixture allow the experimental determination of heat absorbed or released during the corresponding chemical reaction. Indeed the amount of heat required to change the temperature of any substance X from T_1 to T_2 is proportional to $(T_2 - T_1)$ and the quantity of X:

$$Q = mC(T_2 - T_1)$$

or

$$Q = nc(T_2 - T_1)$$

where m is the mass of X, n the number of moles. The constant C or c is called the <u>heat capacity</u>. The standard units for C and c are, respectively, the $Jkg^{-1}K^{-1}$ and the $Jmol^{-1}K^{-1}$. C which is the heat capacity per <u>unit mass</u> is also referred to as the <u>specific heat capacity</u>. If you refer back to the definition of the calorie (see CHM 7.3) you will understand that the specific heat of water is necessarily: $1\ cal\ g^{-1}\ °C^{-1}$.

Note that heat can be absorbed or released without a change in temperature (CHM 4.3.3). In fact, this situation occurs whenever a phase change takes place for a pure compound. For instance, ice melts at a constant temperature of 0 °C in order to break the forces that keep the water molecules in a crystal of ice we need to supply an amount of heat of 6.01 kJ/mol. There is no direct way of calculating the heat corresponding to a phase change.

Heats of phase changes (heat of fusion, heat of vaporization, heat of sublimation) are generally tabulated and indirectly determined in calorimetric experiments. For instance, if a block of ice is allowed to melt in a bucket of warm water, we can determine the heat of fusion of ice by measuring the temperature drop in the bucket of water and applying the law of conservation of energy. The relevant equation is:

$$Q = m L$$

where L is the latent heat which is a constant.

Calorimetry is the science of measuring the heat evolved or exchanged due to a chemical reaction. The thermal energy of a reaction (defined as the system) is measured as a function of its surroundings by observing a temperature change (ΔT) on the surroundings due to the system. The magnitude in temperature change is essentially a measure of a system's or sample's energy content which is measured either while keeping a volume constant (bomb calorimetry) or while keeping a pressure constant (coffee-cup calorimetry).

In a constant volume calorimetry measurement, the bomb calorimeter is kept at a constant volume and there is essentially no heat exchange between the calorimeter and the surroundings and thus, the net heat exchange for the system is zero. The heat exchange for the reaction is then compensated for by the heat change for the water and bomb calorimeter material steel (or surroundings). Thus, $\Delta q_{system} = \Delta q_{reaction} + \Delta q_{water} + \Delta q_{steel} = 0$ in bomb calorimetry, and so $q_{cal} = -q_{reaction}$ in which the temperature change is related to the heat absorbed by the calorimeter (q_{cal}) and if no heat escapes the constant volume calorimeter, the amount of heat gained by the calorimeter then equals that released by the system and so, $q_{cal} = -q_{reaction}$ as stated previously. Note that since $Q = mc\Delta T$ as previously defined, and $q_{reaction} = -(q_{water} + q_{steel})$ therefore, $q_{reaction} = -(m_{water})(c_{water})\Delta T + (m_{steel})(c_{steel})\Delta T$.

For aqueous solutions, a coffee-cup calorimeter is usually used to measure the enthalpy change of the system. This is simply a polystyrene (Styrofoam) cup with a lid and a thermometer. The cup is partially filled with a known volume of water. When a chemical reaction occurs in the coffee-cup calorimeter, the heat of the reaction is absorbed by the water. The change in water temperature is used to calculate the amount of heat that has been absorbed (used to make products, so water temperature decreases) or evolved (lost to the water, so its temperature increases) in the reaction.

8.8 The Second Law of Thermodynamics

The first law of thermodynamics allows us to calculate energy transfers during a given transformation of the system. It does not allow us to predict whether a transformation can or cannot occur spontaneously. Yet our daily observations tell us that certain transformations always occur in a given direction. For instance, heat flows from a hot source to a cold source. We cannot spontaneously transfer heat in the other direction to make the hot source hotter and the cold source colder. The second law of thermodynamics states that entropy (S) of an isolated system will never decrease. In order for a reaction to proceed, the entropy of the system must increase. For any spontaneous process, the entropy of the universe increases which results in a greater dispersal or randomization of the energy ($\Delta S > 0$). The second law of thermodynamics allows the determination of the preferred direction of a given transformation. Transformations which require the smallest amount of energy and lead to the largest disorder of the system are the most spontaneous.

8.9 Entropy

Entropy is regarded as the main driving force behind all the chemical and physical changes known within the universe. All natural processes tend toward an increase in energy dispersal or, in other words, an entropy increase within our universe. Thus, a chemical system or reaction proceeds in a direction of universal entropy increase.

Entropy S is the state function which measures the degree of "disorder" in a system. For instance, the entropy of ice is lower than the entropy of liquid water since ice corresponds to an organized crystalline structure (virtually no disorder). In fact, generally speaking, the entropy increases as we go from a solid to a liquid to a gas. For similar reasons, the entropy decreases when an elastic band is stretched. Indeed, in the "unstretched" elastic band the molecules of the rubber polymer are coiled up and form a disorganized structure. As the rubber is stretched these molecules will tend to line up with each other and adopt a more organized structure.

Entropy has the dimension of energy as a function of temperature as J/K or cal/K. Entropy can therefore be related to temperature and is thus a measure of energy dispersal (in joules) per unit of temperature (in kelvins).

The second law of thermodynamics can be expressed in the alternative form: a spontaneous transformation corresponds to an increase of the entropy of the system plus its surroundings. Hence, a chemical system is known to proceed in a direction that increases the entropy of the universe. As a result, ΔS must be incorporated in an expression that includes both the system and its surroundings so that, $\Delta S_{universe} = \Delta S_{surroundings} + \Delta S_{system} > 0$. When a system reaches a certain temperature equilibrium, it then also reaches its maximal entropy and so, $\Delta S_{universe} = \Delta S_{surroundings} + \Delta S_{system} = 0$. The entropy of the thermodynamic system is therefore a measure of how far the equalization has progressed.

Entropy, like enthalpy, is a state function and is therefore path independent. Hence, a change in entropy depends only on the initial and final states ($\Delta S = S_{final} - S_{initial}$) and not on how the system arrived at that state. Under standard conditions, for any process or reaction, the entropy change for that reaction will be the difference between the entropies of products and reactants as follows:

$$\Delta S°_{reaction} = \Delta S°_{products} - \Delta S°_{reactants}$$

8.10 Free Energy

The Gibbs free energy G is another state function which can be used as a criterion for spontaneity. This function is defined as:

$$G = H - T \cdot S$$

where: H is the enthalpy of the system in a given state,

T is the temperature,

and S is the entropy of the system.

Consequently, Gibbs Free Energy (G) also determines the direction of a spontaneous change for a chemical system. The derivation for the formulation thus incorporates both the entropy and enthalpy parameters studied in the previous sections. Following various manipulations and derivations, one can then note that Gibbs Free Energy is an alternative form of both enthalpy and the entropy changes of a chemical process.

The standard Gibbs Free Energy of a reaction ($\Delta G°_{rxn}$), is determined at 25°C and a pressure of 1 atm. For a reaction carried out at constant temperature we can write that the change in the Gibbs free energy is:

$$\Delta G = \Delta H - T \Delta S$$

A reaction carried out at constant pressure is spontaneous if

$$\Delta G < 0$$

It is not spontaneous if:

$$\Delta G > 0$$

and it is in a ==state of equilibrium== (reaction spontaneous in both directions) if:

$$\Delta G = 0.$$

As noted in the previous chapter, the study of thermodynamics generally describes the spontaneity or the direction and extent to which a reaction will proceed. It therefore enables one to predict if a reaction will occur spontaneously or not. Note that non spontaneous processes may turn into spontaneous processes if coupled to another spontaneous process or more specifically by the addition of some external energy.

Thermochemistry then can be used to essentially calculate how much work a system can do or require. Thermodynamics basically then deals with the relative potentials of both the reactants and products of a chemical system. The next chapter will describe the actual rate (or chemical kinetics or speed) of a chemical reaction. In chemical kinetics, the chemical potential of intermediate states of a chemical reaction may also be described and thus enabling one to determine why a reaction may be slow or fast.

GOLD NOTES

THE PHYSICAL SCIENCES CHM-111

GOLD NOTES

RATE PROCESSES IN CHEMICAL REACTIONS
Chapter 9

Memorize	Understand	Not Required*
ction order ne: rate determining step eralized potential energy diagrams ne: activation energy, catalysis ne: saturation kinetics, substrate	* Reaction rates, rate law, determine exponents * Reaction mechanism for free radicals * Rate constant equation; apply Le Chatelier's * Kinetic vs. thermodynamic control * Law of mass action, equations for Gibbs free E., saturation kinetics, Keq	* Advanced level college info * Memorizing the rate constant equation

GAMSAT-Prep.com

Introduction

Rate processes involve the study of the velocity (speed) and mechanisms of chemical reactions. **Reaction rate** (= *velocity*) tells us how fast the concentrations of reactants change with time. **Reaction mechanisms** show the sequence of steps to get to the overall change. Experiments show that 4 important factors generally influence reaction rates: (1) the nature of the reactants, (2) their concentration, (3) temperature, and (4) catalysis.

Additional Resources

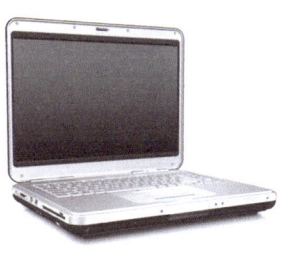

Free Online Q&A + Forum

Video: Online or DVD

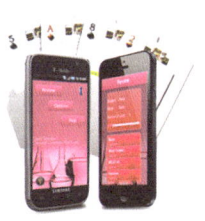

Flashcards

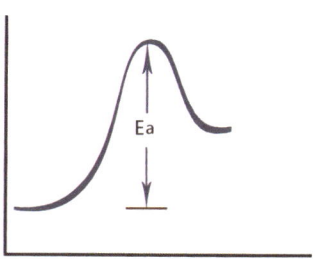

Special Guest

THE PHYSICAL SCIENCES CHM-113

* The real GAMSAT may have advanced level information presented (ie. in a passage) but previous knowledge of said information is not required to answer the questions that would follow. Practice ACER and GS practice GAMSATs can help you clarify this point.

9.1 Reaction Rate

Consider a general reaction

$$2A + 3B \rightarrow C + D$$

The rate or the velocity at which this reaction proceeds can be expressed by one of the following:

(i) rate of disappearance of A: $-\Delta[A]/\Delta t$

(ii) rate of disappearance of B: $-\Delta[B]/\Delta t$

(iii) rate of appearance or formation of C: $\Delta[C]/\Delta t$

(iv) rate of appearance or formation of D: $\Delta[D]/\Delta t$

Where [ ] denotes the concentration of a reactant or a product in moles/liter. Thus, the reaction rate measure is usually expressed as a change in reactant or product concentration ($\Delta_{conc.}$) per unit change in time (Δt).

Since A and B are disappearing in this reaction, [A] and [B] are decreasing with time, i.e. $\Delta[A]/\Delta t$ and $\Delta[B]/\Delta t$ are negative quantities. On the other hand, the quantities $\Delta[C]/\Delta t$ and $\Delta[D]/\Delta t$ are positive since both C and D are being formed during the process of this reaction. By convention: rates of reactions are expressed as positive numbers; as a result, a negative sign is necessary in the first two expressions.

Suppose that A disappears at a rate of 6 (moles/liter)/s. In the same time interval (1s), in a total volume of 1L we have:

(3 mol B/2 mol A) × 6 mol A
= 9 moles of B disappearing
(1 mol C/2 mol A) × 6 mol A
= 3 moles of C being formed
(1 mol D/2 mol A) × 6 mol A
= 3 moles of D being formed

Therefore <u>individual rates of formation or disappearance</u> are not convenient ways to express the rate of a reaction. Indeed, depending on the reactant or product considered the rate will be given by a different numerical value unless the stoichiometric coefficients are equal (e.g. for C and D in our case).

A more convenient expression of the rate of a reaction is the <u>overall rate</u>. This rate is simply obtained by dividing the rate of formation or disappearance of a given reactant or product by the corresponding stoichiometric coefficient, i.e.:

overall rate = $-(1/2) \Delta[A]/\Delta t$, or
$-(1/3) \Delta[B]/\Delta t$,

or $\Delta[C]/\Delta t$, or $\Delta[D]/\Delta t$.

A simple verification on our example will show you that these expressions all lead to the same numerical value for the overall rate: 3 (moles/L)/s. Therefore for a generic equation such as, $aA + bB \rightarrow cC + dD$, a generalization of the overall reaction rate would be as follows:

$$\text{Rate} = \frac{-1}{a}\frac{\Delta[A]}{\Delta t} = \frac{-1}{b}\frac{\Delta[B]}{\Delta t} = \frac{+1}{c}\frac{\Delta[C]}{\Delta t} = \frac{+1}{d}\frac{\Delta[D]}{\Delta t}$$

GENERAL CHEMISTRY

It can be seen from the preceding overall rate relationship that the rate is the same whether we use one of the reactants or one of the products to calculate the rates. Generally, one can see that knowing the rate of change in the concentration of any one reactant or product at a certain time point allows one to invariably determine the rate of change in the concentration of any other reactant or product at the same time point using the stoichiometrically balanced equation.

Whenever the term "rate" is used (with no other specification) it refers to the "overall rate" unless individual and overall rates are equal.

9.2 Dependence of Reaction Rates on Concentration of Reactants

The rate of a reaction (given in moles per liter per second) can be expressed as a function of the concentration of the reactants. In the previous chemical reaction we would have:

$$\text{rate} = k\,[A]^m\,[B]^n$$

where [ ] is the concentration of the corresponding reactant in moles per liter

k is referred to as the rate constant
m is the order of the reaction with respect to A
n is the order of the reaction with respect to B
m+n is the overall reaction order.

The rate constant k is reaction specific. It is directly proportional to the rate of a reaction. It increases with increasing temperature since the proportion of molecules with energies greater than the activation energy E_a of a reaction increases with higher temperatures.

According to the rate law above, the reaction is said to be an (m + n)th order reaction, or, an mth order reaction with respect to A, or, an nth order reaction with respect to B.

The value of the m or nth rate orders of the reaction describes how the rate of the reaction depends on the concentration of the reactant(s).

For example, a zero rate order for reactant A (where m = 0), would indicate that the rate of the reaction is independent of the concentration of reactant A and therefore has a constant reaction rate (this is also applicable to reactant B). The rate equation can therefore be expressed as a rate constant k or the rate = k. The rate probably depends on temperature or other factors excluding concentration.

A first rate order for reactant A (where m = 1) would indicate that the rate of the reaction is directly proportional to the concentration of the reactant A (or B, where n = 1). Thus, the rate equation can be expressed as follows: rate = $k[A]^1$ or rate = $k[B]^1$.

A second rate order for reactant A (m = 2) would indicate that the rate is proportional to the square of the reactant concentration. The

THE PHYSICAL SCIENCES CHM-115

rate equation can thus be expressed as follows: rate = k[A]^2.

Hence, the rate orders or exponents in the rate law equation can be integers, fractions, or zeros and are not necessarily equal to the stoichiometric coefficients in the given reaction except when a reaction is the rate-determining step (or elementary step). Consequently, although there are other orders, including both higher and mixed orders or fractions that are possible as described, the three described orders (0, 1st and 2nd), are amongst the most common orders studied.

As shown by the graphical representation below, for the zero order reactant, as the concentration of reactant A decreases over time, the slope of the line is constant and thus the rate is constant. Moreover, the rate does not change regardless of the decrease in reactant A concentration over time and thus the zero order rate order. For the first order, the decrease in reactant A concentration is shown to affect the rate of reaction in direct proportion. Thus, as the concentration decreases, the rate decreases proportionally. Lastly, for the second order, the rate of the reaction is shown to decrease proportionally to the square of the reactant A concentration. In fact, the curves for 1st and 2nd order reactions resemble exponential decay.

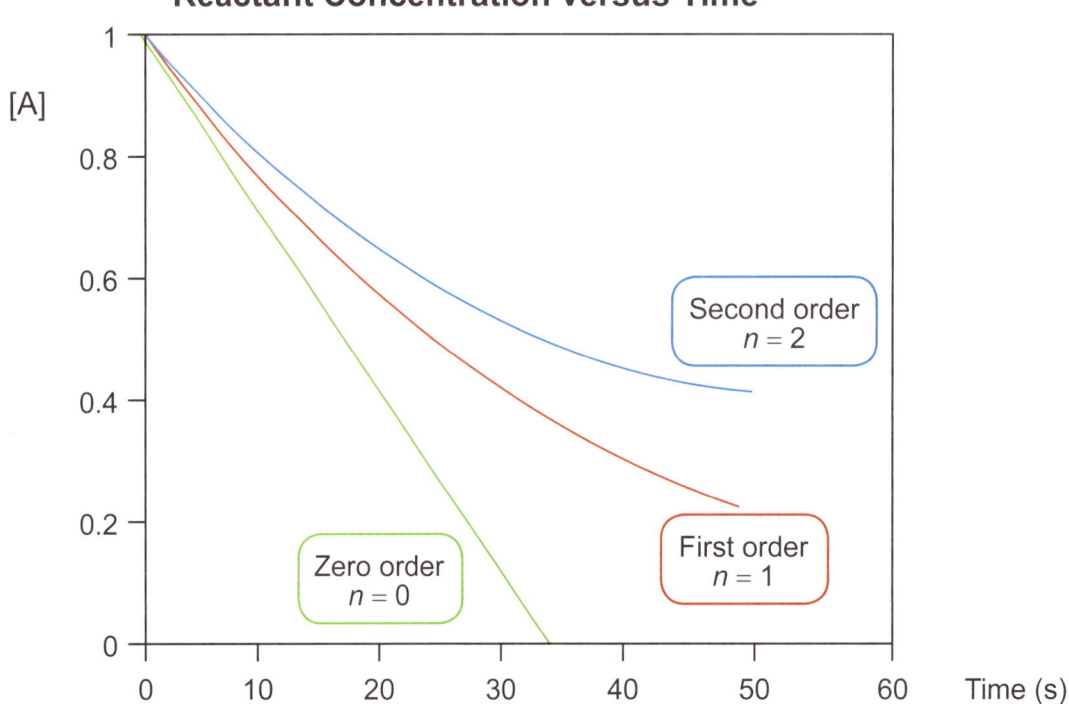

Figure III.A.9.0: Reactant concentration vs. time curves. Notice that first and second order reactions have exponential decay curves (PHY 10.5) but, of course, second order reactions decay faster. It is expected that you can recognize the graphs above and those in the next section (CHM 9.2.1).

GENERAL CHEMISTRY

9.2.1 Differential Rate Law vs. Integrated Rate Law

Rate laws may be expressed as differential equations or as integrated rate laws. As differential equations, the relationship is shown between the rate of a reaction and the concentration of a reactant. Alternatively, the integrated rate law expresses a rate as a function of concentration of a reactant or reactants and time.

For example, for a zero order rate, Rate = $k[A]^0$ = k and since Rate = $-\Delta[A]/\Delta t$, then $-\Delta[A]/\Delta t$ = k and following the integration of the differential function, the following zero-order integrated rate law is obtained: $[A]_t = -kt + [A]_o$, where $[A]_t$ = is the concentration of A at a particular time point t and $[A]_o$ is the initial concentration of A and k is the rate constant.

The following table summarizes the main rate laws of the 0, 1st and 2nd rate orders and their respective relationships.

Table 9.2.1: The graphs below do not need to be memorized but you may be expected to match any Integrated Rate Law equation with its graph since they follow the simple standard of y = mx + b (GM 3.4.4, 3.5.1).

Reaction Order	Rate Law	Units of k	Integrated Rate Law	Straight-Line Plot	Half-Life Equation
0	Rate = $k[A]^0$	$M \cdot s^{-1}$	$[A]_t = -kt + [A]_o$	[A] vs Time t; y-intercept = $[A]_o$, slope = $-k$	$t_{1/2} = \dfrac{[A]_0}{2k} = \dfrac{1}{k}\dfrac{[A]_0}{2}$
1	Rate = $k[A]^1$	s^{-1}	$\ln[A]_t = -kt + \ln[A]_o$ $\ln \dfrac{[A]_t}{[A]_0} = -kt$	ln[A] vs Time t; y-intercept = $\ln[A]_o$, slope = $-k$	$t_{1/2} = \dfrac{0.693}{k} = \dfrac{1}{k}(0.693)$
2	Rate = $k[A]^2$	$M^{-1} \cdot s^{-1}$	$\dfrac{1}{[A]_t} = kt + \dfrac{1}{[A]_0}$	1/[A] vs Time t; slope = k, y-intercept = $1/[A]_o$	$t_{1/2} = \dfrac{1}{k[A]_0} = \dfrac{1}{k}\dfrac{1}{[A]_0}$

THE PHYSICAL SCIENCES

As depicted by the table, the first and second order rate laws are also derived in a similar manner as the zero order rate law.

Included within the table is also the half-life's of the three described rate laws. The half-life of a reaction is defined as the time needed to decrease the concentration of the reactant to one-half of the original starting concentration (PHY 12.4). Note that each rate order has its own respective half-life.

The rate order of a reactant may be determined experimentally by either the isolation or initial rates method as described in the following section or by plotting concentration, or some function of concentration such as ln[ ] or 1/[ ] of reactant as a function of time. A linear relationship between the dependent concentration variable of reactant and the independent time variable will then delineate the actual order of the reactant. Moreover, if a linear curve is obtained when plotting [reactant] versus time, the order would be zero whereas, if a linear relationship is noted when plotting ln [reactant] versus time, this would be first order and second order would be for a linear relationship between 1/[reactant] versus time.

Therefore, the rate law of a reaction with a multi-step mechanism cannot be deduced from the stoichiometric coefficients of the overall reaction; it must be determined experimentally for a given reaction at a given temperature as will be described in the following section.

9.3 Determining Exponents of the Rate Law

The only way to determine the exponents with certainty is via experimentation. The rate law for any reaction must therefore always be determined by experimentation, often by a method known as the "initial rates method or the isolation method".

In the initial rates method, if there are two or more reactants involved in the reaction, the reactant concentrations are usually varied independent of each other so that, for example, in a two reactant reaction, if one reactant concentration is altered the other reactant concentration would be kept constant and the effect on the initial rate of the reaction would be measured. Consider the following five experiments varying the concentrations of reactants A and B with resulting initial rates of reaction:

$$A + B \rightarrow products$$

In the first three experiments the concentration of A changes but B remains the same. Thus the resultant changes in rate only depend on the concentration of A. Note that when [A] doubles (Exp. 1, 2) the reaction rate doubles, and when [A] triples (Exp. 1, 3) the reaction

GENERAL CHEMISTRY

Exp. #	Initial Concentration [A]	Initial Concentration [B]	Initial Rate (mol L^{-1} s^{-1})
1	0.10	0.10	0.20
2	0.20	0.10	0.40
3	0.30	0.10	0.60
4	0.30	0.20	2.40
5	0.30	0.30	5.40

rate triples. Because it is directly proportional, the exponent of [A] must be 1. Thus the rate of reaction is first order with respect to A.

In the final three sets of experiments, [B] changes while [A] remains the same. When [B] doubles (Exp. 3, 4) the rate increases by a factor of 4 (= 2^2). When [B] triples (Exp. 3, 5) the rate increases by a factor of 9 (= 3^2). Thus the relation is exponential where the exponent of [B] is 2. The rate of reaction is second order with respect to B.

$$\text{initial rate} = k[A]^1[B]^2$$

The overall rate of reaction (n+m) is third order. The value of the rate constant k can be easily calculated by substituting the results from any of the five experiments. For example, using experiment #1:

$$k = \frac{\text{initial rate}}{[A]^1 [B]^2}$$

$$k = \frac{0.20 \text{ mol } L^{-1} \text{ s}^{-1}}{(0.10 \text{ mol } L^{-1})(0.10 \text{ mol } L^{-1})^2}$$

$$= 2.0 \times 10^2 \text{ L}^2\text{mol}^{-2}\text{s}^{-1}$$

k is the rate constant for the reaction which includes all five experiments.

Note: The units of the resultant rate constant "k" will differ depending on the overall rate order of a reaction.

9.4 Reaction Mechanism - Rate-determining Step

Chemical equations fail to describe the detailed process through which the reactants are transformed into the products. For instance, consider the reaction of formation of hydrogen chloride from hydrogen and chlorine:

$$Cl_2(g) + H_2(g) \rightarrow 2\ HCl(g)$$

The equation above fails to mention that in fact this reaction is the result of a chain of reactions proceeding in three steps:

Initiation step: formation of free chlorine radicals by photon irradiation or introduction of heat (= *radicals*, the mechanism will be discussed in organic chemistry):

$$1/2\ Cl_2 \rightleftharpoons Cl\cdot$$

The double arrow indicates that in fact some of the Cl free radicals recombine to form chlorine molecules, the whole process eventually reaches a state of equilibrium where the following ratio is constant:

$$K = [Cl\cdot]/[Cl_2]^{1/2}$$

The determination of such a constant will be dealt with in the sub-section on "equilibrium constants."

Propagation step: formation of reactive hydrogen free radicals and reaction between hydrogen free radicals and chlorine molecules:

$$Cl\cdot + H_2 \rightarrow HCl + H\cdot$$

$$H\cdot + Cl_2 \rightarrow HCl + Cl\cdot$$

Termination step: Formation of hydrogen chloride by reaction between hydrogen free radicals and chlorine free radicals.

$$H\cdot + Cl\cdot \rightarrow HCl$$

The detailed chain reaction process above is called the mechanism of the reaction. Each individual step in a detailed mechanism is called an elementary step. Any reaction proceeds through some mechanism which is generally impossible to predict from its chemical equation. Such mechanisms are usually determined through an experimental procedure. Generally speaking each step proceeds at its own rate.

The rate of the overall reaction is naturally limited by the slowest step; therefore, the rate-determining step in the mechanism of a reaction is the slowest step. In other words, the overall rate law of a reaction is basically equal to the rate law of the slowest step. The faster processes have an indirect influence on the rate: they regulate the concentrations of the reactants and products. The chemical equation of an elementary step reflects the exact molecular process that transforms its reactants into its products. For this reason its rate law can be predicted from its chemical equation: in an elementary process, the orders with respect to the reactants are equal to the corresponding stoichiometric coefficients.

In our example, experiments show that the rate-determining step is the reaction between chlorine radicals and hydrogen molecules, all the other steps are much faster. According to the principles stated, the rate law of the overall reaction is equal to the rate law of this rate-determining step. Therefore, the rate of the overall reaction is proportional to the concentration of hydrogen molecules and chlorine radicals but is not directly proportional to the concentration of chlorine molecules. However, since the ratio of concentrations of Cl and Cl_2 is regulated by the initiation step concentration, it can be shown that according to the mechanism provided the rate law is:

$$\text{rate} = k[H_2] \cdot [Cl_2]^{1/2}$$

It is important to note that the individual orders of a reaction are generally not equal to the stoichiometric coefficients.

9.5 Dependence of Reaction Rates upon Temperature

Rates of chemical reactions are generally very sensitive to temperature fluctuations. In particular, many reactions are known to slow down by decreasing the temperature or vise versa. How does one therefore explain the temperature dependence on reaction rates? The rate of a reaction is essentially equal to the reactant concentration raised to a reaction order (n) times the rate constant k or rate = $k[A]^x$. From the collision theory of chemical kinetics it was established that the rate constant of a reaction can be expressed as follows:

$$k = A\,e^{-Ea/RT}$$

- A is a constant referred to as the "Arrhenius constant" or the frequency factor which includes two separate components known as, the orientation factor (p) and the collision frequency (z). More specifically, the collision frequency (z) is defined as the number of collisions that molecules acquire per unit time and the orientation factor (p) is defined as the proper orientation reactant molecules require for product formation. Thus, the Arrhenius constant, A, is related to both the frequency of collisions (z) and the proper orientation (p) of the molecular collisions required for final product formation and so A = pz.
- e is the base of natural logarithms,
- E_a is the activation energy, it is the energy required to get a reaction started. For reactants to transform into products, the reactants must go through a high energy state or "transition state" which is the minimum energy (activation energy) required for reactants to transform into products. If two molecules of reactants collide with proper orientation and sufficient energy

or force in such a way that the molecules acquire a total energy content surpassing the activation energy, E_a, the collisions will result in a complete chemical reaction and the formation of products. Note: only a fraction of colliding reactant molecules will have sufficient kinetic energy to exceed an activation energy barrier.
- R is the ideal gas constant (1.99 cal mol^{-1} K^{-1})
- *T* is the absolute temperature.

It can therefore be seen that the rate constant, k, contains the temperature component as an exponent and thus, temperature affects a reaction rate by affecting the actual rate constant k. Note: A rate constant remains constant only when temperature remains constant. The rate constant equation otherwise known as the "Arrhenius equation" thus describes the relationship between the rate constant (k) and temperature.

Either an increase in temperature or decrease in activation energy will result in an increase in the reaction constant k and thus an increase in the reaction rate. The species formed during an efficient collision, before the reactants transform into the final product(s) is called the activated complex or the transition state.

Within the framework of this theory, when a single step reaction proceeds, the potential energy of the system varies according to Figure III.A.9.1.

The change in enthalpy (*ΔH*) during the reaction is the difference between the total energy of the products and the reactants.

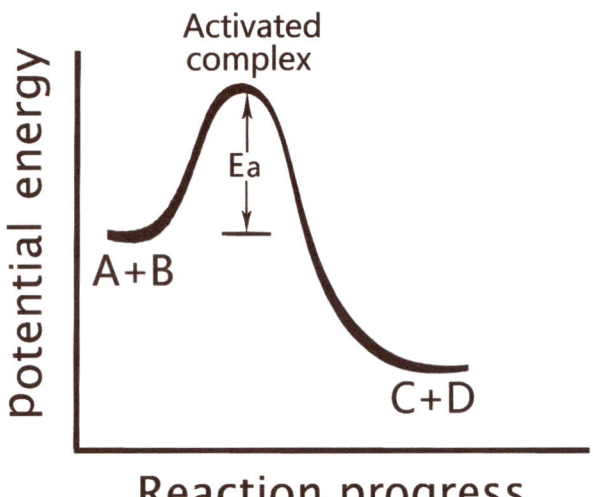 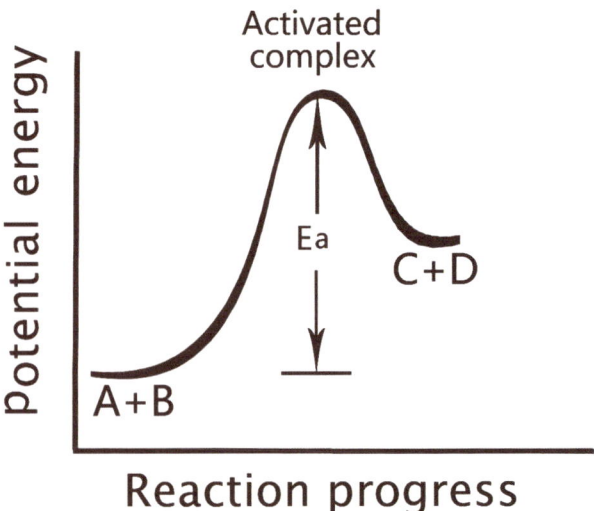

Figure III.A.9.1: Potential energy diagrams: exothermic vs. endothermic reactions.

The left curve of Figure III.A.9.1 shows that the total energy of the reactants is higher than the total energy of the products: this is obviously the case for an exothermic reaction. The right curve of Figure III.A.9.1, shows the profile of an endothermic reaction. A negative enthalpy change indicates an exothermic reaction and a positive enthalpy change depicts an endothermic reaction. The difference in potential energy between the reactant(s) and the activated complex is the activation energy of the forward reaction and the difference between the product(s) and the activated complex is the activation energy of the reverse reaction. Also note that the bigger the difference between the total energy of the reactants and the activated complex, i.e. the activation energy E_a, the slower the reaction.

If a reaction proceeds through several steps one can construct a diagram for each step and combine the single-step diagrams to obtain the energy profile of the overall reaction.

9.6 Kinetic Control vs. Thermodynamic Control

Consider the case where two molecules A and B can react to form either products C or D. Suppose that C has the lowest Gibbs free energy (i.e. the most thermodynamically stable product). Also suppose that product D requires the smallest activation energy and is therefore formed faster than C. If it is product C which is exclusively observed when the reaction is actually performed, the reaction is said to be thermodynamically controlled (i.e. out of a list of possible pathways the reactants choose the one leading to the most stable product). If on the other hand the reactants choose the pathway leading to the product which is produced more quickly it is said to be kinetically controlled.

9.7 Catalysis

A catalyst is a compound that does not directly participate in a reaction (the initial number of moles of this compound in the reaction mixture is equal to the number of moles of this compound once the reaction is completed). Catalysts work by providing an alternative mechanism for a reaction that involves a different transition state, one in which a lower activation energy occurs at the rate-determining step. Catalysts help lower the activation energy of a reaction and help the reaction to proceed. Enzymes are the typical biological catalysts. They are protein molecules with very large molar masses containing one or more active sites (BIO 4.1-4.4). Enzymes are very specialized catalysts. They are generally specific and operate only on certain biological reactants called substrates. They also generally increase the rate of reactions by large factors. The general mechanism of operation of enzymes is as follows:

Enzyme (E) + Substrate (S) → ES (complex)

ES → Product (P) + Enzyme (E)

If we were to compare the energy profile of a reaction performed in the absence of an enzyme to that of the same reaction performed with the addition of an enzyme we would obtain Figure III.A.9.2.

As you can see from Figure III.A.9.2, the reaction from the substrate to the product is facilitated by the presence of the enzyme because the reaction proceeds in two fast steps (low E_a's). Generally, catalysts (or enzymes) stabilize the transition state of a reaction by lowering the energy barrier between reactants and the transition state. Catalysts (or enzymes) do not change the energy difference between reactants and products. Therefore, catalysts do not alter the extent of a reaction or the chemical equilibrium itself. Generally, the rate of an enzyme-catalysed reaction is:

$$\text{rate} = k[ES]$$

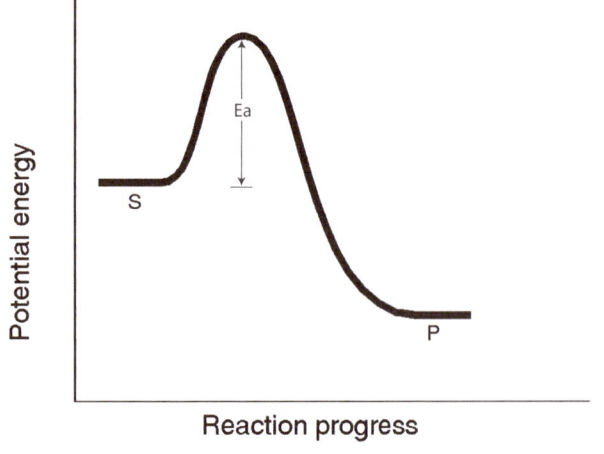 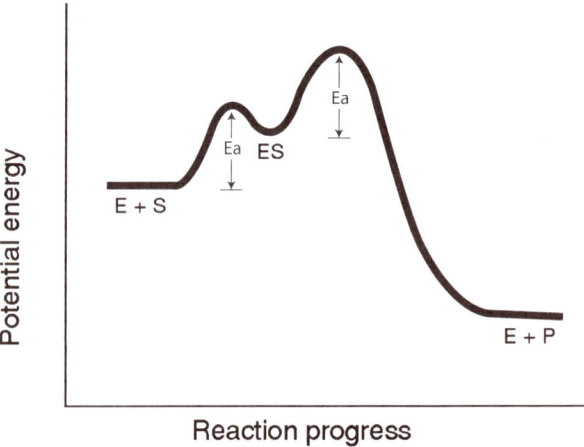

Figure III.A.9.2: Potential energy diagrams: without and with a catalyst.

The rate of formation of the product $\Delta[P]/\Delta t$ vs. the concentration of the substrate [S] yields a plot as in Figure III.A.9.3.

When the concentration of the substrate is large enough for the substrate to occupy all the available active sites on the enzyme, any further increase would have no effect on the rate of the reaction. This is called *saturation kinetics* (BIO 1.1.2).

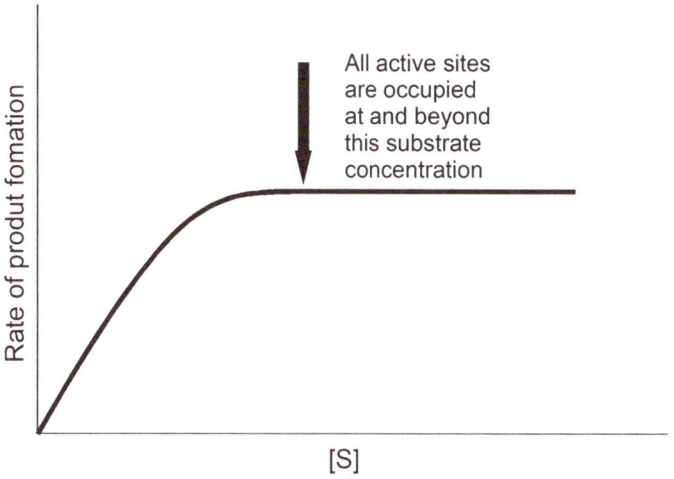

Figure III.A.9.3: Saturation kinetics.

9.8 Equilibrium in Reversible Chemical Reactions

In most chemical reactions once the product is formed, it reacts in such a way to yield back the initial reactants. Eventually, the system reaches a state where there are as many molecules of products being formed as there are molecules of reactants being generated through the reverse reaction. At equilibrium, the concentrations of reactants and products will not necessarily be equal, however, the concentrations remain the same. Hence, the relative concentrations of all components of the forward and reverse reactions become constant at equilibrium. This is called a state of "dynamic equilibrium". It is characterized by a constant K:

$$aA + bB \rightleftharpoons cC + dD$$

where a, b, c and d are the corresponding stoichiometric coefficients:

$$K = \frac{[C]^c [D]^d}{[A]^a [B]^b}$$

The equilibrium constant K (sometimes symbolized as K_{eq}) has a given value at a given temperature. If the temperature changes the value of K changes. At a given temperature, if we change the concentration of A, B, C or D, the system evolves in such a way as to re-establish the value of K. This is called the law of mass action. {Note: catalysts speed up the rate of reaction without affecting K_{eq}}

The following is an example of how an equilibrium constant K is calculated based on a chemical reaction at equilibrium. Remember that the equilibrium constant K can be directly calculated only when the equilibrium concentrations of reactants and products are known or obtained.

As an example, suppose that initially, 5 moles of reactant X are mixed with 12 moles of Y and both are added into an empty 1 liter container. Following their reaction, the system eventually reaches equilibrium with 4 moles of Z formed according to the following reaction:

$$X(g) + 2Y(g) \rightleftharpoons Z(g)$$

For this gaseous, homogeneous mixture (CHM 1.7), what is the value of the equilibrium constant K?

At equilibrium, 4 moles of Z are formed and therefore, 4 moles of X and 8 moles of Y are consumed based on the mole:mole ratio of the balanced equation. Since 5 moles X and 12 moles Y were initially available prior to equilibrium, at equilibrium following the reaction, there remains 1 mol X and 4 moles Y. Since all of the reaction takes place in a 1 L volume, the equilibrium concentrations are therefore, 1 mol/L for X, 4 mol/L for Y and Z, respectively.

Thus, the equilibrium constant can then be calculated as follows:

$$K = [Z]/[X][Y]^2 = [4]/[1][4]^2 = 0.25.$$

The K value is an indication of where the equilibrium point of a reaction actually lies, either far to the right or far to the left or somewhere in between. The following is a summary of the significance of the magnitude of an equilibrium constant K and its meaning:

1. If $K > 1$, this means that the forward reaction is favored and thus, the reaction favors product formation. If K is very large, the equilibrium mixture will then contain very little reactant compared to product.

2. If $K < 1$, the reverse reaction is favored and so the reaction does not proceed very far towards product formation and thus very little product is formed.

3. If $K = 1$, neither forward nor reverse directions are favored.

Note: Pure solids and pure liquids do not appear in the equilibrium constant. Thus in heterogeneous equilibria, since the liquid and solid phases are not sensitive to pressure, their "concentrations" remain constant throughout the reaction and so, mathematically, their values are denoted as 1.

Naturally, H_2O is one of the most common liquids dealt with in reactions. Remember to set its activity equal to 1 when it is a liquid but, if H_2O is written as a gas, then its concentration must be considered.

GENERAL CHEMISTRY

9.8.1 The Reaction Quotient Q to Predict Reaction Direction

The reaction quotient Q is the same ratio as the equilibrium constant K. Q defines all reaction progresses including the K value. In other words, the equilibrium constant K is a special case of the reaction quotient Q.

Thus, the Q ratio has many values dependent on where the reaction lies prior to or subsequent to the concentrations at equilibrium. One may therefore determine if a reaction is going towards an equilibrium by making more products or, alternatively, if a reaction is moving towards equilibrium by making more reactants. The following is a summary of what Q means in relation to K.

Consider the following reaction:

$$aA + bB \rightleftharpoons cC + dD,$$

$$Q = [C]^c[D]^d/[A]^a[B]^b$$

The reaction quotient Q relative to the equilibrium constant K is essentially a mea-

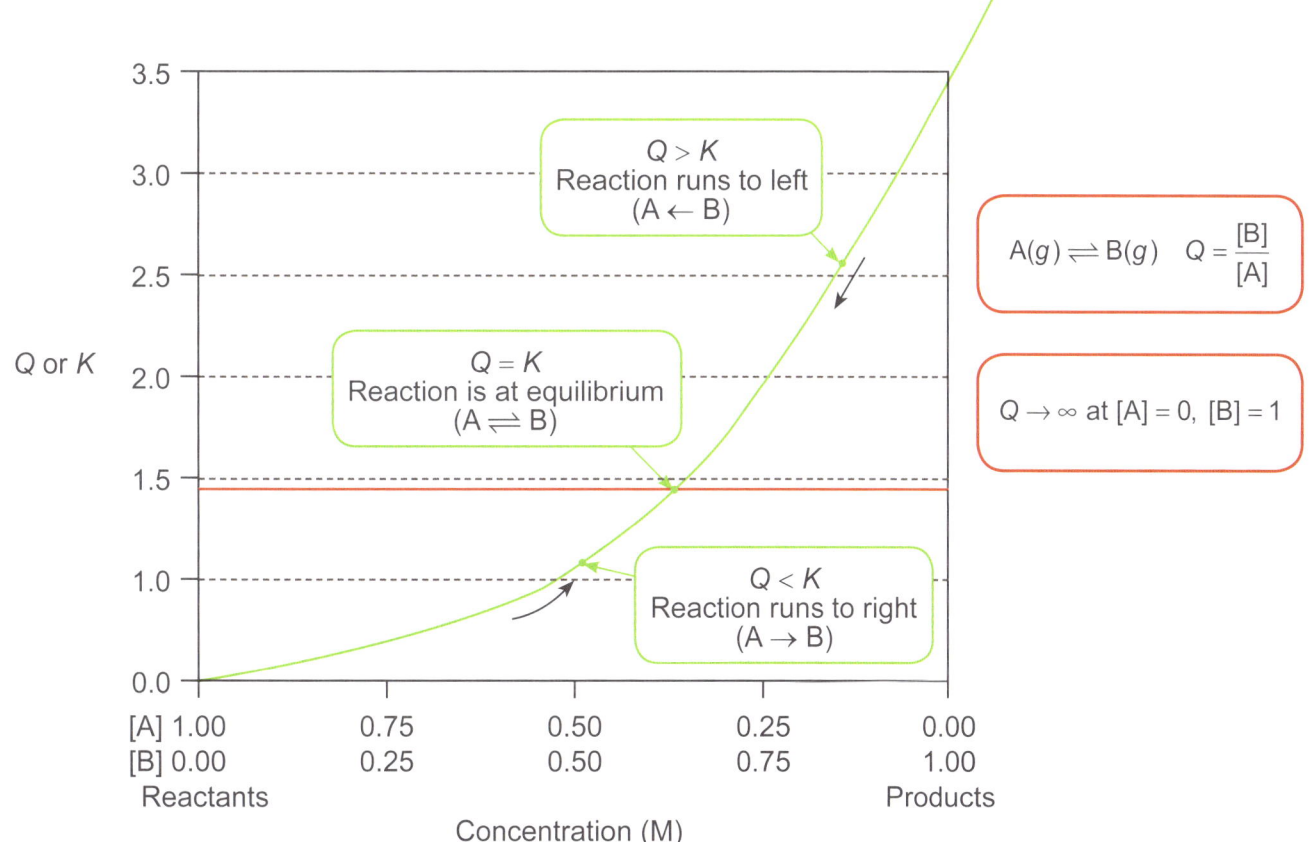

THE PHYSICAL SCIENCES   CHM-127

sure of the progress of a reaction toward equilibrium. The reaction quotient Q has many different values and changes continuously as a reaction progresses and depends on the current state of a reaction mixture. However, once all equilibrium concentrations have been reached, Q = K.

If Q = K, the reaction is at equilibrium and all concentrations are at equilibrium. If Q > K, there are more products initially than there are reactants so the reaction proceeds in reverse direction towards a decrease in product concentrations and a simultaneous increase in reactant concentrations until equilibrium is reached. If Q < K, there are more reactants then products and so the reaction proceeds forward towards product formation until equilibrium is reached.

9.9 Le Chatelier's Principle

Le Chatelier's principle states that whenever a perturbation is applied to a system at equilibrium, the system evolves in such a way as to compensate for the applied perturbation. For instance, consider the following equilibrium:

$$N_2 + 3H_2 \rightleftharpoons 2NH_3$$

If we introduce some more hydrogen in the reaction mixture at equilibrium, i.e. if we increase the concentration of hydrogen, the system will evolve in the direction that will decrease the concentration of hydrogen (from left to right). If more ammonia is introduced, the equilibrium shifts from the right-hand side to the left-hand side, while the removal of ammonia from the reaction vessel would do the opposite (i.e. shifts equilibrium from the left-hand side to the right-hand side).

In a similar fashion, an <u>increase in total pressure (decrease in volume) favors the direction which decreases the total number of compressible (i.e. gases) moles</u> (from the left-hand side where there are 4 moles to the right-hand side where there are 2 moles). It can also be said that when there are different forms of a gaseous substance, an increase in total pressure (decrease in volume) favors the form with the greatest density, and a decrease in total pressure (increase in volume) favors the form with the lowest density.

Finally, if the temperature of a reaction mixture at equilibrium is increased, the equilibrium evolves in the direction of the endothermic (heat-absorbing) reaction. For instance, the forward reaction of the equilibrium:

$$N_2O_4(g) \rightleftharpoons 2NO_2(g)$$

is endothermic; therefore, an increase in temperature favors the forward reaction over the backward reaction. In other words, the dissociation of N_2O_4 increases with temperature.

GENERAL CHEMISTRY

9.10 Relationship between the Equilibrium Constant and the Change in the Gibbs Free Energy

In the "thermodynamics" section we defined the Gibbs free energy. The *standard* Gibbs free energy ($G°$) is determined at 25 °C (298 K) and 1 atm. The change in the standard Gibbs free energy for a given reaction can be calculated from the change in the standard enthalpy and entropy of the reaction using:

$$\Delta G° = \Delta H - T \Delta S°$$

where T is the temperature at which the reaction is carried out. If this reaction happens to be the forward reaction of an equilibrium, the equilibrium constant associated with this equilibrium is simply given by:

$$\Delta G° = -R\, T \ln K_{eq}$$

where R is the ideal gas constant (1.99 cal mol^{-1} K^{-1}) and ln is the natural logarithm (i.e. log to the base *e*; see QR Appendix).

It is important to remember the sign for Gibbs free energy when the reaction is not spontaneous, spontaneous and at equilibrium (CHM 8.10).

After acid-bases, questions based on the information provided in this chapter (Chapter 9) would be the 2nd most frequently tested amongst ACER's practice materials for General Chemistry.

Go online to GAMSAT-prep.com for free chapter review Q&A and forum.

GOLD NOTES

ELECTROCHEMISTRY

Chapter 10

Memorize
- Define: anode, cathode, anion, cation
- Define: standard half-cell potentials
- Define: strong/weak oxidizing/reducing agents

Understand
* Electrolytic cell, electrolysis
* Calculation involving Faraday's law
* Galvanic (voltaic) cell, purpose of salt bridge
* Half reaction, reduction potentials
* Direction of electron flow

Not Required*
* Advanced level college info
* Memorizing the value of a faraday
* Frost diagram

GAMSAT-Prep.com

Introduction

Electrochemistry links chemistry with electricity (the movement of electrons through a conductor). If a chemical reaction produces electricity (i.e. a battery or galvanic/voltaic cell) then it is an **electrochemical cell**. If electricity is applied externally to drive the chemical reaction then it is **electrolysis**. In general, oxidation/reduction reactions occur and are separated in space or time, connected by an external circuit. If you need to balance redox reactions using the "half-reaction method of balancing" (CHM 10.1) during the GAMSAT, you will be reminded of the rules (i.e. do not memorize them).

Additional Resources

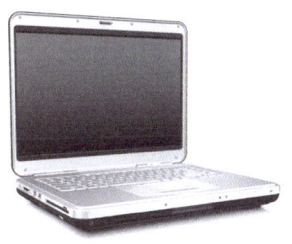

Free Online Q & A

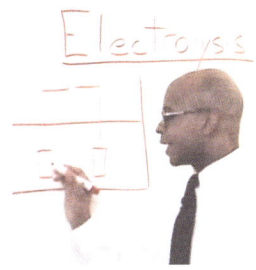

Video: Online or DVD

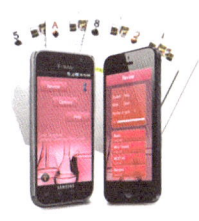

Flashcards

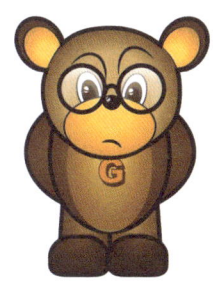

Special Guest

THE PHYSICAL SCIENCES   CHM-131

* The real GAMSAT may have advanced level information presented (ie. in a passage) but previous knowledge of said information is not required to answer the questions that would follow. Practice ACER and GS practice GAMSATs can help you clarify this point.

GAMSAT-Prep.com
THE GOLD STANDARD

10.1 Generalities

Electrochemistry is based on oxidation-reduction or redox reactions in which one or more electrons are transferred from one ionic species to another. Recall that oxidation is defined as the loss of one or more electrons and reduction is defined as the gain in electron(s). In a redox reaction, reduction and oxidation must occur simultaneously. Before you read this section you should review the rules that allow the determination of the oxidation state of an element in a polyatomic molecule or ion and the definition of oxidation and reduction processes. We had previously applied the rules for the determination of oxidation numbers in the case of the following overall reaction (see CHM 1.6):

$$CuSO_4(aq) + Zn(s) \rightleftharpoons$$
Oxid.#:   +2   0
$$Cu(s) + ZnSO_4(aq)$$
Oxid.#:   0   +2

The reduction and oxidation half-reactions of the forward process are:

reduction half-reaction:
$Cu^{2+}(aq) + 2e^- \rightarrow Cu(s)$

oxidation half-reaction:
$Zn(s) \rightarrow Zn^{2+}(aq) + 2e^-$

A half reaction does not occur on its own merit. Any reduction half reaction must be accompanied by an associated oxidation half reaction or vise versa, as electrons need to be transferred accordingly from one reactant to another. To determine the number and the side on which to put the electrons one follows the simple rules:

(i) The electrons are always on the left-hand side of a reduction half-reaction.

(ii) The electrons are always on the right-hand side of an oxidation half-reaction.

(iii) For a reduction half-reaction:

\# of electrons required = initial oxidation #
  − final oxidation #

(iv) For an oxidation half-reaction:
\# of electrons required = final oxidation #
  − initial oxidation #

The next step is to balance each half-reaction, i.e. the charges and the number of atoms of all the elements involved have to be equal on both sides. The preceding example is very simple since the number of electrons required in the two half-reactions is the same. Consider the following more complicated example:

reduction: $Sn^{2+}(aq) + 2e^- \rightarrow Sn(s)$
oxidation: $Al(s) \rightarrow Al^{3+}(aq) + 3e^-$

to balance the overall reaction you need to multiply the first half-reaction by a factor of 3 and the second by a factor of 2.

Balancing redox reactions in aqueous solutions may not always be as straight forward as balancing other types of chemical reactions. For redox type reactions, both the mass and the charge must be balanced. In addition, when looking at redox reactions occurring in aqueous solutions one must also consider at times if the solution is acidic or basic. The procedure used to balance redox reactions in acidic versus basic solutions is slightly different. Generally, the recommended steps used in balancing redox reactions is as follows and the method used is called the "*half-reaction method of balancing*":

1) Identify all the oxidation states of all elements within the redox reaction.

2) Identify the elements being oxidized and those being reduced.

3) Separate the overall redox reaction into its corresponding oxidation and reduction half reactions.

4) Balance all elements for each half reaction excluding hydrogen and oxygen.

5) Balance oxygen by the addition of water to the side missing the oxygen and balance the oxygen atoms by adding the appropriate coefficients in front of water.

6) Balance hydrogen by the addition of H^+ ion to the side missing the hydrogen atoms until hydrogen is balanced with the appropriate coefficients added. Note that the difference in balancing redox reactions in acidic versus basic aqueous solutions is at this step. In basic solutions, an additional step is required to neutralize the H^+ ions with the addition of OH^- ions so that both may then combine to form water.

7) Balance the half reactions with respect to charge by the addition of electrons on the appropriate side.

8) Balance the number of electrons for each half reaction by multiplying each of the half reactions (if required) with the appropriate coefficient.

9) Add the two half reactions making sure that all electrons are cancelled.

10) Finally, as a check: you should always verify that all elements and charges are balanced on both sides of the overall reaction and that the final overall reaction *never contains any free electrons.*

Example: In acidic solution, balance the following redox reaction:

Step 1:
$$Fe^{2+} (aq) + MnO_4^- (aq) \rightarrow Fe^{3+} (aq) + Mn^{2+} (aq)$$
$$+2 \quad\quad +7\; -2 \quad\quad +3 \quad\quad +2$$

Step 2: Fe is oxidized (+2 to +3)
Mn in MnO_4^- is reduced to Mn^{2+}
(+7 to +2, oxygen will be balanced with water)

Step 3: Oxidation: $Fe^{2+} (aq) \rightarrow Fe^{3+} (aq)$
Reduction: $MnO_4^- (aq) \rightarrow Mn^{2+} (aq)$

Step 4, 5 and 6:
Oxidation: $Fe^{2+} (aq) \rightarrow Fe^{3+} (aq)$
Reduction: $8H^+ (aq) + MnO_4^- (aq) \rightarrow Mn^{2+} (aq) + 4H_2O (l)$

Step 7:
Oxidation: $Fe^{2+} (aq) \rightarrow Fe^{3+} (aq) + 1e^-$
Reduction: $5e^- + 8H^+ (aq) + MnO_4^- (aq) \rightarrow Mn^{2+} (aq) + 4H_2O (l)$

Step 8:
Oxidation: $5[Fe^{2+} (aq) \rightarrow Fe^{3+} (aq) + 1e^-]$
$5Fe^{2+} (aq) \rightarrow 5Fe^{3+} (aq) + 5e^-$
Reduction: $5e^- + 8H^+ (aq) + MnO_4^- (aq) \rightarrow Mn^{2+} (aq) + 4H_2O (l)$

Step 9:
Overall: $5Fe^{2+} (aq) + 8H^+ (aq) + MnO_4^- (aq) \rightarrow 5Fe^{3+} (aq) + Mn^{2+} (aq) + 4H_2O (l)$

Step 10: Check if all is balanced.

The oxidation/reduction capabilities of substances are measured by their standard reduction half reaction potentials E°(V). The reduction potential E°(V) is a measure of the tendency of a chemical species to acquire electrons and thereby be reduced. The more positive the reduction potential, the more likely the species is to be reduced. Thus, the species would be regarded as a strong oxidizing agent. These potentials are relative. The reference half-cell electrode chosen to measure the relative potential of all other half cells is known as the **s**tandard **h**ydrogen **e**lectrode or SHE and it corresponds to the following half-reaction:

$$2H^+(1 \text{ molar}) + 2e^- \rightarrow H_2(1 \text{ atm}) \quad E° = 0.00 \text{ (V)}.$$

As the reference SHE cell potential is defined as 0.00 V, any half-cell system that accepts electrons from a SHE cell is reduced and therefore defined by a positive redox potential. Alternatively, any half-cell that donates electrons to a SHE cell is defined by a negative redox potential. Thus, the larger the reduction potential value of a half-cell, the greater the tendency for that half-cell to gain electrons and become reduced. Standard half-cell potentials for other half-reactions have been tabulated and you will see examples to follow, and more in the chapter review Warm-Up Exercises. They are defined for standard conditions, i.e., concentration of all ionic species equal to 1 molar and pressure of all gases involved, if any, equal to 1 atm. The standard temperature is taken as 25 °C. In the case of the Cu^{2+}/Zn reaction the relevant data is tabulated as reduction potentials as follows:

$$Zn^{2+}(aq) + 2e^- \rightarrow Zn(s) \quad E° = -0.76 \text{ volts}$$
$$Cu^{2+}(aq) + 2e^- \rightarrow Cu(s) \quad E° = +0.34 \text{ volts}$$

As shown, it can be seen that the Cu/Cu^{2+} electrode is positive relative to the SHE and that the Zn/Zn^{2+} is negative relative to the SHE. The more positive the E° value, the more likely the reaction will occur spontaneously as written. The strongest reducing agents have large negative E° values. The strongest oxidizing agents have large positive E° values. Therefore, in our example Cu^{2+} is a stronger oxidizing agent than Zn^{2+}. This conclusion can be expressed in the following practical terms:

(i) If you put Zn in contact with a solution containing Cu^{2+} ions a spontaneous redox reaction will occur.

$$Zn(s) \rightarrow Zn^{2+}(aq) + 2e^-; \quad E°(V) = +0.76$$
$$Cu^{2+}(aq) + 2e^- \rightarrow Cu(s); \quad E°(V) = +0.34$$
$$E°_{cell} = E°_{red} + E°_{ox} = +0.34 + 0.76 = +1.10 \text{ V}.$$

(ii) If you put Cu directly in contact with a solution containing Zn^{2+} ions, no reaction takes place spontaneously.

$$Cu(s) \rightarrow Cu^{2+}(aq) + 2e^-; \quad E°(V) = -0.34$$
$$Zn^{2+}(aq) + 2e^- \rightarrow Zn(s); \quad E°(V) = -0.76$$
$$E°_{cell} = E°_{red} + E°_{ox} = -0.76 + (-0.34) = -1.10 \text{ V}.$$

Thus for the spontaneous reaction:

(1) $E° = E°_{red} - E°_{ox}$

$$E° = E°_{red} - E°_{ox} = +0.34 - (-0.76) = 1.10 \text{ V}.$$

or (2) $E°_{cell} = E°_{red} + E°_{ox} = +0.34 + 0.76 = 1.10 \text{ V}.$

The positive value confirms the spontaneous nature of the reaction. {The theme of many exam questions: ==the oxidizing agent is *reduced*; the reducing agent is *oxidized*==}

For a cell potential (E°) calculation, if one is to calculate it using the formula (1) should use the tabulated reduction potentials for both half cell reduction reactions. Alternatively, if one were to calculate the cell potential using the second formula (2), the half cell potential that has the lower potential value or the oxidized half cell (more negative value), needs to be reversed to have it in an oxidized format and therefore the electromotive (E°) potential sign itself is also inverted accordingly and the sum of the two half cells is then calculated. Also, note that the stoichiometric factors are <u>not</u> used if one is simply calculating the E° of the cell (because the concentrations are, of course, standard at 1 M).

10.2 Galvanic Cells

As a result of a redox reaction, one may harvest a substantial amount of energy and the energy generated is usually carried out in what is known as an electrochemical cell. There are two types of electrochemical cells: a galvanic (or voltaic) cell and an electrolytic cell. A galvanic cell produces electrical energy from a spontaneous chemical reaction that takes place within an electrochemical cell. On the other hand, an electrolytic cell induces a nonspontaneous chemical reaction within an electrochemical cell by the consumption of electrical energy.

Batteries are self-contained galvanic cells. A <u>galvanic cell</u> uses a <u>spontaneous redox reaction</u> to <u>produce electricity</u>. For instance, one can design a galvanic cell based on the spontaneous reaction:

$$Zn(s) + CuSO_4(aq) \rightarrow Cu(s) + ZnSO_4(aq)$$

An actual view of a galvanic cell is depicted in Figure III.A.10.1a. In addition, Figure III.A.10.1b shows a sketch of a line diagram of the same galvanic cell outlining all the different parts. Note that in Figure III.A.10.1b, Zn is not in direct contact with the Cu^{2+} solution; otherwise electrons will be directly transferred from Zn to Cu^{2+} and no electricity will be produced to an external circuit.

The half-reaction occurring in the left-hand (anode) compartment is the oxidation:

$$Zn(s) \rightarrow Zn^{2+}(aq) + 2e^-$$

The half-reaction occurring in the right-hand (cathode) compartment is the reduction:

$$Cu^{2+}(aq) + 2e^- \rightarrow Cu(s)$$

Therefore, <u>electrons flow</u> out of the compartment where the <u>oxidation</u> occurs to the compartment where the <u>reduction</u> takes place.

GAMSAT-Prep.com
THE GOLD STANDARD

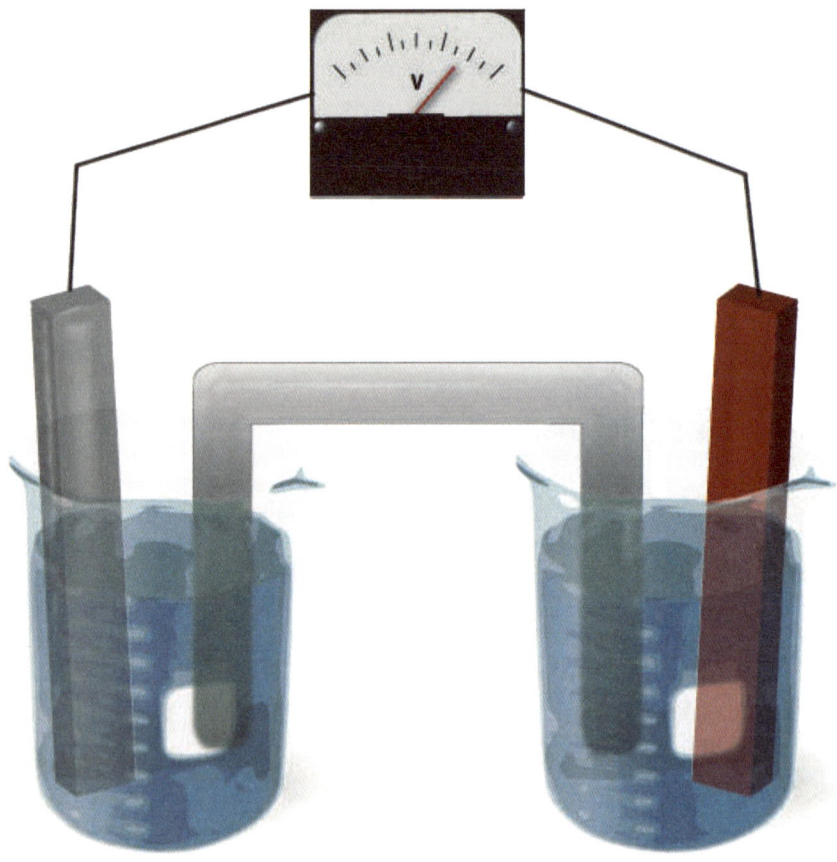

Figure III.A.10.1a: A galvanic (electrochemical) cell. As shown by the displacement in voltage via the voltmeter, the energy of a spontaneous redox reaction is essentially captured within the galvanic cell. A galvanic cell consists mainly of the following parts: **1)** Two separate half cells; **2)** Two solid element electrodes with differing redox potentials; **3)** Two opposing aqueous solutions each in contact with opposing solid electrodes; **4)** One salt bridge with an embedded salt solution; **5)** One ammeter or voltmeter and; **6)** An electrical solid element or wire to allow conductivity of electrons from anode to cathode.

The metallic parts (Cu(s) and Zn(s) in our example) of the galvanic cell which allow its connection to an external circuit are called electrodes. The electrode out of which electrons flow is the anode, the electrode receiving these electrons is the cathode. In a galvanic cell the oxidation occurs in the anodic compartment and the reduction in the cathodic compartment. The voltage difference between the two electrodes is called the electromotive force (*emf*) of the cell. The voltage is measured by the voltmeter.

All of the participants belonging to each of the half cells are included within their respective half cell. Consequently, one half of the electrochemical cell consists of an appropriate metal (Zn) immersed within a solution containing the ionic form of the same metal ($ZnSO_4$). The other half then contains the

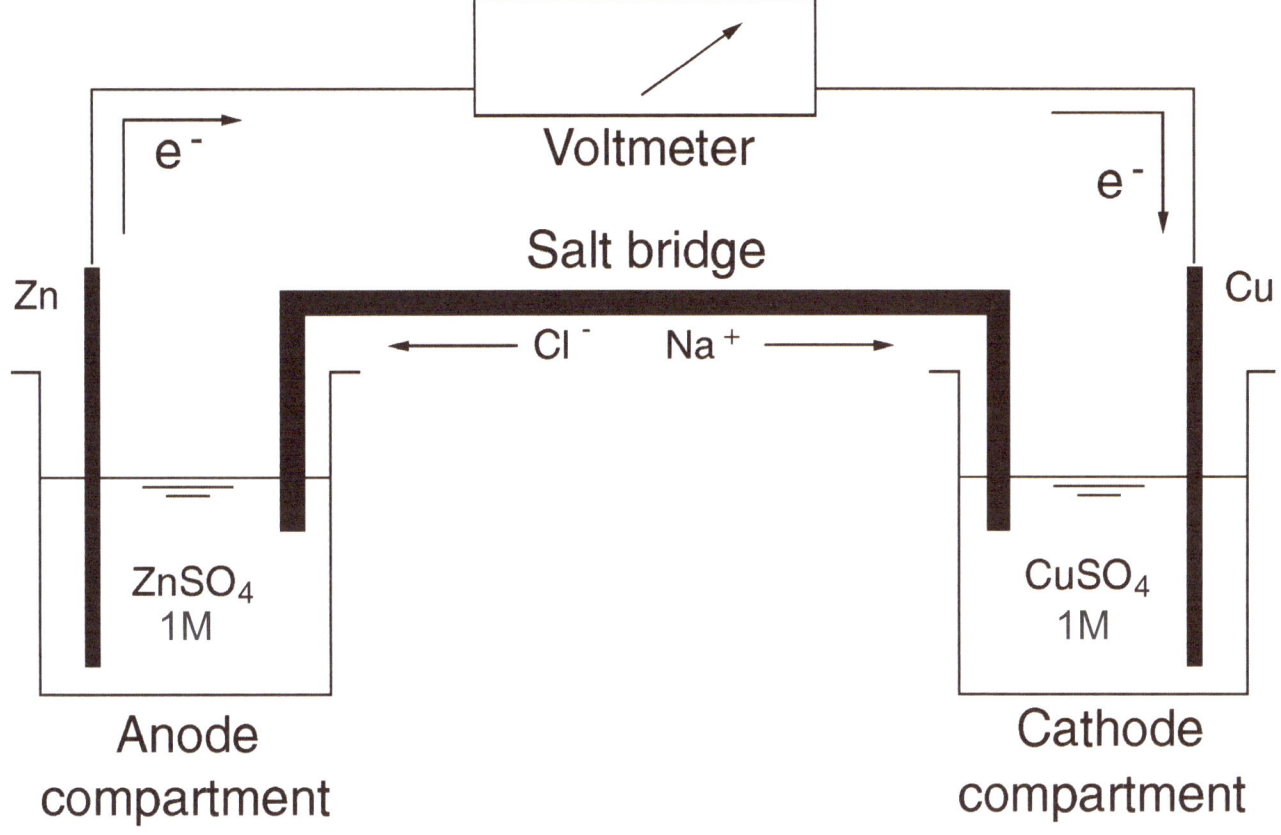

Figure III.A.10.1b: Line diagram of a galvanic (electrochemical) cell.

complementary metal (Cu) immersed into an aqueous solution consisting of its metal ion ($CuSO_4$) (Figure III.A.10.1b).

In certain cells, however, the participants involved in the reduction half reaction may all be part of the aqueous solution; in such a case, an inert electrode would replace the respective metal electrode. The inert electrode such as graphite or platinum would act as a conductive surface for electron transfer. An example of such a half-cell would be one where the reduction of manganese (Mn^{7+}) as MnO_4^- occurs in a solution which also contains manganese as ions (Mn^{2+}). To complete the electrochemical circuit, the two half-cells are then connected with a conducting wire which provides a means for electron flow. Electrons always flow from the anode (oxidation half-cell) to the cathode (reduction half-cell). The electrical energy from the flow of electrons may then be harvested and transformed into some alternative form of energy or mechanical work (as required). In order to prevent an excessive charge build up within each of the half-cell solutions as a result of oxidation and reduction reactions at the anode and cathode, a salt bridge is constructed and used to connect both half-cell solutions.

> **Mnemonic:** LEO is A GERC
> - Lose Electrons Oxidation is Anode
> - Gain Electrons Reduction at Cathode

Electrochemical cells are usually represented as a cell diagram or a compact notation denoting all the parts of the cell. For example, the cell diagram of the cell that was previously discussed in which Zn is oxidized and Cu reduced would be represented as follows:

$$Zn(s) \mid Zn^{2+}(aq) \parallel Cu^{2+}(aq) \mid Cu(s).$$

The oxidation half reaction is on the left and the reduction half reaction is on the right side of the cell diagram. The single vertical lines represent the substances of each half-cell in different phases (solid and aqueous) and the double vertical line represents the salt bridge.

10.2.1 The Salt Bridge

A salt bridge is a U-shaped tube with a strong electrolyte suspended in a gel allowing the flow of the ions into the half-cell solutions. The salt bridge connects the two compartments chemically (for example, with Na^+ and Cl^-). It has two important functions:

1) Maintenance of Neutrality: As $Zn(s)$ becomes $Zn^{2+}(aq)$, the net charge in the anode compartment becomes positive. To maintain neutrality, Cl^- ions migrate to the anode compartment. The reverse occurs in the cathode compartment: positive ions are lost (Cu^{2+}), therefore positive ions must be gained (Na^+).

2) Completing the Circuit: Imagine the galvanic cell as a circuit. Negative charge leaves the anode compartment via *electrons* in a wire and then returns via *chemicals* (i.e. Cl^-) in the salt bridge. Thus the galvanic cell is an *electrochemical* cell.

As an alternative to a salt bridge, the solutions (i.e. $ZnSO_4$ and $CuSO_4$) can be placed in one container separated by a porous material which allows certain ions to cross (i.e. SO_4^{2-}, Zn^{2+}). Thus it would serve the same functions as the salt bridge.

GENERAL CHEMISTRY

10.3 Concentration Cell

If the concentration of the ions in one of the compartments of a galvanic cell is not 1 molar, the half-cell potential E is either higher or lower than E°. Therefore, in principle one could use the same substance in both compartments but with different concentrations to produce electricity.

Thus, one may construct a galvanic cell in which both half-cell reactions are the same however, the difference in concentration is the driving force for the flow of current. The emf is equal in this case to the difference between the two potentials E. Such a cell is called a <u>concentration cell</u>.

To determine the direction of electron flow the same rules as previously described are used. The cathodic compartment, in which the reduction takes place is the one corresponding to the largest positive (smallest negative) E.

The electromotive force varies with the differences in concentration of solutions in the half-cells. When the concentration of solution is not equal to 1M, the emf or E_{cell} can be determined by the use of the Nernst equation as follows:

$$E_{cell} = E°_{cell} - (RT/nF)(\ln Q)$$

or

$$E_{cell} = E°_{cell} - 0.0592V/n (\log Q)$$

where; $E°_{cell}$ is the standard electromotive force, R is the gas constant 8.314J/Kmol, T is the absolute temperature in K, F is the Faraday's constant (CHM 10.5), n is the number of moles of electrons exchanged or transferred in the redox reaction, and Q is the reaction quotient (CHM 9.8.1).

Under standard conditions, Q = 1.00 as all concentrations are at 1.00 M and since log 1 = 0, $E_{cell} = E°_{cell}$.

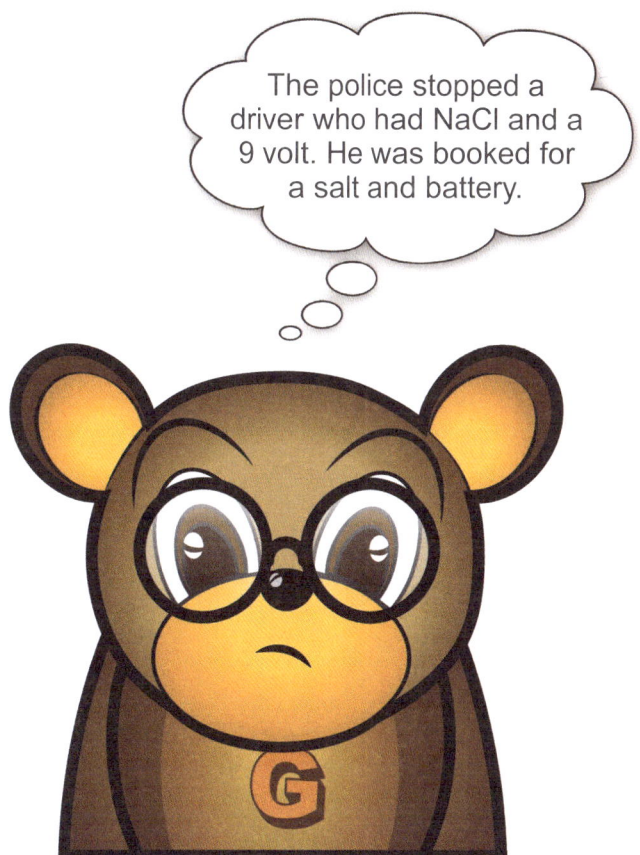

10.4 Electrolytic Cell

There is a fundamental difference between a galvanic cell or a concentration cell and an electrolytic cell: in the first type of electrochemical cell a spontaneous redox reaction is used to produce a current, in the second type a current is actually imposed on the system to drive a non-spontaneous redox reaction. A cathode is defined as the electrode to which cations flow to and an anode is defined as the electrode to which anions flow. Thus, a similarity between the two cells is that the cathode attracts cations, whereas the anode attracts anions. In both the galvanic cell and the electrolytic cell, reduction occurs always at the cathode and oxidation always occurs at the anode.

Remember the following key concepts:

(i) generally a battery is used to produce a current which is imposed on the electrolytic cell.

(ii) the battery acts as an electron pump: electrons flow into the electrolytic cell at the cathode and flow out of it at the anode.

(iii) the half-reaction occurring at the cathode is a reduction since it requires electrons.

(iv) the half-reaction occurring at the anode is an oxidation since it produces electrons.

In galvanic cells, a spontaneous oxidation reaction takes place at the cell's anode creating a source of electrons. For this reason, the anode is considered the negative electrode. However, in electrolytic cells, a non-spontaneous reduction reaction takes place at the cell's cathode using an external electrical energy as the source of electrons such as a battery. For this reason, the cathode is considered the negative electrode.

An electrolytic cell is composed of three parts: an electrolyte solution and two electrodes made from an inert material (i.e. platinum). The oxidation and reduction half reactions are usually placed in one container.

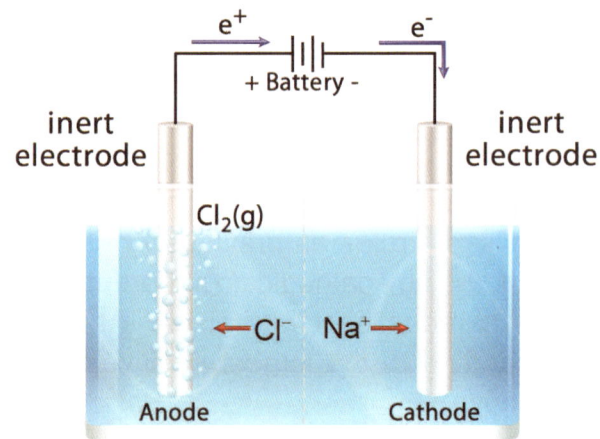

The diagram is a depiction of the electrolysis of molten NaCl. As such, the Na^+ and Cl^- ions are the only species that are present in the electrolytic cell. Thus, the chloride anion (Cl^-) cannot be reduced any further and so it is oxidized at the anode and the sodium cation (Na^+) is therefore reduced. The final products are sodium solid formation at the cathode and chlorine (Cl_2) gas formation at the anode.

Note: the flow of electrons is still from anode to cathode as is for galvanic cells.

GENERAL CHEMISTRY

10.5 Faraday's Law

Faraday's law relates the amount of elements deposited or gas liberated at an electrode due to current.

We have seen that in a galvanic cell $Cu^{2+}(aq)$ can accept electrons to become $Cu(s)$ which will actually plate onto the electrode. Faraday's Law allows us to calculate the amount of $Cu(s)$. In fact, the law states that the weight of product formed at an electrode is proportional to the amount of electricity transferred at the electrode and to the equivalent weight of the material. Thus we can conclude that 1 mole of $Cu^{2+}(aq)$ + 2 moles of electrons will leave 1 mole of $Cu(s)$ at the electrode. One mole (= Avogadro's number) of electrons is called a *faraday* ($\mathcal{F}$). A faraday is equivalent to 96 500 coulombs. A coulomb is the amount of electricity that is transferred when a current of one ampere flows for one second (1C = 1A · S).

10.5.1 Electrolysis Problem

How many grams of copper would be deposited on the cathode of an electrolytic cell if, for a period of 20 minutes, a current of 2.0 amperes is run through a solution of $CuSO_4$? {The molecular weight of copper is 63.5.}

Calculate the number of coulombs:

$$Q = It = 2.0 \text{ A} \times 20 \text{ min} \times 60 \text{ sec/min}$$
$$= 2400 \text{ C}$$

Thus

$$\text{Faradays} = 2400 \text{ C} \times 1\mathcal{F}/96\,500 \text{ C}$$
$$= 0.025\mathcal{F}$$

Faradays can be related to moles of copper since

$$Cu^{2+} + 2e^- \rightarrow Cu$$

Since 1 mol Cu : 2 mol e^- we can write

$$0.025\mathcal{F} \times (1 \text{ mol Cu}/2\mathcal{F}) \times (63.5 \text{g Cu/mol Cu})$$
$$= 0.79\text{g Cu}$$

Electrolysis would deposit 0.79 g of copper at the cathode.

To do the previous problem, you must know the definition of current and charge (CHM 10.5) but the value of the constant (a Faraday) would be given on the exam. You should be able to perform the preceding calculation quickly and efficiently because it involves dimensional analysis.

> "A diamond is merely a lump of coal that did well under pressure." If you have completed all previous chapters then you are more than half way finished your GAMSAT review. Good luck!

> Go online to GAMSAT-prep.com for free chapter review Q&A and forum.

THE PHYSICAL SCIENCES   CHM-141

GOLD NOTES

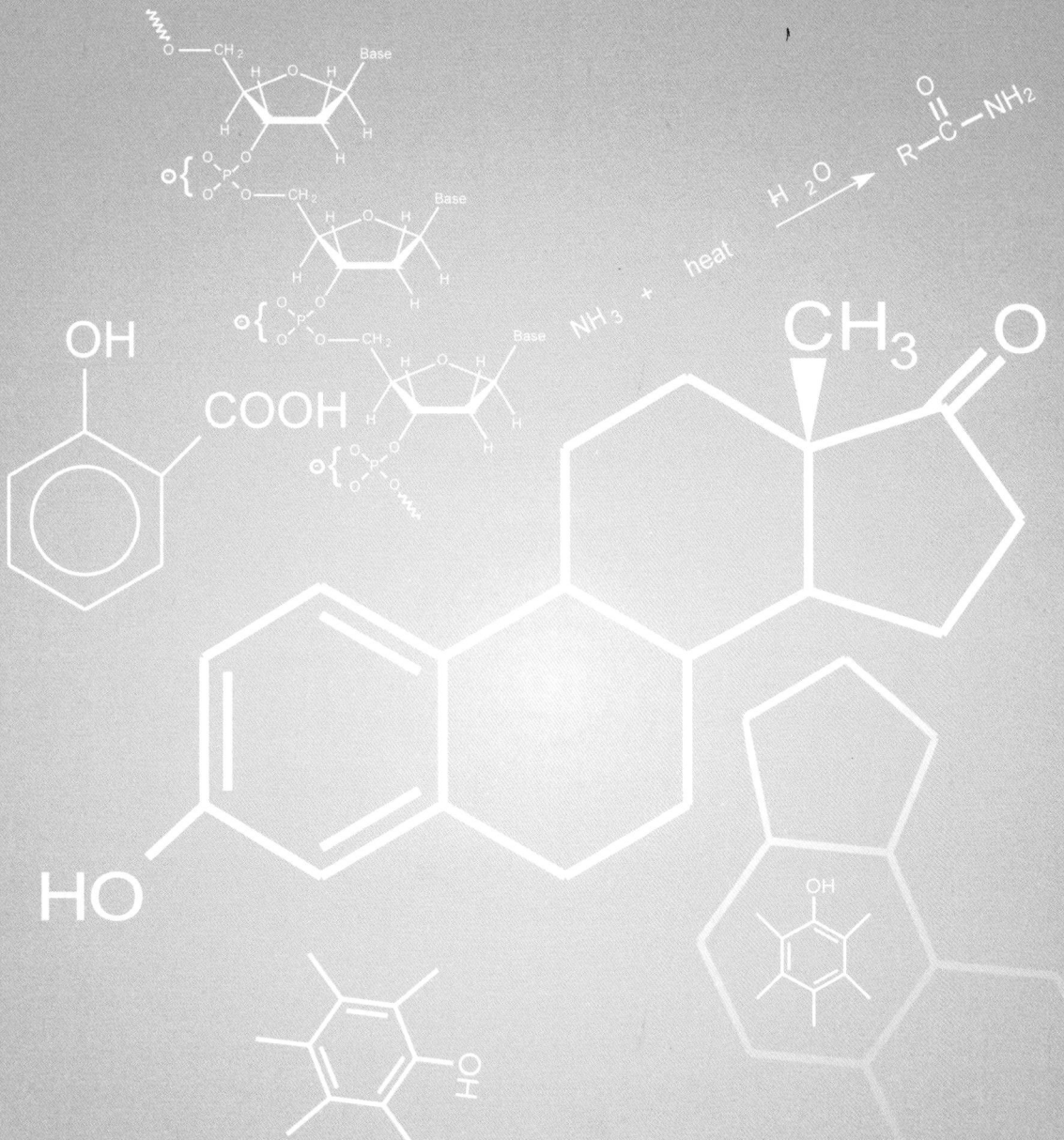

GAMSAT-Prep.com
ORGANIC CHEMISTRY
PART IV.B: BIOLOGICAL SCIENCES

IMPORTANT: Before doing your science survey for the GAMSAT, be sure you have read the Preface, Introduction and Part II, Chapter 2. The beginning of each science chapter provides guidelines as to what you should Memorize, Understand and what is Not Required. These are guides to get you a top score without getting lost in the details. Our guides have been determined from an analysis of all ACER materials plus student surveys. Additionally, the original owner of this book gets a full year access to many online features described in the Preface and Introduction including an online Forum where each chapter can be discussed.

MOLECULAR STRUCTURE OF ORGANIC COMPOUNDS
Chapter 1

Memorize
* brid orbitals and geometries
* riodic table trends
* fine: Lewis, dipole moments
* ound rules for reaction mechanisms

Understand
* Delocalized electrons and resonance
* Multiple bonds, length, energies
* Basic stereochemistry
* Principles for reaction mechanisms

Not Required*
* Advanced level college info
* Hybrids involving d, f, etc.

GAMSAT-Prep.com

Introduction

Organic chemistry is the study of the structure, properties, composition, reactions, and preparation (i.e. synthesis) of chemical compounds containing carbon. Such compounds may contain hydrogen, nitrogen, oxygen, the halogens as well as phosphorus, silicon and sulfur. To give some perspective, it is interesting to note that almost 99% of the mass of the human body is made up of just six elements: carbon, hydrogen, oxygen, nitrogen, phosphorus, and calcium. If you master the basic rules in this chapter, you will be able to conquer GAMSAT Organic Chemistry with little or no further memorization.

Additional Resources

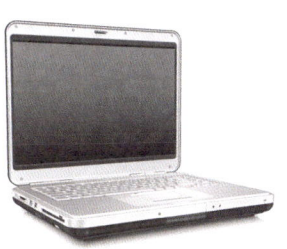

Free Online Q&A + Forum

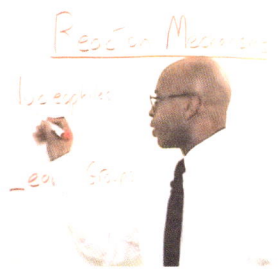

Video: Online or DVD

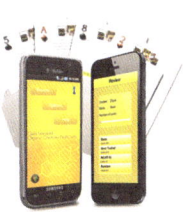

Flashcards

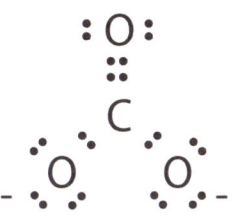

Special Guest

THE BIOLOGICAL SCIENCES   ORG-03

* The real GAMSAT may have advanced level information presented (ie. in a passage) but previous knowledge of said information is not required to answer the questions that would follow. Practice ACER and GS practice GAMSATs can help you clarify this point.

1.1 Overview: The Atoms of Organic Chemistry

Organic chemistry may be defined as the chemistry of the compounds of carbon. Organic chemistry is very important, as living systems are composed mainly of water and organic compounds. Other important organic molecules form essential components of fuels, plastics and other petroleum derivatives.

Carbon (C), hydrogen (H), oxygen (O), nitrogen (N) and the halides (i.e. fluorine – F, chlorine – Cl, bromine – Br, etc.) are the most common atoms found in organic compounds. The atoms in most organic compounds are held together by covalent bonds (*the sharing of an electron pair between two atoms*). Some ionic bonding (*the transfer of electrons from one atom to another*) does exist. Common to both types of chemical bonds is the fact that the atoms bond such that they can achieve the electron configuration of the nearest noble gas, usually eight electrons. This is known as the *octet rule*.

A **carbon** atom has one s and three p orbitals in its outermost shell, allowing it to form 4 single bonds. As well, a carbon atom may be involved in a double bond, where two electron pairs are shared, or a triple bond, where three electron pairs are shared. An **oxygen** atom may form 2 single bonds, or one double bond. It has 2 unshared (lone) electron pairs. A **hydrogen** atom will form only one single bond. A **nitrogen** atom may form 3 single bonds. As well, it is capable of double and triple bonds. It has one unshared electron pair. The **halides** are all able to form only one (single) bond. Halides all have three unshared electron pairs.

Throughout the following chapters we will be examining the structural formulas of molecules involving H, C, N, O, halides and phosphorus (P). However it should be noted that less common atoms often have similar structural formulas within molecules as compared to common atoms. For example, silicon (Si) is found in the same group as carbon in the periodic table; thus they have similar properties. In fact, Si can also form 4 single bonds leading to a tetrahedral structure (i.e. SiH_4, SiO_4). Likewise sulfur (S) is found in the same group as oxygen. Though it can be found as a solid (S_8), it still has many properties similar to those of oxygen. For example, like O in H_2O, sulfur can form a bent, polar molecule which can hydrogen bond (H_2S). We will later see that sulfur is an important component in the amino acid cysteine. {*To learn more about molecular structure, hybrid orbitals, polarity and bonding, review General Chemistry chapters 2 and 3*}

Mnemonic: **HONC** increasing bonds for neutrality . . .
H requires 1 more electron in its outer shell to become stable:
    thus hydrogen is neutral when bonded once
O requires 2: thus oxygen is neutral when bonded twice
N requires 3: thus nitrogen is neutral when bonded 3 times
C requires 4: thus carbon is neutral when bonded 4 times

ORGANIC CHEMISTRY

1.2 Hybrid Orbitals

In organic molecules, the orbitals of the atoms are combined to form **hybrid orbitals**, consisting of a mixture of the s and p orbitals. In a carbon atom, if the one s and three p orbitals are mixed, the result is four hybrid sp^3 orbitals. Three hybridized sp^2 orbitals result from the mixing of one s and two p orbitals, and two hybridized sp orbitals result from the mixing of one s and one p. The geometry of the hybridized orbitals is shown in Figure IV.B.1.1.

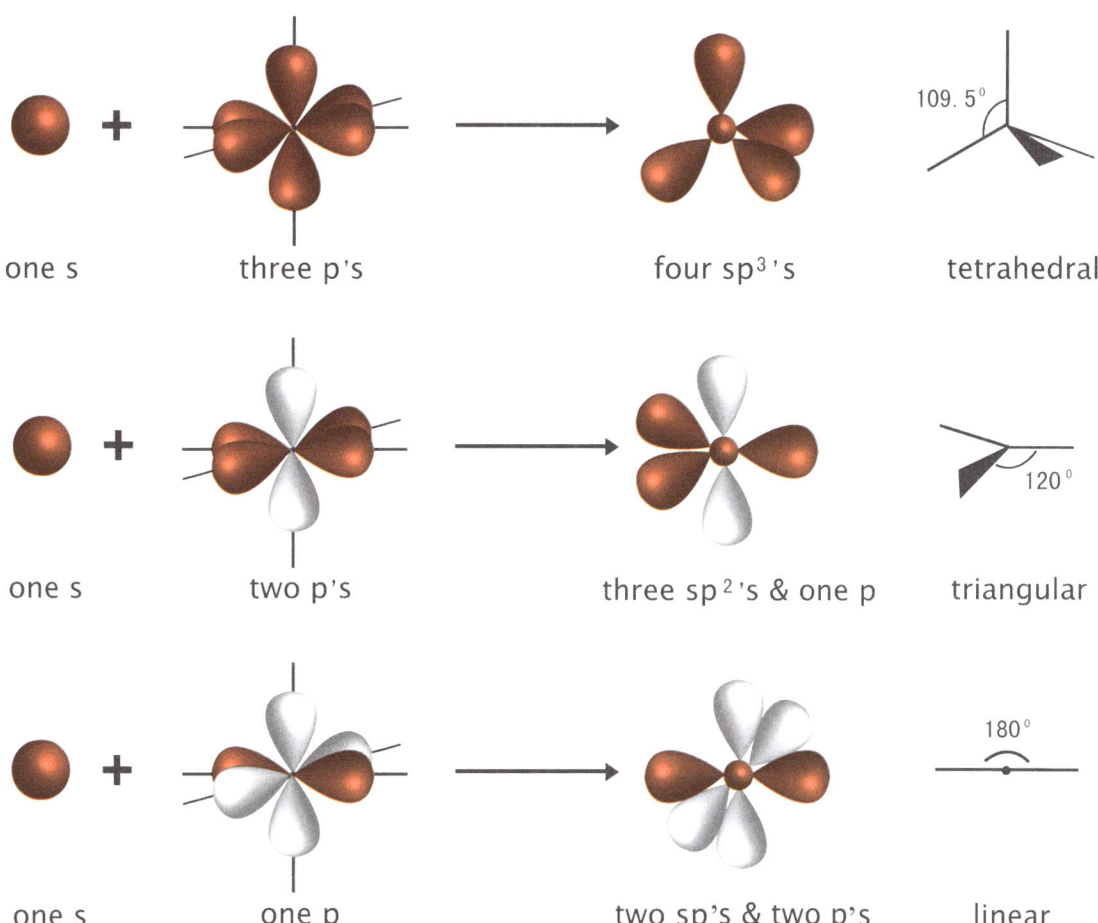

Figure IV.B.1.1: Hybrid orbital geometry

NOTE: For details regarding atomic structure and orbitals, see General Chemistry (CHM) sections 2.1, 2.2. For more details regarding hybridized bonds and bond angles (especially for carbon, nitrogen, oxygen and sulfur), see CHM 3.5. Notice in the first line of the image there are three p orbitals occupying the x, y and z axes (GM 3.6) thus p_x, p_y and p_z.

1.3 Bonding

Sigma (or single) bonds are those in which the electron density is between the nuclei. They are symmetric about the axis, can freely rotate, and are formed when orbitals (regular or hybridized) overlap directly. They are characterized by the fact that they are circular when a cross section is taken and the bond is viewed along the bond axis. The electron density in pi bonds overlaps both above and below the plane of the atoms. A single bond is a sigma bond; a double bond is one sigma and one pi bond; a triple bond is one sigma (σ) and two pi (π) bonds.

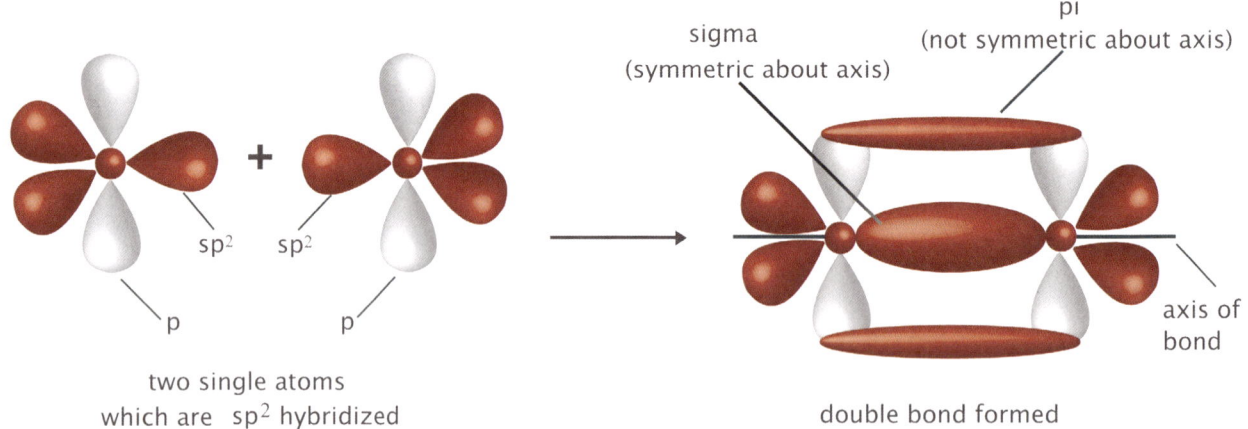

Figure IV.B.1.2: Sigma and pi bonds. The sp^2 hybrids overlap between the nuclei to form a σ bond; the p orbitals overlap above and below the axis between the nuclei to form a π bond.

1.3.1 The Effects of Multiple Bonds

The pi bonds in doubly and triply bonded molecules create a barrier to free rotation about the axis of the bond. Thus multiple bonds create molecules which are much more rigid than a molecule with only a single bond which can freely rotate about its axis.

As a rule, the length of a bond decreases with multiple bonds. For example, the carbon-carbon triple bond is shorter than the carbon-carbon double bond which is shorter than the carbon-carbon single bond.

Bond strength and thus the amount of energy required to break a bond (= *BE, the bond dissociation energy*) varies with the number of bonds. One σ bond has a BE $\approx$ 110 kcal/mole and one π bond has a BE $\approx$ 60 kcal/mole. Thus a single bond (one σ) has a BE $\approx$ 110 kcal/mole while a double bond (one σ + one π) has a BE $\approx$ 170 kcal/mole. Hence multiple bonds have greater bond strength than single bonds.

ORGANIC CHEMISTRY

1.4 Delocalized Electrons and Resonance

Delocalization of charges in the pi bonds is possible when there are hybridized orbitals in adjacent atoms. This delocalization may be represented in two different ways, the molecular orbital (MO) approach or the resonance (*valence bond*) approach. See the diagram below and consider reviewing CHM 3.2.

The MO approach takes a linear combination of atomic orbitals to form molecular orbitals, in which electrons form the bonds. These molecular orbitals cover the whole molecule, and thus the delocalization of electrons is depicted. In the resonance approach, there is a linear combination of different structures with localized pi bonds and electrons, which together depict the true molecule, or **resonance hybrid**. There is no single structure that represents the molecule.

For example, a 'diene' is a hydrocarbon (hydrogen + carbon) chain that has two double bonds that may or may not be adjacent to each other (ORG 4.1). Conjugated dienes (i.e. butadiene) have two double bonds separated by a single bond and are more stable than non conjugated dienes because: (1) the delocalization of charge through resonance and (2) hybridization energy. Basically, the positioning and overlap of the pi orbitals strengthen the single bond between the two double bonds.

Along with resonance, hybridization energy affects the stability of the compound. For example in 1,3-butadiene (Fig IV.B.1.3) the carbons with the single bond are sp^2 hybridized, unlike in non conjugated dienes where the carbons with single bonds are sp^3 hybridized. This difference in hybridization shows that the conjugated dienes have more 's' character and draw in more of the pi electrons, thus making the single bond stronger and shorter than an ordinary alkane C-C bond. Questions on this concept would always be preceded by an explanatory passage so we will explore s character in the online practice questions.

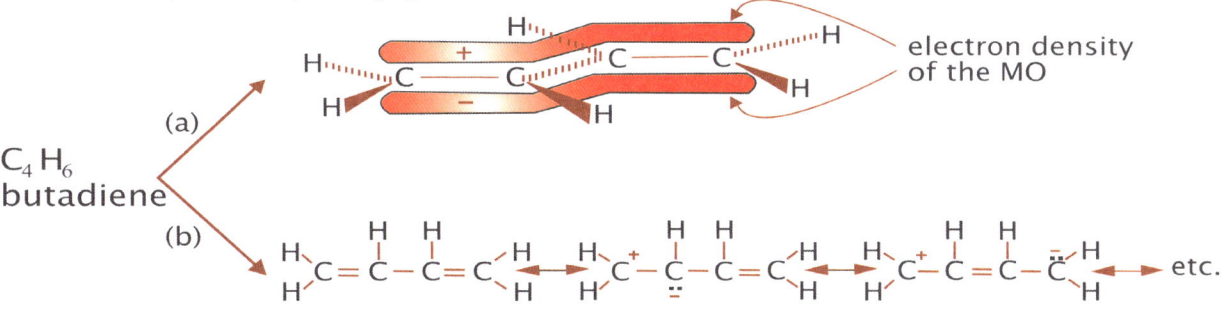

Figure IV.B.1.3: A comparison of MO and resonance approaches. (a) The electron density of the MO covers the entire molecule such that π bonds and p orbitals are not distinguishable. (b) No singular resonance structure accurately portrays butadiene; rather, the true molecule is a composite of all of its resonance structures. Notice that although the bonds can change, atoms do not move in resonance structures. We will be examining resonance structures repeatedly throughout the following chapters because they represent typical exam questions.

1.5 Lewis Structures, Charge Separation and Dipole Moments

The outer shell (or **valence**) electrons are those that form chemical bonds. **Lewis dot structures** are a method of showing the valence electrons and how they form bonds. These electrons, along with the octet rule (*which states that a maximum of eight electrons are allowed in the outermost shell of an atom*) holds only for the elements in the second row of the periodic table (C,N,O,F). The elements of the third row (Si, P, S, Cl) use d orbitals, and thus can have more than eight electrons in their outer shell.

Let us use CO_2 as an example. Carbon has four valence electrons and oxygen has six. By covalently bonding, electrons are shared and the octet rule is followed,

·C· + 2 :O: ⟶

:O::C::O: or :O=C=O:

Carbon and oxygen can form resonance structures in the molecule CO_3^{-2}. The -2 denotes two extra electrons to place in the molecule. Once again the octet rule is followed,

In the final structure, each element counts one half of the electrons in a bond as its own, and any unpaired electrons are counted as its own. The sum of these two quantities should equal the number of valence electrons that were originally around the atom.

If the chemical bond is made up of atoms of different electronegativity, there is a **charge separation:**

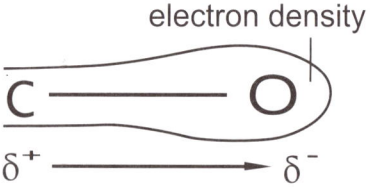

There is a slight pulling of electron density by the more electronegative atom (oxygen in the preceding example) from the less electronegative atom (carbon in the preceding example). This results in the C–O bond having **partial ionic character** (i.e. *a polar bond; see* CHM 3.3). The charge separation also causes an <u>electrical dipole</u> to be set up in the direction of the arrow. A dipole has a positive end (carbon) and a negative end (oxygen). A dipole will line up in an electric field.

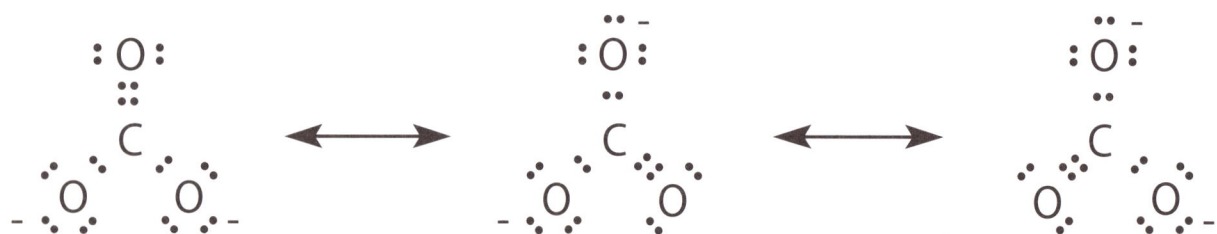

The most electronegative elements (in order, with electronegativities in brackets) are fluorine (4.0), oxygen (3.5), nitrogen (3.0), and chlorine (3.0) [To examine trends, see the periodic table in CHM 2.3]. These elements will often be paired with hydrogen (2.1) and carbon (2.5), resulting in bonds with partial ionic character. The **dipole moment** is a measure of the charge separation and thus, the electronegativities of the elements that make up the bond; the larger the dipole moment, the larger the charge separation.

No dipole moment is found in molecules with no charge separation between atoms (i.e. Cl_2, Br_2), or, when the charge separation is symmetric resulting in a cancellation of bond polarity like vector addition in physics (i.e. CH_4, CO_2).

A molecule where the charge separation between atoms is not symmetric will have a non-zero dipole moment (i.e. CH_3F, H_2O, NH_3 - see ORG 11.1.2). It is important to note that lone pair electrons make large contributions to the overall dipole moment of a molecule.

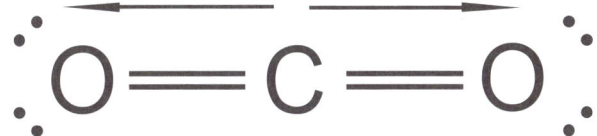

Figure IV.B.1.4: CO_2 - polar bonds but overall it is a non-polar molecule; therefore, CO_2 has a zero dipole moment. Notice that the arrows add to zero like typical vectors (PHY 1.1).

Note: Up to the time of publication, a periodic table has never been provided in a real GAMSAT. One of the purposes of completing the hundreds of chapter review practice questions, that are part of the online features of this textbook, is to increase your familiarity with the trends in the periodic table (CHM 2.3) for the most frequently encountered atoms in GAMSAT Organic Chemistry.

1.5.1 Strength of Polar vs. Non-Polar Bonds

Non-polar bonds are generally stronger than polar covalent and ionic bonds, with ionic bonds being the weakest. However, in compounds with ionic bonding, there is generally a large number of bonds between molecules and this makes the compound as a whole very strong. For instance, although the ionic bonds in one compound are weaker than the non-polar covalent bonds in another compound, the ionic compound's melting point will be higher than the melting point of the covalent compound. Polar covalent bonds have a partially ionic character, and thus the bond strength is usually intermediate between that of ionic and that of non-polar covalent bonds. The strength of bonds generally decreases with increasing ionic character.

1.6 Ground Rules

Opposites attract. Like charges repel. Such simple statements are fundamental in solving over 90% of mechanisms in organic chemistry. Once you are comfortable with the basics - electronegativity, polarity and resonance - you will not need to memorize the grand majority of outcomes of given reactions. You will be capable of quickly deducing the answer even when new scenarios are presented.

A substance which has a formal positive charge (+) or a partial positive charge ("delta+" or δ^+) is attracted to a substance with a formal negative charge (−) or a partial negative charge (δ^-). In general, a substance with a formal charge would have a greater force of attraction than one with a partial charge when faced with an oppositely charged species. There is an important exception: spectator ions. Ions formed by elements in the first two groups of the periodic table (i.e. Na$^+$, K$^+$, Ca^{++}) do not actively engage in reactions in organic chemistry. They simply watch the reaction occur then at the very end they associate with the negatively charged product.

In most carbon-based compounds the carbon atom is bonded to a more electronegative atom. For example, in a carbon-oxygen bond the oxygen is δ^- resulting in a δ^+ carbon (see ORG 1.5). Because opposites attract, a δ^- carbon (which is unusual) could create a carbon-carbon bond with a δ^+ carbon (which is common). There are two important categories of compounds which can create a carbon-carbon bond; a) alkyl lithiums (RLi) and b) Grignard reagents (RMgBr), because they each have a δ^- carbon. Note that the carbon is δ^- since lithium is to the left of carbon on the periodic table (for electronegativity trends see CHM 2.3). {The letter R typically stands for any hydrocarbon group like alkyl (ORG 3.1), phenyl (ORG 5.1), etc.}

The expressions "like charges repel" and "opposites attract" are the basic rules of electrostatics. "Opposites attract" is translated in Organic Chemistry to mean "nucleophile attacks electrophile". The nucleophile is "nucleus loving" and so it is negatively charged or partially negative, and we follow its electrons using arrows in reaction mechanisms as it attacks the "electron loving" electrophile which is positively charged or partially positively charged. Sometimes we will use color, or an asterix*, or a "prime" symbol on the letter R (i.e. R vs R' vs R'' vs R'''), or a superscript on the letter R (R^1, R^2, etc.), during reaction mechanisms to help you follow the movement of atoms or groups of atoms (the latter may be called *ligands* or *substituents*). Alternatively, an isotope of an atom is used (PHY 12.2). For example, instead of hydrogen, deuterium (^{2}H or D; PHY 12.2; ORG 14.2.1), or instead of 'normal' oxygen (O-16; ^{16}O), the stable isotope O-18 (^{18}O) is used. Any of the techniques above can be used on an exam question.

For nucleophiles, the general trend is that the stronger the nucleophile, the stronger the base it is. For example:

RO$^-$ > HO$^-$ >> RCOO$^-$ > ROH > H$_2$O

For information on the quality of leaving groups, see ORG 6.2.4.

ORGANIC CHEMISTRY

In organic chemistry, functional groups are specific groups of atoms or bonds within molecules that are responsible for the characteristic chemical reactions of those molecules. The same functional group will undergo the same or similar chemical reaction(s) regardless of the size of the molecule that it is in.

You will find the most common functional groups illustrated below. The short hand for a carbon atom is each corner of a geometric figure as well as the end of a line. Hydrogens are presumed to be present such that each carbon is bonded 4 times (see ORG 1.1). We will be exploring the functional groups below and many others over the following chapters.

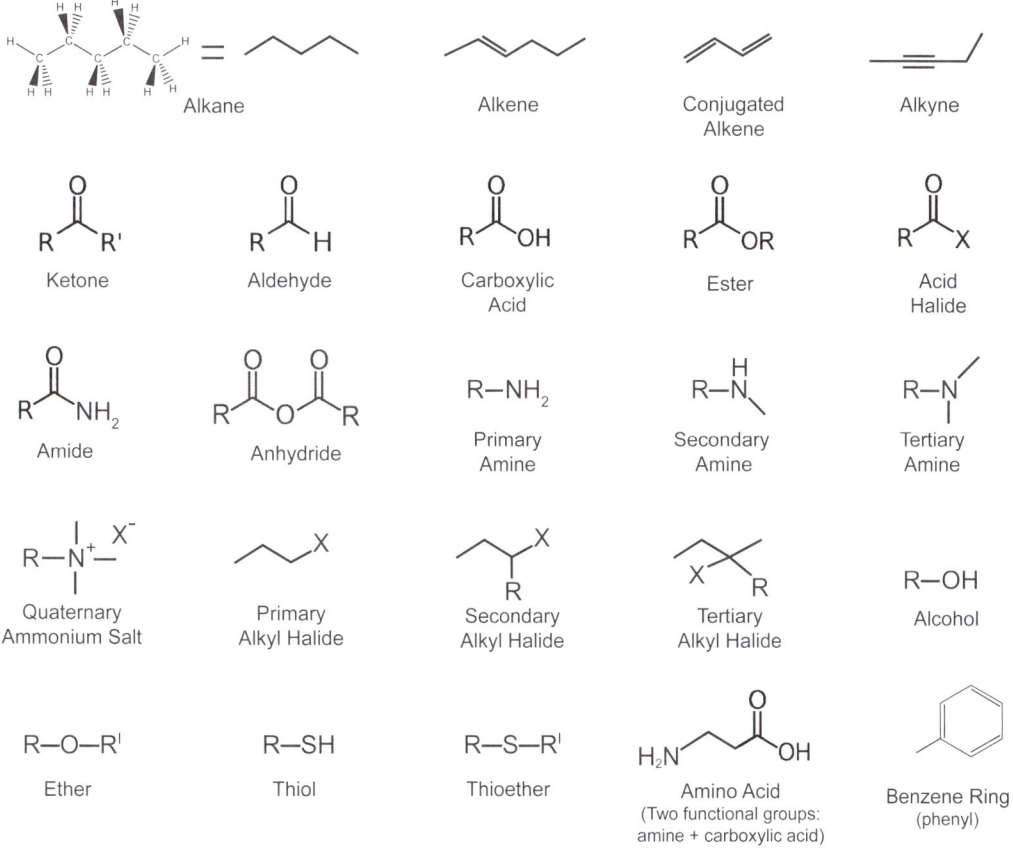

Reminder: Chapter review questions are available online for the original owner of this textbook. Doing practice questions will help clarify concepts and ensure that you study in a targeted way. First, register at gamsat-prep.com, then login and click on GAMSAT Textbook Owners in the right column so you can use your Online Access Card to have access to the Lessons section.

No science background? Consider watching the relevant videos at gamsat-prep.com and you have support at gamsat-prep.com/forum. Don't forget to check the Index at the beginning of this book to see which chapters are HIGH, MEDIUM and LOW relative importance for the GAMSAT.

Your online access continues for one full year from your online registration.

THE BIOLOGICAL SCIENCES   ORG-11

GOLD NOTES

STEREOCHEMISTRY

Chapter 2

Memorize	Understand	Not Required*
• categories of stereoisomers • define enantiomers, diastereomers • define ligand, chiral, racemic mixture	* Basic stereochemistry * Identify meso compounds * Assign R/S/E/Z * Fischer projections	* Advanced level college info * Memorize specific rotation equation

GAMSAT-Prep.com

Introduction

Stereochemistry is the study of the relative spatial (3-D) arrangement of atoms within molecules. An important branch of stereochemistry, and most relevant to the GAMSAT, is the study of chiral molecules.

More than 1/3 of organic chemistry questions from ACER practice materials test content presented in this chapter. Of course, this does not guarantee the balance of questions on your upcoming exam but it underlines the relative importance of this chapter. Normally, but not always, ACER will reiterate - in the exam's stimulus material - the rules for assigning R/S/E/Z configuration ("stimulus material" refers to the passage, article, graphs, tables or diagrams that precede multiple-choice questions).

Additional Resources

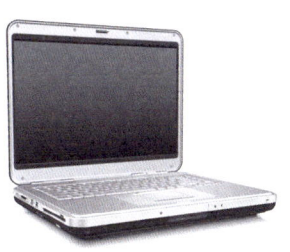

Free Online Q&A + Forum

Video: Online or DVD

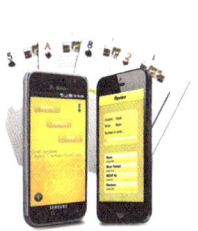

Flashcards

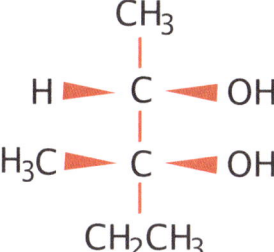

Special Guest

THE BIOLOGICAL SCIENCES   ORG-13

* The real GAMSAT may have advanced level information presented (ie. in a passage) but previous knowledge of said information is not required to answer the questions that would follow. Practice ACER and GS practice GAMSATs can help you clarify this point.

GAMSAT-Prep.com
THE GOLD STANDARD

2.1 Isomers

Stereochemistry is the study of the arrangement of atoms in a molecule, in three dimensions. Two *different molecules* with the same number and type of atoms (= *the same molecular formula*) are called isomers. Isomers fall into two main categories: *structural* (constitutional) isomers and *stereoisomers* (spatial isomers). Structural isomers differ by the way their atoms are connected and stereoisomers differ in the way their atoms are arranged in space (enantiomers and diastereomers; see Figure IV.B.2.1.1).

2.1.1 Structural (Constitutional) Isomers

Structural isomers have different atoms and/or bonding patterns in relation to each other like the following *chain* or *skeletal* isomers:

$$H_3C-\underset{\underset{H}{|}}{\overset{\overset{CH_3}{|}}{C}}-CH_2CH_2CH_3 \quad \text{and} \quad H_3C-\underset{\underset{CH_2}{|}}{\overset{\overset{H}{|}}{C}}-CH_2CH_3$$
$$\phantom{H_3C-\overset{H}{C}-CH_2CH_3\ \text{and}\ H_3C-}\underset{CH_3}{|}$$

Functional isomers are structural isomers that have the same molecular formula but have different functional groups or *moieties*. For example, the following alcohol (ORG 6.1) and ether (ORG 10.1):

butan-1-ol (n-butanol)

ethoxyethane (diethyl ether)

Positional or regioisomers are structural isomers where the functional group changes position on the parent structure. For example, the hydroxyl group (-OH) occupying 3 different positions on the n-pentane (= normal, non-branched alkane with 5 carbons) chain resulting in 3 different compounds:

pentan-1-ol (1-pentanol)

2-pentanol

3-pentanol

ORG-14   STEREOCHEMISTRY

2.2 Spatial/Stereoisomers

2.2.1 Geometric Isomers *cis/trans*, E/Z

Geometric isomers occur because carbons that are in a ring or double bond structure are *unable* to freely rotate (see conformation of cycloalkane; ORG 3.3, 3.3.1). This results in *cis* and *trans* compounds. When the substituents (i.e. Br) are on the same side of the ring or double bond, it is designated *cis*. When they are on opposite sides, it is designated *trans*. The *trans* isomer is more stable since the substituents are further apart, thus electron shell repulsion is minimized.

cis-dibromoethene   *trans*-dibromoethene

In general, structural and geometric isomers have different reactivity, spectra and physical properties (i.e. boiling points, melting points, etc.). Geometric isomers may have different physical properties but, in general, tend to have similar chemical reactivity.

The E, Z notation is the IUPAC preferred method for designating the stereochemistry of double bonds. E, Z is particularly used for isomeric compounds with 4 different substituent groups bonded to the two *ethenyl* or *vinyl* carbons (i.e. C=C which are sp^2 hybridized carbon atoms). We have just reviewed how to use *cis/trans*. The E, Z notation is used on more complex molecules and, as described, on situations were 4 different substituents are present.

To begin with, each substituent at the double bond is assigned a priority (see 2.3.1 for rules). If the two groups of higher priority are on opposite sides of the double bond, the bond is assigned the configuration E, (from *entgegen*, the German word for "opposite"). If the two groups of higher priority are on the same side of the double bond, the bond is assigned the configuration Z, (from *zusammen*, the German word for "together"). {Generally speaking, learning German is NOT required for the GAMSAT!}

cis-2-bromobut-2-ene
(2 methyl groups on same side)
BUT
(*E*)-2-bromobut-2-ene
(Br is higher priority than methyl)

Mnemonic: Z = Zame Zide; E = Epposites.

2.2.2 Enantiomers and Diastereomers

Stereoisomers are different compounds with the same structure, differing only in the spatial orientation of the atoms (= *configuration*). Stereoisomers may be further divided into enantiomers and diastereomers. Enantiomers must have opposite absolute configurations at each and every chiral carbon.

We will soon highlight the easy way to remember the meaning of a *chiral molecule*, however, the formal definition of chirality is of an object that is not identical with its mirror image and thus exists in two enantiomeric forms. A molecule cannot be chiral if it contains a plane of symmetry. A molecule that has a plane of symmetry must be superposable on its mirror image and thus must be *achiral*. The most common chirality encountered in organic chemistry is when the carbon atom is bonded to four different groups. Such a carbon lacks a plane of symmetry and is referred to as a *chiral center*. When a carbon atom has only three different substituents, such as the central carbon in methylcyclohexane, it has a plane of symmetry and is therefore achiral.

methylcyclohexane
line of symmetry

A stereocenter (= stereogenic center) is an atom bearing attachments such that interchanging any two groups produces a stereoisomer. If a molecule has n stereocenters, then it can have up to 2^n different non-superimposable (non-superposable) structures (= enantiomers).

Enantiomers come in pairs. They are two non-superposable molecules, which are mirror images of each other. In order to have an enantiomer, a molecule must be chiral. Chiral molecules contain at least one chiral carbon which is a carbon atom that has four different substituents attached. For the purposes of the GAMSAT, the concepts of a chiral carbon, asymmetric carbon and stereocenter are interchangeable.

Enantiomers have the same chemical and physical properties. The only difference is with their interactions with other chiral molecules, and their rotation of plane polarized light.

Conversely, diastereomers are any pair of stereoisomers that are not enantiomers. Diastereomers are both chemically and physically different from each other.

Superimposable vs Superposable: Most exams and many textbooks use these terms interchangeably. On the real GAMSAT, unless the question is preceded by their definitions, then the 2 words have the same meaning. Technically, "superimposable" is to lay or place (something, i.e. a molecule) on or over something else (i.e. another molecule). If the preceding proves that the 2 molecules are identical, then they are "superposable".

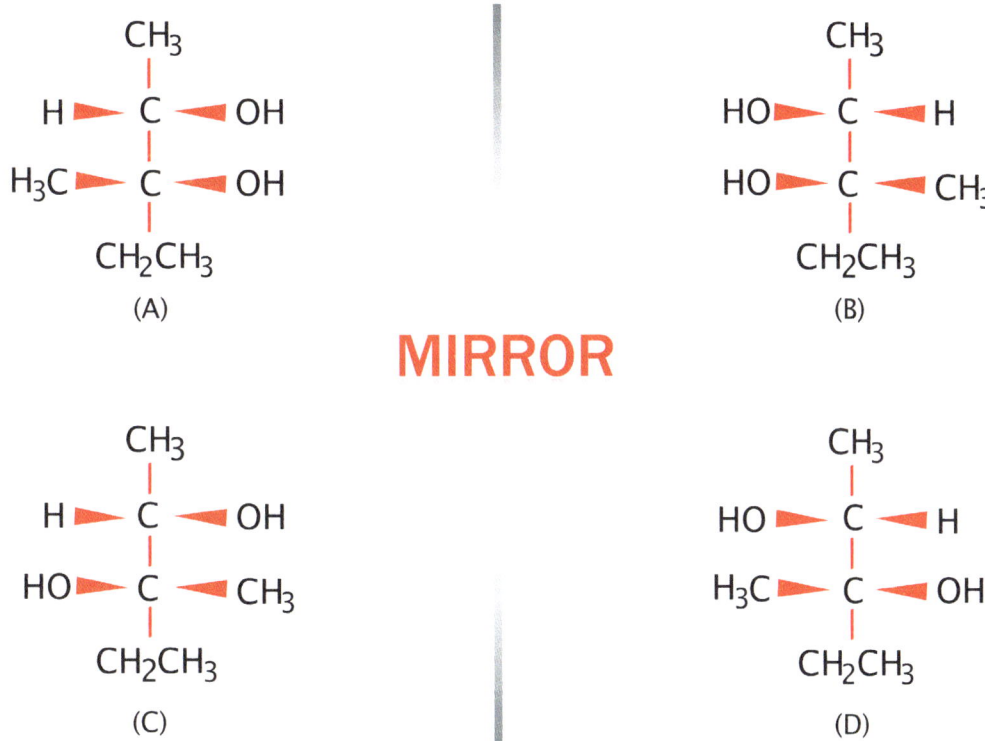

Figure IV.B.2.1: Enantiomers and diastereomers. The enantiomers are A & B, C & D. The diastereomers are A & C, A & D, B & D, B & C. Thus there are 2 pairs of enantiomers. This is consistent with the 2^n equation since each of the structures above have exactly 2 chiral carbons (stereocenters) and thus $2^2 = 4$ enantiomers.

2.3 Absolute and Relative Configuration

Absolute configuration uses the R, S system of naming compounds (*nomenclature*; ORG 2.3.1) and relative configuration uses the D, L system (ORG 2.3.2).

Before 1951, the absolute three dimensional arrangement or configuration of chiral molecules was not known. Instead chiral molecules were compared to an arbitrary standard (*glyceraldehyde*). Thus the *relative* configuration could be determined. Once the actual spatial arrangements of groups in molecules were finally determined, the *absolute* configuration could be known.

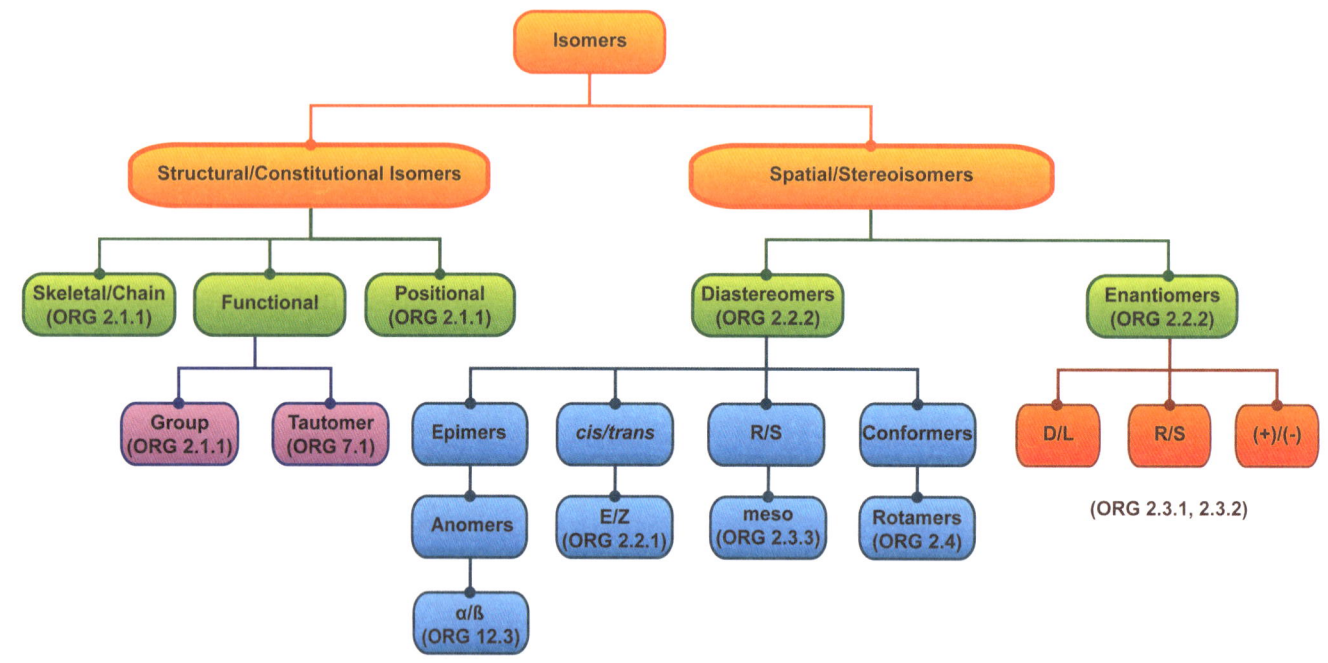

Figure IV.B.2.1.1: Categories of isomers.

2.3.1 The R, S System and Fischer Projections

One consequence of the existence of enantiomers, is a special system of nomenclature: the R, S system. This system provides information about the absolute configuration of a molecule. This is done by assigning a stereochemical configuration at each asymmetric (*chiral*) carbon in the molecule by using the following steps:

1. Identify an asymmetric carbon, and the four attached groups.

2. Assign priorities to the four groups, using the following rules (Cahn–Ingold–Prelog priority rules = CIP system):

i. Atoms of higher atomic number have higher priority.
ii. An isotope of higher atomic mass receives higher priority.
iii. The higher priority is assigned to the group with the atom of higher atomic number or mass at the first point of difference.
iv. If the difference between the two groups is due to the number of otherwise identical atoms, the higher priority is assigned to the group with the greater number of atoms of higher atomic number or mass.

ORG-18 STEREOCHEMISTRY

ORGANIC CHEMISTRY

v. To assign priority of double or triple bonded groups, multiple-bonded atoms are considered as equivalent number of single bonded atoms:

–CH=CH is taken as
```
          –CH–CH
            |   |
            C   C
```

>C=O is taken as
```
         O
        /
    >C
        \
         O
```

–CH≡CH is taken as
```
          C   C
          |   |
         –C—CH
          |   |
          C   C
```

3. In other words, you must re-orient the molecule in space so that the group of lowest priority is pointing directly back, away from you. The remaining three substituents with higher priority should radiate from the asymmetric carbon atom like the spoke on a steering wheel.

4. Consider the clockwise or counterclockwise order of the priorities of the remaining groups. If they increase in a clockwise direction, the asymmetric carbon is said to have the R configuration. If they decrease in a clockwise direction, the asymmetric carbon is said to have the S configuration {Mnemonic: Clockwise means that when you get to the top of the molecule, you must turn to the Right = R}.

A stereoisomer is named by indicating the configurations of each of the asymmetric carbons.

A **Fischer projection is a 2-D way of looking at 3-D structures**. All horizontal bonds project toward the viewer, while vertical bonds project away from the viewer. In organic chemistry, Fischer projections are used mostly for carbohydrates (*see* ORG 12.3.1, 12.3.2). To determine if 2 Fischer projections are superposable (i.e. identical), you can: (1) rotate one projection 180° or (2) keep one substituent in a fixed position and then you can rotate the other 3 groups either clockwise or counterclockwise (3-D configuration preserved):

```
      OH              OH              OH
      |               |               |
H₃C—–—CO₂H  =  HO₂C—–—H   =   H—–—CH₃
      |               |               |
      H               CH₃             CO₂H
```

(3) interchange (switch) the positions of all 4 substituents, in any direction, at the same time:

```
      OH                      CO₂H
      |                       |
H₃C—–—CO₂H     =    H—–—OH
      |                       |
      H                       CH₃
```

Assigning R, S configurations to Fischer projections:

1. Assign priorities to the four substituents.

2. If the lowest priority group is on the vertical axis, determine the direction of rotation by going from priority 1 to 2 to 3, and then assign R or S configuration.

3. If the lowest priority group is on the horizontal axis, determine the direction of rotation by going from priority 1 to 2 to 3, obtain the R or S configuration, now the TRUE configuration will be the opposite of what you have just obtained.

THE BIOLOGICAL SCIENCES   ORG-19

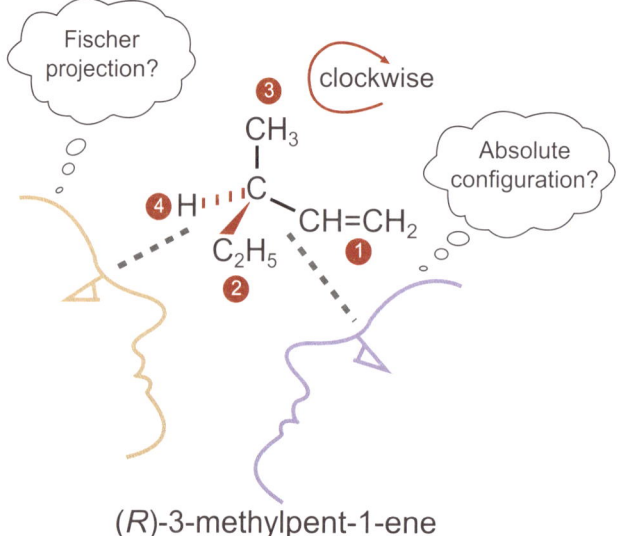

(R)-3-methylpent-1-ene

Figure IV.B.2.2(a): Assigning Absolute Configuration. In organic chemistry, the directions of the bonds are symbolized as follows: a broken line extends away from the viewer (i.e. INTO the page), a solid triangle projects towards the viewer, and a straight line extends in the plane of the paper. According to rule #3, we must imagine that the lowest priority group (H) points away from the viewer.

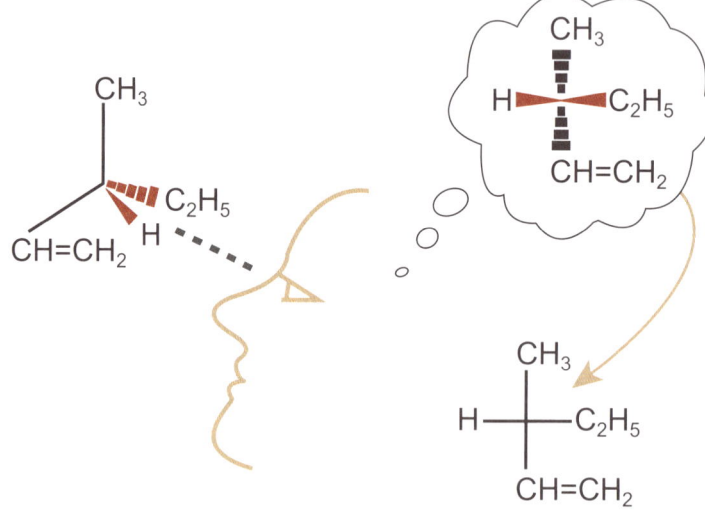

Fischer Projection

Figure IV.B.2.2(b): Creating the Fischer projection of (R)-3-methyl-1-pentene. Notice that the perspective of the viewer in the image is the identical perspective of the viewer on the left of Figure IV.B.2.2(a). In either case, a perspective is chosen so that the horizontal groups project towards the viewer.

> **Note:** For the GAMSAT, it is not normally expected that you have memorized the rules to assign R, S configurations. They would normally provide the rules before asking questions to confirm that you know how to apply the rules. However, it is normally expected that you know the rules to compare different Fischer projections (ORG 2.3.1).

ORG-20   STEREOCHEMISTRY

ORGANIC CHEMISTRY

2.3.2 Optical Isomers and the D, L System

Optical isomers are enantiomers and thus are stereoisomers that differ by different spatial orientations about a chiral carbon atom. Light is an electromagnetic wave that contains oscillating fields. In ordinary light, the electric field oscillates in all directions. However, it is possible to obtain light with an electric field that oscillates in only one plane. This type of light is known as **plane polarized light**. When plane polarized light is passed through a sample of a chiral substance, it will emerge vibrating in a different plane than it started. Optical isomers differ only in this rotation. If the light is rotated in a clockwise direction, the compound is dextrorotary, and is designated by a D or (+). If the light is rotated in a counterclockwise direction, the compound is levrorotary, and is designated by an L or (−). All L compounds have the same relative configuration as L-glyceraldehyde.

A racemic mixture will show no rotation of plane polarized light. This is a consequence of the fact that a racemate is a mixture with equal amounts of the D and L forms of a substance.

Specific rotation (α) is an inherent physical property of a molecule. It is defined as follows:

$$\alpha = \frac{\text{Observed rotation in degrees}}{(\text{tube length in dm})(\text{concentration in g/ml})}$$

The observed rotation is the rotation of the light passed through the substance. The tube length is the length of the tube that contains the sample in question. The specific rotation is dependent on the solvent used,

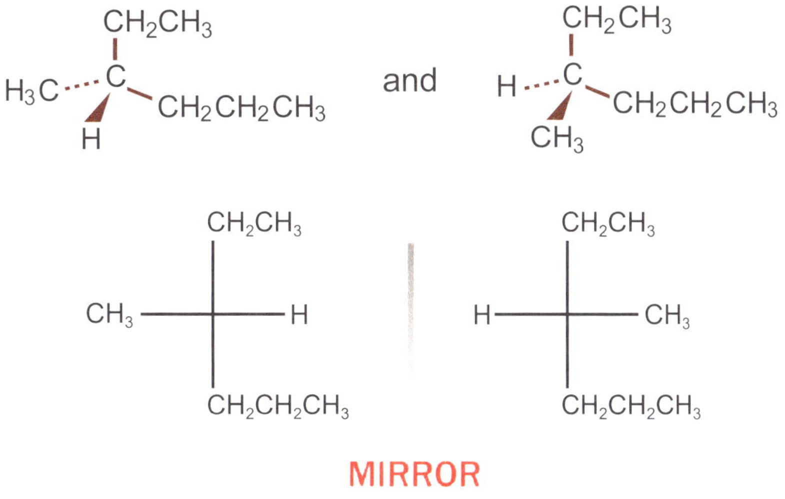

MIRROR

Figure IV.B.2.3: Optical isomers and their Fischer projections. To prove to yourself that the 2 molecules are non-superposable mirror images (enantiomers), review the rules for Fischer projections (ORG 2.3.1) and compare.

THE BIOLOGICAL SCIENCES ORG-21

the temperature of the sample, and the wavelength of the light.

It should be noted that there is no clear correlation between the absolute configuration (i.e. R, S) and the direction of rotation of plane polarized light, designated by D/(+) or L (-). Therefore, the direction of optical rotation cannot be determined from the structure of a molecule and must be determined experimentally.

2.3.3 Meso Compounds

Tartaric acid (= 2,3-dihydroxybutanedioic acid which, in the chapters to come, is a compound that you will be able to name systematically = using IUPAC rules) has two chiral centers that have the same four substituents and are equivalent. As a result, two of the four possible stereoisomers of this compound are identical due to a plane of symmetry. Thus there are only three stereoisomeric tartaric acids. Two of these stereoisomers are enantiomers and the third is an achiral diastereomer, called a meso compound. Meso compounds are achiral (optically inactive) diastereomers of chiral stereoisomers.

In a *meso compound*, an internal plane of symmetry exists by drawing a line that will cut the molecule in half. For example, notice that in *meso*-tartaric acid, you can draw a line perpendicular to the vertical carbon chain creating 2 symmetric halves {**MeSo** = **M**irror of **S**ymmetry}.

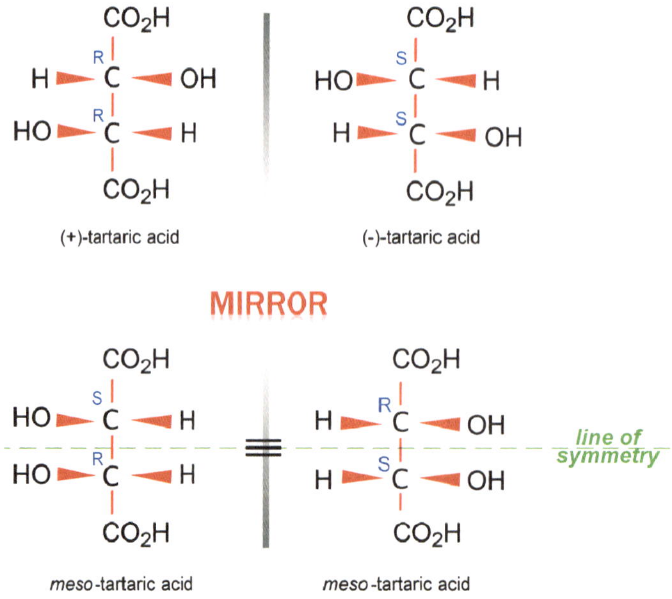

(+)-tartaric acid   (-)-tartaric acid

MIRROR

meso-tartaric acid ≡ *meso*-tartaric acid

line of symmetry

2.4 Conformational Isomers

Conformational isomers are isomers which differ only by the rotation about single bonds. As a result, substituents (= *ligands* = *attached atoms or groups*) can be maximally close (*eclipsed conformation*), maximally apart (*anti or staggered conformation*) or anywhere in between (i.e. *gauche conformation*). Though all conformations occur at room temperature, anti is most stable since it minimizes electron shell repulsion. Conformational isomers are not true isomers. Conformers are different spatial orientations of the same molecules.

Different conformations can be seen when a molecule is depicted from above and from the right, sawhorse projection, or where the line of sight extends along a carbon-carbon bond axis, a Newman projection. The different conformations occur as the molecule is rotated about its axis.

Example 1: Ethane

The lowest energy, most stable conformation, of ethane is the one in which all six carbon-hydrogen bonds are as far away from each other as possible: *staggered*. The reason, of course, is that atoms are surrounded by an outer shell of negatively charged electrons and, the basic rule of electrostatics is that, like charges repel (= electron shell repulsion = **ESR**). The highest energy, or least stable conformation, of ethane is the one in which all six carbon-hydrogen bonds are as close as possible: *eclipsed*. In between these two extremes are an infinite number of possibilities. As we have previously reviewed, when carbon is bonded to four different atoms (i.e. ethane), its bonds are sp^3 hybridized and the carbon atom sits in the center of a tetrahedron (ORG 1.2, CHM 3.5).

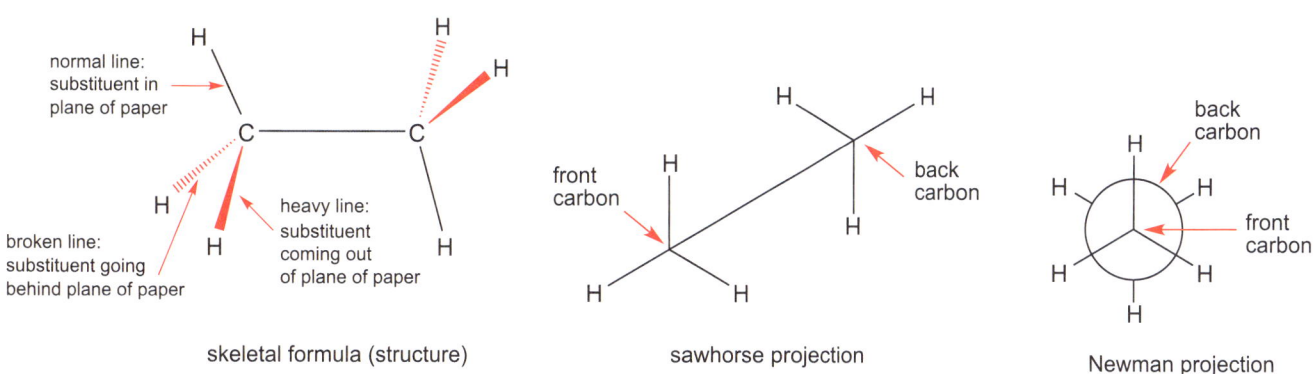

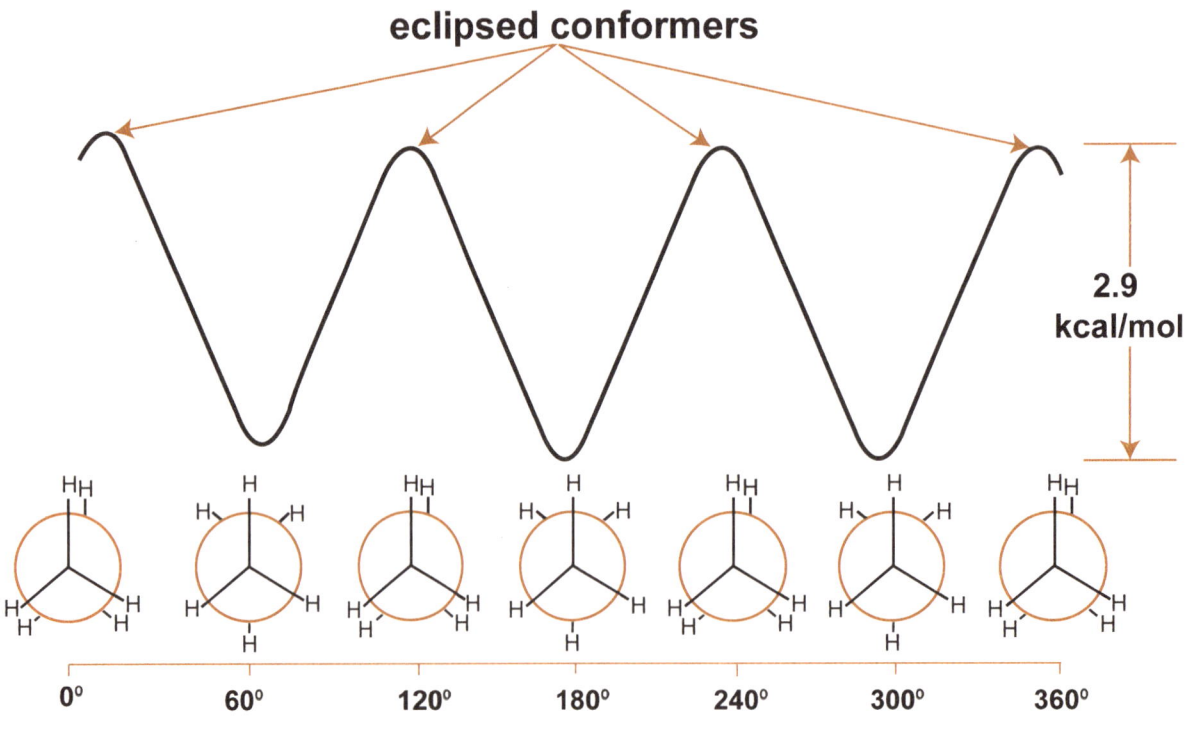

ORGANIC CHEMISTRY

Example 2: Butane

anti conformation

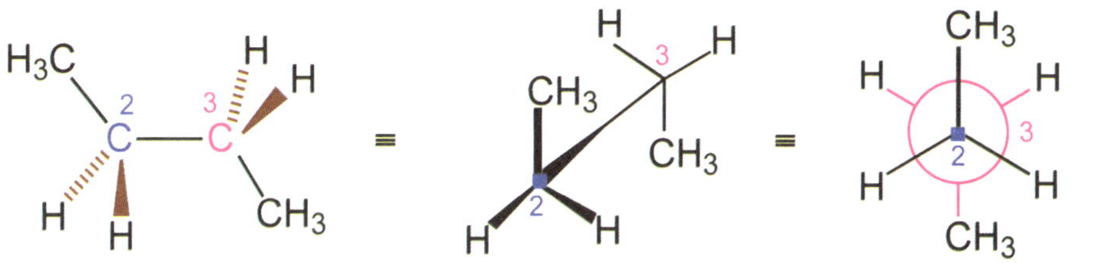

eclipsed conformation

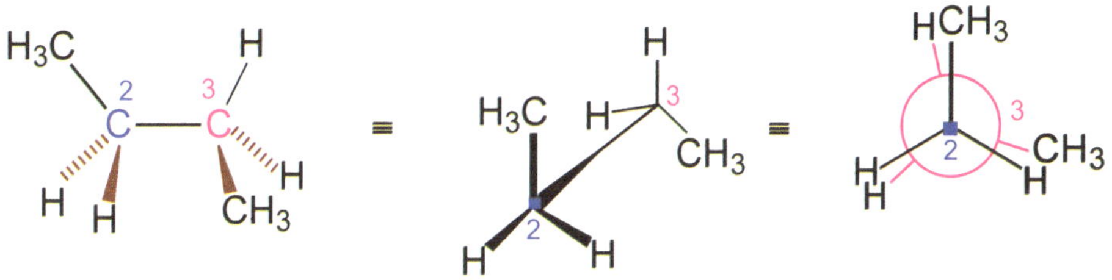

gauche conformation

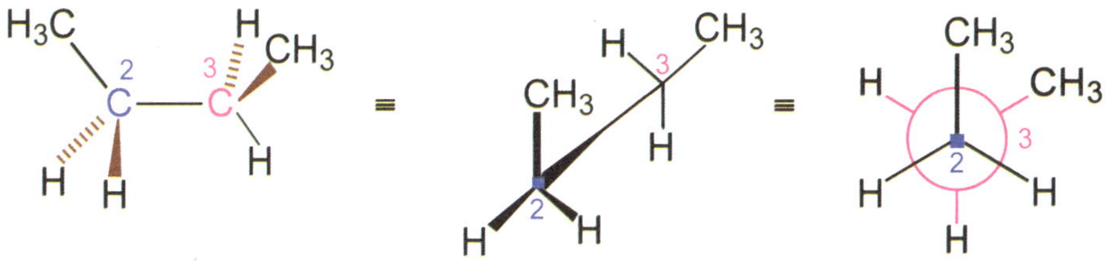

eclipsed conformation

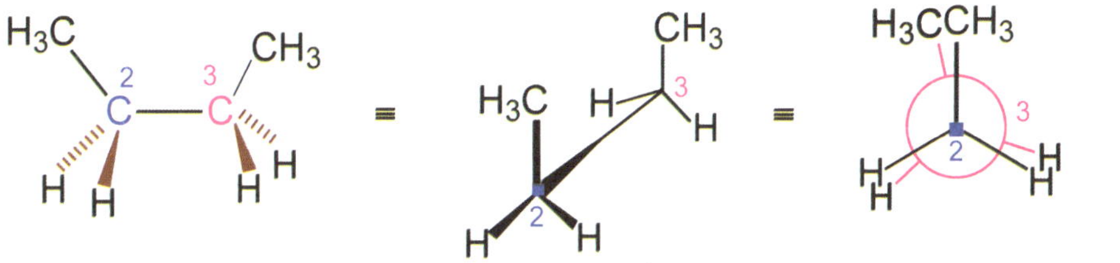

    The preceding illustration is a plot of potential energy versus rotation about the C2-C3 bond of butane.

    The lowest energy arrangement, the anti conformation, is the one in which two methyl groups (C1 and C4) are as far apart as possible, that is, 180 degrees from each other. When two substituents (i.e. the two methyl groups) are anti and in the same plane, they are *antiperiplanar* to each other.

    As rotation around the C2-C3 bond occurs, an eclipsed conformation is reached when there are two methyl-hydrogen interactions and one hydrogen-hydrogen interaction. When the rotation continues, the two methyl groups are 60 degrees apart, thus the gauche conformation. It is still higher in energy than the anti conformation even though it has no eclipsing interactions. The reason, again, is ESR. Because ESR is occurring due to the relative bulkiness (i.e. big size)

THE BIOLOGICAL SCIENCES ORG-25

of the methyl group compared to hydrogens in this molecule, we say that steric strain exists between the two close methyl groups.

When two methyl groups completely overlap with each other, the molecule is said to be totally eclipsed and is in its highest energy state (least stable).

At room temperature, these forms easily interconvert: all forms are present to some degree, though the most stable forms dominate.

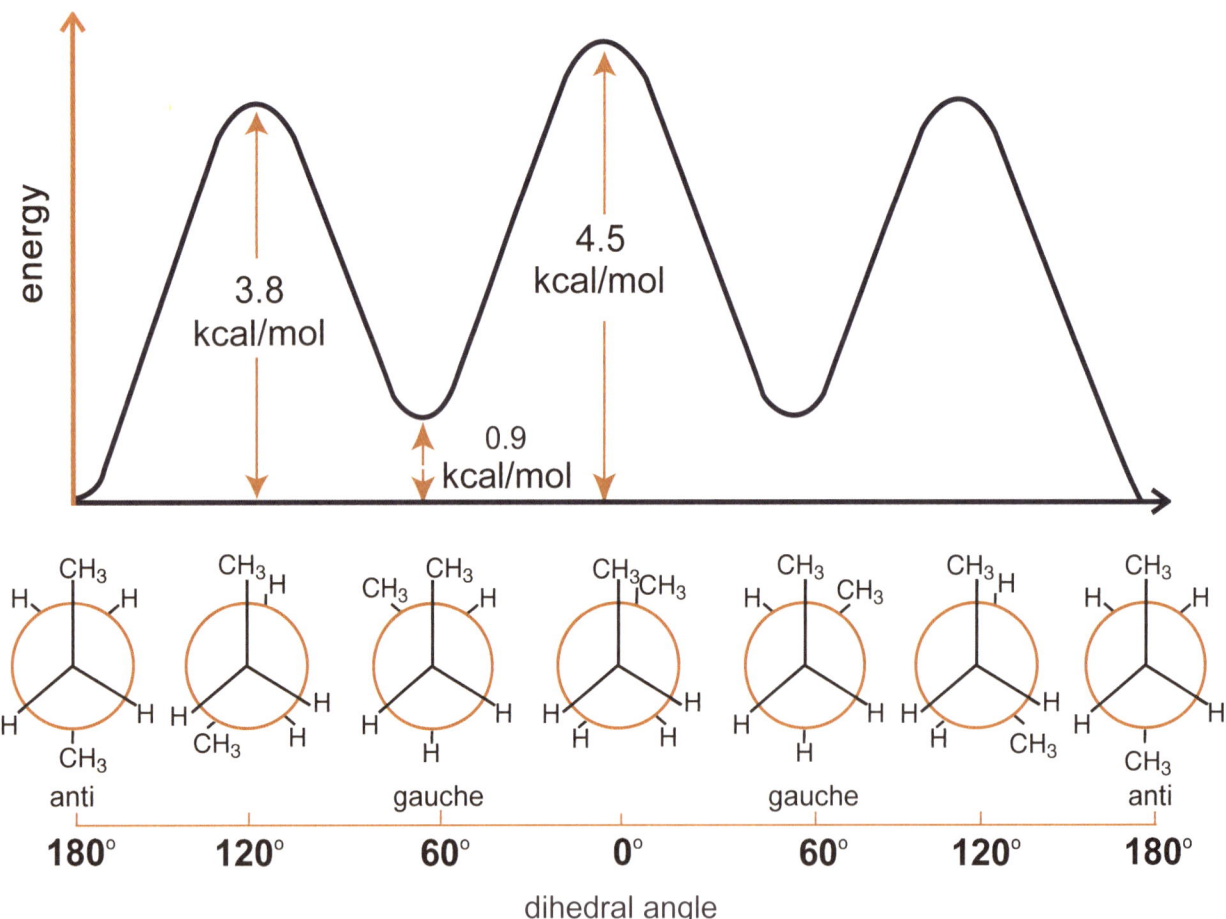

We have seen that conformers rotate about their single bonds. The rotational barrier, or barrier to rotation, is the <u>activation energy</u> (CHM 9.5) required to interconvert a subset of the possible conformations called rotamers. Butane has three rotamers: two gauche conformers and an anti conformer, where the four carbon centers are coplanar. The three eclipsed conformations with angles between the planes (= dihedral angles) of 120°, 0°, and 120° (which is 240° from the first), are not considered to be rotamers, but are instead <u>transition states</u>.

Common Terms

- dihedral angle: torsion (turn/twist) angle
- gauche: skew, synclinal
- **anti**: *trans*, antiperiplanar
- eclipsed: **syn**, *cis*, synperiplanar, torsion angle = 0°

"anti" and "syn" are IUPAC preferred descriptors.

There is no need to try to memorize the terms above. If they are required during the exam, the term(s) will be repeated with some context (image or explanatory text). The key is to understand the ideas behind these terms which have been described in this section (ORG 2.4). Again, chapter review practice questions and/or videos will help clarify any doubts and, thereafter, we also have the free forum.

Go online to GAMSAT-prep.com for chapter review Q&A and forum.

GOLD NOTES

ALKANES

Chapter 3

Memorize	Understand	Not Required*
* IUPAC nomenclature * Physical properties	* Trends based on length, branching * Ring strain, ESR * Complete combustion * Free Radicals	* Advanced level college info * Technical categorization of "cyclic alkanes"

GAMSAT-Prep.com

Introduction

Alkanes (a.k.a. paraffins) are compounds that consist only of the elements carbon (C) and hydrogen (H) (i.e. hydrocarbons). In addition, C and H are linked together exclusively by single bonds (i.e. they are saturated compounds). Methane is the simplest possible alkane while saturated oils and fats are much larger.

Additional Resources

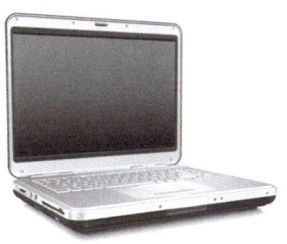

Free Online Q&A + Forum

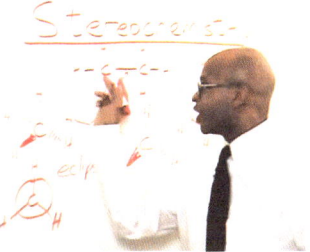

Video: Online or DVD

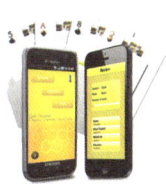

Flashcards

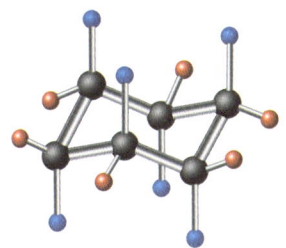

Special Guest

---

* The real GAMSAT may have advanced level information presented (ie. in a passage) but previous knowledge of said information is not required to answer the questions that would follow. Practice ACER and GS practice GAMSATs can help you clarify this point.

3.1 Description and Nomenclature

Alkanes are hydrocarbon molecules containing only sp³ hybridized carbon atoms (single bonds). They may be unbranched, branched or cyclic. Their general formula is C_nH_{2n+2} for a straight chain molecule; 2 hydrogen (H) atoms are subtracted for each ring. They contain no functional groups and are fully saturated molecules (= *no double or triple bonds*). As a result, they are chemically unreactive except when exposed to heat or light.

Systematic naming of compounds (= *nomenclature*) has evolved from the International Union of Pure and Applied Chemistry (IUPAC). **The nomenclature of alkanes is the basis of that for many other organic molecules.** The root of the compound is named according to the number of carbons in the longest carbon chain:

C_1 = meth	C_5 = pent	C_8 = oct
C_2 = eth	C_6 = hex	C_9 = non
C_3 = prop	C_7 = hept	C_{10} = dec
C_4 = but		

When naming these as fragments, (alkyl fragments: *the alkane minus one H atom*, symbol: R), the suffix '–yl' is used. If naming the alkane, the suffix '-ane' is used. Some prefixes result from the fact that a carbon with *one* R group attached is a *primary* (normal or n –) carbon, *two* R groups is *secondary* (sec) and with *three* R groups it is a *tertiary* (tert or t –) carbon. Some alkyl groups have special names:

C–C–C– n-propyl (= propyl)

C–C–C–C– n-butyl (= butyl)

isopropyl (= 2-propyl or propan-2-yl)

sec-butyl (= 1-methylpropyl)

tert-butyl (= 1,1-dimethylethyl)

neopentyl (= dimethylpropyl)

Cyclic alkanes are named in the same way (according to the number of carbons), but the prefix 'cyclo' is added. The shorthand for organic compounds is a geometric figure where each corner represents a carbon; hydrogens need not be written, though it should be remembered that the number of hydrogens would exist such that the number of bonds at each carbon is four.

cyclobutane

cyclohexane

ORG-30 ALKANES

As mentioned, carbon atoms can be characterized by the number of other carbon atoms to which they are directly bonded. It is very important for you to train your eyes to quickly indentify a primary carbon atom (**1°**), which is bonded to only one other carbon; a secondary carbon atom (**2°**), which is bonded to two other carbons; a tertiary carbon atom (**3°**), which is bonded to three other carbons; and a quaternary carbon atom (**4°**), which is bonded to four other carbons.

For example:

CH_3CH_2—C(CH_3)—C(CH_3)—C(CH_2CHCH_3 / CH_3)—CH_2CH_3 with CH and H_3C, CH_3 substituents

4,6-Diethyl-2,5,5,6,7-pentamethyl octane (7 substituents) or 3,5-Diethyl-2,3,4,4,7-pentamethyl octane (a bit better for keeners!) NOT 2,5,5,6-Tetramethyl-4-ethyl-6-isopropyl octane (6 substituents)

Naming cycloalkanes:

1. Use the cycloalkane name as the parent name. The only exception is when the alkyl side chain contains a larger number of carbons than the ring. In that case, the ring is considered as a substituent to the parent alkane.

The nomenclature for <u>branched-chain alkanes</u> begins by determining the longest <u>straight chain</u> (i.e. *the highest number of carbons attached in a row*). The groups attached to the straight or *main* chain are numbered so as to achieve the lowest set of numbers. Groups are cited in alphabetical order. If a group appears more than once, the prefixes di-(2), tri-(3), tetra-(4) are used. Prefixes such as di-, tri-, tetra- as well as tert-, sec-, n- are not used for alphabetizing purposes. However, cyclo-, iso-, and neo- are considered part of the group name and are used for alphabetizing purposes. If two chains of equal length compete for selection as the main chain, choose the chain with the most substituents.

2. Number the substituents on the ring to arrive at the lowest sum. When two or more different alkyl groups are present, they are numbered by an alphabetical order.

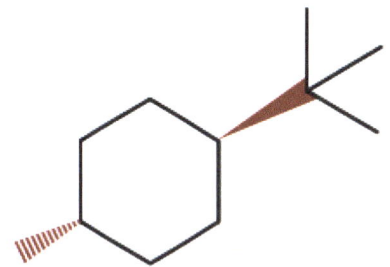

trans-1-tert-butyl-4-methylcyclohexane

THE BIOLOGICAL SCIENCES ORG-31

3.1.1 Physical Properties of Alkanes

At room temperature and one atmosphere of pressure straight chain alkanes with 1 to 4 carbons are gases (i.e. CH_4 – methane, CH_3CH_3 – ethane, etc.), 5 to 17 carbons are liquids, and more than 17 carbons are solid. Boiling points of straight chain alkanes (= *aliphatic*) show a regular increase with increasing number of carbons. This is because they are nonpolar molecules, and have weak intermolecular forces. Branching of alkanes leads to a dramatic decrease in the boiling point. As a rule, as the number of carbons increase the melting points also increase.

Alkanes are soluble in nonpolar solvents (i.e. benzene, CCl_4 – carbon tetrachloride, etc.), and not in aqueous solvents (= *hydrophobic*). They are insoluble in water because of their low polarity and their inability to hydrogen bond. Alkanes are the least dense of all classes of organic compounds (<< ρ_{water}, 1 g/ml). Thus petroleum, a mixture of hydrocarbons rich in alkanes, floats on water.

3.2 Important Reactions of Alkanes

3.2.1 Combustion

Combustion (CHM 1.4) is typically when a substance reacts with oxygen, releasing energy in the form of heat and light. Combustion includes the burning of hydrocarbons found in fossil fuels like gasoline (i.e. octane and other alkanes for internal combustion engines) and natural gas (i.e. methane and other alkanes for heating, cooking, and electricity generation).

Note that the "heat of combustion" is the change in enthalpy of a combustion reaction. Therefore, the higher the heat of combustion, the higher the energy level of the molecule, the less stable the molecule was prior to combustion.

Combustion may be either complete or incomplete. In complete combustion, the hydrocarbon is converted to carbon dioxide (CO_2) and water (H_2O). If there is insufficient oxygen for complete combustion, the reaction gives other products, such as carbon monoxide (CO) and soot (molecular C). This strongly exothermic reaction may be summarized:

$$C_nH_{2n+2} + \text{excess } O_2 \rightarrow nCO_2 + (n+1)H_2O$$

3.2.2 Radical Substitution Reactions

Radical substitution reactions with halogens may be summarized (recall E = hf, see PHY 9.2.4; also see CHM 9.4):

RH + X$_2$ + uv light(*hf*) or heat → RX + HX

The halogen X$_2$, may be F$_2$, Cl$_2$, or Br$_2$. I$_2$ does not react. The mechanism of *halogenation* may be explained and summarized by example:

i. Initiation: This step involves the formation of *free radicals* (highly reactive substances which contain an unpaired electron, which is symbolized by a single dot):

Cl:Cl + uv light or heat → 2Cl•

ii. Propagation: In this step, the chlorine free radical begins a series of reactions that form new free radicals:

CH$_4$ + Cl• → •CH$_3$ + HCl
•CH$_3$ + Cl$_2$ → CH$_3$Cl + Cl•

iii. Termination: These reactions end the radical propagation steps. Termination reactions destroy the free radicals (coupling).

Cl• + •CH$_3$ → CH$_3$Cl

•CH$_3$ + •CH$_3$ → CH$_3$CH$_3$

Cl• + Cl• → Cl$_2$

Radical substitution reactions can also occur with halide acids (i.e. HCl, HBr) and peroxides (i.e. HOOH – hydrogen peroxide). Chain propagation (step ii) can destroy many organic compounds fairly quick. This step can be inhibited by using a resonance stabilized free radical to "mop up" (*termination*) other destructive free radicals in the medium. For example, BHT is a resonance stabilized free radical added to packaging of many breakfast cereals in order to inhibit free radical destruction of the cereal (= *spoiling*).

The stability of a free radical depends on the ability of the compound to stabilize the unpaired electron. This is analogous to stabilizing a positively charged carbon (= *carbocation*). Thus, in both cases, a tertiary compound is more stable than secondary which, in turn, is more stable than a primary compound.

Also in both cases, the reason for the trend is the same: the charge on the carbon is stabilized by the electron donating effect of the presence of alkyl groups. Alkyl groups are not strongly electron donating, they are normally described as "somewhat" electron donating; however, the combined effect of multiple R groups has an important stabilizing effect that we will see as a critical feature in many reaction types.

Pyrolysis occurs when a molecule is broken down by heat (*pyro* = fire, *lysis* = separate). C-C bonds are cleaved and smaller chain alkyl radicals often recombine in termination steps creating a variety of alkanes.

$$•CR_3 > •CR_2H > •CRH_2 > •CH_3$$
$$3° > 2° > 1° > \text{methyl}$$

Please note that the rate law for free radical substitution reactions was discussed in CHM 9.4.

3.3 Ring Strain in Cyclic Alkanes

Cyclic alkanes are strained compounds. This **ring strain** results from the bending of the bond angles in greater amounts than normal. This strain causes cyclic compounds of 3 and 4 carbons to be unstable, and thus not often found in nature. The usual angle between bonds in an sp^3 hybridized carbon is 109.5° (= *the normal tetrahedral angle*).

The expected angles in some cyclic compounds can be determined geometrically: 60° in cyclopropane; 90° in cyclobutane and 108° in cyclopentane. Cyclohexane, in the chair conformation, has normal bond angles of 109.5°. The closer the angle is to the normal tetrahedral angle of 109.5°, the more stable the compound. In fact, cyclohexane can be found in a chair or boat conformation or any conformation in between; however, at any given moment, 99% of the cyclohexane molecules would be found in the chair conformation because it is the most stable (lower energy).

It is important to have a clear understanding of electron shell repulsion (ESR). Essentially all atoms and molecules are surrounded by an electron shell (CHM 2.1, ORG 1.2) which is more like a cloud of electrons. Because like charges repel, when there are options, atoms and molecules assume the conformation which minimizes ESR.

For example, when substituents are added to a cyclic compound (i.e. *see* ORG 12.3.1, Fig. IV.B.12.1 Part II) the most stable position is equatorial (equivalent to the anti conformation, ORG 2.1) which minimizes ESR.

This conformation is most pronounced when the substituent is bulky (i.e. isopropyl, t-butyl, phenyl, etc.). In other words, a large substituent takes up more space thus ESR has a more prominent effect.

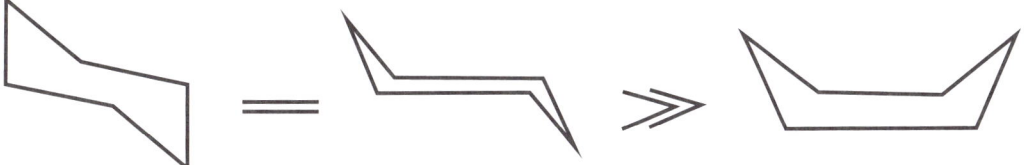

Figure IV.B.3.1: The chair and boat conformations of cyclohexane. Some students like to remember that you sit in a chair because a chair is stable. However, a boat can be tippy and so it's less stable.

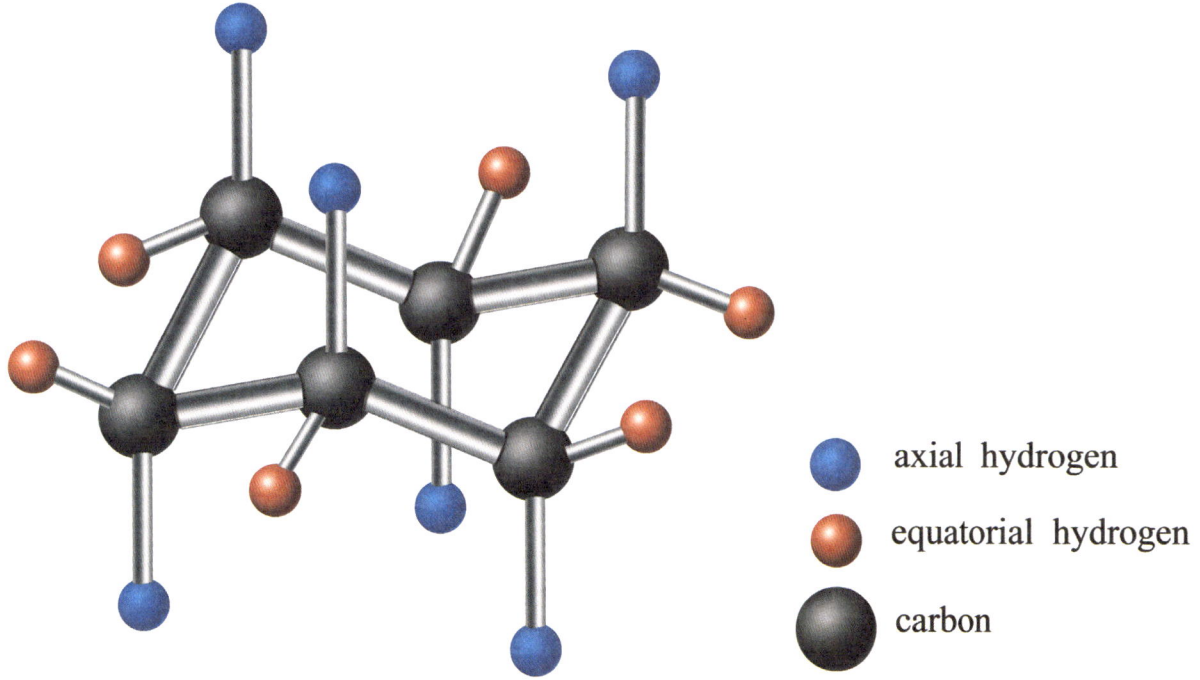

Figure IV.B.3.2: The chair conformation of cyclohexane. The hydrogens which are generally in the same plane as the ring are <u>equatorial</u>. The hydrogens which are generally perpendicular to the ring are <u>axial</u>. The hydrogen atoms are maximally separated and staggered to minimize electron shell repulsion.

Go online to GAMSAT-prep.com for chapter review Q&A and forum.

GOLD NOTES

… ALKENES

Chapter 4

Memorize	Understand	Not Required*
* Basic nomenclature	* Electrophilic addition, hydrogenation, Markovnikoff's rule, oxidation	* Advanced level college info

GAMSAT-Prep.com

Introduction

An alkene (a.k.a. olefin) is an unsaturated chemical compound containing at least one carbon-to-carbon double bond.

Additional Resources

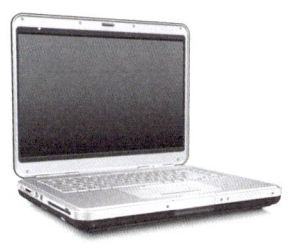   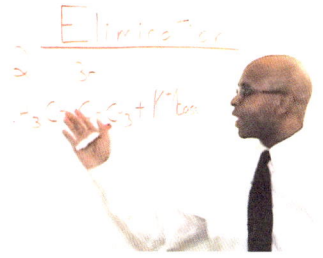   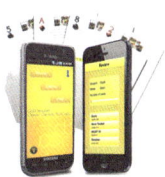   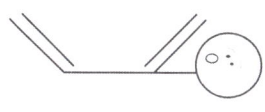

Free Online Q&A + Forum   Video: Online or DVD   Flashcards   Special Guest

THE BIOLOGICAL SCIENCES   ORG-37

* The real GAMSAT may have advanced level information presented (ie. in a passage) but previous knowledge of said information is not required to answer the questions that would follow. Practice ACER and GS practice GAMSATs can help you clarify this point.

4.1 Description and Nomenclature

Alkenes *(olefins)* are unsaturated hydrocarbon molecules containing carbon-carbon double bonds. Their general formula is C_nH_{2n} for a straight chain molecule; 2 hydrogen (H) atoms are subtracted for each ring. The *functional group* in these molecules is the double bond which determines the chemical properties of alkenes. Double bonds are sp^2 hybridized (see ORG 1.2, 1.3). The nomenclature is the same as that for alkanes, except that i) the suffix 'ene' replaces 'ane' and ii) the double bond is (are) numbered in the molecule, trying to get the smallest number for the double bond(s). Always select the longest chain that contains the double bond or the greatest number of double bonds as the parent hydrocarbon. For cycloalkenes, the carbons of the double bond are given the 1– and 2– positions.

$CH_3-CH=CHCH_2-C(CH_3)(CH_3)-CH_3$

5,5-Dimethyl-2-hexene

1-methylcyclopentene

Two frequently encountered groups are sometimes named as if they were substituents.

$CH_2=CH-$

the vinyl group

$CH_2=CHCH_2-$

the allyl group

Alkenes have similar physical properties to alkanes. *Trans* compounds tend to have higher melting points (due to better symmetry), and lower boiling points (due to less polarity) than its corresponding *cis* isomer. Alkenes, however, due to the nature of the double bond may be polar. The dipole moment is oriented from the electropositive alkyl group toward the electronegative alkene.

has a small dipole moment

has no dipole moment

(cis) small dipole moment

(trans) no dipole moment

ORGANIC CHEMISTRY

The greater the number of attached alkyl groups (i.e. *the more highly substituted the double bond*), the greater is the alkene's stability. The reason is that alkyl groups are somewhat electron donating, thus they stabilize the double bond.

An alkene with 2 double bonds is a diene, 3 is a triene. A diene with one single bond in between is a conjugated diene. Conjugated dienes are more stable than non-conjugated dienes primarily due to resonance stabilization (see the resonance stabilized conjugated molecule 1,3-butadiene in ORG 1.4). Alkenes, including polyenes (multiple double bonds), can engage in addition reactions (ORG 4.2.1). The notable exceptions include aromatic compounds (conjugated double bonds in a ring; ORG 5.1) which cannot engage in addition reactions which will be discussed in the next chapter.

• Synthesis of Alkenes: The two most common alkene-forming reactions involve elimination reactions of either HX from an alkyl halide or H_2O from alcohol. Dehydrohalogenation occurs by the reaction of an alkyl halide with a strong base. Dehydration occurs by reacting an alcohol with a strong acid.

We will discuss elimination reactions (E1 and E2), which can be used to synthesize alkenes, in the chapter reviewing alcohols (ORG 6.2.4).

4.2 Important Chemical Reactions

4.2.1 Electrophilic Addition

The chemistry of alkenes may be understood in terms of their functional group, the double bond. When electrophiles (*substances which seek electrons*) add to alkenes, carbocations (= *carbonium ions*) are formed. An important electrophile is H^+ (i.e. in HBr, H_2O, etc.). A nucleophile is a molecule with a free pair of electrons, and sometimes a negative charge, that seeks out partially or completely positively charged species (i.e. a carbon nucleus). Some important nucleophiles are OH⁻ and CN⁻.

E = electrophile   carbocation (intermediate)

Nu = nucleophile

Note that the carbon-carbon double bond is electron rich (nucleophilic) and can donate a pair of electrons to an electrophile (= "electron loving") during reactions. Electrons from the π bond attack the electrophile. As the π bond is weaker than the σ bond, it can be broken without breaking the σ bond. As a result, the carbon skeleton can remain intact. Electrophilic addition to an unsymmetrically substituted alkene gives the more highly substituted carbocation (i.e. the most stable intermediate). We will soon see that Markovnikoff's rule (or Markovnikov's rule) is a guide to determine the outcome of addition reactions.

Another important property of the double bond is its ability to stabilize carbocations, carbanions or radicals attached to adjacent carbons (*allylic carbons*). Note that all the following are resonance stabilized:

carbocation

carbanion

carbon radical

The stability of the intermediate carbocation depends on the groups attached to it, which can either stabilize or destabilize it. As well, groups which place a partial or total positive charge adjacent to the carbocation withdraw electrons inductively, by sigma bonds, to destabilize it. More highly substituted carbocations are more stable than less highly substituted ones.

These points are useful in predicting which carbon will become the carbocation, and to which carbon the electrophile and nucleophile will bond. The intermediate carbocation formed must be the most stable. **Markovnikoff's rule** is a result of this, and it states: *the nucleophile will be bonded to the most substituted carbon* (fewest hydrogens attached) *in the product. Equivalently, the electrophile will be bonded to the least sub* *stituted carbon* (most hydrogens attached) *in the product*. An example of this is:

$$H_3C\underset{H_3C}{\diagdown}C\!=\!C\underset{H}{\overset{CH_3}{\diagup}} + HBr$$
              ① ②

$$\xrightarrow{H^+} \underset{H_3C}{\overset{H_3C}{\diagdown}}\underset{①}{\overset{+}{C}}\!\!-\!\!\underset{②}{\overset{CH_3}{\underset{H}{C}}}\!\!-\!\!H$$

$$\xrightarrow{Br^-} H_3C\!-\!\underset{\underset{CH_3}{|}}{\overset{\overset{Br}{|}}{C}}\!\!-\!\!\underset{\underset{H}{|}}{\overset{CH_3}{C}}\!\!-\!\!H$$
                   ①   ②

$\overset{+}{H}$ = electrophile
$\overset{-}{Br}$ = nucleophile
① most substituted carbon
② least substituted carbon
① forms the most stable carbonium ion.

The product, 2-bromo-2-methyl butane, is the more likely or major product (*the Markovnikoff product*). Had the H⁺ added to the most substituted carbon (which has a much lower probability of occurrence) the less likely or minor product would be formed (*the anti-Markovnikoff product*). {Memory guide for Markovnikoff's rule: "Hydrogen prefers to add to the carbon in the double bond where most of its friends are" (this works because the least substituted carbon has the most bonds to hydrogen atoms)}

Carbocation intermediate rearrangement: In both *hydride shift* and *alkyl group shift*, H or CH₃ moves to a positively charged carbon, tak-

ing its electron pair with it. As a result, a less stable carbocation rearranges to a more stable one (more substituted).

secondary carbocation → tertiary carbocation

secondary carbocation → tertiary carbocation

Markovnikoff's rule is true for the ionic conditions presented in the preceding reaction. However, for radical conditions the reverse occurs. Thus *anti-Markovnikoff* products are the major products under free radical conditions.

• Addition of halogens: This is a simple and rapid laboratory diagnostic tool to test for the presence of unsaturation (C=C). Immediate disappearance of the reddish Br₂ color indicates that the sample is an alkene. The general chemical formula of the halogen addition reaction is:

$$C=C + X_2 \rightarrow X-C-C-X$$

The π electron pair of the double bond attacks the bromine, or X₂ molecule, setting up an induced dipole (*see* CHM 4.2) and then displacing the bromide ion. The intermediate forms a cyclic bromonium ion R₂Br⁺, which is then attacked by Br⁻, giving the di-bromo addition product.

Since the intermediate is a bromonium ion, the bromide anion can only attack from the opposite side, yielding an anti product.

RDS = rate determining step (CHM 9.4)

cyclohexane → trans-1,2-dibromocyclohexane (enantiomers)

cyclohexane or toluene $\xrightarrow{Br_2}$ no reaction

Halogen addition does not occur in saturated hydrocarbons (i.e. cyclohexane) which lack the electron rich double bond, nor do the reactions occur within an aromatic ring because of the increased stability afforded by conjugation in a ring system due to resonance.

- Halohydrin formation reaction: A halohydrin (or haloalcohol) is a functional group where one carbon atom has a halogen substituent and an adjacent carbon atom has a hydroxyl substituent. This addition, which produces a halohydrin, is done by reacting an alkene with a halogen X_2 in the presence of water. The intermediate forms a cyclic bromonium ion R_2Br. The water molecule competes with the bromide ion as a nucleophile and reacts with the bromonium ion to form the halohydrin. The net effect is the addition of HO-X to the alkene.

In practice, the bromohydrin reaction is carried out using a reagent called NBS. Markovnikoff regiochemistry and anti addition is observed.

alkene $\xrightarrow{X_2, H_2O}$ halohydrin + HX

ORG-42 ALKENES

ORGANIC CHEMISTRY

> **"Should I memorize these reaction mechanisms and the ones on the way?"**
>
> That would not be very helpful. If a related question were asked, normally the passage or question stem would begin by spelling out the mechanism and then the questions would lean towards your skills involving nomenclature, geometry, pattern recognition and time efficiency. Mechanisms should be followed like a good story that contains a consistent, reasonable plot. The key is to follow the plot, not to memorize it. If the plot can be reasoned then, if given a blueprint and different characters during an exam (or practice), you should be able to determine the conclusion, and how the examiners arrived at that conclusion (i.e. the intermediates when necessary).
>
> Geometry and pattern recognition allow you to follow if an addition is cis (= syn) or trans (= anti, i.e. halohydrin formation). They also help you: follow where the different R groups end up (i.e. alkene oxidation; ORG 4.2.2); recognize unusual product geometries once you have a blueprint (i.e. Diels-Alder reaction; ORG 4.2.4); etc. As often as possible, get in the habit of drawing molecules shorthand while completing your online chapter review practice questions. Drawing and practice questions are important components of GAMSAT Organic Chemistry preparation.

- **Addition of HX**: As we have seen earlier in this section, this reaction occurs via a carbocation intermediate. The halide ion then combines with the carbocation to give an alkyl halide. The proton will add to the less substituted carbon atom, yielding a more substituted (stabilized) carbocation. Markovnikoff regiochemistry is observed. This can be seen in the first two mechanisms shown in this section (ORG 4.2.1).

- **Free radical addition of HBr to alkenes**: Once a bromine free radical has formed in an initiation step (ORG 3.2.2), it adds to the alkene double bond, yielding an alkyl radical. The regiochemistry of this free radical addition is determined in the first propagation step because, instead of H attacking first in electrophilic addition, the bromine radical adds first to the alkene. Thus anti-Markovnikoff addition is observed.

The stability order of radicals is identical to the stability order of carbocations, tertiary being the most stable and methyl the least. Notice that the free radical reaction mechanism that follows uses single headed (blue) arrows to follow the movement of single electrons, as opposed to the normal arrows that we have seen which follow the movement of electron pairs.

THE BIOLOGICAL SCIENCES   ORG-43

4.2.2 Oxidation

Alkenes can undergo a variety of reactions in which the carbon-carbon double bond is oxidized. Using potassium permanganate (KMnO$_4$) under mild conditions (*no heat*), or osmium tetroxide (OsO$_4$), a glycol (= *a dialcohol*) can be produced.

In the following chapters, you will learn how to derive systematic nomenclature (these are names of compounds based on rules as opposed to "common" names often based on tradition). IUPAC (official) nomenclature is usually systematic (i.e. ethane-1,2-diol) but sometimes it is not (i.e. acetic acid). Knowing both the common and the systematic names is the safest way to approach the GAMSAT.

The first reaction that follows is the oxidation of ethene (= ethylene) under mild conditions and the second is the oxidation of 2-butene under abrasive conditions.

$$CH_2 = CH_2 + KMnO_4 \xrightarrow[OH^-]{Cold} \underset{\underset{OH}{|}}{CH_2} - \underset{\underset{OH}{|}}{CH_2}$$

Ethylene glycol
(1,2-ethanediol or ethane-1,2-diol)

Using KMnO$_4$ under more abrasive conditions leads to an oxidative cleavage of the double bond:

$$CH_3 CH = CHCH_3 \xrightarrow[heat]{KMnO_4, OH^-} 2CH_3C(=O)O^- \xrightarrow{H^+} 2CH_3C(=O)OH$$

Acetate ion (ethanoate ion) → Acetic acid (ethanoic acid)

Specifically, cold dilute KMnO$_4$ produces 1,2-diols with the syn orientation. Hot, basic KMnO$_4$ leads to oxidative cleavage of the double bonds with the double bond being replaced with a C=O bond and an O atom added to each H atom.

$$CH_3 - CH = CH_2 \xrightarrow{KMnO_4} CH_3 - C(=O)OH + CO_2$$
acetic acid

$$CH_3 - CH = C(CH_3)_2 \xrightarrow{KMnO_4} CH_3 - C(=O)OH + O = C(CH_3)_2$$
acetic acid   acetone

$$CH_2 = CH - CH = CH_2 \xrightarrow{KMnO_4} CO_2 \text{ only}$$

Ozone (O$_3$) reacts vigorously with alkenes. The reaction (= *ozonolysis*) leads to an oxidative cleavage of the double bond which can produce a ketone and an aldehyde:

$$\underset{\text{2-Methyl-2-butene}}{CH_3\underset{\underset{CH_3}{|}}{C} = CHCH_3} \xrightarrow[(2) Zn, H_2O]{(1) O_3}$$

$$\underset{\underset{\text{Acetone (propanone)}}{}}{CH_3\underset{\underset{CH_3}{|}}{C}=O} + \underset{\underset{\text{Acetaldehyde (ethanal)}}{}}{CH_3CH(=O)}$$

THE BIOLOGICAL SCIENCES ORG-45

Note that the second step in the reaction uses a reducing agent such as zinc metal. If the starting alkene has a tetra-substituted double bond (i.e. 4 R groups), two ketones will be formed. If it has a tri-substituted double bond, a ketone and an aldehyde will be formed as in the reaction shown. If it has a di-substituted double bond, two aldehydes will be formed.

The hydroboration–oxidation reaction is a two-step organic reaction that converts an alkene into an alcohol by the addition of water across the double bond. The hydrogen and hydroxyl group are added in a syn addition leading to *cis* stereochemistry. Hydroboration–oxidation is an anti-Markovnikoff reaction since the hydroxyl group (not the hydrogen) attaches to the less substituted carbon.

- Epoxide Formation: Alkenes can be oxidized with peroxycarboxylic acids (i.e. CH_3CO_3H or mCPBA). The product is an oxirane (discussed in ORG 10.1.1, ethers).

ORG-46   ALKENES

4.2.3 Hydrogenation

Alkenes react with hydrogen in the presence of a variety of metal catalysts (i.e. Ni – nickel, Pd – palladium, Pt – platinum). The reaction that occurs is an *addition* reaction since one atom of hydrogen adds to each carbon of the double bond (= hydrogenation). Both hydrogens add to the double bond from the same metal catalyst surface, thus syn addition is observed. Since there are two phases present in the process of hydrogenation (the hydrogen and the metal catalyst), the process is referred to as a heterogenous catalysis.

A carbon with multiple bonds is not bonded to the maximum number of atoms that potentially that carbon could possess. Thus it is *unsaturated*. Alkanes, which can be formed by hydrogenation, are *saturated* since each carbon is bonded to the maximum number of atoms it could possess (= *four*). Thus hydrogenation is sometimes called the process of saturation.

$$CH_3CH = CH_2 + H_2 \longrightarrow CH_3CH_2-CH_3$$

Alkenes are much more reactive than other functional groups towards hydrogenation. As a result, other functional groups such as ketones, aldehydes, esters and nitriles are usually unchanged during the alkene hydrogenation process.

4.2.4 The Diels–Alder Reaction

The Diels–Alder reaction is a cycloaddition reaction between a conjugated diene and a substituted alkene (= the dienophile) to form a substituted cyclohexene system.

Diene + Dienophile = Cyclohexene

All Diels-Alder reactions have four common features: (1) the reaction is initiated by heat; (2) the reaction forms new six-membered rings; (3) three π bonds break and two new C-C σ bonds and one new C-C π bond are formed; (4) all bonds break and form in a single step.

The Diels Alder diene must have the two double bonds on the same side of the single bond in one of the structures, which is called the s-*cis* conformation (s-*cis*: *cis* with respect to the single bond). If double bonds are on the opposite sides of the single bond in the Lewis structure, this is called the s-*trans* conformation (s-*trans*: *trans* with respect to the single bond).

The Diels-Alder reaction is useful because it sometimes creates stereocenters, it always forms a ring, and the reaction is stereospecific (i.e. the reaction mechanism dictates the stereoisomers). For example, a *cis* dienophile generates a ring with *cis* substitution, while a *trans* dienophile generates a ring with *trans* substitution.

Diels-Alder reactions are reversible (= "Retro-Diels-Alder").

ORG-48 ALKENES

4.2.5 Resonance Revisited

General Chemistry section 3.2 and Organic Chemistry section 1.4 are important to review before you move on to the next chapter on Aromatics. Many exam questions rely on your understanding of resonance and how it affects stability and reactions. It is helpful to remember that the only difference between different resonance forms is the placement of π or non-bonding electrons. The atoms themselves do not change positions, create new bonds nor are they "resonating" back and forth. The resonance hybrid with its electrons delocalized is more stable than any single resonance form. The greater the numbers of authentic resonance forms possible, the more stable the molecule.

4.3 Alkynes

Alkynes are unsaturated hydrocarbon molecules containing carbon-carbon triple bonds. The nomenclature is the same as that for alkenes, except that the suffix 'yne' replaces 'ene'. Alkynes have a higher boiling point than alkenes or alkanes. Internal alkynes, where the triple bond is in the middle of the compound, boil at higher temperatures than terminal alkynes. Terminal alkynes are relatively acidic.

Basic reactions such as reduction, electrophilic addition, free radical addition and hydroboration proceed in a similar manner to alkenes. Oxidation also follows the same rules and uses the same reactants and catalysts. However, unlike alkenes, alkynes can be partially hydrogenated yielding alkenes with just one equivalent of H_2. The reaction with palladium in Lindlar's catalyst produces the *cis* alkene while sodium or lithium in liquid ammonia will produce the *trans* alkene via a free radical mechanism.

Go online to GAMSAT-prep.com for chapter review Q&A and forum.

GOLD NOTES

AROMATICS

Chapter 5

Memorize	Understand	Not Required*
sic nomenclature	* Electrophilic aromatic substitution * How to apply Hückel's rule	* Advanced level college info * Memorizing O-P or meta directors

GAMSAT-Prep.com

Introduction

Aromatics are cyclic compounds with unusual stability due to cyclic delocalization and resonance.

Additional Resources

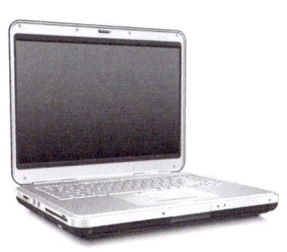

Free Online Q&A + Forum

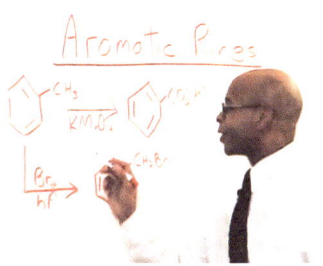

Video: Online or DVD

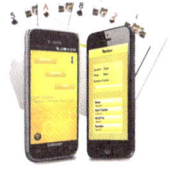

Flashcards

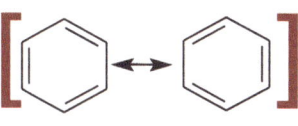

Special Guest

THE BIOLOGICAL SCIENCES   ORG-51

* The real GAMSAT may have advanced level information presented (ie. in a passage) but previous knowledge of said information is not required to answer the questions that would follow. Practice ACER and GS practice GAMSATs can help you clarify this point.

5.1 Description and Nomenclature

Aromatic compounds are cyclic and have their π electrons delocalized over the entire ring and are thus stabilized by π-electron delocalization. Benzene is the simplest of all the aromatic hydrocarbons. The term *aromatic* has historical significance in that many well known fragrant compounds were found to be derivatives of benzene. Although at present, it is known that not all benzene derivatives have fragrance, the term remains in use today to describe benzene derivatives and related compounds.

Benzene is known to have only one type of carbon-carbon bond, with a bond length of ≈ 1.4 Å (angstroms, 10^{-10}m) somewhere between that of a single and double bond. Benzene is a hexagonal, flat symmetrical molecule. All C-C-C bond angles are 120° and all C-C bonds are of equal length - a value between a normal single and double bond length; all six carbon atoms are sp^2 hybridized; and, all carbons have a p orbital perpendicular to the benzene ring, leading to six π electrons delocalized around the ring. The benzene molecule may thus be represented by two different resonance structures, showing it to be the average of the two:

Many monosubstituted benzenes have common names by which they are known.

Others are named by substituents attached to the aromatic ring. Some of these are:

phenol   toluene   aniline

nitrobenzene   benzoic acid

Disubstituted benzenes are named as derivatives of their primary substituents. In this case, either the usual numbering or the ortho-meta-para system may be used. Ortho (*o*) substituents are at the 2nd position from the primary substituent; meta (*m*) substituents are at the 3rd position; para (*p*) substituents are at the 4th position. If there are more than two substituents on the aromatic ring, the numbering system is used. Some examples are:

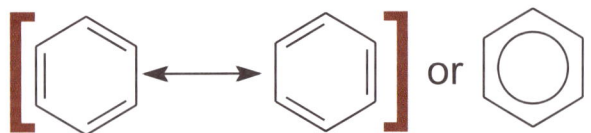

m - Nitrotoluene   o - Dinitrobenzene

o - Methylaniline
o - Aminotoluene

3 - nitro - 4 - hydroxy benzoic acid

When benzene is a substituent, it is called a *phenyl or aryl group*. The shorthand for phenyl is Ph. Toluene without a hydrogen on the methyl substituent is called a *benzyl group*.

phenyl group

benzyl group

Benzene undergoes substitution reactions that retain the cyclic conjugation as opposed to electrophilic addition reactions.

5.1.1 Hückel's Rule

If a compound does not meet all the following criteria, it is likely not aromatic.

1. The molecule is cyclic.
2. The molecule is planar.
3. The molecule is fully conjugated (i.e. p orbitals at every atom in the ring; ORG 1.4).
4. The molecule has $4n + 2$ π electrons.

If rules 1., 2. and/or 3. are broken, then the molecule is non-aromatic. If rule 4. is broken then the molecule is antiaromatic.

Notice that the number of π delocalized electrons must be even but NOT a multiple of 4. So $4n + 2$ number of π electrons, where n = 0, 1, 2, 3, and so on, is known as Hückel's Rule. Thus the number of pi electrons can be 2, 6, 10, etc. Of course, benzene is aromatic (6 electrons, from 3 double bonds), but cyclobutadiene is not, since the number of π delocalized electrons is 4. Note that a cyclic molecule with conjugated double bonds in a monocyclic (= 1 ring) hydrocarbon is called an annulene. So cyclobutadiene can be called [4]annulene.

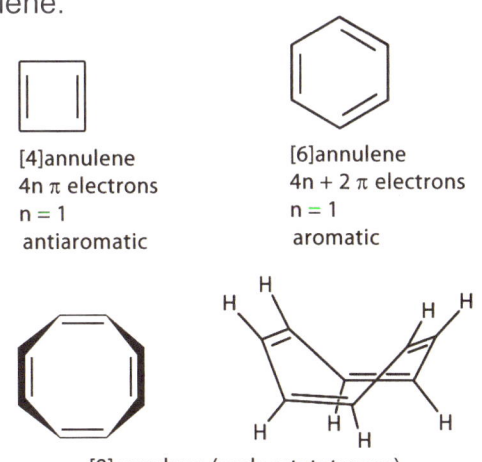

[4]annulene
$4n$ π electrons
n = 1
antiaromatic

[6]annulene
$4n + 2$ π electrons
n = 1
aromatic

[8]annulene (cyclooctatetraene)
$4n$ π electrons, n = 2
non-planar "tub shape"
non-aromatic

A GAMSAT question on Hückel's rule would normally be preceded by Hückel's rule. The point is to verify that you understand its application. There is no need to memorize Hückel's rule.

THE BIOLOGICAL SCIENCES ORG-53

The number of p orbitals and the number of π electrons can be different, which means, whether a molecule is neutral, a cation or an anion, it can be aromatic. Note that aliphatic describes all compounds that are aromatic. A cyclic compound containing only 4n electrons is said to be anti-aromatic.

- Cyclopentadienide anion:

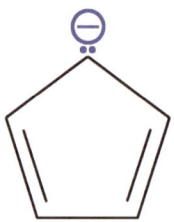

Because of the lone pair, there are 6 π electrons, which meets Hückel's number, so it is aromatic. Thus you can see that if an electron pair is added, or subtracted, a molecule can then become aromatic by fulfilling Hückel's rule. Therefore, if 2 electrons are added to [8]annalene, it will then become a more stable molecule. Specifically, the cyclooctatetraenide dianion ($C_8H_8^{2-}$) is aromatic (thus it has increased stability), and planar, like the cyclopentadienide anion, and both fulfill Hückel's rule.

- Cycloheptatrienyl cation:

6 π electrons with conjugation through resonance because of the cation, meets Hückel's number, so it is aromatic.

Heterocyclic compounds (usu. = a ring with C + another atom) can also be aromatic.

- Pyridine:

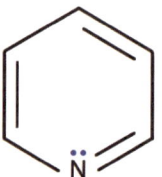

Each sp^2 hybridized carbon atom has a p orbital and contains one π electron. The nitrogen atom is also sp^2 hybridized and has one electron in the p orbital, bringing the total to six π electrons. The nitrogen nonbonding electron pair is in a sp^2 orbital perpendicular to other p orbitals and is not involved with the π system. Thus pyridine is aromatic.

- Pyrrole:

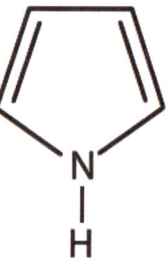

Each sp^2 hybridized carbon atom has a p orbital and contains one π electron. The nitrogen atom is also sp^2 hybridized with its nonbonding electron pair sitting in the p orbital, bringing the total to six π electrons. Thus pyrrole is aromatic.

5.2 Electrophilic Aromatic Substitution

One important reaction of aromatic compounds is known as electrophilic aromatic substitution, which occurs with electrophilic reagents. The reaction is similar to a S_N1 mechanism in that an addition leads to a rearrangement which produces a substitution. However, in this case it is the electrophile (*not a nucleophile*) which substitutes for an atom in the original molecule. The reaction may be summarized:

Note that the intermediate positive charge is stabilized by resonance.

It is important to understand that the electrophile used in electrophilic aromatic substitution must always be a powerful electrophile. After all, the resonance stabilized aromatic ring is resistant to many types of routine chemical reactions (i.e. oxidation with $KMnO_4$ – ORG 4.2.2, electrophilic addition with acid - ORG 4.2.1, and hydrogenation - ORG 4.2.3). Remembering that Br, a halide, is already very electronegative (CHM 2.3), Br^+ is an example of a powerful electrophile. In a reaction called bromination, $Br_2/FeBr_3$ is used to generate the Br^+ species which adds to the aromatic ring. Similar reactions are performed to "juice up" other potential substituents (i.e. alkyl, acyl, iodine, etc.) to become powerful electrophiles to add to the aromatic ring.

- Aromatic halogenation: The benzene ring with its 6 π electrons in a conjugated system acts as an electron nucleophile (electron donor) in most chemical reactions. It reacts with bromine, chlorine or iodine to produce mono-substituted products. Fluorine is too reactive and tends to produce multi-substituted products. Therefore, the electrophilic substitution reaction is characteristic of aromaticity and can be used as a diagnostic tool to test the presence of an aromatic ring.

benzene + X₂ →(Fe or FeX₃) halobenzene-X + HX

(X = Cl or Br)

- **Aromatic nitration**: The aromatic ring can be nitrated when reacted with a mixture of nitric and sulfuric acid. The benzene ring reacts with the electrophile in this reaction, the nitronium ion NO_2^+, yielding a carbocation intermediate in a similar way as the aromatic halogenation reaction.

benzene + HNO_3 →(H_2SO_4 catalyst, 50 °C) nitrobenzene (NO_2)

- **Aromatic sulfonation**: Aromatic rings can react with a mixture of sulfuric acid and sulfur trioxide (H_2SO_4/SO_3) to form sulfonic acid. The electrophile in this reaction is either HSO_3 or SO_3.

benzene →(H_2SO_4/SO_3, $-H_2O$) benzenesulfonic acid (SO_3H)

- **Friedel-Crafts alkylation**: This is an electrophilic aromatic substitution in which the benzene ring is alkylated when it reacts with an alkyl halide. The benzene ring attacks the alkyl cation electrophile, yielding an alkyl-substituted benzene product.

There are several limitations to this reaction:

1. The reaction does not proceed on an aromatic ring that has a strong deactivating substituent group.
2. Because the product is attacked even faster by alkyl carbocations than the starting material, poly-alkylation is often observed.
3. Skeletal rearrangement of the alkyl group sometimes occurs. A hydride shift or an alkyl shift may produce a more stable carbocation (see ORG 4.2.1).

$R-Cl + FeCl_3 \longrightarrow R^+ + FeCl_4^-$

→(- HCl, catalyst regenerated)

- **Friedel-Crafts acylation**: An electrophilic aromatic substitution in which the benzene ring is acylated when an acyl group is introduced to the ring. The mechanism is similar to that of Friedel-Crafts alkylation. The electrophile is an acyl cation generated by the reaction between the acyl halide and $AlCl_3$. Because the product is less reactive than the starting material, only mono-substitution is observed.

CHEMISTRY

When groups are attached to the aromatic ring, the intermediate charge delocalization is affected. Thus nature of first substituent on the ring determines the position of the second substituent. Substituents can be classified into three classes: ortho-para (o-p) directing activators, ortho-para directing deactivators, and meta-directing deactivators. As implied, these groups indicate where most of the electrophile will end up in the reaction.

5.2.1 O-P Directors

If a substituted benzene reacts more rapidly than a benzene alone, the substituent group is said to be an <u>activating group</u>. Activating groups can *donate* electrons to the ring.

Thus the ring is more attractive to an electrophile. All activating groups are o/p directors. Some examples are $-OH, -NH_2, -OR, -NR_2$, -OCOR and alkyl groups.

Note that the partial electron density (δ^-) is at the ortho and para positions, so the electrophile favors attack at these positions. Good stabilization results with a substituent at the ortho or para positions:

THE BIOLOGICAL SCIENCES ORG-57

When there is a substituent at the meta position, the –OH can no longer help to delocalize the positive charge, so the o-p positions are favored over the meta:

Note that even though the substituents are o-p directors, probability suggests that there will still be a small percentage of the electrophile that will add at the meta position.

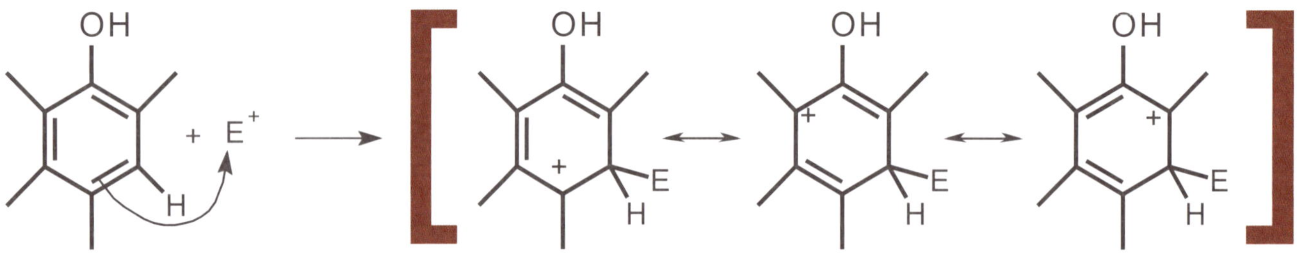

5.2.2 Meta Directors

If a substituted benzene reacts more slowly than the benzene alone, the substituent group is said to be a <u>deactivating group</u>. Deactivating groups can *withdraw* electrons from the ring. Thus the ring is less attractive to an electrophile. All deactivating groups are meta directors, with the exception of the weakly deactivating halides which are o–p directors (-F, -Cl, -Br, -I). Some examples of meta directors are $-NO_2$, $-SO_2$, $-CN$, $-SO_3H$, $-COOH$, -COOR, -COR, CHO.

Without any substituents, the partial positive charge density (δ+) will be at the o–p positions. Thus the electrophile avoids the positive charge and favors attack at the meta position:

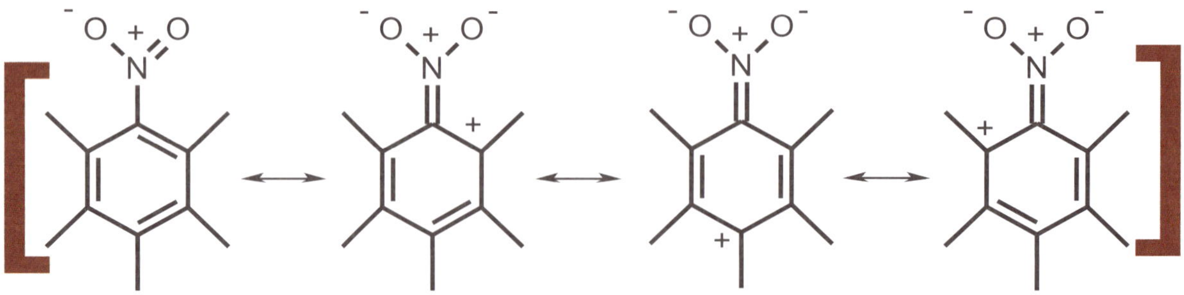

If you are seeking another way to learn, consider logging into your GAMSAT-prep.com account and clicking on Videos to choose the Aromatic Chemistry videos.

With a substituent at the meta position:

Note that even though the substituents are meta directors, probability suggests that there will still be a smaller percentage of the electrophile that will add at the o–p positions.

5.2.3 Reactions with the Alkylbenzene Side Chain

- Oxidation: Alkyl groups on the benzene ring react rapidly with oxidizing agents and are converted into a carboxyl group. The net result is the conversion of an alkylbenzene into benzoic acid.

aromatic ring with alkyl substituent → benzoic acid

- Bromination: NBS (N-bromosuccinimide) reacts with alkylbenzene through a radical chain mechanism (ORG 3.2.2): the benzyl radical generated from NBS in the presence of benzoyl peroxide reacts with Br_2 to yield the final product and bromine radical, which will cycle back into the reaction to act as a radical initiator. The reaction occurs exclusively at the benzyl position because the benzyl radical is highly stabilized through different forms of resonance.

- Reduction: Reductions of aryl alkyl ketones in the presence of H_2 and Pd/C can be used to convert the aryl alkyl ketone generated by the Friedel-Crafts acylation reaction into an alkylbenzene.

Go online to GAMSAT-prep.com for chapter review Q&A and forum.

GOLD NOTES

ALCOHOLS

Chapter 6

Memorize	Understand	Not Required*
AC nomenclature ical properties ucts of oxidation ne: steric hindrance	* Trends based on length, branching * Effect of hydrogen bonds * Mechanisms of reactions * Nucleophilic substitution	* Advanced level college info

GAMSAT-Prep.com

Introduction

An alcohol is any organic compound in which a hydroxyl group (-OH) is bound to a carbon atom of an alkyl or substituted alkyl group.

Additional Resources

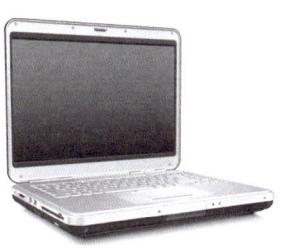

Free Online Q&A + Forum

Video: Online or DVD

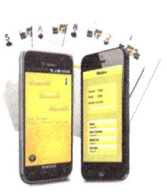

Flashcards

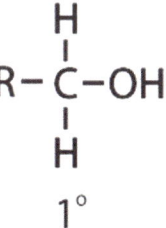

Special Guest

THE BIOLOGICAL SCIENCES   ORG-61

* The real GAMSAT may have advanced level information presented (ie. in a passage) but previous knowledge of said information is not required to answer the questions that would follow. Practice ACER and GS practice GAMSATs can help you clarify this point.

6.1 Description and Nomenclature

The systematic naming of alcohols is accomplished by replacing the –e of the corresponding alkane with –ol.

Alcohols are compounds that have hydroxyl groups bonded to a saturated carbon atom with the general formula ROH. It can be thought of as a substituted water molecule, with one of the water hydrogens replaced with an alkyl group R. Alcohols are classified as primary (1°), secondary (2°) or tertiary (3°):

```
    H              H              R
    |              |              |
R – C – OH    R – C – OH    R – C – OH
    |              |              |
    H              R              R
    1°             2°             3°
```

As with alkanes, special names are used for branched groups:

```
         OH                         OH
         |                          |
CH₃ — CH — CH₃              CH₃ — C — CH₃
                                   |
                                   CH₃
IUPAC: propan-2-ol          IUPAC: 2-methylpropan-2-ol
 • Isopropanol              • 2-methyl-2-propanol
 • Isopropyl alcohol        • tert-butanol
```

The alcohols are always numbered to give the carbon with the attached hydroxy (–OH) group the lowest number (choose the longest carbon chain that contains the hydroxyl group as the parent):

```
              OH
              |
CH₃CH₂CH₂CHCH₂CH₃
3-hexanol NOT 4-hexanol
```

```
         CH₃    OH     CH₃
         |      |      |
CH₃CH₂CH₂ CHCH₂ CHCH₂ CHCH₃
         2,6-dimethyl-4-nonanol
```

The shorthand for methanol is MeOH, and the shorthand for ethanol is EtOH. Alcohols are weak acids ($K_a \approx 10^{-18}$), being weaker acids than water. Their conjugate bases are called alkoxides, very little of which will be present in solution:

$$C_2H_5OH + OH^- \rightleftharpoons C_2H_5O^- + H_2O$$
ethanol   *ethoxide*

The acidity of an alcohol decreases with increasing number of attached carbons. Thus CH_3OH is more acidic than CH_3CH_2OH; and CH_3CH_2OH (a primary alcohol) is more acidic than $(CH_3)_2CHOH$ (a secondary alcohol), which is, in turn, more acidic than $(CH_3)_3COH$ (a tertiary alcohol).

Alcohols have higher boiling points and a greater solubility than comparable alkanes, alkenes, aldehydes, ketones and alkyl halides. The higher boiling point and greater solubility is due to the greater polarity and hydrogen bonding of the alcohol. In alcohols, hydrogen bonding is a weak association of the –OH proton of one molecule, with the oxygen of another. To form the hydrogen bond, both a donor, and an acceptor are required:

```
donor                              H    acceptor
                                   |
            O — H - - - O
            |      δ⁺    δ⁻    |
            CH₃                CH₃
```

ORG-62   ALCOHOLS

Sometimes an atom may act as both a donor and acceptor of hydrogen bonds. One example of this is the oxygen atom in an alcohol:

$$\begin{array}{c} R \quad\quad R \quad\quad R \\ | \quad\quad | \quad\quad | \\ O \quad\quad O \quad\quad O \\ \cdots H \quad H \quad H \cdots \end{array}$$

hydrogen bonds

As the length of the carbon chain (= R) of the alcohol molecule increases, the nonpolar chain becomes more meaningful, and the alcohol becomes less water soluble. The hydroxyl group of a primary alcohol is able to form hydrogen bonds with molecules such as water more easily than the hydroxyl group of a tertiary alcohol. The hydroxyl group of a tertiary alcohol is crowded by the surrounding methyl groups and thus its ability to participate in hydrogen bonds is lessened. As well, in solution, primary alcohols are more acidic than secondary alcohols, and secondary alcohols are more acidic than tertiary alcohols. In the gas phase, however, the order of acidity is reversed.

6.1.1 Acidity and Basicity of Alcohols

Alcohols are both weakly acidic and weakly basic. Alcohols can dissociate into a proton and its conjugate base, the alkoxy ion (alkoxide, RO⁻), just as water dissociates into a proton and a hydroxide ion. As weak acids, alcohols act as proton donors, thus $ROH + H_2O \rightarrow RO^- + H_3O^+$. As weak bases, alcohols act as proton acceptors, thus $ROH + HX \rightarrow ROH_2^+ + X^-$.

Substituent effects are important in determining alcohol acidity. The more easily the alkoxide ion is accessible to a water molecule, the easier it is stabilized through solvation (CHM 5.3), the more its formation is favored, and the greater the acidity of the alcohol molecule. For example $(CH_3)_3COH$ is less acidic than CH_3OH.

Inductive effects are also important in determining alcohol acidity. Electron-withdrawing groups stabilize an alkoxide anion by spreading out the charge, thus making the alcohol molecule more acidic. Vice versa, electron-donating groups destabilize an alkoxide anion, thus making the alcohol molecule less acidic. For example $(CH_3)_3COH$ is less acidic than $(CF_3)_3OH$.

Since alcohols are weak acids, they do not react with weak bases. However, they do react with strong bases such as NaH, NaNH₂, or sodium or potassium metal.

$CH_3CH_2OH + NaH \rightarrow CH_3CH_2O^-Na^+ + H_2$

$CH_3CH_2OH + NaNH_2 \rightarrow CH_3CH_2OH + NH_3$

$2CH_3CH_2OH + 2Na \rightarrow 2CH_3CH_2O^-Na^+ + H_2$

6.1.2 Synthesis of Alcohols

1. **Hydration of alkenes:** Alcohols can be prepared through the hydration of alkenes: **(1)** Halohydrin (one carbon with a halogen and an adjacent carbon with a hydroxyl substituent) formation yields a Markovnikoff hydration product with anti stereospecificity (i.e. the OH nucleophile adds to the most substituted carbon but *opposite* to the halide); **(2)** Hydroboration-oxidation yields a syn stereospecific anti-Markovnikoff hydration product (the OH adds to the least substituted carbon); **(3)** Oxymercuration-reduction yields a Markovnikoff hydration product.

2. **Reduction of carbonyl compounds:** An alcohol can be prepared through the reduction of an aldehyde, ketone, carboxylic acid or ester. Aldehydes are converted into primary alcohols and ketones are converted into secondary alcohols in the presence of reducing agents $NaBH_4$ or $LiAlH_4$ (also symbolized as LAH or LithAl). Since $LiAlH_4$ is more powerful and more reactive than $NaBH_4$, it can be used as a reducing agent for the reduction of carboxylic acids and esters to give primary alcohols (see ORG 6.2.2).

3. **Addition reaction with Grignard reagents:** Grignard reagents (RMgX) react with carbonyl compounds to give alcohols. Grignard reagents are created by reacting Mg metal with alkyl (aryl or vinyl) halide.

$$R\text{-}X + Mg \longrightarrow RMgX$$

A number of different alcohol products can be obtained from Grignard reactions with formaldehyde, other aldehydes, ketones or esters. A carboxylic acid does not give an alcohol product because, instead of addition reaction, the carboxylic acid reacts with the Grignard reagent giving a hydrocarbon and magnesium salt of the acid.

- <u>Formaldehyde</u>: Primary alcohol

For alkene hydration, reduction of carbonyl, addition with Grignards, and the other reactions, follow the story, follow the geometry, follow the substituents (R, R', R'', etc.) as you have been doing with the other chapters. It is extremely unlikely to be asked a GAMSAT question that requires the memorization of a reagent (= the chemical added to bring about the reaction, i.e. Grignard, ether, catalysts, etc.).

ORGANIC CHEMISTRY

- Aldehyde: Secondary alcohol

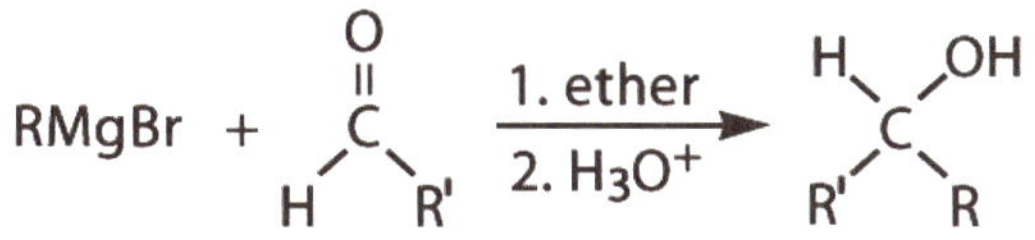

  RMgBr + [aldehyde structure] →(1. ether, 2. H₃O⁺) secondary alcohol

- Ketone: Tertiary alcohol

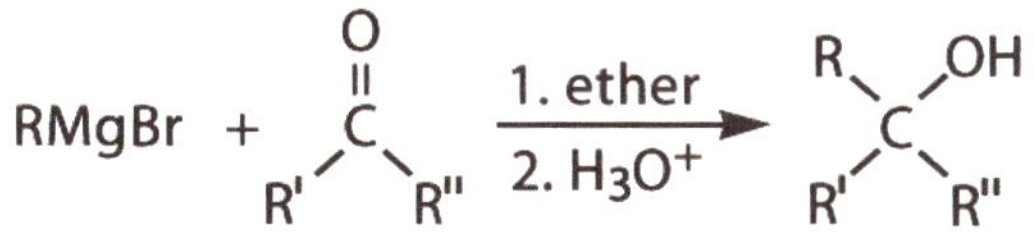

  RMgBr + [ketone structure] →(1. ether, 2. H₃O⁺) tertiary alcohol

- Ester: Tertiary alcohol

  Two substituents from the Grignard reagent are added to the carbonyl-bearing carbon, giving a tertiary alcohol.

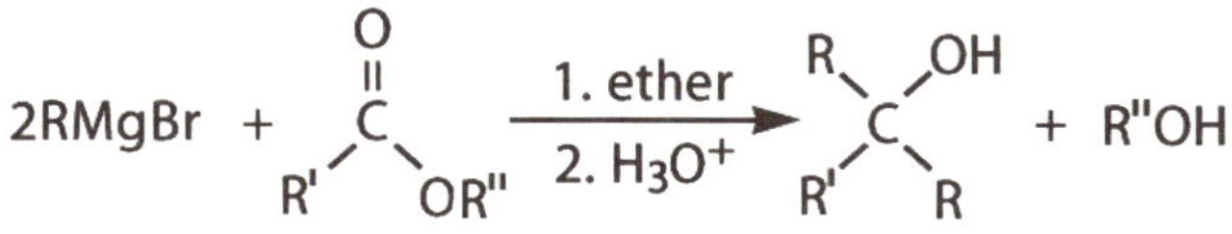

  2 RMgBr + [ester structure] →(1. ether, 2. H₃O⁺) tertiary alcohol + R"OH

6.2 Important Reactions of Alcohols

6.2.1 Dehydration

Dehydration (= *loss of water*) reactions of alcohols produce alkenes. The general dehydration reaction is shown in Figure IV.B.6.1.

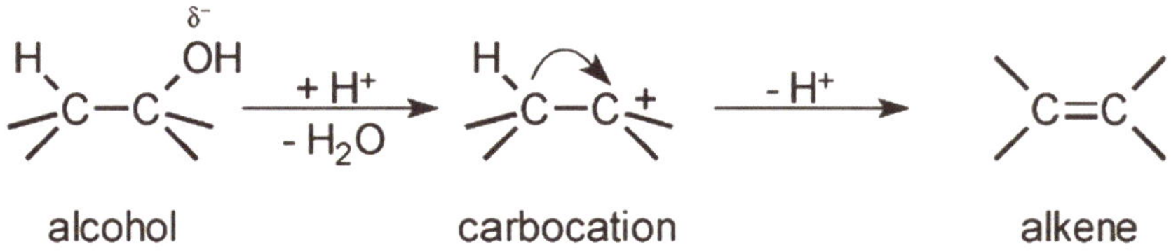

alcohol →(+H⁺, −H₂O) carbocation →(−H⁺) alkene

Figure IV.B.6.1: Dehydration of an alcohol. The proton (H⁺) is attracted to the partial negative charge of –OH thus water is formed which is a good leaving group. Then electrons are attracted to the positively charged carbon causing a proton to leave. Thus the acid (i.e. proton) increases the reaction rate and is regenerated (= *catalyst;* CHM 9.7).

For the preceding reaction to occur, the temperature must be between 300 and 400 degrees Celsius, and the vapors must be passed over a metal oxide catalyst. Alternatively, strong, hot acids, such as H_2SO_4 or H_3PO_4 at 100 to 200 degrees Celsius may be used.

The reactivity depends upon the type of alcohol. A tertiary alcohol is more reactive than a secondary alcohol which is, in turn, more reactive than a primary alcohol. The faster reactions have the most stable carbocation intermediates. The alkene that is formed is the most stable one. A phenyl group will take preference over one or two alkyl groups, otherwise the most substituted double bond is the most stable (= *major product*) and the least substituted is less stable (= *minor product*).

THE BIOLOGICAL SCIENCES ORG-65

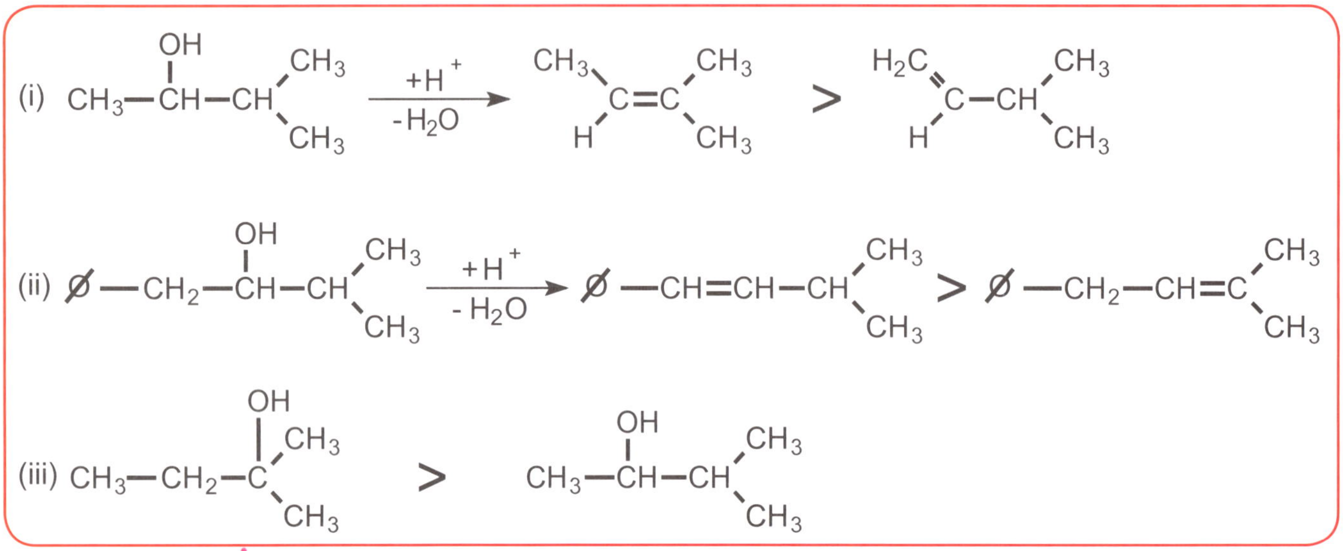

Figure IV.B.6.2: Dehydration of substituted alcohols. Major and minor products, respectively, are represented in reactions (i) and (ii). An example of a reactant with a greater reaction rate due to more substituents as an intermediate is represented by (iii). φ = a phenyl group.

6.2.2 Oxidation-Reduction

In organic chemistry, oxidation (O) is the increasing of oxygen or decreasing of hydrogen content, and reduction (H) is the opposite. Primary alcohols are converted to aldehydes using PCC or $KMnO_4$, under mild conditions (i.e. room temperature, neutral pH). Primary alcohols are converted to carboxylic acids using CrO_3 (the mixture is called a Jones'

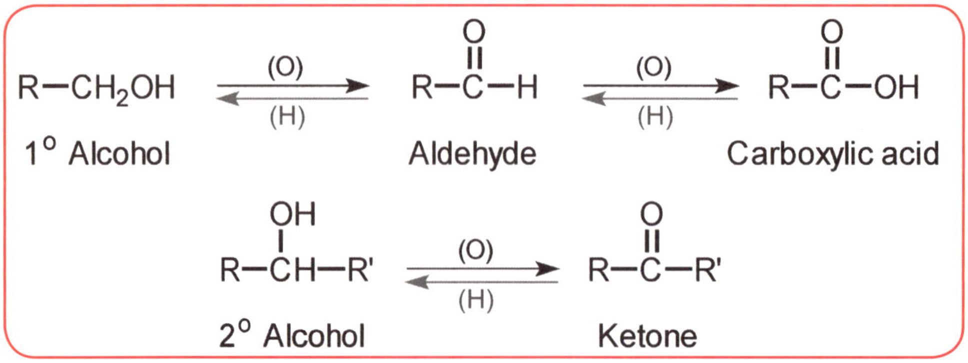

Figure IV.B.6.3: Oxidation-Reduction. In organic chemistry, traditionally the symbols R and R' denote an attached hydrogen, or a hydrocarbon side chain of any length (which are consistent with the reactions above), but sometimes these symbols refer to any group of atoms.

ORG-66 ALCOHOLS

reagent), $K_2Cr_2O_7$, or $KMnO_4$ under abrasive conditions (i.e. increased temperature, presence of OH-). Secondary alcohols are converted to ketones by any of the preceding oxidizing agents. It is *very* difficult to oxidize a tertiary alcohol. Under acidic conditions, tertiary alcohols are unaffected; they may be oxidized under acidic conditions by dehydration and *then* oxidizing the double bond of the resultant alkene. Classic reducing agents (H) include $LiAlH_4$ (strong), H_2/metals (strong) and $NaBH_4$ (mild).

6.2.3 Substitution

In a substitution reaction one atom or group is *substituted* or replaced by another atom or group. For an alcohol, the –OH group is replaced (*substituted*) by a halide (usually chlorine or bromine). A variety of reagents may be used, such as HCl, HBr or PCl_3. There are two different types of substitution reactions, S_N1 and S_N2.

In the S_N1 (*1st order or monomolecular nucleophilic substitution*) reaction, the transition state involves a carbocation, the formation of which is the rate-determining step. Alcohol substitutions that proceed by this mechanism are those involving benzyl groups, allyl groups, tertiary and secondary alcohols. The mechanism of this reaction is:

(i) $R–L \rightarrow R^+ + L^-$
(ii) $Nu^- + R^+ \rightarrow Nu–R$

The important features of this reaction are:

- The reaction is first order (this means that the rate of the reaction depends only on the concentration of one compound); the rate depends on [R–L], where R represents an alkyl group, and L represents a substituent or ligand.

- There is a racemization of configuration, when a chiral molecule is involved.

- A stable carbonium ion should be formed; thus in terms of reaction rate, benzyl groups = allyl groups > tertiary alcohols > secondary alcohols >> primary alcohols.

- The stability of alkyl groups is as follows: primary alkyl groups < secondary alkyl groups < tertiary alkyl groups.

The mechanism of the S_N2 (*2nd order or bimolecular nucleophilic substitution*) reaction is:

$Nu^- + R–L \rightarrow [Nu----R----L]^- \rightarrow Nu–R + L^-$

There are several important points to know about this reaction:

- The reaction rate is second order overall (the rate depends on the concentration of two compounds); first order with respect to [R-L] and first order with respect to the concentration of the nucleophile [Nu⁻].

- Note that the nucleophile adds to the alkyl group by *backside displacement* (i.e. Nu must add to the *opposite* site to the ligand). Thus optically active alcohols react to give an inversion of configuration, forming the opposite enantiomer.

- Large or bulky groups near or at the reacting site may hinder or retard a reaction. This is called *steric hindrance*. Size or steric factors are important since they affect S_N2 reaction rates; in terms of reaction rates, CH_3^- > primary alcohols > secondary alcohols >> tertiary alcohols.

The substitution reactions for methanol (CH_3OH) and other primary alcohols are by the S_N2 reaction mechanism.

6.2.4 Elimination

Elimination reactions occur when an atom or a group of atoms is removed (*eliminated*) from adjacent carbons leaving a multiple bond:

There are two different types of elimination reactions, E1 and E2. In the E1 (Elimination, 1st order) reaction, the rate of reaction depends on the concentration of one compound. E1 often occurs as minor products alongside S_N2 reactions. E1 can occur as major products in alkyl halides or, as in the following example, to an alcohol:

cyclohexanol

2° carbocation   cyclohexene

The acid-catalyzed dehydration of alcohols is thus an E1 reaction which yields the more highly substituted alkene as the major product. There is a carbocation intermediate formed during the preceding reaction, thus a tertiary alcohol will react faster and yield an alkene in a more stable way than a secondary or primary alcohol.

Secondary and primary alcohols will only react with acids in very harsh condition (75%-95% H_2SO_4, 100 °C). However, they will react with $POCl_3$ converting the –OH into a good leaving group to yield an alkene. This reaction takes place with an E2 mechanism.

In the E2 (Elimination, 2nd order)

ORG-68   ALCOHOLS

ORGANIC CHEMISTRY

reaction, the rate of reaction depends on the concentration of two compounds. E2 reactions require strong bases like KOH or the salt of an alcohol (i.e. *sodium alkoxide*). An alkoxide can be synthesized from an alcohol using either Na(s) or NaH (*sodium hydride*) as reducing agents. The hydride ion H⁻ is a powerful base:

$$R\text{-}OH + NaH \longrightarrow \underset{\text{sodium alkoxide}}{R\text{-}O^-Na^+} + H_2$$

Now the alkoxide can be used as a proton acceptor in an E2 reaction involving an alkyl halide:

$$C_2H_5O^- + H-\underset{H}{\overset{H}{C}}-\underset{Br}{\overset{H}{C}}-CH_3$$
ethoxide   2-bromopropane

$$\longrightarrow \underset{H}{\overset{H}{C}}=\underset{CH_3}{\overset{H}{C}} + C_2H_5OH + Br^-$$
propene   ehanol

In the preceding reaction, the first step (1) involves the base (ethoxide) removing (*elimination*) a proton, thus carbon has a negative charge (*primary carbanion*, <u>very unstable</u>). The electron pair is quickly attracted to the δ⁺ neighboring carbon (2) forming a double bond (note that the carbon was δ⁺ because it was attached to the electronegative atom Br, see ORG 1.5). Simultaneously, Br (*a halide, which are good leaving groups*) is bumped (3) from the carbon as carbon can have only four bonds. {Notice that in organic chemistry the curved arrows always follow the movement of electrons}

The determination of the quality of a leaving group is quite simple: <u>good leaving groups</u> have *strong* conjugate acids. As examples, H_2O is a good leaving group because H_3O^+ is a strong acid, likewise for Br^-/HBr, Cl^-/HCl, HSO_4^-/H_2SO_4, etc.

> Substitution and elimination reactions are the most important mechanisms to understand in GAMSAT Organic Chemistry.

6.2.5 Conversion of Alcohols to Alkyl Halides

Alcohols can participate in substitution reactions only if the hydroxyl group is converted into a better leaving group by either protonation or the formation of an inorganic ester. Tertiary alcohols can be converted into alkyl halides by a reaction with HCl or HBr. This reaction occurs in an S_N1 mechanism.

Primary and secondary alcohols do not react with HCl or HBr readily and are converted into halides by $SOCl_2$ or PBr_3. This reaction occurs in an S_N2 mechanism.

$$RCH_2OH + SOCl_2 \longrightarrow RCH_2Cl + SO_2 + HCl$$
$$RCH_2OH + PBr_3 \longrightarrow RCH_2Br + HOPBr_2$$

> Go online to GAMSAT-prep.com for chapter review Q&A and forum.

THE BIOLOGICAL SCIENCES   ORG-69

GOLD NOTES

ALDEHYDES AND KETONES

Chapter 7

Memorize	Understand	Not Required*
AC nomenclature ox reactions	* Effect of hydrogen bonds * Mechanisms of reactions * Acidity of the alpha H * Resonance, polarity * Grignards, organometallic reagents	* Advanced level college info

GAMSAT-Prep.com

Introduction

An aldehyde contains a terminal carbonyl group. The functional group is a carbon atom bonded to a hydrogen atom and double-bonded to an oxygen atom (O=CH-) and is called the aldehyde group. A ketone contains a carbonyl group (C=O) bonded to two other carbon atoms: R(CO)R'.

Additional Resources

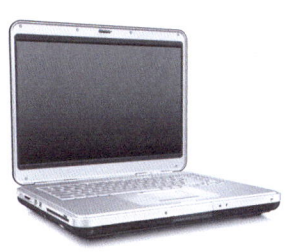

Free Online Q&A + Forum

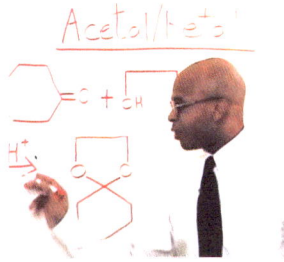

Video: Online or DVD

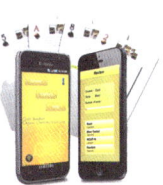

Flashcards

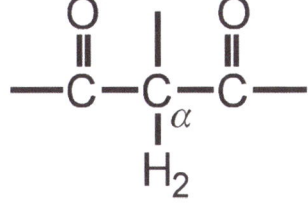

Special Guest

THE BIOLOGICAL SCIENCES   ORG-71

* The real GAMSAT may have advanced level information presented (ie. in a passage) but previous knowledge of said information is not required to answer the questions that would follow. Practice ACER and GS practice GAMSATs can help you clarify this point.

GAMSAT-Prep.com
THE GOLD STANDARD

7.1 Description and Nomenclature

Aldehydes and ketones are two types of molecules, both containing the carbonyl group, C=O, which is the basis for their chemistry.

The carbonyl functional group is planar with bond angles of approximately 120°. The carbonyl carbon atom is sp^2 hybridized and forms three σ bonds. The C=O double bond is both stronger and shorter than the C-O single bond.

The general structure of aldehydes and ketones is:

$$R-\underset{\text{Aldehyde}}{\overset{O}{\underset{\|}{C}}}-H \qquad R-\underset{\text{Ketone}}{\overset{O}{\underset{\|}{C}}}-R'$$

Aldehydes have at least one hydrogen bonded to the carbonyl carbon, as well as a second hydrogen (= *formaldehyde*) or either an alkyl or an aryl group (= *benzene minus one hydrogen*). Ketones have two alkyl or aryl groups bound to the carbonyl carbon (i.e. the carbon forming the double bond with oxygen).

Systematic naming of these compounds is done by replacing the '–e' of the corresponding alkane with '–al' for aldehydes, and '-one' for ketones. For aldehydes, the longest chain chosen as the parent name must contain -CHO group and the -CHO group must occupy the terminal (C1) position. For ketones, the longest chain chosen as the parent name must contain the ketone group and give the lowest possible number to the carbonyl carbon. Common names are given in brackets:

$$\underset{\substack{\text{ethanal}\\\text{(acetaldehyde)}}}{CH_3\overset{O}{\underset{\|}{C}}-H} \qquad \underset{\substack{\text{propanone}\\\text{(acetone)}}}{CH_3\overset{O}{\underset{\|}{C}}CH_3} \qquad \underset{\substack{\text{2-pentanone}\\\text{(methyl propyl ketone)}}}{CH_3\overset{O}{\underset{\|}{C}}CH_2CH_2CH_3}$$

The important features of the carbonyl group are:

- Resonance: There are two resonance forms of the carbonyl group:

$$R-\overset{\overset{\delta^-}{O}}{\underset{\underset{\delta^+}{\|}}{C}}-R' \longleftrightarrow R-\overset{\overset{-}{O}}{\underset{\underset{+}{|}}{C}}-R'$$

- Polarity: Reactions about this group may be either nucleophilic, or electrophilic. Since opposite charges attract, nucleophiles (Nu⁻) attack the δ⁺ carbon, and electrophiles (E⁺) attack the δ⁻ oxygen. In both of these types of reactions, the character of the double bond is altered:

$$R-\overset{\overset{\delta^-}{O}}{\underset{\underset{\delta^+}{\|}}{C}}-R \xrightarrow{E^+} \text{Electrophilic}$$

$$\left[R-\overset{\overset{+O-E}{}}{\underset{\|}{C}}-R \longleftrightarrow R-\overset{\overset{O-E}{}}{\underset{\underset{+}{|}}{C}}-R \right]$$

$$\underset{Nu^-}{} R-\overset{\overset{\delta^-}{O}}{\underset{\underset{\delta^+}{\|}}{C}}-R \xrightarrow{\text{Nucleophilic}} R-\overset{\overset{-}{O}}{\underset{\underset{Nu}{|}}{C}}-R$$

ORG-72   ALDEHYDES AND KETONES

- **Acidity of the α-hydrogen**: The α-hydrogen is the hydrogen attached to the carbon next to the carbonyl group (the α-carbon). The β-carbon is the carbon adjacent to the α-carbon. The α-hydrogen may be removed by a base. The acidity of this hydrogen is increased if it is between 2 carbonyl groups:

$$-\overset{|}{\underset{|}{C}}_\beta-\overset{|}{\underset{H_1}{C}}_\alpha-\overset{O}{\overset{\|}{C}}- \qquad -\overset{O}{\overset{\|}{C}}-\overset{|}{\underset{H_2}{C}}_\alpha-\overset{O}{\overset{\|}{C}}-$$

$$H_2 > H_1 \text{ in acidity}$$

This acidity is a result of the resonance stabilization of the α-carbanion formed. This stabilization will also permit addition at the β-carbon in α-β unsaturated carbonyls (*those with double or triple bonds*):

$$\left[-\overset{|}{\underset{-}{C}}-\overset{O}{\overset{\|}{C}}- \longleftrightarrow -\overset{|}{C}=\overset{O^-}{\underset{|}{C}}- \right]$$

carbanion

resonance stabilization

$$\overset{\diagdown}{\underset{\diagup}{C}}=\overset{|}{\underset{\beta}{C}}_\alpha-\overset{O}{\overset{\|}{C}}- \rightleftharpoons$$

$$\uparrow$$
Nu⁻

α, β unsaturated carbonyl

$$\left[\overset{\diagdown}{\underset{\diagup}{\underset{Nu}{C}}}-\overset{|}{\underset{-}{C}}-\overset{O}{\overset{\|}{C}}- \longleftrightarrow \overset{\diagdown}{\underset{\diagup}{\underset{Nu}{C}}}-\overset{|}{C}=\overset{O^-}{\underset{|}{C}}- \right]$$

Note that only protons at the α position of carbonyl compounds are acidic. Protons further from the carbonyl carbon (β, gamma - γ, and so on, positions) are not acidic.

- **Keto-enol tautomerization**: Tautomers are constitutional isomers (ORG 2.1-2.3) that readily interconvert (= *tautomerization*). Because the interconversion is so fast, they are usually considered to be the same chemical compound. The carbonyl exists in equilibrium with the enol form of the molecule (enol = alk*ene* + alco*hol*). The carbonyl exists in equilibrium with the enol form of the molecule. Although the carbonyl is usually the predominant one, if the enol double bond can be conjugated with other double bonds, it becomes stable (conjugated double bonds are those which are separated by a single bond):

$$-\overset{H}{\underset{|}{\overset{|}{C}}}-\overset{O}{\overset{\|}{C}}- \rightleftharpoons \overset{\diagdown}{\diagup}C=C\overset{OH}{\underset{|}{\diagdown}}-$$

carbonyl   enol

- **Hydrogen bonds**: The O of the carbonyl forms hydrogen bonds with the hydrogens attached to other electronegative atoms, such as O's or N's:

$$\begin{array}{cc} \overset{H-O-H}{\underset{\diagup}{O}} & \overset{H-N-H}{\underset{\diagup}{\underset{|}{O}}} \\ \overset{\|}{\underset{R-C-R'}{}} \quad \text{or} & \overset{\|}{\underset{R-C-R'}{}}\,H \end{array}$$

Since there is no hydrogen on the carbonyl oxygen, aldehydes and ketones do not form hydrogen bonds with themselves.

7.2 Important Reactions of Aldehydes & Ketones

7.2.1 Overview

Since the carbonyl group is the functional group of aldehydes and ketones, groups adjacent to the carbonyl group affect the rate of reaction for the molecule. For example, an electron withdrawing ligand adjacent to the carbonyl group will increase the partial positive charge on the carbon making the carbonyl group more attractive to a nucleophile. Conversely, an electron donating ligand would decrease the reactivity of the carbonyl group.

Generally, aldehydes oxidize easier, and undergo nucleophilic additions easier than ketones. This is a consequence of steric hindrance.

Aldehydes will be oxidized to carboxylic acids with the standard oxidizing agents such as $KMnO_4$, CrO_3 (Jones reagent), HNO_3, Ag_2O (Tollens' reagent). Ketones rarely oxidize. When the Tollens' reagent is used, metallic silver Ag is produced if the aldehyde functional group is present in a molecule of unknown structure, thus making it useful as a diagnostic tool. Therefore, the aldehyde will form a silver precipitate while a ketone will not because ketones cannot be oxidized to carboxylic acid.

There are several methods for preparing aldehydes and ketones. We have already seen ozonolysis (ORG 4.2.2) and the classic redox series of reactions (please review ORG 6.2.2). To add to the preceding is a reaction called "hydroformylation" shown for the generation of butyraldehyde by the hydroformylation of propene:

$$H_2 + CO + CH_3CH=CH_2 \longrightarrow CH_3CH_2CH_2CHO$$

Primary alcohols can be oxidized to yield aldehydes. The reaction is performed with the mild oxidation reagent PCC.

$$CH_3-CH_2-OH \xrightarrow[CH_2Cl_2]{C_5H_5NH^+[CrO_3Cl]^- \text{ (PCC)}} CH_3-\overset{O}{\overset{\|}{C}}H$$

ethanol → ethanal

Secondary alcohols can be oxidized to yield ketones. These reactions are usually performed with PCC, Jones' reagent (CrO_3), and sodium dichromate.

Other reagents include: $K_2Cr_2O_7/H_2SO_4$ or CrO_3/H_2SO_4 or $KMnO_4/OH^-$ or $KMnO_4/H_3O^+$.

Alkenes can be oxidatively cleaved to yield aldehydes when treated with ozone (ORG 4.2.2).

Alkenes can be oxidatively cleaved to

ORGANIC CHEMISTRY

yield ketones when treated with ozone if one of the double bond carbon atoms is di-substituted.

$$CH_3-\underset{CH_3}{\underset{|}{C}}=CH-CH_3 \xrightarrow{\text{1. } O_3}{\text{2. } H^+} CH_3-\overset{O}{\underset{\|}{C}}-CH_3 + CH_3-\overset{O}{\underset{\|}{C}}-H$$

Ketones can also be prepared by Friedel-Crafts acylation of a benzene ring with acyl halide in the presence of an AlCl₃ catalyst (ORG 5.2).

Hydration of terminal alkynes will yield methyl ketones in the presence of mercuric ion as catalyst and strong acids. The formation of an unstable vinyl alcohol undergoes keto-enol tautomerization (ORG 7.1) to form ketones.

$$R-C\equiv C-R \xrightarrow[\text{HgSO}_4]{\text{H}_2\text{O} + \text{H}^\oplus} \left[\underset{H}{\overset{R}{C}}=\underset{R}{\overset{\ddot{O}-H}{C}} \right]$$
addition → enol tautomer

tautomerization ⇌ $R-\underset{H}{\overset{H}{\underset{|}{\overset{|}{C}}}}-\underset{R}{\overset{\ddot{O}}{\underset{\|}{C}}}$
keto tautomer

There are two classes of reactions that will be investigated: nucleophilic addition reactions at C=O bond, and reactions at adjacent positions.

The most important reaction of aldehydes and ketones is the nucleophilic addition reaction. A nucleophile attacks the electrophilic carbonyl carbon atom and a tetrahedral alkoxide ion intermediate is formed. The intermediate can lead to the protonation of the carbonyl oxygen atom to form an alcohol or expel the carbonyl oxygen atom as H_2O or OH^- to form a carbon-nucleophile double bond.

Aldehydes and ketones react with water in the presence of acid or base catalyst to form 1,1-diols, or gem-diols. Water acts as the nucleophile here attacking the carbonyl carbon.

$$CH_3-\overset{O}{\underset{\|}{C}}-H \xrightarrow[H^+]{H_2O} CH_3-\underset{OH}{\overset{OH}{\underset{|}{\overset{|}{C}}}}-H$$

THE BIOLOGICAL SCIENCES   ORG-75

Aldehydes and ketones react with HCN to form cyanohydrin. CN⁻ attacks the carbonyl carbon atom and protonation of O⁻ foms tetrahedral cyanohydrin product.

$$CH_3-CH_2-\overset{O}{\overset{\|}{C}}H + HCN \rightleftharpoons CH_3CH_2\underset{CN}{\overset{OH}{\underset{|}{\overset{|}{C}}}}-H$$
propanal

$$CH_3-\overset{O}{\overset{\|}{C}}-CH_3 + HCN \rightleftharpoons CH_3\underset{CN}{\overset{OH}{\underset{|}{\overset{|}{C}}}}-CH_3$$
acetone

Reduction of aldehydes and ketones with Grignard reagents yields alcohols. Grignard reagents react with formaldehyde to produce primary alcohols, all other aldehydes to produce secondary alcohols, and ketones to produce tertiary alcohols.

$$\overset{\delta^-}{R}-\overset{\delta^+}{MgX} + R-\overset{O}{\overset{\|}{C}}-H(R) \xrightarrow{H^+} R-\underset{R}{\overset{OH}{\underset{|}{\overset{|}{C}}}}-H(R)$$

$$\overset{\delta^-}{R}-\overset{\delta^+}{Li} + R-\overset{O}{\overset{\|}{C}}-H(R) \xrightarrow{H^+} R-\underset{R}{\overset{OH}{\underset{|}{\overset{|}{C}}}}-H(R)$$

$$R-C\equiv C^-Na^+ + R-\overset{O}{\overset{\|}{C}}-H(R)$$

$$\xrightarrow{H^+} R-C\equiv C-\underset{H}{\overset{OH}{\underset{|}{\overset{|}{C}}}}-H(R)$$

Reducing agents such as NaBH₄ and LiAlH₄ react with aldehydes and ketones to form alcohols (ORG 6.2.2). The reducing agent functions as if they are hydride ion equivalents and the H:⁻ attacks the carbonyl carbon atom to form the product.

LiAlH₄ or NaBH₄

$$+ \overset{O}{\underset{H\quad H}{\overset{\|}{C}}} \longrightarrow H-\underset{H}{\overset{OH}{\underset{|}{\overset{|}{C}}}}-H$$

$$+ \overset{O}{\underset{R'\quad H}{\overset{\|}{C}}} \longrightarrow H-\underset{R'}{\overset{OH}{\underset{|}{\overset{|}{C}}}}-H$$

$$+ \overset{O}{\underset{R'\quad R''}{\overset{\|}{C}}} \longrightarrow H-\underset{R'}{\overset{OH}{\underset{|}{\overset{|}{C}}}}-R''$$

7.2.2 Acetal (ketal) and Hemiacetal (hemiketal) Formation

Aldehydes and ketones will form hemiacetals and hemiketals, respectively, when dissolved in an excess of a primary alcohol. In addition, if this mixture contains a trace of an acid catalyst, the hemiacetal (hemiketal) will react further to form acetals and ketals.

An acetal is a composite functional group in which two ether functions are joined to a carbon bearing a hydrogen and an alkyl group. A ketal is a composite functional group in which two ether functions are joined to a carbon bearing two alkyl groups.

This reaction may be summarised:

$$R-\underset{\underset{}{\overset{\overset{O}{\|}}{C}}}{}-R' + R''OH \underset{-H^+}{\overset{+H^+}{\rightleftharpoons}}$$

aldehyde (R' = H)   excess
or ketone (R' = alkyl) alcohol

$$R-\underset{OR''}{\overset{OH}{\underset{|}{\overset{|}{C}}}}-R' \underset{+H_2O}{\overset{+H^+/-H_2O}{\rightleftharpoons}} R-\underset{OR''}{\overset{OR''}{\underset{|}{\overset{|}{C}}}}-R'$$

hemiacetal   acetal
or   or
hemiketal   ketal

The <u>first step</u> in the above reaction is that the most charged species (+, the hydrogen) attracts electrons from the δ⁻ oxygen, leaving a carbocation intermediate. The <u>second step</u> involves the δ⁻ oxygen from the alcohol *quickly* attracted to the current most charged species (+, carbon). A proton is lost which regenerates the catalyst, and produces the hemiacetal or hemiketal. Now the proton may attract electrons from -OH forming H_2O, a good leaving group. Again the δ⁻ oxygen on the alcohol is attracted to the positive carbocation. And again the alcohol releases its proton, regenerating the catalyst, producing an acetal or ketal.

Aldehydes and ketones can also react with HCN (hydrogen cyanide) to produce stable compounds called cyanohydrins which owe their stability to the newly formed C-C bond.

7.2.3 Imine and Enamine Formation

Imines and enamines are formed when aldehydes and ketones are allowed to react with amines.

When an aldehyde or ketone reacts with a primary amine, an <u>imine</u> (or Schiff base) is formed. A primary amine is a nitrogen compound with the general formula $R-NH_2$, where R represents an alkyl or aryl group. In an imine the carbonyl group of the aldehyde or ketone is replaced with a C=N-R group.

The reaction may be summarised:

When an aldehyde or ketone reacts with a secondary amine, an <u>enamine</u> is formed. A secondary amine is a nitrogen with the general formula R_2N-H, where R represents aryl or alkyl groups (these groups need not be identical).

Tertiary amines (of the general form R_3N) do not react with the aldehydes or ketones.

7.2.4 Aldol Condensation

<u>Aldol condensation</u> is a base catalyzed reaction of aldehydes and ketones that have α-hydrogens. The intermediate, an aldol, is both an <u>ald</u>*ehyde* and a *alcoh*<u>ol</u>. The aldol undergoes a dehydration reaction producing a carbon-carbon bond in the condensation product, an *enal* (= alk<u>en</u>e + al<u>dehyde</u>).

The reaction may be summarised:

$$\underset{\text{Aldol}}{-\overset{OH}{\underset{|}{C}}-\overset{H}{\underset{|}{C}}-C=O} \xrightarrow[-H_2O]{H^+} \underset{\text{condensation product}}{-C=C-C=O}$$

Starting materials:
$$-\overset{O}{\overset{\|}{C}}- \;+\; -\overset{|}{\underset{H}{C}}-\overset{|}{C}=O \xrightarrow{NaOH}$$

The reaction mechanism:

$$H-\overset{H}{\underset{H}{\overset{|}{C}}}-\overset{H}{\underset{}{\overset{|}{C}}}=O \;+\; :\overset{-}{\ddot{O}}H$$

$$\longrightarrow H-\overset{H}{\underset{H}{\overset{|}{C}}}-\overset{\cdot\cdot^-}{\underset{}{\overset{|}{C}}}=O$$

$$H-\overset{H}{\underset{H}{\overset{|}{C}}}-\overset{H}{\underset{}{\overset{|}{C}}}=O^{\delta-} \;+\; :CH_2-\overset{H}{\underset{}{\overset{|}{C}}}=O$$

$$\longrightarrow H-\overset{H}{\underset{H}{\overset{|}{C}}}-\overset{:\ddot{O}:^-}{\underset{H}{\overset{|}{C}}}-CH_2-\overset{H}{\underset{}{\overset{|}{C}}}=O$$

$$\longrightarrow H-\overset{H}{\underset{H}{\overset{|}{C}}}-\overset{:\ddot{O}:^-}{\underset{H}{\overset{|}{C}}}-CH_2-\overset{H}{\underset{}{\overset{|}{C}}}=O \;+\; HOH$$

$$\longrightarrow H-\overset{H}{\underset{H}{\overset{|}{C}}}-\overset{OH}{\underset{H}{\overset{|}{C}}}-CH_2-\overset{H}{\underset{}{\overset{|}{C}}}=O \;+\; \overline{O}H$$

An aldol can now lose H_2O to form a β-unsaturated aldehyde via an E1 mechanism.

$$CH_3-\overset{OH}{\underset{H}{\overset{|}{C}}}-CH_2-\overset{H}{\underset{}{\overset{|}{C}}}=O$$

$$\xrightarrow[\Delta]{^-OH} CH_3-C=\underset{H}{\overset{|}{C}}-\overset{H}{\underset{H}{\overset{|}{C}}}=O$$

ORG-78   ALDEHYDES AND KETONES

7.2.5 Conjugate Addition to α-β Unsaturated Carbonyls

α-β unsaturated carbonyls are unusually reactive with nucleophiles. This is best illustrated by example:

Examples of relevant nucleophiles includes CN⁻ from HCN, and R⁻ which can be generated by a Grignard Reagent (= RMgX) or as an alkyl lithium (= RLi).

For example:

Go online to GAMSAT-prep.com for chapter review Q&A and forum.

GOLD NOTES

CARBOXYLIC ACIDS

Chapter 8

Memorize	Understand	Not Required*
IUPAC nomenclature Redox reactions	* Hydrogen bonding * Mechanisms of reactions * Relative acid strength * Resonance, inductive effects * Grignards, organometallic reagents	* Advanced level college info

GAMSAT-Prep.com

Introduction

Carboxylic acids are organic acids with a carboxyl group, which has the formula -C(=O)OH, usually written -COOH or -CO$_2$H. Carboxylic acids are Brønsted-Lowry acids (proton donors) that are actually, in the grand scheme of chemistry, weak acids. Salts and anions of carboxylic acids are called carboxylates.

Additional Resources

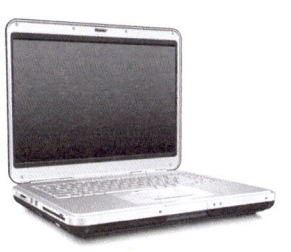

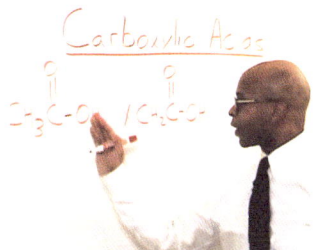

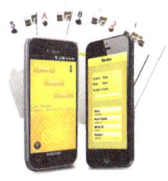

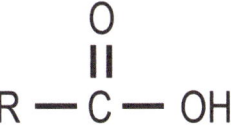

Free Online Q&A + Forum | Video: Online or DVD | Flashcards | Special Guest

THE BIOLOGICAL SCIENCES ORG-81

* The real GAMSAT may have advanced level information presented (ie. in a passage) but previous knowledge of said information is not required to answer the questions that would follow. Practice ACER and GS practice GAMSATs can help you clarify this point.

8.1 Description and Nomenclature

Carboxylic acids are molecules containing the *carboxylic group* (carbonyl + hydroxyl), which is the basis of their chemistry. The general structure of a carboxylic acid is:

$$R-\underset{\underset{\displaystyle OH}{|}}{\overset{\overset{\displaystyle O}{\|}}{C}}$$

Systematic naming of these compounds is done by replacing the '–e' of the corresponding alkane with '–oic acid'. The molecule is numbered such that the carbonyl carbon is carbon number one. Many carboxylic acids have common names by which they are usually known (systematic names in italics):

formic acid / *methanoic acid*
acetic acid / *ethanoic acid*
carbonic acid / *hydroxymethanoic acid*

succinic acid / *butanedioic acid*

benzoic acid / same: *benzoic acid*

Low molecular weight carboxylic acids are liquids with strong odours and high boiling points. The high boiling point is due to the polarity and the hydrogen bonding capability of the molecule. Strong hydrogen bonding has a noticeable effect on boiling points and makes carboxylic acids boil at much higher temperatures than corresponding alcohols. Because of this hydrogen bonding, these molecules are water soluble. Carboxylic acids with more than 6 carbons are only slightly soluble in water, however, their alkali salts are quite soluble due to ionic properties. As well, carboxylic acids are soluble in dilute bases (NaOH or $NaHCO_3$), because of their acid properties. The carboxyl group is the basis of carboxylic acid chemistry, and there are four important features to remember. Looking at a general carboxylic acid:

- The hydrogen (H) is weakly acidic. This is due to its attachment to the oxygen atom, and because the carboxylate anion is resonance stabilized:

resonance forms

- The carboxyl carbon is very susceptible to nucleophilic attack. This is due to the attached oxygen atom, and the carbonyl oxygen, both atoms being electronegative:

- In basic conditions, the hydroxyl group, as is, is a good leaving group. In acidic conditions, the protonated hydroxyl (i.e. water) is an excellent leaving group. This promotes nucleophilic substitution:

$$Nu^- + R-C(=O)-O^+H_2 \longrightarrow R-C(=O)-Nu + HOH$$

- Because of the carbonyl and hydroxyl moieties (i.e. parts), hydrogen bonding is possible both inter- and intramolecularly:

intermolecular (dimerization)

intramolecular

As implied by their name, carboxylic acids are acidic - the most common acid of all organic compounds. In fact, they are colloquially known as organic acids. Organic classes of molecules in order of increasing acid strength are:

alkanes < ammonia < alkynes < alcohols < water < carboxylic acids

In terms of substituents added to benzoic acid, electron-withdrawing groups such as $-Cl$ or $-NO_2$ inductively withdraw electrons and delocalize the negative charge, thereby stabilizing the carboxylate anion and increasing acidity. Electron-donating groups such as $-NH_2$ or $-OCH_3$ donate electrons and concentrate the negative charge, thereby destabilizing the carboxylate anion and decreasing acidity.

The relative acid strength among carboxylic acids depends on the <u>inductive effects</u> of the attached groups, and their proximity to the carboxyl. For example:

$CH_3CH_2-C(Cl)_2-COOH$ *is a stronger acid than* $CH_3CH_2-CH(Cl)-COOH$.

The reason for this is that chlorine, which is electronegative, withdraws electron density and stabilizes the carboxylate anion. Proximity is important, as:

$CH_3CH_2-C(Cl)_2-COOH$ *is a stronger acid than* $CH_3-C(Cl)_2-CH_2COOH$.

Thus the effect of halogen substitution decreases as the substituent moves further away from the carbonyl carbon atom.

8.1.1 Carboxylic Acid Formation

A carboxylic acid can be formed by reacting a Grignard reagent with carbon dioxide, or by reacting an aldehyde with KMnO₄ (*see* ORG 6.2.2). Carboxylic acids are also formed by reacting a nitrile (in which nitrogen shares a triple bond with a carbon) with aqueous acid.

Mechanisms to synthesize carboxylic acids:

- Oxidative cleavage of alkenes/alkynes gives carboxylic acids in the presence of oxidizing reagents such as NaCr₂O₇ or KMnO₄ or ozone.

- Oxidation of primary alcohols and aldehydes gives carboxylic acids. Primary alcohols often react with an oxidant such as the Jones' reagent (CrO₃, H₂SO₄). Aldehydes often react with oxidants such as the Jones' reagent or Tollens' reagent [Ag(NH₃)₂]⁺, also symbolized Ag₂O. Other reagents include: K₂Cr₂O₇/H₂SO₄ or CrO₃/H₂SO₄ or KMnO₄.

- Hydrolysis of nitriles, RCN, under either strong acid or base conditions can yield carboxylic acids and ammonia (or ammonium salts). Since cyanide anion CN⁻ is a good nucleophile in S$_N$2 reactions with primary and secondary alkyl halides, it allows the preparation of carboxylic acids from alkyl halides through cyanide displacement followed by hydrolysis of nitriles. Note that a nitrile hydrolysis reaction increases chain length by one carbon.

$$RCH_2X \xrightarrow{Na^{+-}CN} RCH_2C \equiv N \xrightarrow{H_3O^+} RCH_2COOH + NH_3$$

- Carboxylation of Grignards or other organometallic reagents react with carbon dioxide CO₂ to form carboxylic acids. Alkyl halides react with metal magnesium to form organomagnesium halide, which then reacts with carbon dioxide in a nucleophilic addition mechanism. Protonation of the carboxylate ion forms the final carboxylic acid product. Note that the carboxylation of a Grignard reagent increases chain length by one carbon.

$$RX + Mg \longrightarrow R-Mg-X$$

$$\xrightarrow{CO_2} R-CO_2^- {}^+MgX$$

$$\xrightarrow{H^+} \underset{R}{\overset{O}{\underset{\|}{C}}}-OH$$

Grignard reagents are particularly useful in converting tertiary alkyl halides into carboxylic acids, which otherwise is very difficult.

$$\text{>-Br} \xrightarrow[\substack{2)\ CO_2 \\ 3)\ H_3O^+}]{1)\ Mg,\ ether} \text{>-CO_2H}$$

8.2 Important Reactions of Carboxylic Acids

Carboxylic acids undergo nucleophilic substitution reactions with many different nucleophiles, under a variety of conditions:

$$Nu^- + R-\overset{O}{\underset{\|}{C}}-OH \longrightarrow R-\overset{O}{\underset{\|}{C}}-Nu + OH^-$$

If the nucleophile is –OR, the resulting compound is an ester. If it is –NH$_2$, the resulting compound is an amide. If it is Cl from SOCl$_2$, or PCl$_5$, the resulting compound is an acid chloride.

The typical esterification reaction may be summarized:

$$R'O^*H + R-\overset{O}{\underset{\|}{C}}-OH$$
alcohol acid

$$\longrightarrow R-\overset{O}{\underset{\|}{C}}-O^*R' + H_2O$$
ester

Notice that an asterix* was added to the oxygen of the alcohol so that you can tell where that oxygen ended up in the product (i.e. the ester). In the lab, instead of an asterix (!), an isotope (CHM 1.3) of oxygen is used as a tracer or label.

The decarboxylation reaction involves the loss of the carboxyl group as CO_2:

$$HO-\underset{\underset{R}{|}}{\overset{\overset{O}{\|}}{C}}-\underset{\underset{R}{|}}{\overset{\overset{H}{|}}{C}}-\overset{\overset{O}{\|}}{C}-OH \xrightarrow[\text{heat}]{\text{base}} H-\underset{\underset{R}{|}}{\overset{\overset{H}{|}}{C}}-\overset{\overset{O}{\|}}{C}-OH + CO_2$$

β – diacid

$$R-\overset{\overset{O}{\|}}{C}-\underset{\underset{H}{|}}{\overset{\overset{H}{|}}{C}}-\overset{\overset{O}{\|}}{C}-OH \xrightarrow[\text{heat}]{\text{base}} R-\overset{\overset{O}{\|}}{C}-CH_3 + CO_2$$

β – keto acid

$$LiAlH_4 + R-\overset{\overset{O}{\|}}{C}-OH$$
$$\longrightarrow R-CH_2-OH$$
alcohol

This reaction is not important for most ordinary carboxylic acids. There are certain types of carboxylic acids that decarboxylate easily, mainly:

- Those which have a keto group at the β position, known as β-keto acids.
- Malonic acids and its derivatives (i.e. β-diacids: those with two carboxyl groups, separated by one carbon).
- Carbonic acid and its derivatives.

Carboxylic acids are reduced to alcohols with lithium aluminum hydride, $LiAlH_4$, or H_2/metals (see ORG 6.2.2). Sodium borohydride, $NaBH_4$, being a milder reducing agent, only reduces aldehydes and ketones. Carboxylic acids may also be converted to esters or amides first, and then reduced:

ORGANIC CHEMISTRY

GOLD NOTES

CARBOXYLIC ACID DERIVATIVES
Chapter 9

Memorize	Understand	Not Required*
C nomenclature	* Mechanisms of reactions * Relative reactivity * Steric, inductive effects	* Advanced level college info

GAMSAT-Prep.com

Introduction

Carboxylic acid derivatives are a series of compounds that can be synthesized using carboxylic acid. For the GAMSAT, this includes acid chlorides, anhydrides, amides and esters.

Additional Resources

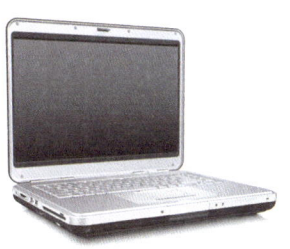

Free Online Q&A + Forum

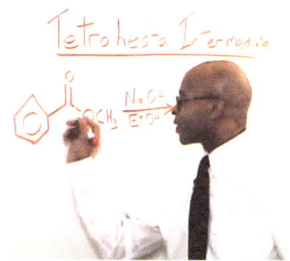

Video: Online or DVD

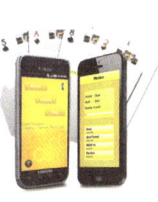

Flashcards

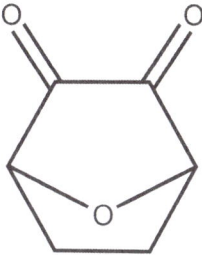

Special Guest

THE BIOLOGICAL SCIENCES   ORG-89

* The real GAMSAT may have advanced level information presented (ie. in a passage) but previous knowledge of said information is not required to answer the questions that would follow. Practice ACER and GS practice GAMSATs can help you clarify this point.

9.1 Acid Halides

The general structure of an acid halide is:

$$R-\overset{\overset{O}{\|}}{C}-X \quad X = \text{Halide}$$

These are named by replacing the 'ic acid' of the parent carboxylic acid with the suffix 'yl halide.' For example:

$$CH_3CH_2CH_2-\overset{\overset{O}{\|}}{C}-Br \quad \text{Butanoyl bromide}$$

$$CH_3-\overset{\overset{O}{\|}}{C}-Cl \quad \text{Acetyl chloride (ethanoyl chloride)}$$

An "acyl" group (IUPAC name: alkanoyl) refers to the functional group RCO-.

Acid chlorides are synthesized by reacting the parent carboxylic acid with PCl_5 or $SOCl_2$. Acid chlorides react with $NaBH_4$ to form alcohols. This can be done in one or two steps. In one step, the acid chloride reacts with $NaBH_4$ to immediately form an alcohol. In two steps, the acid chloride can react first with H_2/Pd/C to form a carboxylic acid; reaction of the carboxylic acid with $NaBH_4$ then produces an alcohol.

Acid halides can engage in nucleophilic reactions similar to carboxylic acids (see ORG 8.2); however, acid halides are more reactive (see ORG 9.6).

Acyl halides can be converted back to carboxylic acids through simple hydrolysis with H_2O. They can also be converted to esters by a reaction with alcohols. Lastly, acyl halides can be converted to amides ($RCONR_2$) by a reaction with amines.

9.1.1 Acid Anhydrides

The general structure of an acid anhydride is:

$$R-\overset{\overset{O}{\|}}{C}-O-\overset{\overset{O}{\|}}{C}-R$$

These are named by replacing the 'acid' of the parent carboxylic acid with the word 'anhydride.' For example:

$$CH_3-\overset{\overset{O}{\|}}{C}-O-\overset{\overset{O}{\|}}{C}-CH_3$$
acetic anhydride
(ethanoic anhydride)

$$CH_3-\overset{\overset{O}{\|}}{C}-O-\overset{\overset{O}{\|}}{C}-H$$
acetic formic anhydride
(ethanoic methanoic anhydride)

Anhydrides can be synthesized by the reaction of an acyl halide with a carboxylate salt and are a bit less reactive than acyl chlorides.

Both acid chlorides and acid anhydrides have boiling points comparable to esters of similar molecular weight.

ORGANIC CHEMISTRY

9.2 Important Reactions of Carboxylic Acid Derivatives

- Nucleophilic acyl substitution reaction: Carboxylic acid derivatives undergo nucleophilic acyl substitution reactions in which a potential leaving group is substituted by the nucleophile, thereby generating a new carbonyl compound. Relative reactivity of carboxylic acid derivatives toward a nucleophilic acyl substitution reaction is amide < ester < acid anhydride < acid chloride. Note that it is possible to convert a more reactive carboxylic acid derivative to a less reactive one, but not the opposite.

- Synthesis of acid halides: Acid halides are synthesized from carboxylic acids by the reaction with thionyl chloride (SOCl$_2$), phosphorus trichloride (PCl$_3$) or phosphorus pentachloride (PCl$_5$). Reaction with phosphorus tribromide PBr$_3$ produces an acid bromide.

- Reactions of acid halides:

1. **Friedel-Crafts reaction:** A benzene ring attacks a carbocation electrophile -COR which is generated by the reaction with the AlCl$_3$ catalyst, yielding the final product Ar-COR.

2. **Conversion into acids:** Acid chlorides react with water to yield carboxylic acids. The attack of the nucleophile water followed by elimination of the chloride ion gives the product carboxylic acid and HCl.

3. **Conversion into esters:** Acid chlorides react with alcohol to yield esters. The same type of nucleophilic acyl substitution mechanism is observed here. The alkoxide ion attacks the acid chloride while chloride is displaced.

4. **Conversion into amides:** Acid chlorides react with ammonia or amines to yield amides. Both mono- and di-substituted amines react well with acid chlorides, but not tri-substituted amines. Two equivalents of ammonia or amine must be used, one reacting with the acid chloride while the other reacting with HCl to form the ammonium chloride salt.

5. **Conversion into alcohols:** Acid chlorides are reduced by LiAlH₄ to yield primary alcohols. The reaction is a substitution reaction of -H for -Cl, which is then further reduced to yield the final product alcohol.

$$\underset{R\ Cl}{\overset{O}{\underset{\|}{C}}} \xrightarrow{LiAlH_4} \underset{R\ H}{\overset{O}{\underset{\|}{C}}} \xrightarrow{LiAlH_4} RCH_2OH$$

Acid chlorides react with Grignard reagents to yield tertiary alcohols. Two equivalents of the Grignard reagent attack the acid chloride yielding the final product, the tertiary alcohol.

$$\underset{R\ Cl}{\overset{O}{\underset{\|}{C}}} + 2\ R'MgX \longrightarrow \underset{R\ OH}{\overset{R'\ R'}{\underset{}{C}}}$$

Acid chlorides also react with H₂ in the presence of Lindlar's catalyst (Pd/BaSO₄, quinoline) to yield an aldehyde intermediate which can then be further reduced to yield an alcohol.

$$\underset{R\ Cl}{\overset{O}{\underset{\|}{C}}} \xrightarrow{\underset{Pd/BaSO_4}{H_2}} \underset{R\ H}{\overset{O}{\underset{\|}{C}}}$$

6. **Synthesis of acid anhydrides:** Acid anhydrides can be synthesized by a nucleophilic acyl substitution reaction of an acid chloride with a carboxylate anion.

- **Reactions of acid anhydrides:** The chemistry of acid anhydrides is similar to that of acid chlorides. Since they are more stable, acid anhydrides react more slowly.

1. **Conversion into acids:** Acid anhydrides react with water to yield carboxylic acids. The nucleophile in this reaction is water and the leaving group is a carboxylic acid.

2. **Conversion into esters:** Acid anhydrides react with alcohols to form esters and acids as in the following example with ethanoic anhydride.

3. **Conversion into amides:** Ammonia attacks the acid anhydride, yielding an amide and the leaving group carboxylic acid, which is reacted with another molecule of ammonia to give the ammonium salt of the carboxylate anion.

ORG-92 CARBOXYLIC ACID DERIVATIVES

ORGANIC CHEMISTRY

4. **Conversion into alcohols:** Acid anhydrides are reduced by LiAlH$_4$ to yield primary alcohols.

$$\underset{R}{\overset{O}{\overset{\|}{C}}}-O-\underset{R}{\overset{O}{\overset{\|}{C}}} \xrightarrow{[H]} RCH_2OH$$

9.3 Amides

The general structure of an amide is:

$$R-\overset{O}{\overset{\|}{C}}-NR'_2$$

These are named by replacing the '-ic (oic) acid' of the parent anhydride with the suffix '-amide.' If there are alkyl groups attached to the nitrogen, they are named as substituents, and designated by the letter N. For example:

$$CH_3-\overset{O}{\overset{\|}{C}}-N\underset{C_2H_5}{\overset{C_2H_5}{\diagup}} \quad \text{N,N-diethylacetamide}$$

$$CH_3CH_2-\overset{O}{\overset{\|}{C}}-NH_2 \quad \text{propanamide}$$

Unsubstituted and monosubstituted amides form very strong intermolecular hydrogen bonds, and as a result, they have very high boiling and melting points. The boiling points of disubstituted amides are similar to those of aldehydes and ketones. Amides are essentially neutral (no acidity, as compared to carboxylic acids, and no basicity, as compared to amines).

Amides may be prepared by reacting carboxylic acids (or other carboxylic acid derivatives) with ammonia:

$$R-\overset{O}{\overset{\|}{C}}-OH + NH_3 + \text{heat} \xrightarrow{-H_2O} R-\overset{O}{\overset{\|}{C}}-NH_2$$

As well, amides undergo nucleophilic substitution reactions at the carbonyl carbon:

$$R-\overset{O}{\overset{\|}{C}}-NH_2 + NuH \longrightarrow R-\overset{O}{\overset{\|}{C}}-Nu + NH_3$$

Amides can be hydrolyzed to yield the parent carboxylic acid and amine. This reaction may take place under acidic or basic conditions:

$$\underset{\text{amide}}{R-\overset{O}{\overset{\|}{C}}-NHR} + H_2O \xrightarrow{H^+} \underset{\text{acid}}{R-\overset{O}{\overset{\|}{C}}-OH} + \underset{\text{amine}}{RNH_2}$$

$$\underset{\text{amide}}{R-\overset{O}{\overset{\|}{C}}-NHR} + H_2O \xrightarrow{OH^-}$$

$$\underset{\text{carboxylate}}{R-\overset{O}{\overset{\|}{C}}-O^-} + \underset{\text{amine}}{RNH_2} \xrightarrow{H^+} \underset{\text{acid}}{R-\overset{O}{\overset{\|}{C}}-OH}$$

Amides can also form amines by reacting with LiAlH$_4$.

Amides can also be converted to primary amines with the loss of the carbonyl carbon. This is known as a <u>Hofmann rearrangement</u>:

$$R-C(=O)-NH_2 \xrightarrow[NaOH]{Br_2} [R-N=C=O] \xrightarrow[-CO_2]{H_2O} R-NH_2$$

9.3.1 Important Reactions of Amides

Amides are much less reactive than acid chlorides, acid anhydrides or esters.

1. **Conversion into acids:** Amides react with water to yield carboxylic acids in acidic conditions or carboxylate anions in basic conditions.

$$R-C(=O)-NR'_2 \xrightarrow[heat]{H_2O} R-C(=O)-OH + R'_2NH$$

2. **Conversion into alcohols:** Amides can be reduced by LiAlH$_4$ to give amines. The net effect of this reaction is to convert an amide carbonyl group into a methylene group (C=O → CH$_2$).

$$LiAlH_4 + R-C(=O)-NH_2 \longrightarrow R-CH(H)-NH_2$$

9.4 Esters

The general structure of an ester is:

$$R-C(=O)-O-R'$$

These are named by first citing the name of the alkyl group, followed by the parent acid, with the 'ic acid' replaced by 'ate.' For example:

$$CH_3-C(=O)-O-CH_3$$
methyl acetate
(methyl ethanoate)

The boiling points of esters are lower than those of comparable acids or alcohols, and similar to comparable aldehydes and ketones, because they are polar compounds, without hydrogens to form hydrogen bonds. Esters with

ORG-94   CARBOXYLIC ACID DERIVATIVES

ORGANIC CHEMISTRY

longer side chains (R-groups) are more nonpolar than esters with shorter side chains (R-groups). Esters usually have pleasing, fruity odors.

Esters may be synthesized by reacting carboxylic acids or their derivatives with alcohols under either basic or acidic conditions:

$$R'O^*H + R-\underset{\underset{O}{\|}}{C}-OH \longrightarrow R-\underset{\underset{O}{\|}}{C}-O^*R' + H_2O$$
alcohol   acid   ester

As well, esters undergo nucleophilic substitution reactions at the carbonyl carbon:

$$R-\underset{\underset{O}{\|}}{C}-OR' + NuH \longrightarrow R-\underset{\underset{O}{\|}}{C}-Nu + R'OH$$

Esters may also be hydrolyzed, to yield the parent carboxylic acid and alcohol. This reaction may take place under acidic or basic conditions.

$$R-\underset{\underset{O}{\|}}{C}-O^*R' + H_2O \xrightarrow{H^+}$$
ester

$$R-\underset{\underset{O}{\|}}{C}-OH + R'O^*H$$
acid   alcohol

Esters can be transformed from one ester into another by using alcohols as nucleophiles. This process is known as <u>transesterification</u>:

[structure: H₂C=C(R¹)-C(=O)-OR²] + [structure: R³R⁴N-R⁵-OH]

$$\xrightarrow[-R^2OH]{catalyst}$$

[structure: H₂C=C(R¹)-C(=O)-O-R⁵-NR³R⁴]

Another reaction type involves the formation of ketones using Grignard reagents. The ketone formed is usually only temporary and is further reduced to a tertiary alcohol due to the reactive nature of the newly formed ketone:

$$CH_3-\underset{\underset{O}{\|}}{C}-OC_2H_5 \xrightarrow{CH_3MgI} \left[CH_3-\underset{\underset{CH_3}{|}}{\overset{\overset{OMgI}{|}}{C}}-OC_2H_5\right] \xrightarrow{-C_2H_5OMgI}$$

$$CH_3-C=O \atop CH_3$$

$$\xrightarrow{CH_3MgI} \left[CH_3-\underset{\underset{CH_3}{|}}{\overset{\overset{OMgI}{|}}{C}}-CH_3\right] \xrightarrow{HOH} CH_3-\underset{\underset{CH_3}{|}}{\overset{\overset{OH}{|}}{C}}-CH_3$$

2-methylpropan-2-ol (*tert*-butanol)

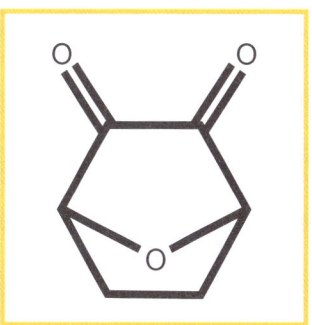

The Ester Bunny

NB: The Ester Bunny is NOT GAMSAT material. In fact for you super-keeners: is the Ester Bunny a real ester? Find out in our Forum!

An important reaction of esters involves the combination of two ester molecules to form an acetoacetic ester (when two moles of ethyl acetate are combined). This is known as the Claisen condensation and is similar to the aldol condensation seen in ORG 7.2.4:

- More reactions with esters: Esters have similar chemistry to acid chlorides and acid anhydrides; however, they are less reactive toward nucleophilic substitution reactions.

1. **Conversion into amides**: Esters can react with ammonia or amines to give amides and an alcohol side product.

$$R-CO-OR' \xrightarrow[\text{base}]{R_2NH} R-CO-NR_2$$

2. **Conversion into alcohols**: Esters can be easily reduced by $LiAlH_4$ to form primary alcohols. A hydride ion attacks the ester carbonyl carbon to form a tetrahedral intermediate. Loss of the alkoxide ion from the intermediate yields an aldehyde intermediate, which is further reduced by another hydride ion to give a primary alcohol final product.

$$LiAlH_4 + R'-CO-OR'' \longrightarrow H-C(OH)(H)-R' + R''O-H$$

Esters can also be reduced to tertiary alcohols by reacting with a Grignard reagent (or alkyl lithium). Grignard reagents add to the ester carbonyl carbon to form ketone intermediates, which are further attacked by the next equivalent of the Grignard reagent. Thus two equivalents of the Grignard reagent (or alkyl lithium) are used to produce tertiary alcohols.

$$2RLi \text{ or } 2RMgX + R'-CO-OR'' \longrightarrow R-C(OH)(R')-R$$

ORG-96   CARBOXYLIC ACID DERIVATIVES

ORGANIC CHEMISTRY

9.4.1 Fats, Glycerides and Saponification

A special class of esters is known as fats (i.e. mono-, di-, and triglycerides). These are biologically important molecules, and they are formed in the following reaction:

$$CH_3(CH_2)_{14}\overset{O}{\underset{||}{C}}O^*H \; + \; \begin{matrix}CH_2OH\\|\\CHOH\\|\\CH_2OH\end{matrix} \xrightarrow{-H_2O^*} \begin{matrix}CH_2O-\overset{O}{\underset{||}{C}}-(CH_2)_{14}CH_3\\|\\CHOH\\|\\CH_2OH\end{matrix} \xrightarrow{-H_2O} || \xrightarrow{-H_2O} |||$$

fatty acid   glycerol   monoglyceride

Fatty acids (= *long chain carboxylic acids*) are formed through the condensation of C2 units derived from acetate, and may be added to the monoglyceride formed in the above reaction, forming diglycerides, and triglycerides. Fats may be hydrolyzed by a base to the components glycerol and the salt of the fatty acids. The salts of long chain carboxylic acids are called <u>soaps</u>. Thus this process is called *saponification*:

$$\begin{matrix}CH_2O-\overset{O}{\underset{||}{C}}-(CH_2)_{14}CH_3\\|\\CHO-\overset{O}{\underset{||}{C}}-(CH_2)_{14}CH_3\\|\\CH_2O-\overset{O}{\underset{||}{C}}-(CH_2)_{14}CH_3\end{matrix} \xrightarrow{3\,NaOH} \begin{matrix}CH_2OH\\|\\CHOH\\|\\CH_2OH\end{matrix} \; + \; 3\,CH_3(CH_2)_{14}CO_2^-Na^+$$

a triglyceride (a fat)   glycerol   salt of the fatty acid

9.5 β-Keto Acids

β-keto acids are carboxylic acids with a keto group (i.e. *ketone*) at the β position. Thus it is an acid with a carbonyl group one carbon removed from a carboxylic acid group.

Upon heating the carboxyl group can be readily removed as CO_2. This process is called *decarboxylation*. For example:

THE BIOLOGICAL SCIENCES   ORG-97

$$\underset{\beta-\text{keto acid}}{R-\overset{O}{\underset{\|}{C}}-CH_2-\overset{O}{\underset{\|}{C}}-OH} \xrightarrow{\text{heat}} \underset{\text{ketone}}{R\overset{O}{\underset{\|}{C}}CH_3} + CO_2$$

9.6 Relative Reactivity of Carboxylic Acid Derivatives

Any factors that make the carbonyl group more easily attacked by nucleophiles favor the nucleophilic acyl substitution reaction. In terms of nucleophilic substitution, generally, carboxylic acid derivatives are more reactive than comparable non-carboxylic acid derivatives. One important reason for the preceding is that the carbon in carboxylic acids is also attached to the electronegative oxygen atom of the carbonyl group; therefore, carbon is more δ^+, thus being more attractive to a nucleophile. Hence an acid chloride (R-COCl) is more reactive than a comparable alkyl chloride (R-Cl); an ester (R-COOR') is more reactive than a comparable ether (R-OR'); and an amide (R-CONH$_2$) is more reactive than a comparable amine (R-NH$_2$).

Amongst carboxylic acid derivatives, the carbonyl reactivity in order from most to least reactive is:

acid chlorides > anhydrides >> esters
> acids > amides > nitriles

The reasons for this may be attributed to resonance effects and inductive effects. The <u>resonance effect</u> is the ability of the substituent to stabilize the carbocation intermediate by delocalization of electrons. The <u>inductive effect</u> is the substituent group, by virtue of its electronegativity, to pull electrons away increasing the partial positivity of the carbonyl carbon.

Within each carboxylic acid derivative, <u>steric or bulk effects</u> also play an important role. The less the steric hindrance, the more access a nucleophile will have to attack the carbonyl carbon, and vice versa.

9.7 Phosphate Esters

Phosphoric acid derivatives have similar features to those of carboxylic acid derivatives. Phosphoric acid and mono- or di-phosphoric esters are acidic. Under acidic condition, these phosphoric esters can be converted to the parent acid H_3PO_4 and alcohols. To see the structure of phosphate esters, see ORG 12.5.

Go online to GAMSAT-prep.com for chapter review Q&A and forum.

ORGANIC CHEMISTRY

GOLD NOTES

ETHERS AND PHENOLS

Chapter 10

Memorize	Understand	Not Required*
nomenclature	* Ether synthesis, electrophilic aromatic substitution	* Advanced level college info

GAMSAT-Prep.com

Introduction

Ethers are composed of an oxygen atom connected to two alkyl or aryl groups of the general formula R–O–R'. A classic example is the solvent and anesthetic diethyl ether, often just called "ether." Phenol is a toxic, white crystalline solid with a sweet tarry odor often referred to as a "hospital smell"! Its chemical formula is C_6H_5OH and its structure is that of a hydroxyl group (-OH) bonded to a phenyl ring thus it is an aromatic compound.

Additional Resources

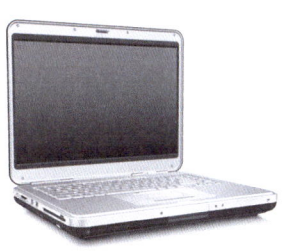

Free Online Q&A + Forum

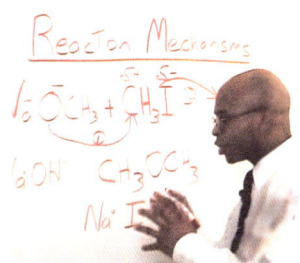

Video: Online or DVD

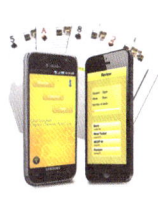

Flashcards

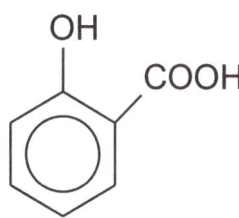

Special Guest

* The real GAMSAT may have advanced level information presented (ie. in a passage) but previous knowledge of said information is not required to answer the questions that would follow. Practice ACER and GS practice GAMSATs can help you clarify this point.

10.1 Description and Nomenclature of Ethers

The general structure of an ether is R-O-R', where the R's may be either aromatic or aliphatic (= *containing only carbon and hydrogen atoms*). In the common system of nomenclature, the two groups on either side of the oxygen are named, followed by the word ether:

$$CH_3-O-CH_3 \qquad CH_3-O-\underset{\underset{CH_3}{|}}{C}HCH_3$$
$$\text{dimethyl ether} \qquad \text{methyl isopropyl ether}$$

In the systematic system of nomenclature, the alkoxy (RO-) groups are always named as substituents:

$$CH_3-O-CH_3 \qquad CH_3-O-\underset{\underset{CH_3}{|}}{C}HCH_3$$
$$\text{methoxy methane} \qquad \text{methoxy isopropane}$$

The boiling points of ethers are comparable to that of other hydrocarbons, which is regarded as relatively low temperatures when compared to alcohols. Ethers are more polar than other hydrocarbons, but are not capable of forming intermolecular hydrogen bonds (those between two ether molecules). Ethers are only slightly soluble in water. However, they can form intermolecular hydrogen bonds between the ether and the water molecules.

Ethers are <u>good solvents</u>, as the ether linkage is inert to many chemical reagents. Ethers are weak Lewis bases and can be protonated to form positively charged conjugate acids. In the presence of a high concentration of a strong acid (especially HI or HBr), the ether linkage will be cleaved, to form an alcohol and an alkyl halide:

$$CH_3-O-CH_3 + HI \longrightarrow$$
$$CH_3-OH + CH_3-I$$

10.1.1 Important Reactions of Ethers

- <u>Williamson ether synthesis</u>: A metal alkoxide can react with a primary alkyl halide to yield an ether in an S_N2 mechanism. The alkoxide, which is prepared by the reaction of an alcohol with a strong base (ORG 6.2.4), acts as a nucleophile and displaces the halide. Since primary halides work best in an S_N2 mechanism, asymmetrical ethers will be synthesized by the reaction between non-hindered halides and more hindered alkoxides. This reaction will not proceed with a hindered alkyl halide substrate:

$$Na^+ \; {}^-OCH_3 + {}^{\delta+}CH_3\text{-}I^{\delta-} \longrightarrow$$
$$CH_3\text{-}O\text{-}CH_3 + Na^+I^-$$

ORG-102   ETHERS AND PHENOLS

ORGANIC CHEMISTRY

Cyclic ethers can also be prepared by reacting an alkene with m-CPBA (meta-chloroperoxybenzoic acid) which can also form an oxirane:

cyclohexene → 1,2-epoxycyclohexane (cyclohexene epoxide)

cyclohexyl methyl ether (methoxycyclohexane)

In a variant of the Williamson ether synthesis, an alkoxide ion displaces a chloride atom within the same molecule. The precursor compounds are called halohydrins. For example, with 2-chloropropanol, an intramolecular epoxide formation reaction is possible creating the cyclic ether called oxirane (C_2H_4O). Note that oxirane is a three-membered cyclic ether (epoxide).

- **Acidic Cleavage**: Cleavage reactions of straight chain ethers takes place in the presence of HBr or HI (or even H_2SO_4) and is initiated by protonation of the ether oxygen.

Primary or secondary ethers react by an S_N2 mechanism in which I⁻ or Br⁻ attacks the protonated ether at the less hindered site. Tertiary, benzylic and allylic ethers react by an S_N1 or E1 mechanism because these substrates can produce stable intermediate carbocations. Please see the following mechanism:

THE BIOLOGICAL SCIENCES ORG-103

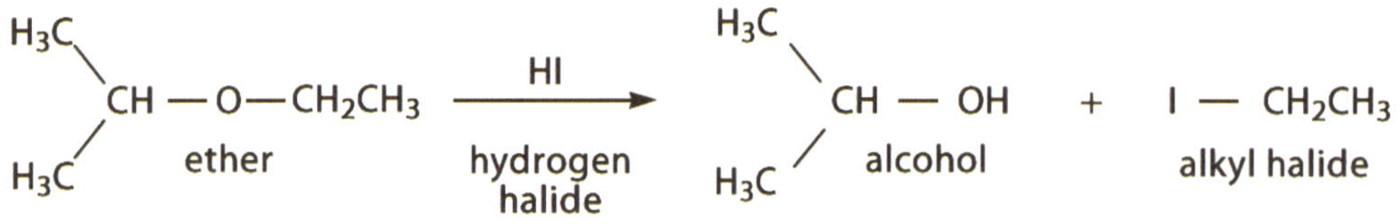

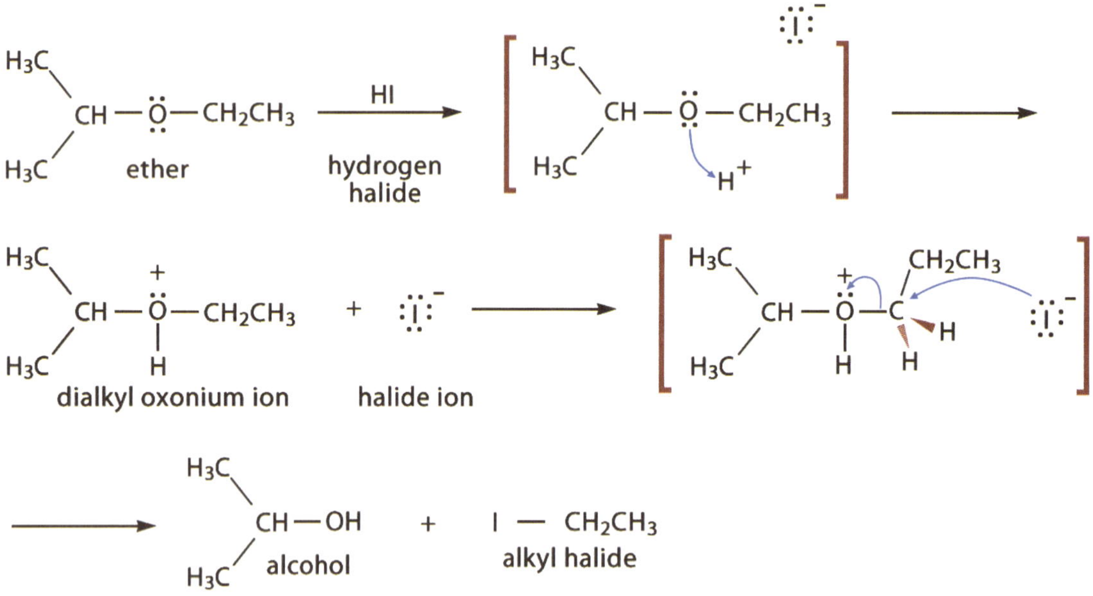

10.2 Phenols

A phenol is a molecule consisting of a hydroxyl (–OH) group attached to a benzene (aromatic) ring. The following are some phenols and derivatives which are important to biochemistry, medicine and nature:

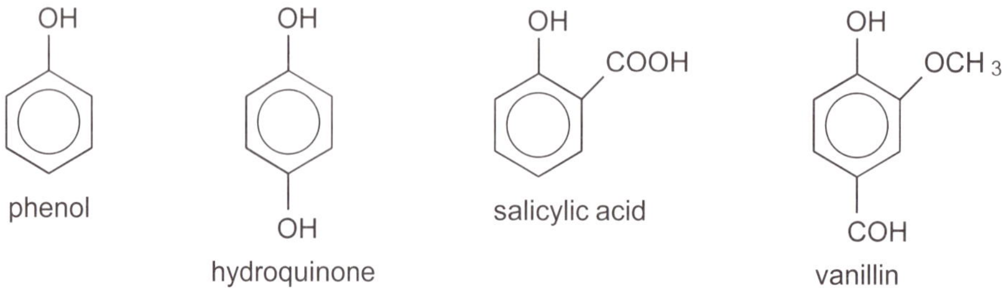

phenol

hydroquinone

salicylic acid

vanillin

Phenols are more acidic than their corresponding alcohols. This is due mainly to the electron withdrawing and resonance stabilization effects of the aromatic ring in the conjugate base anion (the phenoxide ion):

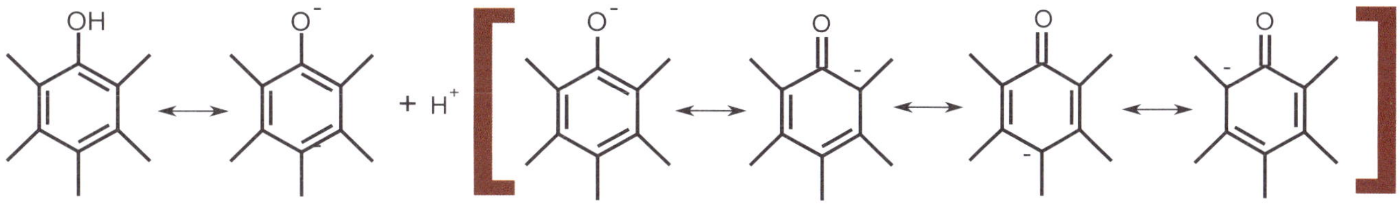

ORGANIC CHEMISTRY

Substituent groups on the ring affect the acidity of phenols by both inductive effects (as with alcohols) and resonance effects. The resonance structures show that electron stabilizing (*withdrawing* or *meta directing*) groups at the ortho or para positions should increase the acidity of the phenol. Examples of these groups include the nitro group ($-NO_2$), $-CN$, $-CO_2H$, and the weakly deactivating o-p directors - the halogens. Destabilizing groups, such as alkyl groups, or other ortho-para directors, will make the compound less acidic. Phenols are ortho-para directors (see ORG Chapter 5).

Phenols can form hydrogen bonds, resulting in fairly high boiling points. Their solubility in water, however, is limited, because of the hydrophobic nature of the aromatic ring. Ortho phenols have lower boiling points than meta and para phenols, as they can form intramolecular hydrogen bonds. However, the para and even the ortho compounds can sometimes form intermolecular hydrogen bonds:

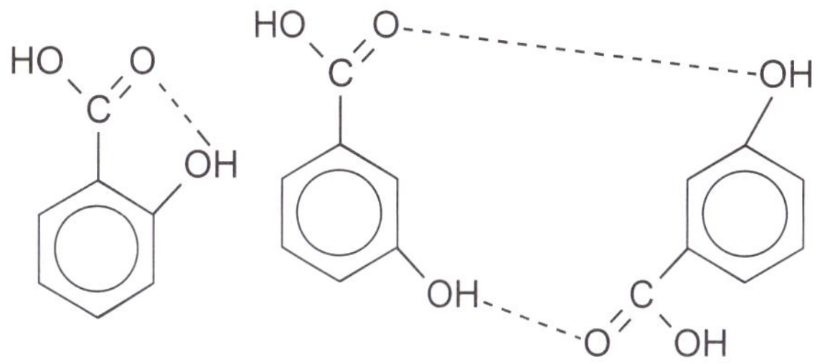

10.2.1 Electrophilic Aromatic Substitution for Phenols

The hydroxyl group is a powerful activating group and an ortho-para director in electrophilic substitutions. Thus phenols can brominate three times in bromine water as follows:

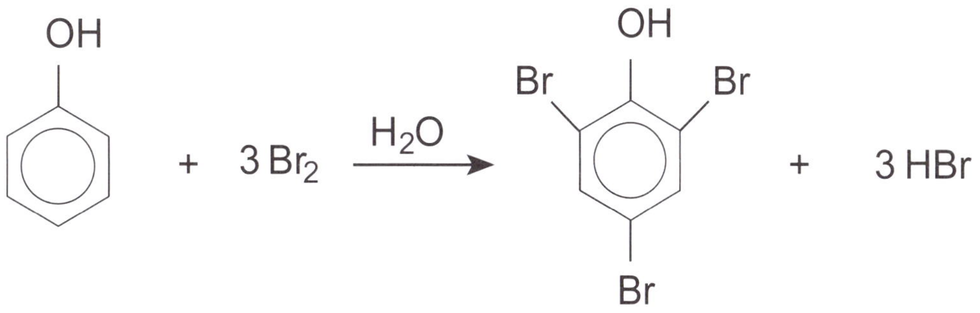

Go online to GAMSAT-prep.com for chapter review Q&A and forum.

THE BIOLOGICAL SCIENCES   ORG-105

GOLD NOTES

AMINES

Chapter 11

Memorize	Understand	Not Required*
IUPAC nomenclature	* Effect of hydrogen bonds * Mechanisms of reactions * Trends in basicity * Resonance, delocalization of electrons	* Advanced level college info

GAMSAT-Prep.com

Introduction

Amines are compounds and functional groups that contain a basic nitrogen atom with a lone pair. Amines are derivatives of ammonia (NH_3), where one or more hydrogen atoms are replaced by organic substituents such as alkyl and aryl groups.

Additional Resources

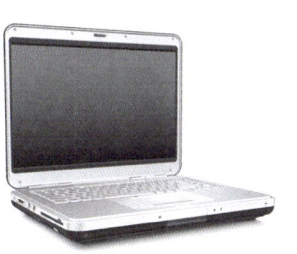

Free Online Q & A

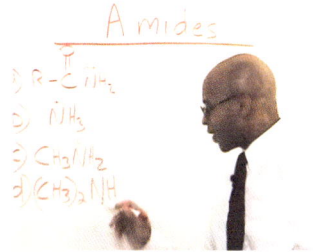

Video: Online or DVD

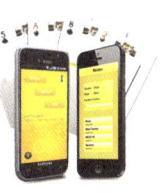

Flashcards

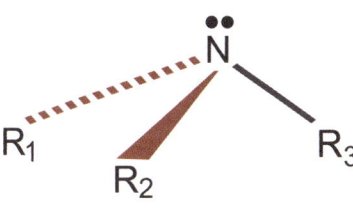

Special Guest

THE BIOLOGICAL SCIENCES   ORG-107

* The real GAMSAT may have advanced level information presented (ie. in a passage) but previous knowledge of said information is not required to answer the questions that would follow. Practice ACER and GS practice GAMSATs can help you clarify this point.

11.1 Description and Nomenclature

Organic compounds with a trivalent nitrogen atom bonded to one or more carbon atoms are called amines. These are organic derivatives of ammonia. They may be classified depending on the number of carbon atoms bonded to the nitrogen:

Primary Amine:	RNH_2
Secondary Amine:	R_2NH
Tertiary Amine:	R_3N
Quaternary Salt:	$R_4N^+ \, X^-$

In the common system of nomenclature, amines are named by adding the suffix '-amine' to the name of the alkyl group. In a secondary or tertiary amine, where there is more than one alkyl group, the groups are named as N-substituted derivatives of the larger group:

$$CH_3 - CH(CH_3) - N(CH_3) - CH_2 - CH_3$$

N, N-methyl ethyl isopropylamine

In the systematic system of nomenclature, amines are named analagous to alcohols, except the suffix '-amine' is used instead of the suffix '-ol'.

When amines are present with multiple asymmetric substituents, they are named by considering the largest group as the parent name and the other alkyl groups as N-substituents of the parent:

N, N-dimethyl-2-butanamine

The $-NH_2$ group is named as an amino substituent on a parent molecule when amines are present with more than one functional group:

4-aminobutanoic acid

The bonding in amines is similar to the bonding in ammonia. The nitrogen atom is sp^3 hybridized (ORG 1.1, 1.2, CHM 3.5). Primary, secondary and tertiary amines have a trigonal pyramidal shape (CHM 3.5). The C-N-C bond angle is approximately 108°. Quaternary amines have a tetrahedral shape and a normal tetrahedral bond angle of 109.5°.

With its tetrahedral geometry, amines with three different substituents are considered chiral. Such amines are analogous to chiral alkanes in that the nitrogen atom will possess four different substituents - considering the lone pair of electrons to be the fourth substituent. However, unlike chiral alkanes, chiral amines do not exist in two separate enantiomers. Pyramidal nitrogen inversion between the two enantiomeric forms occurs so rapidly at room temperature that the two forms cannot be isolated.

11.1.1 The Basicity of Amines

Along with the three attached groups, amines have an unbonded electron pair. Most of the chemistry of amines depends on this unbonded electron pair:

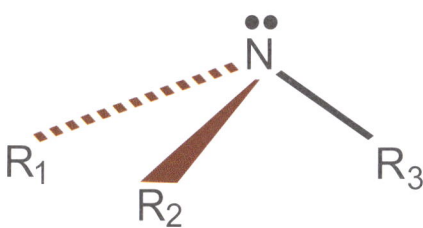

The electron pair is stabilized by the electron donating effects of alkyl groups. Thus the lone pair in tertiary amines is more stable than in secondary amines which, in turn, is more stable than in primary amines. As a result of this electron pair, amines are Lewis bases (see CHM 3.4), and good nucleophiles. In aqueous solution, amines are weak bases, and can accept a proton:

$$R_3N + H_2O \longrightarrow R_3NH^+ + OH^-$$

The ammonium cation in the preceding reaction is stabilized, once again, by the electron donating effects of the alkyl groups. Conversely, should the nitrogen be adjacent to a carbocation, the lone pair can stabilize the carbocation by delocalizing the charge.

The relative basicity of amines is determined by the following:

- If the free amine is stabilized relative to the cation, the amine is less basic.
- If the cation is stabilized relative to the free amine, the amine is more stable, thus the stronger base.

Groups that withdraw electron density (such as halides or aromatics) decrease the availability of the unbonded electron pair. Electron releasing groups (such as alkyl groups) increase the availability of the unbonded electron pair. The base strength then increases in the following series (where Ø represents a phenyl group):

$NO_2-Ø-NH_2 < Ø-NH_2 < Ø-CH_2-NH_2 < NH_3 < CH_3-NH_2 < (CH_3)_2-N-H < (CH_3)_3-N$

Note that a substituent attached to an aromatic ring can greatly affect the basicity of the amine. For example, electron withdrawing groups (i.e. $-NO_2$) withdraw electrons from the ring which, in turn, withdraws the lone electron pair (*delocalization*) from nitrogen. Thus the lone pair is less available to bond with a proton; consequently, it is a weaker base. The opposite occurs with an electron donating group, making the amine, relatively, a better base (see ORG Chapter 5).

11.1.2 More Properties of Amines

- The nitrogen atom can hydrogen bond (using its electron pair) to hydrogens attached to other N's or O's. It can also form hydrogen bonds from hydrogens attached to it with electron pairs of N, O, F or Cl:

```
        H
        |
—N—H ·········· O—H
  |
                 H
                 |
or —N—  ········ O—H
   |
```

Note that primary or secondary amines can hydrogen bond with each other, but tertiary amines cannot. This leads to boiling points which are higher than would be expected for compounds of similar molecular weight, like alkanes, but lower than similar alcohols or carboxylic acids. The hydrogen bonding also renders low weight amines soluble in water.

- A dipole moment is possible:

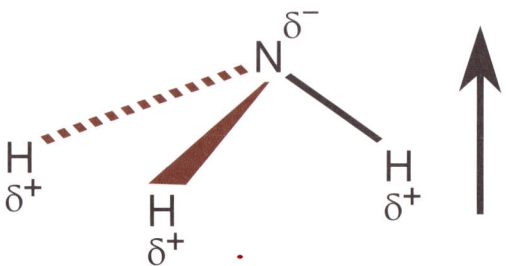

- The nitrogen in amines can contribute its lone pair electrons to activate a benzene ring. Thus amines are ortho-para directors.

- The solubility of quaternary salts decreases with increasing molecular weight. The quaternary structure has steric hindrance and the lone pair electrons on N is not available for H-bonding, thus their solubility is much less than other amines or even alkyl ammonium salts (i.e. $R-NH_3^+X^-$, $R_2-NH_2^+X^-$, $R_3-NH^+X^-$). Quaternary ammonium salts can be synthesized from ammonium hydroxides which are very strong bases.

$$(CH_3)_4N^+OH^- + HCl \longrightarrow (CH_3)_4N^+Cl^- + H_2O$$
Quaternary hydroxide → Quaternary salt

11.2 Important Reactions of Amines

- **Amide formation** is an important reaction for protein synthesis. Primary and secondary amines will react with carboxylic acids and their derivatives to form *amides*:

$$R'NH_2 + R-\underset{\underset{O}{\|}}{C}-OH$$

primary or secondary amine   acid

$$\longrightarrow R-\underset{\underset{O}{\|}}{C}-NHR' + H_2O$$

amide

Amides can engage in resonance such that the lone pair electrons on the nitrogen is delocalized. Thus amides are by far <u>less basic</u> than amines.

$$\left[R-\underset{\underset{O}{\|}}{C}-NR_2 \longleftrightarrow R-\underset{\underset{O^-}{|}}{C}=NR_2^+ \right]$$

As can be seen, the C–N bond has a partial double bond character. Thus there is restricted rotation about the C–N bond.

- **Alkylation** is another important reaction which involves amines with alkyl halides:

$$RCH_2Cl + R'NH_2 \longrightarrow RCH_2NHR' + HCl$$

1°, 2° or 3° amine

Both amide formation and alkylation make use of the nucleophilic character of the electrons on nitrogen.

Thus ammonia or an alkyl amine reacts with an alkyl halide to yield an amine in an S_N2 mechanism. Ammonia produces a primary amine; a primary amine produces a secondary amine; a secondary amine produces a tertiary amine; and tertiary amine produces a quaternary ammonium salt.

$$H-\underset{\underset{R^2}{|}}{\overset{\overset{R^1}{|}}{N:}} + R^3X$$

primary or secondary amine   halogenoalkane

$$\longrightarrow :\underset{\underset{R^2}{|}}{\overset{\overset{R^1}{|}}{N}}-R^3 + HX$$

alkyl-substituted amine   halogen acid
(secondary or tertiary)

> **Note:** Standard notation for R dictates that when you see a subscript (i.e. 2), just like for other atoms or groups, it means that 2 R groups are present. This has a different meaning than a superscript 2 (ORG 1.6) which means that there is only 1 R group at that position but it is different from any other R group with a different superscript. You will also notice on this page: the R prime notation (R') indicating a single R group different from R without the prime symbol (ORG 1.6). Any of the above notations could be used during the GAMSAT.

GAMSAT-Prep.com
THE GOLD STANDARD

$R^3 - \underset{\underset{R^2}{|}}{\overset{\overset{R^1}{|}}{N:}} \quad + \quad R^4X$

tertiary amine   halogenoalkane

$\longrightarrow \quad R^3 - \underset{\underset{R^2}{|}}{\overset{\overset{R^1}{|}}{N^+}} - R^4 \quad + \quad X^-$

halide anion

quaternary ammonium cation

$\underbrace{\qquad\qquad\qquad\qquad\qquad}$
quaternary ammonium salt

- **Gabriel synthesis:** Primary amines can also be obtained from azide synthesis and Gabriel synthesis in an S_N2 mechanism. The azide ion N_3^-, acting as a nucleophile, displaces the halide ion from the alkyl halide to form RN_3, which is then reduced by $LiAlH_4$ to form the desired primary amine.

$R-Cl \xrightarrow[\text{2. LiAlH}_4]{\text{1. NaN}_3} R-NH_2$

Gabriel amine synthesis occurs via a phthalimide ion displacing the halide from the alkyl halide followed by basic hydrolysis of the N-alkyl phthalimide yielding a primary amine.

$\xrightarrow{NH_2NH_2} R-NH_2$

- **Reductive amination:** Amines can also be synthesized by reductive amination in which an aldehyde or ketone reacts with ammonia, a primary amine or a secondary amine to form a corresponding primary amine, secondary amine or tertiary amine.

ORG-112   AMINES

ORGANIC CHEMISTRY

- **Reduction of nitriles:** Nitriles can be reduced by LiAlH$_4$ to produce primary amines. This offers a way to convert alkyl halides into primary amines with one more carbon atom.

- **Reduction of amides:** Amides can also be reduced by LiAlH$_4$ to produce primary amines. Thus carboxylic acids can be converted into primary amines with the same number of carbon atoms.

$$RX \xrightarrow{NaCN} R-C\equiv N \xrightarrow[Pt]{H_2(g)} R-CH_2NH_2$$

$$RCOOH \xrightarrow[\text{2. NH}_3]{\text{1. SOCl}_2} R-\underset{NH_2}{\overset{O}{C}}\!- \xrightarrow[\text{2. H}^+/H_2O]{\text{1. LiAlH}_4/\text{ether}} R-CH_2NH_2$$

Free Gold Standard GAMSAT Organic Chemistry Reactions Summary
Yes, it's online, it's free and it summarizes the most important reactions. You can find the link on the Members home page when you log into your gamsat-prep.com account or you can google it. You can choose to print the page and work through examples changing the different R groups to H's, secondary alkyl groups, aryl groups, etc. to see if you are really following what is happening and that you can name the products. Our Summary page also includes a free YouTube video by Dr. Ferdinand explaining each reaction. Each reaction is also cross-referenced (at the bottom of the page) to a specific section of this textbook for further reading should you wish.

Go online to GAMSAT-prep.com for chapter review Q&A and forum.

GOLD NOTES

BIOLOGICAL MOLECULES

Chapter 12

Memorize
sic structures
electric point equation
fine: amphoteric, zwitterions

Understand
* Effect of H, S, hydrophobic bonds
* Basic mechanisms of reactions
* Effect of pH, isoelectric point
* Protein structure
* Different ways of drawing structures

Not Required*
* Advanced level college info
* Memorizing all the names of amino acids
* Detailed mech. specific to bio molecules

GAMSAT-Prep.com

Introduction

Biological molecules truly involve the chemistry of life. Such molecules include amino acids and proteins, carbohydrates (glucose, disaccharides, polysaccharides), lipids (triglycerides, steroids) and nucleic acids (DNA, RNA).

Additional Resources

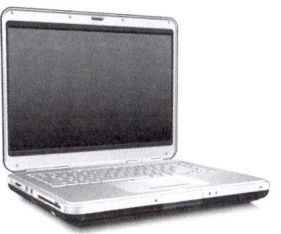

Free Online Q & A

Video: Online or DVD

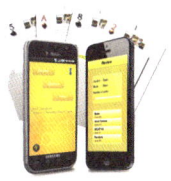

Flashcards

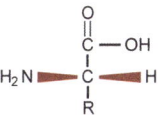

Special Guest

THE BIOLOGICAL SCIENCES ORG-115

* The real GAMSAT may have advanced level information presented (ie. in a passage) but previous knowledge of said information is not required to answer the questions that would follow. Practice ACER and GS practice GAMSATs can help you clarify this point.

GAMSAT-Prep.com
THE GOLD STANDARD

12.1 Amino Acids

Protein-building <u>amino acids</u> are molecules that contain a side chain (R), a carboxylic acid, and an amino group at the α carbon. Thus the general structure of α-amino acids is:

L - amino acid
"left-handed" isomer

D - amino acid
"right-handed" isomer

From your GAMSAT Organic Chemistry review, you should remember that the carbonyl carbon (C=O) is carbon-1 and the adjacent carbon (carbon-2) is the alpha position, carbon-3 is the beta position and carbon-4 is thus the gamma position.

Amino acids may be named systematically as substituted carboxylic acids, however, there are 20 important α-amino acids that are known by common names. These are naturally occurring and they form the building blocks of most proteins found in humans. The following are a few examples of α-amino acids:

Glycine

Alanine

Serine

Aspartic acid

Note that the D/L system is commonly used for amino acid and carbohydrate chemistry. The reason is that naturally occurring amino acids have the same relative configuration, the <u>L-configuration</u>, while naturally occurring carbohydrates are nearly all <u>D-configuration</u>. However, the absolute configuration (i.e. R/S) depends on the priority assigned to the side group (*see* ORG 2.3.1 *for rules*).

In the preceding amino acids, the <u>S-configuration</u> prevails (*except glycine which cannot be assigned any configuration since it is not chiral*).

The following mnemonic is helpful for determining the D/L isomeric form of an amino acid: the "CORN" rule. The substituents **CO**OH, **R**, **N**H$_2$, and H are arranged around the chiral center. Starting with H away from the viewer, if these groups are arranged clockwise around the chiral carbon, then it is the D-form. If counter-clockwise, it is the L-form.

Also note that, except for glycine, the α-carbon of all amino acids are chiral indicating that there must be at least two different enantiomeric forms. Notice in the preceding

ORG-116   BIOLOGICAL MOLECULES

illustrations that the alpha carbon in glycine is not bonded to 4 different substitutents since it is bonded to hydrogen twice; however, the alpha carbon in alanine, serine and aspartic acid has 4 different substituents in each case meaning that carbon is chiral. Notice that chirality of carbon hinges on its attachment to 4 different substituents (i.e. groups/ligands) and NOT necessarily 4 different atoms. A chiral carbon is sometimes referred to as a stereocenter or as a stereogenic or asymmetric carbon.

Many important amino acids can play critical non-protein roles within the body. For example, glutamate and gamma-aminobutyric acid ("GABA", a non-standard gamma-amino acid) are, respectively, the main excitatory and inhibitory neurotransmitters in the human brain (BIO 5.1).

Unless specified otherwise, the following sections will be exploring features of alpha amino acids.

GABA: A gamma-amino acid.
Notice that the amino group is attached to the 3rd carbon from the carbonyl carbon (C=O).

12.1.1 Hydrophilic vs. Hydrophobic

Different types of amino acids tend to be found in different areas of the proteins that they make up. Amino acids which are ionic and/or polar are hydrophilic, and tend to be found on the exterior of proteins (i.e. *exposed to water*). These include aspartic acid and its amide, glutamic acid and its amide, lysine, arginine and histidine. Certain other polar amino acids are found on either the interior or exterior of proteins. These include serine, threonine, and tyrosine. Hydrophobic ('water-fearing") amino acids which may be found on the interior of proteins include methionine, leucine, tryptophan, valine and phenylalanine. Hydrophobic molecules tend to cluster in aqueous solutions (= *hydrophobic bonding*). Alanine is a nonpolar amino acid which is unusual because it is less hydrophobic than most nonpolar amino acids. This is because its nonpolar side chain is very short.

Glycine is the smallest amino acid, and the only one that is not optically active. It is often found at the 'corners' of proteins. Alanine is small and, although hydrophobic, is found on the surface of proteins.

12.1.2 Acidic vs. Basic

Amino acids have both acid and basic components (= *amphoteric*). The amino acids with the R group containing an amino (–NH$_2$) group, are basic. The two basic amino acids are lysine and arginine. Amino acids with an R group containing a carboxyl (–COOH) group are acidic. The two acidic amino acids are aspartic acid and glutamic acid. One amino acid, histidine, may act as either an acid or a base, depending upon the pH of the resident solution. This makes histidine a very good physiologic buffer. The rest of the amino acids are considered to be neutral.

The basic –NH$_2$ group in the amino acid is present as an ammonium ion, –NH$_3^+$. The acidic carboxyl –COOH group is present as a carboxylate ion, –COO$^-$. As a result, amino acids are <u>dipolar ions</u>, or *zwitterions*. In an aqueous solution, there is an equilibrium present between the dipolar, the anionic, and the cationic forms of the amino acid:

Therefore the charge on the amino acid will vary with the pH of the solution, and with the <u>isoelectric point</u>. This point is the pH where a given amino acid will be neutral (i.e. have no net charge). This isoelectric point is the average of the two pK$_a$ values of an amino acid (*depending on the dissociated group*):

isoelectric point = pI = (pK$_{a1}$ + pK$_{a2}$)/2

Since this is a commonly tested GAMSAT concept, let's further summarize for the average amino acid: When in a relatively acidic solution, the amino acid is fully protonated and exists as a cation, that is, it has two protons available for dissociation, one from the carboxyl group and one from the amino group. When in a relatively basic solution, the amino acid is fully deprotonated and exists as an anion, that is, it has two proton accepting groups, the carboxyl group and the amino group. At the isoelectric point, the amino acid exists as a neutral, dipolar zwitterion, which means that the carboxyl group is deprotonated while the amino group is protonated.

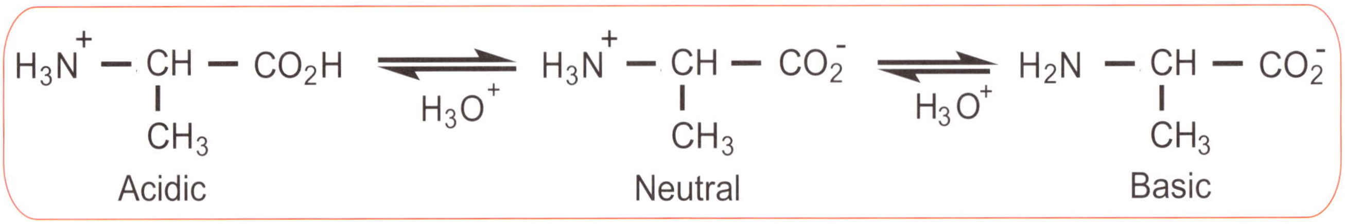

H$_3$N$^+$ – CH – CO$_2$H ⇌ (H$_3$O$^+$) H$_3$N$^+$ – CH – CO$_2^-$ ⇌ (H$_3$O$^+$) H$_2$N – CH – CO$_2^-$
         | | |
        CH$_3$ CH$_3$ CH$_3$
      Acidic   Neutral   Basic

12.1.3 The 20 Alpha-Amino Acids

Approximately 500 amino acids are known - of these, only 22 are proteinogenic ("protein building") amino acids. Of these, 20 amino acids are known as "standard" and are found in human beings and other eukaryotes, and are encoded directly by the universal genetic code (BIO 3). The 2 exceptions are the "non-standard" pyrrolysine — found only in some methanogenic organisms but not humans — and selenocysteine which is present in humans and a wide range of other organisms.

Of the 20 standard amino acids, 9 are called "essential" for humans because they cannot be created from other compounds by the human body, and so must be taken in as food.

The following summarizes the categories of amino acids based on side chains, pK_a and charges at physiological pH:

1. **Nonpolar amino acids:** R groups are hydrophobic and thus decrease solubility. These amino acids are usually found within the interior of the protein molecule.

2. **Polar amino acids:** R groups are hydrophilic and thus increase the solubility. These amino acids are usually found on the protein's surface.

3. **Acidic amino acids:** R groups contain an additional carboxyl group. These amino acids have a negative charge at physiological pH.

4. **Basic amino acids:** R groups contain an additional amine group. These amino acids have a positive charge at physiological pH. Note that asparagine and glutamine have amide side chains and are thus not considered basic (see ORG 9.3).

Table IV.A.1.1: Basic Nomenclature for Biological Molecules. The exception to the monomer/polymer rule is lipids since lipid base units are not generally considered monomers.

Building block	Polymerizes to form…	Chemical bonds	Macromolecule
Monomers	Dimer, trimer, tetramer, oligomers, etc.	Covalent* bonds	Polymer
Amino acids	Dipeptide, tripeptide, tetra/oligopeptide, etc	Peptide bonds	Polypeptide, protein
Monosaccharides ('simple sugars'**)	Disaccharide, tri/tetra/oligosaccharide, etc.	Glycosidic bonds	Polysaccharide
Nucleotides	Nucleotide dimer, tri/tetra/oligomer, etc.	Phosphodiester bonds	Polynucleotides, nucleic acids

*There are exceptions. For example, in certain circumstances polypeptides are considered monomers and they may bond non-covalently to form dimers (i.e. higher orders of protein structure which will be discussed in following sections).
**Note that disaccharides are also sugars (i.e. sucrose is a glucose-fructose dimer known as 'table sugar'; lactose is a glucose-galactose dimer known as 'milk sugar').

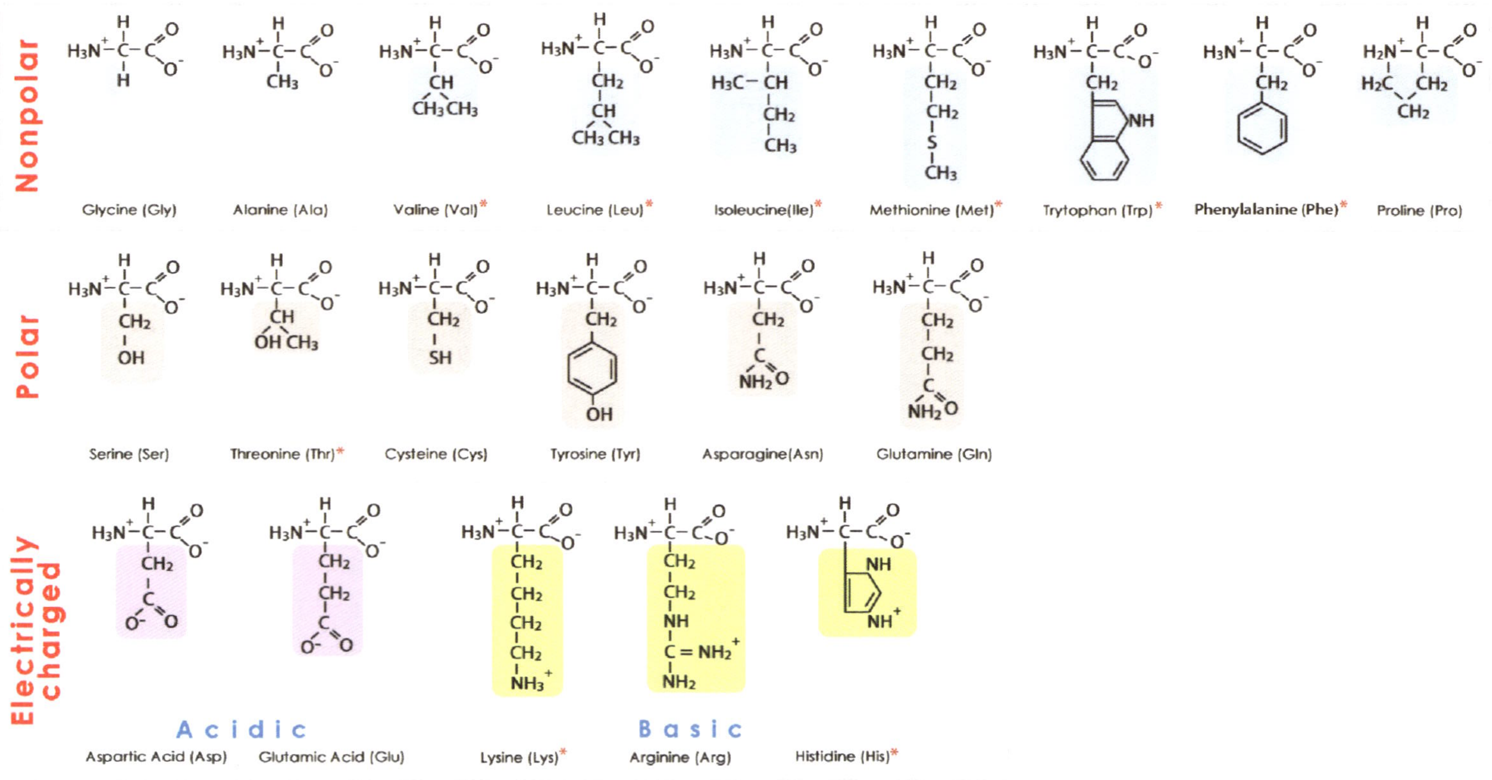

GAMSAT-Prep.com
THE GOLD STANDARD

Nonpolar: Glycine (Gly), Alanine (Ala), Valine (Val)*, Leucine (Leu)*, Isoleucine (Ile)*, Methionine (Met)*, Tryptophan (Trp)*, Phenylalanine (Phe)*, Proline (Pro)

Polar: Serine (Ser), Threonine (Thr)*, Cysteine (Cys), Tyrosine (Tyr), Asparagine (Asn), Glutamine (Gln)

Electrically charged

Acidic: Aspartic Acid (Asp), Glutamic Acid (Glu)

Basic: Lysine (Lys)*, Arginine (Arg), Histidine (His)*

Figure IV.A.1.1: The 20 Standard Amino Acids. A red asterix * is used to indicate the 9 essential amino acids. Notice that if the acidic electrically charged amino acids are fully protonated, the overall charge would be +1 but if fully deprotonated, the overall charge would be -2. The opposite being true for basic amino acids: If fully protonated, the overall charge would be +2 but if fully deprotonated, the overall charge would be -1. These cases are different than for the average amino acid described at the end of section ORG 12.1.2. Skim through the names and structures of the 20 standard amino acids but please do not memorize.

ORG-120 BIOLOGICAL MOLECULES

12.2 Proteins

12.2.1 General Principles

An <u>oligopeptide</u> consists of between 2 and 20 amino acids joined together by amide *(peptide)* bonds. Oligopeptides include dipeptides (2 amino acids), tripeptides (3), tetrapeptides (4), pentapeptides (5), etc. <u>Polypeptides</u> - generally regarded to be between the size of oligopeptides and proteins - are polymers of up to 100 or even 1000 α-amino acids (depending on the molecule and the reference). <u>Proteins</u> are long chain polypeptides which often form higher order structures. These peptide bonds are derived from the amino group of one amino acid, and the acid group of another. When a peptide bond is formed, a molecule of water is released *(condensation = dehydration = water loss)*. The bond can be broken by adding water *(hydrolysis = water lyses = water 'breaks apart' another molecule)*.

Since proteins are polymers of amino acids, they also have isoelectric points. Classification as to the acidity or basicity of a protein depends on the numbers of acidic and basic amino acids it contains. If there is an excess of acidic amino acids, the isoelectric point will be at a pH of less than 7. At pH = 7, these proteins will have a net negative charge. Similarly, those with an excess of basic amino acids will have an isoelectric point at a pH of greater than 7. Therefore, at pH = 7, these proteins will have a net positive charge. Proteins can be separated according to their isoelectric point on a polyacrylamide gel *(electrophoresis;* ORG 13). We will be discussing protein synthesis in Biology Chapter 3.

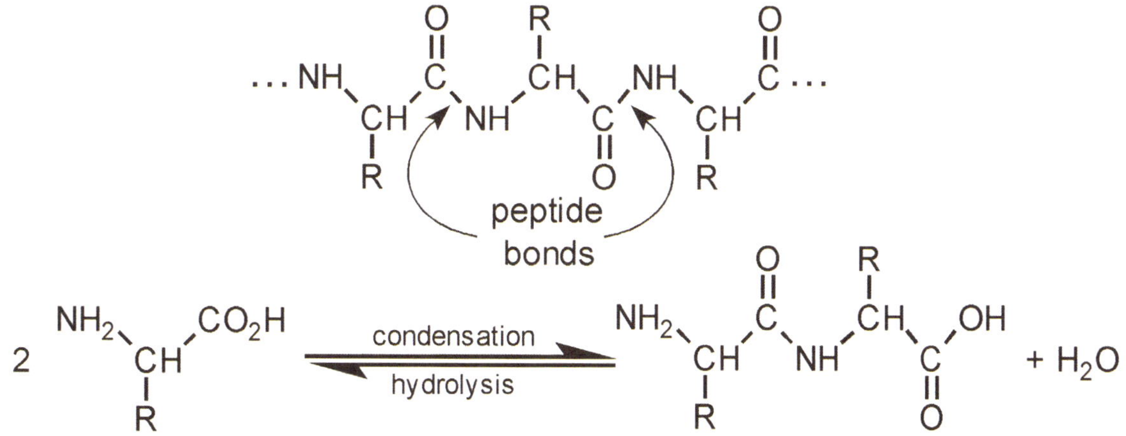

Figure IV.A.1.2: Condensation and hydrolysis. Note that the forward reaction shows 2 moles of amino acid producing a dipeptide and water. The dipeptide is composed of 2 amino acid 'residues' (i.e. what is left over once water is removed). By convention, the amino group (N-terminus) is on the left and the carboxyl group (C-terminus) on the right.

12.2.2 Protein Structure

Protein structure may be divided into primary, secondary, tertiary and quaternary structures. The *primary structure* is the sequence of amino acids as determined by the DNA and the location of covalent bonds (*including disulfide bonds*). This structure determines the higher order structures.

The primary structure is usually shown using 3-letter abbreviations for the amino acid residues as shown in Fig IV.A.1.1. By convention, the amino group (N-terminus) is on the left and the carboxyl group (C-terminus) on the right. For example, insulin (BIO 6.3.4) is composed of 51 amino acids in 2 chains. One chain has 30 amino acids, and the other has 21 amino acids with the following primary structure: GLY-ILE-VAL-GLU-GLN-CYS-CYS-THR-SER-ILE-CYS-SER-LEU-TYR-GLN-LEU-GLU-ASN-TYR-CYS-ASN.

The *secondary structure* is the orderly inter- or intramolecular *hydrogen bonding* of the protein chain. The resultant structure may be the more stable α-helix (e.g. keratin), or a β-pleated sheet (e.g. silk). Proline is an amino acid which cannot participate in the regular array of H-bonding in an α-helix. Proline disrupts the α-helix, thus it is usually found at the beginning or end of a molecule (i.e. hemoglobin).

The *tertiary structure* is the further folding of the protein molecule onto itself. This is the 3D shape (spatial organization) of an entire protein molecule. Protein folding is largely self-organising mainly based on the protein's primary structure. The tertiary structure is maintained by *noncovalent bonds* like hydrogen bonding, Van der Waals forces, hydrophobic bonding and electrostatic bonding (CHM 4.2). The resultant structure is a globular protein with a hydrophobic interior and hydrophilic exterior. Enzymes are classical examples of such a structure. In fact, enzyme activity often depends on tertiary structure.

The covalent bonding of cysteine (*disulfide bonds or bridge*) helps to stabilize the tertiary structure of proteins. Cysteine will form sulfur-sulfur covalent bonds with itself, producing *cystine*. For example, insulin is composed of 2 polypeptide chains, an A-chain and a B-chain (2 = a dimer), which are linked together by disulfide bonds.

$$2\,H_2N-CH(CH_2SH)-CO_2H \xrightarrow{-H_2}$$

cysteine

$$H_2N-CH(CO_2H)-CH_2-S-S-CH_2-CH(CO_2H)-NH_2$$

cystine

The *quaternary structure* is when there are two or more protein chains bonded together by noncovalent bonds. For example, hemoglobin (BIO 7.5.1) consists of four polypeptide subunits (*globin*) held together by hydrophobic bonds forming a globular almost tetrahedryl arrangement.

The secondary, tertiary, and quaternary structures of a protein may be destroyed in a number of ways (= *denaturation*). For example, heating (cooking) can break hydrogen bonds. Altering the pH can protonate or deprotonate the molecule and interrupt ionic interactions. Reducing agents can break disulfide bonds. Depending on the conditions, denaturation may be reversible.

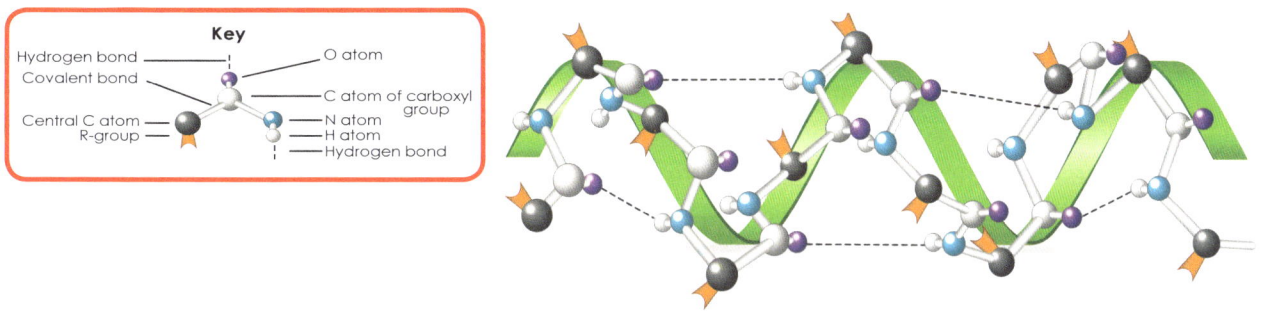

Figure IV.A.1.3: Secondary Structure: α-helix. This is a structure in which the peptide chain is coiled into a helical structure around a central axis. This helix is stabilized by hydrogen bonding between the N-H group and C=O group four residues away. A typical example with this secondary structure is keratin. Keratin is a fibrous, structural protein found in skin, hair and nails (BIO 13.2, 13.3.1).

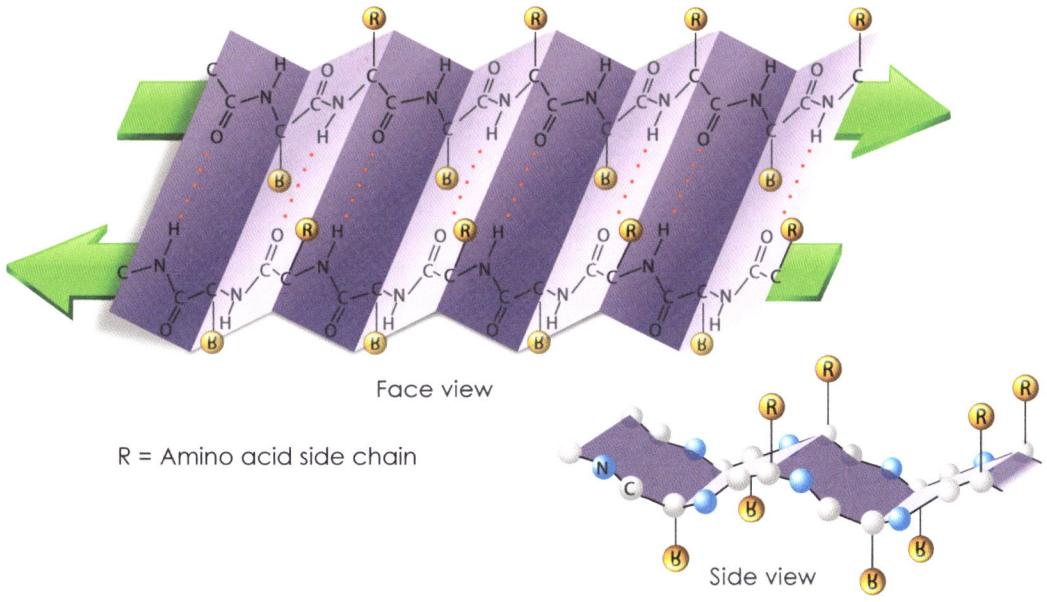

Figure IV.A.1.4: Secondary Structure: β-pleated sheet. Peptide chains lie alongside each other in a parallel manner. This structure is stabilized by hydrogen bonding between the N-H group on one peptide chain and C=O group on another. A typical example with this secondary structure is produced by some insect larvae: the protein fiber "silk" which is mostly composed of fibroin.

12.2.3 Protein Function and Detection

Over the chapters to come, we will be exploring many of the specific functions of proteins. Suffice to say for now that proteins are involved in virtually every process within cells. Proteins include the enzymes that catalyze biochemical reactions. Proteins also have both structural (cytoskeleton) and mechanical functions (actin and myosin). Other protein functions include cell signaling, immune responses, cell adhesion and the cell cycle. Proteins are a necessary component of our diets since we cannot synthesize all the amino acids we need and thus must obtain essential amino acids from food.

During the GAMSAT, it is likely that you will read passages that describe various methods in which proteins can be purified from other cellular components. These techniques include ultracentrifugation, precipitation, electrophoresis and chromatography (ORG 13). Protein structure and function are often studied using immunohistochemistry, site-directed mutagenesis, X-ray crystallography, nuclear magnetic resonance (NMR) and mass spectrometry (ORG 14).

12.3 Carbohydrates

12.3.1 Description and Nomenclature

In general, the names of most carbohydrates are recognizable by an -ose suffix. Carbohydrates are sugars and their derivatives. Formally they are 'carbon hydrates,' that is, they have the general formula $C_m(H_2O)_n$. Usually they are defined as polyhydroxy aldehydes and ketones, or substances that hydrolyze to yield polyhydroxy aldehydes and ketones. The basic units of carbohydrates are monosaccharides (sugars).

There are two ways to classify sugars. One way is to classify the molecule based on the type of carbonyl group it contains: one with an aldehyde carbonyl group is an *aldose*; one with a ketone carbonyl group is a *ketose*. The second method of classification depends on the number of carbons in the molecule: those with 6 carbons are hexoses, with 5 carbons are pentoses, with 4 carbons are tetroses, and with 3 carbons are trioses. Sugars may exist in either the ring form, as hemiacetals, or in the straight chain form, as polyhydroxy aldehydes. *Pyranoses* are 6 carbon sugars in the ring form; *furanoses* are 5 carbon sugars in the ring form.

In the ring form, there is the possibility of α or β *anomers*. Anomers occur when 2 cyclic forms of the molecule differ in conformation only at the hemiacetal carbon (carbon 1). Generally, pyranoses take the 'chair' conformation, as it is very stable, with all (usually) hydroxyl groups at the equatorial position. *Epimers* are diastereomers that differ in the configuration of only one stereogenic center. For carbohy-

ORG-124 BIOLOGICAL MOLECULES

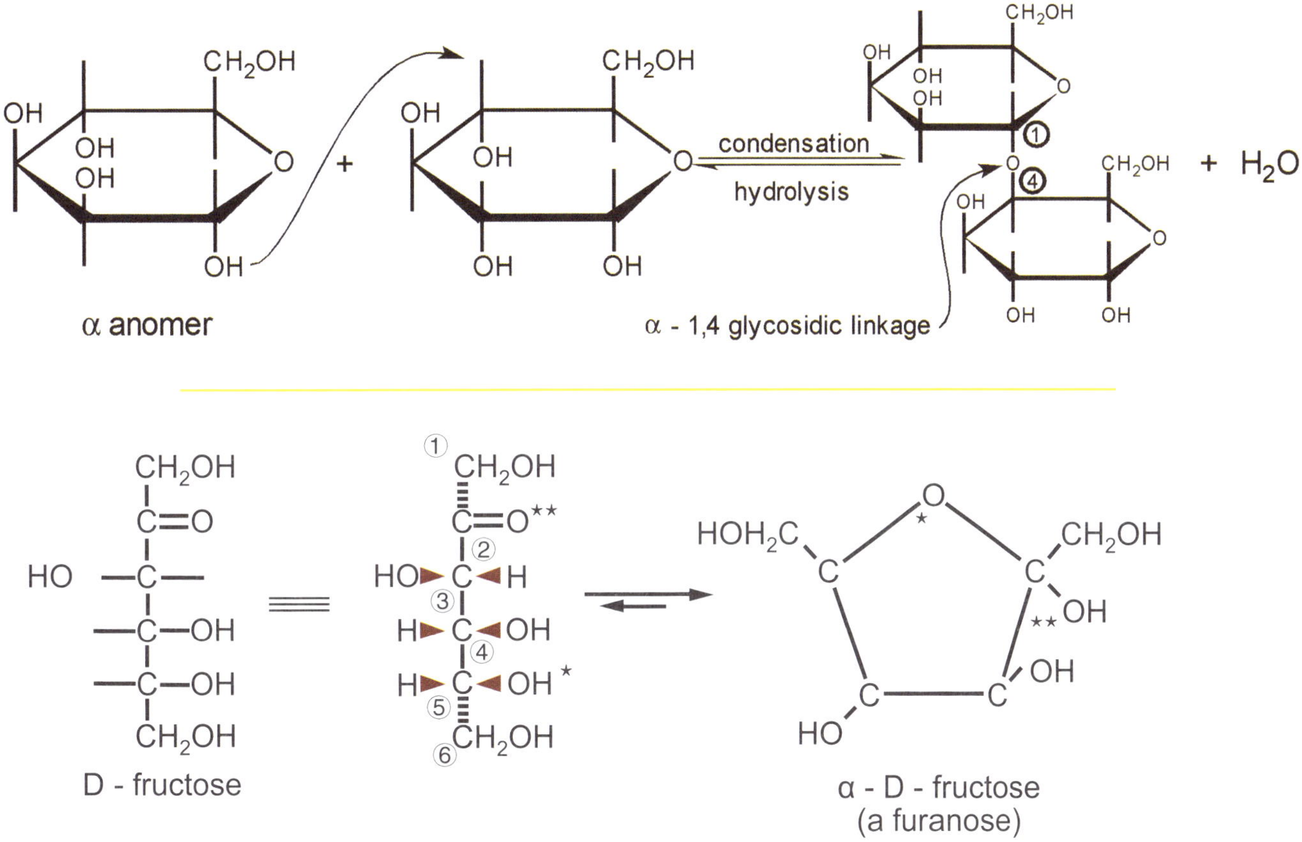

Figure IV.A.1.5 Part I: Names and configurations of common sugars. Notice that the asterix * and ** allow you to follow a specific oxygen atom. Following atoms through a reaction is a common GAMSAT-type question. An asterix, a prime symbol (') or a labelled isotope are examples of techniques that may be used to identify the atom that you must follow.

drates, epimers are 2 monosaccharides which differ in the conformation of one hydroxyl group.

To determine the number of possible optical isomers, one need only know the number of asymmetric carbons, normally 4 for hexoses and 3 for pentoses, designated as n. The number of optical isomers is then 2^n, where n is the number of asymmetric carbons (ORG 2.2.2).

Most but not all of the naturally occurring aldoses have the D-configuration. Thus they have the same *relative* configuration as D-glyceraldehyde. The configuration (D or L) is *only* assigned to the highest numbered chiral carbon. The *absolute* configuration can be determined for any chiral carbon. For example, using the rules from Section 2.3.1, it can be determined that the absolute configuration of D-glyceraldehyde is the R-configuration.

Most carbohydrates contain one or more chiral carbons. For this reason, they are optically active. The names and structures of some common sugars are shown in Figure IV.A.1.5.

THE BIOLOGICAL SCIENCES ORG-125

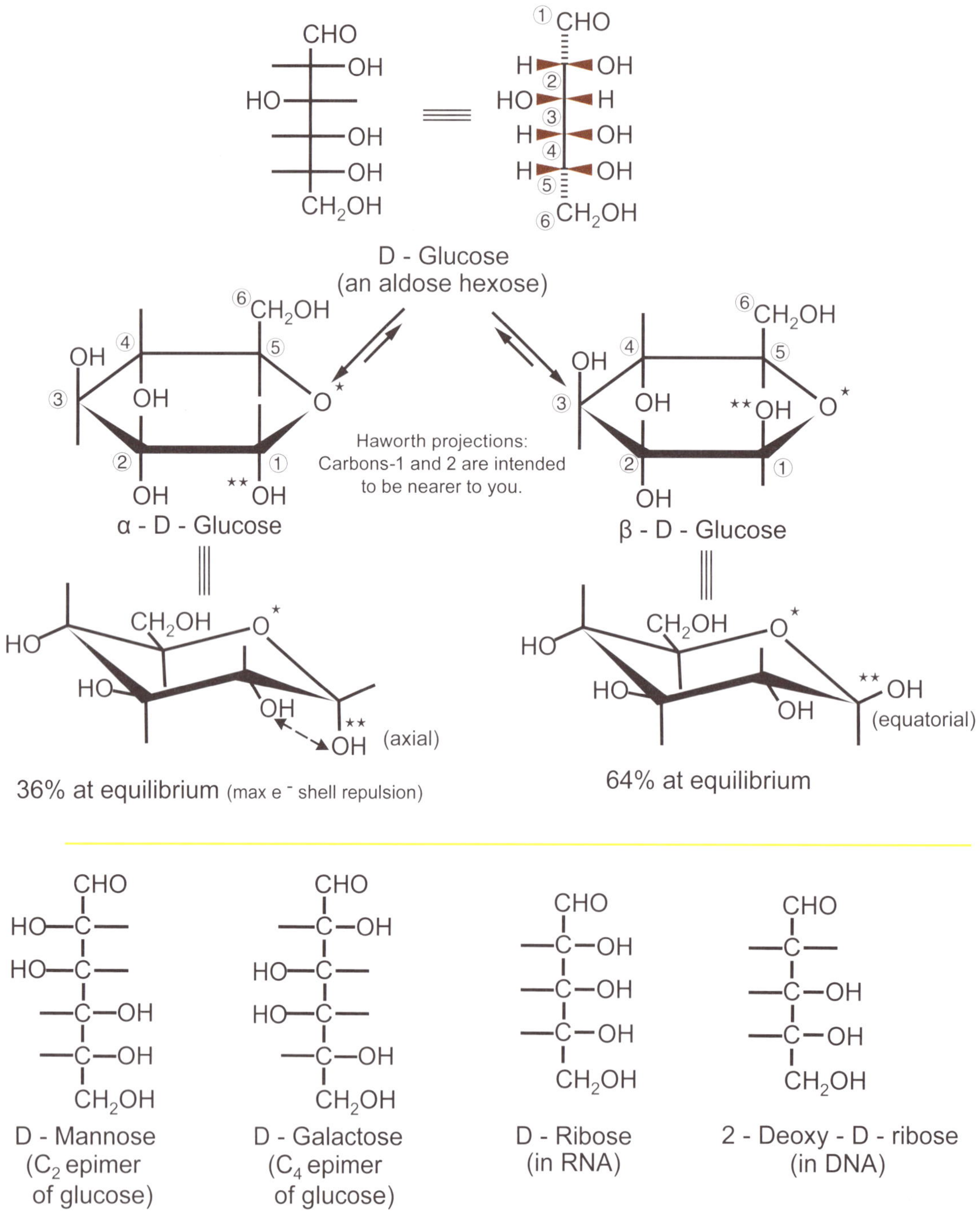

GAMSAT-Prep.com
THE GOLD STANDARD

D - Glucose
(an aldose hexose)

Haworth projections: Carbons-1 and 2 are intended to be nearer to you.

α - D - Glucose

β - D - Glucose

36% at equilibrium (max e⁻ shell repulsion)   (axial)

64% at equilibrium   (equatorial)

D - Mannose
(C₂ epimer of glucose)

D - Galactose
(C₄ epimer of glucose)

D - Ribose
(in RNA)

2 - Deoxy - D - ribose
(in DNA)

Figure IV.A.1.5 Part II: Names, structures and configurations of common sugars. Though not by convention, H belongs to the end of all empty bonds in the diagrams above. Note the following equivalent positions for substituents with glucose as an example: Right on Fischer = down on Hawthorne = alpha configuration = axial in the chair confirmation, and the opposite if on the left for a Fischer projection.

BIOLOGICAL MOLECULES

In the diagram that follows, you will notice a Fischer projection to the far left (see ORG 2.3.1). You will also find Fischer projections throughout this chapter since they are a common way to represent carbohydrates. Recall that the horizontal lines in a Fischer projection are projecting towards you.

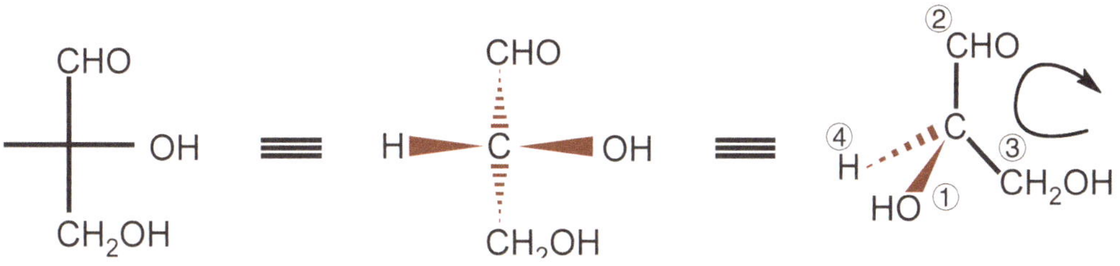

Fischer projection and 3-dimensional representation of D-glyceraldehyde, R-glyceraldehyde (see ORG 2.1, 2.2, 2.3 for rules).

12.3.2 Important Reactions of Carbohydrates

Hemiacetal Reaction

Monosaccharides can undergo an intramolecular nucleophilic addition reaction to form cyclic hemiacetals (see ORG 7.2.2). For example, the hydroxyl group on C4 of ribose attacks the aldehyde group on C1 forming a five-membered ring called furanose.

Diastereomers differing in configuration at this newly formed chiral carbon (= C1 where the straight chain monosaccharide converted into a furanose or pyranose) are known as anomers. This newly chiral carbon, which used to be a carbonyl carbon, is known as the

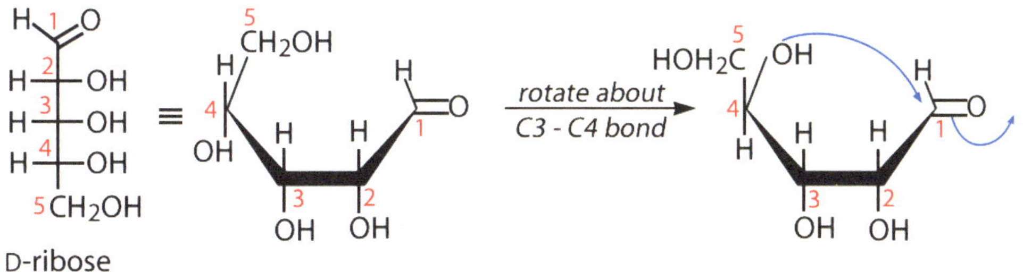

D-ribose

α & β-D-ribofuranose

Note: It is not necessary to memorize the names of products in this section (ORG 12.3.2). However, you are expected to be able to follow what goes where. Of course during the real exam, there will be no color and it is unlikely that they would politely number all the carbons to make it easy for you to follow! ACER practice materials have several passages based on carbohydrates including the "Red" booklet current units 8 and 14.

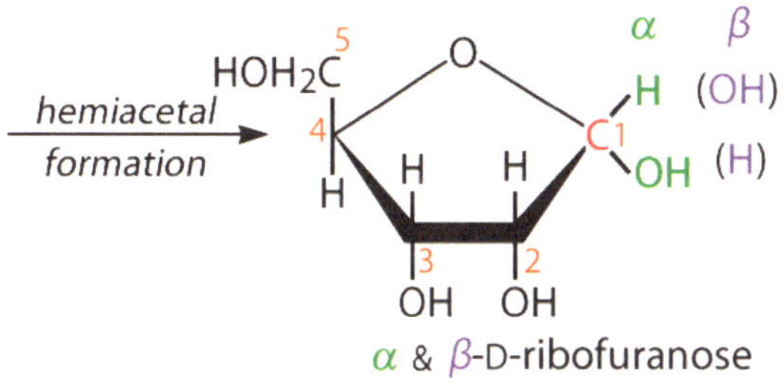

THE BIOLOGICAL SCIENCES   ORG-127

anomeric center. When the OH group on C1 is *trans* to CH₂OH, it is called an α anomer. When the OH group on C1 is *cis* to CH₂OH, it is called a β anomer.

Mutarotation is the formation of both anomers into an equilibrium mixture when exposed to water.

Glycosidic Bonds

A **disaccharide** is a molecule made up of two monosaccharides, joined by a *glycosidic bond* between the hemiacetal carbon of one molecule, and the hydroxyl group of another. The glycosidic bond forms an α-1,4-glycosidic linkage if the reactant is an α anomer. A β-1,4-glycosidic linkage is formed if the reactant is a β anomer. When the bond is formed, one molecule of water is released (condensation). In order to break the bond, water must be added (hydrolysis):

- Sucrose (common sugar or table sugar) = glucose + fructose
- Lactose (milk sugar) = glucose + galactose
- Maltose (α-1,4 bond) = glucose + glucose
- Cellobiose (β-1,4 bond) = glucose + glucose

Ester Formation

Monosaccharides react with acid chloride or acid anhydride to form esters (see ORG 9.4, 9.4.1). All of the hydroxyl groups can be esterified.

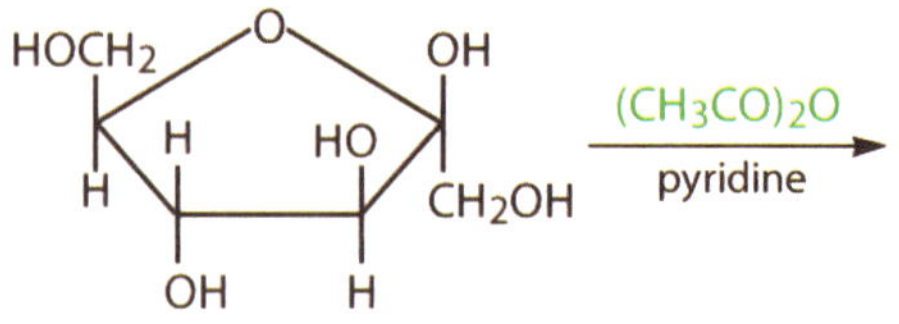

β-D-fructofuranose

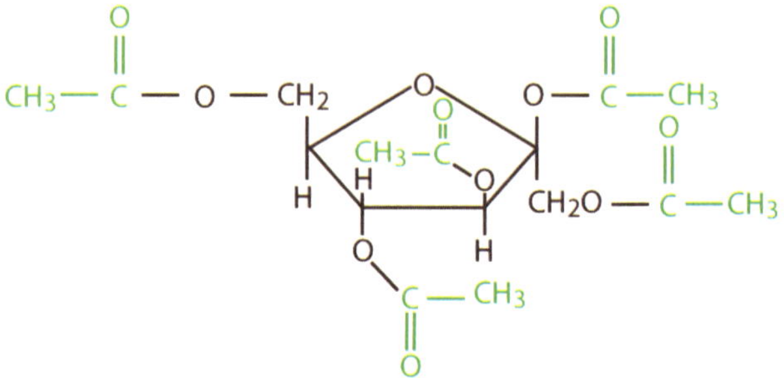

penta-O-acetyl-β-D-fructofuranoside

Ether Formation

Monosaccharides react with alkyl halide in the presence of silver oxide to form ethers. All of the hydroxyl groups are converted to -OR groups.

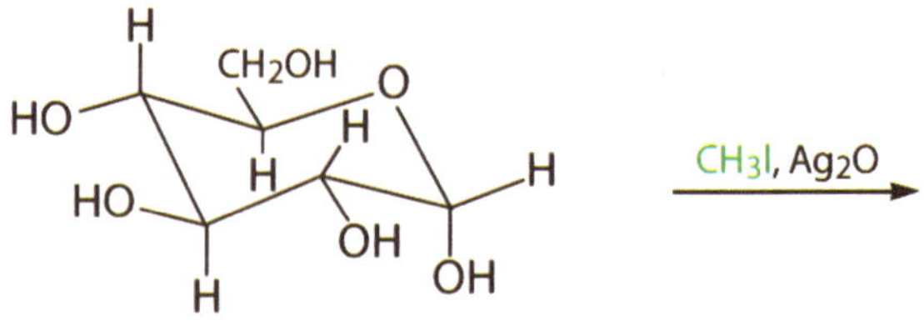

α-D-glucopyranose

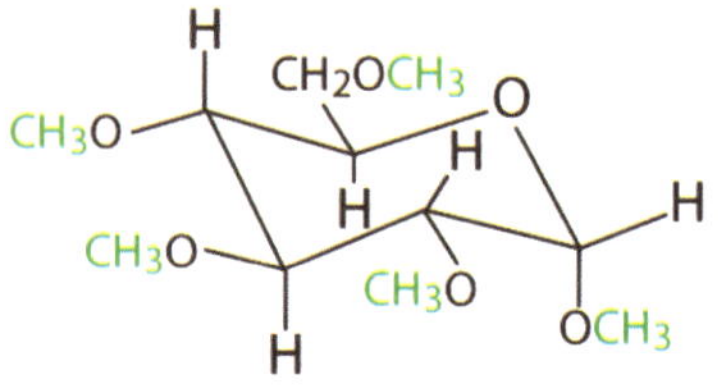

methyl 2, 3, 4, 6-tetra-O-methyl-α-D-glucopyranoside

Ether synthesis can also proceed using alcohols (see ORG 10.1):

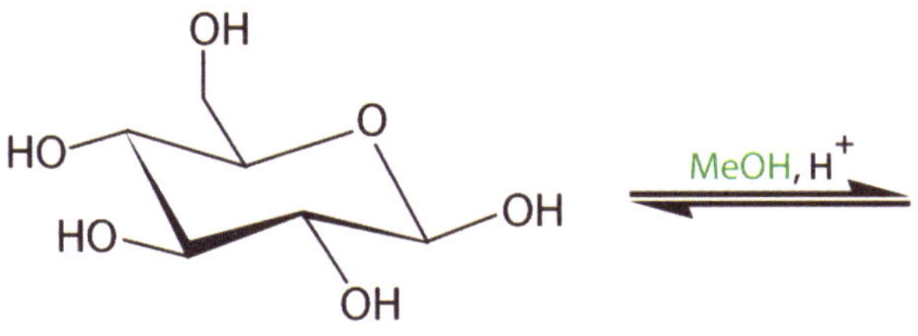

β-D-glucopyranose

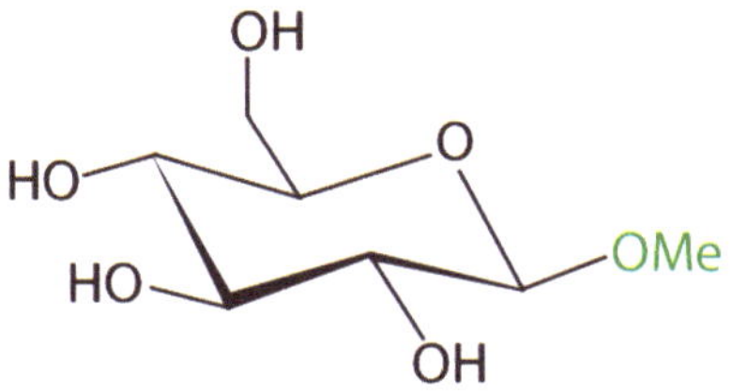

⇌ MeOH, H⁺

methyl-β-D-glucopyranoside

Oxidation Reaction

Again, the hemiacetal ring form is in equilibrium with the open chain aldehyde/ketone form. Aldoses can be oxidized by the Tollens' reagent [Ag(NH$_3$)$_2$]⁺, Fehling's reagent (Cu^{2+}/Na$_2$C$_4$H$_4$O$_6$), and Benedict's reagent (Cu^{2+}/Na$_3$C$_6$H$_5$O$_7$) to yield carboxylic acids. If the Tollens' reagent is used, metallic silver is produced as a shiny mirror. If the Fehling's reagent or Benedict's reagent is used, cuprous oxide is produced as a reddish precipitate.

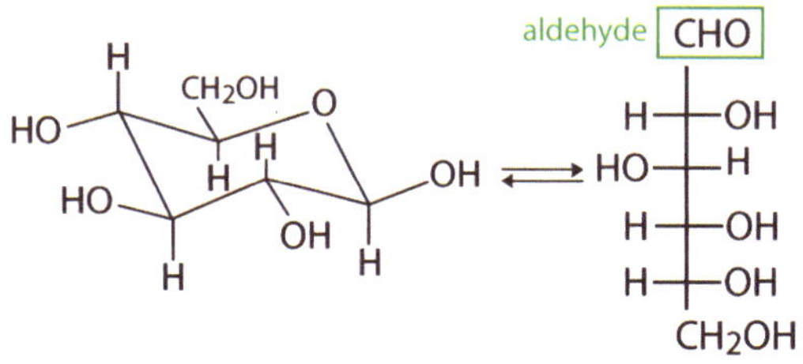

β-D-glucose ⇌ open-chain form

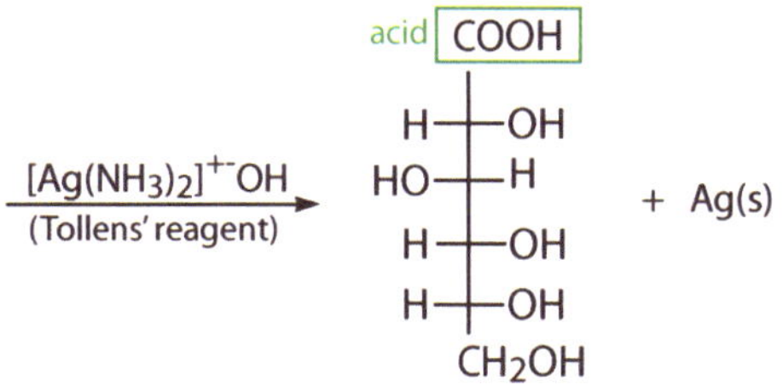

[Ag(NH$_3$)$_2$]⁺ ⁻OH (Tollens' reagent) → D-gluconic acid (+ side products) + Ag(s)

Reduction Reaction

Open chain monosaccharides are present in equilibrium between the aldehyde/ketone and the hemiacetal form. Therefore, monosaccharides can be reduced by NaBH$_4$ to form polyalcohols (see ORG 6.2.2).

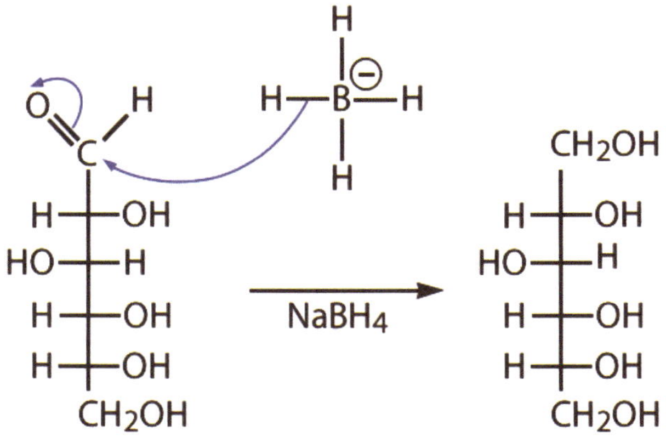

D-glucose →(NaBH$_4$)→ D-sorbitol

Redox (reduction/oxidation) and chain extending GAMSAT questions are usually easily solved by noticing that the stereochemistry of groups that are not directly involved in the reaction remain unchanged. For these substituents, the integrity of the Fischer projection is intact (in other words, whether the H or OH is on the left or right of the structure does not change).

When aldoses are treated with bromine water, the aldehyde is oxidized to a carboxylic acid group, resulting in a product known as an *aldonic acid*:

D- glucose (an aldose) + Br$_2$ $\xrightarrow{\text{H}_2\text{O}, \text{CaCO}_3, \text{pH 5-6}}$ D-Gluconic acid (an aldonic acid) + HBr

Aldoses treated with dilute nitric acid will have both the primary alcohol and aldehyde groups oxidize to carboxylic acid groups, resulting in a product known as an *aldaric acid*:

D-glucose (an aldose) $\xrightarrow{\text{HNO}_3, 55\text{-}60°}$ D-Glucaric acid (an aldaric acid)

Reducing Sugars/Non-reducing Sugars

All aldoses are reducing sugars because they contain an aldehyde carbonyl group. Some ketoses such as fructose are reducing sugars as well. They can be isomerized through keto-enol tautomerization (ORG 7.1) to an aldose, which can be oxidized normally. Glycosides are non-reducing sugars because the acetal group cannot be hydrolyzed to aldehydes. Thus they do not react with the Tollens' reagent.

12.3.3 Polysaccharides

Polymers of many monosaccharides are called polysaccharides. As in disaccharides, they are joined by glycosidic linkages. They may be straight chains, or branched chains. Some common polysaccharides are:

- Starch (plant energy storage)
- Cellulose (plant structural component)
- Glycocalyx (associated with the plasma membrane)
- Glycogen (animal energy storage in the form of glucose)
- Chitin (structural component found in shells or arthropods)

Carbohydrates are the most abundant organic constituents of plants. They are the source of chemical energy in living organisms, and, in plants, they are used in making the support structures. Cellulose consists of β(1→4) linked D-glucose. Starch and glycogen are mostly α(1→4) glycosidic linkages of D-glucose.

12.4 Lipids

Lipids are a class of organic molecules containing many different types of substances, such as fatty acids, fats, waxes, triacyl glycerols, terpenes and steroids. The main biological functions of lipids include storing energy, signaling and acting as structural components of cell membranes.

Lipids are relatively water-insoluble or nonpolar. Lipids can be linear or ring in structure, and may or may not be aromatic. In general, the bulk of lipid structure is nonpolar or hydrophobic; however, often a part of their structure is polar or hydrophilic. This duality makes many lipids amphipathic (= amphiphilic) molecules (having both hydrophobic and hydrophilic portions).

Triacyl glycerols are oils and fats of either animal or plant origin. In general, fats are solid at room temperature, and oils are liquid at room temperature.

Triacyl glycerols are also commonly referred to as triglycerides (= triacylglycerides) and are, by definition, fatty acid triesters of the trihydroxy alcohol glycerol. {Note: "triacyl" refers to the presence of 3 acyl substituents (RCO-, ORG 9.1)}

Glycerol + 3 Fatty acids = Triglyceride

The general structure of a triacyl glycerol is:

$$CH_2O-\overset{O}{\underset{\|}{C}}-R$$
$$CHO-\overset{O}{\underset{\|}{C}}-R'$$
$$CH_2O-\overset{O}{\underset{\|}{C}}-R''$$

The R groups may be the same or different, and are usually long chain alkyl groups. Upon hydrolysis of a triacyl glycerol, the products are three fatty acids and glycerol. The fatty acids may be saturated (= no multiple bonds, i.e. *palmitic acid*) or unsaturated (= containing double or triple bonds, i.e. *oleic acid*). Unsaturated fatty acids are usually in the cis configuration. Saturated fatty acids have a higher melting point than unsaturated fatty acids. Some common fatty acids are:

$$CH_3(CH_2)_{14}COOH$$
palmitic acid

$$CH_3(CH_2)_{16}COOH$$
stearic acid

$$CH_3(CH_2)_7 \underset{H}{\overset{}{\diagdown}} C=C \underset{H}{\overset{(CH_2)_7CO_2H}{\diagup}}$$
oleic acid

General formula for a saturated fatty acid = $C_nH_{2n+1}COOH = CH_3(CH_2)_nCOOH$

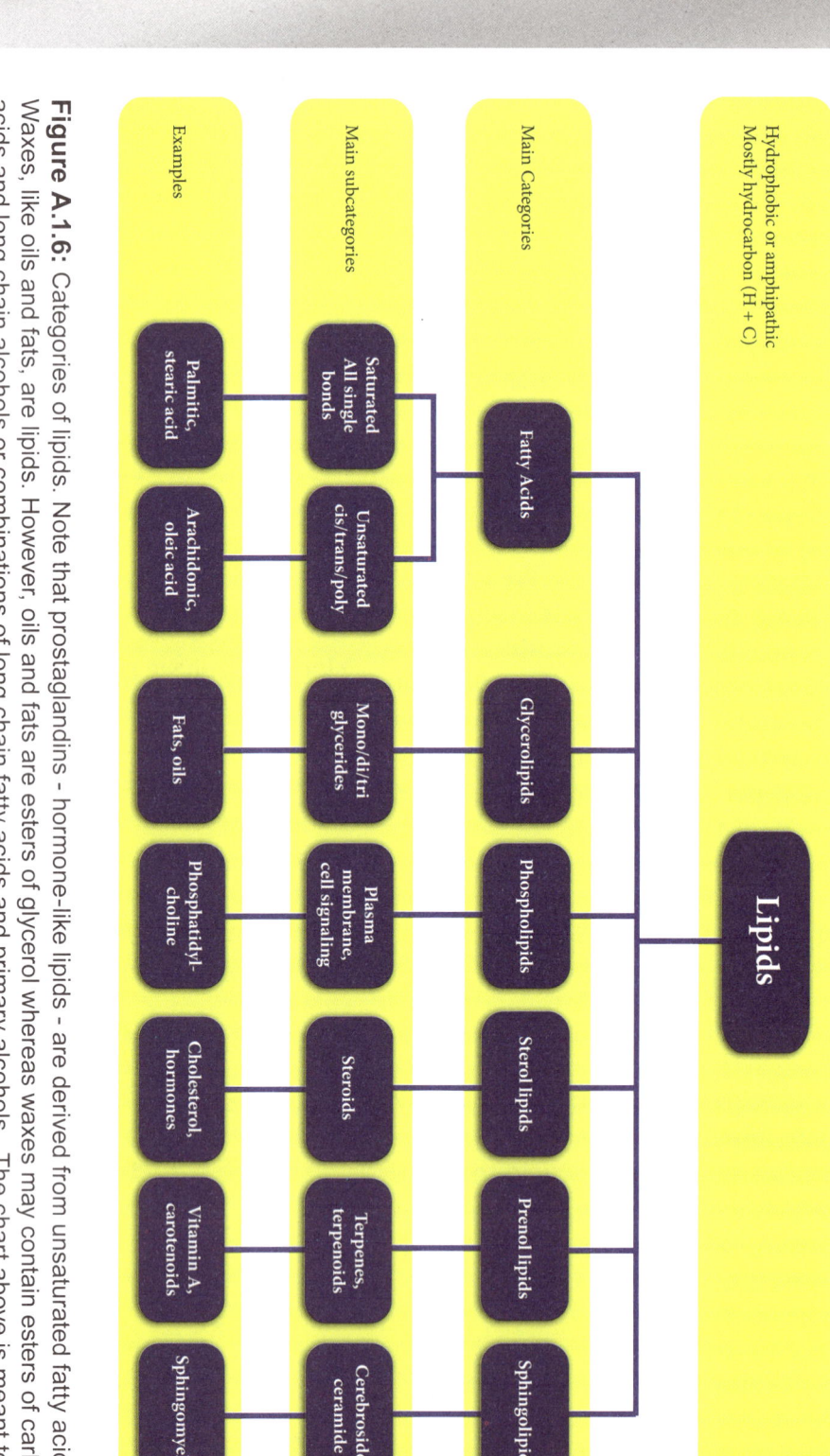

Figure A.1.6: Categories of lipids. Note that prostaglandins - hormone-like lipids - are derived from unsaturated fatty acids. Waxes, like oils and fats, are lipids. However, oils and fats are esters of glycerol whereas waxes may contain esters of carboxylic acids and long chain alcohols or combinations of long chain fatty acids and primary alcohols. The chart above is meant to give you an overview of lipids but please do not memorize.

ORGANIC CHEMISTRY

$$CH_3(CH_2)_{14}\overset{O}{\underset{}{C}}O^*H \;+\; \begin{matrix}CH_2OH\\|\\CHOH\\|\\CH_2OH\end{matrix} \xrightarrow{-H_2O^*} \begin{matrix}CH_2O-\overset{O}{\underset{}{C}}-(CH_2)_{14}CH_3\\|\\CHOH\\|\\CH_2OH\end{matrix} \xrightarrow{-H_2O} \; || \; \xrightarrow{-H_2O} \; |||$$

fatty acid — glycerol — monoglyceride

Biosynthesis of fats and oils. Fats and oils are a special class of esters (i.e. mono-, di-, and triglycerides). Fatty acids (= long chain carboxylic acids) may be added to the monoglyceride formed in the above reaction, forming diglycerides, and triglycerides.

"Essential" fatty acids are fatty acids that humans - and other animals - must ingest because the body requires them but cannot synthesize them. Only two are known in humans: alpha-linolenic acid and linoleic acid. Because they have multiple double bonds that begin near the methyl end, they are both known as polyunsaturated omega fatty acids (omega is the last letter of the Greek alphabet thus signifying the methyl end).

A wax is a simple ester of a fatty acid and a long-chain alcohol. In general, a wax, such as the wax in your ears, serves as a protective coating.

Soap is a mixture of salts of long chain fatty acids formed by the hydrolysis of fat. This process is called saponification. Soap possesses both a nonpolar hydrocarbon tail and a polar carboxylate head. When soaps are dispersed in aqueous solution, the long nonpolar tails are inside the sphere while the polar heads face outward. Recall that a sphere is the shape that minimizes surface tension (i.e. the smallest surface area relative to volume; CHM 4.2).

Soaps are surfactants (BIO 12.3). They are compounds that lower the surface tension of a liquid because of their amphipathic nature

$$\begin{matrix}CH_2O-\overset{O}{\underset{}{C}}-(CH_2)_{14}CH_3\\|\\CHO-\overset{O}{\underset{}{C}}-(CH_2)_{14}CH_3\\|\\CH_2O-\overset{O}{\underset{}{C}}-(CH_2)_{14}CH_3\end{matrix} \xrightarrow{3NaOH} \begin{matrix}CH_2OH\\|\\CHOH\\|\\CH_2OH\end{matrix} \;+\; 3\,CH_3(CH_2)_{14}\,CO_2^-\,Na^+$$

a triglyceride (a fat) — glycerol — salt of the fatty acid

Saponification. Fats may be hydrolyzed by a base to the components glycerol and the salt of the fatty acids. The salts of long chain carboxylic acids are called soaps. Thus this process is called saponification.

THE BIOLOGICAL SCIENCES ORG-133

(i.e. they contain both hydrophobic tails and hydrophilic heads; see BIO 1.1).

Of course, the cellular membrane is a lipid bilayer (Biology Chapter 1). The polar heads of the lipids align towards the aqueous environment, while the hydrophobic tails minimize their contact with water and tend to cluster together. Depending on the concentration of the lipid, this interaction may result in micelles (spherical), liposomes (spherical) or other lipid bilayers.

Micelles are closed lipid monolayers with a fatty acid core and polar surface. The main function of bile (BIO 9.4.1) is to facilitate the formation of micelles, which promotes the processing or emulsification of dietary fat and fat-soluble vitamins.

Liposomes are composed of a lipid bilayer separating an aqueous internal compartment from the bulk aqueous environment. Liposomes can be used as a vehicle for the administration of nutrients or pharmaceutical drugs.

The dual solubility nature of soap is why it removes oil or grease from skin or clothes. The soap forms a micelle that surrounds the nonpolar oil/grease in the nonpolar 'center' of the micelle. The polar end of the soap micelle is soluble in water, allowing the oil/grease to be removed during rinsing.

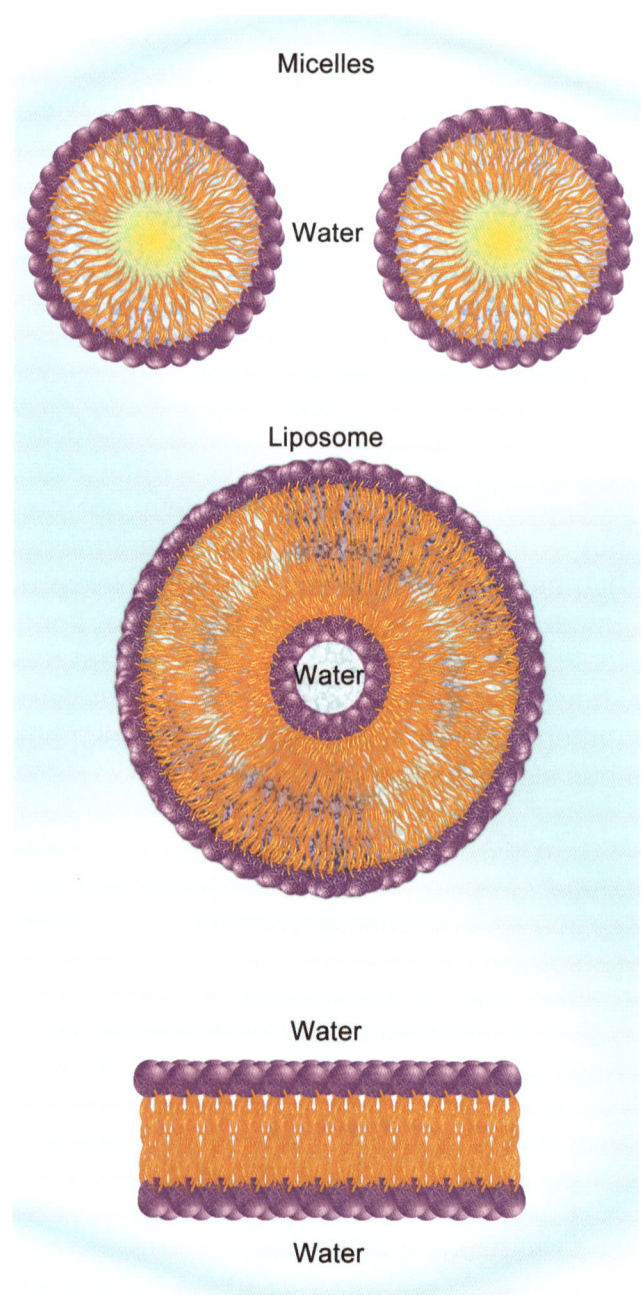

Figure IV.A.1.7. Amphipathic molecules arranged in micelles, a liposome and a bilipid layer.

12.4.1 Steroids

Steroids are a class of lipids which are derivatives of the basic ring structure:

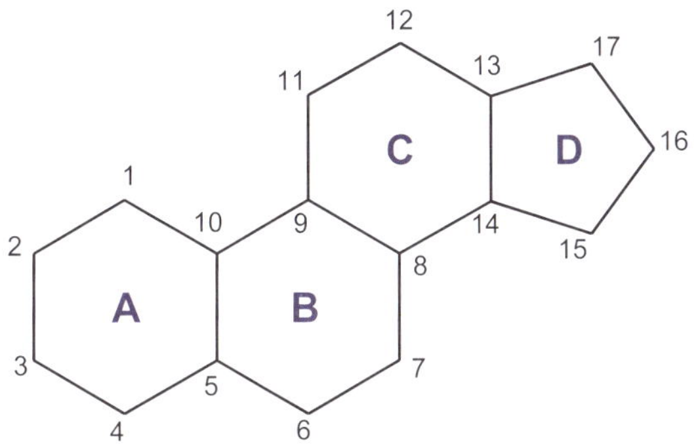

The IUPAC-recommended ring-lettering and the carbon atoms are numbered as shown. Many important substances are steroids, some examples include: cholesterol, D vitamins, bile acids, adrenocortical hormones, and male and female sex hormones.

Cholesterol is the most abundant steroid. It is a component of the plasma membrane and can serve as a building block to produce other steroids (including hormones) and related molecules. Cholesterol comes from the diet, but may be synthesized by the liver if necessary.

The rate limiting step in the production of steroids (= *steroidogenesis*) in humans is the conversion of cholesterol to pregnenolone, which is in the same family as progesterone. This occurs inside of mitochondria and serves as the precursor for all human steroids.

Since such a significant portion of a steroid contains hydrocarbons, which are hydrophobic, steroids can dissolve through the hydrophobic interior of a cell's plasma membrane (BIO 1.1, 6.3). Furthermore, steroid hormones contain polar side groups which allow the hormone to easily dissolve in water. Thus steroid hormones are well designed to be transported through the vascular space, to cross the plasma membranes of cells, and to have an effect either in the cell's cytosol or, as is usually the case, in the nucleus.

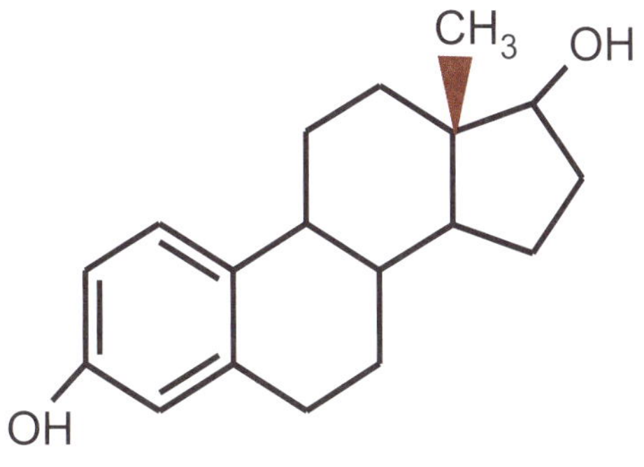

Estradiol
(an estrogen)

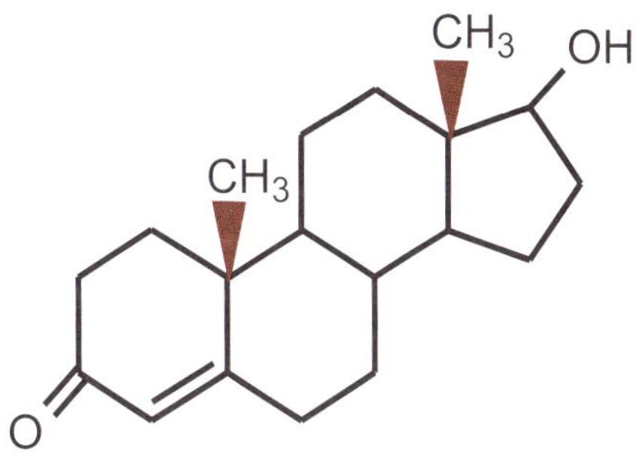

Testosterone
(an androgen)

THE BIOLOGICAL SCIENCES   ORG-135

12.4.2 Lipoproteins

Most biological molecules are proteins, followed by lipids. In fact, proteins and lipids by far dominate the biological molecules in the human body. Lipoproteins comprise unique biochemical assemblies (aggregates) containing both proteins and lipids, bound to the proteins, which allow lipids to move through hydrophilic intracellular and extracellular spaces. Many enzymes, structural proteins, transporters, antigens and toxins are lipoproteins.

Using electrophoresis and ultracentrifugation, lipoproteins can be classified according to size and density. Lipoproteins are larger and less dense when the fat to protein ratio is increased. Thus there are four major classes of plasma lipoproteins which enable lipids to be carried in the blood stream: (1) chylomicrons carry triglycerides from the intestines to the liver, to skeletal muscle, and to adipose tissue ("body fat"); (2) very low-density lipoproteins (VLDL) carry liver-synthesized triglycerides to adipose tissue; (3) low-density lipoproteins (LDL = "bad cholesterol") carry cholesterol from the liver to cells of the body; (4) and high-density lipoproteins (HDL = "good cholesterol") collect cholesterol from the body's tissues, and take it back to the liver.

12.5 Phosphorous in Biological Molecules

Phosphorous is an essential component of various biological molecules including adenosine triphosphate (ATP), phospholipids in cell membranes (BIO 1.1), and the nucleic acids which form DNA (BIO 1.2.2). Phosphorus can also form phosphoric acid (key to making the phosphate buffer in plasma; CHM 6.8), and several phosphate esters.

A phospholipid is produced from three ester linkages to glycerol. Phosphoric acid is ester linked to the terminal hydroxyl group and two fatty acids are ester linked to the two remaining hydroxyl groups of glycerol (*see Biology Section 1.1 for a schematic view of a phospholipid*).

Among the following Biology chapters, the production of ATP will be discussed. The

phosphoric acid   phosphate esters

ORG-136 BIOLOGICAL MOLECULES

ORGANIC CHEMISTRY

components ADP and P$_i$ (= *inorganic phosphate*) combine using the energy generated from a coupled reaction to produce ATP. We will be discussing the bioenergetics of ATP in the Biology Chapter 4. The linkage between the phosphate groups are via *anhydride bonds*:

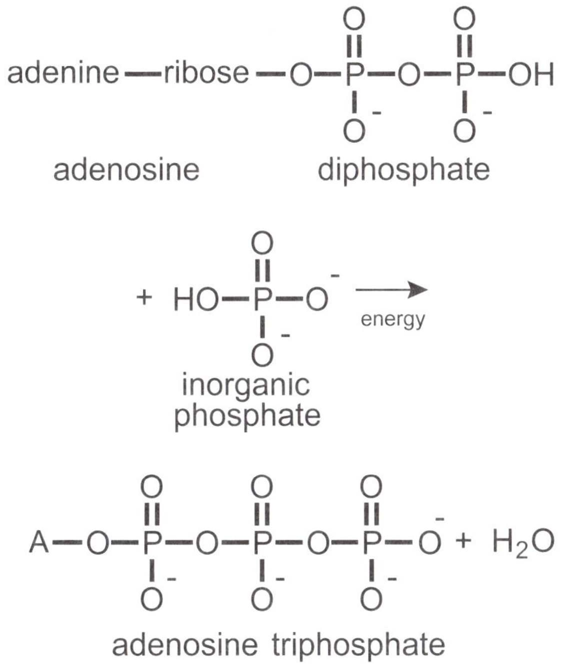

adenine—ribose—O—P(=O)(O⁻)—O—P(=O)(O⁻)—OH

adenosine diphosphate

+ HO—P(=O)(O⁻)—O⁻ → energy

inorganic phosphate

A—O—P(=O)(O⁻)—O—P(=O)(O⁻)—O—P(=O)(O⁻)—O⁻ + H$_2$O

adenosine triphosphate

In DNA, the phosphate groups engage in two ester linkages creating phosphodiester bonds. It is the 5' phosphorylated position of one pentose ring which is linked to the 3' position of the next pentose ring (*see* BIO 1.2.2):

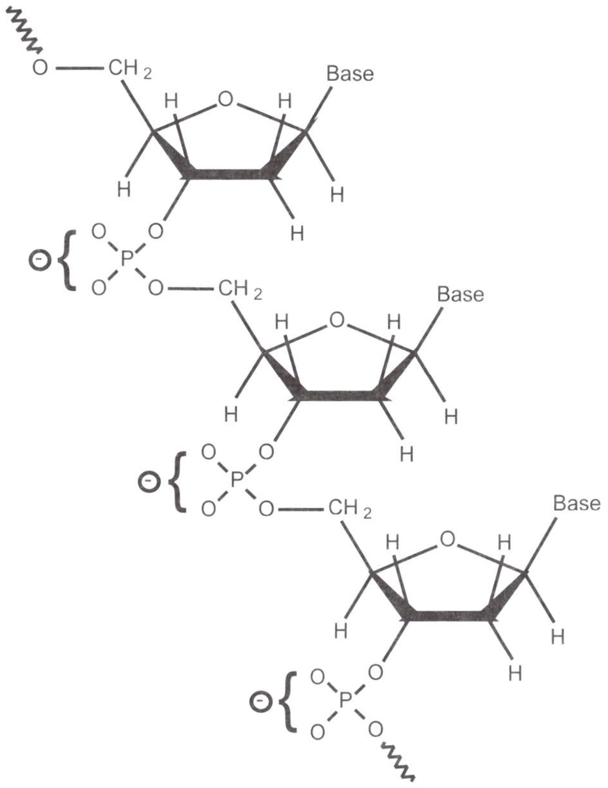

Go online to GAMSAT-prep.com for chapter review Q&A and forum.

GOLD NOTES

SEPARATIONS AND PURIFICATIONS
Chapter 13

Memorize
* Definitions of the major techniques
* Interactions between organic molecules

Understand
* Different phases in the various techniques
* How to improve separation, purification
* How to avoid overheating (distillation)

Not Required*
* Advanced level college info
* Electrolysis, affinity purification
* Refining, smelting

GAMSAT-Prep.com

Introduction

Separation techniques are used to transform a mixture of substances into two or more distinct products. The separated products may be different in chemical properties or some physical property (i.e. size). Purification in organic chemistry is the physical separation of a chemical substance of interest from foreign or contaminating substances.

Additional Resources

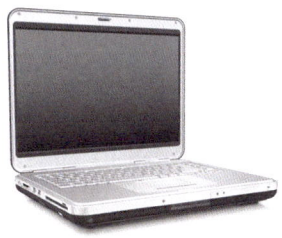

Free Online Q & A

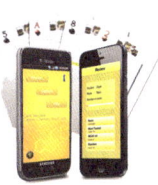

Flashcards

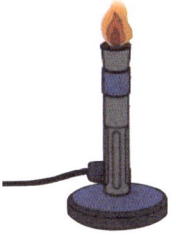

Special Guest

THE BIOLOGICAL SCIENCES   ORG-139

* The real GAMSAT may have advanced level information presented (ie. in a passage) but previous knowledge of said information is not required to answer the questions that would follow. Practice ACER and GS practice GAMSATs can help you clarify this point.

13.1 Separation Techniques

Extraction is the process by which a solute is transferred (*extracted*) from one solvent and placed in another. This procedure is possible if the two solvents used cannot mix (= *immiscible*) and if the solute is more soluble in the solvent used for the extraction.

For example, consider the extraction of solute A which is dissolved in solvent X. We choose solvent Y for the extraction since solute A is highly soluble in it and because solvent Y is immiscible with solvent X. We now add solvent Y to the solution involving solute A and solvent X. The container is agitated. Solute A begins to dissolve in the solvent where it is most soluble, solvent Y. The container is left to stand, thus the two immiscible solvents separate. The phase containing solute A can now be removed.

In practice, solvent Y would be chosen such that it would be sufficiently easy to evaporate (= *volatile*) after the extraction so solute A can be easily recovered. Also, it is more efficient to perform several extractions using a small amount of solvent each time, rather than one extraction using a large amount of solvent.

The main purpose of filtration is to isolate a solid from a liquid. There are two basic types of filtration: gravity filtration and vacuum filtration. In gravity filtration the solution containing the substance of interest is poured through the filter paper with the solvent's own weight responsible for pulling it through. This is often done using a hot solvent to ensure that the product remains dissolved. In vacuum filtration the solvent is forced through the filter with a vacuum on the other side. This is helpful when it is necessary to isolate large quantities of solid.

Sublimation is a process which goes from a heated solid directly into the gas phase without passing through the intermediate liquid phase (CHM 4.3.1). Low pressure reduces the temperature required for sublimation. The substance in question is heated and then condensed on a cool surface (cold finger), leaving the non-volatile impurities behind.

Centrifugation is a separation process that involves the use of centrifugal forces for the sedimentation of mixtures. Particles settle at different rates depending on their size, viscosity, density and shape. Compounds of greater mass and density settle toward the bottom while compounds of lighter mass and density remain on top. This process is most useful in separating polymeric materials such as biological macromolecules.

Distillation is the process by which compounds are separated based on differences in boiling points. Compounds with a lower boiling point are preferably vaporized, condensed on a water cooler, and are separated from compounds with higher boiling points.

For instance, a classic example of simple distillation is the separation of salt from water. The solution is heated. Water will boil and vaporize at a far lower temperature than salt. Hence the water boils away leaving salt behind. Water vapor can now be condensed into pure liquid water (distilled water).

ORGANIC CHEMISTRY

As long as one compound is more volatile (CHM 4.4.2, 5.1.1), the distillation process is quite simple. If the difference between the two boiling points is low, it will be more difficult to separate the compounds by this method. Here are 3 standard ways to separate compounds using distillation:

1. **Simple distillation** is used to separate liquids whose boiling points differ by at least 25 °C and that boil below 150 °C. The composition of the distillate depends on the composition of the vapors at a given temperature and pressure.

2. **Vacuum distillation** is used to separate liquids whose boiling points differ by at least 25 °C and that boil above 150 °C. The vacuum environment prevents compounds from decomposition because the low pressure reduces the temperature required for distillation.

3. **Fractional distillation** is used to separate liquids whose boiling points are less than 25 °C apart. The repeated vaporization-condensation cycle of compounds will eventually yield vapors that contain a greater and greater proportion of the lower boiling point component.

The fractional distillation apparatus can include a column filled with glass beads which is placed between the distillation flask and the condenser (see Figure IV.B.13.0). The glass beads increase the surface area over which the less volatile compound can condense and drip back down to the distillation (distilling) flask below. The more volatile compound boils away and condenses. Thus the two compounds are separated.

The efficiency of the distillation process in producing a pure product is improved by repeating the distillation process, increasing the length of the fractionating column and avoiding overheating. Overheating may destroy the pure compounds or increase the percent of impurities. Some of the methods which are used to prevent overheating include boiling slowly, the use of boiling chips (= *ebulliator*, which makes bubbles) and the use of a vacuum which decreases the vapor pressure and thus the boiling point.

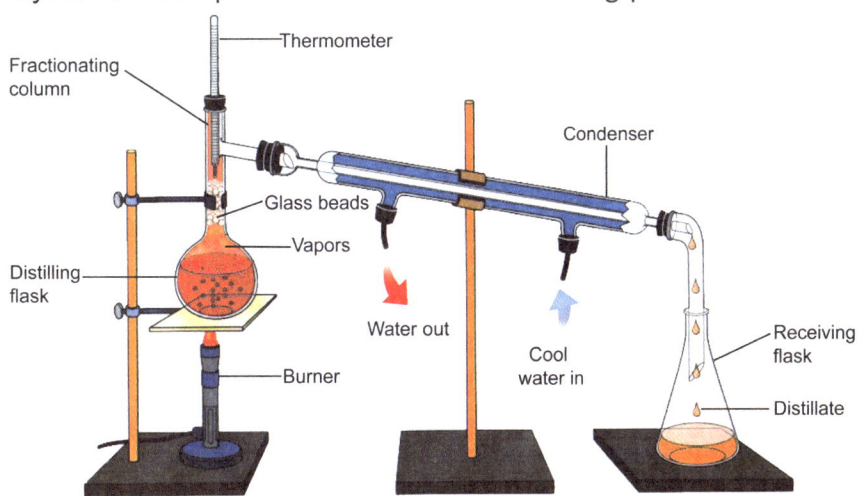

Figure IV.B.13.0: Standard fractional distillation apparatus heated with Bunsen burner.

13.2 Chromatography

Chromatography is the separation of a mixture of compounds by their distribution between two phases: one stationary and one moving. The mobile phase is run through the stationary phase. Different substances distribute themselves according to their relative affinities for the two phases. This causes the separation of the different compounds. Molecules are separated based on differences in polarity and molecular weight.

13.2.1 Gas-Liquid Chromatography

In gas-liquid chromatography, the *stationary phase* is a liquid absorbed to an inert solid. The liquid can be polyethylene glycol, squalene, or others, depending on the polarity of the substances being separated.

The mobile phase is a gas (i.e. He, N_2) which is unreactive both to the stationary phase and to the substances being separated. The sample being analyzed can be injected in the direction of gas flow into one end of a column packed with the stationary phase. As the sample migrates through the column certain molecules will move faster than others. As mentioned the separation of the different types of molecules is dependent on size (*molecular weight*) and charge (*polarity*). Once the molecules reach the end of the column special detectors signal their arrival.

13.2.2 Thin-Layer Chromatography

Thin-layer chromatography (TLC) is a solid-liquid technique, based on adsorptivity and solubility. The *stationary phase* is a type of finely divided polar material, usually silica gel or alumina, which is thinly coated onto a glass plate.

A mixture of compounds is placed on the stationary phase, either a thin layer of silica gel or alumina on glass sheet. Silica gel is a very polar and hydrophobic substance. The mobile phase is usually of low polarity and moves by capillary action. Therefore, if silica gel is used as the stationary phase, nonpolar compounds move quickly while polar compounds have strong interaction with the gel and are stuck tightly to it. In reverse-phase chromatography, the stationary phase is nonpolar and the mobile phase is polar; as a result, polar compounds move quickly while nonpolar compounds stick more tightly to the adsorbant.

There are several types of interactions that may occur between the organic molecules in the sample and the silica gel, in order from weakest to strongest (see CHM 3.4, 4.2):

- Van der Waals force (nonpolar molecules)

- Dipole-dipole interaction (polar molecules)
- Hydrogen bonding (hydroxylic compounds)
- Coordination (Lewis bases)

Molecules with functional groups with the greatest polarity will bind more strongly to the stationary phase and thus will not rise as high on the glass plate.

Organic molecules will also interact with the *mobile phase* (= a solvent), or *eluent* used in the process. The more polar the solvent, the more easily it will dissolve polar molecules. The mobile phase usually contains organic solvents like ethanol, benzene, chloroform, acetone, etc.

As a result of the interactions of the organic molecules with the stationary and moving phases, for any adsorbed compound there is a dynamic distribution equilibrium between these phases. The different molecules will rise to different heights on the plate. Their presence can be detected using special stains (i.e. pH indicators, $KMnO_4$) or uv light (*if the compound can fluoresce; PHY 12.6*).

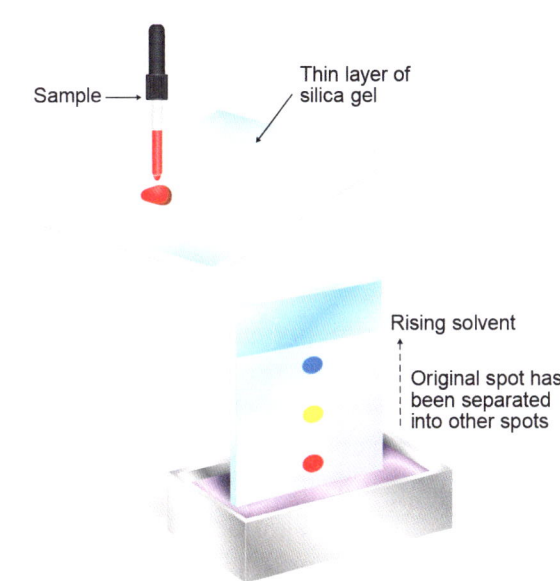

Figure IV.B.13.1: Thin-layer Chromatography.

13.2.3 Column Chromatography

Column chromatography is similar to TLC in principle; however, column chromatography uses silica gel or alumina as an adsorbant in the form of a column rather than TLC which uses paper in a layer-like form. The solvent and compounds move down the column (by gravity) allowing much more separation. The solvent drips out into a waiting flask where fractions containing bands corresponding to the different compounds are collected. After the solvent has evaporated, the compounds can then be isolated. Often the desired compounds are proteins or nucleic acids for which several techniques exist:

1. Ion exchange chromatography – Beads coated with charged substances are placed in the column so that they will attract compounds with an opposing charge.

2. Size exclusion chromatography – The column contains beads with tiny pores which allow small substances to enter, leaving larger molecules to pass through the column faster.

3. Affinity chromatography – Columns are customized to bind a substance of interest (e.g. a receptor or antibody) which allows it to bind very tightly.

13.3 Gel Electrophoresis

Gel electrophoresis is an important method to separate biological macromolecules (i.e. protein and DNA) based on size and charge of molecules. Molecules are made to move through a gel which is placed in an electrophoresis chamber. When an electric current is applied, molecules move at different velocities. These molecules will move towards either the cathode or anode depending on their size and charge (anions move towards anode while cations move towards the cathode. The migration velocity is proportional to the net charge on the molecule and inversely proportional to a coefficient dependent on the size of the molecule. Highly charged, small molecules will move the quickest with size being the most important factor.

There are three main types of electrophoresis:

1. Agarose gel electrophoresis – Used to separate pieces of negatively charged nucleic acids based on their size.

2. SDS-polyacrylamide gel electrophoresis (SDS-PAGE) – Separates proteins on the basis of mass and not charge. The SDS (sodium dodecyl sulfate) binds to proteins and creates a large negative charge such that the only variable effecting their movement is the frictional coefficient which is solely dependent on mass.

3. Isoelectric focusing – The isoelectric point is the pH at which the net charge of a protein is zero (ORG Chapter 12.1.2). A mixture of proteins can be separated by placing them in an electric field with a pH gradient. The proteins will lose their charge and come to a stop when the pH is equal to their isoelectric point.

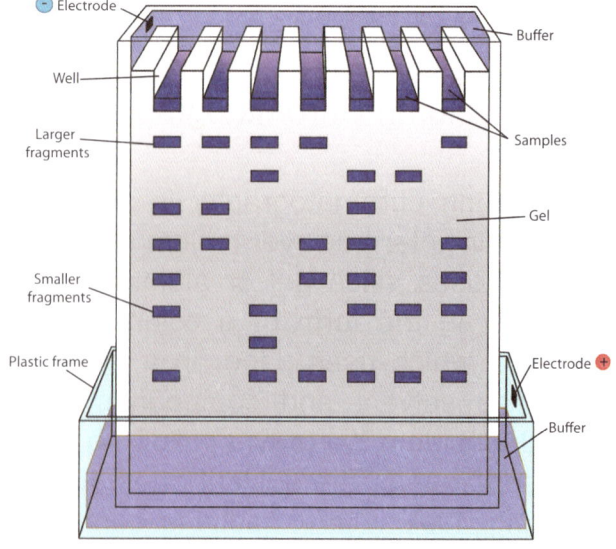

Figure IV.B.13.2: Gel Electrophoresis.

13.4 Recrystallization

Recrystallization is a useful purification technique. A solid organic compound with some impurity is dissolved in a hot solvent, and then the solvent is slowly cooled to allow the pure compound to reform or *recrystallize*, while leaving the impurities behind in the solvent. This is possible because the impurities do not normally fit within the crystal structure of the compound.

In choosing a solvent, solubility data (e.g. K_{sp} at various temperatures, etc.) regarding both the compound to be purified and the impurities should be known. The data should be analyzed such that the solvent would:

- have the capability to dissolve alot of the compound (to be purified) at or near the boiling point of the solvent, while being able to dissolve little of the compound at room temperature. As well, the impurities should be soluble in the cold solvent.

- have a low boiling point, so as to be easily removed from the solid in a drying process.

- not react with the solid.

GOLD NOTES

SPECTROSCOPY

Chapter 14

Memorize	Understand	Not Required*
•thing	* Basic theory: IR spect., NMR, mass spectrometry * Very basic spectrum (graph) analysis	* Advanced level college info * Interpreting the results of spectroscopy without first being given clues or being reminded of the rules.

GAMSAT-Prep.com

Introduction

Spectroscopy is the use of the absorption, emission, or scattering of electromagnetic radiation by matter to study the matter or to study physical processes. The matter can be atoms, molecules, atomic or molecular ions, or solids.

Consider the hundreds of molecules and dozens of functional groups that we have already seen in this textbook. Spectroscopy can provide evidence for which atoms compose those molecules, and how those atoms are arranged in those molecules.

Additional Resources

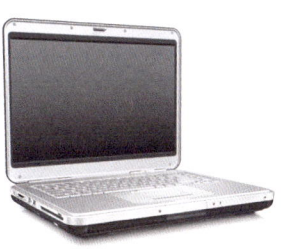 Free Online Q & A

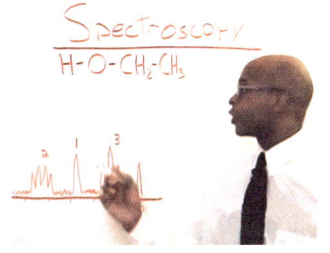 Video: Online or DVD

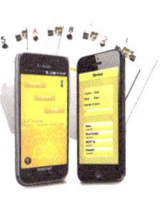 Flashcards

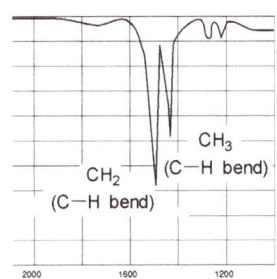 Special Guest

THE BIOLOGICAL SCIENCES   ORG-147

* The real GAMSAT may have advanced level information presented (ie. in a passage) but previous knowledge of said information is not required to answer the questions that would follow. Practice ACER and GS practice GAMSATs can help you clarify this point.

14.1 IR Spectroscopy

In an infrared spectrometer, a beam of infrared (IR) radiation is passed through a sample. The spectrometer will then analyze the amount of radiation transmitted (= % *transmittance*) through the sample as the incident radiation is varied. Ultimately, a plot results as a graph showing the transmittance or absorption (*the inverse of transmittance*) versus the frequency or wavelength of the incident radiation or the wavenumber (= the reciprocal of the wavelength). IR spectroscopy is best used for the identification of functional groups.

The location of an IR absorption band (*or peak*) can be specified in *frequency units* by its wavenumber, measured in cm^{-1}. As the wave number decreases, the wavelength increases, thus the energy decreases (this can be determined using two physics equations which we have already seen, PHY 7.1.2, 9.2.4: $v = \lambda f$ and $E = hf$). A schematic representation of the IR spectrum of octane is:

Electromagnetic radiation consists of discrete units of energy called *quanta* or *photons* (PHY 7.1.3, 11.1). All organic compounds are capable of absorbing many types of electromagnetic energy. The absorption of energy leads to an increase in the amplitude of intramolecular rotations and vibrations.

Intramolecular rotations are the rotations of a molecule about its center of gravity. The difference in rotational energy levels is inversely proportional to the moment of inertia of a molecule. Rotational energy is quantized and gives rise to absorption spectra in the microwave region of the electromagnetic spectrum.

Intramolecular vibrations are the bending and stretching motions of bonds within a molecule. The relative spacing between vibrational energy levels increases with the increasing strength of an intramolecular bond. Vibrational energy is quantized and gives rise

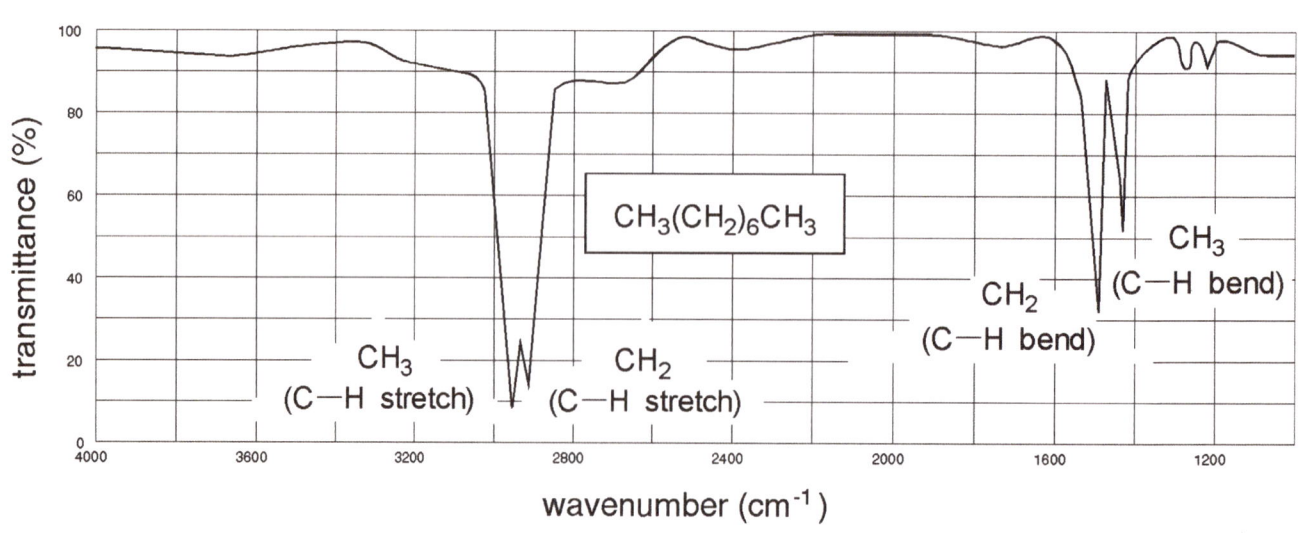

to absorption spectra in the infrared region of the electromagnetic spectrum.

Thus there are two types of bond vibration: stretching and bending. That is, after exposure to the IR radiation the bonds stretch and bend (*or contract*) to a greater degree once energy is absorbed. In general, bending vibrations will occur at lower frequencies (higher wavelengths) than stretching vibrations of the same groups. So, as seen in the sample spectra for octane, each group will have two characteristic peaks, one due to stretching, and one due to bending.

Different functional groups will have transmittances at characteristic wave numbers, which is why IR spectroscopy is useful. Some examples (*approximate values*) of characteristic absorbances are shown in the table.

By looking at the characteristic transmittances of a compound's spectrum, it is possible to identify the functional groups present in the molecule.

Symmetrical molecules or molecules composed of the same atoms do not exhibit

Group	Frequency Range (cm^{-1})
Alkyl (C–H)	2850 – 2960
Alkene (C=C)	1620 – 1680
Alkyne (C≡C)	2100 – 2260
Alcohol (O–H)	3200 – 3650
Benzene (Ar–H)	3030
Carbonyl (C=O)	1630 – 1780
▸ Aldehyde	1680 – 1750
▸ Ketone	1735 – 1750
▸ Carboxylic Acid	1710 – 1780
▸ Amide	1630 – 1690
Amine (N–H)	3300 – 3500
Nitriles (C≡N)	2220 – 2260

a change in dipole moment under IR radiation and thus absorptions do not show up in IR spectra.

Most introductory level courses require students to memorize at least the absorbances for, arguably, the two most important functional groups at the introductory level: carbonyl (around 1700) and alcohol (around 3300). Knowing these 2 benchmarks may be helpful but there is no evidence that even these 2 values are required knowledge for the GAMSAT.

14.2 Proton NMR Spectroscopy

Nuclear Magnetic Resonance (NMR) spectroscopy can be used to examine the environments of the hydrogen atoms in a molecule. In fact, using a (*proton*) NMR or

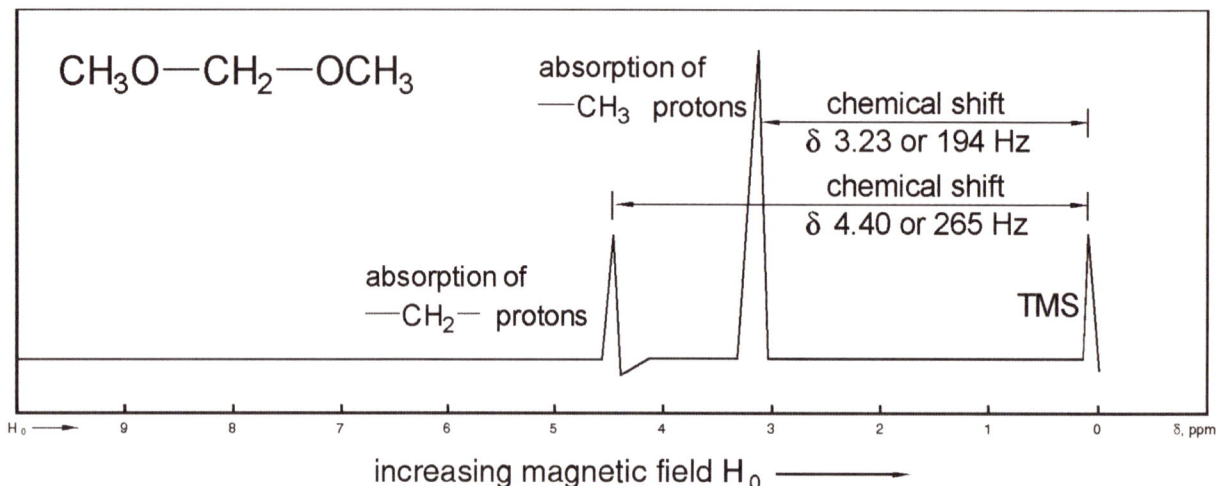

¹HNMR, one can determine both the number and types of hydrogens in a molecule. The basis of this stems from the magnetic properties of the hydrogen nucleus (proton). Similar to electrons, the hydrogen proton has a nuclear spin, able to take either of two values. These values are designated as +1/2 and –1/2. As a result of this spin, the nucleus will respond to a magnetic field by being oriented in the direction of the field. NMR spectrometers measure the absorption of energy by the hydrogen nuclei in an organic compound.

A schematic representation of an NMR spectrum, that of dimethoxymethane is shown in the diagram above.

The small peak at the right is that of TMS, tetramethylsilane, shown here:

$$CH_3-Si(CH_3)_2-CH_3$$

This compound is added to the sample to be used as a reference, or standard. It is volatile, inert and absorbs at a higher field than most other organic chemicals.

The position of a peak relative to the standard is referred to as its *chemical shift*. Since NMR spectroscopy differentiates between types of protons, each type will have a different chemical shift, as shown. Protons in the same environment, like the three hydrogens in $-CH_3$, are called *equivalent protons*.

Dimethoxymethane is a symmetric molecule, thus the protons on either methyl group are equivalent. So, in the example above, the absorption of $-CH_3$ protons occurs at one peak (*a singlet*) 3.23 ppm downfield from TMS. In most organic molecules, the range of absorption will be in the 0–10 ppm (= *parts per million*) range.

The area under each peak is directly related to the number of protons contributing to it, and thus may be used to determine the

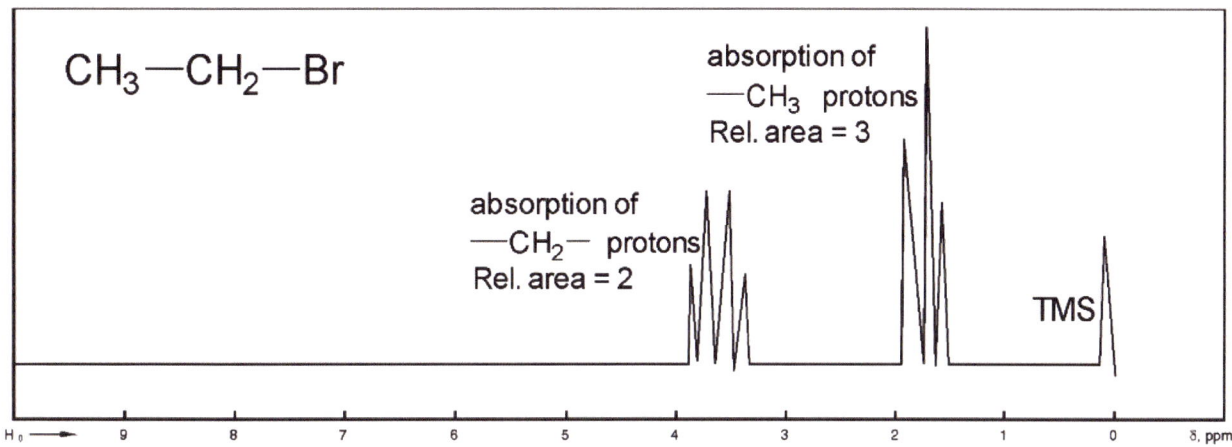

relative number of protons in the molecule. Accurate measurements of the area under the two peaks above yield the ratio 1:3 which represents the relative number of hydrogens (i.e. 1:3 = 2:6).

Let us now examine a schematic representation of the NMR spectrum of ethyl bromide shown in the diagram above.

It is obvious that something is different. Looking at the molecule, one can see that there are two different types of protons (*either far from Br or near to Br*). However, there are more than two signals in the spectrum. As such, the NMR signal for each group is said to be split. This type of splitting is called spin-spin splitting (= *spin-spin coupling*) and is caused by the presence of neighboring protons (*protons on an adjacent or vicinal carbon*) that are not equivalent to the proton in question. Note that protons that are farther than two carbons apart do not exhibit a coupling effect.

The number of lines in the splitting pattern for a given set of equivalent protons depends on the number of adjacent protons according to the following rule: if there are n equivalent protons in adjacent positions, a proton NMR signal is split into $n + 1$ lines.

Therefore the NMR spectrum for ethyl bromide can be interpreted thus:

- There are two groups of lines (*two split peaks*), therefore there are two different environments for protons.

- The relative areas under each peak is 2:3, which represents the relative number of hydrogens in the molecule.

- There are 4 splits (*quartet*) in the peak which has relatively two hydrogens ($-CH_2$). Thus the number of adjacent hydrogens is $n + 1 = 4$; therefore, there are 3 hydrogens on the carbon adjacent to $-CH_2$.

- There are 3 splits (*triplet*) in the peak which has relatively three hydrogens ($-CH_3$).

Thus the number of adjacent hydrogens is $n + 1 = 3$; therefore, there are 2 hydrogens on the carbon adjacent to $-CH_3$.

The relative areas under each peak may be expressed in three ways: (i) the information may simply be provided to you (*too easy!*); (ii) the integers may be written above the signals (= *integration integers*, i.e. 2,3 in the previous example); or (iii) a step-like *integration curve* above the signals where the relative height of each step equals the relative number of hydrogens.

14.2.1 Deuterium Exchange

Deuterium, the hydrogen isotope ^2H or D, can be used to identify substances with readily exchangeable or acidic hydrogens. Rather than H_2O, D_2O is used to identify the chemical exchange:

$$ROH + DOD \rightleftharpoons ROD + HOD$$

The previous signal due to the acidic $-O\boxed{H}$ would now disappear. However, if excess D_2O is used, a signal as a result of HOD may be observed.

Solvents may also be involved in exchange phenomena. The solvents carbon tetrachloride (CCl_4) and deuteriochloroform ($CDCl_3$) can also engage in exchange-induced decoupling of acidic hydrogens (usu. in alcohols).

14.2.2 ^{13}C NMR

The main difference between proton NMR and ^{13}C NMR is that most carbon 13 signals occur 0–200 δ downfield from the carbon peak of TMS. There is also very little coupling between carbon atoms as only 1.1% of carbon atoms are ^{13}C. There is coupling between carbon atoms and their adjacent protons which are directly attached to them. This coupling of one bond is similar to the three bond coupling exhibited by proton NMR.

Signals will be split into a triplet with an area of 1:2:1 when a carbon atom is attached to two protons. Another unique feature of ^{13}C NMR is a phenomenon called spin decoupling where a spectrum of singlets can be recorded - each corresponding to a singular carbon atom. This allows one to accurately determine the number of different carbons in their respective chemical environments as well as the number of adjacent hydrogens (spin-coupled only).

To remind yourself of the isotopes deuterium and carbon-13, consider reviewing PHY 12.2.

ORGANIC CHEMISTRY

14.3 Mass Spectrometry

Mass spectrometry (the former expression "mass spectroscopy" is discouraged), unlike other forms of NMR we have seen, destroys the sample during its analysis. The analysis is carried out using a beam of electrons which ionize the sample and a detector to measure the number of particles that are deflected due to the presence of a magnetic field. The reflected particle is usually an unstable species which decomposes rapidly into a cationic fragment and a radical fragment.

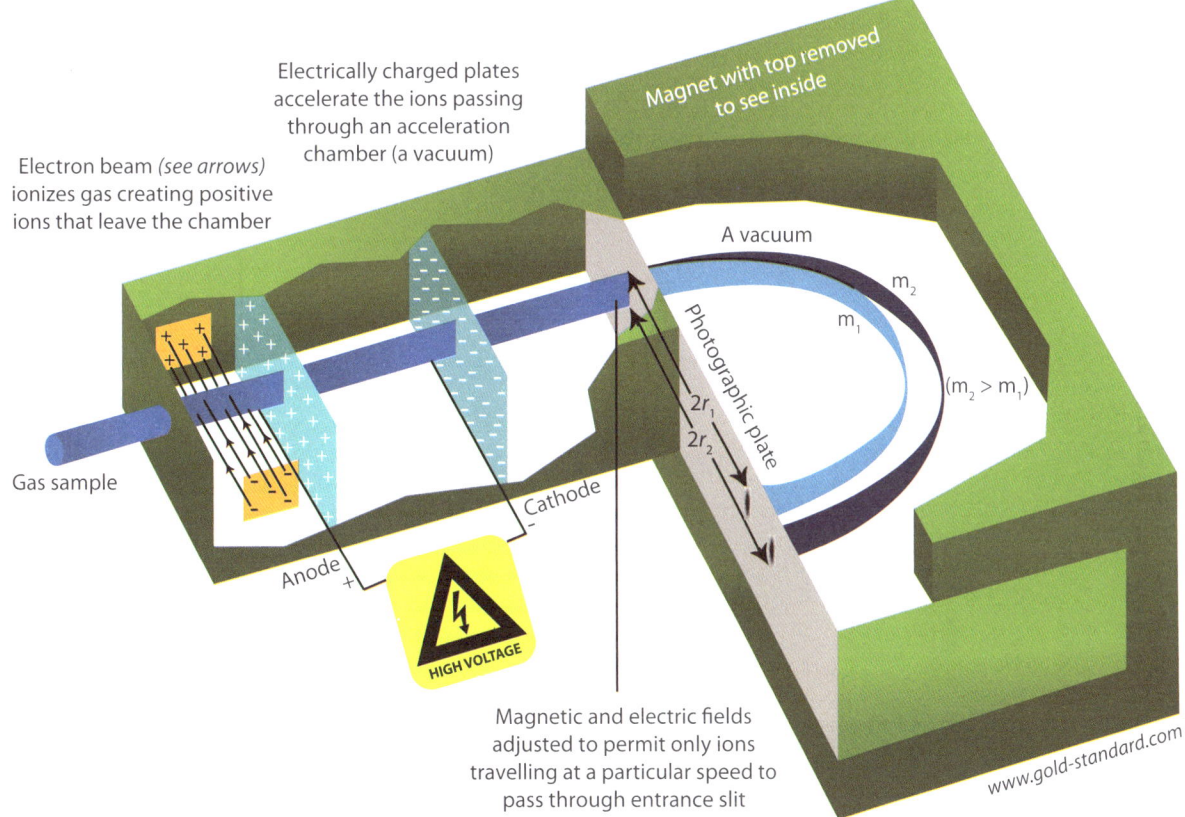

Figure IV.B.14.1: Diagrammatic representation of a mass spectrometer. Electrons stream out (beam) from a heated cathode (negatively charged orange plate) towards the anode (positively charged orange plate) thus bombarding the gas creating cations. The cations are accelerated by a high voltage electric field. Magnetic and electric fields are adjusted to permit only ions traveling at a particular speed to pass through the entrance slit (i.e. to pass through the slit between the acceleration chamber and the magnetic chamber). Notice that the heavier particles are less deviated (more inertia; PHY 4.2) and thus have a larger diameter (= 2r) from the slit to the photographic plate. ACER's GAMSAT "Red" Booklet (GAMSAT Practice Questions, currently Unit 15) has a series of questions based on the mass spectrometer requiring an integration of concepts including electromagnetic fields (PHY 9.1, 9.2) and, because of the path of the ions in the magnetic chamber, circular motion (PHY 3.3). (adapted from chemeddl.org)

THE BIOLOGICAL SCIENCES ORG-153

Since there are many ways in which the particle can decompose, a typical mass spectrum is often composed of numerous lines, with each one corresponding to a specific mass/charge ratio (m/z, sometimes symbolized as m/e or m/q). It is important to note that only cations are deflected by the magnetic field, thus only cations will appear on the spectrum which plots m/z (x-axis) vs. the abundance of the cationic fragments (y-axis). See the figure provided.

The tallest peak represents the most common ion and is also referred to as the base peak. The molecular weight can be obtained not from the base peak but rather from the peak with the highest m/z ratio, 129 in this case. This is called the parent ion peak and is designated by M+. By looking at the fragmentation pattern we can ascertain information regarding the compound's structure, something that IR spectroscopy is incapable of achieving. Note that if the charge on the ion has a magnitude of 1 (which is usually the case) then the magnitude on the x axis is simply the mass (i.e. m/z = m/1 = m = atomic mass units = amu; PHY 12.2, CHM 1.3).

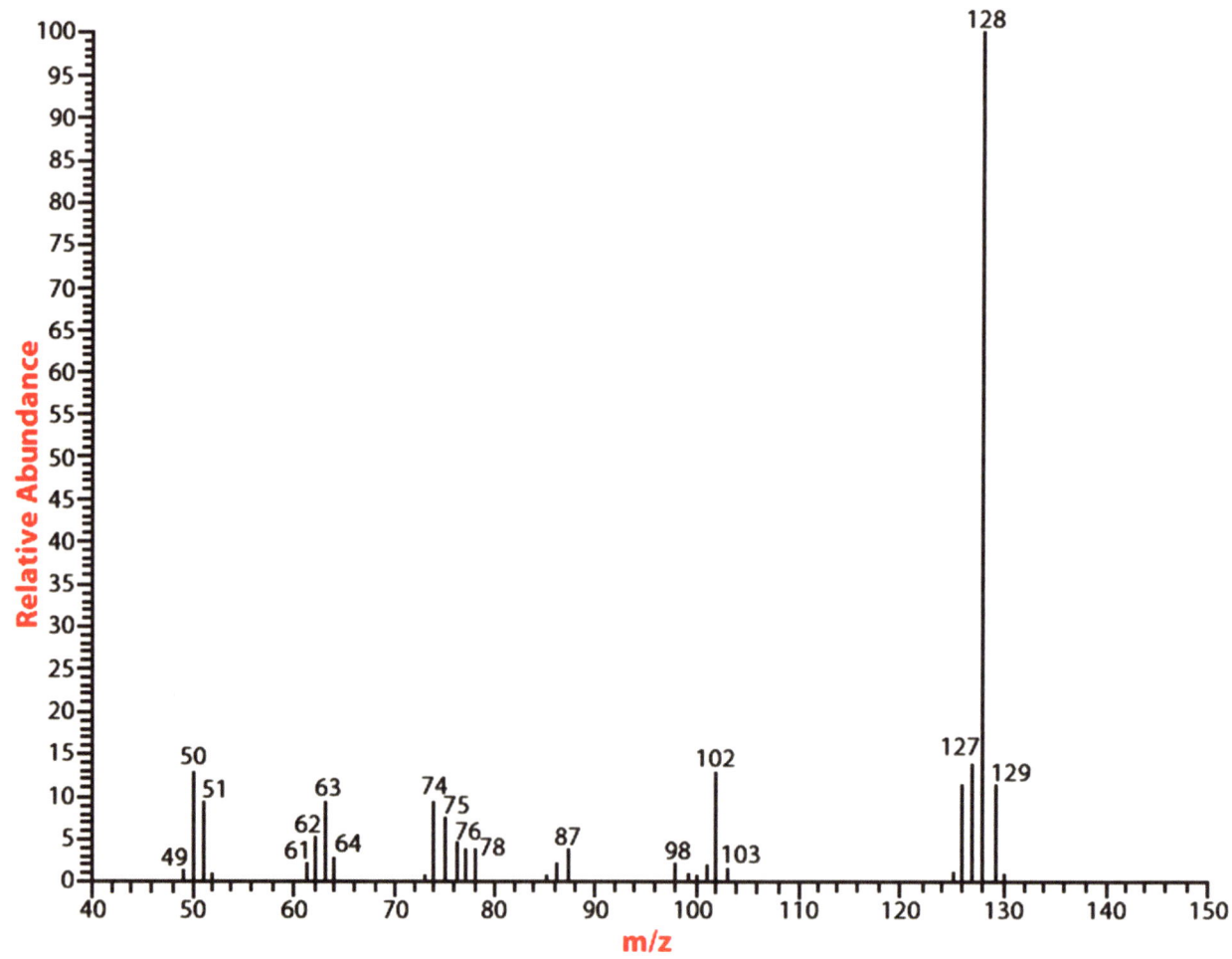

ORGANIC CHEMISTRY

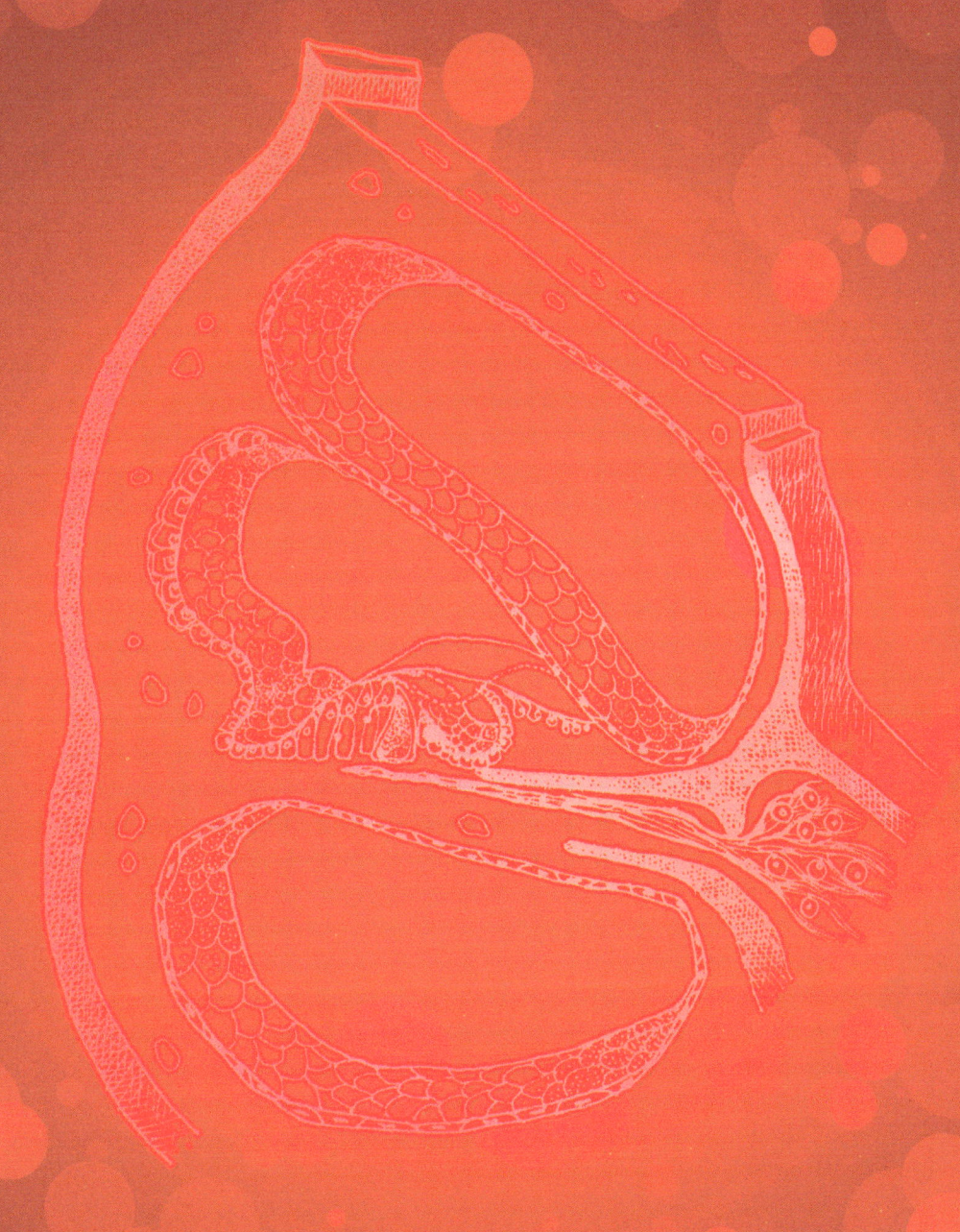

GAMSAT-Prep.com
BIOLOGY
PART IV.A: BIOLOGICAL SCIENCES

IMPORTANT: Before doing your science survey for the GAMSAT, be sure you have read the Preface, Introduction and Part II, Chapter 2. The beginning of each science chapter provides guidelines as to what you should Memorize, Understand and what is Not Required. These are guides to get you a top score without getting lost in the details. Our guides have been determined from an analysis of all ACER materials plus student surveys. Additionally, the original owner of this book gets a full year access to many online features described in the Preface and Introduction including an online Forum where each chapter can be discussed.

GENERALIZED EUKARYOTIC CELL
Chapter 1

Memorize	Understand	Not Required*
ucture/function: cell/components mponents and function: cytoskeleton A structure and function nsmission of genetic information osis, events of the cell cycle	* Intro level college info * Membrane transport * Hyper/hypotonic solutions * Saturation kinetics: graphs * Unique features of eukaryotes * Basics: Cell junctions, microscopy	* Advanced level college info * Molecular bio., detailed mechanisms * Plant cells, chloroplasts * Experiments in genetics * Specify polymerases or such details

GAMSAT-Prep.com

Introduction

Cells are the basic organizational unit of living organisms. They are contained by a plasma membrane and/or cell wall. Eukaryotic cells (*eu* = true; *karyote* refers to nucleus) are cells with a true nucleus found in all multicellular and nonbacterial unicellular organisms including animal, fungal and plant cells. The nucleus contains genetic information, DNA, which can divide into 2 cells by mitosis.

Get ready to waste some time! Glad to have your attention! Our experience is that most students 'overstudy' Biology and underperform in Biology when they see the types of questions that are asked on the GAMSAT. Please do not get trapped in details. We'll guide you as much as we can but in the end, it's up to you: color-coded table of contents, yellow highlighter, underline, online practice questions, etc. For now, enjoy the story that you are expected to be exposed to for the GAMSAT, but generally the content will likely be more helpful to you in medical school.

Additional Resources

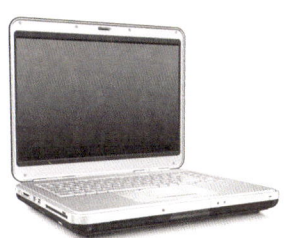
Free Online Q&A + Forum

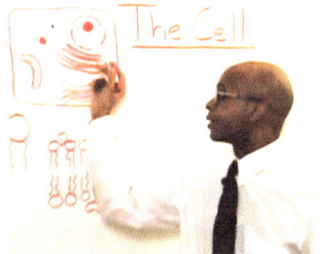
Video: Online or DVD

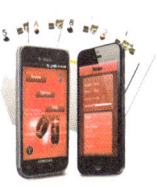
Flashcards

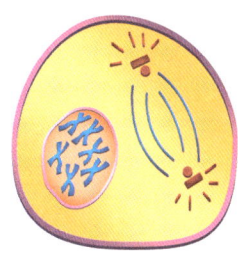
Special Guest

THE BIOLOGICAL SCIENCES   BIO-03

* The real GAMSAT may have advanced level information presented (ie. in a passage) but previous knowledge of said information is not required to answer the questions that would follow. Practice ACER and GS practice GAMSATs can help you clarify this point.

GAMSAT-Prep.com
THE GOLD STANDARD

1.1 Plasma Membrane: Structure and Functions

The plasma membrane is a semipermeable barrier that defines the outer perimeter of the cell. It is composed of lipids (fats) and protein. The membrane is dynamic, selective, active, and fluid. It contains phospholipids which are <u>amphipathic</u> molecules. They are amphipathic because their tail end contains fatty acids which are insoluble in water (*hydrophobic*), the opposite end contains a charged phosphate head which is soluble in water (*hydrophilic*). The plasma membrane contains two layers or "leaflets" of phospholipids thus it is called a bilipid layer. Unlike eukaryotic membranes, prokaryotic membranes do not contain steroids such as cholesterol.

The <u>Fluid Mosaic Model</u> tells us that the hydrophilic heads project to the outside and the hydrophobic tails project towards the inside of the membrane. Further, these phospholipids are <u>fluid</u> - thus they move freely from place to place in the membrane. Fluidity of the membrane increases with increased temperature and with decreased saturation of fatty acyl tails. Fluidity of the membrane decreases with decreased temperature, increased saturation of fatty acyl tails and increase in the membrane's cholesterol content. The structures of these and other biological molecules were discussed in Organic Chemistry Chapter 12.

Glycolipids are limited to the extracellular aspect of the membrane or outer leaflet. The carbohydrate portion of glycolipids extends from the outer leaflet into the extracellular space and forms part of the glycocalyx. "Glycocalyx" is the sugar coat on the outer surface of the outer leaflet of plasma membrane. It consists of oligosaccharide linked to

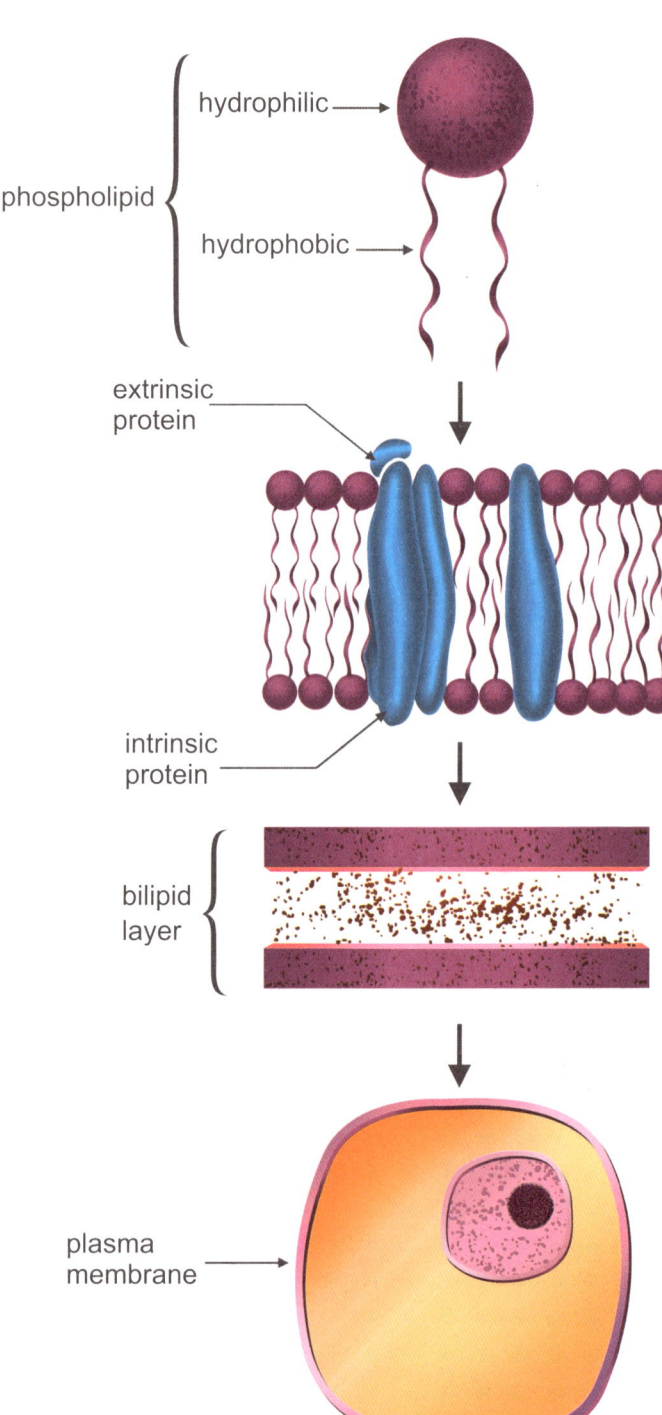

Figure IV.A.1.1: Structure of the plasma membrane. Note that: hydro = water, phobic = fearing, philic = loving

BIO-04 GENERALIZED EUKARYOTIC CELL

protein or lipids of the plasma membrane. The glycocalyx aids in attachment of some cells, facilitates cell recognition, helps bind antigen and antigen-presenting cells to the cell surface. Distributed throughout the membrane is a mosaic of proteins with limited mobility.

Proteins can be found associated with the outside of the membrane (extrinsic or peripheral) or may be found spanning the membrane (intrinsic or integral). Integral proteins are dissolved in the lipid bilayer. Transmembrane proteins contain hydrophilic and hydrophobic amino acids and cross the entire plasma membrane. Most transmembrane proteins are glycoproteins. They usually function as membrane receptors and transport proteins.

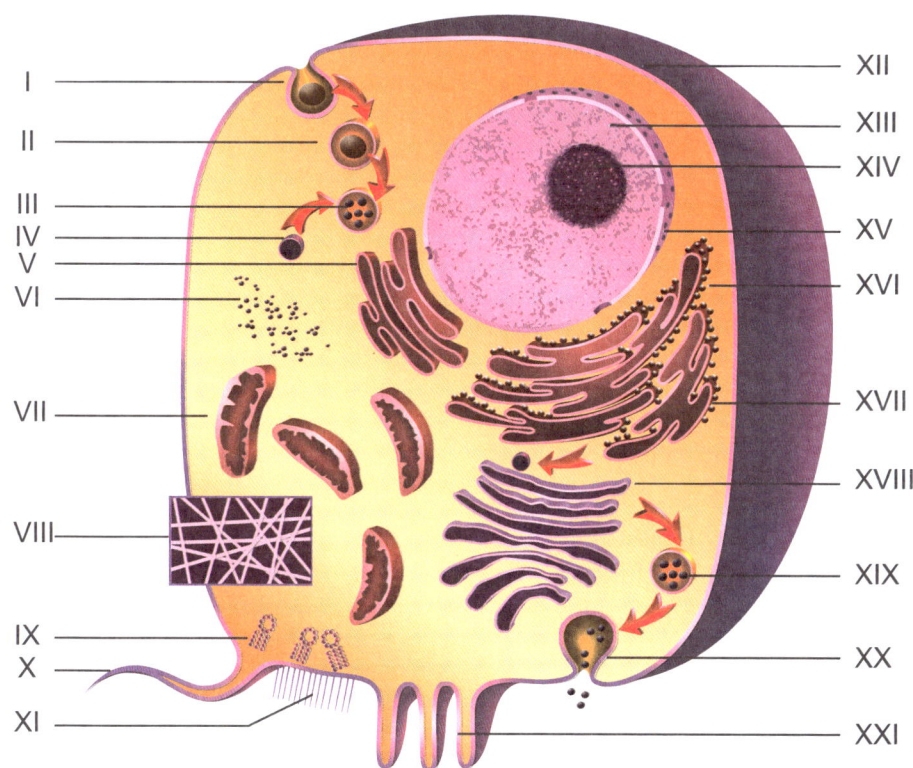

Figure IV.A.1.2: The generalized eukaryotic cell

I	endocytosis	VIII	cytoskeleton (further magnified)	XV	nuclear envelope
II	endocytotic vesicle	IX	basal body (magnified)	XVI	cytosol
III	secondary lysosome	X	flagellum	XVII	rough endoplasmic reticulum
IV	primary lysosome	XI	cilia	XVIII	Golgi apparatus
V	smooth endoplasmic reticulum	XII	plasma membrane	XIX	exocytotic vesicle
VI	free ribosomes	XIII	nucleus	XX	exocytosis
VII	mitochondrion	XIV	nucleolus	XXI	microvillus

Peripheral proteins do not extend into the lipid bilayer but can temporarily adhere to either side of the plasma membrane. They bond to phospholipid groups or integral proteins of the membrane via noncovalent interactions. Common functions include regulatory protein subunits of ion channels or transmembrane receptors, associations with the cytoskeleton and extracellular matrix, and as part of the intracellular second messenger system.

The plasma membrane is semipermeable. In other words, it is permeable to small uncharged substances which can freely diffuse across the membrane (i.e. O_2, CO_2, urea). The eukaryotic plasma membrane does not have pores, as pores would destroy the barrier function. On the other hand, it is relatively impermeable to charged or large substances which may require transport proteins to cross the membrane (i.e. ions, amino acids, sugars) or cannot cross the membrane at all (i.e. protein hormones, intracellular enzymes). Substances which can cross the membrane may do so by simple diffusion, carrier-mediated transport, or by endo/exocytosis.

1.1.1 Simple Diffusion

Simple diffusion is the spontaneous spreading of a substance going from an area of higher concentration to an area of lower concentration (i.e. a concentration gradient exists). Gradients can be of a chemical or electrical nature. A chemical gradient arises as a result of an unequal distribution of molecules and is often called a concentration gradient. In a chemical (or concentration) gradient, there is a higher concentration of molecules in one area than there is in another area, and molecules tend to diffuse from areas of high concentration to areas of lower concentration.

An electrical gradient arises as a result of an unequal distribution of charge. In an electrical gradient, there is a higher concentration of charged molecules in one area than in another (this is independent of

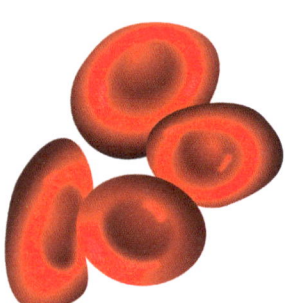

Figure IV.A.1.2.1a: Isotonic Solution. The fluid bathing the cell (i.e. red blood cell or RBC in this case; see BIO 7.5) contains the same concentration of solute as the cell's inside or cytoplasm. When a cell is placed in an isotonic solution, the water diffuses into and out of the cell at the same rate.

the concentration of all molecules in the area). Molecules tend to move from areas of higher concentration of charge to areas of lower concentration of charge.

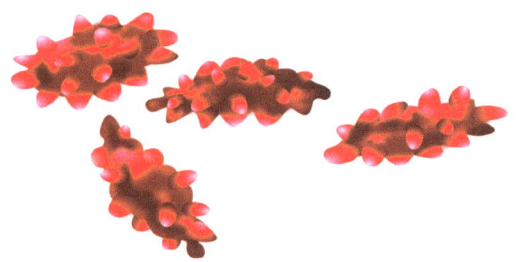

Figure IV.A.1.2.1b: Hypertonic Solution. Here the fluid bathing the RBC contains a high concentration of solute relative to the cell's cytoplasm. When a cell is placed in a hypertonic solution, the water diffuses out of the cell, causing the cell to shrivel (crenation).

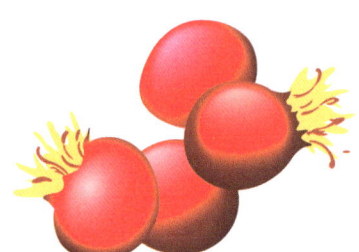

Figure IV.A.1.2.1c: Hypotonic Solution. Here the surrounding fluid has a low concentration of solute relative to the cell's cytoplasm. When a cell is placed in a hypotonic solution, the water diffuses into the cell, causing the cell to swell and possibly rupture (lyse).

Osmosis is the diffusion of water across a semipermeable membrane moving from an area of higher water concentration (i.e. lower solute concentration = hypotonic) to an area of lower water concentration (i.e. higher solute concentration = hypertonic). The hydrostatic pressure needed to oppose the movement of water is called the osmotic pressure. Thus, an isotonic solution (i.e. the concentration of solute on both sides of the membrane is equal), would have an osmotic pressure of zero.

{Memory guide: notice that the "O" in hyp-O-tonic looks like a swollen cell. The O is also a circle which makes you think of the word "around." So IF the environment is hypOtonic AROUND the cell, then fluid rushes in and the cell swells like the letter O}.

1.1.2 Carrier-mediated Transport

Amino acids, sugars and other solutes need to reversibly bind to proteins (carriers) in the membrane in order to get across. Because there are a limited amount of carriers, if the concentration of solute is too high, the carriers would be saturated, thus the rate of crossing the membrane would level off (= saturation kinetics).

The two carrier-mediated transport systems are:

(i) <u>facilitated transport</u> where the carrier helps a solute diffuse across a membrane it could not otherwise penetrate. Facilitated diffusion occurs via ion channels or carrier proteins and transport molecules down a concentration of electrochemical gradient. Ions and large molecules are therefore able to cross the membrane that would otherwise be impermeable to them.

ii) <u>active transport</u> where energy (i.e. ATP) is used to transport solutes <u>against</u> their

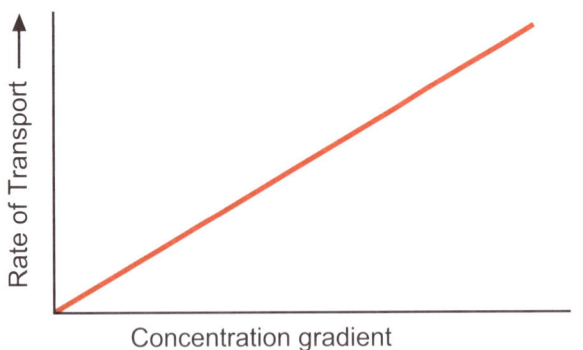

Simple Diffusion: the greater the concentration gradient, the greater the rate of transport across the plasma membrane.

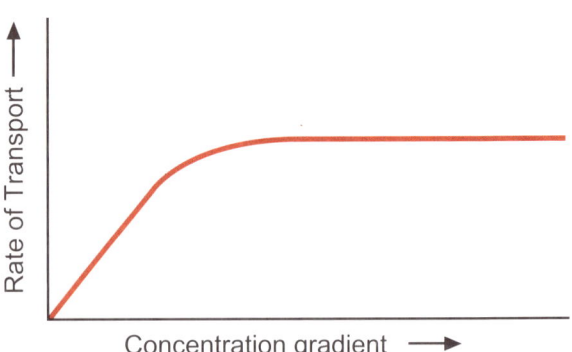

Carrier-mediated Transport: increasing the concentration gradient increases the rate of transport up to a maximum rate, at which point all membrane carriers are saturated.

Figure IV.A.1.3: Simple diffusion versus Carrier-mediated transport.

concentration gradients. The Na^+-K^+ exchange pump uses ATP to actively pump Na^+ to where its concentration is highest (outside the cell) and K^+ is brought within the cell where its concentration is highest (see Neural Cells and Tissues, BIO 5.1.1).

1.1.3 Endo/Exocytosis

Endocytosis is the process by which the cell membrane actually invaginates, pinches off and is released intracellularly (endocytotic vesicle). If a solid particle was ingested by the cell (i.e. a bacterium), it is called phagocytosis. If fluid was ingested, it is pinocytosis.

The receptor-mediated endocytosis of ligands (e.g. low density lipoprotein, transferrin, growth factors, antibodies, etc.) are mediated by clathrin-coated vesicles (CCVs). CCVs are found in virtually all cells and form areas in the plasma membrane termed clathrin-coated pits. Caveolae are the most common reported non-clathrin-coated plasma membrane buds, which exist on the surface of many, but not all cell types. They consist of the cholesterol-binding protein caveolin with a bilayer enriched in cholesterol and glycolipids.

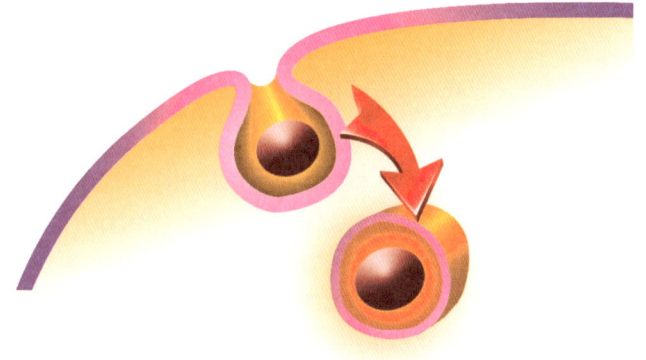

Figure IV.A.1.4: Endocytosis.

Exocytosis is, essentially, the reverse process. The cell directs an intracellular vesicle to fuse with the plasma membrane thus releasing its contents to the exterior (i.e. neurotransmitters, pancreatic enzymes, cell membrane proteins/lipids, etc.).

The transient vesicle fusion with the cell membrane forms a structure shaped like a pore (= *porosome*). Thus porosomes are cup-shaped structures where vesicles dock in the process of fusion and secretion. Porosomes contain many different types of protein including chloride and calcium channels, actin, and SNARE proteins that mediate the docking and fusion of vesicles with the cell membrane. The primary role of SNARE proteins is to mediate vesicle fusion through

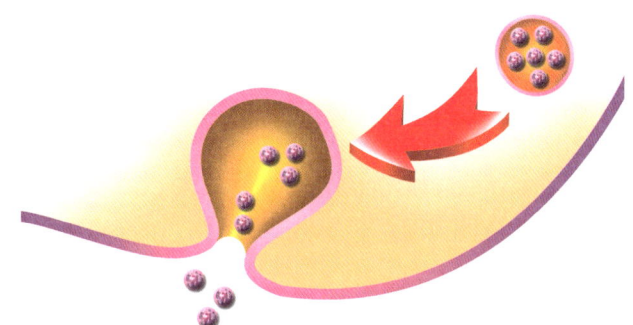

Figure IV.A.1.5: Exocytosis.

full fusion exocytosis or open and close exocytosis. The former is where the vesicle collapses fully into the plasma membrane; in the latter, the vesicle docks transiently with the membrane (= "kiss-and-run") and is recycled (i.e. in the synaptic terminal; BIO 1.5.1, 5.1).

1.2 The Interior of a Eukaryotic Cell

Cytoplasm is the interior of the cell. It refers to all cell components enclosed by the cell's membrane which includes the cytosol, the cytoskeleton, and the membrane bound organelles. Transport within the cytoplasm occurs by cyclosis (circular motion of cytoplasm around the cell).

Cytosol is the solution which bathes the organelles and contains numerous solutes like amino acids, sugars, proteins, etc.

Cytoskeleton extends throughout the entire cell and has particular importance in shape and intracellular transportation. The cytoskeleton also makes extracellular complexes with other proteins forming a matrix so that cells can "stick" together. This is called cellular adhesion.

The components of the cytoskeleton in increasing order of size are: microfilaments, intermediate filaments, and microtubules. Microfilaments are important for cell movement and contraction (i.e. actin and myosin. See Contractile Cells and Tissues, BIO 5.2). Microfilaments, also known as actin filaments, are composed of actin monomer (G actin) linked into a double helix. They display polarity (= having distinct and opposite poles), with polymerization and depolymerization occuring preferentially at the barbed end [also called the plus (+) end which is where ATP is bound to G actin; BIO 5.2]. Microfilaments squeeze the membrane together in phagocytosis and cytokinesis. They are also important for muscle contraction and microvilli movement.

Intermediate filaments and microtubules extend along axons and dendrites of neurons acting like railroad tracks, so organelles or protein particles can shuttle to or from the cell body. Microtubules also form:

(i) the core of cilia and flagella (see the 9 doublet + 2 structure in BIO 1.5);
(ii) the mitotic spindles which we shall soon discuss; and
(iii) centrioles.

A flagellum is an organelle of locomotion found in sperm and bacteria. Eukaryotic flagella are made from microtubule configurations while prokaryotic flagella are thin strands of a single protein called flagellin. Thus, eukaryotic flagella move in a whip-like motion while prokaryotic flagella rotate. Cilia are hair-like vibrating organelles which can be used to move particles along the surface of the cell (e.g., in the fallopian tubes cilia can help the egg move toward the uterus). Microtubules are composed of tubulin subunits. They display polarity, with polymerization and depolymerization occuring preferentially at the plus end where GTP is bound to the tubulin subunit. Microtubules are involved in flagella and cilia construction, and the spindle apparatus. Centrioles are cylinder-shaped complexes of microtubules associated with the mitotic spindle (MTOC, see later). At the base of flagella and cilia, two centrioles can be found at right angles to each other: this is called a basal body.

Microvilli are regularly arranged finger-like projections with a core of cytoplasm (see BIO 9.5). They are commonly found in the small intestine where they help to increase the absorptive and digestive surfaces (= brush border).

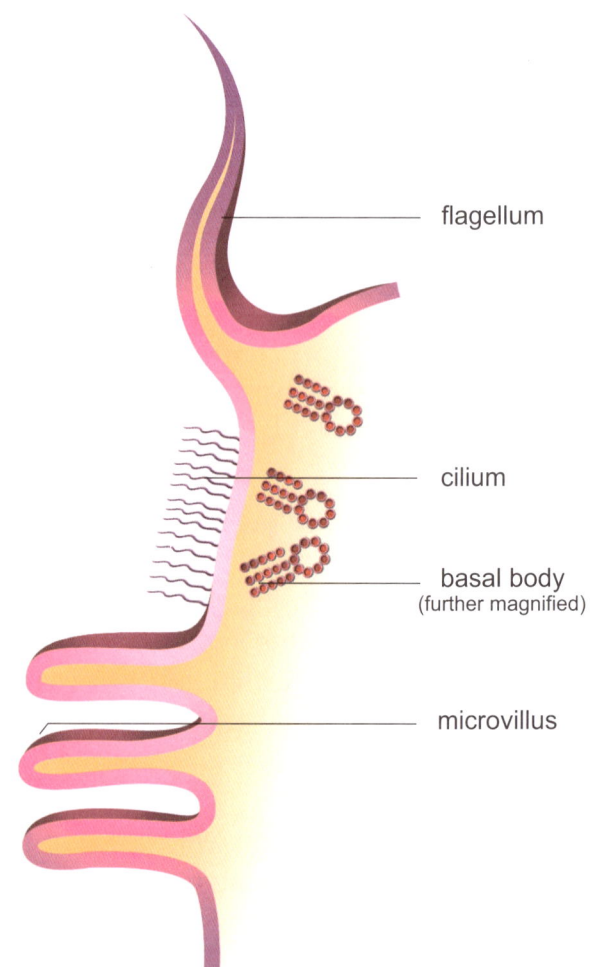

Figure IV.A.1.6: Cytoskeletal elements and the plasma membrane. The core of cilia and flagella is composed of 9 doublet or pairs of microtubules with another *doublet* in the center (= *axoneme*; see BIO 1.5).

BIOLOGY

1.2.1 Membrane Bound Organelles

Mitochondrion: The Power House

Mitochondria produce energy (i.e. ATP) for the cell through aerobic respiration (BIO 4.4). It is a double membraned organelle whose inner membrane has shelf-like folds which are called cristae. The matrix, the fluid within the inner membrane, contains the enzymes for the Krebs cycle and circular DNA. The latter is the only cellular DNA found outside of the nucleus with the exception of chloroplasts (= the organelle capable of photosynthesis, the conversion of light into chemical energy, in plant cells). There are numerous mitochondria in muscle cells. Mitochondria synthesize ATP via the Krebs cycle via oxidation of glucose, amino acids or fatty acids (BIO 4.4-4.10).

Mitochondria have their own DNA and ribosomes and replicate independently from eukaryotic cells. However, most proteins used in mitochondria are coded by nuclear DNA, not mitochondrial DNA (BIO 15.6.1).

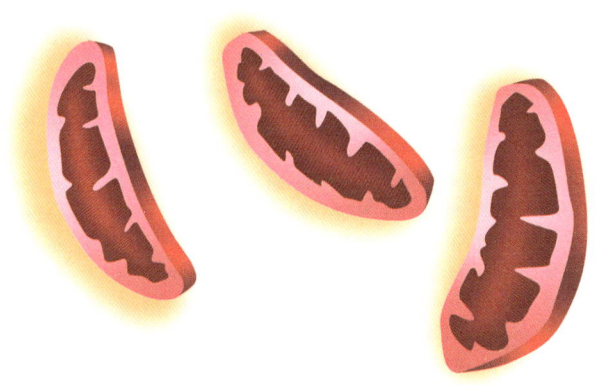

Figure IV.A.1.7: Mitochondria.

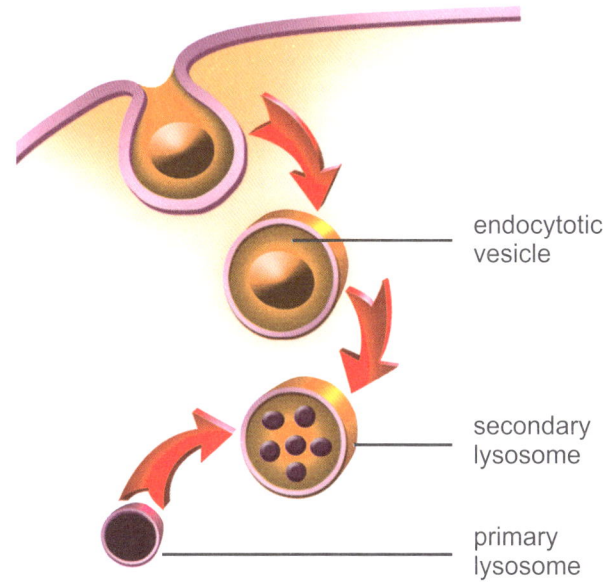

Figure IV.A.1.8: Heterolysis.

Lysosomes: Suicide Sacs

In a diseased cell, lysosomes may release their powerful acid hydrolases to digest away the cell (autolysis). In normal cells, a primary (normal) lysosome can fuse with an endocytotic vesicle to form a secondary lysosome where the phagocytosed particle (i.e. a bacterium) can be digested. This is called heterolysis. There are numerous lysosomes in phagocytic cells of the immune system (i.e. macrophages, neutrophils; BIO 7.5).

Endoplasmic Reticulum: Synthesis Center

The endoplasmic reticulum (ER) is an interconnected membraned system resembling flattened sacs and extends from the cell membrane to the nuclear membrane.

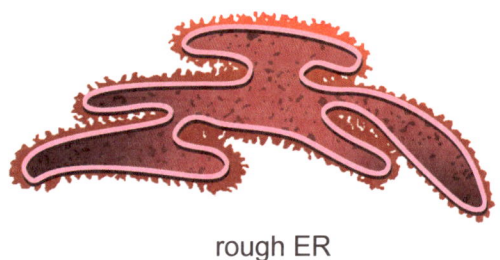
rough ER

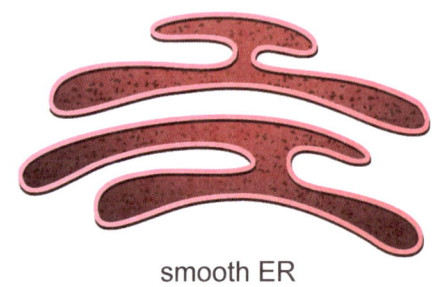
smooth ER

Figure IV.A.1.9: The endoplasmic reticulum.

There are two kinds: (i) dotted with ribosomes on its surface which is called rough ER and (ii) without ribosomes which is smooth ER.

The ribosomes are composed of ribosomal RNA (rRNA) and numerous proteins. It may exist freely in the cytosol or bound to the rough ER or outer nuclear membrane. The ribosome is a site where mRNA is translated into protein.

Rough ER is important in protein synthesis and is abundant in cells synthesizing secretory proteins. It is associated with the synthesis of secretory protein, plasma membrane protein, and lysosomal protein. Smooth ER is abundant in cells synthesizing steroids, triglycerides and cholesterol. It is associated with the synthesis and transport of lipids such as steroid hormone and detoxification of a variety of chemicals. It is also common in skeletal muscle cells involving muscle contraction and relaxation. It is a factor in phospholipid and fatty acid synthesis and metabolism.

Golgi Apparatus: The Export Department

The Golgi apparatus forms a stack of smooth membranous sacs or *cisternae* that function in protein modification, such as the addition of polysaccharides (i.e. glycosylation). The Golgi also packages secretory proteins in membrane bound vesicles which can be exocytosed.

The Golgi apparatus has a distinct polarity with one end being the "cis" face and the other being "trans". The cis face lies close to a separate vesicular-tubular cluster (VTC) also referred to as the ER-Golgi intermediate compartment (ERGIC) which is an organelle. The ERGIC mediates trafficking between the ER and Golgi complex, facilitating the sorting of 'cargo'. The medial (middle) compartment of the Golgi lies between the cis and trans faces. The trans face is oriented towards vacuoles

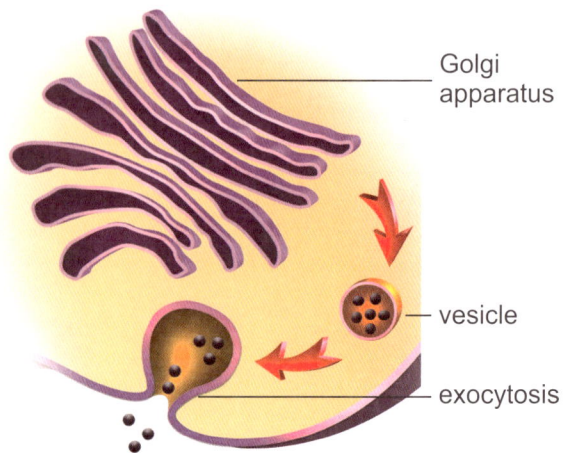

Figure IV.A.1.10: Golgi apparatus.

and secretory granules. The trans Golgi network separates from the trans face and sorts proteins for their final destination.

An abundant amount of rER and Golgi is found in cells which produce and secrete protein. For example, *B-cells* of the immune system which secrete antibodies, *acinar cells* in the pancreas which secrete digestive enzymes into the intestines, and *goblet cells* of the intestine which secrete mucus into the lumen.

Peroxisomes (Microbodies)

Peroxisomes are membrane bound organelles that contain enzymes whose functions include oxidative deamination of amino acids, oxidation of long chain fatty acids and synthesis of cholesterol.

The name "*perox*isome" comes from the fact that it is an organelle with enzymes that can transfer hydrogen from various substrates to oxygen, producing and then degrading hydrogen *perox*ide (H_2O_2).

The Nucleus

The nucleus is surrounded by a double membrane called the nuclear envelope. Throughout the membrane are nuclear pores which selectively allow the transportation of large particles to and from the nucleus. The nucleus is responsible for protein synthesis in the cytoplasm via ribosomal RNA (rRNA), messenger RNA (mRNA), and transfer RNA (tRNA).

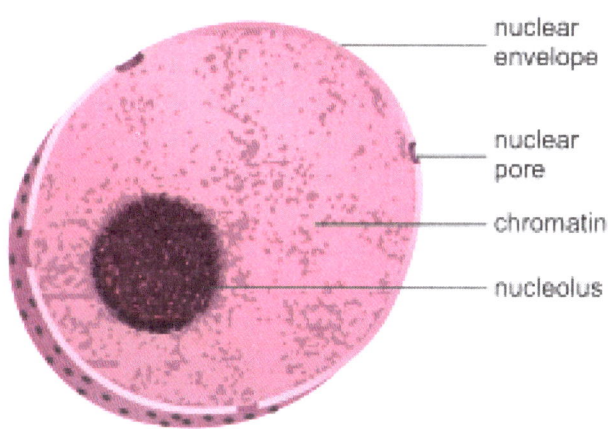

Figure IV.A.1.11: The nucleus.

DNA can be found within the nucleus as chromatin (DNA complexed to proteins like *histones*) or as chromosomes which are more clearly visible in a light microscope. The nucleolus is not membrane bound. It contains mostly ribosomal RNA and protein as well as the DNA necessary to synthesize ribosomal RNA.

The nucleolus is associated with the synthesis of ribosomal RNA (rRNA) and its assembly into ribosome precursors.

Chromosomes are basically extensively folded chromatin maintained by histone proteins. Each chromosome is composed of DNA and associated proteins, forming a nucleosome, the basic structural unit of chromatin. Chromatin exists as heterochromatin and euchromatin. Heterochromatin is a transcriptionally inactive form of chromatin while euchromatin is a transcriptionally active form of chromatin. Chromatin is responsible for RNA synthesis.

1.2.2 DNA: The Cell's Architect

Deoxyribonucleic Acid (DNA) and ribonucleic acid (RNA) are essential components in constructing the proteins which act as the cytoskeleton, enzymes, membrane channels, antibodies, etc. It is the DNA which contains the genetic information of the cell.

DNA and RNA are both important nucleic acids. Nucleotides are the subunits which attach in sequence or in other words polymerize via phosphodiester bonds to form nucleic acids. A nucleotide (also called a *nucleoside phosphate*) is composed of a five carbon sugar, a nitrogen base, and an inorganic phosphate.

The sugar in RNA is ribose but for DNA an oxygen atom is missing in the second position of the sugar thus it is 2-deoxyribose.

There are two categories of nitrogen bases: *purines* and *pyrimidines*. The purines have two rings and include adenine (A) and guanine (G). The pyrimidines contain one ring and include thymine (T), cytosine (C), and uracil (U).

DNA contains the following four bases: adenine, guanine, thymine, and cytosine. RNA contains the same bases except uracil is substituted for thymine.

Watson and Crick's model of DNA has allowed us to get insight into what takes shape as the nucleotides polymerize to form this special nucleic acid. The result is a double *helical* or *stranded* structure.

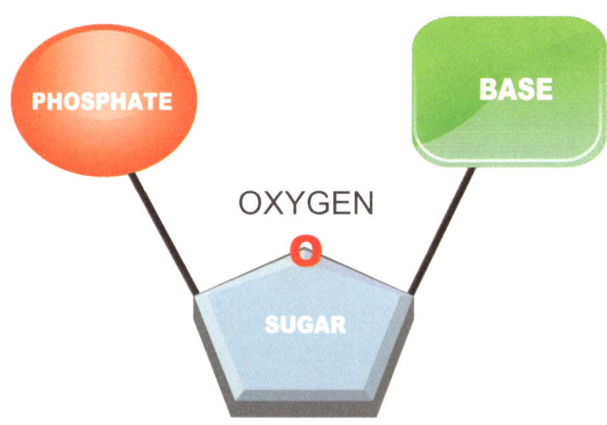

Figure IV.A.1.12: Nucleotide.

The DNA double helix is composed of two complementary and anti-parallel DNA strands held together by hydrogen bonds between base pairing A-T and G-C.

DNA is made from deoxyribose while RNA is made from ribose. DNA is double stranded while RNA is single stranded. DNA contains thymine while RNA contains uracil.

The backbone of each helix is the 2-deoxyribose phosphates. The nitrogen bases project to the center of the double helix in order to hydrogen bond with each other (imagine the double helix as a winding staircase: each stair would represent a pair of bases binding to keep the shape of the double helix intact).

There is specificity in the binding of the bases: one purine binds one pyrimidine. In fact, adenine only binds thymine (through two hydrogen bonds) and guanine only binds cytosine (through three hydrogen bonds).

BIOLOGY

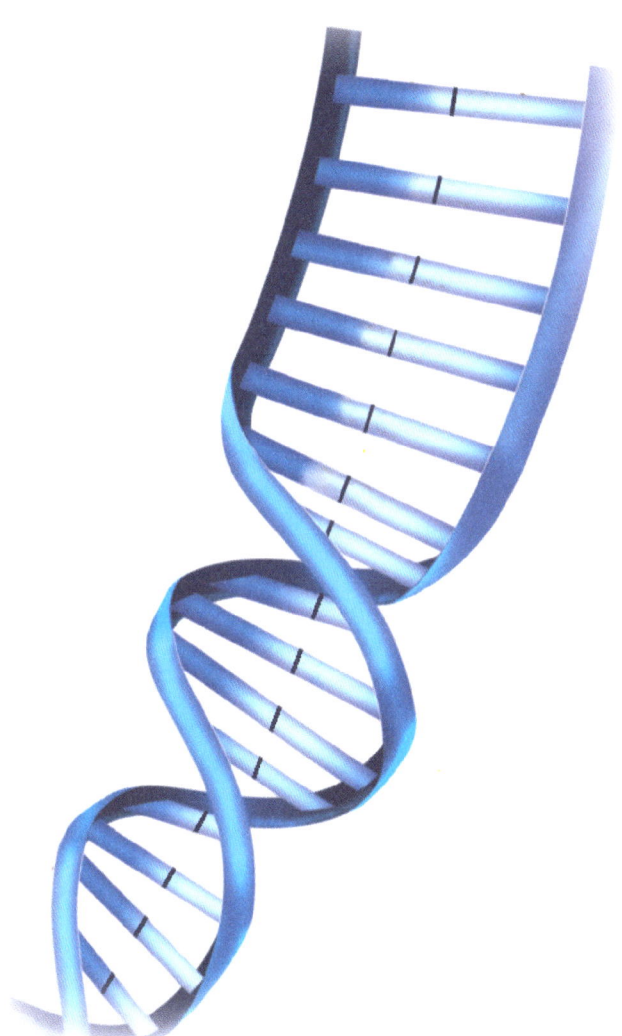

The more the H-bonds (i.e. the more G-C), the more stable the helix will be.

The *replication* (duplication) of DNA is semi-conservative: each strand of the double helix can serve as a template to generate a complementary strand. Thus for each double helix there is one parent strand (*old*) and one daughter strand (*new*). The latter is synthesized using one nucleotide at a time, enzymes including DNA polymerase, and the parent strand as a template. The preceding is termed "DNA Synthesis" and occurs in the S stage of interphase during the cell cycle.

Each nucleotide has a hydroxyl or phosphate group at the 3rd and 5th carbons designated the 3' and 5' positions (see ORG 12.3.2, 12.5). Phosphodiester bonds can be formed between a free 3' hydroxyl group and a free 5' phosphate group. Thus the DNA strand has *polarity* since one end of the molecule will have a free 3' hydroxyl while the other terminal nucleotide will have a free 5' phosphate group. Polymerization of the two strands occurs in opposite directions (= *antiparallel*). In other words, one strand runs in the 5' - 3' direction, while its partner runs in the 3' - 5' direction.

DNA replication is semi-discontinuous. DNA polymerase can only synthesize DNA in the 5' to 3' direction. As a result of the anti-parallel nature of DNA, the 5' - 3' strand is replicated continuously (the *leading strand*), while the 3' - 5' strand is replicated discontinuously (the *lagging strand*) in the reverse direction. The short, newly synthesized DNA fragments that are formed on the lagging strand are called *Okazaki fragments*. DNA synthesis begins at a specific site called the replication origin (*replicon*) and proceeds in both directions. Eukaryotic chromosomes contain multiple origins while prokaryotic chromosomes contain a single origin. The parental strand is always read in the 3' - 5' direction and the daughter strand is always synthesized in the 5' - 3' direction.

THE BIOLOGICAL SCIENCES BIO-15

GAMSAT-Prep.com
THE GOLD STANDARD

Previous knowledge of recombinant DNA techniques, restriction enzymes, hybridization, DNA repair mechanisms, etc., is not normally required for the GAMSAT. However, because these topics do occasionally show up on the exam, they are discussed here and in BIO 2.2.1 and BIO 15.7. The following is an overview regarding DNA repair.

Because of environmental factors including chemicals and UV radiation, any one of the trillions of cells in our bodies may undergo as many as 1 million individual molecular "injuries" per day. Structural damage to DNA may result and could have many effects such as inducing mutation. Thus our DNA repair system is constantly active as it responds to damage in DNA structure.

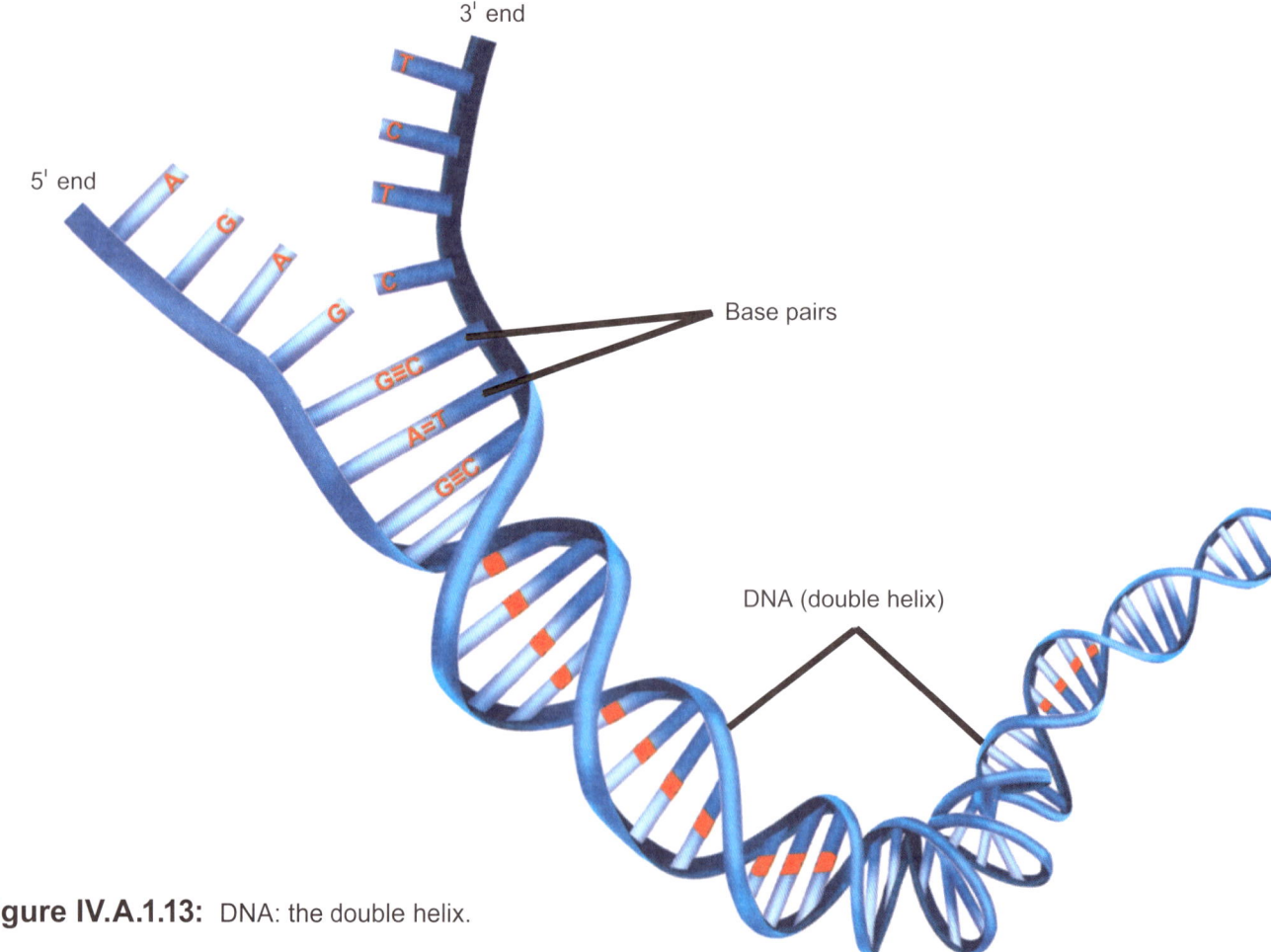

Figure IV.A.1.13: DNA: the double helix.

BIOLOGY

A cell that has accumulated a large amount of DNA damage, or one that no longer effectively repairs damage to its DNA, can: (1) become permanently dormant; (2) exhibit unregulated cell division which could lead to cancer; (3) succumb to cell suicide, also known as *apoptosis* or programmed cell death.

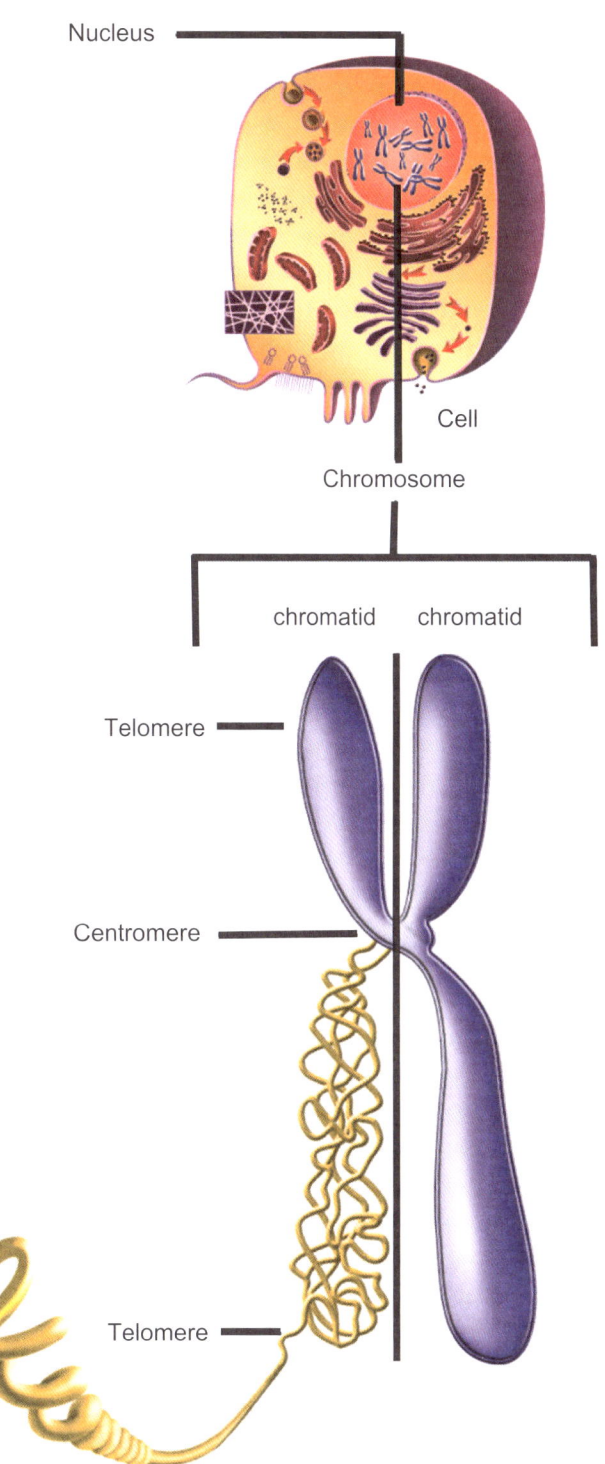

1.3 The Cell Cycle

The cell cycle is a period of approximately 18 - 22 hours during which the cell can synthesize new DNA and partition the DNA equally; thus the cell can divide. Mitosis involves nuclear division (*karyokinesis*) which is usually followed by cell division (*cytokinesis*). Mitosis and cytokinesis together define the mitotic (M) phase of the cell cycle - the division of the mother cell into two daughter cells, genetically identical to each other and to their parent cell. The cell cycle is divided into a number of phases: interphase (G_1, S, G_2) and mitosis (prophase, metaphase, anaphase and telophase).

The cell cycle is temporarily suspended in resting cells. These cells stay in the G_0 state but may reenter the cell cycle and start to divide again. The cell cycle is permanently suspended in non-dividing differentiated cells such as cardiac muscle cells.

Interphase occupies about 90% of the cell cycle. During interphase, the cell prepares for DNA synthesis (G_1), synthesizes or replicates DNA (S) resulting in duplication of chromosomes, and ultimately begins preparing for mitosis (G_2). During interphase, the DNA is not folded and the individual chromosomes are not visible. Also, centrioles grow to maturity, RNA and protein for mitosis are synthesized. Mitosis begins with prophase.

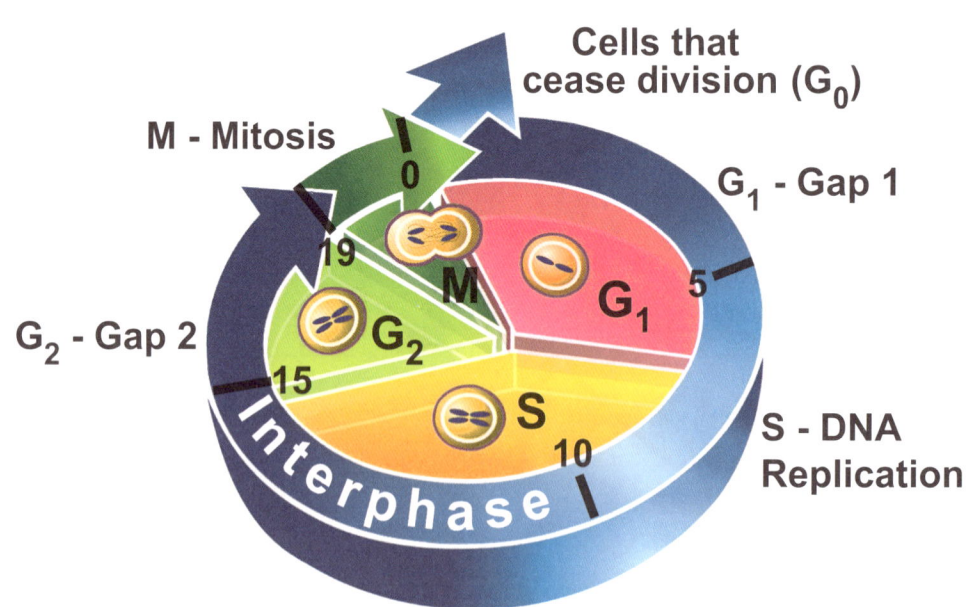

Figure IV.A.1.14: The cell cycle. The numbers represent time in hours. Note how mitosis (M) represents the shortest period of the cycle.

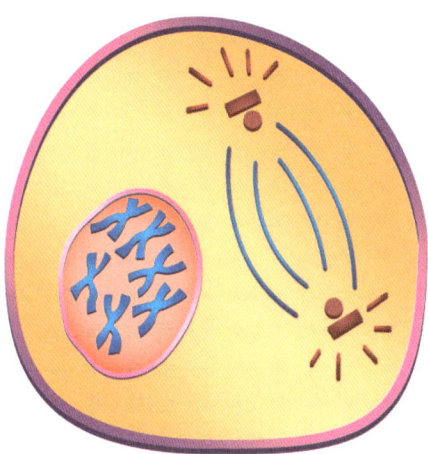

Figure IV.A.1.15: Prophase.

Prophase: pairs of centrioles migrate away from each other while microtubules appear in between forming a spindle. Other microtubules emanating from the centrioles give a radiating star-like appearance; thus they are called asters. Therefore, centrioles form the core of the Microtubule Organizing Centers (MTOC). The MTOC is a structure found in eukaryotic cells from which microtubules emerge and associated with the protein tubulin.

Simultaneously, the diffuse nuclear chromatin condenses into the visible chromosomes which consist of two sister chromatids - each being identical copies of each other. Each chromatid consists of a complete double stranded DNA helix. The area of constriction where the two chromatids are attached is the *centromere*. Kinetochores develop at the centromere region and function as MTOC. Just as centromere refers to the center, *telomere* refers to the ends of the chromosome (note: as cells divide and we age, telomeres progressively shorten). Ultimately, the nuclear envelope disappears at the end of prophase.

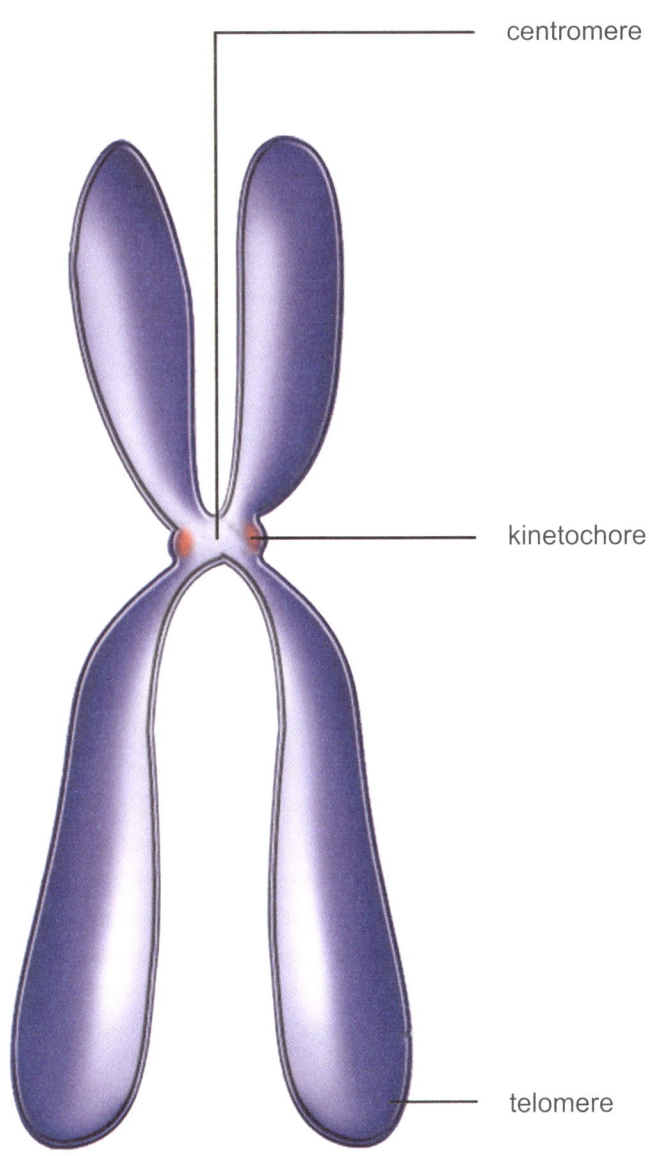

Figure IV.A.1.16: Chromosome Anatomy. Each chromosome has two arms separated by the centromere, labeled p (the shorter, named for 'petit' meaning 'small') and q (the longer of the two). The telomeres contain repetitive nucleotide sequences which protect the end of the chromosome. Over time, due to each cell division, the telomeres become shorter.

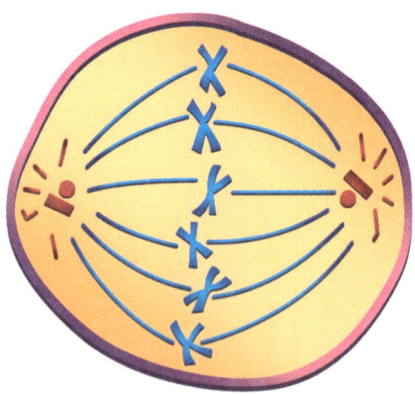

Figure IV.A.1.17: Metaphase.

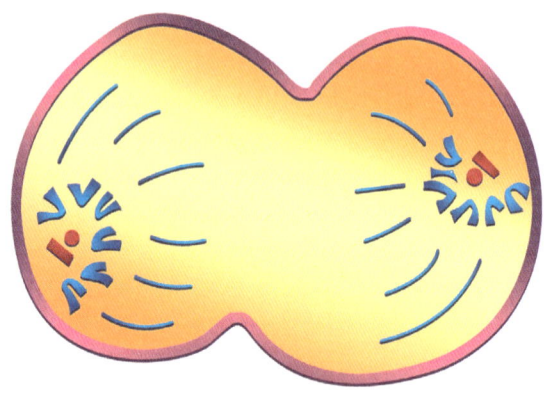

Figure IV.A.1.19: Telophase.

Metaphase: centromeres line up along the equatorial plate. At or near the centromeres are the *kinetochores* which are proteins that face the spindle poles (asters). Microtubules, from the spindle, attach to the kinetochores of each chromosome.

Anaphase: sister chromatids are pulled apart such that each migrates to opposite poles being guided by spindle microtubules. At the end of anaphase, a cleavage furrow forms around the cell due to contraction of actin filaments called the contractile ring.

Telophase: new membranes form around the daughter nuclei; nucleoli reappear; the chromosomes uncoil and become less distinct (decondense). At the end of telophase, the cleavage furrow becomes deepened, facilitating the division of cytoplasm into two new daughter cells - each with a nucleus and organelles.

Finally, *cytokinesis* (cell separation) occurs. The cell cycle continues with the next interphase. {Mnemonic for the sequence of phases: P. MATI}

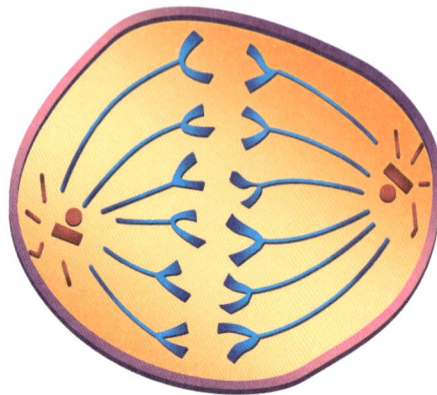

Figure IV.A.1.18: Anaphase.

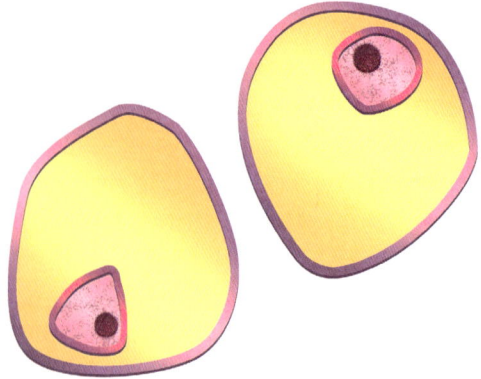

Figure IV.A.1.20: Interphase.

BIO-20   GENERALIZED EUKARYOTIC CELL

BIOLOGY

1.4 Cell Junctions

Multicellular organisms (i.e. animals) have cell junctions or intercellular bridges. They are especially abundant in epithelial tissues and serve as points of contact between cells and/or the extracellular matrix (BIO 4.3, 4.4). The multiprotein complex that comprise cell junctions can also build up the barrier around epithelial cells (*paracellular*) and control paracellular transport.

The molecules responsible for creating cell junctions include various cell adhesion molecules (CAMs). CAMs help cells stick to each other and to their surroundings. There are four main types: selectins, cadherins, integrins, and the immunoglobulin superfamily.

> You are expected to have been exposed to these topics but please do not try to memorize details: BIO 1.4.1, 1.5, 1.5.1.

1.4.1 Types of Cell Junctions

There are three major types of cell junctions in vertebrates:

1. **Anchoring junctions**: (note: "adherens" means "to adhere to"): (i) Adherens junctions, AKA "belt desmosome" because they can appear as bands encircling the cell (= zonula adherens); they link to the actin cytoskeleton; (ii) desmosomes, AKA macula (= "spot") adherens analogous to spot welding. Desmosomes include cell adhesion proteins like cadherins which can bind intermediate filaments and provide mechanical support and stability; and (iii) hemidesmosomes ("hemi" = "half"), whereas desmosomes link two cells together, hemidesmosomes attach one cell to the extracellular matrix (usually anchoring the 'bottom' or basal aspect of the epithelial cell or keratinocyte to the basement membrane; see Fig. IV.A.1.21 and BIO 5.3).

2. **Communicating junctions**: Gap junctions which are narrow tunnels which allow the free passage of small molecules and ions. One gap junction channel is composed of two connexons (or hemichannels) which connect across the intercellular space.

3. **Occluding junctions**: Tight junctions, AKA zonula occludens, as suggested by the name, are a junctional complex that join together forming a virtually impermeable barrier to fluid. These associate with different peripheral membrane proteins located on the intracellular side of the plasma membrane which anchor the strands to the actin component of the cytoskeleton. Thus, tight junctions join together the cytoskeletons of adjacent cells. Often tight junctions form narrow belts that circumferentially surround the upper part of the lateral (i.e. "side") surfaces of adjacent epithelial cells.

GAMSAT-Prep.com
THE GOLD STANDARD

Invertebrates have several other types of specific junctions; for example, the septate junction which is analogous to the tight junction in vertebrates.

In multicellular plants, the structural functions of cell junctions are instead provided for by cell walls. The analogues of communicating cell junctions in plants are called plasmodesmata.

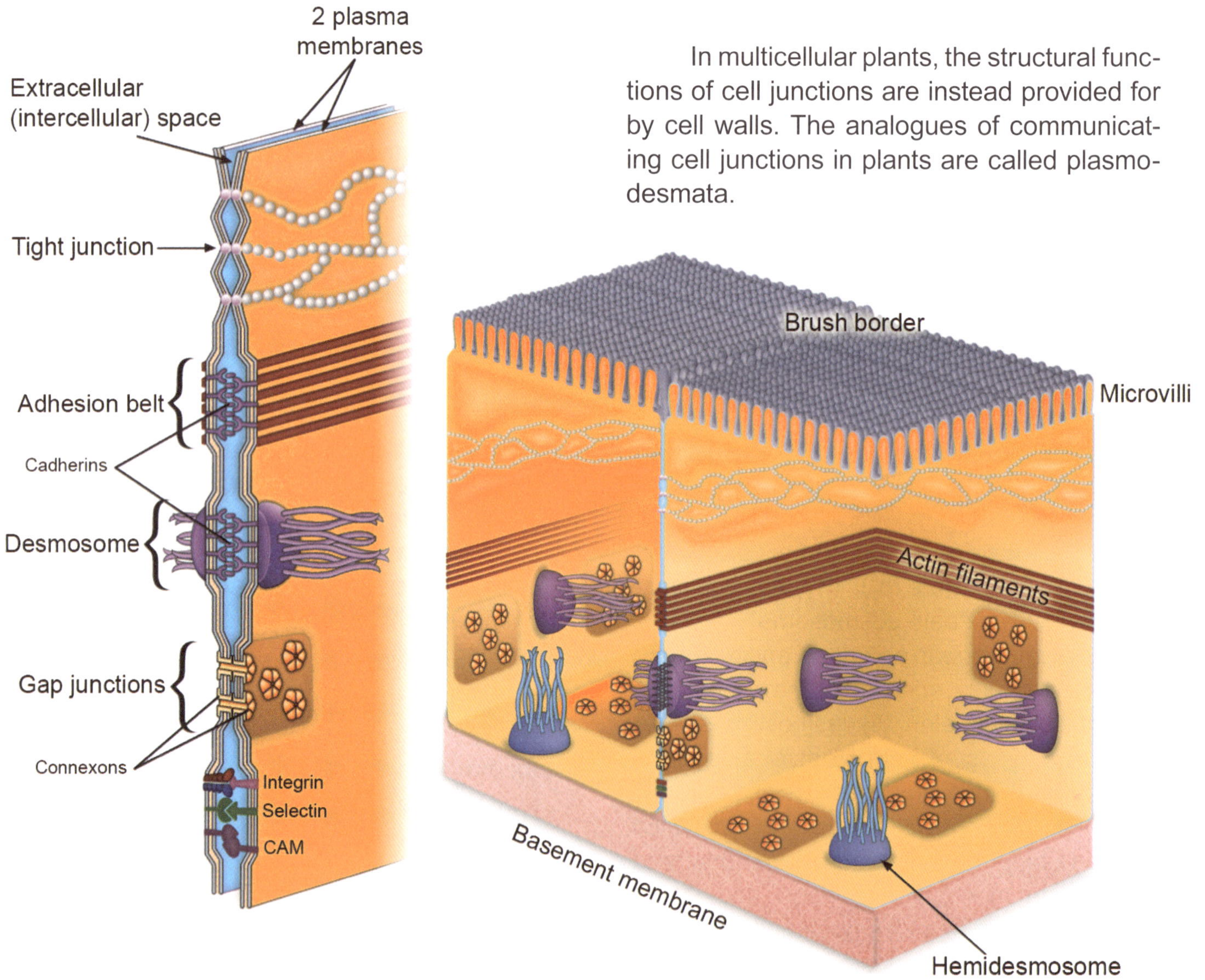

Figure IV.A.1.21: Various cell junctions in epithelia with microvilli at the surface (brush border, BIO 9.5).

BIO-22   GENERALIZED EUKARYOTIC CELL

BIOLOGY

1.5 Microscopy

A natural question about cells would be: if they are so small, how do we know what the inside of a cell really looks like? The story begins with the instrument used to produce magnified images of objects too small to be seen by the naked eye: the microscope.

Let us compare the basic principles of two popular methods of microscopy utilized by the vast majority of molecular biology research scientists: (1) the optical or light microscope; and (2) the electron microscope (the transmission electron microscope or TEM and the scanning electron microscope or SEM).

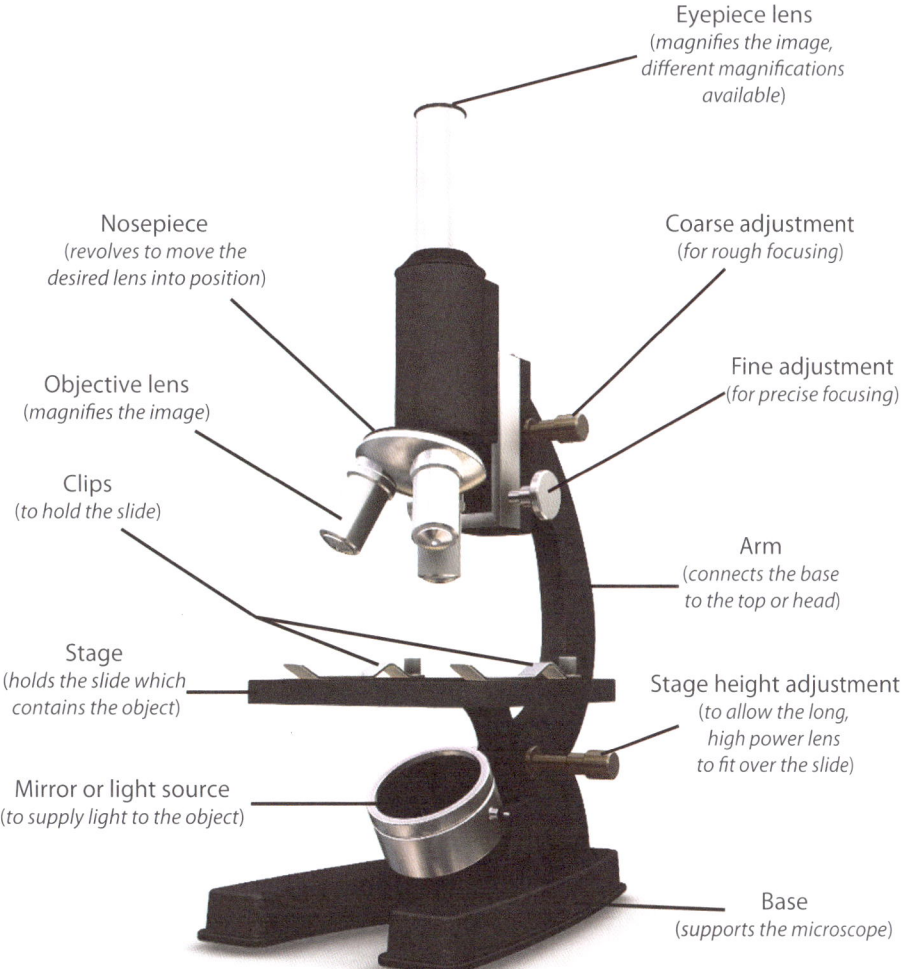

Figure IV.A.1.21: Compound light microscope. Typical magnification for the eyepiece is 10x and for the objective: 10x, 40x or 100x.

GAMSAT-Prep.com
THE GOLD STANDARD

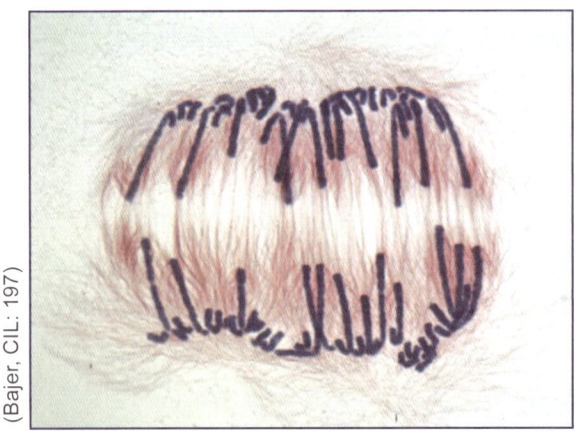

Figure IV.A.1.22: Light microscope image of a cell from the endosperm (= tissue in the seed) of an African lily. Staining shows microtubules in red and chromosomes in blue during late anaphase (BIO 1.3).

Light microscopy involves the use of an external or internal light source. The light first passes through the *iris* which controls the amount of light reaching the specimen. The light then passes through a *condenser* which is a lens that focuses the light beam through the specimen before it ultimately meets the *objective lens* which magnifies the image depending on your chosen magnification factor. Two terms you should be familiar with are *magnification* (how much bigger the image appears) and *resolution* (the ability to distinguish between two points on an image).

Magnification (PHY 11.3, 11.5) is the ratio between the apparent size of an object (or its size in an image) and its true size, and thus it is a dimensionless number usually followed by the letter "x". A compound microscope uses multiple lenses to collect light from the sample or specimen (this lens is the objective with a magnification of up to 100x), and then a separate set of lenses to focus the light into the eye or camera (the eyepiece, magnification up to 10x). So the total magnification can be 100 x 10 = 1000 times the size of the specimen (1000x makes a 100 nanometer object visible).

Light microscopes enjoy their popularity thanks to their relative low cost and ease of use. A very important feature is that they can be used to view live specimens. Their shortfall is that the magnification is limited.

> **Common Units of Length in Biology**
> *For details on units, see GM 2.1.2, 2.1.3*
>
> - m = meter(s)
> - cm = centimeter(s) (1 cm = 10^{-2} m)
> - mm = millimeter(s) (1 mm = 10^{-3} m)
> - µm = micrometer(s) (1 µm = 10^{-6} m)
>   NOT micron or µ
> - nm = nanometer(s) (1 nm = 10^{-9} m)
> - Å = angstrom(s) (1 Å = 10^{-10} m)
> - pm = picometer(s) (1 pm = 10^{-12} m)
>
> *The term "micron" is no longer in technical use.*

Electron microscopy is less commonly used due to its high price and associated scarcity. It also cannot observe live organisms as a vacuum is required and the specimen is flooded with electrons. All images being produced are in black and white though color is sometimes added to the raw images. Its primary advantage lies in the fact that it is possible to achieve a magnification up to 10,000,000x and it is the obvious choice when a high level of detail is required using an extremely small specimen. In fact, an object as tiny as a small fraction of a nanometer becomes visible with an incredible 50 picometer resolution. TEM shows the interior of the cell while SEM shows the surface of the specimen.

BIOLOGY

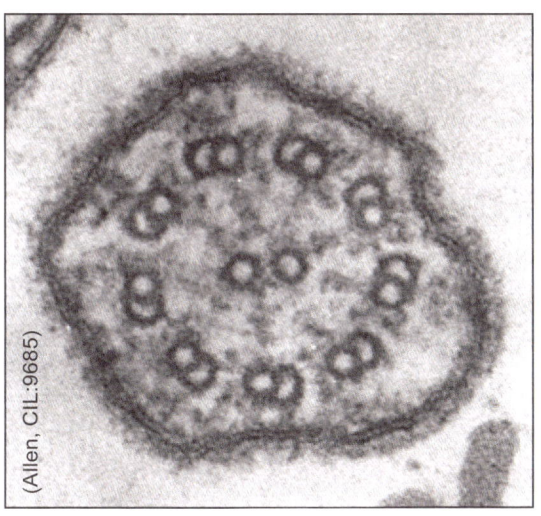

Figure IV.A.1.23: TEM of the cross section of a cilium (BIO 1.2) showing an axoneme consisting of 9 doublet and 2 central microtubules (= 9x2 + 2). Each doublet is composed of 2 subfibers: a complete A subfiber with dynein and an attached B subfiber. Eukaryotic flagella are also 9x2 + 2.

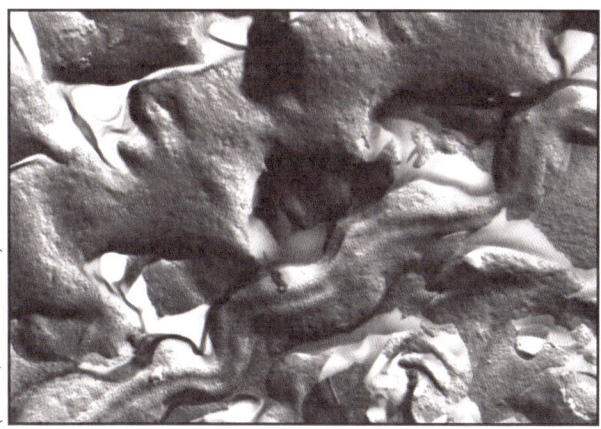

Figure IV.A.1.24: TEM freeze fracture of the plasma membrane which is cleaved between the acyl tails of membrane phospholipids (BIO 1.1; ORG 12.4), leaving a monolayer on each half of the specimen. The "E" face is the inner face of the outer lipid monolayer. The complementary surface is the "P" face (the inner surface of the inner leaflet of the bilayer shown above). The 2 large ribbons are intrinsic proteins.

1.5.1 Fluorescent Microscopy and Immunofluorescence

Lastly, you should be familiar with <u>fluorescent microscopy</u> which is commonly used to identify cellular components (organelles, cytoskeleton, etc.) and microbes with a high degree of specificity and color. The fluorescent microscope makes use of a special filter that only permits certain radiation wavelengths that matches the fluorescing material being analyzed. It is an optical microscope and very similar to the light microscope except that a highly intensive light source is used to excite a fluorescent species in the sample of interest.

<u>Immunofluorescence</u> is a technique that uses the specificity of the antibody-antigen interaction (BIO 8.2) to target fluorescent dyes to specific molecules in a cell. Immunofluorescence can be used on tissue sections, cultured cell lines or individual cells. This can be called *immunostaining*, or specifically, *immunohistochemistry* where the location of the antibodies can be seen using fluorophores (= a fluorescent chemical that can re-emit light upon light excitation; PHY 12.5, 12.6).

There are two classes of immunofluorescence: direct (= primary) and indirect (= secondary).

<u>Direct immunofluorescence</u> uses a single antibody linked to a fluorophore. The antibody binds to the target molecule (antigen),

THE BIOLOGICAL SCIENCES BIO-25

and the fluorophore attached to the antibody can be detected with a microscope. This technique is cheaper, faster but less sensitive than indirect immunofluorescence.

Indirect immunofluorescence uses two antibodies: (1) the unlabeled first, or primary, antibody binds the antigen; and (2) the secondary antibody, which carries the fluorophore and recognizes the primary antibody and binds to it.

Photobleaching is the photochemical destruction of a dye or a fluorophore. Thus the fluorescent molecules are sometimes destroyed by the light exposure necessary to stimulate them into fluorescing. On the other hand, photobleaching can be fine tuned to improve the signal-to-noise ratio (like seeing the tree from the forest). Photobleaching can also be used to study the motion of molecules (i.e. FRAP).

Immunofluorescence samples can be seen through a simple fluorescent microscope (*epifluorescence*) or through the more complex *confocal* microscope.

A confocal microscope is a state-of-the-art fluorescent microscope which uses a laser as the light source. The confocal microscope is used in FRAP, fluorescence recovery after photobleaching, which is an optical technique used to "view" the movement of proteins or molecules. FRAP is capable of quantifying the 2D diffusion of a thin film of molecules containing fluorescently labeled probes, or to examine single cells. FRAP has had many uses including: studies of cell membrane diffusion and protein binding; determining if axonal transport is retrograde or anterograde, meaning towards or away from the neuron's cell body (soma), respectively.

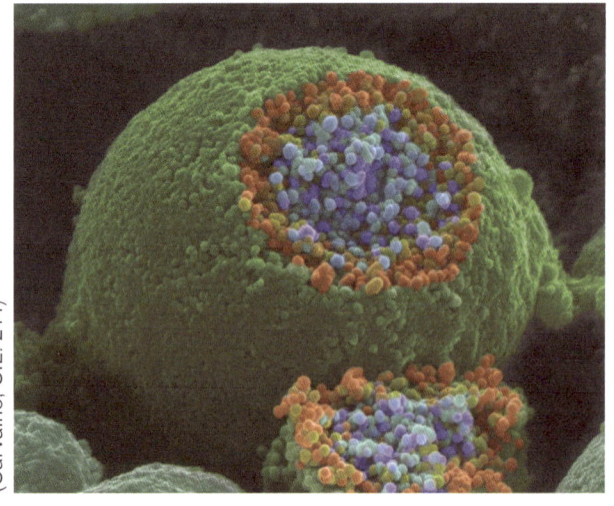

Figure IV.A.1.25: SEM colorized image of a neuron's presynaptic terminal (BIO 5.1) that has been broken open to reveal the synaptic vesicles (orange and blue) beneath the cell membrane.

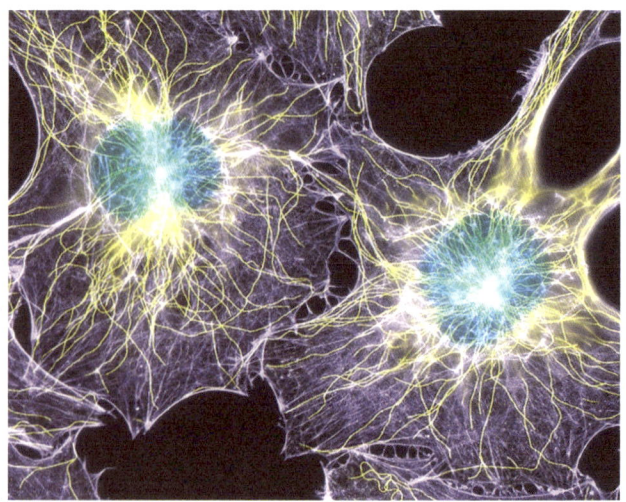

Figure IV.A.1.26: Fluorescence microscopy of two interphase cells with immunofluorescence labeling of actin filaments (purple), microtubules (yellow), and nuclei (green).

GOLD NOTES

GOLD NOTES

MICROBIOLOGY

Chapter 2

Memorize	Understand	Not Required*
uctures, functions, life cycles neralized viral life cycle sic categories of bacteria uation for bacterial doubling ferences, similarities	* Eukaryotes vs. Prokaryotes * General aspects of life cycles * Gen. aspects of genetics/reproduction * Calculation of exponential growth * Scientific method	* Advanced level college info * Evolutionary history, habitats * Taxonomic (scientific) classification * Role in infectious diseases

GAMSAT-Prep.com

Introduction

Microbiology is the study of microscopic organisms including viruses, bacteria and fungi. It is important to be able to focus on the differences and similarities between these microorganisms and the generalized eukaryotic cell you have just studied.

Additional Resources

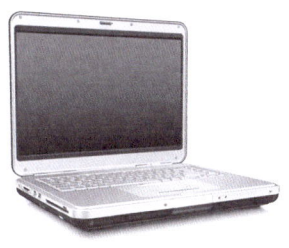
Free Online Q&A + Forum

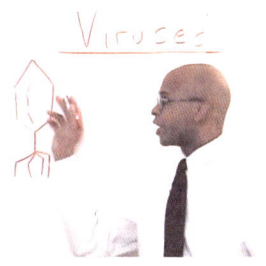
Video: Online or DVD

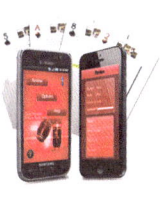
Flashcards

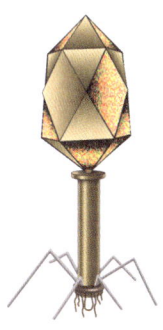
Special Guest

SURVEY OF THE NATURAL SCIENCES   BIO-29

* The real GAMSAT may have advanced level information presented (ie. in a passage) but previous knowledge of said information is not required to answer the questions that would follow. Practice ACER and GS practice GAMSATs can help you clarify this point.

GAMSAT-Prep.com
THE GOLD STANDARD

2.1 Viruses

Unlike cells, viruses are too small to be seen directly with a light microscope. Viruses infect all types of organisms, from animals and plants to bacteria and archaea (BIO 2.2). Only a very basic and general understanding of viruses is required for the GAMSAT.

Viruses are obligate intracellular parasites; in other words, in order to replicate their genetic material and thus multiply, they must gain access to the inside of a cell. Replication of a virus takes place when the virus takes control of the host cell's synthetic machinery. Viruses are often considered non-living for several reasons:

(i) they do not grow by increasing in size

(ii) they cannot carry out independent metabolism

(iii) they do not respond to external stimuli

(iv) they have no cellular structure.

The genetic material for viruses may be either DNA or RNA, never both. Viruses do not have organelles or ribosomes. The nucleic acid core is encapsulated by a protein coat (capsid) which together forms the head region in some viruses. The tail region helps to anchor the virus to a cell. An extracellular viral particle is called a *virion*.

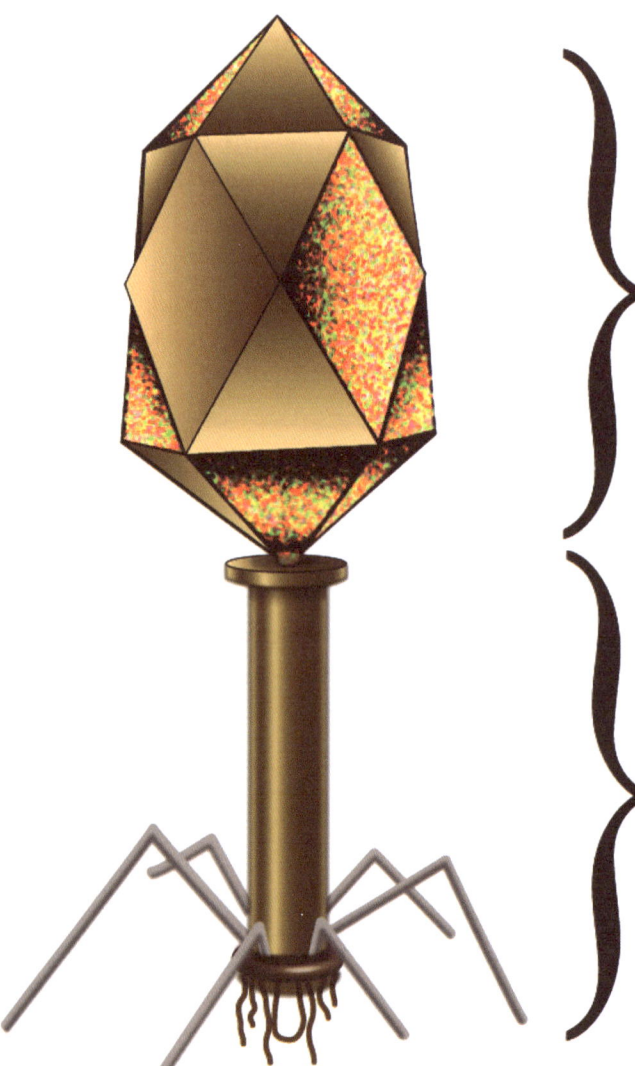

Figure IV.A.2.1: A virus.

BIOLOGY

Viruses are much smaller than prokaryotic cells (i.e. bacteria) which, in turn, are much smaller than eukaryotes (i.e. animal cells, fungi). A virus which infects bacteria is called a bacteriophage or simply a phage.

The life cycle of viruses has many variants; the following represents the main themes for GAMSAT purposes. A virus attaches to a specific receptor on a cell. Some viruses may now enter the cell; others, as in the diagram, will simply inject their nucleic acid. Either way, viral molecules induce the metabolic machinery of the host cell to produce more viruses.

The new viral particles may now exit the cell by lysing (bursting). This is also a feature of many bacteria. The preceding is deemed lytic or virulent. Some virus lie latent for long periods of time without lysing the host and its genome becomes incorporated by genetic recombination into the host's chromosome. Therefore, whenever the host replicates, the viral genome is also replicated. These are called lysogenic or temperate viruses. Eventually, at some point, the virus may become activated and lyse the host cell.

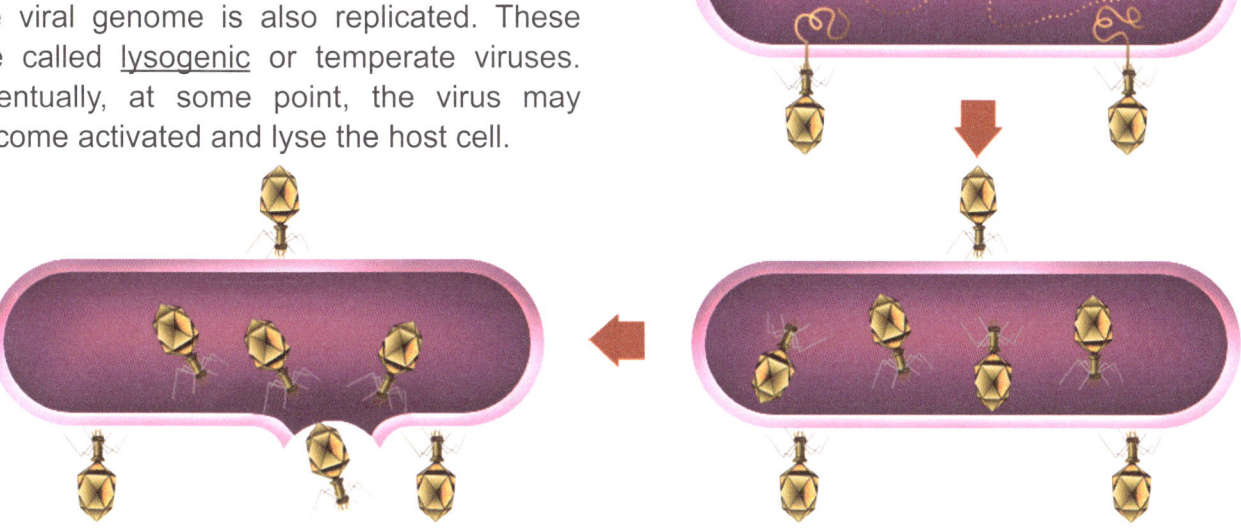

Figure IV.A.2.2: Lytic viral life cycle in a rod shaped bacterium (bacilli).

2.1.1 Retroviruses

A retrovirus uses RNA as its genetic material. It is called a retrovirus because of an enzyme (reverse transcriptase) that gives these viruses the unique ability of transcribing RNA (their RNA) into DNA (see Biology Chapter 3 for the central dogma regarding protein synthesis). The retroviral DNA can then integrate into the chromosomal DNA of the host cell to be expressed there. The human immunodeficiency virus (HIV), the cause of AIDS, is a retrovirus.

Retroviruses are used, in genetics, to deliver DNA to a cell (= a vector); in medicine, they are used for gene therapy.

2.2 Prokaryotes

Prokaryotes (= pre-nucleus) are organisms without a membrane bound nucleus which includes 2 types of organisms: bacteria (= Eubacteria) and archaea (= bacteria-like organisms that live in extreme environments). For the purposes of the GAMSAT, we will focus on bacteria. They are haploid and have a long circular strand of DNA in a region called the nucleoid.

The nucleoid is a region in a bacterium that contains DNA but is not surrounded by a nuclear membrane. Because bacterial DNA is not surrounded by a nuclear membrane, transcription and translation can occur at the same time, that is, protein synthesis can begin while mRNA is being produced. Bacteria also have smaller circular DNA called plasmid, which is extra chromosomal genetic element that can replicate independently of the bacterial chromosome and helps to confer resistance to antibiotics.

Bacteria do not have mitochondria, Golgi apparatus, lysosomes, nor endoplasmic reticulum. Instead, metabolic processes can

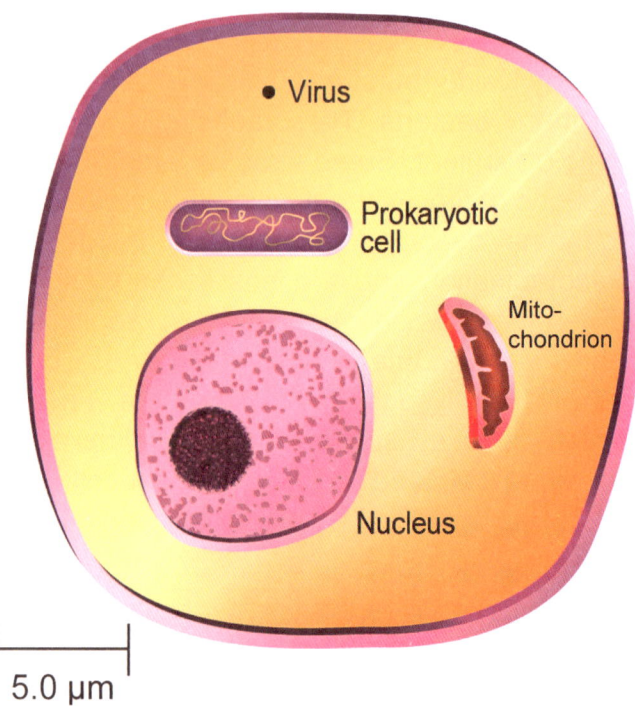

Figure IV.A.2.3
Comparing the size of a typical eukaryote, prokaryote and virus. Note that both the prokaryote and mitochondrion are similar in size and both contain circular DNA suggesting an evolutionary link.

be carried out in the cytoplasm or associated with bacterial membranes. Bacteria have ribosomes (smaller than eukaryotes), plasma membrane, and a cell wall. The cell wall, made of peptidoglycans, helps to prevent the hypertonic bacterium from bursting. Some bacteria have a slimy polysaccharide mucoid-like capsule on the outer surface for protection.

Bacteria can achieve movement with their flagella. Bacterial flagella are helical filaments, each with a rotary motor at its base which can turn clockwise or counterclockwise.

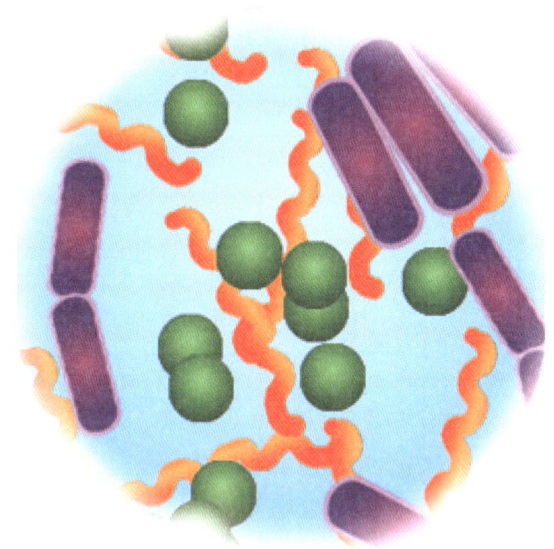

Figure IV.A.2.5
Schematic representation of bacteria colored for the purpose of identification: cocci (spherical, green), bacilli (cylindrical, purple) and spirilli (helical, orange).

The form and rotary engine of flagella are maintained by proteins (i.e. flagellin) which interact with the plasma membrane and the basal body (BIO 1.2). Power is generated by a proton motive force similar to the proton pump in metabolism (Biology, Chapter 4).

Bacteria also have short, hairlike filaments called pili (also called fimbriae) arising from the bacterial cell wall. These pili are much shorter than flagella. Common pili can serve as adherence factors which promote binding of bacteria to host cells. Sex pili, encoded by a self-transmissible plasmid, are involved in transferring of DNA from one bacterium to another via conjugation.

Bacteria are partially classified according to their shapes: cocci which are spheri-

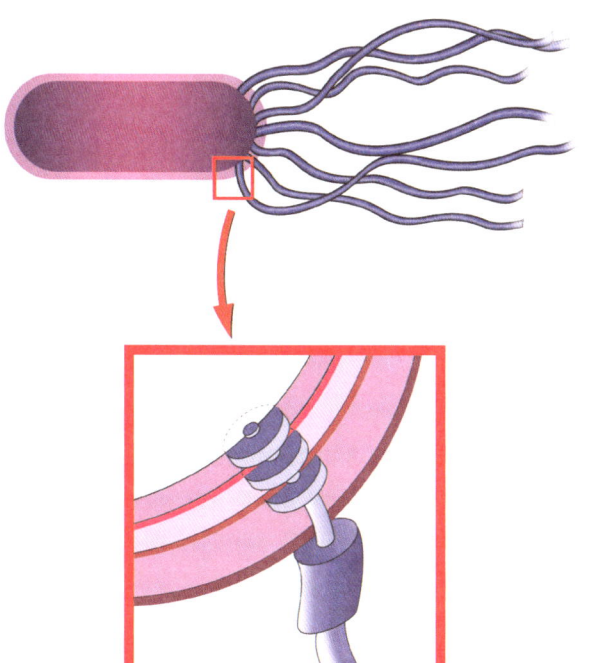

Figure IV.A.2.4
Schematic representation of the basis for flagellar propulsion. The flagellum, similar to a flexible hook, is anchored to the membrane and cell wall by a series of protein rings forming a motor. Powered by the flow of protons, the motor can rotate the flagellum more than 100 revolutions per second.

Prokaryotic Cells	Eukaryotic Cells
Small cells (1-10 μm)	Larger cells (10-100 μm)
Always unicellular	Often multicellular
No nuclei or any membrane-bound organelles, such as mitochondria	Always have nuclei and other membrane-bound organelles
DNA is circular, without proteins	DNA is linear and associated with proteins to form chromatin
Ribosomes are small (70S)	Ribosomes are large (80S)
No cytoskeleton	Always has a cytoskeleton
Motility by rigid rotating flagellum made of flagellin)	Motility by flexible waving cilia or flagellae (made of tubulin)
Cell division is by binary fission	Cell division is by mitosis or meiosis
Reproduction is always asexual	Reproduction is asexual or sexual
Great variety of metabolic pathways	Common metabolic pathways

Table IV.A.2.1: Summary of the differences between prokaryotic and eukaryotic cells.

cal or sometimes elliptical; <u>bacilli</u> which are rod shaped or cylindrical (Fig. IV.A.2.2 in BIO 2.1 showed phages attacking a bacillus bacterium); <u>spirilli</u> which are helical or spiral. They are also classified according to whether or not their cell wall reacts to a special dye called a Gram stain; thus they are gram-positive if they retain the stain and gram-negative if they do not.

Most bacteria engage in a form of asexual reproduction called binary fission. Two identical DNA molecules migrate to opposite ends of a cell as a transverse wall forms, dividing the cell in two. The cells can now separate and enlarge to the original size. Under ideal conditions, a bacterium can undergo fission every 10-20 minutes producing over 10^{30} progeny in a day and a half. If resources are unlimited, exponential growth would be expected. The doubling time of bacterial populations can be calculated as follows:

$$b = B \times 2^n$$

where b is the number of bacteria at the end of the time interval, B is the number of bacteria at the beginning of the time interval and n is the number of generations. Thus if we start with 2 bacteria and follow for 3 generations then we get:

$$b = B \times 2^n = 2 \times 2^3 = 2 \times 8 = 16$$
bacteria after 3 generations.

{Note: bacterial doubling time is a relatively popular question type.}

Bacteria do not produce gametes nor zygotes, nor do they undergo meiosis; however, four forms of genetic recombination do occur: <u>transduction</u>, <u>transformation</u>, <u>conjugation</u> and <u>transposon</u> <u>insertion</u>.

In transduction, fragments of bacterial chromosome accidentally become packaged into virus during a viral infection. These viruses may then infect another bacterium. A piece of bacterial DNA that the virus is accidentally carrying will be injected and incorporated into the host chromosome if there is homology between the newly injected piece of DNA and the recipient bacterial genome.

In transformation, a foreign chromosome fragment (plasmid) is released from one bacterium during cell lysis and enters into another bacterium. The DNA can then become incorporated into the recipient's genome if there is homology between the newly incorporated genome and the recipient one.

In conjugation, DNA is transferred directly by cell-to-cell contact formed by a conjugation bridge called the sex pilus. For conjugation to occur, one bacterium must have the sex factor called F plasmid. Bacteria that carry F plasmids are called F^+ cells. During conjugation, a F^+ cell replicates its F factor and will pass its F plasmid to an F^- cell, converting it to an F^+ cell. This type of exchange is the major mechanism for transfer of antibiotic resistance.

In transposon insertion, mobile genetic elements called transposons move from one position to another in a bacterial chromosome or between different molecules of DNA without having DNA homology.

Most bacteria cannot synthesize their own food and thus depend on other organisms for it; such a bacterium is heterotrophic. Most heterotrophic bacteria obtain their food from dead organic matter; this is called saprophytic. Some bacteria are autotrophic meaning they can synthesize organic compounds from simple inorganic substances. Thus some are photosynthetic producing carbohydrate and releasing oxygen, while others are chemoautotrophic obtaining energy via chemical reactions including the oxidation of iron, sulfur, nitrogen, or hydrogen gas.

Bacteria can be either aerobic or anaerobic. The former refers to metabolism in the presence of oxygen and the latter in the absence of oxygen (i.e. fermentation).

Based on variations in the oxygen requirement, bacteria are divided into four types:

1) Obligate aerobes: require oxygen for growth

2) Facultative anaerobes: are aerobic; however, can grow in the absence of oxygen by undergoing fermentation
3) Aerotolerant anaerobes: use fermentation for energy; however, can tolerate low amounts of oxygen
4) Obligate anaerobes: are anaerobic, can be damaged by oxygen

Symbiosis generally refers to close and often long term interactions between different biological species. Bacteria have various symbiotic relationships with, for example, humans. These include mutualism (both benefit: GI tract bacteria, BIO 9.5), parasitism (parasite benefits over the host: tuberculosis, appendicitis) and commensalism (one benefits and the other is not significantly harmed or benefited: some skin bacteria).

2.2.1 Operons

E. coli is a gram-negative, rod-shaped intestinal bacterium with DNA sequences called *operons* that direct biosynthetic pathways. Operons are composed of:

1. A repressor which can bind to an operator and prevent gene expression by blocking RNA polymerase. However, in the presence of an inducer, a repressor will be bound to the inducer instead, forming an inducer-repressor complex. This complex cannot bind to an operator and thus gene expression is permitted.
2. A promoter which is a sequence of DNA where RNA polymerase attaches to begin transcription.
3. Operators which can block the action of RNA polymerase if there is a repressor present.
4. A regulator which codes for the synthesis of a repressor that can bind to the operator and block gene transcription.
5. Structural genes that code for several related enzymes that are responsible for production of a specific end product.

The *lac operon* controls the breakdown of lactose and is the simplest way of illustrating how gene regulation in bacteria works. In the lac operon system there is an active repressor that binds to the operator. In this scenario RNA polymerase is unable to transcribe the structural genes necessary to control the uptake and subsequent breakdown of lactose. When the repressor is inactivated (in the presence of lactose) the RNA polymerase is now able to transcribe the genes that code for the required enzymes. These enzymes are said to be *inducible* as it is the lactose that is required to turn on the operon.

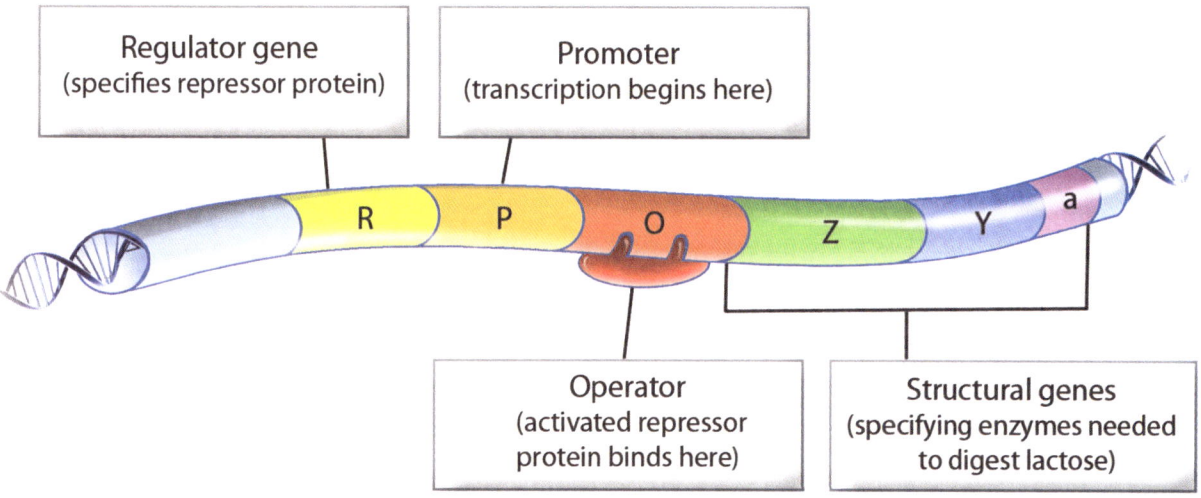

Lac Operon

2.3 Fungi

Fungi are eukaryotic (= true nucleus) organisms which absorb their food through their chitinous cell walls. They may either be unicellular (i.e. yeast) or filamentous (i.e. mushrooms, molds) with individual filaments called hyphae which collectively form a mycelium. Fungal cell membranes contain ergosterol rather than cholesterol found in cell membranes of other eukaryotes.

Fungi often reproduce asexually. In molds, spores can be produced and then liberated from outside of a sporangium; or, as in yeast, a simple asexual budding process may be used. Sexual reproduction can involve the fusion of opposite mating types to produce asci (singular: ascus), basidia (singular: basidium), or zygotes. All of the three preceding diploid structures must undergo meiosis to produce haploid spores. If resources are unlimited, exponential growth would be expected.

Fungi are relatively important for humans as a source of disease and a decomposer of both food and dead organic matter. On the lighter side, they also serve as food (mushrooms, truffles), for alcohol and food production (cheese molds, bread yeast) and they have given us the breakthrough antibiotic, penicillin (from penicillium molds).

2.4 Vectors

A vector can be a person, animal or microorganism that carries and transmits an infectious organism (i.e. bacteria, viruses, etc.) into another living organism. Examples: the mosquito is a vector for malaria; bats are vectors for rabies and a SARS-like virus.

2.5 The Scientific Method

The scientific method could be used in conjunction with any GAMSAT Biology experiment but microbiology is most common.

The point of the experiment is to test your ability to read scientific material, understand what is being tested, and determine if the hypothesis has been proved, refuted or neither. When a hypothesis survives rigorous testing, it graduates to a *theory*.

Observation, formulation of a theory, and testing of a theory by additional observation is called the scientific method. In biology, a key aspect to evaluate the validity of a trial or experiment is the presence of a *control group*. Generally, treatment is withheld from the control group but given to the *experimental group*.

First we will make an observation and then use deductive reasoning to create an appropriate hypothesis which will result in an experimental design. Consider the following: trees grow well in the sunlight. Hypothesis: exposure to light is directly related to tree growth. Experiment: two groups of trees are grown in similar conditions except one group (*experimental*) is exposed to light while the other group (*control*) is not exposed to light. Growth is carefully measured and the two groups are compared. Note that tree growth (*dependent variable*) is dependent on light (*independent variable*).

There are experiments where it is important to expose the control group to some factor different from the factor given to the experimental group (= *positive control*); as opposed to not giving the control group any exposure at all (= *negative control*). Exposure for a control group is used in medicine and dentistry because of the "Placebo Effect."

Experiments have shown that giving a person a pill that contains no biologically active material will cure many illnesses in up to 30% of individuals. Thus if Drug X is developed using a traditional control group, and the "efficacy" is estimated at 32%, it may be that the drug is no more effective than a sugar pill! In this case, the control group must be exposed to an unmedicated preparation to negate the Placebo Effect. To be believable the experiment must be well-grounded in evidence (= *valid,* based on the scientific method) and then one must be able to reproduce the results.

BIOLOGY

2.5.1 The Experiment

A lab in Sydney reports 15% cell death when maximally stimulating the APO-1 receptor. In order to appropriately interpret the results, it must first be compared to:

    A. data from other labs.
    B. the attrition rate of other cell types.
    C. the actual number of APO-1 cells dying in the tissue culture.
    D. the rate of cell death without stimulation of APO-1.

- The experiment: stimulating a specific receptor on cells led to a 15% rate of cell death.
- Treatment is the stimulation of a receptor.
- The control (*group without treatment*): under the same conditions, do not stimulate the receptor (choice **D.**).

Choice **C.** does not answer the question. Choices **A.** and **B.** are most relevant if the initial data is shown to be significant. To prove that the data is significant or valid, one must first compare to a control group (choice **D.**).

GOLD NOTES

PROTEIN SYNTHESIS

Chapter 3

Memorize	Understand	Not Required*
• the genetic code (triplet) • Central Dogma: DNA ➡ RNA ➡ protein • Definitions: mRNA, tRNA, rRNA • Codon-anticodon relationship • Initiation, elongation and termination	* Mechanism of transcription * Mechanism of translation * Roles of mRNA, tRNA, rRNA * Role and structure of ribosomes * One-gene–one-enzyme hypothesis * The biosynthetic pathway	* Advanced level college info * Splicosomes, heterphil nuclear RNA * Inhibitory, signal peptides * Specific post translation changes * Memorizing the ribosomal subunits in Svedberg units * Memorizing stop or start codons

GAMSAT-Prep.com

Introduction

Protein synthesis is the creation of proteins using DNA and RNA. Individual amino acids are connected to each other in peptide linkages in a specific order given by the sequence of nucleotides in DNA. Thus the process occurs through a precise interplay directed by the genetic code and involving mRNA, tRNA and amino acids - all in an environment provided by a ribosome. The "one-gene–one-enzyme hypothesis" and its relation to biosynthetic pathways comprise rather regular GAMSAT questions.

Additional Resources

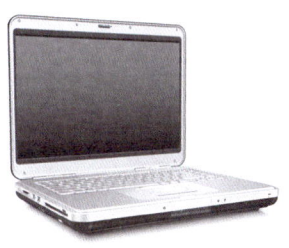

Free Online Q&A + Forum

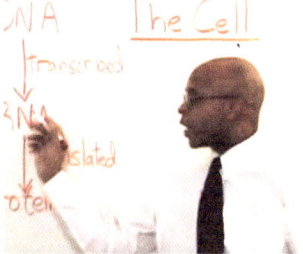

Video: Online or DVD

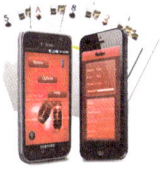

Flashcards

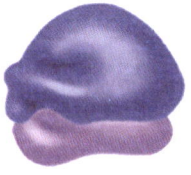

Special Guest

THE BIOLOGICAL SCIENCES   BIO-41

* The real GAMSAT may have advanced level information presented (ie. in a passage) but previous knowledge of said information is not required to answer the questions that would follow. Practice ACER and GS practice GAMSATs can help you clarify this point.

Building Proteins

Proteins (which comprise many hormones, enzymes, antibodies, etc.) are long chains formed by peptide bonds between combinations of twenty amino acid subunits. Each amino acid is encoded in a sequence of three nucleotides (a triplet code = the *genetic code*). A gene is a conglomeration of such codes and thus is a section of DNA which encodes for a protein (or a polypeptide which is exactly like a protein but much smaller).

DNA Transcription

The information in DNA is rewritten (transcribed) into a messenger composed of RNA (= mRNA); the reaction is catalyzed by the enzyme RNA polymerase. The newly synthesized mRNA is elongated in the 5′ to 3′ direction. It carries the complement of a DNA sequence.

Transcription can be summarized in 4 or 5 steps for prokaryotes or eukaryotes, respectively:

1. RNA polymerase moves the transcription bubble, a stretch of unpaired nucleotides, by breaking the hydrogen bonds between complementary nucleotides (see BIO 1.2.2 for nucleoside phosphates - nucleotides - and the binding of nitrogen bases).

2. RNA polymerase adds matching RNA nucleotides that are paired with complementary DNA bases.

3. The extension of the RNA sugar-phosphate backbone is catalyzed by RNA polymerase.

4. Hydrogen bonds of the untwisted RNA +

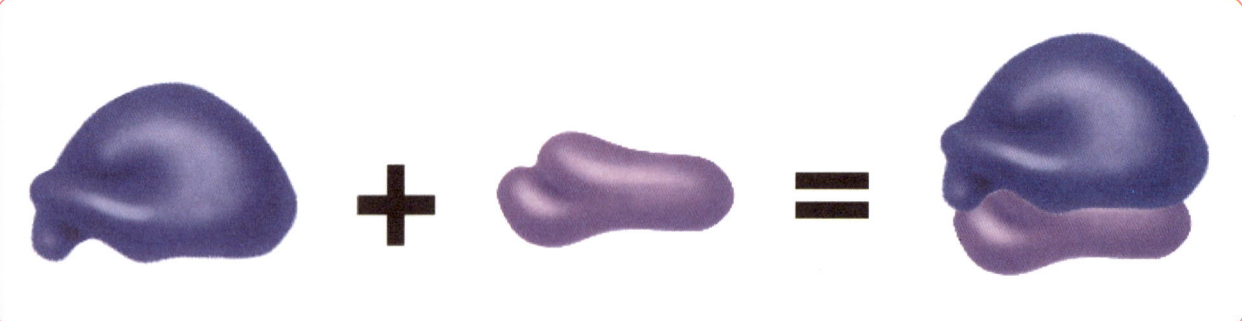

Figure IV.A.3.1: A ribosome provides the environment for protein synthesis. Ribosomes are composed of a large and a small subunit. The unit of measurement used is called the "Svedberg unit" (S) which is a measure of the rate of sedimentation in a centrifuge as opposed to a direct measurement of size. For this reason, fragment names do not add up (70S is made of 50S and 30S). Prokaryotes have 70S ribosomes, each comprised of a small (30S) and a large (50S) subunit. Eukaryotes have 80S ribosomes, each comprised of a small (40S) and large (60S) subunit. The ribosomes found in chloroplasts and mitochondria of eukaryotes also consist of large and small subunits bound together with proteins into one 70S ribosome. These organelles are believed to be descendants of bacteria ("Endosymbiotic theory") thus their ribosomes are similar to those of bacteria (see BIO 16.6.3).

BIOLOGY

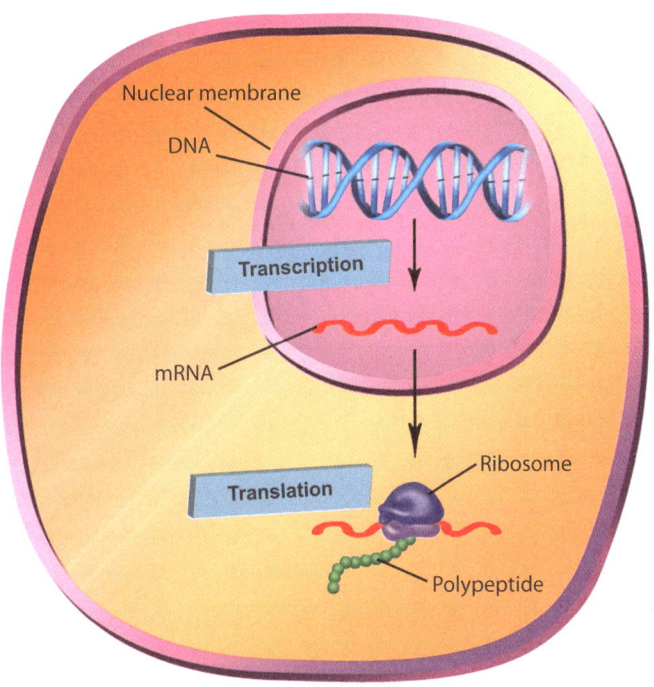

Figure IV.A.3.2: The central dogma of protein synthesis.

DNA helix break, freeing the newly synthesized RNA strand.

5. If the cell has a nucleus, the RNA is further processed [addition of a 5' cap and a 3' poly(A) tail] and then exits through the nuclear pore to the cytoplasm.

The mRNA synthesis in eukaryotes begins with the binding of RNA polymerase at a specific DNA sequence known as promoters. Elongation continues until the RNA polymerase reaches a termination signal. The initially formed primary mRNA transcript, also called pre-mRNA, contains regions called introns that are not expressed in the synthesized protein. The introns are removed and the regions that are expressed (exons) are spliced together to form the final functional mRNA molecule. {EXons EXpressed; INtrons IN the garbage!}

Post-transcriptional processing of mRNA occurs in the nucleus. Even before transcription is completed, a 7-methylguanosine cap is added to the 5' end of the growing mRNA serving as attachment site for protein synthesis and protection against degradation. The 3' end is added with a poly(A) tail consisting of 20 to 250 adenylate residues as protection. Of course, "A" refers to adenine and the nucleotide is thus adenosine monophosphate or AMP (BIO 1.2.2, ORG 12.5) which *polymerizes* to create the tail of residues. The mes-

GAMSAT-Prep.com
THE GOLD STANDARD

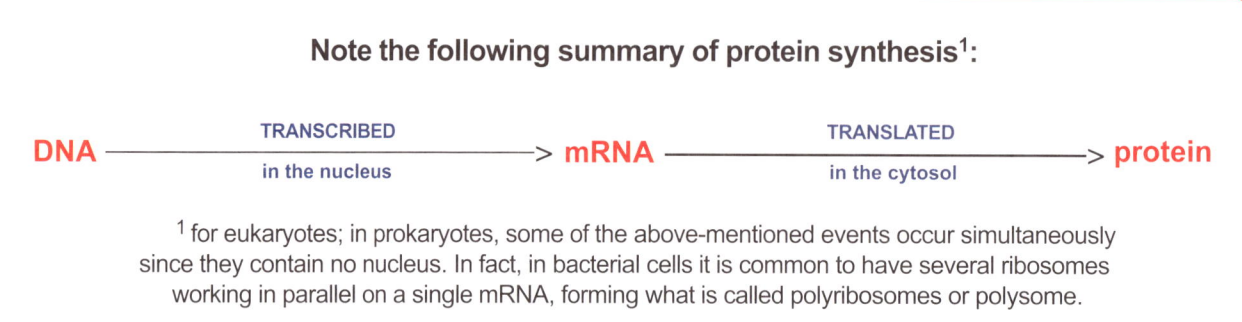

senger then leaves the nucleus with the information necessary to make a protein.

RNA Translation

The mRNA is constantly produced and degraded, which is the main method through which cells regulate the amount of a particular protein they synthesize. It attaches to a small subunit of a ribosome which will then attach to a larger ribosomal subunit thus creating a full ribosome. A ribosome is composed of a complex of protein and ribosomal RNA (= rRNA). The rRNA is the most abundant of all RNA types.

Floating in the cytoplasm is yet another form of RNA; this RNA specializes in taking amino acids and transfering them onto other amino acids when contained within the environment of the ribosome. More specifically, this transfer RNA (tRNA) molecule can be charged with a specific amino acid by aminoacyl-tRNA synthetase enzyme, bring the amino acid to the environment of ribosome, recognize the triplet code (= codon) on mRNA via its own triplet code anticodon, which is a three nucleotide sequence on tRNA that recognizes the complementary codon in mRNA; and finally, tRNA can transfer its amino acid onto the preceding one thus elongating the polypeptide chain. In a way, tRNA translates the code that mRNA carries into a sequence of amino acids which can produce a protein.

Translation of mRNA into a protein involves three stages: initiation, elongation and termination. The direction of synthesis of the protein chain proceeds from the amino end/terminus to the carboxyl end/terminus. Synthesis begins when the ribosome scans the mRNA until it binds to a start codon (AUG), which specifies the amino acid methionine. During elongation, a peptide bond is formed between the existing amino acid in the protein chain and the incoming amino acid. Following peptide bond formation, the ribosome shifts by one codon in the 5′ to 3′ direction along mRNA and the uncharged tRNA is expelled and the peptidyl-tRNA grows by one amino acid. Protein synthesis terminates when the ribosome binds to one of the three mRNA termination codons (UAA, UAG or UGA; notice the similarity with the DNA stop codons in Table IV.A.3.1 except that U replaces T in this RNA molecule).

BIOLOGY

The 20 Amino Acids	The 64 DNA Codons
Alanine	GCT, GCC, GCA, GCG
Arginine	CGT, CGC, CGA, CGG, AGA, AGG
Asparagine	AAT, AAC
Aspartic acid	GAT, GAC
Cysteine	TGT, TGC
Glutamic acid	GAA, GAG
Glutamine	CAA, CAG
Glycine	GGT, GGC, GGA, GGG
Histidine	CAT, CAC
Isoleucine	ATT, ATC, ATA
Leucine	CTT, CTC, CTA, CTG, TTA, TTG
Lysine	AAA, AAG
Methionine	ATG
Phenylalanine	TTT, TTC
Proline	CCT, CCC, CCA, CCG
Serine	TCT, TCC, TCA, TCG, AGT, AGC
Threonine	ACT, ACC, ACA, ACG
Tyrosine	TAT, TAC
Tryptophan	TGG
Valine	GTT, GTC, GTA, GTG
Stop codons	TAA, TAG, TGA

Table IV.A.3.1: The 20 standard amino acids. Do not memorize.

The 20 standard amino acids are encoded by the genetic code of 64 codons. Notice that since there are 4 bases (A, T, G, C), if there were only two bases per codon, then only 16 amino acids could be coded for ($4^2=16$). However, since at least 21 codes are required (20 amino acids plus a stop codon) and the next largest number of bases is three, then 4^3 gives 64 possible codons, meaning that some degeneracy exists.

Degeneracy is the redundancy of the genetic code. Degeneracy occurs because there are more codons than encodable amino acids. This makes the genetic code more tolerant to point mutations (BIO 15.5). For example, in theory, fourfold degenerate codons can tolerate any point mutation at the third position (see valine, alanine, glycine, etc. in Table IV.A.3.1 and notice that any 3rd base codes for the same amino acid). The structure of amino acids will be discussed in ORG 12.1.

A nonsense mutation is a point mutation (BIO 15.5) in a sequence of DNA that results in a premature stop codon (UAA, UAG, UGA), or a nonsense codon in the transcribed mRNA. Either way, an incomplete, and usually nonfunctional protein is the result. A missense mutation is a point mutation where a single nucleotide is changed to cause substitution of a different amino acid. Some genetic disorders (i.e. thalassemia) result from nonsense mutations.

Protein made on free ribosomes in the cytoplasm may be used for intracellular purposes (i.e. enzymes for glycolysis, etc.). Whereas proteins made on rER ribosomes are usually modified by both rER and the Golgi apparatus en route to the plasma membrane or exocytosis (i.e. antibodies, intestinal enzymes, etc.).

Key Points

Note the following: i) the various kinds of RNA are single stranded molecules which are produced using DNA as a template; ii) hormones can have a potent regulatory effect on protein synthesis (esp. enzymes); iii) allosteric enzymes (= proteins with two different configurations - each with different biological

DNA	Coding Strand (codons)	5' → → ------ T T C ------ → → 3'
	Template Strand (anticodons)	3' ← ← ------ A A G ------ ← ← 5'
mRNA	The Message (codons)	5' → → ------ U U C ------ → → 3'
tRNA	The Transfer (anticodons)	3' ← ← A A G ← ← 5'
Protein	Amino Acid	N-terminus → → Phenylalanine → → C-terminus

Table IV.A.3.2. DNA, RNA and protein strands with directions of synthesis. For both DNA and RNA, strands are synthesized from the **5'** ends → → to the **3'** ends. Protein chains are synthesized from the **N-terminus** → → to the **C-terminus**. Color code: the **old** end is **cold blue**; the **new** end is **red hot** where new residues are added. As shown in the table, mRNA is synthesized complementary and antiparallel to the **template strand (anticodons)** of DNA, so the resulting mRNA consists of codons corresponding to those in the coding strand of DNA. The **anticodons of tRNA** read each three-base mRNA codon and thus transfers the corresponding **amino acid** to the growing **polypeptide chain** or **protein** according to the genetic code.

properties) are important regulators of transcription; iv) there are many protein factors which trigger specific events in the initiation (using a start codon, AUG), elongation and termination (using a stop codon) of the synthesis of a protein; v) one end of the protein has an amine group (-NH$_2$, which projects from the first amino acid), while the other end has a carboxylic acid group (-COOH, which projects from the last amino acid). {Amino acids and protein structure will be explored in ORG 12.1 and 12.2}

Note that the free amine group end, the start of the protein, is also referred to as: N-terminus, amino-terminus, NH$_2$-terminus, N-terminal end or amine-terminus. The free carboxylic acid end, which is the end of the protein, is also referred to as: C-terminus, carboxyl-terminus, carboxy-terminus, C-terminal tail, C-terminal end, or COOH-terminus.

Differences in translation between prokaryotes and eukaryotes:

1) Ribosomes: in prokaryotes it is 70S, in eukaryotes it is 80S

2) Start codon: the start codon AUG specifies formyl-methionine [f-Met] in prokaryotes, in eukaryotes it is methionine

Location of translation: in prokaryotes translation occurs at the same compartment and same time as transcription, in eukaryotes transcription occurs in the nucleus while translation occurs in the cytosol.

Because of the incredible variety of organisms that use the genetic code, it was thought to be a *truly* 'universal' code but that is not quite accurate. Variant codes have evolved. For example, protein synthesis in human mitochondria relies on a genetic code that differs from the standard genetic code.

Furthermore, not all genetic information is stored using the genetic code. DNA also has regulatory sequences, chromosomal structural areas and other non-coding DNA that can contribute greatly to phenotype. Such elements operate under sets of rules that are different from the codon-to-amino acid standard underlying the genetic code.

3.1 One Gene, One Enzyme, and the Biosynthetic Pathway

Duchenne muscular dystrophy (DMD) is a disease caused by a mutation in the DNA (X-linked recessive mutation; BIO 15.3). DMD patients have a mutation in the gene coding for the protein dystrophin. This protein connects the cytoskeleton to the extracellular matrix (thus through the plasma membrane) in muscle cells and appears to stabilize the muscle during contraction. Without dystrophin, the plasma membrane ruptures during muscle contraction and degeneration of the muscle tissue occurs (most DMD patients become wheelchair-dependent early in life). One gene, one protein and we can see how it is expressed in the organism (phenotype; BIO 15.1).

Experiments done in the 1940s, that would later give birth to Molecular Biology, used the bread mold *Neurospora* (a fungus; BIO 2.3) to conclude the following:

- Molecules are synthesized in a series of steps (= biosynthetic pathway, or, more generally: metabolic pathway)
- Each step is catalyzed by a unique enzyme (of course, enzymes are proteins)
- Each enzyme is specified by a unique gene ("one gene, one enzyme").

As we will see in Chapter 4, in a metabolic pathway, a principal chemical is modified by a series of chemical reactions. Enzymes catalyze these reactions. Because of the many chemicals (= "metabolites") that may be involved, metabolic pathways can be complex. Consider the following straightforward synthetic pathway (Int = Intermediate):

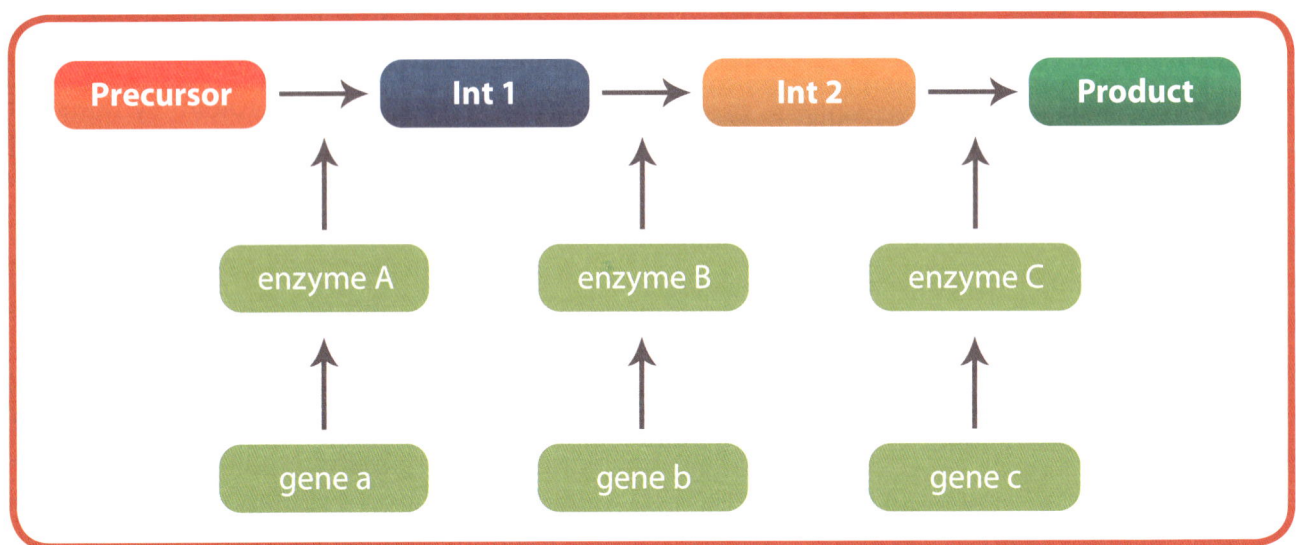

Consider the following questions:

1. Imagine that there was a mutation (or inactivation) in gene c, would any Product be produced? Would you expect the intermediates to be produced? Would their concentrations go up or down?

2. What would be the consequences of a mutation in gene b?

3. What happens if we add Intermediate 1 or Intermediate 2 to the media of a gene b mutation? Would either case result in Product? {Note: "media" is plural and refers to a growth medium or culture medium which is a liquid or gel designed to support the growth of cells}

BIOLOGY

Consider your answers before continuing. You can expect questions like this on the real exam.

1. If there is a mutation at gene c then enzyme C is blocked (i.e. it is either not being produced or it is not functioning normally) which means the Product would not be produced and we would expect Intermediate 2 to increase in concentration (imagine a production line where one worker stops working but there continues to be items arriving at their desk, the result is accumulation at that point and non-production beyond that point).

2. A mutation at gene b stops the function of enzyme B thus the production of Intermediate 2 is blocked thus no Product is formed. Intermediate 1 begins to accumulate.

3. Adding Intermediate 1 just leads to its accumulation since we are presented with one way arrows so the reaction can only move forward but it is blocked because of the gene b mutation [had the arrows been double sided, which is quite normal in nature, then Le Chatelier's principle (CHM 9.9) would suggest that Precursor would be produced because of the stress of increasing Intermediate 1].

However, if Intermediate 2 is added to the media with the gene b mutation, since gene c is not mutated, the Product will be formed. Being beyond the 'blockage' caused by enzyme B dysfunction, the medium supplemented with Intermediate 2 bypasses the problem and is able to produce Product because there are no issues with gene c.

It should be noted that the one gene-one enzyme hypothesis predated the understanding of the genetic code and our modern understanding of enzymes – many of which are composed of multiple polypeptides (ORG 12.2), each of which is coded for by one gene. Thus "one gene-one polypeptide" would be more accurate but even so, remains incomplete because of more recent discoveries outside the scope of this exam.

Peptide: The result of the moon pulling on the Pepsi.   ;)

At the time of publication, the preceding information would be helpful to solve ACER GAMSAT Red Booklet Unit 16, and Blue Booklet Unit 17, and somewhat helpful for Purple Booklet questions 87 and 88. In other words, the reasoning may be helpful during the real exam.

Go online to GAMSAT-prep.com for additional chapter review Q&A and forum.

GOLD NOTES

ENZYMES AND CELLULAR METABOLISM
Chapter 4

Memorize
* fine: catabolism, anabolism, ivation energy
* fine: metabolism, active/ osteric sites

Understand
* Feedback, competitive, non-competitive inhibition
* Krebs cycle, electron transport chain: main features
* Metabolism: carbohydrates (glucose), fats and proteins

Not Required*
* Advanced level college info
* Photosynthesis, gluconeogenesis, fatty acid oxidation
* Knowing the deficiencies in the theoretical yield (36 ATP) calculation

GAMSAT-Prep.com

Introduction

Cells require energy to grow, reproduce, maintain structure, respond to the environment, etc. Biochemical reactions and other energy producing processes that occur in cells, including cellular metabolism, are regulated in part by enzymes. GAMSAT tests almost always include multiple questions exploring your understanding of a cycle or biochemical mechanism with or without negative or positive feedback. The questions do not center on your memorizing details but rather having an understanding of how the presented cycle functions or how it can be stimulated or inhibited. The end of Chapter 6 will focus on feedback loops with respect to hormones. Metabolism can be complex and it forms a story that you should be familiar with but that you should not spend time trying to memorize for the GAMSAT.

Additional Resources

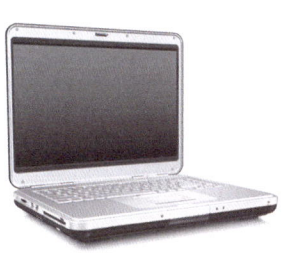
Free Online Q&A + Forum

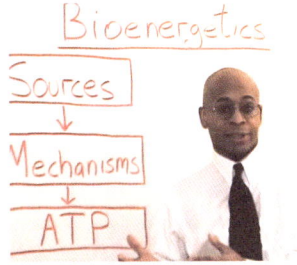
Video: Online or DVD

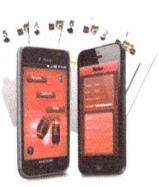
Flashcards

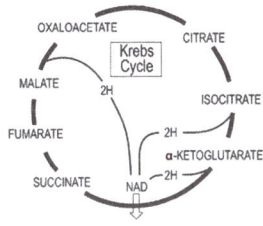
Special Guest

THE BIOLOGICAL SCIENCES   BIO-51

* The real GAMSAT may have advanced level information presented (ie. in a passage) but previous knowledge of said information is not required to answer the questions that would follow. Practice ACER and GS practice GAMSATs can help you clarify this point.

4.1 Overview

In an organism or an individual many biochemical reactions take place. All these biochemical reactions are collectively termed metabolism. In general, metabolism can be broadly divided into two main categories. They are:

(a) Catabolism which is the breakdown of macromolecules (larger molecules) such as glycogen to micromolecules (smaller molecules) such as glucose.

(b) Anabolism which is the building up of macromolecules such as protein using micromolecules such as amino acids.

As we all know, chemical reactions in general involve great energy exchanges when they occur. Similarly most catabolic and anabolic reactions would involve massive amounts of energy if they were to occur in vitro (outside the cell). However, all these reactions could be carried out within an environment of less free energy exchange, using molecules called enzymes.

What is an enzyme?

An enzyme is a protein catalyst. A protein is a large polypeptide made up of amino acid subunits. A catalyst is a substance that alters the rate of a chemical reaction without itself being permanently changed into another compound. A catalyst accelerates a reaction by decreasing the free energy of activation (see diagrams in CHM 9.5, 9.7).

Enzymes fall into two general categories:

(a) Simple proteins which contain only amino acids like the digestive enzymes ribonuclease, trypsin and chymotrypsin.

(b) Complex proteins which contain amino acids and a non-amino acid cofactor. Thus the complete enzyme is called a holoenzyme and it is made up of a protein portion (apoenzyme) and a cofactor.

> Holoenzyme = Apoenzyme + Cofactor.

A metal may serve as a cofactor. Zinc, for example, is a cofactor for the enzymes carbonic anhydrase and carboxypeptidase. An organic molecule such as pyridoxal phosphate or biotin may serve as a cofactor. Cofactors such as biotin, which are covalently linked to the enzyme are called prosthetic groups or ligands.

In addition to their enormous catalytic power which accelerates reaction rates, enzymes exhibit exquisite specificity in the types of reactions that each catalyzes as well as specificity for the substrates upon which they act. Their specificity is linked to the concept of an active site. An active site is a cluster of amino acids within the tertiary (i.e. 3-dimensional) configuration of the enzyme where the actual catalytic event occurs. The active site is often similar to a pocket or groove with properties (chemical or structural) that accommodate the intended substrate with high specificity.

Examples of such specificity are as follows: Phosphofructokinase catalyzes a reaction between ATP and fructose-6-phosphate. The enzyme does not catalyze a reaction between other nucleoside triphosphates. It is worth mentioning the specificity of trypsin and chymotrypsin though both of them are proteolytic (i.e. they degrade or hydrolyse proteins). Trypsin catalyzes the hydrolysis of peptides and proteins only on the carboxyl side of polypeptidic amino acids lysine and arginine. Chymotrypsin catalyzes the hydrolysis of peptides and proteins on the carboxyl side of polypeptidic amino acids phenylalanine, tyrosine and tryptophan. The degree of specificity described in the previous examples originally led to the **Lock and Key Model** which has been generally replaced by the **Induced Fit Hypothesis**. While the former suggests that the spatial structure of the active site of an enzyme fits exactly that of the substrate, the latter is more widely accepted and describes a greater flexibility at the active site and a conformational change in the enzyme to strengthen binding to the substrate.

4.2 Enzyme Kinetics and Inhibition

There is an increase in reaction velocity (= reaction rate) with an increase in the concentration of substrate. At increasingly higher substrate concentrations the increase in activity is progressively smaller. From this, it could be inferred that enzymes exhibit saturation kinetics. The mechanism of the preceding lies largely with saturation of the enzyme's active sites. As substrate concentration increases, more and more enzymes are converted to the substrate bound enzyme complex until all the enzyme active sites are bound to substrate. After this point, further increase in substrate concentration will not increase reaction rate.

Enzyme inhibitors are classified as: competitive inhibitor, noncompetitive inhibitor and irreversible inhibitor. In competitive inhibition, the inhibitor and the substrate are analogues that compete for binding to the active site, forming an unreactive enzyme-inhibitor complex. However, at higher substrate concentration, the inhibition can be reversed. In noncompetitive inhibition, the inhibitor can bind to the enzyme at a site different from the active site where the substrate binds to, thus forming either an unreactive enzyme-inhibitor complex or enzyme-substrate-inhibitor complex. However, a higher substrate concentration does not reverse the inhibition. In irreversible inhibition, the inhibitor binds permanently to the enzyme and inactivates it (e.g. heavy metals, aspirin, organophosphates). The effects caused by irreversible inhibitors are only overcome by synthesis of new enzyme.

4.3 Regulation of Enzyme Activity

The activity of enzymes in the cell is subject to a variety of regulatory mechanisms. The amount of enzyme can be altered by increasing or decreasing its synthesis or degradation. Enzyme induction refers to an enhancement of its synthesis. Repression refers to a decrease in its biosynthesis.

Enzyme activity can also be altered by covalent modification. Phosphorylation of specific serine residues by protein kinases increases or decreases catalytic activity depending upon the enzyme. Proteolytic cleavage of proenzymes (e.g., chymotrypsinogen, trypsinogen, protease and clotting factors) converts an inactive form to an active form (e.g., chymotrypsin, trypsin, etc.).

Enzyme activity can be greatly influenced by its environment (esp. pH and temperature). For example, most enzymes exhibit optimal activity at a pH in the range 6.5 to 7.5. However, pepsin (an enzyme found in the stomach) has an optimum pH

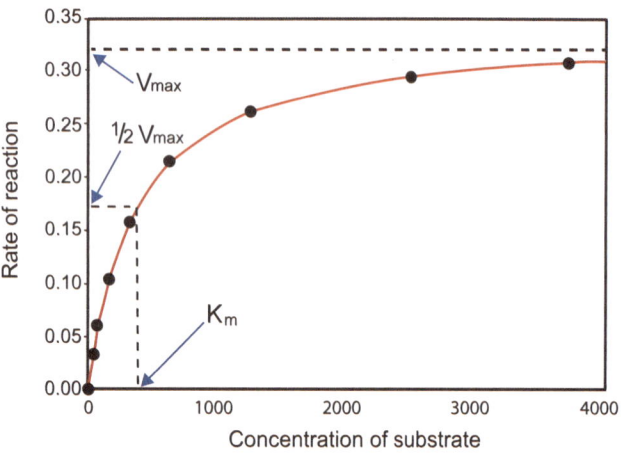
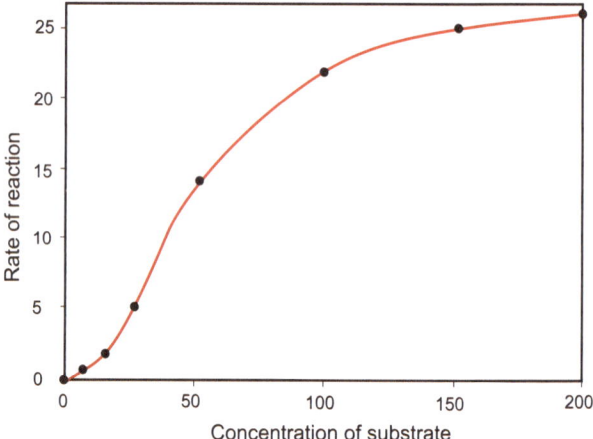

Michaelis-Menten Kinetics: Enzymes with single-substrate mechanisms usually follow the Michaelis-Menten model, in which the plot of velocity vs. substrate concentration [S] produces a rectangular hyperbola. Initially, the reaction rate [V] increases as substrate concentration [S] increases over a range of substrate concentration. However, as [S] gets higher, the enzyme becomes saturated with substrate and eventually the reaction rate [V] reaches maximum velocity V_{max} when the enzyme is fully saturated with substrate. Compare the diagram above with the curve of carrier-mediated transport (i.e. showing saturation kinetics) for solutes crossing the plasma membrane in BIO 1.1.2. The K_m is the substrate concentration at which an enzyme-catalyzed reaction occurs at half its maximal velocity, $V_{max}/2$. K_m is called the Michaelis constant. Each enzyme has a unique K_m value.

Non-Michaelis-Menten Kinetics: Some enzymes with multiple-substrate mechanisms exhibit the non-Michaelis-Menten model, in which the plot of velocity vs. substrate concentration [S] produces a sigmoid curve. This characterizes cooperative binding of substrate to the active site, which means that the binding of one substrate to one subunit affects the binding of subsequent substrate molecules to other subunits. This behavior is most common in multimeric enzymes with several active sites. Positive cooperativity occurs when binding of the first substrate increases the affinity of the other active sites for the following substrates. Negative cooperativity occurs when binding of the first substrate decreases the affinity of the other active site for the following substrates.

Fig. IV. A. 4.1 Enzyme Kinetic Curve Plot.

of ~ 2.0. Thus it cannot function adequately at a higher pH (i.e. in the small intestine). Likewise, enzymes function at an optimal temperature. When the temperature is lowered, kinetic energy decreases and thus the rate of reaction decreases. If the temperature is raised too much then the enzyme may become denatured and thus non-functional.

Enzyme activity can also be modified by an *allosteric* mechanism which involves binding to a site other than the active site. Isocitrate dehydrogenase is an enzyme in the Krebs Tricarboxylic Acid Cycle, which is activated by ADP. ADP is not a substrate or substrate analogue. It is postulated to bind a site *distinct* from the active site called the *allosteric site*. Positive effectors stabilize the more active form of enzyme and enhance enzyme activity while negative effectors stabilize the less active form of enzyme and inhibit enzyme activity.

Some enzymes fail to behave by simple saturation kinetics. In such cases a phenomenon called positive cooperativity is explained in which binding of one substrate or ligand shifts the enzyme from the less active form to the more active form and makes it easier for the second substrate to bind. Instead of a hyperbolic curve of velocity vs. substrate concentration [S] that many enzymes follow, sigmoid curve of velocity vs. [S] characterizes cooperativity (i.e. see the Enzyme Kinetic Curve Plot in this section as well as hemoglobin and myoglobin, BIO 7.5.1).

4.4 Bioenergetics

Biological species must transform energy into readily available sources in order to survive. ATP (adenosine triphosphate) is the body's most important short term energy storage molecule. It can be produced by the breakdown or oxidation of protein, lipids (i.e. fat) or carbohydrates (esp. glucose). If the body is no longer ingesting sources of energy it can access its own stores: glucose is stored in the liver as glycogen, lipids are stored throughout the body as fat, and ultimately, muscle can be catabolized to release protein (esp. amino acids).

We will be examining four key processes that can lead to the production of ATP: glycolysis, Krebs Citric Acid Cycle, the electron transport chain (ETC), and oxidative phosphorylation. Figure IV.A.4.2 is a schematic summary.

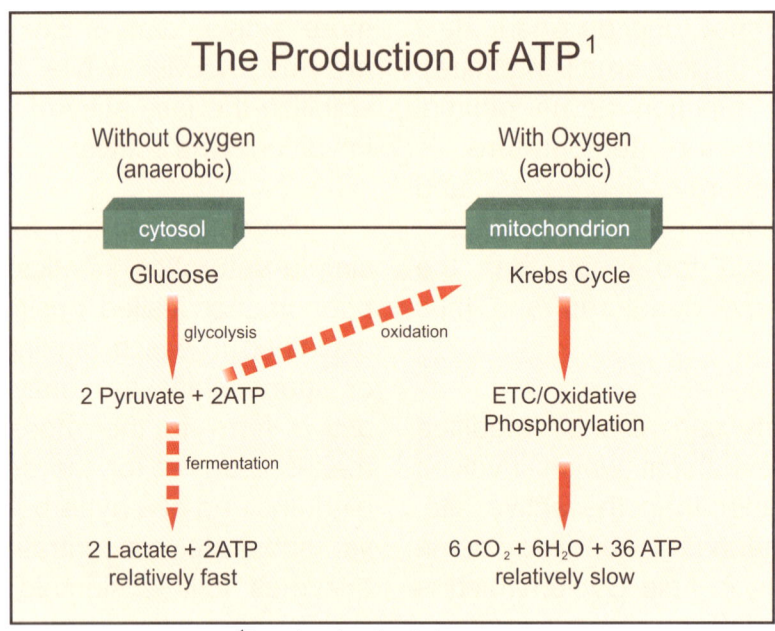

Figure IV.A.4.2: Summary of ATP production.

4.5 Glycolysis

The initial steps in the catabolism or *lysis* of D-glucose constitute the Embden - Meyerhof glyco*lytic* pathway. This pathway can occur in the absence of oxygen (anaerobic). The enzymes for glycolysis are present in all human cells and are located in the cytosol. The overall reaction can be depicted as follows (ADP: adenosine diphosphate, NAD: nicotinamide adenine dinucleotide, P_i: inorganic phosphate):

$$\text{Glucose} + 2\text{ADP} + 2\text{ NAD}^+ + 2P_i \longrightarrow 2\text{Pyruvate} + 2\text{ATP} + 2\text{NADH} + 2\text{H}^+$$

The first step in glycolysis involves the phosphorylation of glucose by ATP. The enzyme that catalyzes this irreversible reaction is either hexokinase or glucokinase. Phosphohexose isomerase then catalyzes the conversion of glucose-6-phosphate to fructose-6-phosphate. Phosphofructokinase (PFK) catalyzes the second phosphorylation. It is an irreversible reaction. This reaction also utilizes 1 ATP. This step, which produces fructose-1,6-diphosphate, is said to be the rate limiting or pacemaker step in glycolysis. Aldolase then catalyzes the cleavage of fructose-1,6-diphosphate to glyceraldehyde-

3-phosphate and dihydroxyacetone phosphate (= 2 triose phosphates). Triose phosphate isomerase catalyzes the interconversion of the two preceding compounds. Glyceraldehyde-3-phosphate dehydrogenase mediates a reaction between the designated triose, NAD$^+$ and P$_i$ to yield 1,3-diphosphoglycerate.

Next, phosphoglycerate kinase catalyzes the reaction of the latter, an energy rich compound, with ADP to yield ATP and phosphoglycerate. This reaction generates 2 ATP per glucose molecule. Phosphoglycerate mutase catalyzes the transfer of the phosphoryl group to carbon two to yield 2-phosphoglycerate. Enolase catalyzes a dehydration reaction to yield phosphoenolpyruvate and water. The enzyme enolase is inhibited by fluoride at high, nonphysiological concentrations. This is why blood samples that are drawn for estimation of glucose are added to fluoride to inhibit glycolysis. Phosphoenolpyruvate is then acted upon by pyruvate kinase to yield pyruvate which is a three carbon compound and 2 ATP.

NADH produced in glycolysis must regenerate NAD$^+$ so that glycolysis can continue. Under **aerobic** conditions (i.e. in the presence of oxygen) pyruvate is converted to Acetyl CoA which will enter the Krebs Cycle followed by oxidative phosphorylation producing a total of 38 ATP per molecule of glucose (i.e. 2 pyruvate). Electrons from NADH are transferred to the electron transfer chain located on the inside of the inner mitochondrial membrane and thus NADH produced during glycolysis in the cytosol is converted back to NAD$^+$.

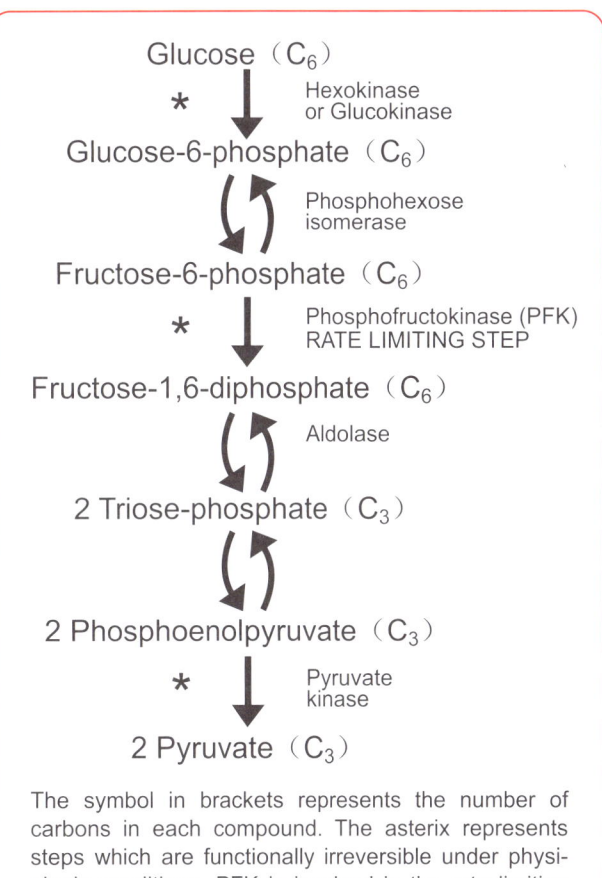

Figure IV.A.4.3: Summary of glycolysis.

Under **anaerobic conditions**, pyruvate is quickly reduced by NADH to lactic acid using the enzyme lactate dehydrogenase and NAD$^+$ is regenerated. A net of only 2 ATP is produced per molecule of glucose (this process is called *fermentation*).

Oxygen Debt: after running a 100m dash you may find yourself gasping for air even if you have completely ceased activity. This is because during the race you could not get an adequate amount of oxygen to your muscles and your muscles needed energy quickly; thus the anaerobic pathway was used. The lactic acid which built up during the race will require you to *pay back* a certain amount of oxygen in order to oxidize lactate to pyruvate and continue along the more energy efficient aerobic pathway.

4.6 Glycolysis: A Negative Perspective

An interesting way to summarize the main events of glycolysis is to follow the fate of the phosphate group which contains a negative charge. Note that *kinases* and *phosphatases* are enzymes that can add or subtract phosphate groups, respectively.

The first event in glycolysis is the phosphorylation of glucose. Thus glucose becomes negatively charged which prevents it from leaking out of the cell. Then glucose-6-phosphate becomes its isomer (= *same* molecular formula, *different* structure) fructose-6-phosphate which is further phosphorylated to fructose-1,6-diphosphate. Imagine that this six carbon sugar (*fructose*) now contains two large negatively charged ligands which repel each other! The six carbon sugar (*hexose*) sensibly breaks into two three-carbon compounds (*triose phosphates*).

A triose phosphate is ultimately converted to 1,3-diphosphoglycerate which is clearly an unstable compound (i.e. *two negative phosphate groups*). Thus it transfers a high energy phosphate group onto ADP to produce ATP. When ATP is produced from a substrate (i.e. 1,3-diphosphoglycerate), the reaction is called *substrate level phosphorylation*.

A closer look at ATP and glycolysis: from one molecule of glucose, 2 molecules of pyruvate are obtained. During the glycolytic reaction, 2 ATP are used (one used in the phosphorylation of glucose to glucose 6-phosphate and one used in the phosphorylation of fructose 6-phosphate to fructose 1,6-bisphosphate) and 4 ATP are generated (two in the conversion of 1,3-bisphophoglycerate to 3-phosphoglycerate and two in the conversion of phosphoenolpyruvate to pyruvate).

4.7 Krebs Citric Acid Cycle

Aerobic conditions: for further breakdown of pyruvate it has to enter the mitochondria where a series of reactions will cleave the molecule to water and carbon dioxide. All these reactions (which were discovered by Hans. A. Krebs) are collectively known as the Tricarboxylic Acid Cycle (TCA) or Krebs Citric Acid Cycle. Not only carbohydrates but also lipids and proteins use the TCA for channelling their metabolic pathways. This is why

TCA is often called the final common pathway of metabolism.

The glycolysis of glucose (C_6) produces 2 pyruvate (C_3) which in turn produces 2 CO_2 and 2 acetyl CoA (C_2). Pyruvate is oxidized to acetyl CoA and CO_2 by the pyruvate dehydrogenase complex (PDC). The PDC is a complex of 3 enzymes located in the mitochondria of eukaryotic cells (and of course, in the cytosol of prokaryotes). This step is also known as the *link reaction* or *transition step* since it links glycolysis and the TCA cycle.

The catabolism of both glucose and fatty acids yield acetyl CoA. Metabolism of amino acids yields acetyl CoA or actual intermediates of the TCA Cycle. The Citric Acid Cycle provides a pathway for the oxidation of acetyl CoA. The pathway includes eight discrete steps. Seven of the enzyme activities are found in the mitochondrial matrix; the eighth (succinate dehydrogenase) is associated with the Electron Transport Chain (ETC) within the inner mitochondrial membrane.

The following includes key points to remember about the TCA Cycle: i) glucose → 2 acetyl CoA → 2 turns around the TCA Cycle; ii) 2 CO_2 per turn is generated as a waste product which will eventually be blown off in the lungs; iii) one GTP (guanosine triphosphate) per turn is produced by substrate level phosphorylation; one GTP is equivalent to one ATP (*GTP + ADP → GDP + ATP*); iv) *reducing equivalents* are hydrogens which are carried by NAD^+ (→ $NADH + H^+$) three times per turn and FAD (→ $FADH_2$) once per turn; v) for each molecule of glucose, 2 pyruvates are produced and oxidized to acetyl CoA in the "fed" state (as opposed to the "fasting" state). The acetyl CoA then enters the TCA cycle, yielding 3 NADH, 1 $FADH_2$, and 1 GTP per acetyl CoA. These reducing equivalents will eventually be oxidized to produce ATP (*oxidative phosphorylation*) and eventually produce H_2O as a waste product (the last step in the ETC); vi) the hydrogens (*H*) which are reducing equivalents are not protons (*H^+*) - quite the contrary! Often the reducing equivalents are simply called electrons.

4.8 Oxidative Phosphorylation

The term oxidative phosphorylation refers to reactions associated with oxygen consumption and the phosphorylation of ADP to yield ATP. The synthesis of ATP is coupled to the flow of electrons from NADH and $FADH_2$ to O_2 in the electron transport chain. Oxidative phosphorylation is associated with an Electron Transport Chain or Respiratory Chain which is found in the inner mitochondrial membrane of eukaryotes. A similar process occurs within the plasma membrane of prokaryotes such as *E.coli*.

The importance of oxidative phosphorylation is that it accounts for the reoxidation of reducing equivalents generated in the reac-

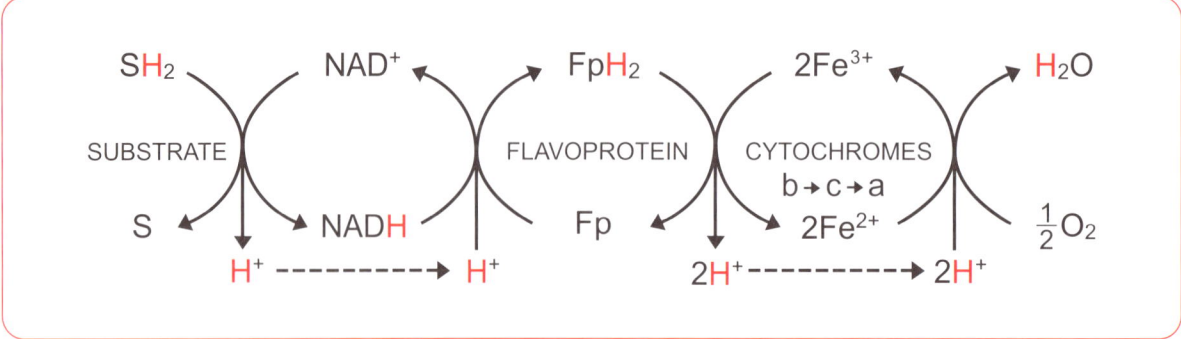

Figure IV.A.4.4: Transport of reducing equivalents through the respiratory chain. Examples of substrates (S) which provide reductants are isocitrate, malate, etc. Cytochromes contain iron (Fe).

tions of the Krebs Cycle as well as in glycolysis. This process accounts for the preponderance of ATP production in humans. The electron flow from NADH and $FADH_2$ to oxygen by a series of carrier molecules located in the inner mitochondrial membrane (IMM) provides energy to pump hydrogens from the mitochondrial matrix to the intermembrane space against the proton electrochemical gradient. The proton motive force then drives the movement of hydrogen back into the matrix thus providing the energy for ATP synthesis by ATP synthase. A schematic summary is in Figure IV.A.4.4.

The term *chemiosmosis* refers to the movement of protons across the IMM (a selectively permeable membrane) down their electrochemical gradient using the kinetic energy to phosphorylate ADP making ATP. The generation of ATP by chemiosmosis occurs in chloroplasts and mitochondria as well as in some bacteria.

4.9 Electron Transport Chain (ETC)

The following are the components of the ETC: iron - sulphur proteins, cytochromes c, b, a and coenzyme Q or *ubiquinone*. The respiratory chain proceeds from NAD specific dehydrogenases through flavoprotein, ubiquinone, then cytochromes and ultimately molecular oxygen. Reducing equivalents can enter the chain at two locations. Electrons from NADH are transferred to NADH dehydrogenase. In reactions involving iron - sulphur proteins electrons are transferred to coenzyme Q; protons are translocated from the mitochondrial matrix to the exterior of the inner membrane during this process. This creates a proton gradient, which is coupled to the production of ATP by ATP synthase.

Electrons entering from succinate dehydrogenase (FADH$_2$) are donated directly to coenzyme Q. Electrons are transported from reduced coenzyme Q to cytochrome b and then cytochrome c. Electrons are then carried by cytochrome c to cytochrome a.

Cytochrome a is also known as *cytochrome oxidase*. It catalyzes the reaction of electrons and protons with molecular oxygen to produce water. Cyanide and carbon monoxide are powerful inhibitors of cytochrome oxidase.

4.10 Summary of Energy Production

Note the following: i) 1 NADH produces 3 ATP molecules while 1 FADH$_2$ produces only 2 ATP; ii) there is a cost of 2 ATP to get the two molecules of NADH generated in the cytoplasm (see the preceding point # 2.) to enter the mitochondrion, thus the *net yield for eukaryotes is 36 ATP*.

The efficiency of ATP production is far from 100%. Energy is lost from the system primarily in the form of heat. Under standard conditions, less than 40% of the energy generated from the complete oxidation of glucose is converted to the production of ATP. As a comparison, a gasoline engine fairs much worse with an efficiency rating generally less than 30%. Further inefficiencies reduce the net theoretical yield in the (non-GAMSAT!) real world.

Process of reaction	ATP yield
1. Glycolysis (Glucose → 2 Pyruvate)	2
2. Glycolysis (2NADH from glyceraldehyde-3-phosphate dehydrogenase)	6
3. Pyruvate dehydrogenase (2NADH)	6
4. Isocitrate dehydrogenase (2NADH)	6
5. Alpha-ketoglutarate dehydrogenase (2NADH)	6
6. Succinate thiokinase (2GTP)	2
7. Succinate dehydrogenase (2FADH$_2$)	4
8. Malate dehydrogenase (2NADH)	6
TOTAL	38 ATP yield per hexose.

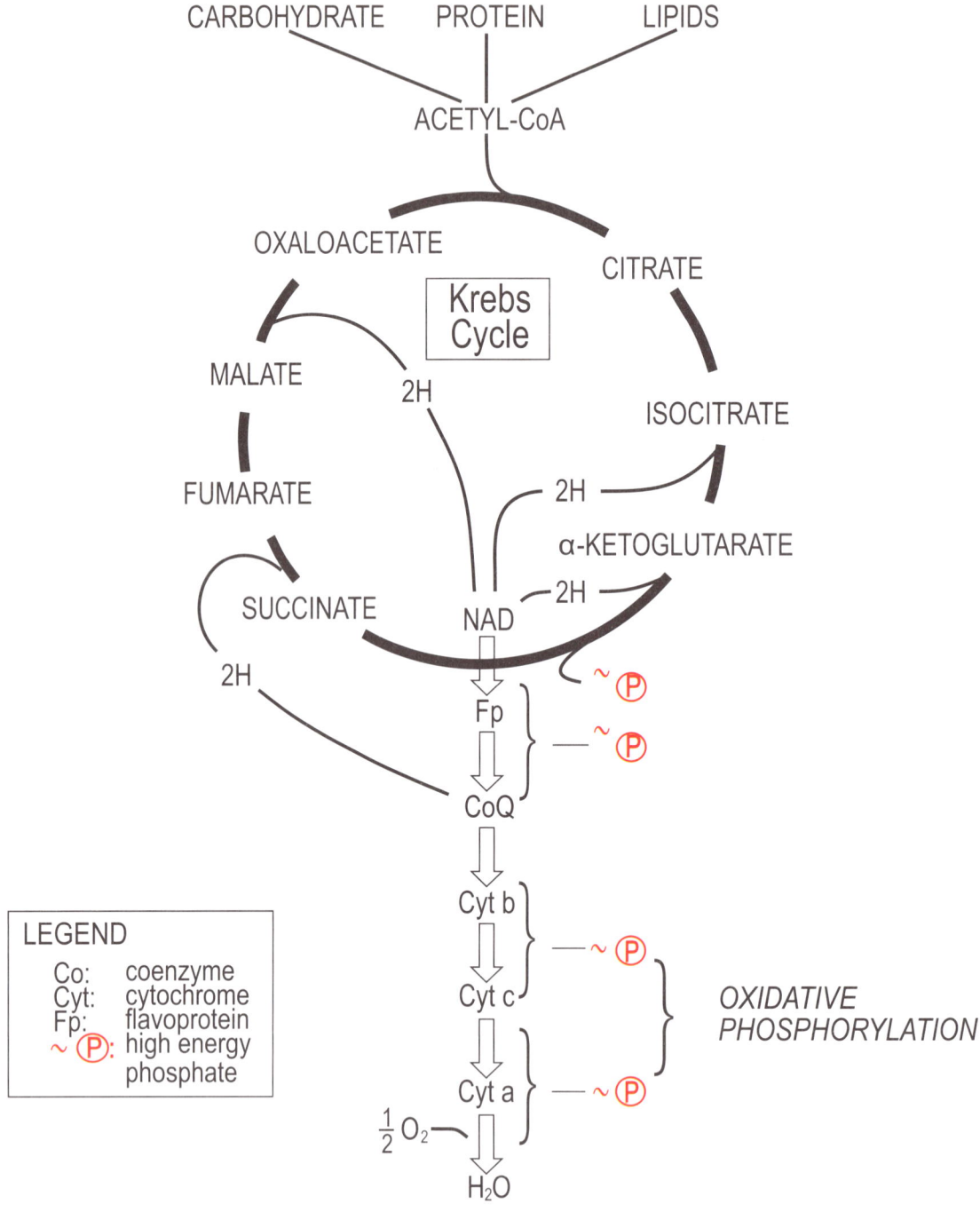

Figure IV.A.4.5: Summary of the Krebs Cycle and the Electron Transport Chain.
Note: Acetyl CoA can be the product of carbohydrate, protein, or lipid metabolism. Thick black arrows represent the Krebs Cycle while white arrows represent the Electron Transport Chain. High energy phosphate groups are transferred from ADP to produce ATP. Ultimately, oxygen accepts electrons and hydrogen from Cyt a to produce water.

GOLD NOTES

GOLD NOTES

SPECIALIZED EUKARYOTIC CELLS AND TISSUES
Chapter 5

Memorize	Understand	Not Required*
ron: basic structure and function sons for the membrane potential	* Resting potential: electrochemical gradient/action potential, graph * Excitatory and inhibitory nerve fibers: summation, frequency of firing * Organization of contractile elements: actin and myosin filaments * Cross bridges, sliding filament model; calcium regulation of contraction	* Advanced level college info * Memorizing details about epithelial cells, connective tissue

GAMSAT-Prep.com

Introduction

To build a living organism, with all the various tissues and organs, cells must specialize. Communication among cells and organs, movement, protection and support are achieved to a great degree by neurons, muscle cells, epithelial cells and the cells of connective tissue, respectively.

Additional Resources

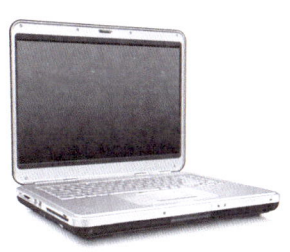

Free Online Q&A + Forum

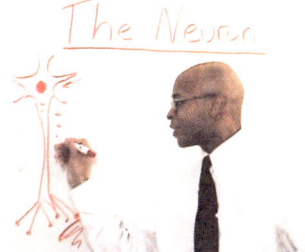

Video: Online or DVD

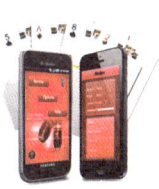

Flashcards

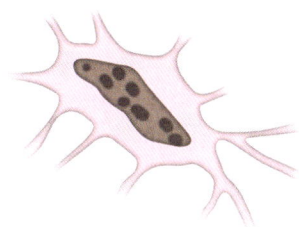

Special Guest

THE BIOLOGICAL SCIENCES   BIO-65

* The real GAMSAT may have advanced level information presented (ie. in a passage) but previous knowledge of said information is not required to answer the questions that would follow. Practice ACER and GS practice GAMSATs can help you clarify this point.

5.1 Neural Cells and Tissues

The brain, spinal cord and peripheral nervous system are composed of nerve tissue. The basic cell types of nerve tissue is the *neuron* and the *glial cell*. Glial cells support and protect neurons and participate in neural activity, nutrition and defense processes. Neurons (= nerve cells) represent the functional unit of the nervous system. They conduct and transmit nerve impulses.

Neurons can be classified based on the shape or *morphology*. Unipolar neurons possess a single process. Bipolar neurons possess a single axon and a single dendrite. Multipolar neurons possess a single axon and more than one dendrite and are the most common type. Pseudounipolar neurons possess a single process that subsequently branches out into an axon and dendrite (note that in biology "pseudo" means "false"). Neurons can also be classified based on function. Sensory neurons receive stimuli from the environment and conduct impulses to the CNS. Motor neurons conduct impulses from the CNS to other neurons, muscles or glands. Interneurons connect other neurons and regulate transmitting signal between neurons.

Each neuron consists of a nerve cell body (*perikaryon or soma*), and its processes, which usually include multiple *dendrites* and a single *axon*. The cell body of a typical neuron contains a nucleus, *Nissl* material which is rough endoplasmic reticulum, free ribosomes, Golgi apparatus, mitochondria, many neurotubules, neurofilaments and pigment inclusions. The cell processes of neurons occur as axons and dendrites.

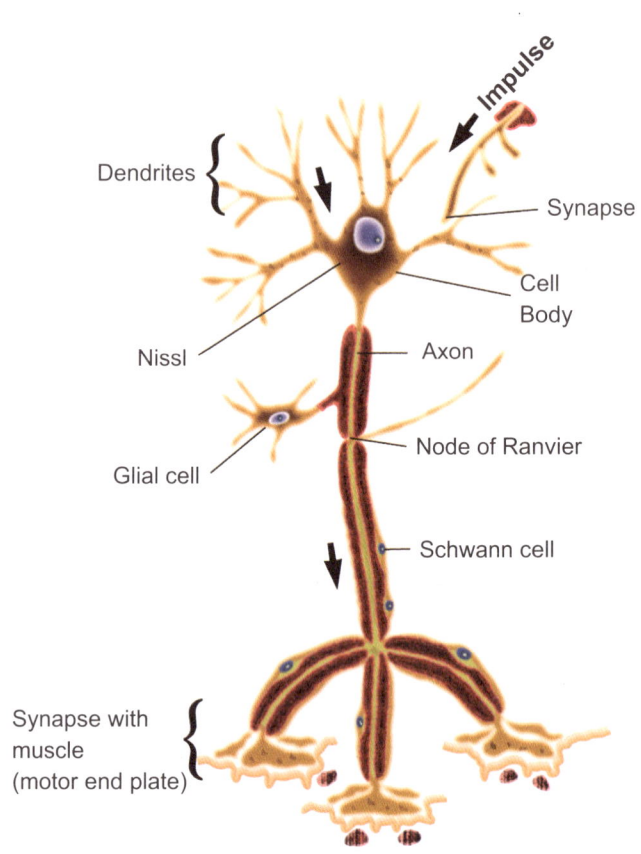

Figure IV.A.5.1: A neuron and other cells of nerve tissue, showing the neuromuscular junction, or motor end plate.

Dendrites contain most of the components of the cell, whereas axons contain major structures found in dendrites except for the Nissl material and Golgi apparatus. As a rule, dendrites receive stimuli from sensory cells, axons, or other neurons and conduct these impulses to the cell body of neurons and ultimately through to the axon. Axons are long cellular processes that conduct impulses away from the cell body of neurons. These originate from the axon hillock, a specialized region that contains many microtubules and neurofilaments. At the synaptic (terminal) ends of axons, the presynaptic process contains vesicles from which are elaborated excitatory or inhibitory substances.

Unmyelinated fibers in peripheral nerves lie in grooves on the surface of the neurolemma (= plasma membrane) of a type of glial cell (*Schwann cell*). **Myelinated** peripheral neurons are invested by numerous layers of plasma membrane of Schwann cells or oligodendrocytes that constitute a *myelin sheath*, which allows axons to conduct impulses faster. The myelin sheath is produced by oligodendrocytes in the CNS and by Schwann cells in the PNS. In junctional areas between adjacent Schwann cells or oligodendrocytes there is a lack of myelin. These junctional areas along the myelinated process constitute the nodes of Ranvier.

The neurons of the nervous system are arranged so that each neuron stimulates or inhibits other neurons and these in turn may stimulate or inhibit others until the functions of the nervous system are performed. The area between a neuron and the successive cell (i.e. another neuron, muscle fiber or gland) is called a *synapse*. Synapses can be classified as either a chemical synapse or an electrical synapse. A chemical synapse involves the release of a neurotransmitter by the presynaptic cell which then diffuses across the synapse and can act on the postsynaptic cell to generate an action potential. Signal transmission is delayed due to the time required for diffusion of the neurotransmitter across the synapse onto the membrane of the postsynaptic cell. An electrical synapse involves the movement of ions from one neuron to another via gap junctions (BIO 1.4.1). Signal transmission is immediate. Electrical synapses are often found in neural systems that require the fastest possible response, such as defensive reflexes.

When a neuron makes a synapse with muscle, it is called a *motor end plate* (see Fig. IV.A.5.1). The terminal endings of the nerve filament that synapse with the next cell are called presynaptic terminals, synaptic knobs, or more commonly - synaptic boutons. The postsynaptic terminal is the membrane part of another neuron or muscle or gland that is receiving the impulse. The synaptic cleft is the narrow space between the presynaptic and postsynaptic membrane.

At the synapse there is no physical contact between the two cells. The space between the dendrite of one neuron and the axon of another neuron is called the synaptic cleft and it measures about 200 - 300 angstroms (1 angstrom = 10^{-10} m) in a chemical synapse and about a tenth of that distance in an electrical synapse. The mediators in a chemical synapse, known as neurotransmitters, are housed in the presynaptic terminal and are exocytosed in response to an increase in intracellular Ca^{2+} concentration. The mediators or transmitters diffuse through the synaptic cleft when an impulse reaches the terminal and bind to receptors in the postsynaptic membrane. This transmitter substance may either excite the *postsynaptic* neuron or inhibit it. They are therefore called either excitatory or inhibitory transmitters (examples include *acetylcholine* and *GABA*, respectively).

5.1.1 The Membrane Potential

A membrane or resting potential (V_m) occurs across the plasma membranes of all cells. In large nerve and muscle cells this potential amounts to about 70 millivolts with positivity outside the cell membrane and negativity inside (V_m = -70 mV). The development of this potential occurs as follows: every cell membrane contains a Na^+ - K^+ ATPase that pumps each ion to where its concentration is highest. The concentration of K^+ is higher inside the neuron and the concentration of Na^+ is higher outside; therefore, Na^+ is pumped to the outside of the cell and K^+ to the inside. However, more Na^+ is pumped outward than K^+ inward ($3Na^+$ per $2K^+$). Also, the membrane is relatively permeable to K^+ so that it can leak out of the cell with relative ease. Therefore, the net effect is a loss of positive charges from inside the membrane and a gain of positive charges on the outside. The resulting membrane potential is the basis of all conduction of impulses by nerve and muscle fibers.

5.1.2 Action Potential

The action potential is a sequence of changes in the electric potential that occurs within a small fraction of a second when a nerve or muscle membrane impulse spreads over the surface of the cell. An excitatory stimulus on a postsynaptic neuron depolarizes the membrane and makes the membrane potential less negative. Once the membrane potential reaches a critical threshold, the voltage-gated Na^+ channels become fully open, permitting the inward flow of Na^+ into the cell. The membrane potential is at the critical threshold when it is in a state where an action potential is inevitable. As a result, the positive sodium ions on the outside of the membrane now flow rapidly to the more negative interior. Therefore, the membrane potential suddenly becomes reversed with positivity on the inside and negativity on the outside. This state is called *depolarization* and is caused by an inward Na^+ current.

Depolarization also leads to the inactivation of the Na^+ channel and slowly opens the K^+ channel. The combined effect of the two preceding events repolarizes the membrane back to its resting potential. This is called *repolarization*. In fact, the neuron may shoot past the resting membrane potential and become even more negative, and this is called hyperpolarization. The depolarized nerve goes on depolarizing the adjacent nerve membrane in a wavy manner which is called an impulse. In other words, an impulse is a wave of depolarization. Different axons can propagate impulses at different speeds. The increasing diameter of a nerve fiber or degree of myelination results in a faster impulse. The impulse is fastest in myelinated fibers since the wave of depolarization "jumps" from node to node of Ranvier: this is called *saltatory* conduction because an action potential can be generated only at nodes of Ranvier.

Immediately following an action potential, the neuron will pass through three stages in the following order: a) it can no longer elicit

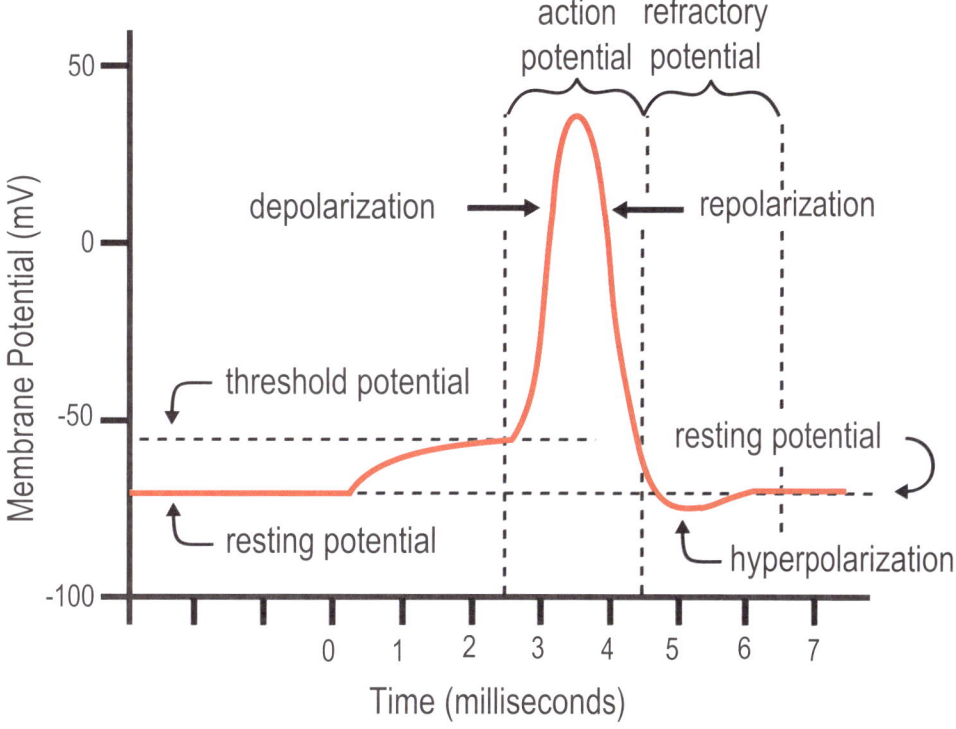

Figure IV.A.5.2: Action potential.

another action potential no matter how large the stimulus is = *absolute refractory period*; b) it can elicit another action potential only if a larger than usual stimulus is provided = *relative refractory period*; c) it returns to its original resting potential and thus can depolarize as easily as it originally did.

The action potential is an all-or-none event. The magnitude or strength of the action potential is not graded according to the strength of the stimulus. It occurs with the same magnitude each time it occurs, or it does not occur at all.

5.1.3 Action Potential: A Positive Perspective

To better understand the action potential it is useful to take a closer look at what occurs to the positive ions Na⁺ and K⁺. To begin with, there are protein channels in the plasma membrane that act like gates which guard the passage of specific ions. Some gates open or close in response to V_m and are thus called *voltage gated channels*.

Once a threshold potential is reached, the voltage gated Na⁺ channels open allowing the permeability or *conductance* of Na⁺ to increase. The Na⁺ ions can now diffuse across their chemical gradient: from an area of high concentration (*outside the membrane*) to an area of low concentration (*inside the membrane*). The Na⁺ ions will also diffuse across their electrical gradient: from an area of relative positivity (*outside the membrane*) to an area of relative negativity (*inside the membrane*). Thus the inside becomes positive and the membrane is depolarized. Repolarization occurs as the Na⁺ channels close and the voltage gated K⁺ channels open. As K⁺ conductance increases to the outside (where K⁺ concentration is lowest), the membrane repolarizes to once again become relatively negative on the inside.

5.2 Contractile Cells and Tissues

There are three types of muscle tissue: smooth, skeletal and cardiac. All three types are composed of muscle cells (fibers) that contain myofibrils possessing contractile filaments of actin and myosin.

Smooth muscle:- Smooth muscle cells are spindle shaped and are organized chiefly into sheets or bands of smooth muscle tissue. They contain a single nucleus and actively divide and regenerate. This tissue is found in blood vessels and other tubular visceral structures (i.e. intestines). Smooth muscles contain both actin and myosin filaments but actin predominates. The filaments are not organized into patterns that give cross striations as in cardiac and skeletal muscle. Filaments course obliquely in the cells and attach to the plasma membrane. Contraction of smooth muscle is involuntary and is innervated by the autonomic nervous system.

Skeletal muscle:- Skeletal muscle fibers are characterized by their peripherally located multiple nuclei and striated myofibrils. Myofibrils are longitudinally arranged bundles of thick and thin myofilaments. Myofilaments are composed of thick and thin filaments present in an alternating arrangement responsible for the cross-striation pattern. The striations in a sarcomere consists of an A-band (dark), which contains both thin and thick filaments. These are bordered toward the Z-lines by I-bands (light), which contain thin filaments only. The mid-region of the A-band contains an H-band (light), which contains thick filaments only and is bisected by an M-line. The Z lines are dense regions bisecting each I-band and anchor the thin filaments. The filaments interdigitate and are cross-bridged in the A-band with myosin filaments forming a hexagonal pattern of one myosin filament surrounded by six actin filaments. In the contraction of a muscle fiber,

BIOLOGY

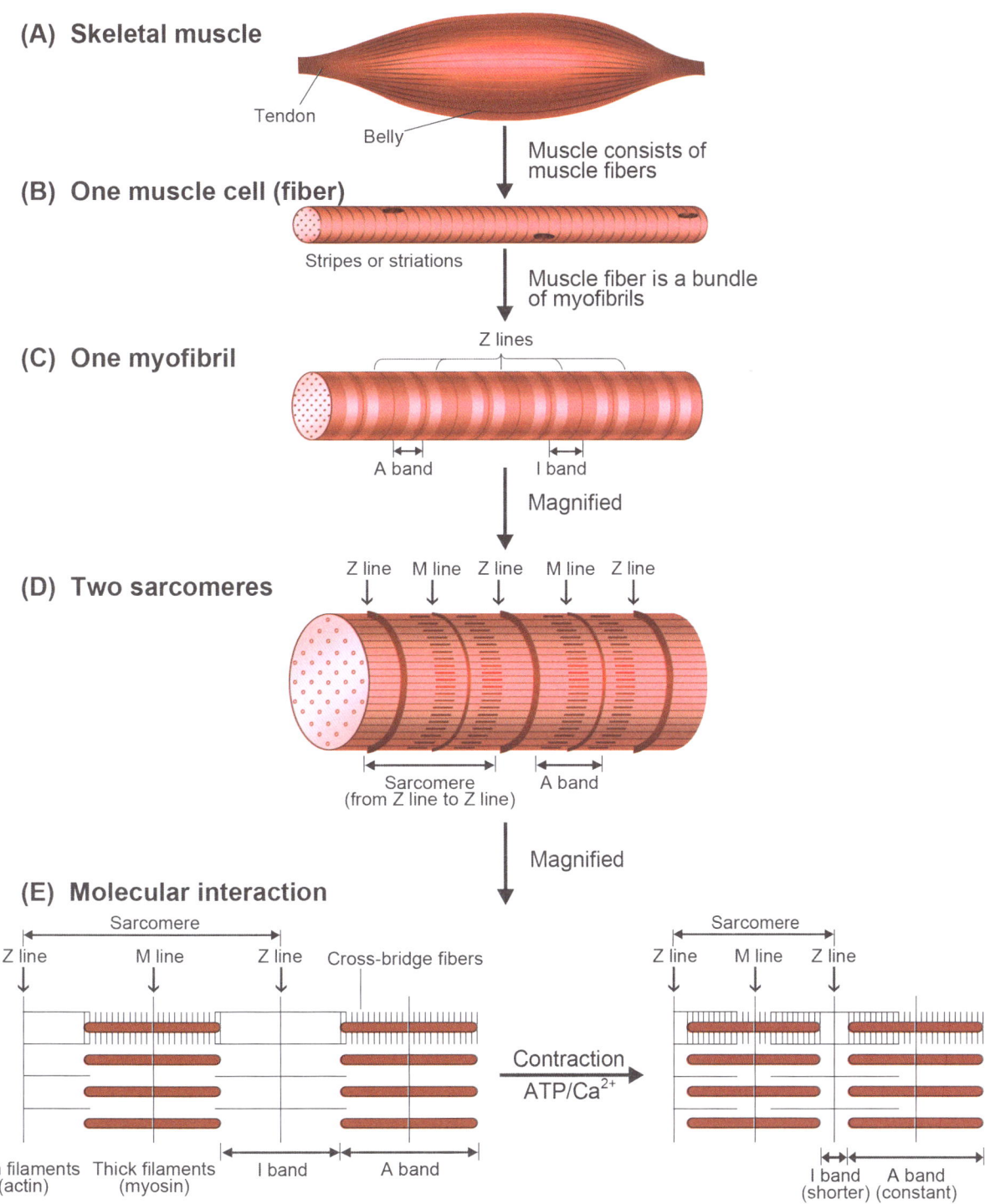

Figure IV.A.5.3: A schematic view of the molecular basis for muscle contraction. Note: the "H zone" is the central portion of an A band and is characterized by the presence of myosin filaments.

thick and thin filaments do not shorten but increase their overlap. The actin filaments of the I-bands move more deeply into the A-band, resulting in a shortening of the H-band and the I-bands as Z disks are brought closer. However, the A-band remains constant in length. {Mnemonic: "HI" bands shorten}

Each skeletal muscle fiber is invested with a sarcolemma (= plasmalemma = plasma membrane) that extends into the fiber as numerous small transverse tubes called T-tubules. These tubules ring the myofibrils at the A-I junction and are bounded on each side by terminal cisternae of the endoplasmic (sarcoplasmic) reticulum. The T-tubules, together with a pair of terminal cisternae form a triad. The triad helps to provide a uniform contraction throughout the muscle cell as it provides channels for ions to flow freely and helps to propagate action potentials. There are thousands of triads per skeletal muscle fiber.

The sarcoplasmic reticulum is a modified endoplasmic reticulum that regulates muscle contraction by either transporting Ca^{2+} into storage (muscle relaxation) or releasing Ca^{2+} during excitation-contraction coupling (muscle contraction).

The thick filaments within a myofibril are composed of about 250 myosin molecules arranged in an antiparallel fashion and some associated proteins. The myosin molecule is composed of two identical heavy chains and two pairs of light chain. The heavy chain consists of two "heads" and one "tail". The head contains an actin binding site which is involved in muscle contraction. The thin filaments within a myofibril are composed of actin and to a lesser degree two smaller proteins: *troponin and tropomyosin*. An action potential in the muscle cell membrane initiates depolarization of the T tubules, which causes the nearby sarcoplasmic reticulum to release its Ca^{2+} ions and thus an increase in intracellular $[Ca^{2+}]$. Calcium then attaches to a subunit of troponin resulting in the movement of tropomyosin and the uncovering of the active sites for the attachment of actin to the cross bridging heads of myosin. Due to this attachment, ATP in the myosin head hydrolyses, producing energy, Pi and ADP which results in a bending of the myosin head and a pulling of the actin filament into the A-band. These actin-myosin bridges detach again when myosin binds a new ATP molecule and attaches to a new site on actin toward the plus end as long as Ca^{2+} is bound to troponin. Finally, relaxation of muscle occurs when Ca^{2+} is sequestered by the sarcoplasmic reticulum. Thus calcium is pumped out of the cytoplasm and calcium levels return to normal, tropomyosin again binds to actin, preventing myosin from binding.

There are three interesting consequences to the preceding:

i) neither actin nor myosin change length during muscle contraction; rather, shortening of the muscle fiber occurs as the filaments slide over each other increasing the area of overlap.

ii) initially a dead person is very stiff (*rigor mortis*) since they can no longer produce the ATP necessary to detach the actin-myosin bridges thus their muscles remain locked in position.

iii) Ca^{2+} is a critical ion both for muscle contraction and for transmitter release from presynaptic neurons.

Cardiac muscle:- Cardiac muscle contains striations and myofibrils that are similar to those of skeletal muscle. Contraction of cardiac muscle is involuntary and is innervated by the autonomic nervous system. It differs from skeletal muscle in several major ways. Cardiac muscle fibers branch and contain centrally located nuclei (characteristically, one nucleus per cell) and large numbers of mitochondria. Individual cardiac muscle cells are attached to each other at their ends by *intercalated* disks. These disks contain several types of membrane junctional complexes, the most important of which is the *gap junction* (BIO 1.4.1). Cardiac muscle cells do not regenerate: injury to cardiac muscle is repaired by fibrous connective tissue.

The gap junction electrically couples one cell to its neighbor (= *syncytium*) so that electric depolarization is propagated throughout the heart by cell-to-cell contact rather than by nerve innervation to each cell. The sarcoplasmic reticulum - T-tubule system is arranged differently in cardiac muscle than in skeletal muscle. In cardiac muscle each T-tubule enters at the Z-line and forms a diad with only one terminal cisterna of sarcoplasmic reticulum.

5.3 Epithelial Cells and Tissues

Epithelia have the following characteristics:

1. they cover all body surfaces (i.e. skin, organs, etc.)
2. they are the principal tissues of glands
3. their cells are anchored by a nonliving layer (= the basement membrane)
4. they lack blood vessels and are thus nourished by diffusion.

Epithelial tissues are classified according to the characteristics of their cells. Tissues with elongated cells are called *columnar*, those with thin flattened cells are *squamous*, and those with cube-like cells are *cuboidal*. They are further classified as **simple** if they have a single layer of cells and **stratified** if they have multiple layers of cells. As examples of the classification, skin is composed of a stratified squamous epithelium while various glands (i.e. thyroid, salivary, etc.) contain a simple cuboidal epithelium. The former epithelium serves to protect against microorganisms, loss of water or heat, while the latter epithelium functions to secrete glandular products.

5.4 Connective Cells and Tissues

Connective tissue connects and joins other body tissue and parts. It also carries substances for processing, nutrition, and waste release. Connective tissue is characterized by the presence of relatively few cells surrounded by an extensive network of extracellular matrix, consisting of ground substance, extracellular fluid, and fibers.

The adult connective tissues are: connective tissue proper, cartilage, bone and blood (see *The Circulatory System*, section 7.5). Connective tissue proper is further classified into loose connective tissue, dense connective tissue, elastic tissue, reticular tissue and adipose tissue.

5.4.1 Loose Connective Tissue

Loose connective tissue is found in the superficial fascia. It is generally considered as the *packaging material* of the body, in part, because it frequently envelopes muscles. Fascia - usually a clear or white sheet (or band) of fibrous connective tissue - helps to bind skin to underlying organs, to fill spaces between muscles, etc. Loose connective tissue contains most of the cell types and all the fiber types found in the other connective tissues. The most common cell types are the fibroblast, macrophage, adipose cell, mast cell, plasma cell and wandering cells from the blood (which include several types of white blood cells).

Fibroblasts are the predominant cell type in connective tissue proper and have the capability to differentiate into other types of cells under certain conditions.

Macrophages are part of the *reticuloendothelial system* (tissue which predominately destroys foreign particles). They are responsible for phagocytosing foreign bodies and assisting the immune response. They possess large lysosomes containing digestive enzymes which are necessary for the digestion of phagocytosed materials. Mast cells reside mostly along blood vessels and contain granules which include *heparin* and *histamine*. Heparin is a compound which prevents blood clotting and histamine is associated with allergic reactions. Mast cells mediate type I hypersensitivity.

Plasma cells are part of the immune system in that they produce circulatory antibodies (BIO 7.5, 8.2). They contain extensive amounts of rough endoplasmic reticulum (rER).

Adipose cells are found in varying quantities, when they predominate, the tissue is called adipose (fat) tissue.

Fibers are long protein polymers present in different types of connective tissue. Common types of fibers include collagen fiber, reticular fiber and elastic fiber.

Collagen fibers are usually found in bundles and provide **strength** to the tissue. Many different types of collagen fibers are identified on the basis of their molecular structure. Of the five most common types, collagen type I is the most abundant, being found in dermis, bone, dentine, tendons, organ capsules, fascia and sclera. Type II is located in hyaline and elastic cartilage. Type III is probably the collagenous component of reticular fibers. Type IV is found in a specific part (*the basal lamina*) of basement membranes. Type V is a component of placental basement membranes. **Reticular fibers** are smaller, more delicate fibers that form the basic framework of reticular connective tissue. **Elastic fibers** branch and provide elasticity and support to connective tissue.

Ground substance is the gelatinous material that fills most of the space between the cells and the fibers. It is composed of acid mucopolysaccharides and structural glycoproteins and its properties are important in determining the permeability and consistency of the connective tissue.

5.4.2 Dense Connective Tissue

Dense irregular connective tissue is found in the dermis, periosteum, perichondrium and capsules of some organs. All of the fiber types are present, but collagenous fibers predominate. Dense regular connective tissue occurs as aponeuroses, ligaments and tendons. In most ligaments and tendons collagenous fibers are most prevalent and are oriented parallel to each other. Fibroblasts are practically the only cell type present.

5.4.3 Cartilage

Cartilage is composed of chondrocytes (= cartilage cells) embedded in an intercellular (= extracellular) matrix, consisting of fibers and an amorphous firm ground substance. In cases of injury, cartilage repairs slowly since it has no direct blood supply. Three types of cartilage are distinguished on the basis of the amount of ground substance and the relative abundance of collagenous and elastic fibers. They are hyaline, elastic and fibrous cartilage.

Hyaline Cartilage is found as costal (rib) cartilage, articular cartilage and cartilage of the nose, larynx, trachea and bronchi. The extracellular matrix consists primarily of collagenous fibers and a ground substance rich in chondromucoprotein, a copolymer of a protein and chondroitin sulphates.

Elastic Cartilage is found in the pinna of the ear, auditory tube and epiglottis, and some laryngeal cartilage. Elastic fibers predominate and thus provide greater flexibility. Calcification of this type of cartilage is rare.

Fibrous Cartilage occurs in the anchorage of tendons and ligaments, in intervertebral disks, in the symphysis pubis, and in some interarticular disks and in some ligaments. Chondrocytes occur singly or in rows between large bundles of collagenous fibers. Compared with hyaline cartilage, only small amounts of hyaline matrix surround the chondrocytes of fibrous cartilage.

5.4.4 Bone

Bone tissue consists of three **cell types** and a calcified **extracellular matrix** that contains organic and inorganic components. The three cell types are: *osteoblasts* which synthesize the organic components of the matrix (osteoid) and become embedded in lacunae; *osteocytes* which are mature bone cells entrapped in their own lacunae within the matrix and maintain communication with each other via gap junctions; and *osteoclasts* which are large multinucleated cells functioning in resorption and remodeling of bone.

The organic matrix consists of dense collagenous fibers (primarily type I collagen) which is important in providing flexibility and tensile strength to bone. The inorganic component is responsible for the *rigidity* of the bone and is composed chiefly of calcium phosphate and calcium carbonate with small amounts of magnesium, fluoride, hydroxide, sulphate and hydroxyapatite.

Compact bone contains haversian systems (osteons), interstitial lamellae and circumferential lamellae. The Haversian system is the structural unit for bone and each osteon consists of a central Haversian canal surrounded by a number of concentric deposits of bony matrix called lamellae. Haversian systems consist of extensively branching haversian canals that are oriented chiefly longitudinally in long bones. Each canal contains blood vessels and is surrounded by 8 to 15 concentric lamellae and osteocytes.

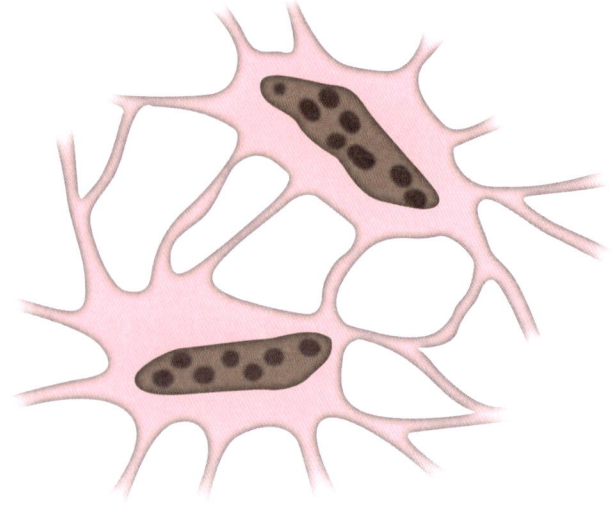

Figure IV.A.5.4: Osteocytes.

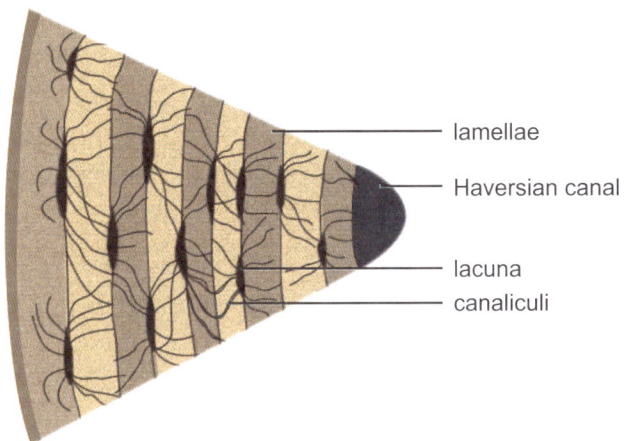

Figure IV.A.5.5: Schematic drawing of part of a haversian system.

Nutrients from blood vessels in the haversian canals pass through canaliculi and lacunae to reach all osteocytes in the system. Volkmann's canals traverse the bone transversely and interconnect the haversian systems. They enter through the outer circumferential lamellae and carry blood vessels and nerves which are continuous with those of the haversian canals and the periosteum. The periosteum is the connective tissue layer which envelopes bone. The endosteum is the connective tissue layer which lines the marrow cavities and supplies osteoprogenitor cells and osteoblasts for bone formation.

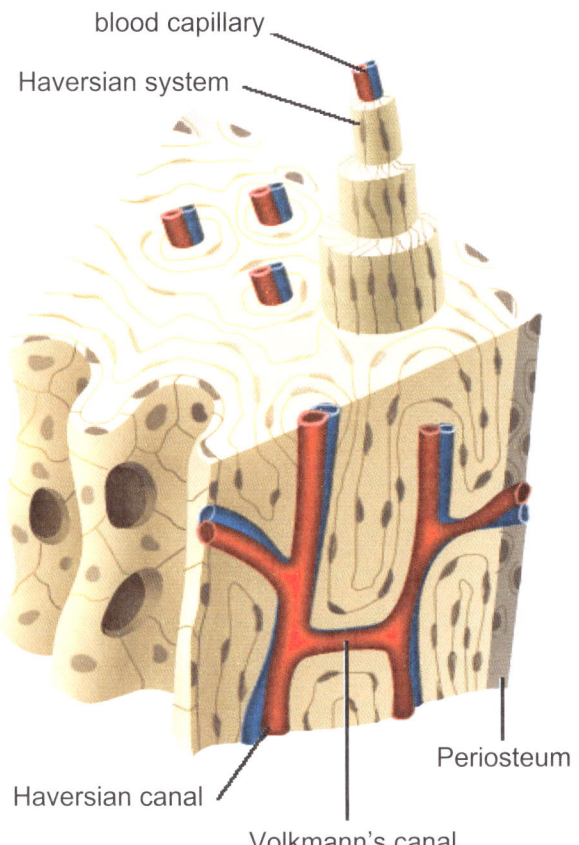

Figure IV.A.5.6
Schematic drawing of the wall of a long bone.

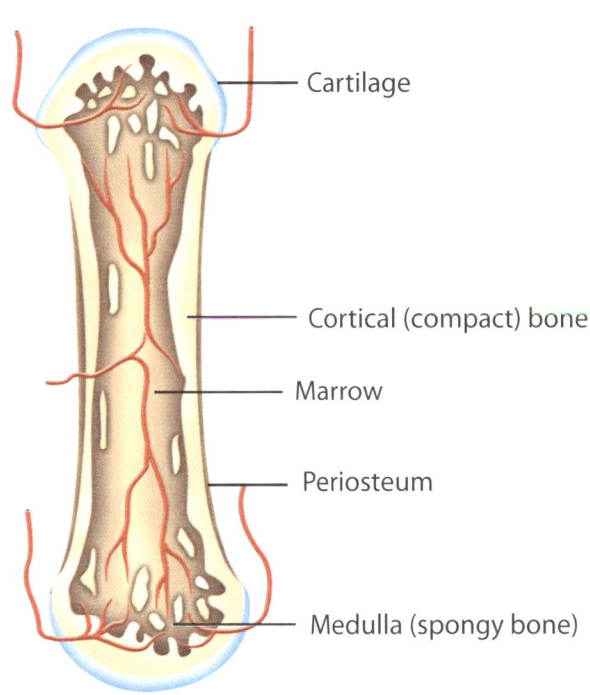

Figure IV.A.5.7
Schematic drawing of adult bone structure.

Bones are supplied by a loop of blood vessels that enter from the periosteal region, penetrate the cortical bone, and enter the medulla before returning to the periphery of the bone. Long bones are specifically supplied by arteries which pass to the marrow through diaphyseal, metaphyseal and epiphyseal arteries (for bone structure, see BIO 11.3.1).

Bone undergoes extensive remodelling, and harvesian systems may break down or be resorbed in order that calcium can be made available to other parts of the body. Bone resorption occurs by osteocytes engaging in osteolysis or by osteoclastic activity.

GOLD NOTES

GOLD NOTES

NERVOUS AND ENDOCRINE SYSTEMS
Chapter 6

Memorize	Understand	Not Required*
nervous system: basic structure, major actions basic sensory reception and processing define: endocrine gland, hormone	* Organization of the nervous system; sensor and effector neurons * Feedback loop, reflex arc: role of spinal cord, brain * Endocrine system: specific chemical control at cell, tissue, and organ level * Cellular mechanisms of hormone action, transport of hormones * Integration with nervous system: feedback control	* Advanced level college info * Memorizing all cranial nerves * Details regarding ear, eye: structure and function * Details regarding endocrine glands: names

GAMSAT-Prep.com

Introduction

The nervous and endocrine systems are composed of a network of highly specialized cells that can communicate information about an organism's surroundings and itself. Thus together, these two systems can process incoming information and then regulate and coordinate responses in other parts of the body.

Additional Resources

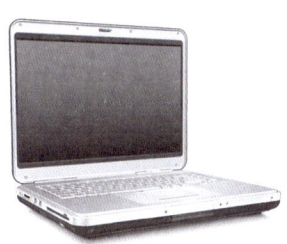

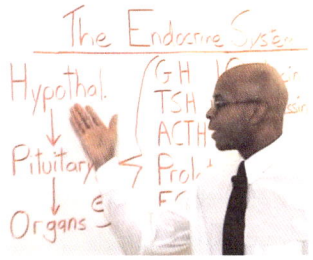

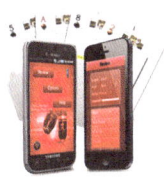

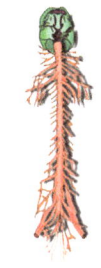

Free Online Q&A + Forum   Video: Online or DVD   Flashcards   Special Guest

THE BIOLOGICAL SCIENCES   BIO-81

* The real GAMSAT may have advanced level information presented (ie. in a passage) but previous knowledge of said information is not required to answer the questions that would follow. Practice ACER and GS practice GAMSATs can help you clarify this point.

6.1 Organisation of the Vertebrate Nervous System

The role of the nervous system is to control and coordinate body activities in a rapid and precise mode of action. The nervous system is composed of central and peripheral nervous systems.

The **central nervous system** (CNS) is enclosed within the cranium (skull) and vertebral (spinal) canal and consists respectively of the brain and spinal cord. The **peripheral nervous system** (PNS) is outside the bony encasement and is composed of peripheral nerves, which are branches or continuations of the spinal or cranial nerves. The PNS can be divided into the **somatic nervous system** and the **autonomic nervous system** which are *anatomically* a portion of both the central and peripheral nervous systems.

The somatic nervous system contains sensory fibers that bring information back to the CNS and motor fibers that innervate skeletal muscles. The autonomic nervous system (ANS) contains motor fibers that innervate smooth muscle, cardiac muscle and glands. The ANS is then divided into *sympathetic* and *parasympathetic* divisions, which generally act against each other. The sympathetic division acts to prepare the body for an emergency situation (fight or flight) while the parasympathetic division acts to conserve energy and restore the body to resting level (rest and digest).

As a rule, a collection of nerve cell bodies in the CNS is called a *nucleus* and outside the CNS it is called a *ganglion*. Neurons that carry information from the environment to the brain or spinal cord are called *afferent neurons*. Neurons that carry motor commands from the brain or spinal cord to the different parts of body are called *efferent neurons*. Neurons that connect sensory and motor neurons in neural pathways are called *interneurons*.

The spinal cord is a long cylindrical structure whose hollow core is called the *central canal*. The central canal is surrounded by a gray matter which is in turn surrounded by a white matter (the reverse is true for the brain: outer gray matter and inner white matter). Basically, the gray matter consists of the cell bodies of neurons whereas the white matter consists of the nerve fibers (axons and dendrites). There are 31 pairs of spinal nerves each leaving the spinal cord at various levels: 8 cervical (neck), 12 thoracic (chest), 5 lumbar (abdomen), 5 sacral and 1 coccygeal (these latter 6 are from the pelvic region). The lower end of the spinal cord is cone shaped and is called the *conus medullaris*.

The brain can be divided into three main regions: the forebrain which contains the telencephalon and the diencephalon; the midbrain; and the hindbrain which contains the cerebellum, the pons and the medulla. The **brain stem** includes the latter two structures and the midbrain.

The telencephalon is the **cerebral hemispheres** (cerebrum) which contain an outer surface (cortex) of gray matter. Its function is in higher order processes (i.e. learning, memory, emotions, voluntary motor activity, processing sensory input, etc.). For

BIOLOGY

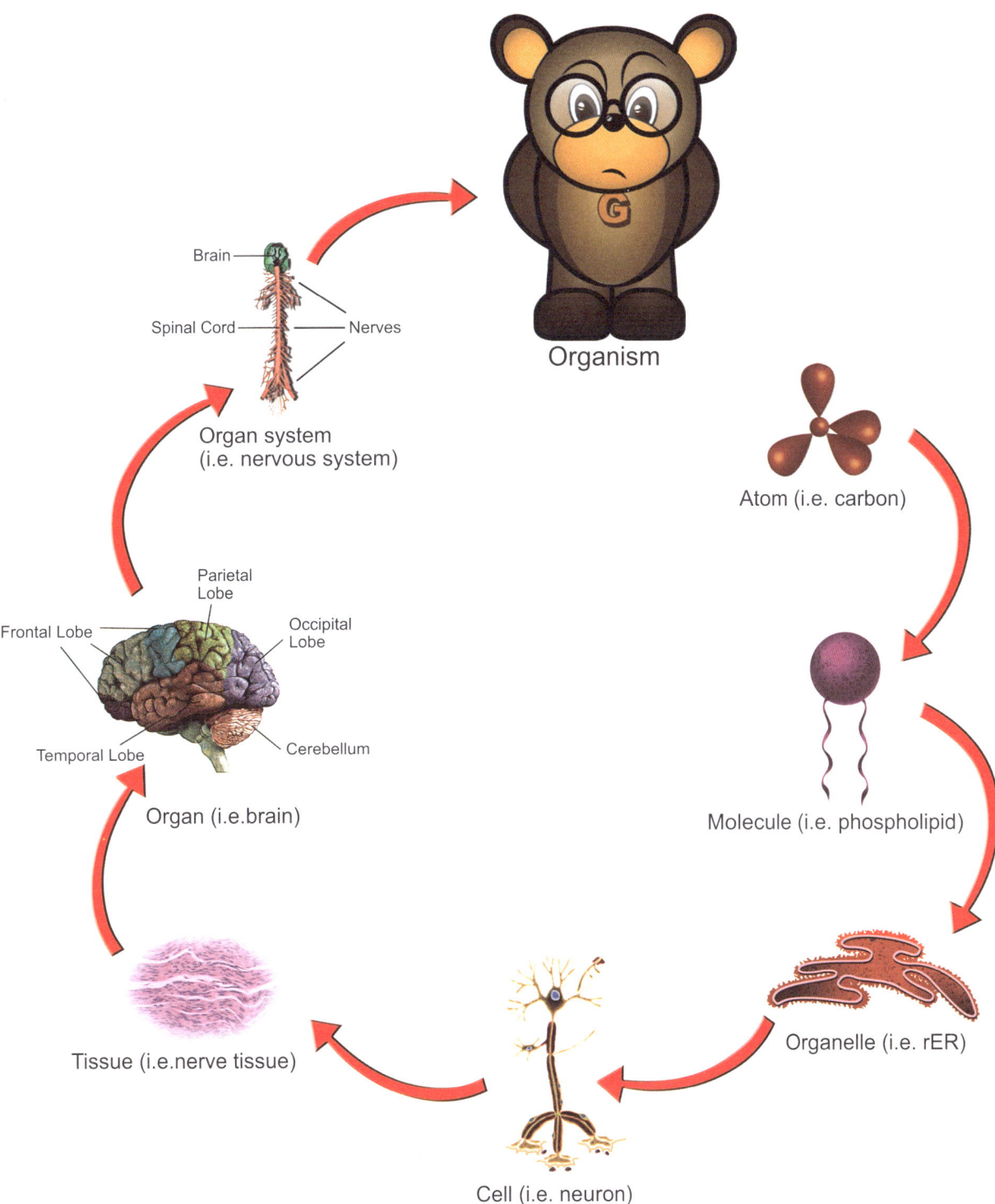

Figure IV.A.6.0: Levels of organization.

most people, the left hemisphere specializes in language, while the right hemisphere specializes in patterns and spatial relationships.

Each hemisphere is subdivided into four lobes: *occipital* which receives input from the optic nerve for vision; *temporal* which receives auditory signals for hearing; *parietal* which receives somatosensory information from the opposite side of the body (= heat, cold, touch, pain, and the sense of body movement); and *frontal* which is involved in problem solving and controls voluntary movements for the opposite side of the body.

The diencephalon contains the **thalamus** which is a relay center for sensory input, and the **hypothalamus** which is crucial for homeostatic controls (heart rate, body temperature, thirst, sex drive, hunger, etc.). Protruding from its base and greatly influenced by the hypothalamus is the **pituitary** which is an endocrine gland. The limbic system, which functions to produce emotions, is composed of the diencephalon and deep structures of the cerebrum (esp. basal ganglia).

The midbrain is a relay center for visual and auditory input and also regulated motor function.

The hindbrain consists of the cerebellum, the pons and the medulla. The cerebellum plays an important role in coordination and the control of muscle tone. The pons acts as a relay center between the cerebral cortex and the cerebellum. The medulla controls many vital functions such as breathing, heart rate, arteriole blood pressure, etc.

There are 12 pairs of cranial nerves which emerge from the base of the brain (esp. the brain stem): *olfactory* (I) for smell; *optic* (II) for vision; *oculomotor* (III), *trochlear* (IV) and *abducens* (VI) for eye movements; *trigeminal* (V) for motor (i.e. *mastication* which is chewing) and sensory activities (i.e. pain, temperature, and pressure for the head and face); *facial* (VII) for taste (sensory) and facial expression (motor); *vestibulo-cochlear* (VIII) for the senses of equilibrium (vestibular branch) and hearing (cochlear branch); *glosso-pharyngeal* (IX) for taste and swallowing; *vagus* (X) for speech, swallowing, slowing the heart rate, and many sensory and motor innervations to smooth muscles of the viscera (internal organs) of the thorax and abdomen; *accessory* (XI) for head rotation and shoulder movement; and *hypoglossal* (XII) for tongue movement.

Both the brain and the spinal cord are surrounded by three membranes (= meninges). The outermost covering is called the dura mater, the innermost is called the pia mater (which is in direct contact with nervous tissue), while the middle layer is called the arachnoid mater. {DAP = **d**ura - **a**rachnoid - **p**ia, repectively, from out to in}.

6.1.1 The Sensory Receptors

The sensory receptors include any type of nerve ending in the body that can be stimulated by some physical or chemical stimulus either outside or within the body. These receptors include the rods and cones of the eye, the cochlear nerve endings of the ear, the taste endings of the mouth, the olfactory endings in the nose, sensory nerve endings in the skin, etc. Afferent neurons carry sense signals to the central nervous system.

6.1.2 The Effector Receptors

These include every organ that can be stimulated by nerve impulses. An important effector system is skeletal muscle. Smooth muscles of the body and the glandular cells are among the important effector organs. Efferent neurons carry motor signals from the CNS to effector receptors. {The term "effector" in biology refers to an organ, cell or molecule that *acts* in response to a stimulus (cause-effect).}

6.1.3 Reflex Arc

One basic means by which the nervous system controls the functions in the body is the reflex arc, in which a stimulus excites a receptor, appropriate impulses are transmitted into the CNS where various nervous reactions take place, and then appropriate effector impulses are transmitted to an effector organ to cause a reflex effect (i.e. removal of one's hand from a hot object, the knee-jerk reflex, etc.). The preceding can be processed at the level of the spinal cord.

Example of knee-jerk reflex: tapping on the patellar tendon causes the thigh muscle (quadriceps) to stretch. The stretching of muscle stimulates the afferent fibers, which synapse on the motoneuron (= motor neuron; BIO 5.1) in the spinal cord. The activation of the motoneuron causes contraction of the muscle that was stretched. This contraction makes the lower leg extend.

GAMSAT-Prep.com
THE GOLD STANDARD

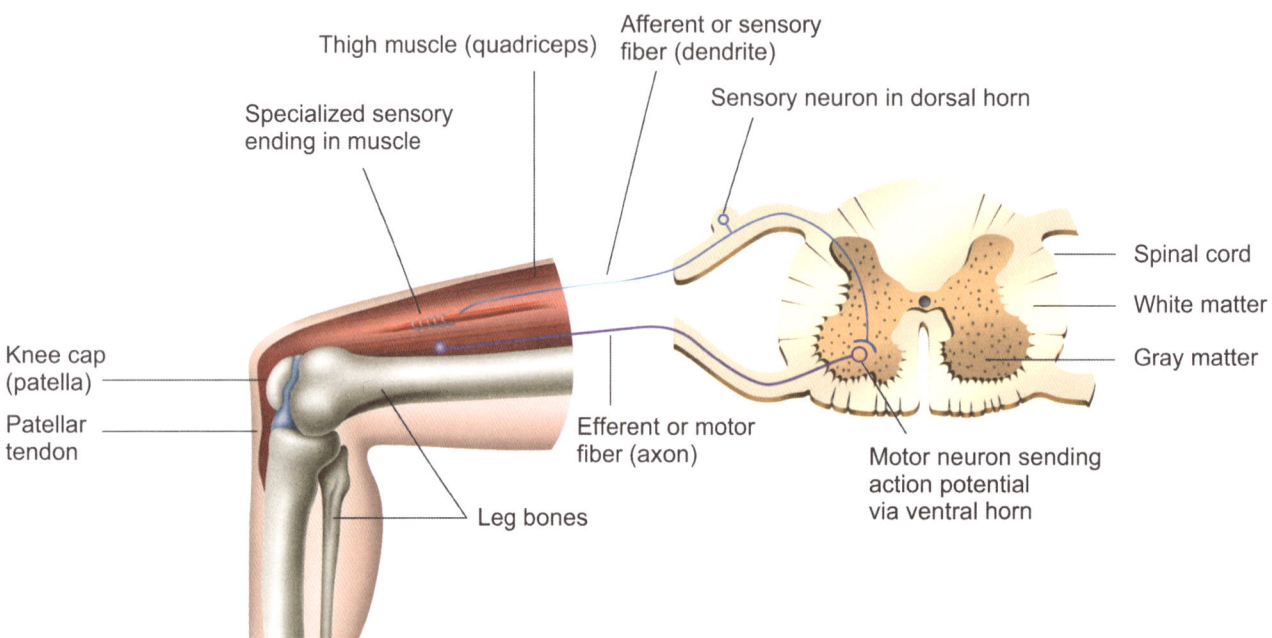

Figure IV.A.6.1: Schematic representation of the basis of the knee jerk reflex.

6.1.4 Autonomic Nervous System

While the Somatic Nervous System controls voluntary activities (i.e. innervates skeletal muscle), the Autonomic Nervous System (ANS) controls involuntary activities. The ANS consists of two components which often antagonize each other: the sympathetic and parasympathetic nervous systems.

The **Sympathetic Nervous System** originates in neurons located in the lateral horns of the gray matter of the spinal cord. Nerve fibers pass by way of anterior (ventral) nerve roots first into the spinal nerves and then immediately into the sympathetic chain. From here fiber pathways are transmitted to all portions of the body, especially to the different visceral organs and to the blood vessels.

The sympathetic nervous system uses norepinephrine as its primary neurotransmitter. This division of the nervous system is crucial in the "fight, fright or flight" responses (i.e. pupillary dilation, increase in breathing, blood pressure and heart rate, increase of blood flow to skeletal muscle, decrease of visceral function, etc.).

Parasympathetic Nervous System: The parasympathetic fibers pass mainly through the *vagus nerves*, though a few fibers pass through several of the other cranial nerves

BIO-86 NERVOUS AND ENDOCRINE SYSTEMS

and through the anterior roots of the sacral segments of the spinal cord. Parasympathetic fibers do not spread as extensively through the body as do sympathetic fibers, but they do innervate some of the thoracic and abdominal organs, as well as the pupillary sphincter and ciliary muscles of the eye and the salivary glands.

The parasympathetic nervous system uses acetylcholine as its primary neurotransmitter. This division of the nervous system is crucial for vegetative responses (i.e. pupillary constriction, decrease in breathing, blood pressure and heart rate, increase in blood flow to the gastro-intestinal tract, etc.).

6.1.5 Autonomic Nerve Fibers

The nerve fibers from the ANS are primarily motor fibers. Unlike the motor pathways of the somatic nervous system, which usually include a single neuron between the CNS and an effector, those of the ANS involve *two* neurons. The first neuron has its cell body in the brain or spinal cord but its axon (= *preganglionic fiber*) extends outside of the CNS. The axon enters adjacent sympathetic chain ganglia, where they synapse with the cell body of a second neuron or travel up or down the chain to synapse with that of a remote second neuron (*recall: a ganglion is a collection of nerve cell bodies outside the CNS*). The axon of the second neuron (= *postganglionic fiber*) extends to a visceral effector.

The sympathetic ganglia form chains which, for example, may extend longitudinally along each side of the vertebral column. Conversely, the parasympathetic ganglia are located *near* or *within* various visceral organs (i.e. bladder, intestine, etc.) thus requiring relatively short postganglionic fibers. Therefore, sympathetic nerve fibers are characterized by short preganglionic fibers and long postganglionic fibers while parasympathetic nerve fibers are characterized by long preganglionic fibers and short postganglionic fibers.

Both divisions of the ANS secrete *acetylcholine* from their preganglionic fibers. Most sympathetic postganglionic fibers secrete *norepinephrine* (= nor*adren*alin), and for this reason they are called **adren**ergic fibers. The parasympathetic postganglionic fibers secrete acetyl**choline** and are called **cholinergic** *fibers*.

There are two types of acetylcholine receptors (AChR) that bind acetylcholine and transmit its signal: muscarinic AChRs and nicotinic AChRs, which are named after the agonists muscarine and nicotine, respectively. The two receptors are functionally different, the muscarinic type is a G-protein coupled receptor that mediates a slow metabolic response via second messenger cascades (involving cAMP), while the nicotinic type is a ligand-gated ionotropic channel that mediates a fast synaptic transmission of the neurotransmitter (no use of second messengers).

6.2 Sensory Reception and Processing

Each modality of sensation is detected by a particular nerve ending. The most common nerve ending is the free nerve ending. Different types of free nerve endings result in different types of sensations such as pain, warmth, pressure, touch, etc. In addition to free nerve endings, skin contains a number of specialized endings that are adapted to respond to some specific type of physical stimulus.

Sensory endings deep in the body are capable of detecting proprioceptive sensations such as joint receptors, which detect the degree of angulation of a joint, Golgi tendon organs which detect the degree of tension in the tendons, and muscle spindles which detect the degree of stretch of a muscle fiber (see diagram of reflex with muscle spindle in BIO 6.1.2).

6.2.1 Olfaction

Olfaction (the sense of smell) is perceived by the brain following the stimulation of the olfactory epithelium located in the nostrils. The olfactory epithelium contain large numbers of neurons with chemoreceptors called olfactory cells which are responsible for the detection of different types of smell. Odorant molecules bind to the receptors located on the cilia of olfactory receptor neurons and produce a depolarizing receptor potential. Once the depolarization passes threshold, an action potential is generated and is conducted into CNS. It is believed that there might be seven or more primary sensations of smell which combine to give various types of smell that we perceive in life.

6.2.2 Taste

Taste buds in combination with olfaction give humans the taste sensation. Taste buds are primarily located on the surface of the tongue with smaller numbers found in the roof of the mouth and the walls of the pharynx (throat). Taste buds contain chemoreceptors which are activated once the chemical is dissolved in saliva which is secreted by the salivary glands. Contrary to olfactory receptor cells, taste receptors are not true neurons: they are chemical receptors only.

Four different types of taste buds are known to exist, each of these responding principally to saltiness, sweetness, sourness and bitterness.

When a stimulus is received by either a taste bud or an olfactory cell for the second time, the intensity of the response is diminished. This is called sensory *adaptation*.

BIOLOGY

6.2.3 Ears: Structure and Function

Ears function in both hearing and balance. It consists of three parts: the *external ear* which receives sound waves; the air-filled *middle ear* which transmits and amplifies sound waves; and the fluid-filled *inner ear* which transduces sound waves into nerve impulse. The vestibular organ, located in the inner ear, is responsible for equilibrium.

The external ear is composed of the external cartilaginous portion, the pinna or *auricle*, and the external auditory meatus or canal. The external auditory meatus connects the auricle and the middle ear or *tympanic cavity*. The tympanic cavity is bordered on the outside by the tympanic membrane, and inside the air-filled cavity are the auditory ossicles - the *malleus* (hammer), *incus* (anvil), and *stapes* (stirrup). The stapes is held by ligaments to a part of inner ear called the *oval window*. The auditory ossicles function in amplifying the sound vibration and transmitting it from the tympanic membrane to the oval window.

The inner ear or *labyrinth* consists of an osseous (= bony) labyrinth containing a membranous labyrinth. The bony labyrinth houses the semicircular canals, the cochlea and the vestibule. The semicircular canals contain the semicircular ducts of the membranous labyrinth, which can detect angular acceleration. The vestibule contains the saccule and utricle, which are sac-like thin connective tissue lined by vestibular hair cells which are responsible for the detection of linear acceleration. Together, the semicircular canals and the vestibule, known as the vestibular system,

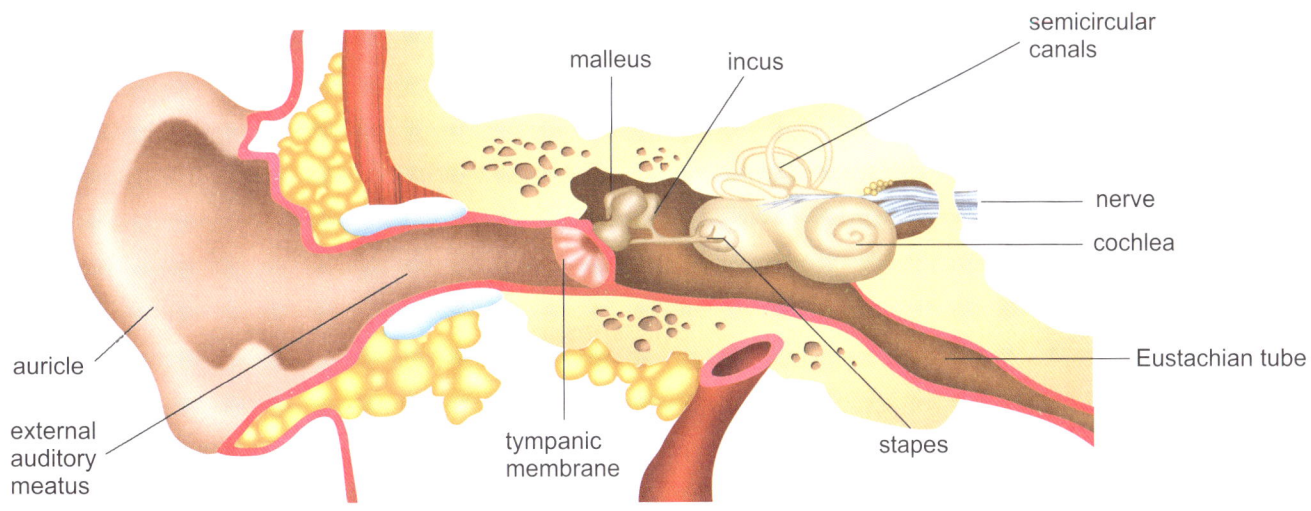

Figure IV.A.6.2: Structure of the external, middle and inner ear.

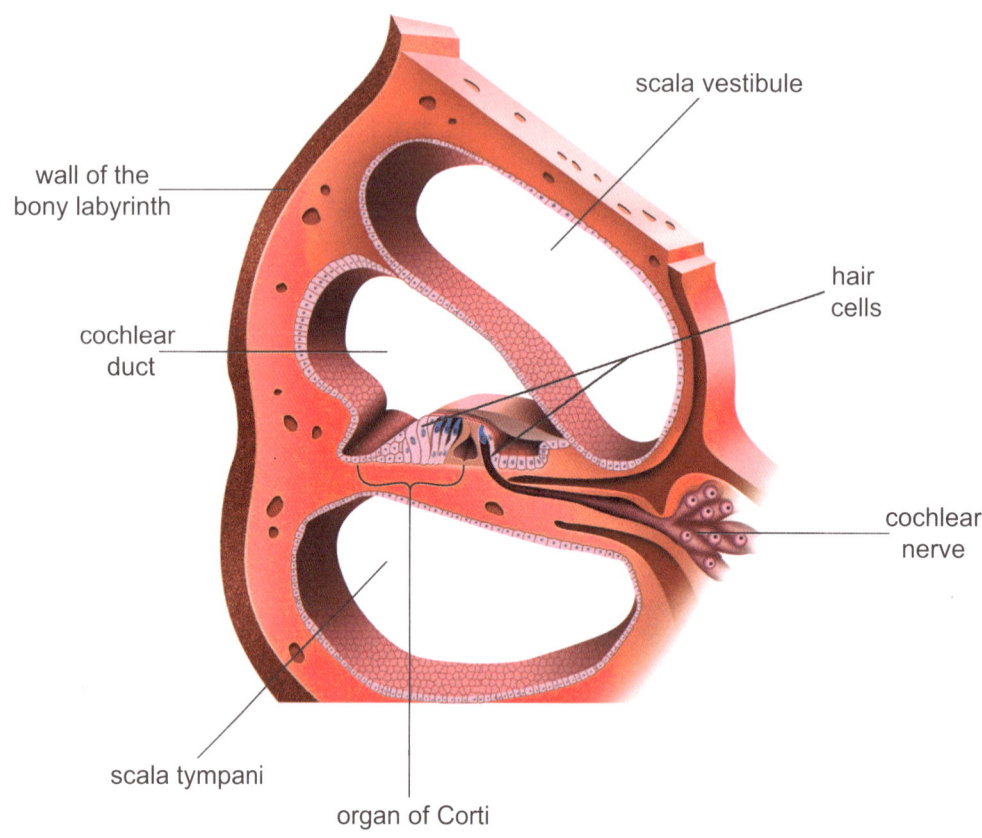

Figure IV.A.6.3: Cross-section of the cochlea.

are responsible for detection of linear and angular acceleration of the head. The cochlea is divided into three spaces: the scala vestibule, scala tympani and the scala media, or cochlear duct. The cochlear duct contains the spiral organ of Corti, which functions in the reception of sound and responds to different sound frequencies.

The eustachian tube connects the middle ear to the pharynx. This tube is important in maintaining equal pressure on both sides of the tympanic membrane. During ascent in an airplane, there is a decrease in cabin air pressure, leading to a relative increase in the pressure of the middle ear. Swallowing or yawning opens the eustachian tube allowing an equalization of pressure in the middle ear.

Mechanism of hearing: Sound is caused by the compression of waves that travel through the air. Each compression wave is funneled by the external ear to strike the tympanic membrane (ear drum). Thus the sound vibrations are transmitted through the osseous system which consists of three tiny bones (the malleus, incus, and stapes) into the cochlea at the oval window. Movement of the stapes at the oval window causes disturbance in the lymph of cochlea and stimulates the hair cells found in the basilar membrane which is called the *organ of Corti*. Bending of the hair cells causes depolarization of the basilar membrane. From here the auditory nerves carry the impulses to the auditory area of the brain (*temporal lobe*) where it is interpreted as sound.

6.2.4 Vision: Eye Structure and Function

The eyeball consists of three layers: i) an outer fibrous tunic composed of the sclera and cornea; ii) a vascular coat (uvea) of choroid, the ciliary body and iris; and iii) the retina formed of pigment and sensory (nervous) layers. The anterior chamber lies between the cornea anteriorly (in front) and the iris and pupil posteriorly (behind); the posterior chamber lies between the iris anteriorly and the ciliary processes and the lens posteriorly.

The transparent cornea constitutes the anterior one sixth of the eye and receives light from external environment. The sclera forms

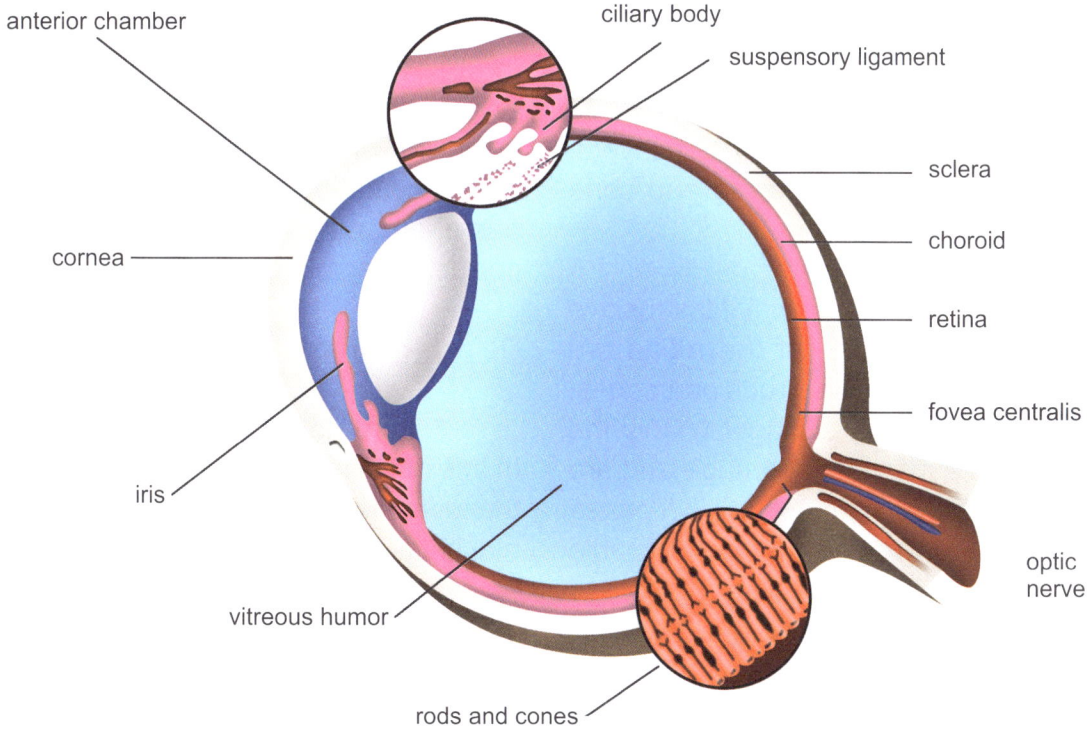

Figure IV.A.6.4: Structure of the eye.

the posterior five sixths of the fibrous tunic and is composed of dense fibrous connective tissue. The choroid layer consists of vascular loose connective tissue. The ciliary body is an anterior expansion of the choroid that encircles the lens. The lens can focus light on the retina by the contraction or relaxation of muscles in the ciliary body which transmit tension along suspensory ligaments to the lens.

Contraction of the ciliary muscle makes the lens become more convex, thereby allowing the eye to focus on nearby objects. Relaxation of the ciliary muscle allows the eye to focus on far objects. The iris separates the anterior and the posterior chamber and forms an aperture called the "pupil" whose diameter is continually adjusted by the pupillary muscles. This helps to control the intensity of light impinging on the retina.

The retina is divisible into ten layers. Layers two to five contain the rod and cone receptors of the light pathway.

Rods and Cones: The light sensitive receptors (*photoreceptors*) of the retina are millions of minute cells called rods and cones. The rods (*"night vision"*) distinguish only the black and white aspects of an image and are sensitive to light of low intensity (*"high sensitivity"*). The cones (*"day vision"*) are capable of distinguishing three colors: red, green and blue and are sensitive to light of high intensity (*"low sensitivity"*). From different combinations of these three colors, all colors can be seen.

Photoreceptors contain photosensitive pigments. For example, rods contain the membrane protein *rhodopsin* which is covalently linked to a form of vitamin A. Light causes an isomerization of *retinal* (an aldehyde form of vitamin A) which can affect Na^+ channels in a manner as to start an action potential.

The central portion of the retina which is called the fovea centralis has only cones, which allows this portion to have very sharp vision, while the peripheral areas, which contain progressively more and more rods, have progressively more diffuse vision. Since acuity and color vision are mediated by the same cells (cones), visual acuity is much better in bright light than dim light.

Each point of the retina connects with a discrete point in the visual cortex which is in the back of the brain (i.e. the occipital lobe). The image that is formed on the retina is upside down and reversed from left to right. This information leaves the eye via the optic nerve en route to the visual cortex which corrects the image.

Defects of vision

1. Myopia (short-sighted or nearsighted): In this condition, an image is formed in front of the retina because the lens converges light too much since the eyeballs are long. A diverging (concave) lens helps focus the image on the retina and it is used for the correction of myopia.

2. Hyperopia (long-sighted or farsighted): In this condition, an image is formed behind the retina since the eyeballs are too short. A converging (convex) lens helps focus the image on the retina.

3. Astigmatism: In this condition, the curvatures of either the cornea or the lens are different at different angles. A cylindrical lens helps to improve this condition.

4. Presbyopia: This condition is characterized by the inability to focus (especially objects which are closer). This condition, which is often seen in the elderly, is corrected by using a converging lens.

6.3 Endocrine Systems

The endocrine system is the set of glands, tissues and cells that secrete hormones directly into circulatory system (ductless). The hormones are transported by the blood system, sometimes bound to plasma proteins, en route to having an effect on the cells of a target organ. Thus hormones control many of the body's functions by acting - predominantly - in one of the following major ways:

1. By controlling transport of substances through cell membranes

2. By controlling the activity of some of the specific genes, which in turn determine the formation of specific enzymes

3. By controlling directly some metabolic systems of cells.

Steroid hormones can diffuse across the plasma membrane and bind to specific receptors in the cytosol or nucleus, thus forming a direct intracellular effect (i.e. on DNA; ORG 12.4.1). Non-steroid hormones do not diffuse across the membrane. They tend to bind plasma membrane receptors, which leads to the production of a second messenger.

Secondary messengers are a component of signal transduction cascades which amplify the strength of a signal (i.e. hormone, growth factors, neurotransmitter, etc.). Examples include cyclic AMP (cAMP), phosphoinositol, cyclic GMP and arachidonic acid systems.

In all four cases, a hormone (= the primary messenger or *agonist*) binds the receptor exposing a binding site for a G-protein (the *transducer*). The G-protein, named for its ability to exchange GDP on its alpha subunit for a GTP (BIO 4.4-4.10), is bound to the inner membrane. Once the exchange for GTP takes place, the alpha subunit of the G-protein transducer breaks free from the beta and gamma subunits, all parts remaining membrane-bound. The alpha subunit is now free to move along the inner membrane and eventually contacts another membrane-bound protein - the *primary effector*.

The primary effector has an action which creates a signal that can diffuse within the cell. This signal is the *secondary messenger*.

Calcium ions are important intracellular messengers which can regulate calmodulin and are responsible for many important physiological functions, such as in muscle contraction (BIO 5.2). The enzyme phospholipase C (primary effector) produces diacylglycerol and inositol trisphosphate (secondary messenger), which increases calcium ion (secondary effector) membrane permeability. Active G-protein can also open calcium channels. The other product of phospholipase C, diacylglycerol (secondary messenger), activates protein kinase C (secondary effector), which assists in the activation of cAMP (another second messenger).

The agonist epinephrine (hormone, BIO 6.1.3) can bind a receptor activating the transducer (G-protein) and using a primary effector (adenylyl cyclase) produces a secondary messenger (cAMP) which, in turn, brings about target cell responses that are recognized as the hormone's actions.

Of the following hormones, if there is no mention as to its chemical nature, then it is a non-steroidal hormone (i.e. protein, polypeptide, etc.).

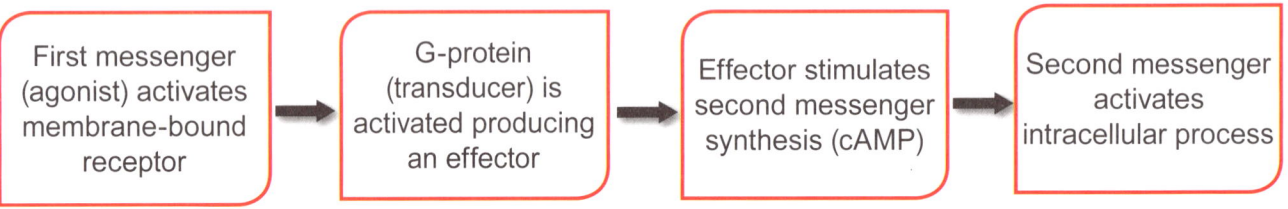

6.3.1 Pituitary Hormones

The **pituitary gland** secretes hormones that regulate a wide variety of functions in the body. This gland is divided into two major divisions: the anterior and the posterior pituitary gland. Six hormones are secreted by the anterior pituitary gland whereas two hormones are secreted by the posterior gland. The **hypothalamus** influences the secretion of hormones from both parts of the pituitary in different ways: i) it secretes specific *releasing factors* into special blood vessels (a *portal system* called hypothalamic-hypophysial portal system) which carries these factors (hormones) that affect the cells in the anterior pituitary by either stimulating or inhibiting the release of anterior pituitary hormones; ii) the hypothalamus contains neurosecretory cell bodies that synthesize, package and transport their products (esp. the two hormones oxytocin and ADH) down the axons directly into the posterior pituitary where they can be released into circulation.

The hormones secreted by the anterior pituitary gland are as follows:

1. Growth hormone (GH)
2. Thyroid Stimulating Hormone (TSH)
3. Adrenocorticotropic hormone (ACTH)
4. Prolactin
5. Follicle Stimulating Hormone (FSH) or Interstitial Cell Stimulating Hormone (ICSH)
6. Luteinizing Hormone (LH)

[N.B. these latter two hormones will be discussed in the section on Reproduction, see BIO 14.2, 14.3]

Growth Hormone causes growth of the body. It causes enlargement and proliferation of cells in all parts of the body. Ultimately, the epiphyses of the long bones unite with the shaft of the bones (BIO 11.3.1). After adolescence, growth hormone continues to be secreted lower than the pre-adolescent rate. Though most of the growth in the body stops at this stage, the metabolic roles of the growth hormone continue such as the enhancement of protein synthesis and lean body mass, increasing blood glucose concentration, increasing lipolysis, etc.

Abnormal increase in the secretion of growth hormone at a young age results in a condition called gigantism, while a reduction in the production of growth hormone leads to dwarfism. Abnormal increase in the secretion of growth hormone in adults results

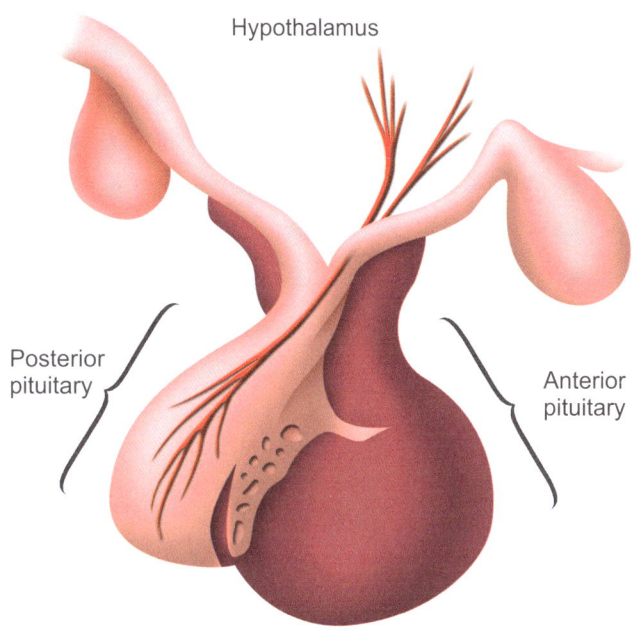

Figure IV.A.6.5: The pituitary gland.

in a condition called acromegaly, a disorder characterized by a disproportionate bone enlargement, especially in the face, hands and feet.

Thyroid Stimulating Hormone stimulates the thyroid gland. The hormones produced by the thyroid gland (*thyroxine:* T_4, *triiodothyronine:* T_3) contain four and three iodine atoms, respectively. They increase the basal metabolic rate of the body (BMR). Therefore, indirectly, TSH increases the overall rate of metabolism of the body.

Adrenocorticotropic hormone strongly stimulates the production of cortisol by the adrenal cortex, and it also stimulates the production of the other adrenocortical hormones, but to a lesser extent.

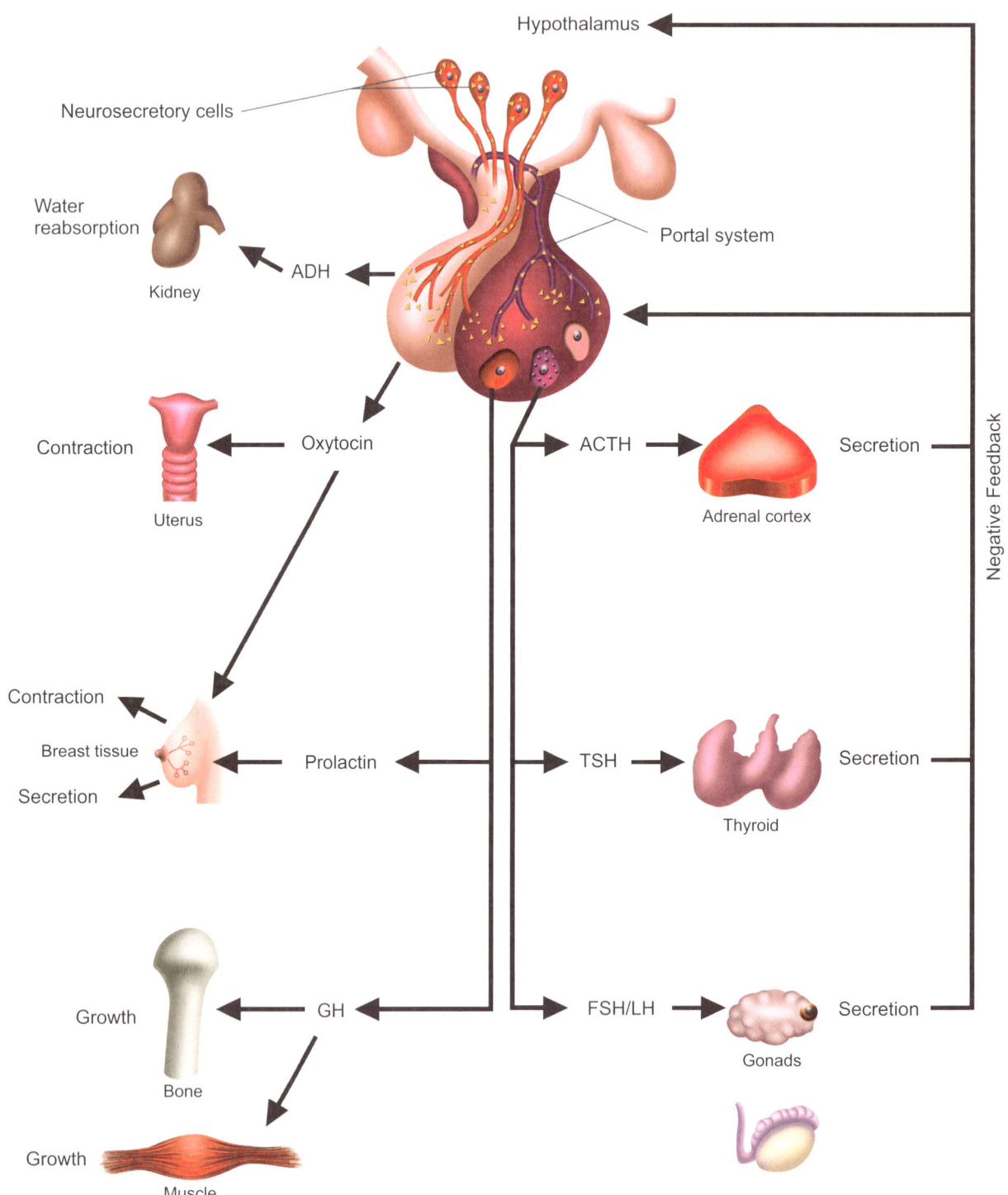

Figure IV.A.6.6: Pituitary hormones and their target organs.

Prolactin plays an important role in the development of the breast during pregnancy and promotes milk production in the breast. In addition, a high level of prolactin can inhibit ovulation.

Antidiuretic hormone (ADH) is synthesized by neurosecretory cells in the hypothalamus and then travels down the axons to the posterior pituitary for secretion. Antidiuretic hormone enhances the rate of water reabsorption from the renal tubules leading to the concentration of urine (BIO 10.3). ADH also constricts the arterioles and causes a rise in arterial pressure and hence it is also called *vasopressin*.

Similar to ADH, *oxytocin* originates in the hypothalamus and then travels down the axons to the posterior pituitary for secretion. Oxytocin causes contraction of the uterus and, to a lesser extent, the other smooth muscles of the body. It also stimulates the myoepithelial cells of the breast in a manner that makes the milk flow into the ducts. This is termed milk ejection or milk *let-down*.

6.3.2 Adrenocortical Hormones

On the top of each kidney lies an adrenal gland which contains an inner region (*medulla*) and an outer region (*cortex*). The adrenal cortex secretes three different types of steroid hormones that are similar chemically but vary widely in a physiological manner.

These are:

1. Mineralocorticoids - e.g., Aldosterone
2. Glucocorticoids - e.g., Cortisol, Cortisone
3. Sex Hormones e.g., Androgens, Estrogens

Mineralocorticoids - Aldosterone

The mineralocorticoids influence the electrolyte balance of the body. Aldosterone is a mineralocorticoid which is secreted and then enhances sodium transport from the renal tubules into the peritubular fluids, and at the same time enhances potassium transport from the peritubular fluids into the tubules. In other words, aldosterone causes conservation of sodium in the body and excretion of potassium in the urine. As a result of sodium retention, there is an increased passive reabsorption of chloride ions and water from the tubules. Overproduction of aldosterone will result in excessive retention of fluid, which leads to hypertension.

Glucocorticoids - Cortisol

Several different glucocorticoids are secreted by the adrenal cortex, but almost all of the glucocorticoid activity is caused by cortisol, also called hydrocortisone. Glucocorticoids affect the metabolism of carbohydrates, proteins and lipids. It causes an increase in the blood concentration of glucose by stimulation of gluconeogenesis (generation of glucose from non-carbohydrate carbon substrates). It causes degradation of proteins and causes increased use of fat for energy. Long term use of glucocorticoids suppresses the immune system. It also has an anti-inflammatory effect by inhibiting the release of inflammatory mediators.

Sex hormones

Androgens (i.e. testosterone) are the masculinizing hormones in the body. They are responsible for the development of the secondary sexual characteristics in a male (i.e. increased body hair). On the contrary estrogens have a feminizing effect in the body and they are responsible for the development of the secondary sexual characteristics in a female (i.e. breast development). The proceeding hormones supplement secretions from the gonads which will be discussed later (see "*Reproduction*"; BIO 14.2, 14.3).

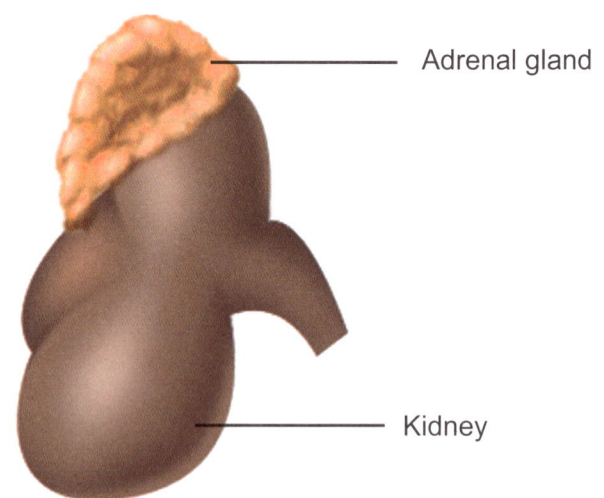

Figure IV.A.6.7: The adrenal gland sits on top of the kidney.

The Adrenal Medulla

The adrenal medulla synthesizes epinephrine (= *adrenaline*) and norepinephrine which: i) are non-steroidal stimulants of the sympathetic nervous system; ii) raise blood glucose concentrations; iii) increase heart rate and blood pressure; iv) increase blood supply to the brain, heart and skeletal muscle; and v) decrease blood supply to the skin, digestive system and renal system.

6.3.3 Thyroid Hormones

The thyroid gland is located anteriorly in the neck and is composed of follicles lined with thyroid glandular cells. These cells secrete a glycoprotein called thyroglobulin. The tyrosine residue of thyroglobulin then reacts with iodine forming mono-iodotyrosine (MIT) and di-iodotyrosine (DIT). When two molecules of DIT combine, thyroxine (T_4) is formed. When one molecule of DIT and one molecule of MIT combine, tri-iodothyronine (T_3) is formed. The rate of synthesis of thyroid hormone is influenced by TSH from the pituitary.

BIOLOGY

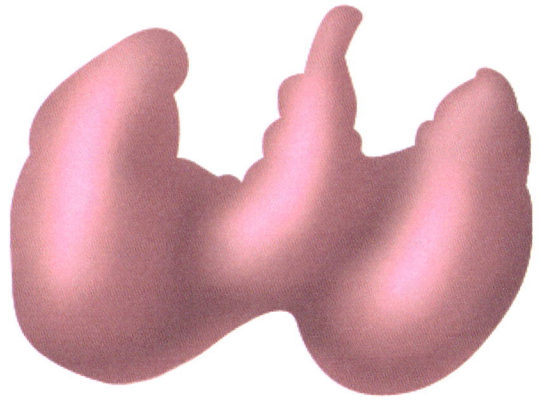

Figure IV.A.6.8: The thyroid gland.

Once thyroid hormones have been released into the blood stream they combine with several different plasma proteins. Then they are released into the cells from the blood stream. They play a vital role in maturation of CNS as thyroid hormone deficiency leads to irreversible mental retardation. They increase heart rate, ventilation rate and O_2 consumption. They also increase the size and numbers of mitochondria and these in turn increase the rate of production of ATP, which is a factor that promotes cellular metabolism; glycogenolysis and gluconeogenesis both increase; lipolysis increases; and protein synthesis also increases. The overall effect of thyroid hormone on metabolism is catabolic.

Hyperthyroidism is an excess of thyroid hormone secretion above that needed for normal function. Basically, an increased rate of metabolism throughout the body is observed. Other symptoms include fast heart rate and respiratory rate, weight loss, sweating, tremor, and protruding eyes.

Hypothyroidism is an inadequate amount of thyroid hormone secreted into the blood stream. Generally it slows down the metabolic rate and enhances the collection of mucinous fluid in the tissue spaces, creating an edematous (fluid filled) state called myxedema. Other symptoms include slowed heart rate and respiratory rate, weight gain, cold intolerance, fatigue, and mental slowness.

The thyroid and parathyroid glands affect blood calcium concentration in different ways. The thyroid produces *calcitonin* which inhibits osteoclast activity and stimulates osteoblasts to form bone tissue; thus blood $[Ca^{2+}]$ decreases. The parathyroid glands produce parathormone (= parathyroid hormone = PTH), which stimulates osteoclasts to break down bone, thus raising $[Ca^{2+}]$ and $[PO_4^{3-}]$ in the blood (BIO 5.4.4).

6.3.4 Pancreatic Hormones

The pancreas contains clusters of cells (= *islets of Langerhans*) closely associated with blood vessels. The islets of Langerhans, which perform the endocrine function of the pancreas, contain alpha cells that secrete *glucagon* and beta cells that secrete *insulin*. Glucagon increases blood glucose concentration by promoting the following events in the liver: the conversion of glycogen to glucose (*glycogenolysis*) and the production of glucose from amino acids (*gluconeogenesis*). Insulin decreases blood glucose by increasing cellular uptake of glucose, promoting glycogen formation and decreasing gluconeogenesis. A deficiency in insulin or insensitivity to insulin results in *diabetes mellitus*.

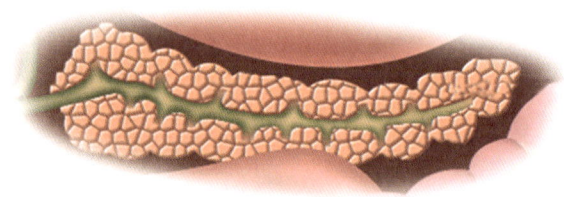

Figure IV.A.6.9: The pancreas.

6.3.5 Kidney Hormones

The kidney produces and secretes *renin*, *erythropoietin* and it helps in the activation of vitamin D. Renin is an enzyme that catalyzes the conversion of angiotensinogen to angiotensin I. Angiotensin I is then converted to angiotensin II by angiotensin-converting enzyme (ACE). Angiotensin II acts on the adrenal cortex to increase the synthesis and release of aldosterone, which increases Na^+ reabsorption, and causes vasoconstriction of arterioles leading to an increase in both blood volume and blood pressure. Erythropoietin increases the production of *erythrocytes* by acting on red bone marrow.

Vitamin D is a steroid which is critical for the proper absorption of calcium from the small intestine; thus it is essential for the normal growth and development of bone and teeth. Vitamin D can either be ingested or produced from a precursor by the activity of ultraviolet light on skin cells. It must be further activated in the liver and kidney by hydroxylation.

6.3.6 A Negative Feedback Loop

In order to maintain the internal environment of the body in equilibrium (= *homeostasis*), our hormones engage in various negative feedback loops. Negative feedback is self-limiting: a hormone produces biologic actions that, in turn, directly or indirectly inhibit further secretion of that hormone.

For example, if the body is exposed to extreme cold, the hypothalamus will activate systems to conserve heat (see *Skin as an Organ System*, BIO 13.1) and to produce heat. Heat production can be attained by increasing the basal metabolic rate. To achieve this, the hypothalamus secretes a releasing factor (thyrotropin releasing factor - TRF) which stimulates the anterior pituitary to secrete TSH. Thus the thyroid gland is stimulated to secrete the thyroid hormones.

Body temperature begins to return to normal. The high levels of circulating thyroid hormones begin to *inhibit* the production of TRF and TSH (= *negative feedback*) which in turn ensures the reduction in the levels of the thyroid hormones. Thus homeostasis is maintained.

6.3.7 A Positive Feedback Loop

As opposed to negative feedback, a positive feedback loop is where the body senses a change and activates mechanisms that accelerate or increase that change. Occasionally this may help homeostasis by working in conjunction with a larger negative feedback loop, but unfortunately it often produces the opposite effect and can be life-threatening.

An example of a beneficial positive feedback loop is seen in childbirth, where stretching of the uterus triggers the secretion of oxytocin (BIO 6.3.1), which stimulates uterine contractions and speeds up labor. Of course, once the baby is out of the mother's body, the loop is broken.

Often, however, positive feedback produces the very opposite of homeostasis: a rapid loss of internal stability with potentially fatal consequences. For example, most human deaths from SARS and the bird flu (H5N1) epidemic were caused by a "cytokine storm" which is a positive feedback loop between immune cells and cytokines (signalling molecules similar to hormones). Thus, in many cases, it is the body's exaggerated response to infection that is the cause of death rather than the direct action of the original infecting agent. Many diseases involve dangerous positive feedback loops.

Go online to GAMSAT-prep.com for additional chapter review Q&A and forum.

GOLD NOTES

THE CIRCULATORY SYSTEM
Chapter 7

Memorize
* c. and lymphatic systems: basic
  uctures and functions
* nposition of blood, lymph, purpose of
  ph nodes
* C production and destruction; spleen,
  e marrow

Understand
* Circ: structure/function; 4 chambered heart: systolic/diastolic pressure
* Oxygen transport; hemoglobin, oxygen content/affinity
* Substances transported by blood, lymph
* Source of lymph: diffusion from capillaries by differential pressure

Not Required*
* Advanced level college info
* Memorizing names of small to medium arteries, veins
* Memorizing Starling's equation

GAMSAT-Prep.com

Introduction

The circulatory system is concerned with the movement of nutrients, gases and wastes to and from cells. The circulatory or cardiovascular system (closed) distributes blood while the lymphatic system (open) distributes lymph.

Additional Resources

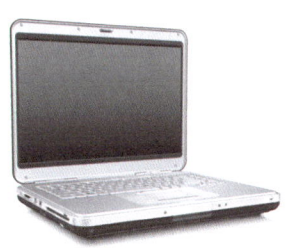
Free Online Q&A + Forum

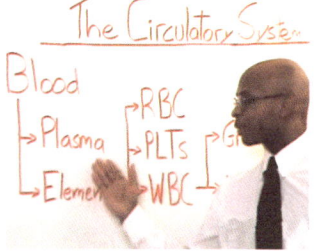
Video: Online or DVD

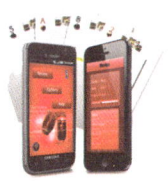
Flashcards

Special Guest

THE BIOLOGICAL SCIENCES   BIO-103

* The real GAMSAT may have advanced level information presented (ie. in a passage) but previous knowledge of said information is not required to answer the questions that would follow. Practice ACER and GS practice GAMSATs can help you clarify this point.

GAMSAT-Prep.com
THE GOLD STANDARD

7.1 Generalities

The circulatory system is composed of the heart, blood, and blood vessels. The heart (which acts like a pump) and its blood vessels (which act like a closed system of ducts) are called the *cardiovascular system* which moves the blood throughout the body.

The following represents some important functions of blood within the circulatory system.

* It transports:
  - hormones from endocrine glands to target tissues
  - molecules and cells which are components of the immune system
  - nutrients from the digestive tract (usu. to the liver)
  - oxygen from the respiratory system to body cells
  - waste from the body cells to the respiratory and excretory systems.

* It aids in temperature control (*thermoregulation*) by:
  - distributing heat from skeletal muscle and other active organs to the rest of the body
  - being directed to or away from the skin depending on whether or not the body wants to release or conserve heat, respectively.

7.2 The Heart

The heart is a muscular, cone-shaped organ about the size of a fist. The heart is composed of connective tissue (BIO 5.4) and cardiac muscle (BIO 5.2) which includes a region that generates electrical signals (see BIO 11.2 for SA node). The heart contains four chambers: two thick muscular walled *ventricles* and two thinner walled *atria*. An inner wall or *septum* separates the heart (and therefore the preceding chambers) into left and right sides. The atria contract or *pump* blood more or less simultaneously and so do the ventricles.

Deoxygenated blood returning to the heart from all body tissues except the lungs (= *systemic circulation*) enters the right atrium through large veins (= *venae cavae*). The blood is then pumped into the right ventricle through the tricuspid valve (which is one of many one-way valves in the cardiovascular system). Next the blood is pumped to the lungs (= *pulmonary circulation*) through semi-lunar valves (pulmonary valves) and pulmonary arteries {remember: blood in arteries goes away from the heart}.

The blood loses CO_2 and is **oxygenated** in the lungs and returns through pulmonary veins to the left atrium. Now the blood is pumped through the mitral (= bicuspid) valve into the largest chamber of the heart: the left ventricle. This ventricle's task is to return

BIO-104   THE CIRCULATORY SYSTEM

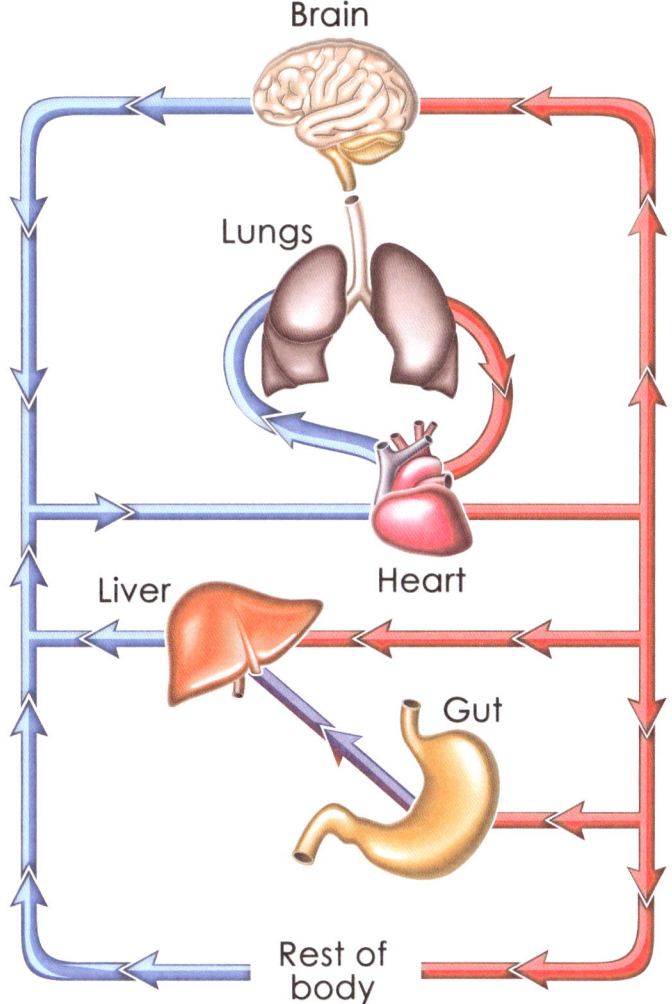

Figure IV.A.7.0: Overview of vascular anatomy.
The vascular anatomy of the human body or for an individual organ is comprised of both in-series and in-parallel vascular components. Blood leaves the heart through the aorta (high in oxygen, red in color) from which it is distributed to major organs by large arteries, each of which originates from the aorta. Therefore, these major distributing arteries are in parallel with each other. Thus the circulations of the head, arms, gastrointestinal systems, kidneys, and legs are all parallel circulations. There are some exceptions, notably the gastrointestinal (gut) and hepatic (liver) circulations, which are partly in series because the venous drainage from the intestines become the hepatic portal vein which supplies most of the blood flow to the liver. Vessels transporting from one capillary bed to another are called portal veins (besides the liver, note the portal system in the anterior pituitary, BIO 6.3.1).

blood into the systemic circulation by pumping into a huge artery: the *aorta* (its valve is the aortic valve).

The mitral (= <u>b</u>icuspid = <u>2</u> leaflets) and tricuspid (<u>tri</u> = <u>3</u> leaflets) valves are prevented from everting into the atria by strong fibrous cords (*chordae tendineae*) which are attached to small mounds of muscle (*papillary muscles*) in their respective ventricles. A major cause of heart murmurs is the inadequate functioning of these valves.

7.3 Blood Vessels

Blood vessels include arteries, arterioles, capillaries, venules and veins. Whereas arteries tend to have thick, smooth muscular walls and contain blood at high pressure, veins have thinner walls and low blood pressure. However, veins contain the highest proportion of blood in the cardiovascular system (about 2/3rds). The wall of a blood vessel is composed of an outer <u>adventitia</u>, an inner <u>intima</u> and a *m*iddle *m*uscle layer, the <u>*m*edia</u>.

Oxygenated blood entering the systemic circulation must get to all the body's tissues. The aorta must divide into smaller and smaller arteries (small artery = **arteriole**) in order to get to the level of the capillary which i) is the smallest blood vessel; ii) often forms branching networks called *capillary beds*; and iii) is the level at which the exchange of wastes and gases (i.e. O_2 and CO_2) occurs by diffusion.

In the next step in circulation, the newly deoxygenated blood enters very small veins (= **venules**) and then into larger and larger veins until the blood enters the venae cavae and then the right atrium. There are two venae cavae: one drains blood from the upper body while the other drains blood from the lower body (*superior* and *inferior* venae cavae, respectively).

Since the walls of veins are thin and somewhat floppy, they are often located in muscles. Thus movement of the leg squeezes the veins, which pushes the blood through 1-way bicuspid valves toward the heart. This is referred to as the *muscle pump*.

<u>Coronary arteries</u> branch off the aorta to supply the heart muscle.

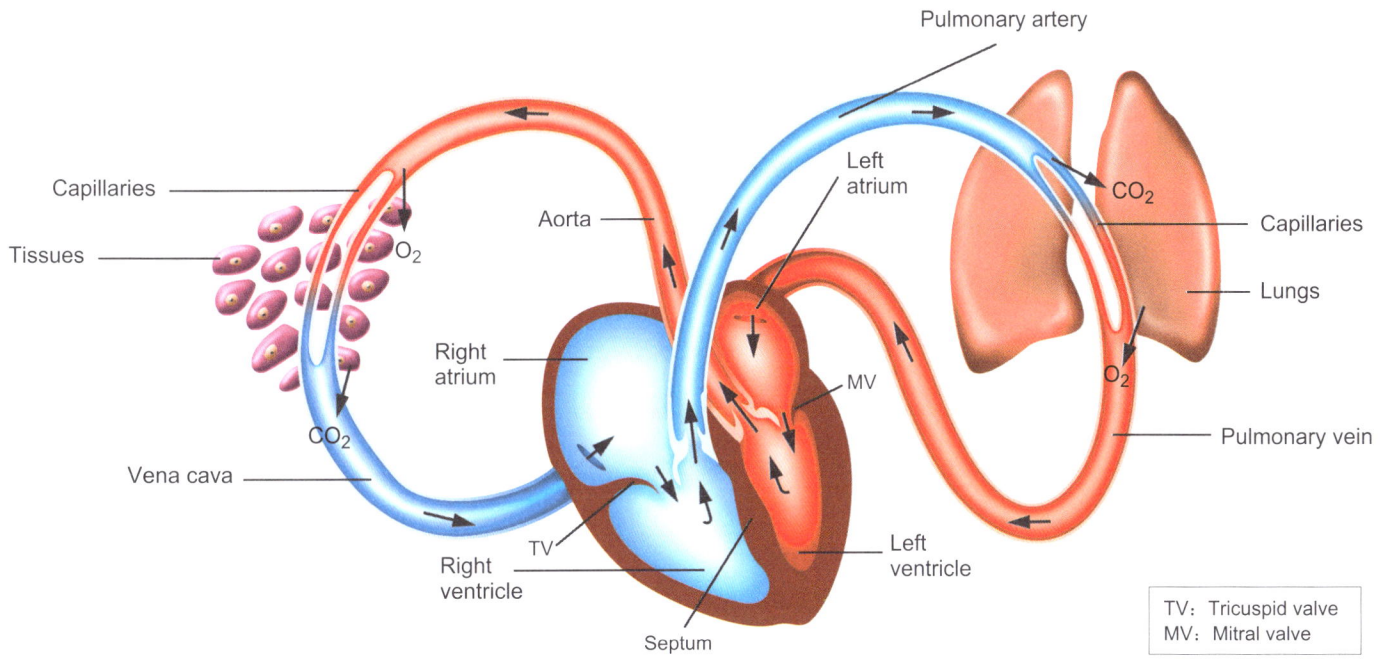

Figure IV.A.7.1: Schematic representation of the circulatory system.
Systemic circulation: transports blood from the left ventricle into the aorta then to all parts of the body and then returns to the right atrium from the superior and inferior venae cavae. *Pulmonary circulation:* transports blood from the right ventricle into pulmonary arteries to the lungs for exchange of oxygen and carbon dioxide and returns blood to the left atrium from pulmonary veins.

7.4 Blood Pressure

Blood pressure is the force exerted by the blood against the inner walls of blood vessels (esp. arteries). Maximum arterial pressure is measured when the ventricle contracts and blood is pumped into the arterial system (= *systolic pressure*). Minimal arterial pressure is measured when the ventricle is relaxed and blood is returned to the heart via veins (= *diastolic pressure*). Pulse pressure is the difference between the systolic pressure and the diastolic pressure. Blood pressure is usually measured in the brachial artery in the arm. A pressure of 120/80 signifies a systolic pressure of 120 mmHg and a diastolic pressure of 80 mmHg. The *pulse pressure* is the difference (i.e. 40 mmHg).

Peripheral resistance is essentially the result of arterioles and capillaries which resist the flow of blood from arteries to veins (the narrower the vessel, the higher the resistance). Arterioles are the site of the highest resistance in the cardiovascular system. An increase in peripheral resistance causes a rise in blood pressure. As blood travels down the systemic circulation, blood pressure decreases progressively due to the peripheral resistance to blood flow.

7.5 Blood Composition

Blood contains plasma (55%) and *formed elements* (45%). Plasma is a straw colored liquid which is mostly composed of water (92%), electrolytes, and the following plasma proteins:

* **Albumin** which is important in maintaining the osmotic pressure and helps to transport many substances in the blood

* **Globulins** which include both transport proteins and the proteins which form antibodies

* **Fibrinogen** which polymerizes to form the insoluble protein *fibrin* which is essential for normal blood clotting. If you take away fibrinogen and some other clotting factors from plasma you will be left with a fluid called *serum*.

The formed elements of the blood originate from precursors in the bone marrow which produce the following for the circulatory system: 99% red blood cells (= *erythrocytes*), then there are platelets (= *thrombocytes*), and white blood cells (= *leukocytes*). Red blood cells (RBCs) are biconcave cells without nuclei (*anucleate*) that circulate for 110-120 days before their components are recycled by macrophages. Interestingly, mature RBCs do not possess most organelles such as mitochondria, Golgi nor ER because RBCs are packed with hemoglobin. The primary function of hemoglobin is the transport of O_2 and CO_2 to and from tissue.

Platelets are cytoplasmic fragments of large bone marrow cells (*megakaryocytes*) which are involved in blood clotting by adhering to the collagen of injured vessels, releasing mediators which cause blood vessels to constrict (= *vasoconstriction*), etc.

Calcium ions (Ca^{2+}) are also important in blood clotting because they help in signaling platelets to aggregate.

White blood cells help in the defense against infection; they are divided into *granulocytes* and *agranulocytes* depending on whether or not the cell does or does not contain granules, respectively.

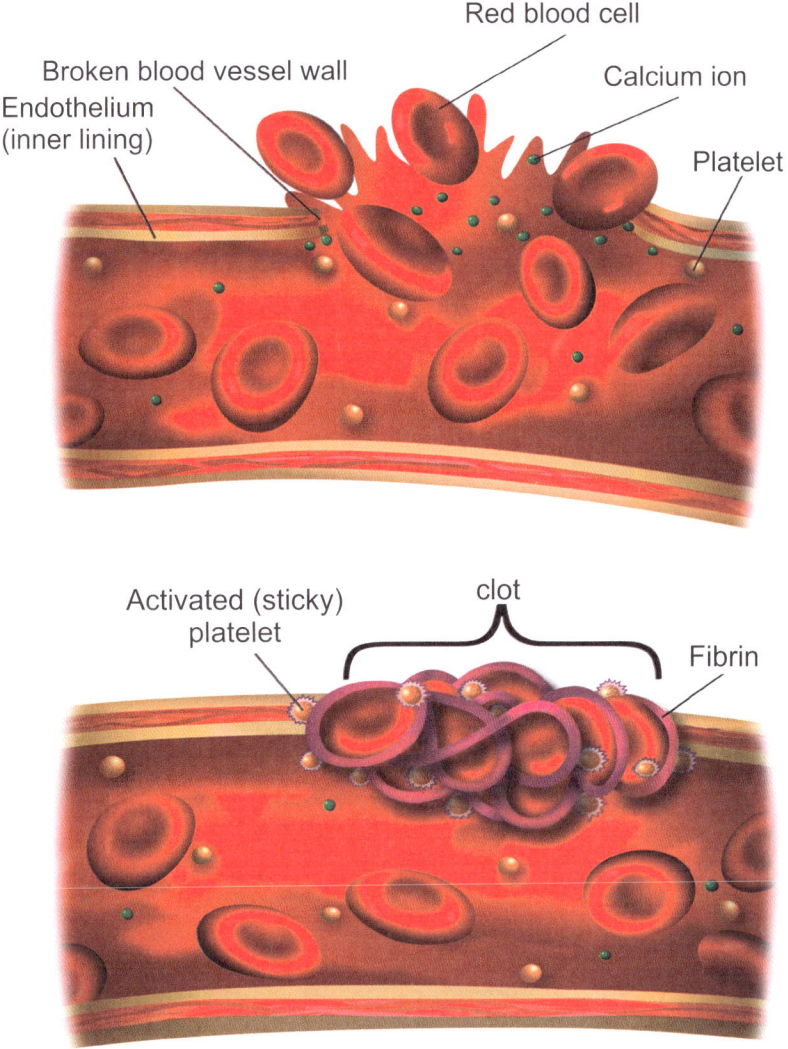

Figure IV.A.7.1.1: Schematic representation of blood clotting.

Granulocytes (= *polymorphonuclear leukocytes*) possess varying number of azurophilic (burgundy when stained) granules and are divided into: i) neutrophils which are the first white blood cells to respond to infection, they are important in controlling bacterial infection by phagocytosis - killing and digesting bacteria - and are the main cellular constituent of pus; ii) eosinophils which, like neutrophils, are phagocytic and also participate in allergic reactions and the destruction of parasites; iii) basophils which can release both anticoagulants (heparin) and substances important in hypersensitivity reactions (histamine).

Agranulocytes (= *mononuclear leukocytes*) lack specific granules and are divided into: i) *lymphocytes* which are vital to the immune system (see *Immune System*, chapter 8); and monocytes (often called *phagocytes* or *macrophages* when they are outside of the circulatory system) which can phagocytose large particles.

The hematocrit measures how much space (volume) in the blood is occupied by red blood cells and is expressed as a percentage. Normal hematocrit in adults is about 45%.

{See BIO 15.2 for ABO Blood Types}

7.5.1 Hemoglobin

Each red blood cell carries hundreds of molecules of a substance which is responsible for their red color: **hemoglobin**. Hemoglobin (Hb) is a complex of *heme*, which is an iron-containing porphyrin ring, and *globin*, which is a tetrameric (= has 4 subunits) protein consisting of two α-subunits and two β-subunits. The iron from the heme group is normally in its reduced state (Fe^{2+}); however, in the presence of O_2, it can be oxidized to Fe^{3+}.

In the lungs, oxygen concentration or *partial pressure* is high, thus O_2 dissolves in the blood; oxygen can then quickly and reversibly combine with the iron in Hb forming bright red *oxyhemoglobin*. The binding of oxygen to hemoglobin is cooperative. In other words, each oxygen that binds to Hb facilitates the binding of the next oxygen. Consequently, the dissociation curve for oxyhemoglobin is sigmoidal as a result of the change in affinity of hemoglobin as each O_2 successively binds to the globin subunit (see BIO 4.3).

Examine Figure IV.A.7.2 carefully. Notice that at a PO_2 of 100 mmHg (e.g. arterial blood), the percentage of saturation of hemoglobin is almost 100%, which means all four heme groups on the four hemoglobin subunits are bound with O_2. At a PO_2 of 40 mmHg (e.g. venous blood), the percentage of saturation of hemoglobin is about 75%, which means three of the four heme groups on the four hemoglobin subunits are bound with O_2. At a PO_2 of 27 mmHg, the percentage of saturation of hemoglobin is only 50%, which means half of the four heme groups on the four hemoglobin subunits are bound with O_2. The partial pressure of oxygen (PO_2) at 50% saturation is called P50.

The curve can: (i) shift to the left which means that for a given PO_2 in the tissue capillary there is decreased unloading (release) of oxygen and that the affinity of hemoglobin for O_2 is increased; or (ii) shift to the right which means that for a given PO_2 in the tissue capillary there is increased

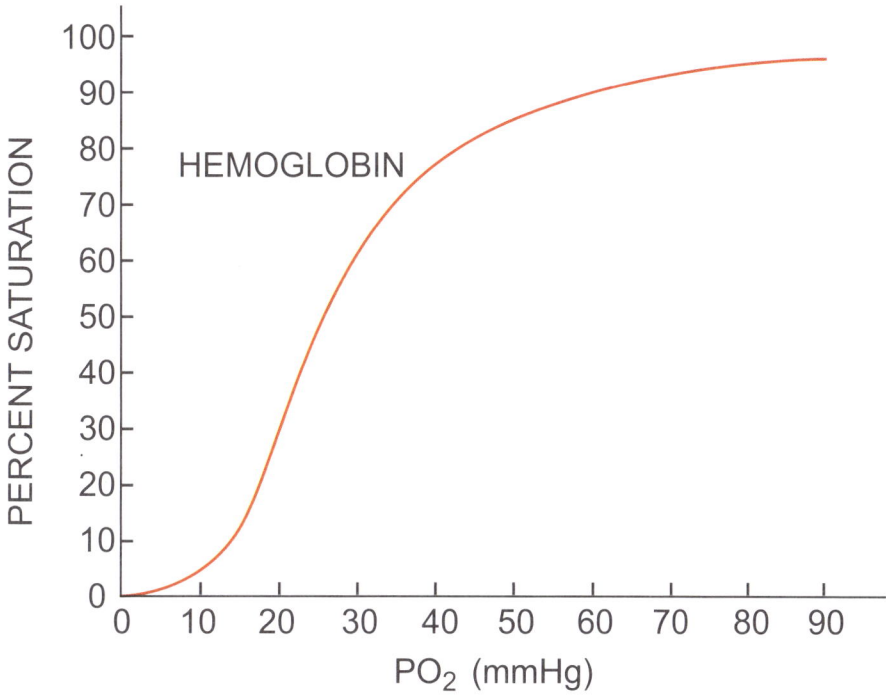

Figure IV.A.7.2: Oxygen dissociation curve: percent O₂ saturation versus O₂ partial pressure.

unloading of oxygen and that the affinity of hemoglobin for O₂ is decreased. The latter occurs when the tissue (i.e. muscle) is very active and thus requires more oxygen.

Thus a right shift occurs when the muscle is hot (↑ temperature during exercise), acid (↓ pH due to lactic acid produced in exercising muscle, see BIO 4.4. and 4.5), hypercarbic (↑CO₂ as during exercise, tissue produces more CO₂, see BIO 4.4. and 12.4.1), or contains high levels of organic phosphates (esp. increased synthesis of 2,3 DPG in red blood cells as a means to adapt to chronic hypoxemia).

In the body tissues where the partial pressure of O₂ is low and CO₂ is high, O₂ is released and CO₂ combines with the protein component of Hb forming the darker colored *carbaminohemoglobin* (also called: deoxyhemoglobin). The red color of muscle is due to a different heme-containing protein concentrated in muscle called myoglobin. Myoglobin is a monomeric protein containing one heme prosthetic group. The O₂ binding curve for myoglobin is hyperbolic, which means that it lacks cooperativity.

7.5.2 Capillaries: A Closer Look

Capillary fluid movement can occur as a result of two processes: diffusion (dominant role) and filtration (secondary role but critical for the proper function of organs, especially the kidney; BIO 10.3). Osmotic pressure (BIO 1.1.1, CHM 5.1.3) due to proteins in blood plasma is sometimes called colloid osmotic pressure or oncotic pressure. The Starling equation is an equation that describes the role of hydrostatic and oncotic forces (= Starling forces) in the movement of fluid across capillary membranes as a result of filtration.

When blood enters the arteriole end of a capillary, it is still under pressure produced by the contraction of the ventricle. As a result of this pressure, a substantial amount of water (hydrostatic) and some plasma proteins filter through the walls of the capillaries into the tissue space. This fluid, called interstitial fluid (BIO 7.6), is simply blood plasma minus most of the proteins.

Interstitial fluid bathes the cells in the tissue space and substances in it can enter the cells by diffusion (mostly) or active transport. Substances, like carbon dioxide, can diffuse out of cells and into the interstitial fluid.

Near the venous end of a capillary, the blood pressure is greatly reduced. Here another force comes into play. Although the composition of interstitial fluid is similar to that of blood plasma, it contains a smaller concentration of proteins than plasma and thus a somewhat greater concentration of water.

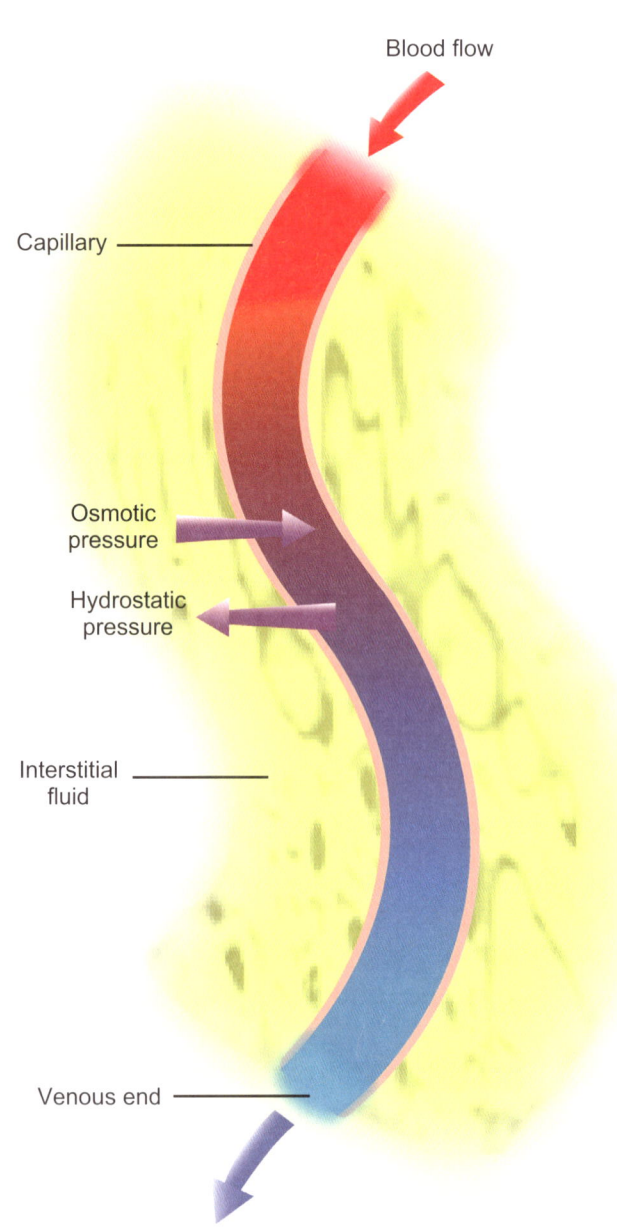

Figure IV.A.7.2b: Circulation at the level of the capillary. The exchange of water, oxygen, carbon dioxide, and many other nutrient and waste chemical substances between blood and surrounding tissues occurs at the level of the capillary.

This difference sets up an osmotic pressure. Although the osmotic pressure is small, it is greater than the blood pressure at the venous end of the capillary. Thus the fluid reenters the capillary here.

To summarize: when the blood pressure is greater than the osmotic pressure, filtration is favored and fluid tends to move out of the capillary; when the blood pressure is less than the osmotic pressure, reabsorption is favored and fluid tends to enter into the capillary.

7.6 The Lymphatic System

Body fluids can exist in blood vessels (intravascular), in cells (intracellular) or in a 3rd space which is intercellular (between cells) or extracellular (outside cells). Such fluids are called interstitial fluids. The **lymphatic system** is a network of vessels which can circulate fluid from the 3rd space to the cardiovascular system.

Aided by osmotic pressure, interstitial fluids enter the lymphatic system via small closed-ended tubes called *lymphatic capillaries* (in the small intestine they are called *lacteals*). Once the fluid enters it is called **lymph**. The lymph continues to flow into larger and larger vessels propelled by muscular contraction (esp. skeletal) and one-way valves. Then the lymph will usually pass through *lymph nodes* and then into a large vessel (esp. *the thoracic duct*) which drains into one of the large veins which eventually leads to the right atrium.

Lymph functions in important ways. Most protein molecules which leak out of blood capillaries are returned to the bloodstream by lymph. Also, microorganisms which invade tissue fluids are carried to lymph nodes by lymph. Lymph nodes contain *lymphocytes* and macrophages which are components of the immune system.

Go online to GAMSAT-prep.com for additional chapter review Q&A and forum.

GOLD NOTES

THE IMMUNE SYSTEM

Chapter 8

Memorize

cells in immunity: T-lymphocytes;
lymphocytes
tissues in the immune system including
bone marrow
spleen, thymus, lymph nodes

Understand

* Concepts of antigen, antibody, interaction
* Structure of antibody molecule
* Mechanism of stimulation by antigen

Not Required*

* Advanced level college info
* The 5 antibody isotypes
* Life cycle of pathogens
* Anatomy of lymph nodes
* Class switching

GAMSAT-Prep.com

Introduction

The immune system protects against disease. Many processes are used in order to identify and kill various microbes (see Microbiology, Chapter 2, for examples) as well as tumor cells (more detail when you get into medical school!). There are 2 acquired responses of the immune system: cell-mediated and humoral.

Additional Resources

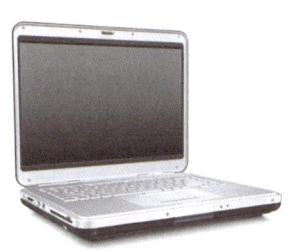

Free Online Q&A + Forum

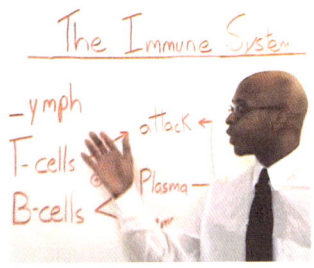

Video: Online or DVD

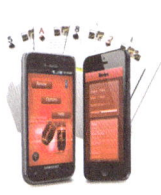

Flashcards

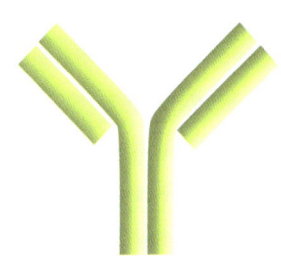

Special Guest

THE BIOLOGICAL SCIENCES BIO-115

* The real GAMSAT may have advanced level information presented (ie. in a passage) but previous knowledge of said information is not required to answer the questions that would follow. Practice ACER and GS practice GAMSATs can help you clarify this point.

GAMSAT-Prep.com
THE GOLD STANDARD

8.1 Overview

The immune system is composed of various cells and organs which defend the body against pathogens, toxins or any other foreign agents. Substances (usu. proteins) on the foreign agent causing an immune response are called **antigens**. There are two acquired responses to an antigen: (1) the **cell mediated response** where T-lymphocytes are the dominant force and act against microorganisms, tumors, and virus infected cells; and (2) the **humoral response** where B-lymphocytes are the dominant force and act against specific proteins present on foreign molecules.

8.2 Cells of the Immune System

B-lymphocytes originate in the bone marrow. Though T-lymphocytes also originate in the bone marrow, they go on to mature in the thymus gland. T-lymphocytes learn with the help of macrophages to recognize and attack only foreign substances (i.e. antigens) in a direct cell to cell manner (= *cell-mediated* or *cellular immunity*). T-lymphocytes have two major subtypes: T-helper cells and T-cytotoxic cells. Some T-cells (T_8, T_C, or T cytotoxic) mediate the apoptosis of foreign cells and virus-infected cells. Some T-cells (T_4, T_H or T *h*elper) mediate the cellular response by secreting substances to activate macrophages, other T-cells and even B-cells. {T_H-cells are specifically targeted and killed by the HIV virus in AIDS patients}

B-lymphocytes act indirectly against the foreign agent by producing and secreting antigen-specific proteins called **antibodies**, which are sometimes called immunoglobulins = *humoral immunity*). Antibodies are "designer" proteins which can specifically attack the antigen for which it was designed. The antibodies along with other proteins (i.e. complement proteins) can attack the antigen-bearing particle in many ways:

• **Lysis** by digesting the plasma membrane of the foreign cell

• **Opsonization** which is the altering of cell membranes so the foreign particle is more susceptible to phagocytosis by neutrophils and macrophages

• **Agglutination** which is the clumping of antigen-bearing cells

• **Chemotaxis** which is the attracting of other cells (i.e. phagocytes) to the area

• **Inflammation** which includes migration of cells, release of fluids and dilatation of blood vessels.

The activated antibody secreting B-lymphocyte is called a *plasma cell*. After the first or *primary* response to an antigen, both T- and B-cells produce *memory cells* which are formed during the initial response to an anti-

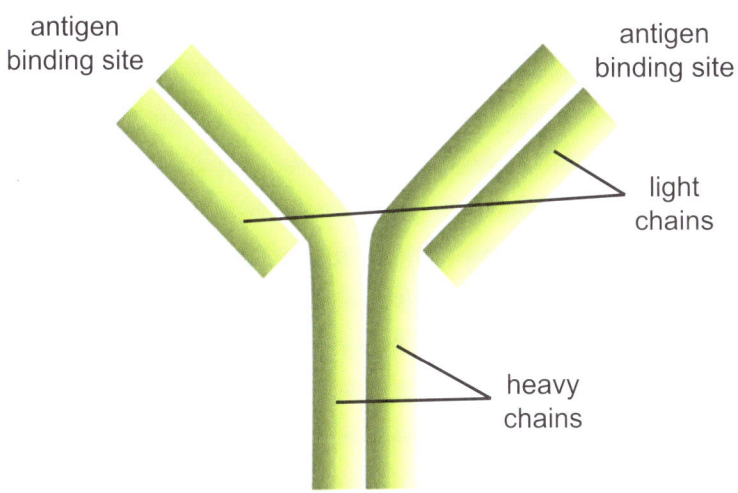

Figure IV.A.8.1: Schematic representation of an antibody. Antibodies are composed of disulfide bond-linked heavy and light chains. The unique part of the antigen recognized by an antibody is called the epitope. The antigen binding site on the antibody is extremely variable (= hypervariable).

Antibody (= Immunoglobulin = Ig)	Description
IgA	Found in saliva, tears and breast milk. Found in mucosal areas, such as the GI, respiratory and urogenital tracts thus prevents colonization by pathogens.
IgD	Functions mainly as an antigen receptor on B-cells that have not been exposed to antigens. Activates mast cells and basophils (BIO 7.5) to produce antimicrobial factors.
IgE	Binds to particles that induce allergic reactions (= allergens) and triggers histamine release from mast cells and basophils. Also protects against parasitic worms.
IgG	In its four forms, provides the majority of antibody-based immunity against invading germs or pathogens. The only antibody capable of crossing the placenta (BIO 14.6) to give passive immunity to the fetus.
IgM	Expressed on the surface of B-cells (monomer) and in a secreted form (pentamer = complex of 5 monomers). Eliminates pathogens in the early stages of B-cell mediated (humoral) immunity before there is sufficient IgG.

Table IV.A.8.1: Antibody isotypes of mammals. Antibodies are grouped into different "isotypes" based on which heavy chain they possess. The five different antibody isotypes known in mammals are displayed in the table.

genic challenge. These memory cells remain in the circulation and will make the next or secondary response much faster and much greater. {Note: though lymphocytes are vital to the immune system, it is the neutrophil which responds to injury first; BIO 7.5}

T-cells cannot recognise, and therefore react to, 'free' floating antigen. T-cells can only recognize an antigen that has been processed and presented by cells in association will a special cell surface molecule called the major histocompatibility complex (MHC). In fact, "antigen presenting cells", through the use of MHC, can teach both B-cells and T-cells which antigens are safe (*self*) and which are dangerous and should be attacked (*nonself*). MHC Class I molecules present to T_C cells while MHC Class II molecules present to T_H cells.

8.3 Tissues of the Immune System

The important tissues of the immune system are the bone marrow, and the lymphatic organs which include the thymus, the lymph nodes and the spleen. The roles of the bone marrow and the thymus have already been discussed. It is of value to add that the thymus secretes a hormone (= *thymosin*) which appears to help stimulate the activity of T-lymphocytes.

Lymph nodes are often the size of a pea and are found in groups or chains along the paths of the larger lymphatic vessels. Their functions can be broken down into three general categories: i) a non-specific filtration of bacteria and other particles from the lymph using the phagocytic activity of macrophages; ii) the storage and proliferation of T-cells, B-cells and antibody production; (iii) initiate immune response on the recognition of antigen.

The **spleen** is the largest lymphatic organ and is situated in the upper left part of the abdominal cavity. Within its lobules it has tissue called red and white pulp. The white pulp of the spleen contains all of the organ's lymphoid tissue (T-cells, B-cells, macrophages, and other antigen presenting cells) and is the site of active immune responses via the proliferation of T- and B-lymphocytes and the production of antibodies by plasma cells. The red pulp is composed of several types of blood cells including red blood cells, platelets and granulocytes. Its main function is to filter the blood of antigen and phagocytose damaged or aged red blood cells (the latter has a lifespan of approximately 110-120 days). In addition, the red pulp of the spleen is a site for red blood cell storage (i.e. a blood storage organ).

BIOLOGY

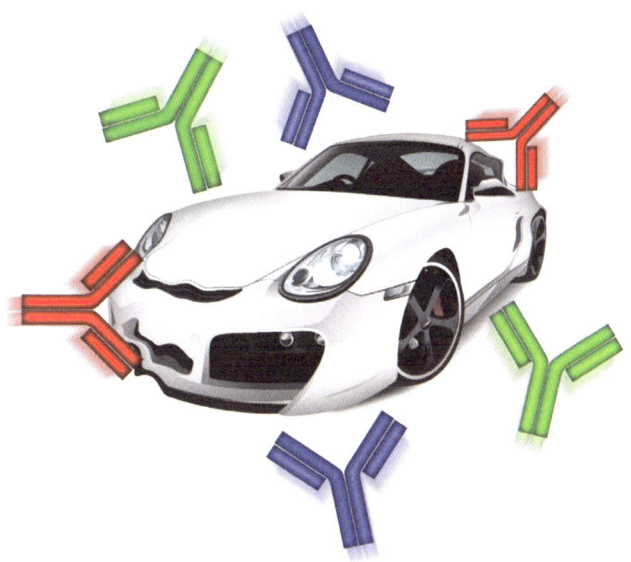

Autoimmunity!

Figure IV.A.8.2: Actually, "autoimmunity" refers to a disease process where the immune system attacks one's own cells and tissues as opposed to one's own car.

8.4 Advanced Topic: ELISA

ELISA, enzyme-linked-immunosorbent serologic assay, is a rapid test used to determine if a particular protein is in a sample and, if so, to quantify it (= assay). ELISA relies on an enzymatic conversion reaction and an antibody-antigen interaction which would lead to a detectable signal – usually a color change. Consequently, ELISA has no need of any radioisotope nor any radiation-counting apparatus.

There are 2 forms of ELISA: (1) direct ELISA uses monoclonal antibodies to detect antigen in a sample; (2) indirect ELISA is used to find a specific antibody in a sample (i.e. HIV antibodies in serum). {Notice the similarity with the concept of "direct" and "indirect" immunofluorescence, BIO 1.5.1}

Go online to GAMSAT-prep.com for additional chapter review Q&A and forum.

GOLD NOTES

THE DIGESTIVE SYSTEM
Chapter 9

Memorize
* ...iva as lubrication and enzyme source
* ...mach low pH, gastric juice, mucal ...otection against self-destruction

Understand
* Basic function of the upper GI and lower GI tracts
* Bile: storage in gallbladder, function
* Pancreas: production of enzymes; transport of enzymes to small intestine
* Small intestine: production of enzymes, site of digestion, neutralize stomach acid
* Peristalsis; structure and function of villi

Not Required*
* Advanced level college info
* Reading dental x-rays!

GAMSAT-Prep.com

Introduction

The digestive system is involved in the mechanical and chemical break down of food into smaller components with the aim of absorption into, for example, blood or lymph. Thus digestion is a form of catabolism.

Additional Resources

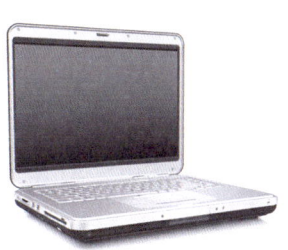
Free Online Q&A + Forum

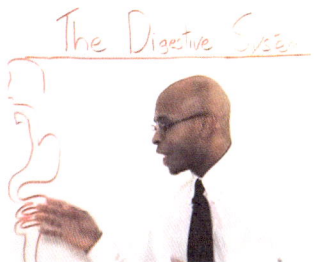
Video: Online or DVD

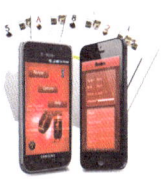
Flashcards

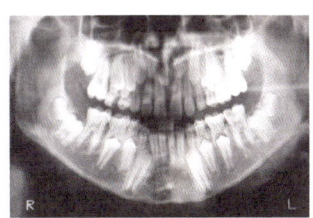
Special Guest

THE BIOLOGICAL SCIENCES BIO-121

* The real GAMSAT may have advanced level information presented (ie. in a passage) but previous knowledge of said information is not required to answer the questions that would follow. Practice ACER and GS practice GAMSATs can help you clarify this point.

9.1 Overview

The digestive or *gastrointestinal* (= GI) system is principally concerned with the intake and reduction of food into subunits for absorption. These events occur in five main phases which are located in specific parts of the GI system: i) **ingestion** which is the taking of food or liquid into the mouth; ii) **fragmentation** which is when larger pieces of food are *mechanically* broken down; iii) **digestion** where macromolecules are *chemically* broken down into subunits which can be absorbed; iv) **absorption** through cell membranes; and v) **elimination** of the waste products. The GI system secretes enzymes and hormones that facilitate in the process of ingestion, digestion, absorption as well as elimination.

The GI tract (gut or *alimentary canal*) is a muscular tract about 9 meters long covered by a layer of mucosa which has definable characteristics in each area along the tract. The GI tract includes the oral cavity (mouth), pharynx, esophagus, stomach, small intestine, large intestine, and anus. The GI system includes the accessory organs which release secretions into the tract: the salivary glands, gallbladder, liver, and pancreas (*see Figure IV.A.9.1*).

9.2 The Oral Cavity and Esophagus

Ingestion, fragmentation and digestion begin in the oral cavity. Teeth are calcified, hard structures in the oral cavity used to fragment food (= *mastication*). Children have twenty teeth (= *deciduous*) and adults have thirty-two (= *permanent*). From front to back, each quadrant (= *quarter*) of the mouth contains: two incisors for cutting, one cuspid (= *canine*) for tearing, two bicuspids (= *premolars*) for crushing, and three molars for grinding.

Digestion of food begins in the oral cavity when the 3 pairs of salivary glands (*parotid, sublingual*, and *submandibular*) synthesize and secrete saliva. Saliva lubricates the oral cavity, assists in the process of deglutition, controls bacterial flora and initiates the process of digestion. Its production is unique in that it is increased by both sympathetic and parasympathetic innervation. Major components of saliva include salivary amylase, lysozyme, lingual lipase and mucus. Amylase is an enzyme which starts the initial digestion of carbohydrates by splitting starch and glycogen into disaccharide subunits. Lipase is an enzyme which starts the initial digestion of triglyceride (fats). The mucous helps to bind food particles together and lubricate it as it is swallowed.

Swallowing (= *deglutition*) occurs in a coordinated manner in which the tongue and pharyngeal muscles propel the bolus of food into the esophagus while at the same time the upper esophageal sphincter relaxes to permit food to enter. The epiglottis is a small flap of

BIOLOGY

Basic Dental Anatomy and Pathology

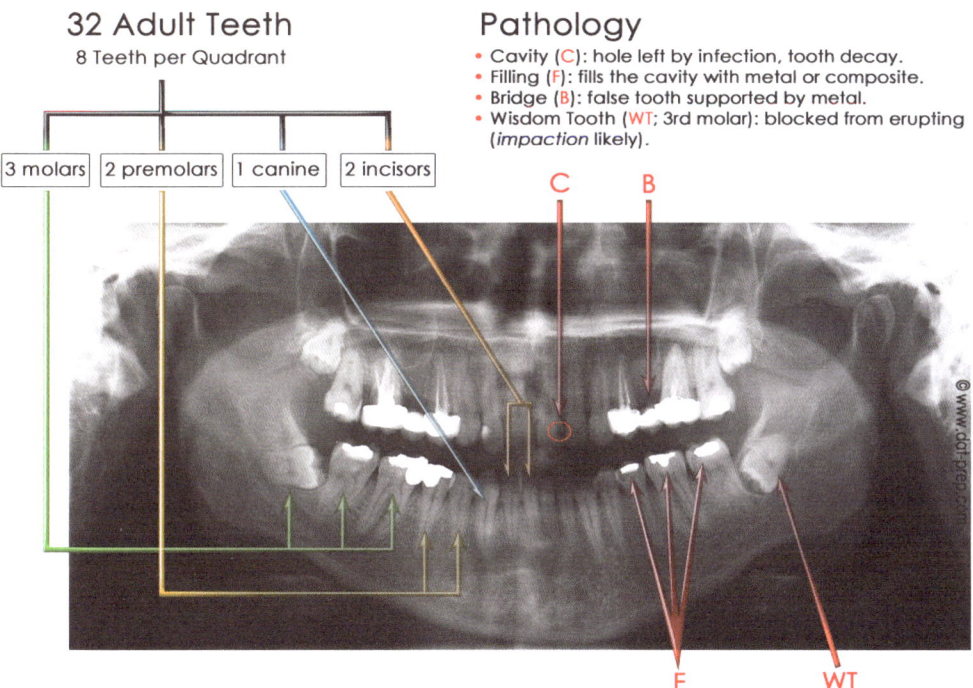

Figure IV.A.9.0a: Dental X-ray of an adult. The pathology of teeth is not prerequisite knowledge for the GAMSAT and is only presented for your interest (and as a minor contribution to the future studies of those of you who are studying GAMSAT for dentistry!).

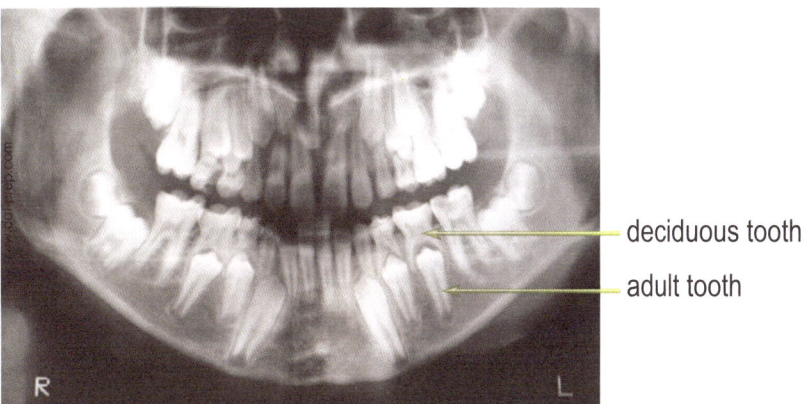

Figure IV.A.9.0b: Dental X-ray of a child showing deciduous (AKA: baby, primary, milk, temporary) teeth and emerging adult (permanent) teeth. Note the "R" on the X-ray indicates the right side of the patient who is facing the observer.

GAMSAT-Prep.com
THE GOLD STANDARD

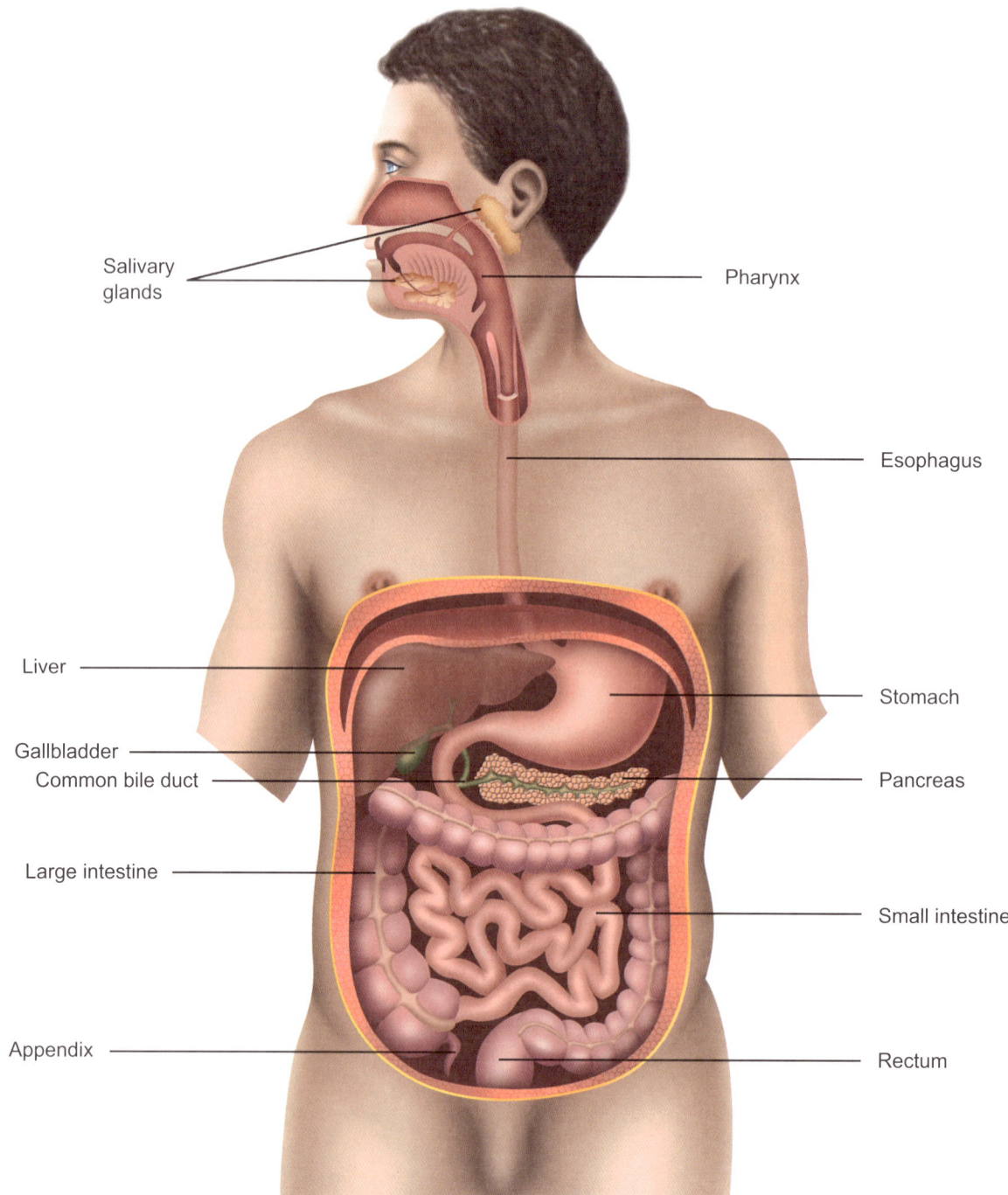

Figure IV.A.9.1: Schematic drawing of the major components of the digestive system.

tissue which covers the opening to the airway (= *glottis*) while swallowing. Gravity and peristalsis help bring the food through the esophagus to the stomach.

The GI system is supplied by both extrinsic innervation and intrinsic innervation. The extrinsic innervation includes the sympathetic and parasympathetic nervous system. The parasympathetic nervous system, mediated by the vagus and pelvic nerves, usually stimulates the functions of the GI tract while the sympathetic nervous system usually inhibits the functions of the GI tract. The intrinsic innervation located in the gut wall includes the *myenteric nerve plexus* and *submucosal nerve plexus* which control GI tract motility including peristalsis.

Peristalsis, which is largely the result of two muscle layers in the GI tract (i.e. the inner circular and outer longitudinal layers), is the sequential wave-like muscular contractions which propell food along the tract. The rate, strength and velocity of muscular contractions are modulated by the ANS.

9.3 The Stomach

The stomach continues in fragmenting and digesting the food with its strong muscular activity, its acidic gastric juice and various digestive enzymes present in the gastric juice. The walls of the stomach are lined by thick mucosa which contains goblet cells. These goblet cells of the GI tract protect the lumen from the acidic environment by secreting mucous.

The important components of gastric juice are: i) HCl which keeps the pH low (approximately = 2) to kill microorganisms, to aid in partial hydrolysis of proteins, and to provide the environment for ii) *pepsinogen*, an inactive form of enzyme (= *zymogen*) secreted by gastric chief cells, which is later converted to its active form *pepsin* in the presence of a low pH. Pepsin is involved in the breakdown of proteins. Both the hormone gastrin, which is produced in the stomach; and parasympathetic impulses can increase the production of gastric juice.

The preceding events turns food into a semi-digested fluid called chyme. Chyme is squirted through a muscular sphincter in the stomach, the *pyloric sphincter*, into the first part of the small intestine, the *duodenum*. Many secretions are produced by exocrine glands in the liver and pancreas and enter the duodenum via the *common bile duct*. Exocrine secretions eventually exit the body through ducts. For example, *goblet cells*, which are found in the stomach and throughout the intestine, are exocrine secretory cells which produce mucus which lines the epithelium of the gastrointestinal tract.

9.4 The Exocrine Roles of the Liver and Pancreas

9.4.1 The Liver

The liver occupies the upper right part of the abdominal cavity. It has many roles including: the conversion of glucose to glycogen; the synthesis of glucose from non-carbohydrates; the production of plasma proteins; the destruction of red blood cells; the deamination of amino acids and the formation of urea; the conversion of toxic ammonia to much less toxic urea (the urea cycle); the storage of iron and certain vitamins; the alteration of toxic substances and most medicinal products (*detoxification*); and its exocrine role - the production of **bile** by liver cells (= *hepatocytes*).

Bile is a yellowish - green fluid mainly composed of water, cholesterol, pigments (from the destruction of red blood cells) and salts. It is the **bile salts** which have a digestive function by the emulsification of fats. Emulsification is the dissolving of fat globules into tiny droplets called *micelles* which have hydrophobic interiors and hydrophilic exteriors (cf. Plasma Membrane, BIO 1.1). Bile salts orient themselves around those lipid droplets with their hydrophilic portions towards the aqueous environment and their hydrophobic portions towards the micelle interior and keep them dispersed. Emulsification also helps in the absorption of the fat soluble vitamins A, D, E, and K.

Thus bile is produced by the liver, stored and concentrated in a small muscular sac, the **gallbladder**, and then secreted into the duodenum via the common bile duct.

9.4.2 The Pancreas

The pancreas is close to the duodenum and extends behind the stomach. The pancreas has both endocrine (*see Endocrine Systems; BIO 6.3.4*) and exocrine functions. It secretes pancreatic juice, which consists of alkaline fluid and digestive enzymes, into the pancreatic duct that joins the common bile duct. Pancreatic juice is secreted both due to parasympathetic and hormonal stimuli. The hormones *secretin* and *CCK* are produced and released by the duodenum in response to the presence of chyme. Secretin acts on the pancreatic ductal cells to stimulate HCO_3^- secretion, whose purpose is to neutralize the acidic chyme. CCK acts on pancreatic acinar cells to stimulate the exocrine pancreatic secretion of digestive enzymes. These enzymes are secreted as enzymes or proenzymes (= *zymogens*; BIO 4.3) that must be activated in the intestinal lumen. The enzymes include pancreatic amylase, which can break down carbohydrates into monosaccharides; pancreatic lipase, which can break down fats into fatty acids and monoglycerides; and nuclease, which can break down nucleic acids. The protein enzymes (proteases) include trypsin, chymotrypsin, carboxypeptidase, which can break down proteins into amino acids, dipeptides or tripeptides.

9.5 The Intestines

The **small intestine** is divided into the duodenum, the jejunum, and the ileum, in that order. It is this part of the GI system that completes the digestion of chyme, absorbs the nutrients (i.e. monosaccharides, amino acids, nucleic acids, etc.), and passes the rest onto the large intestine. Peristalsis is the primary mode of transport. Contraction behind the bolus and simultaneous relaxation in front of the bolus propel chyme forward. Segmentation also aids in small intestine movement - it helps to mix the intestinal contents without any forward movement of chyme. Of course, parasympathetic impulses increase intestinal smooth muscle contraction while sympathetic impulses decrease intestinal smooth muscle contraction.

Absorption is aided by the great surface area involved including the finger-like projections **villi** and **microvilli** (*see the Generalized Eukaryotic Cell*, BIO 1.1F and 1.2). Intestinal villi, which increase the surface area ten-fold, are evaginations into the lumen of the small intestine and contain blood capillaries and a single lacteal (lymphatic capillary). Microvilli, which increase the surface area twenty-fold, contain a dense bundle of actin microfilaments cross-linked by proteins fimbrin and villin.

Absorption of carbohydrates, proteins and lipids is completed in the small intestine. Carbohydrates must be broken down into glucose, galactose and fructose for absorption to occur. In contrast, proteins can be absorbed as amino acids, dipeptides and tripeptides. Specific transporters are required for amino acids and peptides to facilitate the absorption across the luminal membrane. Lipids are absorbed in the form of fatty acids, monoglycerides and cholesterol. In the intestinal cells, they are re-esterified to triglycerides, cholesterol ester and phospholipids.

The lacteals absorb most fat products into the lymphatic system while the blood capillaries absorb the rest taking these nutrients to the liver for processing via a special vein - the *hepatic portal vein* [A portal vein carries blood from one capillary bed to another; BIO 7.3]. Goblet cells secrete a copious amount of mucus in order to lubricate the passage of material through the intestine and to protect the epithelium from abrasive chemicals (i.e. acids, enzymes, etc.).

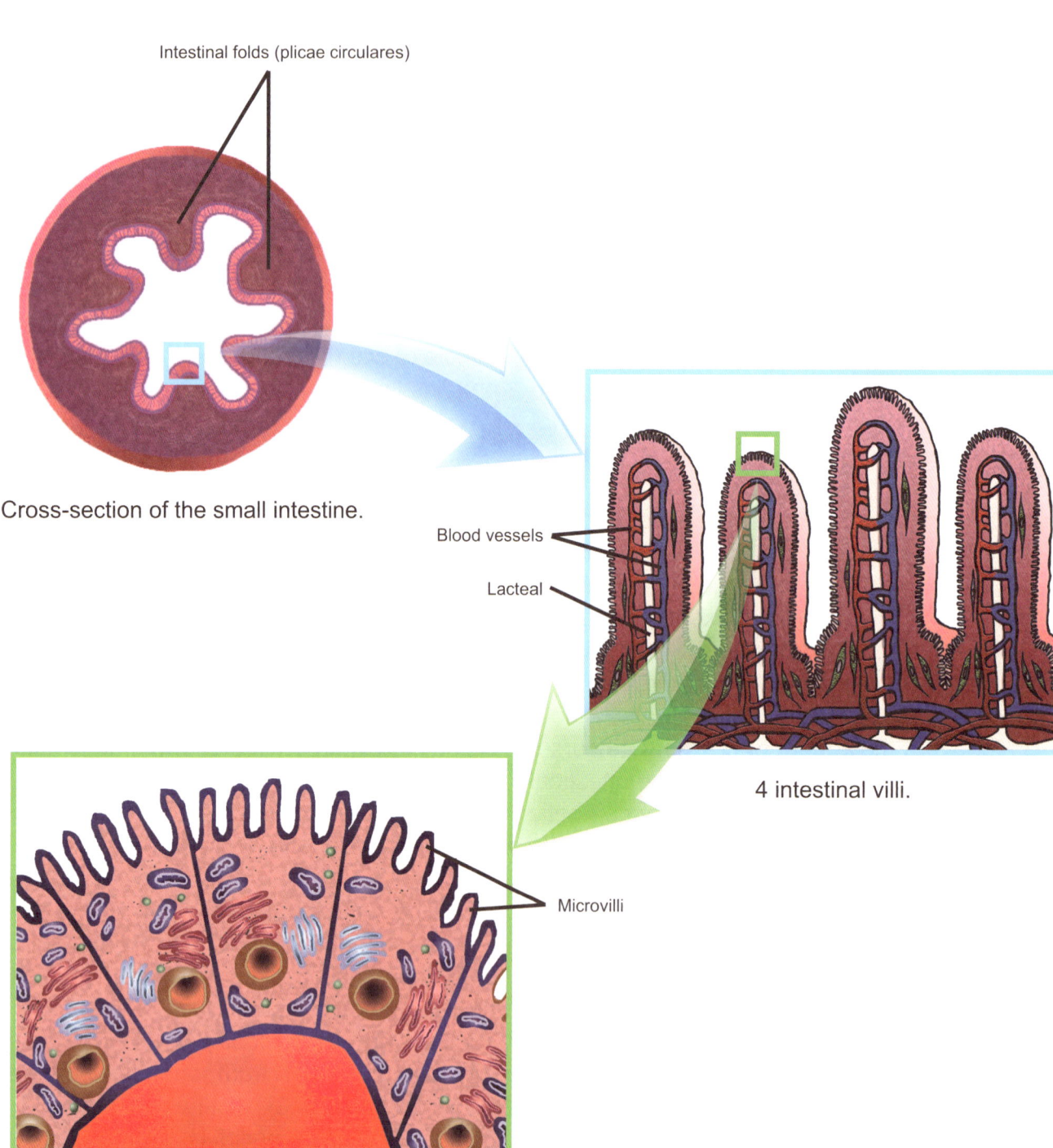

Figure IV.A.9.2: Levels of organization of the small intestine.

9.5.1 The Large Intestines

The large intestine is divided into: the cecum which connects to the ileum and projects a closed-ended tube - the appendix; the <u>colon</u> which is subdivided into ascending, transverse, descending, and sigmoid portions; <u>the rectum</u> which can store feces; and <u>the anal canal</u> which can expel feces (*defecation*) through the anus with the relaxation of the anal sphincter and the increase in abdominal pressure. The large intestine has little or no digestive functions. It absorbs water and electrolytes from the residual chyme and it forms feces. Feces is mostly water, undigested material, mucous, bile pigments (responsible for the characteristic color) and bacteria (= gut flora = 60% of the dry weight of feces).

Essentially, the relationship between the gut and bacteria is mutualistic and symbiotic (BIO 2.2). Though people can survive with no bacterial flora, these microorganisms perform a host of useful functions, such as fermenting unused energy substrates, training the immune system, preventing growth of harmful species, producing vitamins for the host (i.e. vitamin K), and bile pigments.

Go online to GAMSAT-prep.com for additional chapter review Q&A and forum.

GOLD NOTES

THE EXCRETORY SYSTEM
Chapter 10

Memorize	Understand	Not Required*
ney structure: cortex, medulla hron structure: glomerulus, man's capsule, proximal tubule, etc. p of Henle, distal tubule, ecting duct age and elimination: ureter, der, urethra	* Roles of the excretory system in homeostasis * Blood pressure, osmoregulation, acid-base balance, N waste removal * Formation of urine: glomerular filtration, secretion and reabsorption of solutes * Concentration of urine; counter-current multiplier mechanism	*Advanced level college info

GAMSAT-Prep.com

Introduction

The excretory system excretes waste. The focus of this chapter is to examine the kidney's role in excretion. This includes eliminating nitrogen waste products of metabolism such as urea.

Additional Resources

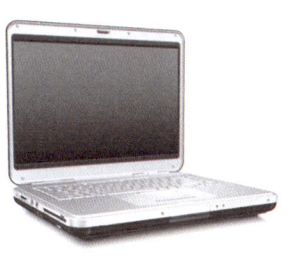 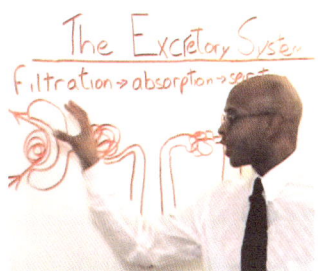 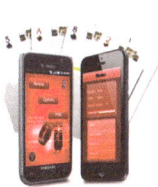 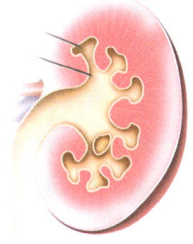

Free Online Q&A + Forum   Video: Online or DVD   Flashcards   Special Guest

THE BIOLOGICAL SCIENCES BIO-131

* The real GAMSAT may have advanced level information presented (ie. in a passage) but previous knowledge of said information is not required to answer the questions that would follow. Practice ACER and GS practice GAMSATs can help you clarify this point.

10.1 Overview

Excretion is the elimination of substances (usu. wastes) from the body. It begins at the level of the cell. Broken down red blood cells are excreted as bile pigments into the GI tract; CO_2, an end product of cellular aerobic respiration, is blown away in the lungs; urea and ammonia (NH_3), breakdown products of amino acid metabolism, creatinine, a product of muscle metabolism, and H_2O, a breakdown product of aerobic metabolism, are eliminated by the urinary system. In fact, the urinary system eliminates such a great quantity of waste it is often called the excretory system. It is composed of a pair of kidneys, a pair of ureters and one bladder and urethra.

The composition of body fluids remains within a fairly narrow range. The urinary system is the dominant organ system involved in electrolyte and water homeostasis (*osmoregulation*). It is also responsible for the excretion of toxic nitrogenous compounds (i.e. urea, uric acid, creatinine) and many drugs into the urine. The urine is produced in the kidneys (mostly by the filtration of blood) and is transported, with the help of peristaltic waves, down the tubular ureters to the muscular sack which can store urine, the bladder. Through the process of urination (= *micturition*), urine is expelled from the bladder to the outside via a tubular urethra.

The amount of volume within blood vessels (= *intravascular* or *blood volume*) and blood pressure are proportional to the rate the kidneys filter blood. Hormones act on the kidney to affect urine formation (see *Endocrine Systems*, BIO 6.3).

10.2 Kidney Structure

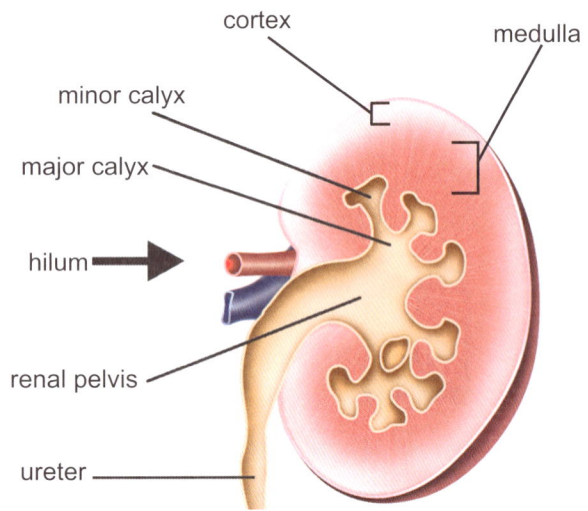

Figure IV.A.10.1: Kidney structure.

The kidney regulates the electrolyte levels in the extracellular fluid and maintains water homeostasis through the production and excretion of urine. The kidney resembles a bean with a concave border (= *the hilum*) where the ureter, nerves, and vessels (blood and lymph) attach. The kidney can be grossly divided into an outer granular-looking **cortex** and an inner dark striated **medulla**. The upper end of the ureter expands into the *renal pelvis* which can be divided into two or three *major calyces*. Each major calyx can be divided into several small branched *minor calyces*. The renal medulla lies deep to the cortex. It is composed of 10-18 medullary pyramids which consist mainly of loop of Henle and collecting tubules. The renal cortex is the superficial layer of the kidney right underneath the capsule. It is composed mainly of renal corpuscles and convoluted tubules.

The kidney is a *filtration-reabsorption-secretion* (excretion) organ. These events are clearly demonstrated at the level of the nephron.

10.3 The Nephron

The nephron is the functional unit of the kidney and consists of the **renal corpuscle** and the **renal tubule**. A renal corpuscle is responsible for the filtration of blood and is composed of a tangled ball of blood capillaries (= *the glomerulus*) and a sac-like structure which surrounds the glomerulus (= *Bowman's capsule*). *Afferent* and *efferent* arterioles lead towards and away from the glomerulus, respectively. The renal tubule is divided into *proximal* and *distal convoluted tubules* with a *loop of Henle* in between. The tube ends in a *collecting duct*.

Blood plasma is **filtered** by the glomerulus through three layers before entering Bowman's capsule. The first layer is formed by the *endothelial cells* of the capillary that possess small holes (= *fenestrae*); the second layer is the *glomerular basement membrane* (BIO 5.3); and the third layer is formed by the negatively charged cells (= *podocytes*) in Bowman's capsule which help repel proteins (most proteins are negatively charged).

The filtration barrier permits passage of water, ions, and small particles from the capillary into Bowman's capsule but prevents pas-

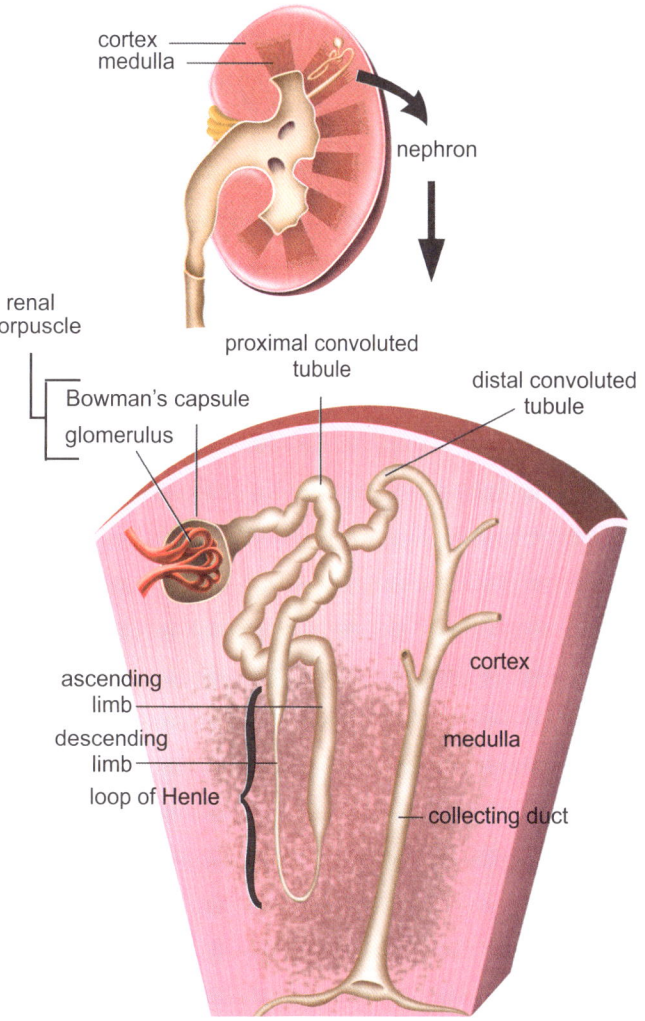

Figure IV.A.10.2: The kidney and its functional unit, the nephron.

GAMSAT-Prep.com
THE GOLD STANDARD

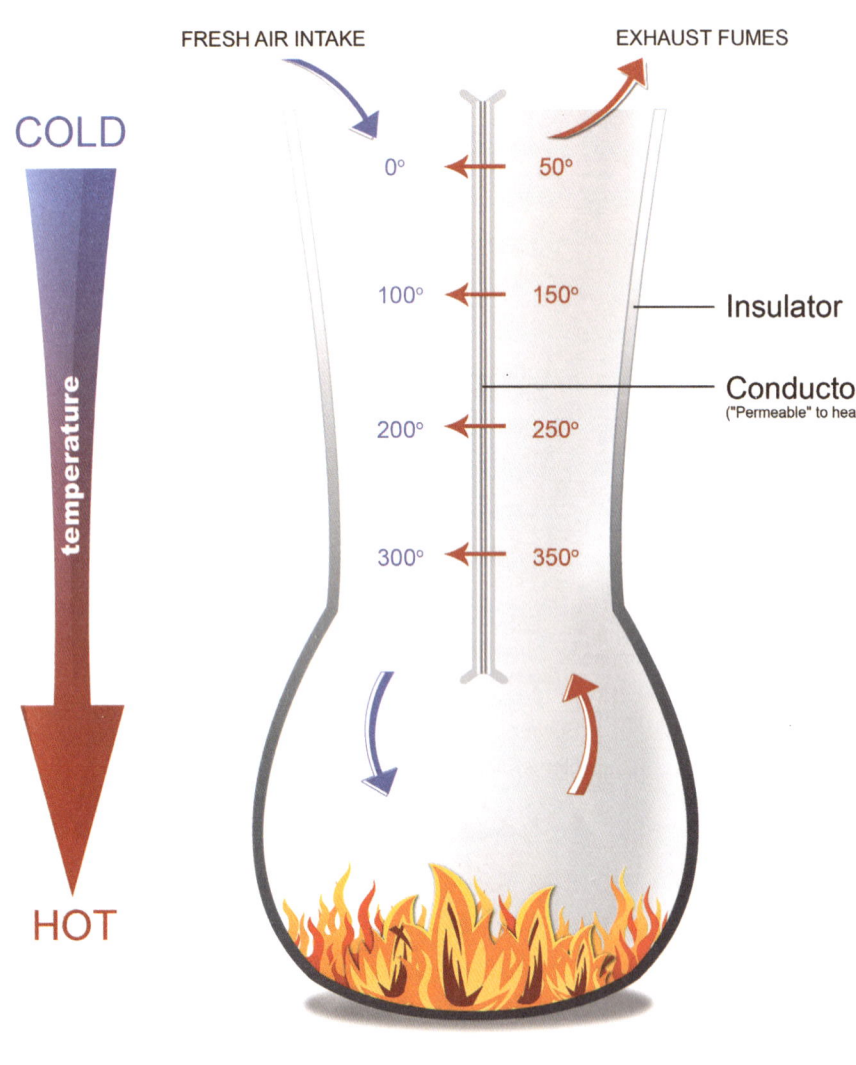

The countercurrent principle depends on a parallel flow arrangement moving in 2 different directions (countercurrent) in close proximity to each other. Our example is that of the air intake and exhaust pipe in this simplified schematic of a furnace.

Heat is transferred from the exhaust fumes to the incoming air.

The small horizontal temperature gradient of only 50° is multiplied longitudinally to a gradient of 300°. This conserves heath that would otherwise be lost.

Figure IV.A.10.3: The countercurrent principle (= counter-current mechanism) using a simplified furnace as an example.

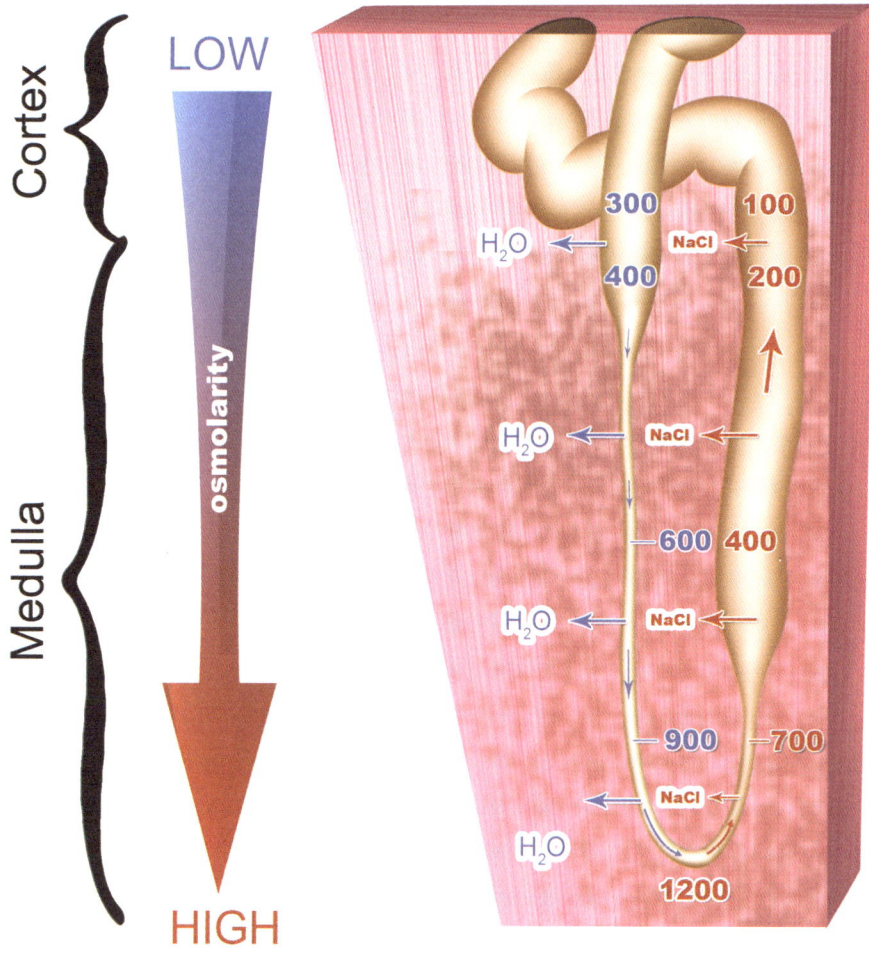

The countercurrent system involving the loop of Henle results in an osmotic gradient increasing from cortex to inner medulla (*juxtamedullary* nephrons). Solutes enter and exit at different segments of the nephron. The descending limb of the loop of Henle is highly permeable to water and relatively impermeable to NaCl (thus the filtrate becomes increasingly hypertonic). The ascending limb is impermeable to water but relatively (through active transport) permeable to NaCl.

Due to the increased osmolarity of the interstitial fluid, water moves out of the descending limb into the interstitial fluid by osmosis. Volume of the filtrate decreases as water leaves. Osmotic concentration of the filtrate increases (1200) as it rounds the hairpin turn of the loop of Henle.

Some of the NaCl leaving the ascending limb moves by diffusion into the descending limb from the interstitial fluid thus increasing the solute concentration in the descending limb. Also, new NaCl in the filtrate continuously enters the tubule inflow to be transported out of the ascending limb into the interstitial fluid. Thus this recycling multiplies NaCl concentration.

Figure IV.A.10.4: The countercurrent principle (= counter-current mechanism) in the loop of Henle.

10.3 The Nephron (cont'd)

sage of large/negatively charged particles (= *ultrafiltration*) and forms a filtrate in the Bowman's space. The rate of filtration is proportional to the net ultrafiltration pressure across the glomerular capillaries. This net pressure, which is usually positive and favors fluid filtration out of the capillary, can be derived from the difference between glomerular capillary hydrostatic pressure, which favors fluid out of the capillary, and the combined effect of glomerular capillary oncotic pressure and Bowman's space *hydrostatic* pressure, which favor fluid back into the capillary. {The oncotic pressure of Bowman's space is typically zero, so it is ignored here; keep in mind that 'oncotic pressure' is simply the osmotic pressure caused by proteins; see BIO 7.5.2}

The filtrate, which is similar to plasma but with minimal proteins, now passes into the proximal convoluted tubule (PCT). It is here that the body actively **reabsorbs** compounds that it needs (i.e. proteins, amino acids, and especially glucose); and over 75% of all ions and water are reabsorbed by *obligate* (= required) reabsorption from the PCT. To increase the surface area for absorption, the cells of the PCT have a lot of microvilli (= *brush border*; cf. BIO 1.2). Some substances like H^+, urea and penicillin are **secreted** into the PCT.

From the PCT the filtrate goes through the descending and ascending limbs of the loop of Henle which extend into the renal medulla. The purpose of the loop of Henle is to concentrate the filtrate by the transport of ions (Na^+ and Cl^-) into the medulla which produces an osmotic gradient (= *a countercurrent mechanism*). As a consequence of this system, the medulla of the kidney becomes concentrated with ions and tends to "pull" water out of the renal tubule by osmosis.

The filtrate now passes on to the distal convoluted tubule (DCT) which reabsorbs ions actively and water passively and secretes various ions (i.e. H^+). Hormones can modulate the reabsorption of substances from the DCT (= *facultative* reabsorption). Aldosterone acts at the DCT to absorb Na^+ which is coupled to the secretion of K^+ and the passive retention of H_2O.

Finally the filtrate, now called urine, passes into the collecting duct which drains into larger and larger ducts which lead to renal papillae, calyces, the renal pelvis, and then the ureter. ADH concentrates urine by increasing the permeability of the DCT and the collecting ducts allowing the medulla to draw water out by osmosis. Water returns to the circulation via a system of vessels called the *vasa recta*.

Renin is a hormone (BIO 6.3.5) which is secreted by cells that are "near the glomerulus" (= *juxtaglomerular cells*). At the beginning of the DCT is a region of modified tubular cells which can influence the secretion of renin (= *macula densa*). The juxtaglomerular cells and the macula densa are collectively known as the juxtaglomerular apparatus.

10.4 The Bladder

Urine flow through the ureters to the bladder is propelled by muscular contractions of the ureter wall - peristalsis. The urine is stored in the bladder and intermittently ejected during urination, termed micturition.

The bladder is a balloon-like chamber with walls of muscle collectively termed the detrusor muscle. The contraction of this muscle squeezes the urine into the lumen (= *space inside*) of the bladder to produce urination. That part of the detrusor muscle at the base of the bladder, where the urethra begins, functions as a sphincter - the internal urethral sphincter. Beyond the outlet of the urethra is the external urethral sphincter, the contraction of which can prevent urination even when the detrusor muscle contracts strongly.

The basic micturition reflex is a spinal reflex (BIO 6.1.3), which can be influenced by descending pathways from the brain. The bladder wall contains stretch receptors whose afferent fibers enter the spinal cord and stimulate the parasympathetic nerves that supply and stimulate the detrusor muscle. As the bladder fills with urine, the pressure within it increases and the stretch receptors are stimulated, thereby reflexively eliciting stimulation of the parasympathetic neurons and contractions of the detrusor muscle. When the bladder reaches a certain volume, the induced contraction of the detrusor muscle becomes strong enough to open the internal urethral sphincter. Simultaneously, the afferent input from the stretch receptors inhibits, within the spinal cord, the motor neurons that tonically stimulate the external urethral sphincter to contract. Both sphincters are now open and the contraction of the detrusor muscle is able to produce urination.

In summary:

- The internal sphincter is a continuation of the detrusor muscle and is thus composed of smooth muscle under involuntary or autonomic control. This is the primary muscle for preventing the release of urine.

- The external sphincter is made of skeletal muscle is thus under voluntary control of the somatic nervous system (BIO 6.1.4, 6.1.5, 11.2).

Go online to GAMSAT-prep.com for additional chapter review Q&A and forum.

GOLD NOTES

THE MUSCULOSKELETAL SYSTEM
Chapter 11

Memorize	Understand	Not Required*
ucture of three basic muscle types: iated, smooth, cardiac untary/involuntary muscles; npathetic/parasympathetic innervation	* Muscle system, important functions * Support, mobility, peripheral circulatory assistance, thermoregulation (shivering reflex) * Control: motor neurons, neuromuscular junctions, motor end plates * Skeletal system: structural rigidity/support, calcium storage, physical protection * Skeletal structure: specialization of bone types, basic joint, endo/exoskeleton	* Advanced level college info

GAMSAT-Prep.com

Introduction

The musculoskeletal system (= locomotor system) permits the movement of organisms with the use of muscle and bone. Other uses include providing form and stability for the organism; protection of vital organs (i.e. skull, rib cage); storage for calcium and phosphorous as well as containing a critical component to the production of blood cells (skeletal system).

Additional Resources

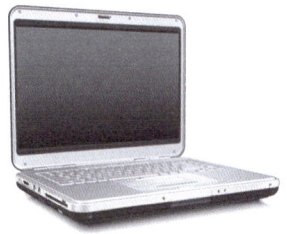

Free Online Q&A + Forum

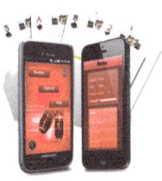

Flashcards

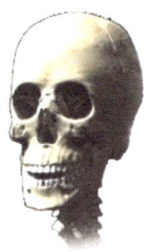

Special Guest

THE BIOLOGICAL SCIENCES   BIO-139

* The real GAMSAT may have advanced level information presented (ie. in a passage) but previous knowledge of said information is not required to answer the questions that would follow. Practice ACER and GS practice GAMSATs can help you clarify this point.

11.1 Overview

The musculoskeletal system supports, protects and enables body parts to move. Muscles convert chemical energy (i.e. ATP, creatine phosphate) into mechanical energy (→ contraction). Thus body heat is produced, body fluids are moved (i.e. lymph), and body parts can move in accordance with lever systems of muscle and bone.

11.2 Muscle

There are many general features of muscle. A latent period is the lag between the stimulation of a muscle and its response. A twitch is a single contraction in response to a brief stimulus which lasts for a fraction of a second. Muscles can either *contract* or *relax* but they cannot actively expand. When muscles are stimulated frequently, they cannot fully relax - this is known as *summation*. Tetany is a sustained contraction (a summation of multiple contractions) that lacks even partial relaxation. If tetany is maintained, the muscle will eventually fatigue or tire. Muscle tone (*tonus*) occurs because even when a muscle appears to be at rest, some degree of sustained contraction is occurring.

The cellular characteristics of muscle have already been described (s*ee Contractile Cells and Tissues,* BIO 5.2). We will now examine the gross features of the three basic muscle types.

Cardiac muscle forms the walls of the heart and is responsible for the pumping action. Its contractions are continuous and are initiated by inherent mechanisms (i.e., they are myogenic) and modulated by the autonomic nervous system. Its activity is decreased by the parasympathetic nervous system and increased by the sympathetic nervous system. The sinoatrial node (SA node) or *pacemaker* contains specialized cardiac muscle cells in the right atrium which initiate the contraction of the heart (BIO 7.2). The electrical signal then progresses to the atrioventricular node (AV node) in the cardiac muscle (myocardium) - between the atria and ventricles - then through the bundle of His which splits and branches out to Purkinje fibers which can then stimulate the contraction of the ventricles (systole; BIO 7.2).

Smooth Muscle has two forms. One type occurs as separate fibers and can contract in response to motor nerve stimuli. These are found in the iris (*pupillary dilation or constriction*) and the walls of blood vessels (*vasodilation or constriction)*. The second and more dominant form occurs as sheets of muscle fibers and is sometimes called *visceral muscle*. It forms the walls of many hollow visceral organs like the stomach, intestines, uterus, and the urinary bladder. Like cardiac muscle, its contractions are inherent, involuntary, and rhythmic. Visceral muscle is responsible for peristalsis. Its contractility is usually slow and can be modulated by the autonomic nervous system, hormones, and local metabolites. The activity of visceral muscle is increased by the parasympathetic nervous system and decreased by the sympathetic nervous system.

Skeletal muscle is responsible for voluntary movements. This includes the skeleton and organs such as the tongue and the globe of the eye. Its cells can form a syncytium which is a mass of cells which merge and can function together. Thus skeletal muscle can contract and relax relatively rapidly (*see the Reflex Arc,* BIO 6.1.3).

It should be noted that there are 2 meanings of the word "syncytium" when describing muscle cells. A classic example is the formation of large multinucleated skeletal muscle cells produced from the fusion of thousands of individual muscle cells (= *myocytes*) as alluded to in the previous paragraph ("true syncytium"). However, "syncytium" can also refer to cells that are interconnected by gap junctions (BIO 1.4), as seen in cardiac muscle cells and certain smooth muscle cells, and are thus synchronized electrically during an action potential ("functional syncytium").

Most skeletal muscles act across joints. Each muscle has a movable end (= *the insertion*) and an immovable end (= *the origin*). When a muscle contracts its insertion is moved towards its origin. When the angle of the joint decreases it is called flexion, when it increases it is called extension. Abduction is movement away from the midline of the body and adduction is movement toward the midline. {Adduction is addicted to the middle (= midline)}

Muscles which assist each other are synergistic (for example: while the deltoid muscle abducts the arm, other muscles hold the shoulder steady). Muscles that can move a joint in opposite directions are antagonistic (for example: at the elbow the biceps can flex while the triceps can extend).

Control of skeletal muscle originates in the cerebral cortex. Skeletal muscle is innervated by the somatic nervous system. Motor (*efferent*) neurons carry nerve impulses from the CNS to synapse with muscle fibers at the *neuro-muscular junction*. The terminal end of the motor neuron (motor end plate) can secrete

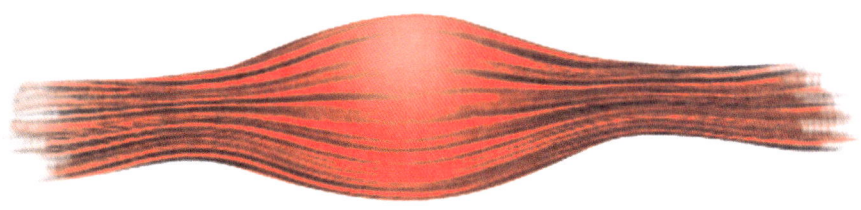

Skeletal muscle

acetylcholine which can depolarize the muscle fiber (BIO 5.1, 5.2). One motor neuron can depolarize many muscle fibers (= *a motor unit*).

The autonomic nervous system can supply skeletal muscle with more oxygenated blood in emergencies (sympathetic response) or redirect the blood to the viscera during relaxed states (parasympathetic response).

Skeletal muscle can be categorized as Type I or Type II. Type I fibers (= *cells*) appear red because of the oxygen-binding protein myoglobin (BIO 7.5.1). These fibers are suited for endurance and are slow to fatigue since they use oxidative metabolism to generate ATP (BIO 4.7-4.10). Type II fibers are white due to the absence of myoglobin and a reliance on glycolytic enzymes (BIO 4.5, 4.6). These fibers are efficient for short bursts of speed and power and use both oxidative metabolism and anaerobic metabolism depending on the particular sub-type. Type II myocytes are quicker to fatigue.

11.3 The Skeletal System

The microscopic features of bone and cartilage have already been described (*see Connective Cells and Tissues*, BIO 5.4.3/4). We will now examine the relevant gross features of the skeletal system.

The bones of the skeleton have many functions: i) acting like levers that aid in **body movement**; ii) the **storage** of inorganic salts like calcium and phosphorus (and to a lesser extent sodium and magnesium); iii) the production of blood cells (= **hematopoiesis**) in the metabolically active red marrow of the spongy parts of many bones. Bone also has a yellow marrow which contains fat storage cells.

11.3.1 Bone Structure and Development

Bone structure can be classified as follows: i) long bones which have a long shaft, the diaphysis, that is made up mostly of compact bone and expanded ends, like arm and leg bones; ii) short bones which are shaped like long bones but are smaller and have only a thin layer of compact bone surrounding a spongy bone interior; iii) flat bones which have broad surfaces like the skull, ribs, and the scapula and have two layers of compact bones with a layer of spongy bone in the middle; iv) irregular bones like the vertebrae and many facial bones and consist of a thin layer of compact bone covering a spongy bone

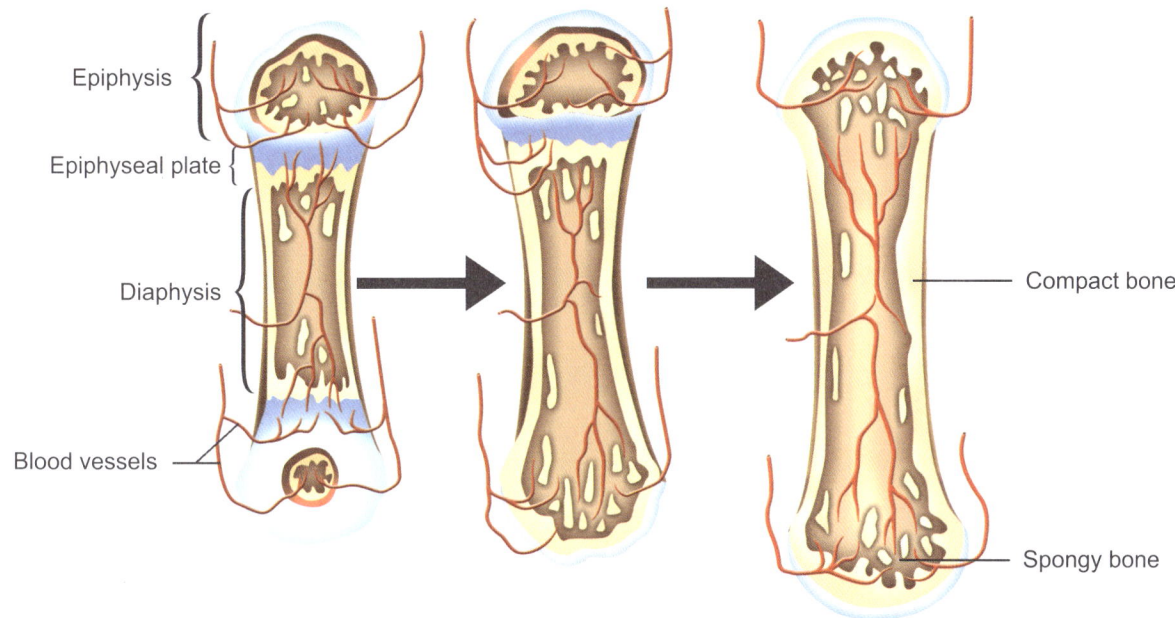

Figure IV.A.11.1: Bone structure and development.

interior. Bone structure can also be classified as: i) <u>primary bone</u>, also known as immature or woven bone, which contains many cells and has a low mineral content; ii) <u>secondary bone</u>, also known as mature or lamellar bone, which has a calcified matrix arranged in regular layers, or lamella.

The rounded expanded end of a long bone is called the *epiphysis* which contains <u>spongy bone</u>. The epiphysis is covered by fibrous tissue (*the periosteum*) and it forms a joint with another bone. Spongy bone contains bony plates called *trabeculae (= spicules)*. The shaft of the bone which connects the expanded ends is called the *diaphysis*. It is predominately composed of <u>compact bone</u>. This kind of bone is very strong and resistant to bending and has no trabeculae or bone marrow cavities.

Animals that fly have less dense, more light bones (spongy bone) in order to facilitate flying. Animals that swim do not need to have as strong bones as land animals as the buoyant force of the water takes away from the everyday stress on the bones. In the adult, yellow marrow is likely to be found in the diaphysis while red marrow is likely to be found in the epiphysis.

Bone growth occurs in two ways, intramembranous and endochondral bone formation. Both formations produce bones that are histologically identical. Intramembranous bone formation begins as layers of membranous connective tissue, which are later calcified by osteoblasts. Most of the flat bones are formed by this process. Endochondral bone formation is the process by which most of long bones are formed. It begins with hyaline cartilage that functions as a template for the bone to grow on.

Vascularizaton of the cartilage causes the transformation of cartilage cells to bone cells (osteoblasts), which later form a cartilage-calcified bone matrix. The osteoblasts continue to replace cartilage with bone and the osteoclasts create perforations to form bone marrow cavities. In children one can detect an **epiphyseal growth plate** on X-ray. This plate is a disk of cartilage between the epiphysis and diaphysis where bone is being actively deposited (= *ossification*).

11.3.2 Joint Structure

Articulations or joints are junctions between bones. They can be **immovable** like the dense connective tissue sutures which hold the flat bones of the skull together; **partly movable** like the hyaline and fibrocartilage joints on disks of the vertebrae; or **freely movable** like the synovial joints which are the most prominent joints in the skeletal system. Synovial joints contain a joint capsule composed of outer ligaments and an inner layer (= *the synovial membrane*) which secretes a lubricant (= *synovial fluid*).

Freely movable joints can be of many types. For example, ball and socket joints have a wide range of motion, like the shoulder and hip joints. On the other hand, hinge joints allow motion in only one plane like a hinged door (i.e. the knee, elbow, and interphalangeal joints).

11.3.3 Cartilage

The microscopic aspects of cartilage have already been discussed (*see Dense Connective Tissue*, BIO 5.4.2/3). Opposing and mobile surfaces of bone are covered by various forms of cartilage. As already mentioned, joints with hyaline or fibrocartilage allow little movement.

Ligaments attach bone to bone. They are formed by dense bands of fibrous connective tissue which reinforce the joint capsule and help to maintain bones in the proper anatomical arrangement.

Tendons connect muscle to bone. They are formed by the densest kind of fibrous connective tissue. Tendons allow muscular forces to be exerted even when the body (*or belly*) of the muscle is at some distance from the action.

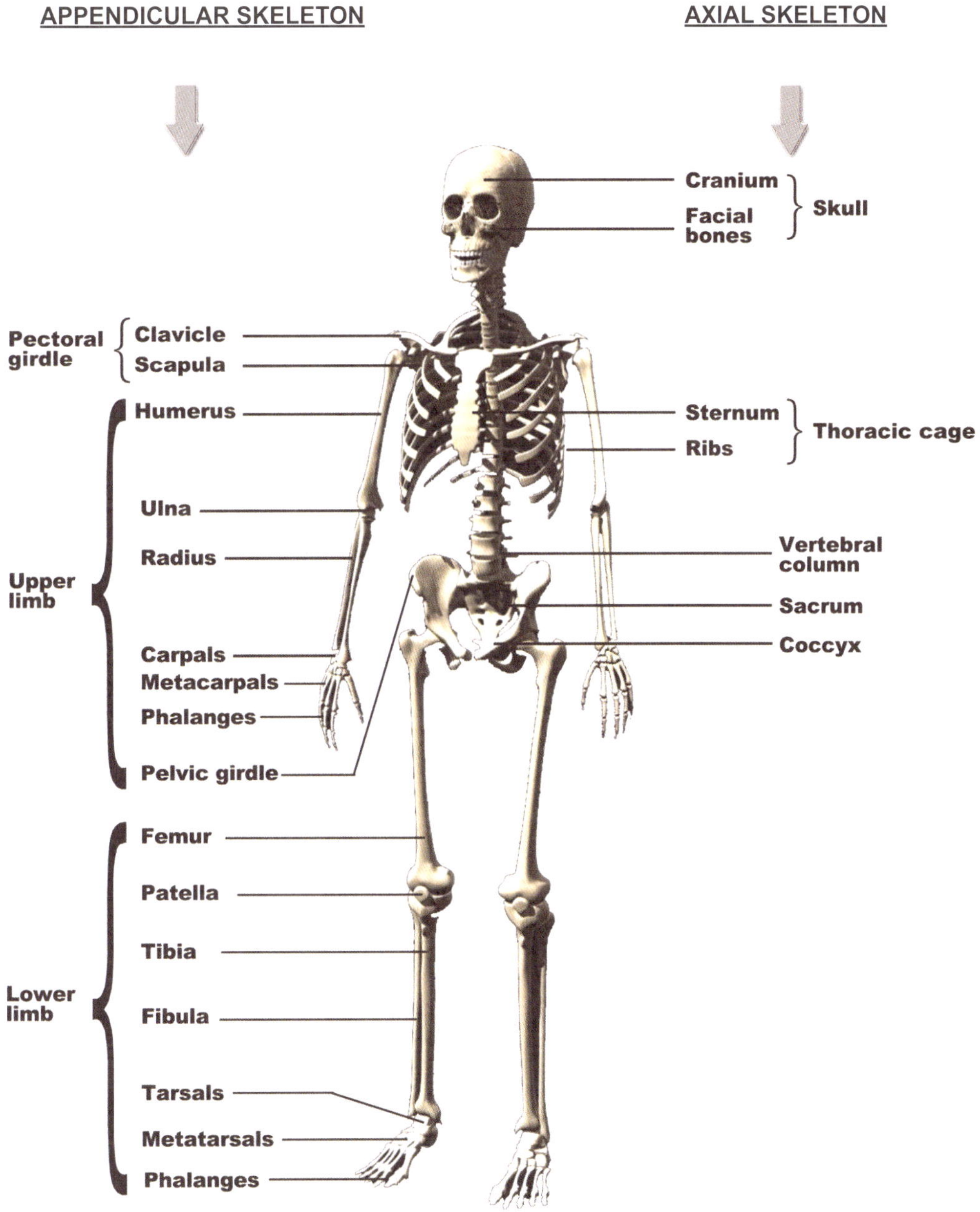

BIOLOGY

APPENDICULAR SKELETON   **AXIAL SKELETON**

- Cranium ⎫
- Facial bones ⎭ Skull

Pectoral girdle { Clavicle, Scapula

- Sternum ⎫
- Ribs ⎭ Thoracic cage

Upper limb { Humerus, Ulna, Radius, Carpals, Metacarpals, Phalanges }

- Vertebral column
- Sacrum
- Coccyx

Pelvic girdle

Lower limb { Femur, Patella, Tibia, Fibula, Tarsals, Metatarsals, Phalanges }

Figure IV.A.11.2: Skeletal structure. Note: in brackets some common relations - scapula (shoulder blade), clavicle (collarbone), carpals (wrist), metacarpals (palm), phalanges (fingers), tibia (shin), patella (kneecap), tarsals (ankle), metatarsals (foot), phalanges (toes), vertebral column (backbone). Note that the appendicular skeleton includes the bones of the appendages and the pectoral and pelvic girdles. The axial skeleton consists of the skull, vertebral column, and the rib cage.

Go online to GAMSAT-prep.com for additional chapter review Q&A and forum.

THE BIOLOGICAL SCIENCES   BIO-145

GOLD NOTES

THE RESPIRATORY SYSTEM
Chapter 12

Memorize
sic anatomy and order

Understand
* Basic functions: gas exchange/thermoreg.
* Protection against disease, particulate matter
* Breathing mechanisms: diaphragm, rib cage, differential pressure
* Resiliency and surface tension effects
* The carbonic acid-bicarbonate buffer
* Henry's Law

Not Required*
* Advanced level college info

GAMSAT-Prep.com

Introduction

The respiratory system permits the exchange of gases with the organism's environment. This critical process occurs in the microscopic space between alveoli and capillaries. It is here where molecules of oxygen and carbon dioxide passively diffuse between the gaseous external environment and the blood.

Additional Resources

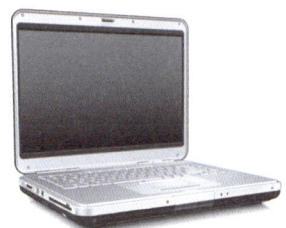

Free Online Q&A + Forum

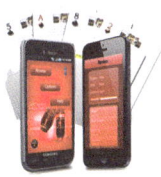

Flashcards

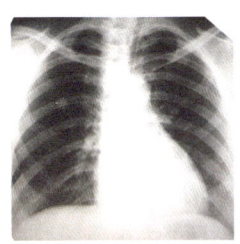

Special Guest

THE BIOLOGICAL SCIENCES   BIO-147

* The real GAMSAT may have advanced level information presented (ie. in a passage) but previous knowledge of said information is not required to answer the questions that would follow. Practice ACER and GS practice GAMSATs can help you clarify this point.

GAMSAT-Prep.com
THE GOLD STANDARD

12.1 Overview

There are two forms of respiration: cellular respiration which refers to the oxidation of organic molecules (see BIO 4.4 - 4.10) and mechanical respiration where the gases related to cellular respiration are exchanged between the atmosphere and the circulatory system (O_2 in and CO_2 out).

The respiratory system, which is concerned with mechanical respiration, has the following principal functions:

- providing a conducting system for the exchange of gases
- the filtration of incoming particles
- to help control the water content and temperature (= *thermoregulation*) of the incoming air
- to assist in speech production, the sense of smell, and the regulation of pH.

The respiratory system is composed of the lungs and a series of airways that connect the lungs to the external environment, deliver air to the lungs and perform gas exchange.

12.2 The Upper Respiratory Tract

The respiratory system can be divided into an *upper* and *lower respiratory tract* which are separated by the pharynx. The **upper respiratory tract** is composed of the nose, the nasal cavity, the sinuses, and the nasopharynx. This portion of the respiratory system warms, moistens and filters the air before it reaches the lower respiratory system. The nose (*nares*) has receptors for the sense of smell. It is guarded by hair to entrap coarse particles. The nasal cavity, the hollow space behind the nose, contains a ciliated mucous membrane (= a form of *respiratory epithelium*) to entrap smaller particles and prevent infection (this arrangement is common throughout the respiratory tract; for cilia see *the Generalized Eukaryotic Cell*, BIO 1.2). The nasal cavity adjusts the humidity and temperature of incoming air. The nasopharynx helps to equilibrate pressure between the environment and the middle ear via the eustachian tube (BIO 6.2.3).

12.3 The Lower Respiratory Tract

The **lower respiratory tract** is composed of the larynx which contains the vocal cords, the trachea which divides into left and right main bronchi which continue to divide into smaller airways (→ 2° bronchi → 3° bronchi → bronchioles → terminal bronchioles). The terminal bronchioles are the most distal part of the conducting portion of the respira-

BIOLOGY

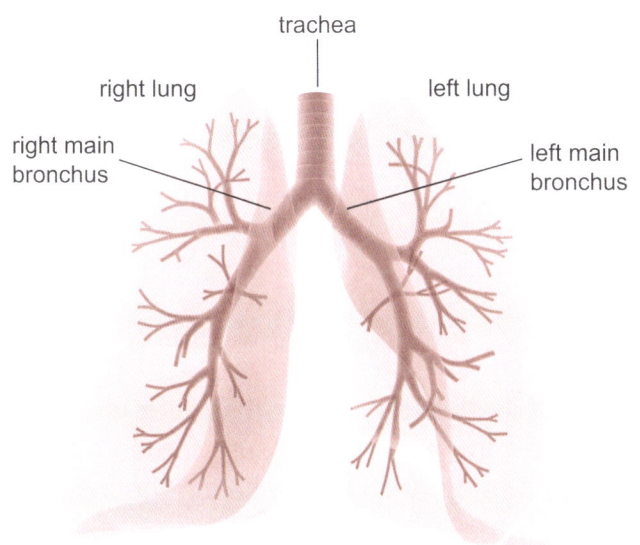

Figure IV.A.12.1: Illustration representing the lower respiratory tract including the dividing bronchial tree and grape-shaped alveoli with blood supply. Note that "right" refers to the patient's perspective which means the left side from your perspective.

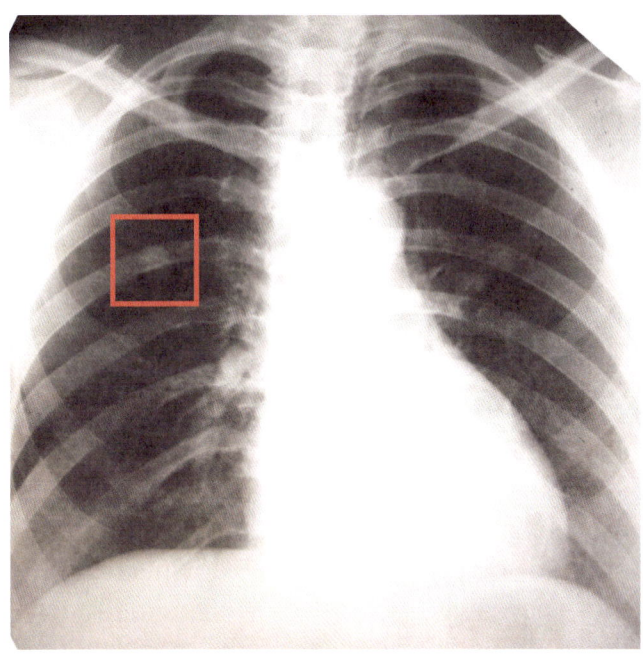

Figure IV.A.12.2: Chest x-ray of an adult male smoker. Notice the coin-shaped shadow in the right lung which presented with coughing blood. Further tests confirmed the presence of a right lung cancer. Cancer-causing chemicals (carcinogens) can irritate any of the cells lining the lower respiratory tract.

tory system. Starting from respiratory bronchioles → alveolar ducts → alveolar sacs until the level of the alveolus, these are considered the respiratory portion of respiratory system, where gas exchange takes place.

It is in these microscopic air sacs called *alveoli* that O_2 diffuses through the alveolar walls and enters the blood in nearby capillaries (where the concentration or *partial pressure* of O_2 is lowest and CO_2 is highest) and CO_2 diffuses from the blood through the walls to enter the alveoli (where the partial pressure of CO_2 is lowest and O_2 is highest). Gas exchange occurs by diffusion across the blood-gas barrier between the alveolar airspace and the capillary lumen. The blood-gas barrier is composed of three layers: type I pneumocyte cells, fused basal laminae and the endothelium of capillaries. *Alveolar macrophages* are phagocytes which help to engulf particles which reach the alveolus. A *surfactant* is secreted into alveoli by special lung cells (*pneumocytes type II*). The surfactant reduces surface tension and prevents the fragile alveoli from collapsing.

Sneezing and coughing, which are reflexes mediated by the medulla, can expel particles from the upper and lower respiratory tract, respectively.

THE BIOLOGICAL SCIENCES   BIO-149

The **lungs** are separated into left and right and are enclosed by the diaphragm and the thoracic cage. It is covered by a membrane (= *pleura*) which secretes a lubricant to reduce friction while breathing. The lungs contain the air passages, nerves, alveoli, blood and lymphatic vessels of the lower respiratory tract.

12.4 Breathing: Structures and Mechanisms

Inspiration is active and occurs according to the following main events: i) nerve impulses from the phrenic nerve cause the muscular diaphragm to contract; as the dome shaped diaphragm moves downward, the thoracic cavity increases; ii) simultaneously, the intercostal (= *between ribs*) muscles and/or certain neck muscles may contract further increasing the thoracic cavity (the muscles mentioned here are called *accessory respiratory muscles* and under normal circumstances the action of the diaphragm is much more important); iii) as the size of the thoracic cavity increases, its internal pressure decreases leaving it relatively negative; iv) the relatively positive atmospheric pressure forces air into the respiratory tract thus inflating the lungs.

Expiration is passive and occurs according to the following main events: i) the diaphragm and the accessory respiratory muscles relax and the chest wall pushed inward; ii) the elastic tissues of the lung, thoracic cage, and the abdominal organs recoil to their original position; iii) this recoil increases the pressure within the lungs (making the pressure relatively positive) thus forcing air out of the lungs and passageways.

12.4.1 Control of Breathing

Though voluntary breathing is possible (!), normally breathing is involuntary, rhythmic, and controlled by the *respiratory center* in the medulla of the brain stem. The respiratory center is sensitive to pH of the cerebrospinal fluid (CSF). An increase in blood CO_2 or consequently, decrease in pH of the CSF, acts on the respiratory center and stimulates breathing, returning the arterial pCO_2 (partial pressure of carbon dioxide) back to normal. The increase in blood CO_2 and the decrease in pH are two interrelated events since CO_2 can be picked up by hemoglobin forming carbamino-hemoglobin (about 20%, BIO 7.5.1), but it can also be converted into carbonic acid by dissolving in blood plasma (about 5%) or by conversion in red blood cells by the enzyme *carbonic anhydrase* (about 75%). The reaction is summarized as follows:

$$CO_2 + H_2O \leftrightarrow \underset{\text{carbonic acid}}{H_2CO_3} \leftrightarrow \underset{\text{bicarbonate}}{HCO_3^-} + H^+$$

According to Henry's Law, the concentration of a gas dissolved in solution is directly proportional to its partial pressure. From the preceding you can see why the respiratory system, through the regulation of the partial pressure of CO_2 in blood, also helps in maintaining pH homeostasis (= a buffer). More generally, the carbonic-acid-bicarbonate buffer is the most important buffer for maintaining acid-base balance in the blood and helps to maintain pH around 7.4.

12.4.2 Henry's Law, Pop and The Bends

Higher gas pressure and lower temperature cause more gas to dissolve in a liquid. When a carbonated drink (soda/pop) is manufactured, water is chilled, optimally to just above freezing, in order to permit the maximum amount of carbon dioxide to dissolve. Then CO_2 is pumped in at high pressure, the pressure is maintained by closing the container (can or bottle), which forces the carbon dioxide to dissolve into the liquid, creating carbonic acid (Le Chatelier's principle; CHM 9.9) and giving 'pop' its tang. Flat soda tastes strange, or at least less pleasant, because of the loss of carbonic acid due to the release of carbon dioxide bubbles/fizz.

So pop is stored in a way to seal pressure, preventing gas escape and maintaining the supersaturation of CO_2 in the solvent. It is pressure and temperature that drive the outgassing process.

Diving underwater exposes the body to increasing pressure (PHY 6.1). A diving cylinder (scuba tank) is used to store and transport high pressure breathing gas. As the dive becomes deeper, inhaled gas is absorbed into body tissue in higher concentrations than normal (Henry's Law). Surfacing from a deep dive underwater, unused gases (inert) like nitrogen try to do the same thing in your bloodstream that happens when you open a container of pop. The release of these bubbles (outgassing) produces the symptoms of decompression sickness (= 'the bends') that can be painful or even fatal. {Breathing (BIO 12.4), carbon dioxide-carbonic acid, and Henry's Law, are the source of the most likely GAMSAT questions from this chapter.}

Go online to GAMSAT-prep.com for additional chapter review Q&A and forum.

GOLD NOTES

THE SKIN AS AN ORGAN SYSTEM
Chapter 13

Memorize
Structure and function of skin, layer differentiation
Sweat glands; nails

Understand
* Skin system: homeostasis and osmoregulation
* Functions in thermoregulation: hair, erectile musculature, fat layer for insulation
* Vasoconstriction and vasodilation in surface capillaries
* Physical protection: nails, calluses, hair; protection against abrasion, disease organisms
* Relative impermeability to water

Not Required*
* Advanced level college info

GAMSAT-Prep.com

Introduction

Skin is composed of layers of epithelial tissues which protect underlying muscle, bone, ligaments and internal organs. Thus skin has many roles including protecting the body from microbes, insulation, temperature regulation, sensation and synthesis of vitamin D.

Additional Resources

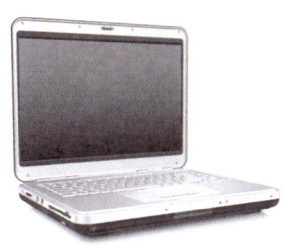

Free Online Q&A + Forum

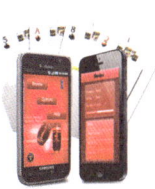

Flashcards

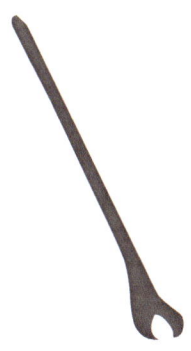

Special Guest

THE BIOLOGICAL SCIENCES BIO-153

* The real GAMSAT may have advanced level information presented (ie. in a passage) but previous knowledge of said information is not required to answer the questions that would follow. Practice ACER and GS practice GAMSATs can help you clarify this point.

GAMSAT-Prep.com
THE GOLD STANDARD

13.1 Overview

The skin, or *integument*, is the body's largest organ. The following represents its major functions:

* **Physical protection:** The skin protects against the onslaught of the environment including uv light, chemical, thermal or even mechanical agents. It also serves as a barrier to the invasion of microorganisms.

* **Sensation:** The skin, being the body's largest sensory organ, contains a wide range of sensory receptors including those for pain, temperature, light touch, and pressure.

* **Metabolism:** Vitamin D synthesis can occur in the epidermis of skin (*see Endocrine Systems*, BIO 6.3). Also, energy is stored as fat in subcutaneous adipose tissue.

* **Thermoregulation and osmoregulation:** Skin is vital for the homeostatic mechanism of thermoregulation and to a lesser degree osmoregulation. Hair (*piloerection*, which can trap a layer of warm air against the skin's surface) and especially subcutaneous fat (*adipose tissue*) insulate the body against heat loss. Shivering, which allows muscle to generate heat, and decreasing blood flow to the skin (= *vasoconstriction*) are important in emergencies.

On the other hand, heat and water loss can be increased by increasing blood flow to the multitude of blood vessels (= *vasodilation*) in the dermis (cooling by radiation), the production of sweat, and the evaporation of sweat due to the heat at the surface of the skin; thus the skin cools. {Remember: the **hypothalamus** also regulates body temperature (*see The Nervous System*, BIO 6.1); it is like a thermostat which uses other organs as tools to maintain our body temperatures at about 37 °C (98.6 °F)}.

13.2 The Structure of Skin

Skin is divided into three layers: i) the outer **epidermis** which contains a stratified squamous keratinized epithelium; ii) the inner **dermis** which contains vessels, nerves, muscle, and connective tissues; iii) the innermost **subcutaneous layer**, known as hypodermis, which contains adipose and a loose connective tissue; this layer binds to any underlying organs.

The epidermis is divided into several different layers or *strata*. The deepest layer, *stratum basale*, contains actively dividing cells (keratinocytes) which are nourished by the vessels in the dermis. The mitotic activity of keratinocytes can keep regenerating epidermis approximately every 30 days. As these cells continue to divide, older epidermal cells are pushed towards the surface of the skin - *away from the nutrient providing dermal layer*; thus in time they die. Simultaneously, these cells are actively producing strands of a tough, fibrous, waterproof protein called keratin. This process is called *keratinization*. The two preceding events lead to the formation of an outermost layer (= *stratum corneum*) of keratin-filled dead cells which are devoid of organelles and are continuously shed by a process called *desquamation*.

Melanin is a dark pigment produced by cells (= *melanocytes*) whose cell bodies are usually found in the stratum basale. Melanin absorbs light thus protects against uv light induced cell damage (i.e. sunburns, skin cancer). Individuals have about the same number of melanocytes - regardless of race. Melanin production depends on genetic factors (i.e. race) and it can be stimulated by exposure to sunlight (i.e. tanning).

Langerhans cells have long processes and contain characteristic tennis-racket-shaped Birbeck granules. They function as antigen presenting cells in the immune response (BIO 8.2, 8.3).

Merkel cells are present in the richly innervated areas of stratum basale. They are responsible for receiving afferent nerve impulses and function as sensory mechano-receptors (BIO 6.1.1).

The dermis is composed of dense irregular connective tissue including type I collagen fibers and a network of elastic fibers. It contains the blood vessels which nourish the various cells in the skin. It also contains motor fibers and many types of sensory nerve fibers such as fine touch receptors, pressure receptors and cold receptors.

13.3 Skin Appendages

The **appendages** of the skin include hair, sebaceous glands and sweat glands. Hair is a modified keratinized structure produced by a cylindrical downgrowth of epithelium (= *hair follicle*). The follicle extends into the dermis (sometimes the subcutaneous tissue as well). The arrector pili muscle attaches to the connective tissue surrounding a hair follicle. When this bundle of smooth muscle contracts (= *piloerection*), it elevates the hair and "goose bumps" are produced.

The sebaceous glands are lobular acinar glands that empty their ducts into the hair follicles. They are most abundant on the face, forehead and scalp. They release an oily/waxy secretion called sebum to lubricate and waterproof the skin.

Sweat glands can be classified as either eccrine sweat glands, which are simple tubular glands present in the skin throughout the body or apocrine sweat glands, which are large specialized glands located only in certain areas of the body (i.e. areola of the nipple, perianal area, axilla which is the "armpit") and will not function until puberty.

We have previously explored endocrine glands and saw how they secrete their products - without the use of a duct - directly into the bloodstream (BIO 6.3). Alternatively, endo-

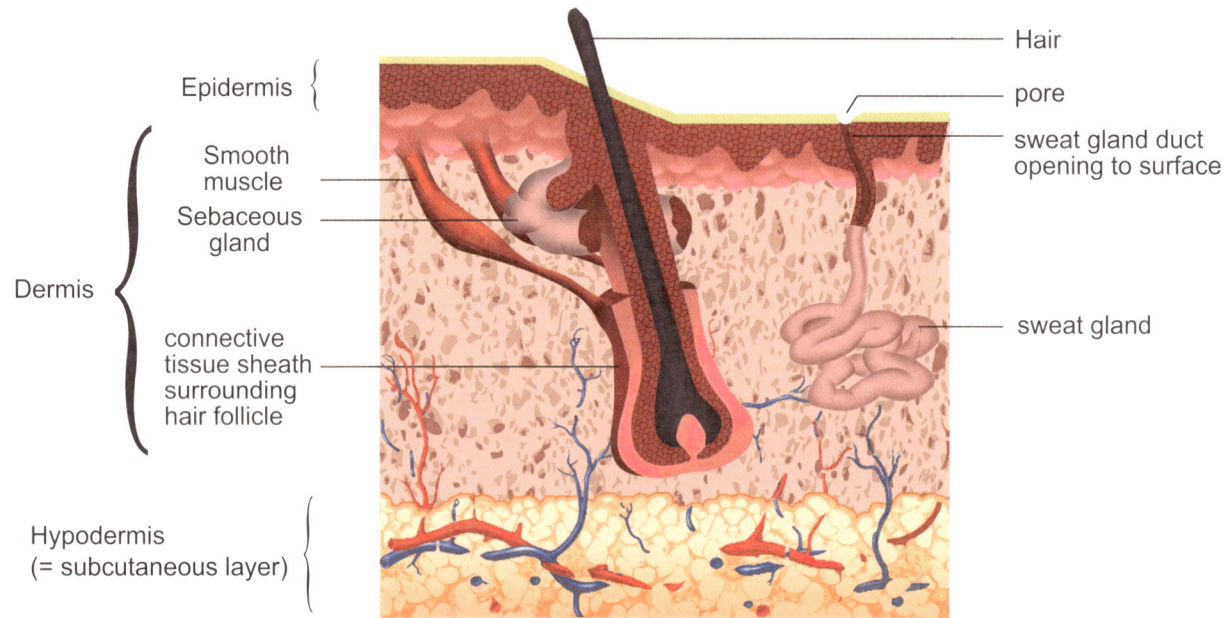

Figure IV.A.13.1: Skin structure with appendages.

crine products may diffuse into surrounding tissue (*paracrine signaling*) where they often affect only target cells near the release site.

An exocrine gland is distinguished by the fact that it excretes its product via a duct to some environment external to itself, either inside the body (BIO 9.3, 9.4) or on a surface of the body. Examples of exocrine glands include the sebaceous glands, sweat glands, salivary glands, mammary glands, pancreas and liver.

Holocrine (= *wholly secretory*) is a type of glandular secretion in which the entire secreting cell, along with its accumulated secretion, forms the secreted matter of the gland; for example, the sebaceous glands. Apocrine concentrates products at the free end of the secreting cell and are thrown off along with a portion of the cytoplasm (i.e. mammary gland, axilla). Eccrine, apocrine and holocrine are subdivisions of exocrine.

13.3.1 Nails, Calluses

Nails are flat, translucent, keratinized coverings near the tip of fingers and toes. In humans, nails grow at an average rate of 3 mm (0.12 in) per month.

A callus is a toughened, thickened area of skin. It is usually created in response to repeated friction or pressure thus they are normally found on the hands or feet.

GOLD NOTES

Go online to GAMSAT-prep.com for additional chapter review Q&A and forum.

GOLD NOTES

REPRODUCTION AND DEVELOPMENT
Chapter 14

Memorize	Understand	Not Required*
ale and female reproductive structures, nctions vum, sperm: differences in formation, lative contribution to next generation eproductive sequence: fertilization; mplantation; development ajor structures arising out of primary rm layers	* Gametogenesis by meiosis * Formation of primary germ layers: endoderm, mesoderm, ectoderm * Embryogenesis: stages of early development: order and general features of each * Cell specialization, communication in development, gene regulation in development * Programmed cell death; basic: the menstrual cycle	* Advanced level college info

GAMSAT-Prep.com

Introduction

Reproduction refers to the process by which new organisms are produced. The process of development follows as the single celled zygote grows into a fully formed adult. These two processes are fundamental to life as we know it.

Additional Resources

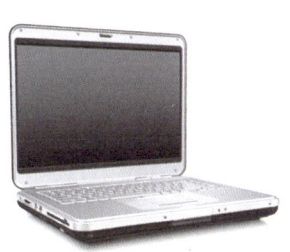

Free Online Q&A + Forum

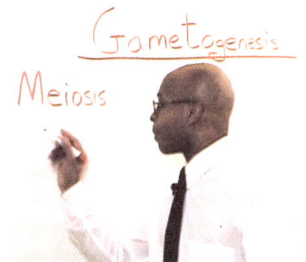

Video: Online or DVD

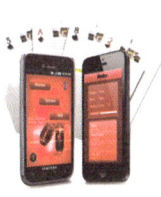

Flashcards

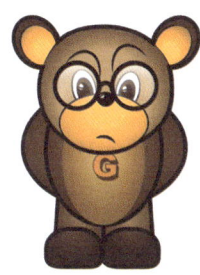

Special Guest

THE BIOLOGICAL SCIENCES   BIO-159

* The real GAMSAT may have advanced level information presented (ie. in a passage) but previous knowledge of said information is not required to answer the questions that would follow. Practice ACER and GS practice GAMSATs can help you clarify this point.

14.1 Organs of the Reproductive System

Gonads are the organs which produce gametes (= germ cells = reproductive cells). The female gonads are the two ovaries which lie in the pelvic cavity. Opening around the ovaries and connecting to the uterus are the Fallopian tubes (= *oviducts*) which conduct the egg (= *ovum*) from the ovary to the uterus. The uterus is a muscular organ. Part of the uterus (= the cervix) protrudes into the vagina or *birth canal*. The vagina leads to the external genitalia. The vulva includes the openings of the vagina, various glands, and folds of skin which are large (= labia majora) and small (= labia minora). The clitoris is found between the labia minora at the anterior end of the vulva. Like the glans penis, it is very sensitive as it is richly innervated. However, the clitoris is unique in being the only organ in the human body devoted solely to sensory pleasure.

The male gonads are the two testicles (= *testes*) which are suspended by spermatic cords in a sac-like scrotum outside the body cavity (this is because the optimal temperature for spermatogenesis is less than body temperature). Sperm (= *spermatozoa*) are produced in the seminiferous tubules in the testes and then continue along a system of ducts including: the epididymis where sperm complete their maturation and are collected and stored; the vas deferens which leads to the ejaculatory duct which in turn leads to the penile urethra which conducts to the exterior. The accessory organs include the seminal vesicles, the bulbourethral and prostate glands. They are exocrine glands whose secretions contribute greatly to the volume of the *ejaculate* (= semen = seminal fluid). The penis is composed of a body or shaft, which contains an erectile tissue which can be engorged by blood; a penile urethra which can conduct either urine or sperm; and a very sensitive head or glans penis which may be covered by foreskin (= *prepuce*, which is removed by circumcision).

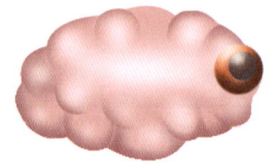 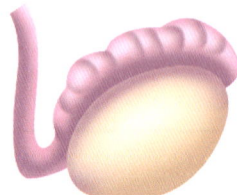

Figure IV.A.14.0: An ovulating ovary and a testicle with spermatic cord.

14.2 Gametogenesis

Gametogenesis refers to the production of gametes (eggs and sperm) which occurs by meiosis (*see Mitosis*, BIO 1.3, *for comparison*). Meiosis involves two successive divisions which can produce four cells from one parent cell. The first division, the reduction division, reduces the number of chromosomes from 2N (= *diploid*) to N (= *haploid*) where N = 23 for humans. This reduction division occurs as follows: i) in **prophase I** the chromosomes appear (= *condensed chromatin*), the nuclear membrane and nucleoli disappear and the spindle fibers become organized. Homologous paternal and maternal chromosomes pair[1] (= *synapsis*) forming a tetrad as each pair of homologous chromosomes consists of four chromatids. The exchange of genetic information (DNA) may occur by crossing over between homologous chromosomes at sites called *chiasmata*, therefore redistributing maternal and paternal genetic information ensuring variability; ii) **in metaphase I** the synaptic pairs of chromosomes line up midway between the poles of the developing spindle (= *the equatorial plate*). Thus each pair consists of 2 chromosomes (= 4 chromatids), each attached to a spindle fiber; iii) in **anaphase I** the homologous chromosomes migrate to opposite poles of the spindle, separating its paternal chromosomes from maternal ones. Thus, each daughter cell will have a unique mixture of paternal and maternal origin of chromosomes. In contrast to anaphase in mitosis, the two chromatids remain held together. Consequently, the centromeres do *not* divide; iv) in **telophase I** the parent cell divides into two daughter cells (= *cytokinesis*), the nuclear membranes and nucleoli reappear, and the spindle fibers are no longer visible. Each daughter cell now contains 23 chromosomes (1N).

The first meiotic division is followed by a short interphase I and then the second meiotic division which proceeds essentially the same as mitosis. Thus prophase II, metaphase II, anaphase II, and telophase II proceed like the corresponding mitotic phases.

Gametogenesis in males (= *spermatogenesis*) proceeds as follows: before the age of sexual maturity only a small number of primordial germ cells (= *spermatogonia*) are present in the testes. There are two types of spermatogonia, type A and type B. Type A spermatogonia (2N) are mitotically active and continuously provide a supply of type A or type B spermatogonia. Type B spermatogonia (2N) undergo meiosis and will give rise to primary spermatocytes. After sexual maturation these cells prolifically multiply throughout a male's life.

In the seminiferous tubules, the type B spermatogonia (2N) enter meiosis I and undergo chromosome replication forming primary spermatocytes with 2N chromosomes. Primary spermatocytes complete meiosis I producing two secondary spermatocytes with 1N chromosomes. Secondary spermatocytes quickly enter meiosis II without an intervening S phase to form four spermatids. Spermatids are haploid (1N) cells.

In summary, each primary spermatocyte results in the production of four spermatids. Spermatids undergo a post-meiotic cytodifferentiation whereby spermatids are transformed into **four** motile sperm (1N) through a process called *spermiogenesis*.

Sperm can be divided into: i) a *head* which is oval and contains the nucleus with its 23 chromosomes {since the nucleus carries either an X or Y sex chromosome, sperm determine the sex of the offspring}. The head is partly surrounded by the acrosome which contains enzymes (esp. hyaluronidase) which help the sperm penetrate the egg. The

---

[1] synapsing homologous chromosomes are often called tetrads or bivalents.

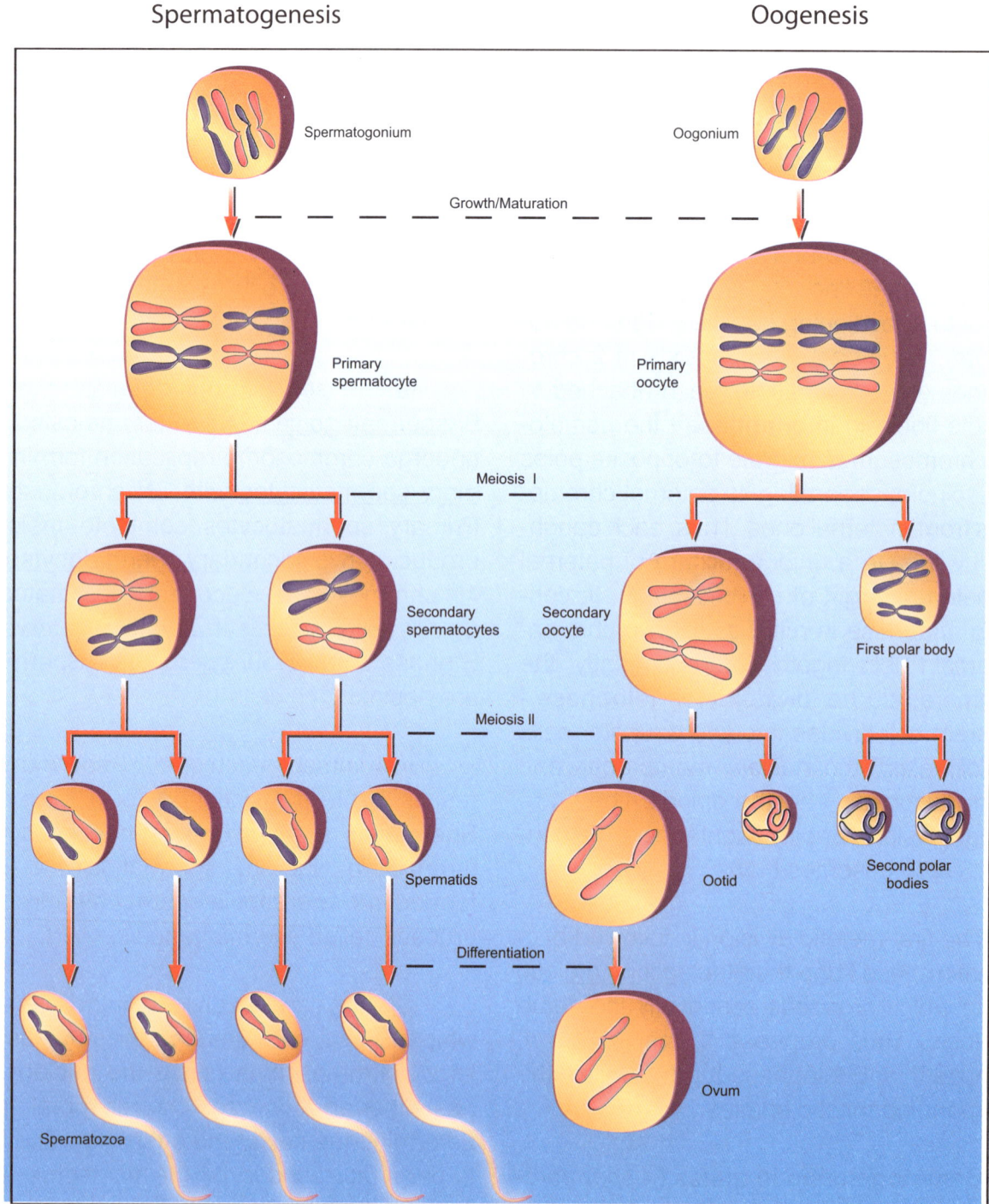

Figure IV.A.14.0a: Gametogenesis.

release of these enzymes is known as the acrosomal reaction; ii) the *body* of the sperm contains a central core surrounded by a large number of mitochondria for power; and iii) the *tail* constitutes a flagellum which is critical for the cell's locomotion. Newly formed sperm are incapable of fertilization until they undergo a process called capacitation, which happens in the female reproductive duct. After removal of its protein coating, the sperm becomes capable of fertilization. Also in the seminiferous tubules are Sertoli cells which support and nourish developing sperm and Leydig cells which produce and secrete testosterone. While LH stimulates the latter, FSH stimulates primary spermatocytes to undergo meiosis. {Remember: LH = Leydig, FSH = spermatogenesis}

Gametogenesis in females (= *oogenesis*) proceeds as follows: in fetal development, groups of cells (= *ovarian or primordial follicles*) develop from the germinal epithelium of the ovary) and differentiate into oogonia (2N). Oogonia (2N) enter meiosis I and undergo DNA replication producing primary oocytes (2N) which are surrounded by epithelia (= *follicular cells*) in the primordial follicle. The oocytes remain arrested in prophase I of meiosis until ovulation which occurs between the ages of about 13 (sexual maturity) and 50 (menopause). Thus, unlike males, all female germ cells are present at birth. Some follicles degenerate and are called *atretic*. During puberty, when the ovarian cycle begins, up to 20 primordial follicles may begin to differentiate to *Graafian follicles*. During this development, meiosis continues. In response to an LH surge from the pituitary gland, the primary oocyte (2N) completes meiosis I just prior to ovulation to form the secondary oocyte (1N) and the first polar body, which will probably degenerate. The secondary oocyte is surrounded by (from the inside out): a thick, tough membrane (= *the zona pellucida*), follicular cells (= *the corona radiata*), and estrogen-secreting thecal cells. It then enters meiosis II and remains arrested in metaphase of meiosis II until fertilization occurs.

Of the twenty or so maturing follicles, all the remaining secondary follicles will degenerate (= *atresia*) except for one which becomes the Graafian (mature) follicle. In response to the LH surge, the secondary oocyte leaves the ruptured Graafian follicle in the process called ovulation. This ovum, along with its zona pellucida and corona radiata, migrate to and through the Fallopian tube (oviduct) where a sperm may penetrate the secondary oocyte (= *fertilization*). If fertilization occurs then the second meiotic division proceeds, forming a mature oocyte, known as ovum, (1N) and a second polar body; if fertilization does not occur, then the ovum degenerates. Unlike in males, each primary germ cell (oocyte) produces one gamete and not four. This is a consequence of the production of *polar bodies* which are degenerated nuclear material. Up to three polar bodies can be formed: one from the division of the primary oocyte, one from the division of the secondary oocyte, and sometimes the first polar body divides.

14.3 The Menstrual Cycle

The "period" or menstrual cycle occurs in about 28 days and can be divided as follows: i) **Menses:** the first four days (days 1-4) of the cycle are notable for the menstrual blood flow. This occurs as a result of an estrogen and progesterone withdrawal which leads to vasoconstriction in the uterus causing the uterine lining (= *endometrium*) to disintegrate and slough away; ii) **Follicular** (ovary) or **Proliferative Phase** (days 5-14): FSH stimulates follicles to mature, and all but one of these follicles will stop growing, and the one dominant follicle in the ovary will continue to mature into a Graafian follicle, which in turn produces and secretes estrogen. Estrogen causes the uterine lining to thicken (= proliferate); iii) **Ovulation**: a very high concentration of estrogen is followed by an LH surge (estrogen-induced LH surge) at about day 15 (midcycle) which stimulates ovulation; iv) **Luteal** or **Secretory Phase** (days 15-28): the follicular cells degenerate into the corpus luteum which secretes estrogen *and* progesterone. Progesterone is responsible for a transient body temperature rise immediately after ovulation and it stimulates the uterine lining to become more vascular and glandular. Estrogen continues to stimulate uterine wall development and, along with progesterone, inhibits the secretion of LH and FSH (= negative feedback).

If the ovum is fertilized, the implanted embryo would produce the hormone *human chorionic gonadotropin* (= hCG) which would stimulate the corpus luteum to continue the secretion of estrogen and progesterone {hCG is the basis for most pregnancy tests}. If there is no fertilization, the corpus luteum degenerates causing a withdrawal of estrogen and progesterone thus the cycle continues [*see* i) *above*].

Estrous vs. menstrual cycles: Mammals with estrous cycles reabsorb the endometrium if conception does not occur during that cycle. Also, they are generally only sexually active during a specific phase of their cycle ("in heat"). In contrast, females of species with menstrual cycles (i.e. humans) can of course be sexually active at any time in their cycle, and the endometrium is shed monthly.

14.4 The Reproductive Sequence

During sexual stimulation parasympathetic impulses in the male lead to the dilation of penile arteries combined with restricted flow in the veins resulting in the engorgement of the penis with blood (= *an erection*). In the female, the preceding occurs in a similar manner to the clitoris, along with the expansion and increase in secretions in the vagina. Intercourse or copulation may lead to orgasm which includes many responses from the sympathetic nervous system. In the male, the ejaculation of semen accompanies orgasm. In the female, orgasm is accompanied by many reflexes including an increase in muscular activity of the uterus and the Fallopian tubes. The latter may help in the transport of the already motile sperm to reach the tubes where the egg might be.

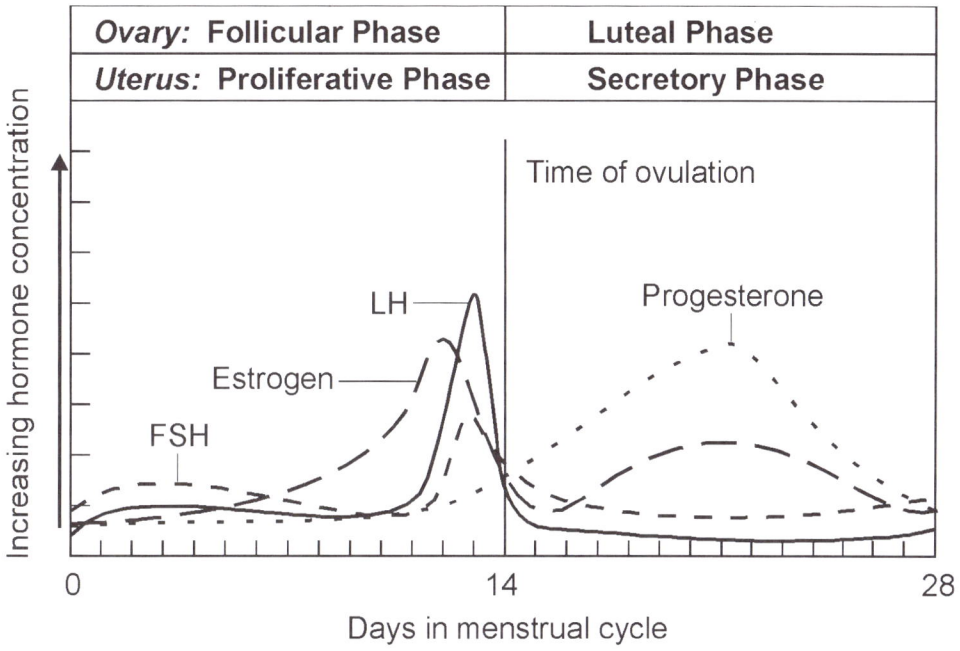

Figure IV.A.14.1: Changing hormone concentration during the menstrual cycle.

14.5 Embryogenesis

The formation of the embryo or *embryogenesis* occurs in a number of steps within two weeks of fertilization. Many parts of the developing embryo take shape during this period (= *morphogenesis*).

Penetration of the zona pellucida leads to the *cortical reaction*, in which the secondary oocyte is no longer permeable to other sperm.

Fertilization is a sequence of events which include: the sperm penetrating the corona radiata and the zona pellucidum due to the release of lytic enzymes from the acrosome known as the acrosome reaction; the fusion of the plasma membranes of the sperm and egg; the egg, which is really a secondary oocyte, becomes a mature ovum by completing the second meiotic division; the nuclei of the ovum and sperm are now called *pronuclei*; the male and female pronuclei fuse forming a zygote (2N). Fertilization, which normally occurs in the Fallopian tubes, is completed within 24 hours of ovulation.

Cleavage consists of rapid, repeated mitotic divisions beginning with the zygote.

Because the resultant daughter cells or blastomeres are still contained within the zona pellucidum, the cytoplasmic mass remains constant. Thus the increasing number of cells requires that each daughter cell be smaller than its parent cell. A morula is a solid ball of about 16 blastomeres which enters the uterus.

Blastulation is the process by which the morula develops a fluid filled cavity (= *blastocoel*) thus converting it to a blastocyst. Since the zona pellucidum degenerates at this point, the blastocyst is free to implant in the uterine lining or endometrium. The blastocyst contains some centrally located cells (= *the inner cell mass*) called the embryoblast which develops into the embryo. The outer cell mass called the trophoblast becomes part of the placenta.

Implantation. The zona pellucida must degenerate before the blastocyst can implant into the endometrium of the uterus. Once implantation is completed, the blastocyst becomes surrounded by layers of cells that further invade the endometrium.

Gastrulation is the process by which the blastula invaginates, and the inner cell mass is converted into a three layered (= *trilaminar*) disk. The trilaminar disk includes the **three primary germ layers**: an outer ectoderm, a middle mesoderm, and an inner endoderm. The ectoderm will develop into the epidermis and the nervous system; the mesoderm will become muscle, connective tissue (incl. blood, bone), and circulatory, reproductive and excretory organs; the endoderm will become the epithelial linings of the respiratory tract, and digestive tract, including the glands of the accessory organs (i.e. the liver and pancreas). During this stage the embryo may be called a gastrula.

Neurulation is the process by which the neural plate and neural folds form and close to produce the neural tube. The neural plate is formed by the thickening of ectoderm which is induced by the developing *notochord*. The notochord is a cellular rod that defines the axis of the embryo and provides some rigidity. Days later, the neural plate invaginates along its central axis producing a central neural groove with neural folds on each side. The neural folds come together and fuse thus converting the neural plate into a neural tube which separates from the surface ectoderm. Special cells on the crest of the neural folds (= *neural crest cells*) migrate to either side of the developing neural tube to a region called the neural crest.

As a consequence, we are left with **three** regions: the surface ectoderm which will become the epidermis; the neural tube which will become the central nervous system (CNS); and the neural crest which will become cranial and spinal ganglia and nerves and the medulla of the adrenal gland. During this stage the embryo may be called a *neurula*.

14.5.1 Mechanisms of Development

Though this is a subject which is still poorly understood, it seems clear that morphogenesis relies on the coordinated interaction of genetic and environmental factors. When the zygote passes through its first few divisions, the blastomeres remain indeterminate or uncommitted to a specific fate. As development proceeds the cells become increasingly committed to a specific outcome (i.e. neural tube cells → CNS). This is called **determination**.

In order for a cell to specialize it must differentiate into a committed or determined cell. Since essentially all cells in a person's body have the same amount of genetic information, differentiation relies on the *difference* in the way these genes are *activated*. For example, though brain cells (neurons) have the same genes as osteoblasts, neurons do not activate such genes (otherwise we would have bone forming in our brains!). The general mechanism by which cells differentiate is called **induction**.

Induction can occur by many means. If two cells divide unevenly, the cell with more cytoplasm might have the necessary amount of a substance which could *induce* its chromosomes to activate cell-specific genes. Furthermore, sometimes a cell, through contact (i.e. *contact inhibition*) or the release of a chemical mediator, can influence the development of nearby cells (*recall that the notochord induces the development of the neural plate*). The physical environment (pH, temperature, etc.) may also influence the development of certain cells. Irrespective of what form of induction is used, the signal must be translated into an intracellular message which influences the genetic activity of the responding cells.

Programmed cell-death (PCD = apoptosis) is death of a cell in any form, which is controlled by an intracellular program. PCD is carried out in a regulated process directed by DNA which normally confers advantage during an organism's life-cycle. PCD serves fundamental functions during tissue development. For example, the development of the spaces between your fingers requires cells to undergo PCD.

Thus cells specialize and develop into organ systems (morphogenesis). The embryo develops from the second to the ninth week, followed by the fetus which develops from the ninth week to birth (*parturition*).

14.6 The Placenta

The **placenta** is a complex vascular structure formed by part of the maternal endometrium (= *the decidua basalis*) and cells of embryonic origin (= *the chorion*). The placenta begins to form when the blastocyst implants in the endometrium. A cell layer from the embryo invades the endometrium with fingerlike bumps (= *chorionic villi*) which project into intervillous spaces which contain maternal blood. Maternal spiral arteries enter the intervillous spaces allowing blood to circulate.

The placenta has three main functions: i) the **transfer** of substances necessary for the development of the embryo or fetus from the mother (O_2, H_2O, carbohydrates, amino acids, IgG antibodies - BIO 8.2, vitamins, etc.) and the **transfer** of wastes from the embryo or fetus to the mother (CO_2, urea, uric acid, etc.); ii) the placenta can synthesize substances (i.e. glycogen, fatty acids) to use as an energy source for itself and the embryo or fetus; iii) the placenta produces and secretes a number of hormones including human chorionic gonadotropin (hCG), estrogen and progesterone. The hCG rescues the corpus luteum from regression and stimulates its production of progesterone.

14.7 Fetal Circulation

Consider the following: the fetus has lungs but does not breathe O_2. In fact, the placenta is, metaphorically, the "fetal lung." Oxygenated and nutrient-rich blood returns to the fetus from the placenta via the left umbilical vein. Most of the blood is directed to the inferior vena cava through the ductus venosus. From there, blood joins the deoxygenated and nutrient-poor blood from the superior vena cava and empties into the right atrium. However, most of the blood is diverted from the pulmonary circulation (bypassing the right ventricle) to the left atrium via a hole in the atrial septum: the patent foramen ovale (for adult circulation and anatomy, see chapter 7). Blood then enters the left ventricle and is distributed through the body (systemic circulation) via the aorta.

Some blood in the right atrium enters into the right ventricle and then proceeds into the pulmonary trunk. However, resistance in the collapsed lung is high and the pulmonary artery pressure is higher than it is in the aorta. Consequently, most of the blood bypasses the lung via the ductus arteriosus back to the aorta.

Blood circulates through the body and is sent back to the placenta via right and left umbilical arteries. The placenta re-oxygenates this deoxygenated and nutrient-poor blood and returns it to the fetus through the umbilical vein and the cardiovascular cycle repeats. Notice that in the fetus, oxygenated and nutrient-rich blood can be carried by veins to the right chambers of the heart which cannot occur in normal adult circulation.

BIOLOGY

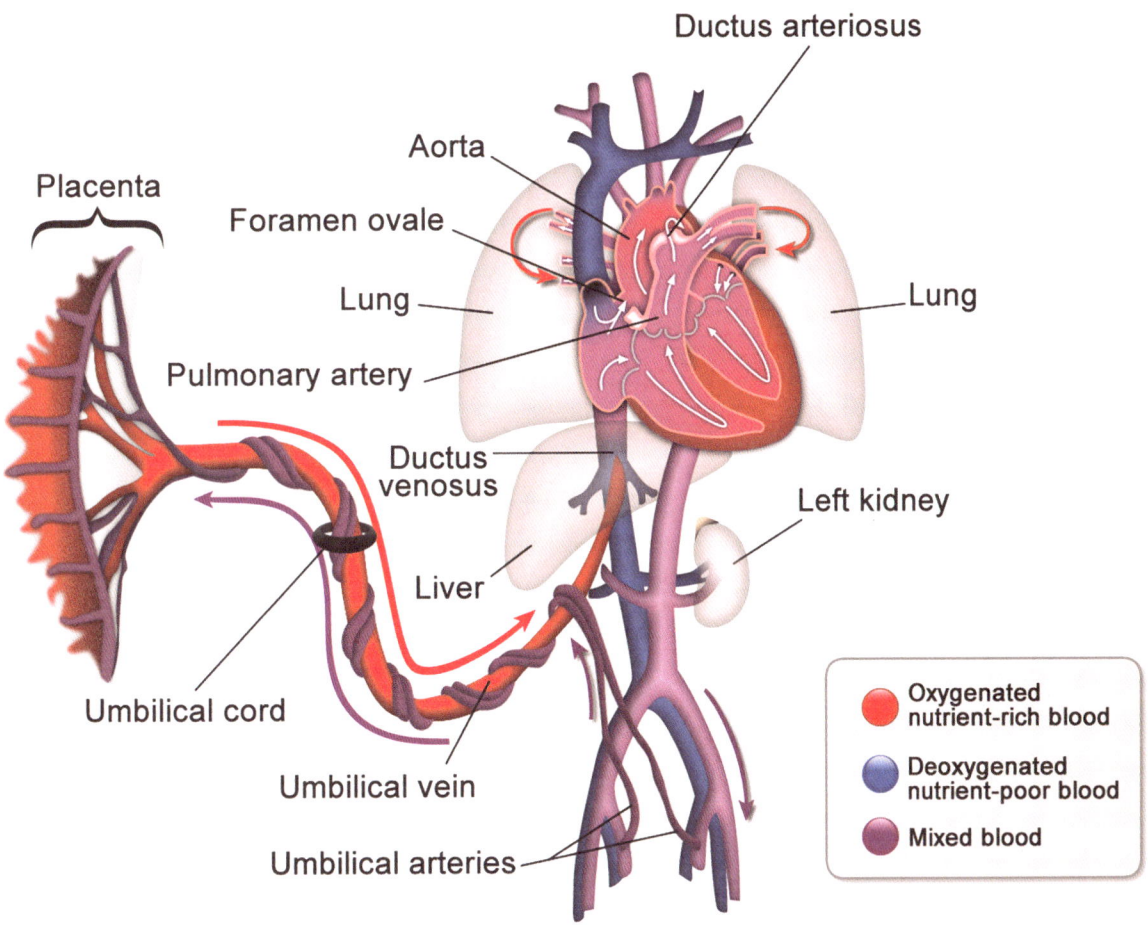

Fig.IV.A.14.2: Fetal circulation.

14.8 Fetal Sexual Development

The normal sexual development of the fetus depends on the genotype (XX female, XY male), the morphology of the internal organs and gonads, and the phenotype or external genitalia. Later, these many factors combine to influence the individual's self-perception along with the development of secondary sexual characteristics (i.e. breast development in females, hair growth and lower pitched voice in males).

Every fetus, regardless of genotype, has the capacity to become a normally formed individual of either sex. Development natu rally proceeds towards "female" unless there is a Y chromosome factor present. Thus the XX genotype leads to the maturation of the Müllerian ducts into the uterus, fallopian tubes, and part of the vagina. The primitive gonad will develop into a testis only if the Y chromosome is present and encodes the appropriate factor and eventually the secretion of testosterone. Thus the XY genotype leads to the involution of the Müllerian ducts and the maturation of the Wolffian ducts into the vas deferens, seminiferous tubules and prostate.

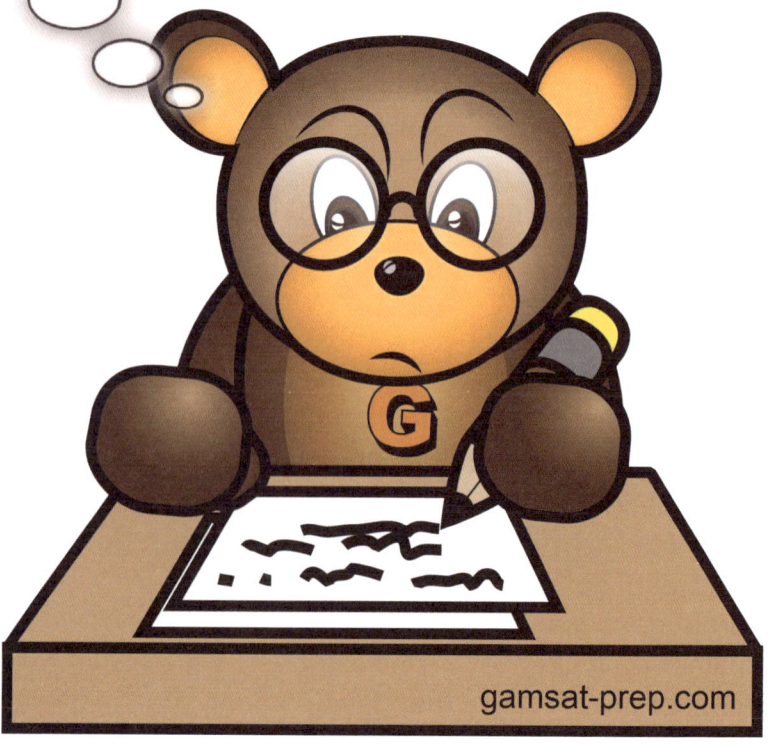

GOLD NOTES

GOLD NOTES

GENETICS

Chapter 15

Memorize
- efine: phenotype, genotype, gene, locus,
- lele: single and multiple
- omo/heterozygosity, wild type, recessiveness, mplete/co-dominance
- complete dominance, gene pool
- x-linked characteristics, sex determination
- pes of mutations: random, translation error, anscription error, base subs., etc.

Understand
* Importance of meiosis; compare/contrast with mitosis
* Segregation of genes, assortment, linkage, recombination
* Single/double crossovers; relationship of mutagens to carcinogens
* Hardy-Weinberg Principle, inborn errors of metabolism
* Test cross: back cross, concepts of parental, F1 and F2 generations

Not Required*
* Advanced level college info

GAMSAT-Prep.com

Introduction

Genetics is the study of heredity and variation in organisms. The observations of Gregor Mendel in the mid-nineteenth century gave birth to the science which would reveal the physical basis for his conclusions, DNA, about 100 years later.

Hopefully you noticed from the Table of Contents that between Biology chapters 8 and 16, by far, this is the most important chapter. Also, be forewarned: despite the fact that a dihybrid cross (BIO 15.3) is time consuming, it appears in 2 separate ACER GAMSAT practice booklets.

Additional Resources

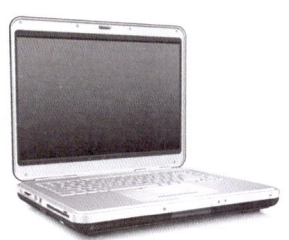

Free Online Q&A + Forum

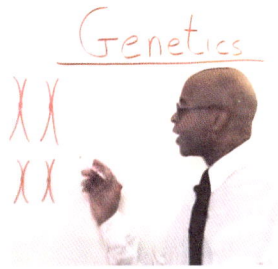

Video: Online or DVD

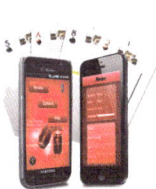

Flashcards

Special Guest

* The real GAMSAT may have advanced level information presented (ie. in a passage) but previous knowledge of said information is not required to answer the questions that would follow. Practice ACER and GS practice GAMSATs can help you clarify this point.

15.1 Background Information

Genetics is a branch of biology which deals with the principles and mechanics of heredity; in other words, the *means* by which *traits* are passed from parents to offspring. To begin, we will first examine some relevant definitions - a few of which we have already discussed.

Chromosomes are a complex of DNA and proteins (incl. histones; BIO 1.2.2). A gene is that sequence of DNA that codes for a protein or polypeptide. A locus is the *position* of the gene on the DNA molecule. Recall that humans inherit 46 chromosomes - 23 from maternal origin and 23 from paternal origin (BIO 14.2). A given chromosome from maternal origin has a counterpart from paternal origin which codes for the same products. This is called a **homologous pair** of chromosomes.

Any homologous pair of chromosomes have a pair of genes which codes for the same product (i.e. hair color). Such pairs of genes are called **alleles**. Thus for one gene product, a nucleus contains one allele from maternal origin and one allele from paternal origin. If both alleles are identical (i.e. they code for the same hair color), then the individual is called **homozygous** for that trait. If the two alleles differ (i.e. one codes for dark hair while the other codes for light hair), then the individual is called **heterozygous** for that trait.

The set of genes possessed by a particular organism is its genotype. The appearance or phenotype of an individual is expressed as a consequence of the genotype and the environment. Consider a heterozygote that expressed one gene (dark hair) but not the other (light hair). The expressed gene would be called dominant while the other unexpressed allele would be called recessive. The individual would have dark hair as their phenotype, yet their genotype would be heterozygous for that trait. The dominant allele is expressed in the phenotype. This is known as Mendel's Law of Dominance.

It is common to symbolize dominant genes with capital letters (A) and recessive genes with small letters (a). From the preceding paragraphs, we can conclude that with two alleles, three genotypes are possible: homozygous dominant (AA), heterozygous (Aa), and homozygous recessive (aa). Note that this only results in two phenotypes since both AA and Aa express the dominant gene, while only aa expresses the recessive gene.

Each individual carries **two** alleles while populations may have many or **multiple alleles**. Sometimes these genes are not strictly dominant or recessive. There may be degrees of blending (= *incomplete dominance*) or sometimes two alleles may be equally dominant (= *codominance*). ABO blood types are an important example of multiple alleles with codominance.

Incomplete dominance occurs when the phenotype of the heterozygote is an intermediate of the phenotypes of the homozygotes. A classic example is flower color in snapdragon: the snapdragon flower color is red for homozygous dominant and white for homozygous recessive. When the red homozygous flower is crossed with the white homozygous flower, the result yields a 100% pink snapdragon flower. The pink snapdragon is the result of the combined effect of both dominant and recessive genes.

15.2 ABO Blood Types

Codominance occurs when multiple alleles exist for a particular gene and more than one is dominant. When a dominant allele is combined with a recessive allele, the phenotype of the recessive allele is completely masked. But when two dominant alleles are present, the contributions of both alleles do not overpower each other and the phenotype is the result of the expression of both alleles. A classic example of codominance is the ABO blood type in humans.

Red blood cells can have various antigens or *agglutinogens* on their plasma membranes which aid in blood typing. The important two are antigens A and B. If the red blood cells have only antigen A, the blood type is A; if they have only antigen B, then the blood type is B; if they have both antigens, the blood type is AB; if neither antigen is present, the blood type is O. There are three allelic genes in the population (I^A, I^B, i^O). Two are codominant (I^A, I^B) and one is recessive (i^O). Thus in a given population, there are six possible genotypes which result in four possible phenotypes:

Genotype	Phenotype
$I^A I^A$, $I^A i^O$	blood type A
$I^B I^B$, $I^B i^O$	blood type B
$I^A I^B$	blood type AB
$i^O i^O$	blood type O

Blood typing is critical before doing a blood transfusion. This is because people with blood type A have anti-B antibodies, those with type B have anti-A, those with type AB have neither antibody, while type O has both anti-A and anti-B antibodies. If a person with type O blood is given types A, B, or AB, the clumping of the red blood cells will occur (= *agglutination*). Though type O can only receive from type O, it can give to the other blood types since its red blood cells have no antigens {type O = universal donor}. Type AB has neither antibody to react against A or B antigens so it can receive blood from all blood types {type AB = universal recipient}.

The only other antigens which have some importance are the Rh factors which are coded by different genes at different loci from the A and B antigens. Rh factors are either there (Rh$^+$) or they are not there (Rh$^-$). 85% of the population are Rh$^+$. The problem occurs when a woman is Rh$^-$ and has been exposed to Rh$^+$ blood and then forms anti-Rh$^+$ antibodies (note: unlike the previous case, exposure is necessary to produce these antibodies). If this woman is pregnant with an Rh$^+$ fetus her antibodies may cross the placenta and cause the fetus' red blood cells to agglutinate (*erythroblastosis fetalis*). This condition is fatal if left untreated.

15.3 Mendelian Genetics

Recall that in gametogenesis homologous chromosomes separate during the first meiotic division. Thus alleles that code for the same trait are segregated: this is **Mendel's First Law of Segregation. Mendel's Second Law of Independent Assortment** states that different chromosomes (*or factors which carry different traits*) separate independently of each other. For example, consider a primary spermatocyte (2N) undergoing its first meiotic division. It is not the case that all 23 chromosomes of paternal origin will end up in one secondary spermatocyte while the other 23 chromosomes of maternal origin ends up in the other. Rather, each chromosome in a homologous pair separates *independently* of any other chromosome in other homologous pairs.

However, it has been noted experimentally that sometimes traits on the same chromosome assort independently! This non-Mendelian concept is a result of *crossing over* (recall that this is when homologous chromosomes exchange parts, BIO 14.2). In fact, it has been shown that two traits located far apart on a chromosome are more likely to cross over and thus assort independently, as compared to two traits that are close. The propensity for some traits to refrain from assorting independently is called linkage. Double crossovers occur when two crossovers happen in a chromosomal region being studied.

Another exception to Mendel's laws involves **sex linkage**. Mendel's laws would predict that the results of a genetic cross should be the same regardless of which parent introduces the allele. However, it can be shown that some traits follow the inheritance of the sex chromosomes. Humans have one pair of sex chromosomes (XX = female, XY = male), and the remaining 22 pairs of homologous chromosomes are called **autosomes**.

Since females have two X chromosomes and males have only one, a single recessive allele carried on an X chromosome could be expressed in a male since there is no second allele present to mask it. When males inherit one copy of the recessive allele from an X chromosome, they will express the trait. In contrast, females must inherit two copies to express the trait. Therefore, an X-linked recessive phenotype is much more frequently found in males than females. In fact, a typical pattern of sex linkage is when a mother passes her phenotype to all her sons but **none** of her daughters. Her daughters become *carriers* for the recessive allele. Certain forms of hemophilia, colorblindness, and one kind of muscular dystrophy are well-known recessive sex-linked traits. {In what was once known as Lyon's Hypothesis, it has been shown that every female has a condensed, inactivated X chromosome in her body or somatic cells called a Barr body.}

Let us examine the predictions of Mendel's First Law. Consider two parents, one homozygous dominant (AA) and the other homozygous recessive (aa). Each parent can only form one type of gamete with respect to that trait (*either* A *or* a, *respectively*). The next generation (*called* first filial *or* **F₁**) must then be uniformly heterozygotes or *hybrids* (Aa). Now the F₁ hybrids can produce gametes that can be either A half the time or a half the time. When the F₁ generation is self-crossed, i.e. Aa X Aa, the F₂ generation will be more genotypically and phenotypically diverse and we can predict the outcome in the next generation (F₂) using a Punnett square:

	1/2 A	1/2 a
1/2 A	1/4 AA	1/4 Aa
1/2 a	1/4 Aa	1/4 aa

Here is an example as to how you derive the information within the square: when you cross A with A you get AA (i.e. 1/2 A × 1/2 A = 1/4 AA). Thus by doing a simple *mono*hybrid cross (Aa × Aa) with random mating, the Punnett square indicates that in the F₂ generation, 1/4 of the population would be AA, 1/2 would be Aa (1/4 + 1/4), and 1/4 would be aa. In other words the *genotypic* ratio of homozygous dominant to heterozygous to homozygous recessive is 1:2:1. However, since AA and Aa demonstrate the same *phenotype* (i.e. dominant) the ratio of dominant phenotype to recessive phenotype is 3:1.

Now we will consider the predictions of Mendel's Second Law. To examine independent assortment, we will have to consider a case with two traits (usu. on different chromosomes) or a *di*hybrid cross. Imagine a parent which is homozygous dominant for two traits (AABB) while the other is homozygous recessive (aabb). Each parent can only form one type of gamete with respect to those traits (*either* AB *or* ab, *respectively*). The F₁ generation will be uniform for the dominant trait (i.e. *the* genotypes *would all be* AaBb). In the gametes of the F₁ generation, the alleles will assort independently.

Consequently, an equal amount of all the possible gametes will form: 1/4 AB, 1/4 Ab, 1/4 aB, and 1/4 ab. When the F₁ generation is self-crossed, i.e. AaBb X AaBb, we can predict the outcome in the F₂ generation using the Punnett square:

	1/4 AB	1/4 Ab	1/4 aB	1/4 ab
1/4 AB	1/16 AABB	1/16 AABb	1/16 AaBB	1/16 AaBb
1/4 Ab	1/16 AABb	1/16 AAbb	1/16 AaBb	1/16 Aabb
1/4 aB	1/16 AaBB	1/16 AaBb	1/16 aaBB	1/16 aaBb
1/4 ab	1/16 AaBb	1/16 Aabb	1/16 aaBb	1/16 aabb

Thus by doing a dihybrid cross with random mating, the Punnett square indicates that there are nine possible genotypes (*the frequency is given in brackets*): AABB (1), AABb (2), AaBb (4), AaBB (2), Aabb (2), aaBb (2), AAbb (1), aaBB (1), and aabb (1). Since A and B are dominant, there are only four phenotypic classes in the ratio 9:3:3:1 which are: the expression of both traits (AABB + AABb + AaBb + AaBB = 9), the expression of only the first trait (AAbb + Aabb = 3), the expression of only the second trait (aaBB + aaBb = 3), and the expression of neither trait (aabb = 1). Now we know, for example, that 9/16 represents that fraction of the population which will have the phenotype of both dominant traits.

15.3.1 A Word about Probability

If you were to flip a quarter, the probability of getting "heads" is 50% (p = 0.5). If you flipped the quarter ten times and each time it came up heads, the probability of getting heads on the next trial is still 50%. After all, previous trials have no effect on the next trial.

Since chance events, such as fertilization of a particular kind of egg by a particular kind of sperm, occur independently, the genotype of one child has no effect on the genotypes of other children produced by a set of parents. Thus in the previous example of the dihybrid cross, the chance of producing the genotype AaBb is 4/16 (25%) irrespective of the genotypes which have already been produced. For more about probability, see GM 6.1.

BIO-178 GENETICS

15.4 The Hardy-Weinberg Law

The Hardy-Weinberg Law deals with population genetics. A **population** includes all the members of a species which occupy a more or less well defined geographical area and have demonstrated the ability to reproduce from generation to generation. A **gene pool** is the sum of all the unique alleles for a given population. A central component to evolution is the changing of alleles in a gene pool from one generation to the next.

Evolution can be viewed as a changing of gene frequencies within a population over successive generations. The Hardy-Weinberg Law or *equilibrium* predicts the outcome of a randomly mating population of sexually reproducing diploid organisms who are not undergoing evolution.

For the Hardy-Weinberg Law to be applied, the idealized population must meet the following conditions: i) **random mating**: the members of the population must have no mating preferences; ii) **no mutations**: there must be no errors in replication nor similar event resulting in a change in the genome; iii) **isolation**: there must be no exchange of genes between the population being considered and any other population; iv) **large population**: since the law is based on statistical probabilities, to avoid sampling errors, the population cannot be small; v) **no selection pressures**: there must be no reproductive advantage of one allele over the other.

To illustrate a use of the law, consider an idealized population that abides by the preceding conditions and have a gene locus occupied by either A or a. Let p = the frequency of allele A in the population and let q = the frequency of allele a. Since they are the only alleles, p + q = 1. Squaring both sides we get:

$$(p + q)^2 = (1)^2$$
$$\text{OR}$$
$$p^2 + 2pq + q^2 = 1$$

The preceding equation (= *the Hardy-Weinberg equation*) can be used to calculate genotype frequencies once the allelic frequencies are given. This can be summarized by the following:

	pA	qa
pA	p^2AA	pqAa
qa	pqAa	q^2aa

The Punnett square illustrates the expected frequencies of the three genotypes in the next generation: AA = p^2, Aa = 2pq, and aa = q^2.

For example, let us calculate the percentage of heterozygous individuals in a population where the recessive allele q has a frequency of 0.2. Since p + q = 1, then p = 0.8. Using the Hardy-Weinberg equation and squaring p and q we get:

$$0.64 + 2pq + 0.04 = 1$$
$$2pq = 1 - 0.68 = 0.32$$

Thus the percentage of heterozygous (2pq) individuals is 32%.

A practical application of the Hardy-Weinberg equation is the prediction of how many people in a generation are carriers for a particular recessive allele. The values would have to be recalculated for every generation since humans do not abide by all the conditions of the Hardy-Weinberg Law (i.e. *humans continually evolve*).

15.4.1 Back Cross, Test Cross

A back cross is the cross of an individual (F_1) with one of its parents (P) or an organism with the same genotype as a parent. Back crosses can be used to help identify the genotypes of the individual in a specific type of back cross called a test cross. A test cross is a cross between an organism whose genotype for a certain trait is unknown and an organism that is homozygous recessive for that trait so the unknown genotype can be determined from that of the offspring. For example, for P: AA x aa and F_1: Aa, we get:

Backcross #1: Aa x AA
Progeny #1: 1/2 Aa and 1/2 AA

Backcross #2: Aa x aa
Progeny #2: 1/2 Aa and 1/2 aa

15.5 Genetic Variability

Meiosis and mutations are sources of genetic variability. During meiosis I, crossing over occurs between the parental and maternal genes which leads to a recombination of parental genes yielding unique haploid gametes. Thus recombination can result in alleles of linked traits separating into different gametes. However, the closer two traits are on a chromosome, the more likely they will be linked and thus remain together, and vice versa.

Further recombination occurs during the random fusion of gametes during fertilization.

Consequently, taking Mendel's two laws and recombination together, we can predict that parents can give their offspring combinations of alleles which the parents never had. This leads to **genetic variability**.

Mutations are rare, inheritable, random changes in the genetic material (DNA) of a cell. Mutations are much more likely to be either neutral (esp. *silent mutations*) or negative (i.e. cancer) than positive for an organism's survival. Nonetheless, such a change in the genome increases genetic variability. Only mutations of gametes, and not somatic cells, are passed on to offspring.

The following are some forms of mutations:

- **Point mutation** is a change affecting a single base pair in a gene
- **Deletion** is the removal of a sequence of DNA, the regions on either side being joined together
- **Inversion** is the reversal of a segment of DNA
- **Translocation** is when one chromosome breaks and attaches to another
- **Duplication** is when a sequence of DNA is repeated.
- **Frame shift mutations** occur when bases are added or deleted in numbers other than multiples of three. Such deletions or additions cause the rest of the sequence to be shifted such that each triplet reading frame is altered.

A mutagen is any substance or agent that can cause a mutation. A mutagen is not the same as a carcinogen. Carcinogens are agents that cause cancer. While many mutagens are carcinogens as well, many others are not. The Ames test is a widely used test to screen chemicals used in foods or medications for mutagenic potential.

Mutations can produce many types of genetic diseases including inborn errors of metabolism. These disorders in normal metabolism are usually due to defects of a single gene that codes for one enzyme.

15.6 Genetics and Heredity: A Closer Look

The rest of this chapter begins to push into more advanced topics in genetics. However, these topics continue to represent legitimate exam material.

Epistasis occurs when one gene masks the phenotype of a second gene. This is often the case in pigmentation where one gene turns on (or off) the production of pigment, while a second gene controls the amount of pigment produced. Such is the case in mice fur where one gene codes for the presence or absence of pigmentation and the other codes for the color. If C and c represent the alleles for the presence or absence of color and B and b represent black and brown then a phenotype of CCbb and Ccbb would both correspond to a brown phenotype. Whenever cc is inherited the fur will be white.

Pleiotropy occurs when a single gene has more than one phenotypic expression. This is often seen in pea plants where the gene that expresses round or wrinkled texture of seeds also influences the expression of starch metabolism. For example, in wrinkled seeds there is more unconverted glucose which leads to an increase of the osmotic gradient. These seeds will subsequently contain more water than round seeds. When they mature they will dehydrate and produce the wrinkled appearance.

Polygenic inheritance refers to traits that cannot be expressed in just a few types but rather as a range of varieties. The most popular example would be human height which ranges from very short to very tall. This phenomenon (many genes shaping one phenotype) is the opposite of pleiotropy.

Penetrance refers to the proportion of individuals carrying a particular variant of a gene (allele or genotype) that also express the associated phenotype. Alleles which are highly penetrant are more likely to be noticed. Penetrance only considers whether individuals express the trait or not. *Expressivity* refers to the variation in the degree of expression of a given trait.

Nondisjunction occurs when the chromosomes do not separate properly and do not migrate to opposite poles as in normal anaphase of meiosis (BIO 14.2). This could arise from a failure of homologous chromosomes to separate in meiosis I, or the failure of sister chromatids to separate during meiosis II or mitosis. Most of the time, gametes produced after nondisjunction are sterile; however, certain imbalances can be fertile and lead to genetic defects. Down Syndrome (Trisomy 21 = 3 copies of chromosome 21 due to its nondisjunction, thus the person has an extra chromosome making a total of 47 chromosomes); Turner and Klinefelter Syndrome (nondisjunction of sex chromosomes); and Cri du Chat (deletion in chromosome 5) are well known genetic disorders. Hemophilia and red-green color blindness are common sex-linked disorders and are recessive.

Phenylketonuria, sickle-cell anemia and Tay-Sachs disease are common autosomal recessive disorders.

Gene linkage refers to genes that reside on the same chromosome and are unable to display independent assortment because they are physically connected (BIO 15.3). The further away the two genes are on the chromosome the higher probability there is that they will crossover during synapsis. In these cases recombination frequencies are used to provide a linkage map where the arrangement of the genes can be ascertained. For example, say you have a fly with genotype BBTTYY and the crossover frequency between B and T is 26%, between Y and T is 18% and between B and Y is 8%. Greater recombination frequencies mean greater distances so you know that B and T are the furthest apart. This corresponds to a gene order of B-Y-T and since frequencies are a direct measure of distance you know exactly how far apart each allele is and can easily calculate the map distances.

Twin studies (nature vs. nurture) help to gauge the relative importance of environmental and genetic influences on individuals in a sample. Twins can either be monozygotic ("identical"), meaning that they develop from one zygote (BIO 14.5) that splits and forms two embryos, or dizygotic ("fraternal"), meaning that they develop from two separate eggs, each fertilized by separate sperm cells. Thus fraternal twins are like any 2 siblings from a genetic point of view, but they may share the same environment as they grow up together.

To control for environment, the classical twin study design compares the similarity of monozygotic and dizygotic twins. If identical twins are considerably more similar than fraternal twins (which is found for most traits), this implies that genes play an important role for those specific traits. By comparing hundreds of families of twins, researchers can then understand more about the roles of genetic effects, shared environment, and unique environment in shaping behavior or in the development of disease.

15.6.1 Mitochondrial DNA

Mitochondrial DNA (mtDNA or mDNA) has become increasingly popular as a tool to determine how closely populations are related as well as to clarify the evolutionary relationships among species (= phylogenetics). Mitochondrial DNA is circular (BIO 1.2.2, 16.6.3) and can be regarded as the smallest chromosome. In most species, including humans, mtDNA is inherited solely from the mother. The DNA sequence of mtDNA has been determined from a large number of organisms and individuals (including some organisms that are extinct).

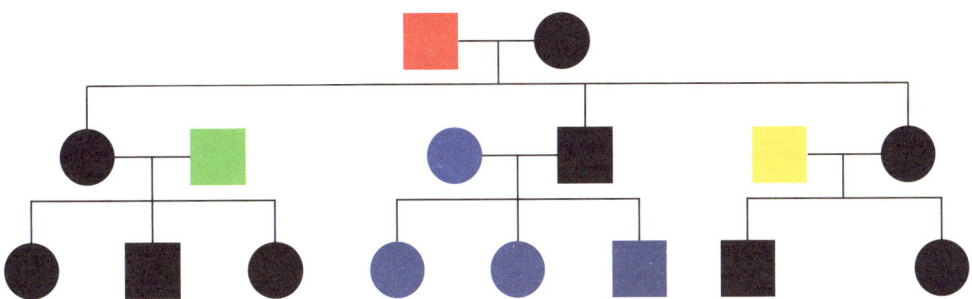

Figure IV.A.15.0: Pedigree ("Family tree"): Maternal inheritance pattern of mtDNA for 3 generations with the grandparents in the top row. As is the standard, circles represent females, squares represent males. Colors show the inheritance of the same mt genome (from mother to offspring, i.e. children). Don't be surprised to see a pedigree of some sort in your practice questions and/or on the real exam.

15.7 DNA Recombination and Genetic Technology

DNA recombination involves DNA that contains segments or genes from different sources. The foreign DNA can come from another DNA molecule, a chromosome or from a complete organism. Most DNA transferred is done artificially using DNA recombination techniques which use restriction enzymes to cut pieces of DNA. These enzymes originate from bacteria and are extremely specific because they only cut DNA at specific recognition sequences along the strand. These recognition sites correspond to different nucleotide sequences and produce sticky and blunt ends when a double stranded DNA segment is cut.

The sticky end is the unpaired part of the DNA that is ready to bind with a complementary codon (sequence of three adjacent nucleotides; BIO 3.0). These cut pieces or **restriction fragments** are often inserted into plasmids (circular piece of DNA that is able to replicate independently of the chromosomal DNA) which are then able to be introduced into the bacteria via transformation (see BIO 2.2).

Treating the plasmid, or replicon, with the same restriction enzymes used on the original fragment produces the same sticky ends in both pieces allowing base pairing to occur when they are mixed together. This attachment is stabilized by DNA ligase. After the ends are joined and the recombinant plasmid is incorporated into bacteria, the bacteria become capable of producing copious amounts of a specific protein that was not native to its species (i.e. bacteria with recombinant DNA producing insulin to treat diabetes).

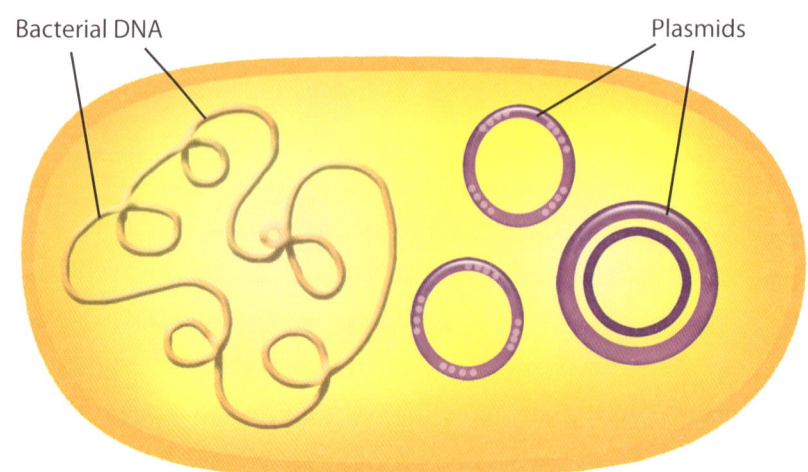

Bacterium and Vector Plasmid

Gel electrophoresis is a method of separating restriction fragments of differing lengths based on their size (as described in the previous section, a restriction fragment is a fragment of DNA cleaved by a restriction enzyme). The DNA fragments are passed through a gel which is under the influence of an electric field. Since DNA is negatively charged it will move towards the cathode (positive electrode). The shorter fragments move faster than the longer ones and can be visualized as a banding pattern using autoradiography techniques.

SDS-PAGE, sodium dodecyl sulfate polyacrylamide gel electrophoresis (ORG 13), also separates proteins according to their electrophoretic mobility. SDS is an anionic detergent (i.e. negatively charged) which has the following effect: (1) linearize proteins and (2) give an additional negative charge to the linearized proteins. In most proteins, the binding of SDS to the polypeptide chain gives an even distribution of charge per unit mass, thus fractionation will approximate size during electrophoresis (i.e. not dependent on charge).

Restriction fragment length polymorphisms or RFLP is a technique that exploits variations in restriction fragments from one individual to another that differ in length due to polymorphisms, or slight differences in DNA sequences. The process involves digesting DNA sequences with different restriction enzymes, detecting the resulting restriction fragments by gel electrophoresis, and comparing their lengths. In DNA fingerprinting, commonly used to analyze DNA left at crime scenes, RFLP's are produced and compared to RFLP's of known suspects in order to catch the perpetrator.

Sometimes it is necessary to obtain the DNA fragment bearing the required gene directly from the mRNA that codes for the polypeptide in question. This is due to the presence of introns (non-coding regions on a DNA molecule; BIO 3.0) which prevent transcription of foreign genes in the genome of bacteria, a common problem in recombinant technology. To carry this out one can use reverse transcriptase producing complementary DNA (cDNA) which lack the problematic introns.

Rather than using a bacterium to clone DNA fragments, sometimes DNA is copied directly using the polymerase chain reaction (PCR). This method allows us to rapidly amplify the DNA content using synthetic primers that initiate replication at specific nucleotide sequences. This method relies on thermal cycling (repeated heating and cooling) of the DNA primers and can lead to thousands and even millions of copies in relatively short periods of time.

GAMSAT-Prep.com
THE GOLD STANDARD

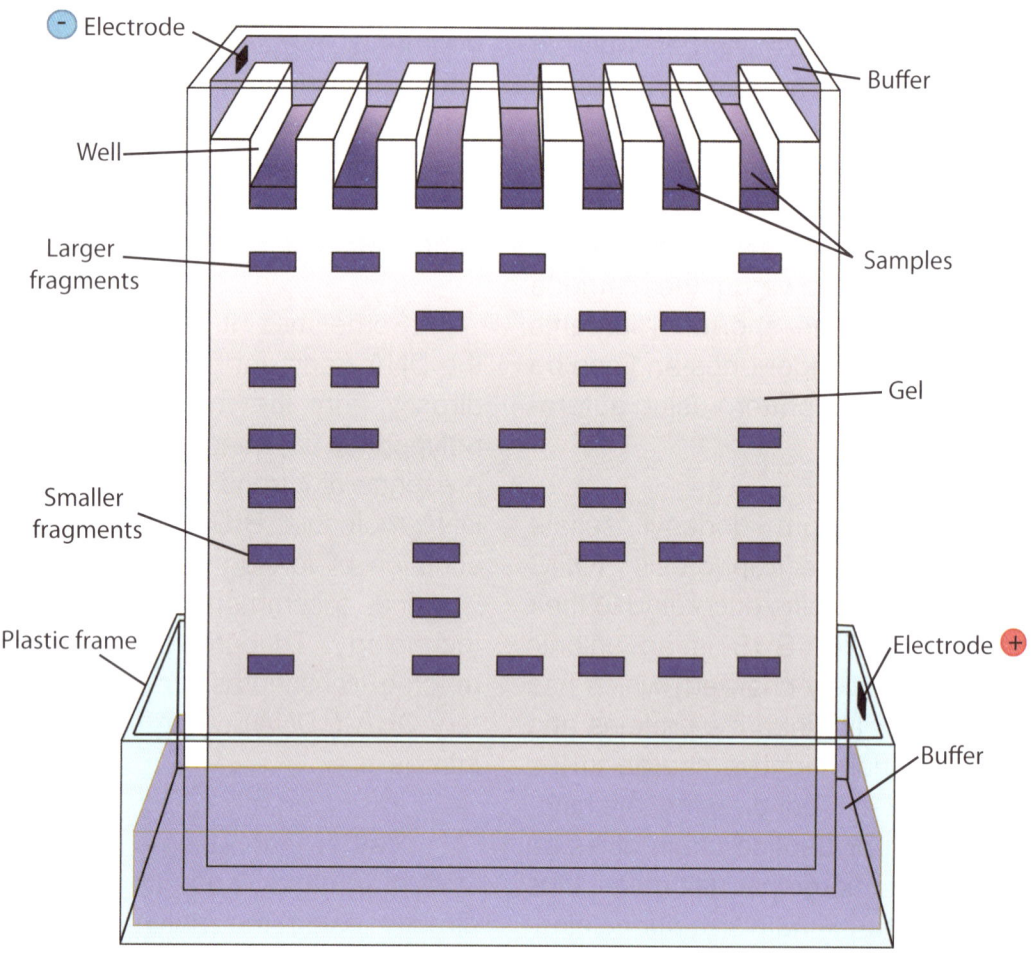

Figure IV.A.15.1: Gel Electrophoresis.

Southern blotting, named after Dr. E. Southern, is the process of transferring DNA fragments from the electrophoresis agarose gel onto filter paper where they are identified with probes. The procedure begins by digesting DNA in a mixture with *restriction endonucleases* to cut out specific pieces of DNA. The DNA fragments are then subjected to gel electrophoresis. The now separated fragments are bathed in an alkaline solution where they immediately begin to denature. These fragments are then placed (or blotted) onto nitrocellulose paper and then incubated with a specific probe whose location can be visualized with autoradiography.

Northern blotting is adapted from the Southern blot to detect specific sequences of RNA by hybridization with cDNA. Similarly, *Western blotting* is used to identify specific amino-acid sequences in proteins. Since this is not required for you to memorize for the GAMSAT, you may want to set aside this mnemonic for when you are attending medical school: SNOW DROP.

SNOW	DROP
Southern	**D**NA
Northern	**R**NA
O	**O**
Western	**P**rotein

DNA microarray technology (= DNA chip or biochip or "laboratory-on-a-chip") helps to determine which genes are active and which are inactive in different cell types. This technology evolved from Southern blotting and can also be used to genotype multiple regions of a genome. DNA microarrays are created by robotic machines that arrange incredibly small amounts of hundreds or thousands of gene sequences on a single microscope slide. These sequences can be a short section of a gene or other DNA element that is used to hybridize a cDNA or cRNA (also called anti-sense RNA) sample. The hybridization is usually observed and quantified by the detection of fluorescent tag.

NB: The molecular biology techniques of FRAP (BIO 1.5) and ELISA (BIO 8.4) were described earlier in this book. Electrophoresis and chromatography are discussed in Organic Chemistry Chapter 13.

GOLD NOTES

EVOLUTION

Chapter 16

Memorize	Understand	Not Required*
* Define: species, genetic drift * Basics: chordates, vertebrates	* Natural selection, speciation * Genetic drift * Basics: origin of life * Basics: comparative anatomy	* Advanced level college info

GAMSAT-Prep.com

Introduction

Evolution is, quite simply, the change in the inherited traits of a population of organisms from one generation to another. This change over time can be traced to 3 main processes: variation, reproduction and selection. The major mechanisms that drive evolution are natural selection and genetic drift.

Additional Resources

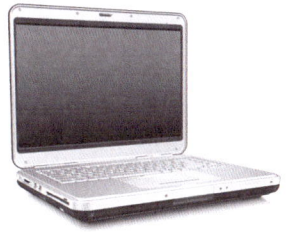

Free Online Q&A + Forum

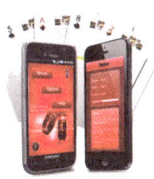

Flashcards

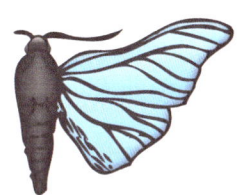

Special Guest

THE BIOLOGICAL SCIENCES   BIO-189

* The real GAMSAT may have advanced level information presented (ie. in a passage) but previous knowledge of said information is not required to answer the questions that would follow. Practice ACER and GS practice GAMSATs can help you clarify this point.

16.1 Overview

Evolution is the change in frequency of one or more alleles in a population's gene pool from one generation to the next. The evidence for evolution lies in the fossil record, biogeography, embryology, comparative anatomy, and experiments from artificial selection. The most important mechanism of evolution is the **selection** of certain phenotypes provided by the **genetic variability** of a population.

16.2 Natural Selection

Natural selection is the non-random differential survival and reproduction from one generation to the next. Natural selection contains the following premises: i) genetic and phenotypic variability exist in populations: offspring show variations compared to parents; ii) more individuals are produced than live to grow up and reproduce; iii) the population competes to survive; iv) individuals with some genes are more likely to survive (greater fitness) than those with other genes; v) individuals that are more likely to survive transmit these favorable variations (genes) to their offspring so that these genes become more dominant in the gene pool.

It is not necessarily true that natural selection leads to the the Darwin-era expression "survival of the fittest"; rather it is the genes, and not necessarily the individual, which are likely to survive.

Evolution goes against the foundations of the Hardy-Weinberg Law. For example, natural selection leads to non-random mating due to phenotypic differences. Evolution occurs when those phenotypic changes depend on an underlying genotype; thus non-random mating can lead to changes in allelic frequencies. Consider an example: if female peacocks decide to only mate with a male with long feathers, then there will be a selection pressure against any male with a genotype which is expressed as short feathers. Because of this differential reproduction, the alleles which are expressed as short feathers will be eliminated from the population. Thus this population evolves.

The three forms of natural selection are: i) **stabilizing selection** in which genetic diversity decreases as the population stabilizes on an average phenotype (*phenotypes have a "bell curve" distribution*). This is the most common form of natural selection. It is basically the opposite of disruptive selection, instead of favoring individuals with extreme phenotypes, it favors the intermediate phenotype; ii) **directional selection** when an extreme phenotype has a selective advantage over the average phenotype causing the allele frequency continually shifting in one direction (*thus the curve can become skewed to the left or right*). It occurs most often when populations migrate to new areas with environmental pressures; iii) **disruptive selection** where both extremes

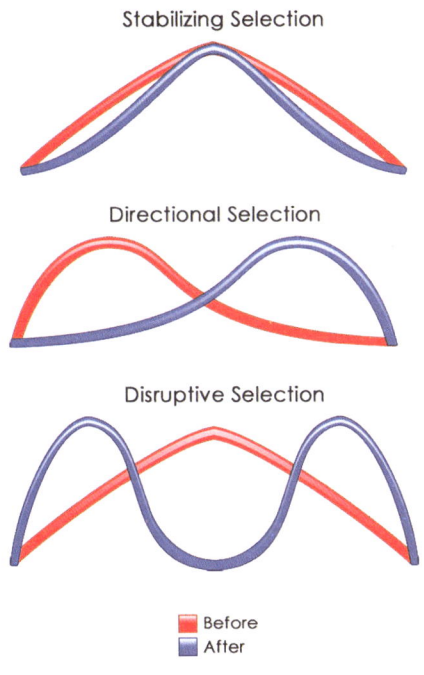

are selected over the average phenotype; this would produce a split down the middle of the "bell curve" such that two new and separate "bell curves" would result. For example, if a bird only ate medium sized seeds and left the large and small ones alone, two new populations or groups of seeds would have a reproductive advantage. Thus by selecting against the group of medium sized seeds, two new groups of large and small seeds will result. This is an example of group selection causing *disruptive selection*.

16.3 Species and Speciation

Species can be defined as the members of populations that interbreed or can interbreed under natural conditions. There are great variations within species. A **cline** is a gradient of variation in a species across a geographical area. **Speciation** is the evolution of new species by the isolation of gene pools of related populations. The isolation of gene pools is typically geographic. An ocean, a glacier, a river or any other physical barrier can isolate a population and prevent it from mating with other populations of the same species. The two populations may begin to differ because their mutations may be different, or, there may be different selection pressures from the two different environments, or, *genetic drift* may play a role.

Genetic drift is the random change in frequencies of alleles or genotypes in a population (recall that this is antagonistic to the Hardy-Weinberg Law). Genetic drift normally occurs when a small population is isolated from a large population. Since the allelic frequencies in the small population may be different from the large population (*sampling error*), the two populations may evolve in different directions.

Populations or species can be sympatric, in which speciation occurs after ecological, genetic or behavioral barriers arise within the same geographical boundary of a single population, or allopatric, in which speciation occurs through geographical isolation of groups from the parent population {Sympatric = live together, Allopatric = live apart}. Mechanisms involved in allopatric speciation are represented in the two preceding paragraphs.

The following represents some isolating mechanisms that prevent sympatric populations of different species from breeding together: i) habitat differences; ii) different breeding times or seasons; iii) mechanical differences (i.e. different anatomy of the genitalia); iv) behavioral specificity (i.e. different courtship behavior); v) gametic isolation (= fertilization cannot occur); vi) hybrid inviability (i.e. the hybrid zygote dies before reaching the age of sexual maturity); vii) hybrid sterility; viii) hybrid breakdown: the hybrid offspring is fertile but produces a next generation (F_2) which is infertile or inviable.

16.4 Origin of Life

Evidence suggests that the primitive earth had a reducing atmosphere with gases such as H_2 and the reduced compounds H_2O (vapor), $NH_{3(g)}$ (ammonia) and $CH_{4(g)}$ (methane). Such an atmosphere has been shown (i.e. Miller, Fox) to be conducive to the formation and stabilization of organic compounds. Such compounds can sometimes polymerize (*possibly due to autocatalysis*) and evolve into living systems with metabolism, reproduction, digestion, excretion, etc.

Critical in the early history of the earth was the evolution of: (1) the reducing atmosphere powered with energy (e.g. lightening, UV radiation, outgassing volcanoes) converting reduced compounds (water, ammonia, methane) into simple organic molecules (the 'primordial soup'); (2) self-replicating molecules surrounded by membranes forming protocells (very primitive microspheres, coacervates assembling into the precursor of prokaryotic cells: protobionts); (3) chemosynthetic bacteria which are anaerobes that used chemicals in the environment to produce energy; (4) photosynthesis which releases O_2 and thus converted the atmosphere into an oxidizing one; (5) respiration, which could use the O_2 to efficiently produce ATP; and (6) the development of membrane bound organelles (*a subset of prokaryotes which evolved into eukaryotes,* BIO 16.6.3) which allowed eukaryotes to develop meiosis, sexual reproduction, and fertilization.

It is important to recognize that throughout the evolution of the earth, organisms and the environment have and will continue to shape each other.

16.5 Comparative Anatomy

Anatomical features of organisms can be compared in order to derive information about their evolutionary histories. Structures which originate from the same part of the embryo are called homologous. **Homologous** structures may have similar anatomical features shared by two different species as a result of a common ancestor but with a late divergent evolutionary pattern in response to different evolutionary forces. Such structures may or may not serve different functions. **Analogous** structures have similar functions in two different species but arise from different evolutionary origins and entirely different developmental patterns (see Figure IV.A.16.1).

Vestigial structures represent further evidence for evolution since they are organs which are useless in their present owners, but are homologous with organs which are important in other species. For example, the appendix in humans is a vestige of an organ that had digestive functions in ancestral species. However, it continues to assist in the digestion of cellulose in herbivores.

Taxonomy is the branch of biology which deals with the classification of organisms. Humans are classified as follows:

Kingdom	Animalia
Phylum (= Division)	Chordata
Subdivision	Vertebrata
Class	Mammalia
Order	Primates
Family	Hominidae
Genus	*Homo*
Species	*Homo sapiens*

{Mnemonic for remembering the taxonomic categories: <u>K</u>ing <u>P</u>hilip <u>c</u>ame <u>o</u>ver for <u>g</u>reat <u>s</u>oup}

The subphyla Vertebrata and Invertebrata are subdivisions of the phylum Chordata. Acorn worms, tunicates, sea squirts and amphioxus are invertebrates. Humans, birds, frogs, fish, and crocodiles are vertebrates. We will examine features of both the chordates and the vertebrates.

Chordates have the following characteristics at some stage of their development: i) a <u>notochord</u>; ii) <u>pharyngeal gill slits</u> which lead from the pharynx to the exterior; iii) a <u>hollow dorsal nerve cord</u>. Other features which are less defining but are nonetheless present in chordates are: i) a more or less segmented anatomy; ii) an internal skeleton (= *endoskeleton*); iii) a tail at some point in their development.

Vertebrates have all the characteristics of chordates. In addition, vertebrates have: i) a vertebral column; ii) well developed sensory and nervous systems; iii) a ventral heart with a closed vascular system; iv) some sort of a liver, endocrine organs, and kidneys; and v) cephalization which is the concentration of sense organs and nerves to the front end of the body producing an obvious head.

16.6 Patterns of Evolution

The evolution of a species can be divided into four main patterns:

1. Divergent evolution – Two or more species originate from a common ancestor.

2. Convergent evolution – Two unrelated species become more alike as they evolve due to similar ecological conditions. The traits that resemble one another are called analogous traits. Similarity in species of different ancestry as a result of convergent evolution is homoplasty. For example, flying insects, birds and bats have evolved wings independently.

3. Parallel evolution – This describes two related species that have evolved similarly after their divergence from a common ancestor. For example, the appearance of similarly shaped leaves in many genera of plant species.

4. Coevolution – This is the evolution of one species in response to adaptations gained by another species. This most often occurs in predator/prey relationships where an adaptation in the prey species that makes them less vulnerable leads to new adaptations in the predator species to help them catch their prey.

16.6.1 Macroevolution

Macroevolution describes patterns of evolution for groups of species rather than individual species. There are two main theories:

1. **Phyletic gradualism** – This theory argues that evolution occurs through gradual accumulation of small changes. They point to fossil evidence as proof that major changes in speciation occur over long periods of geological time and state that the incompleteness of the fossil record is the reason why some intermediate changes are not evidenced.

2. **Punctuated equilibrium** – This theory states that evolutionary history is marked

BIOLOGY

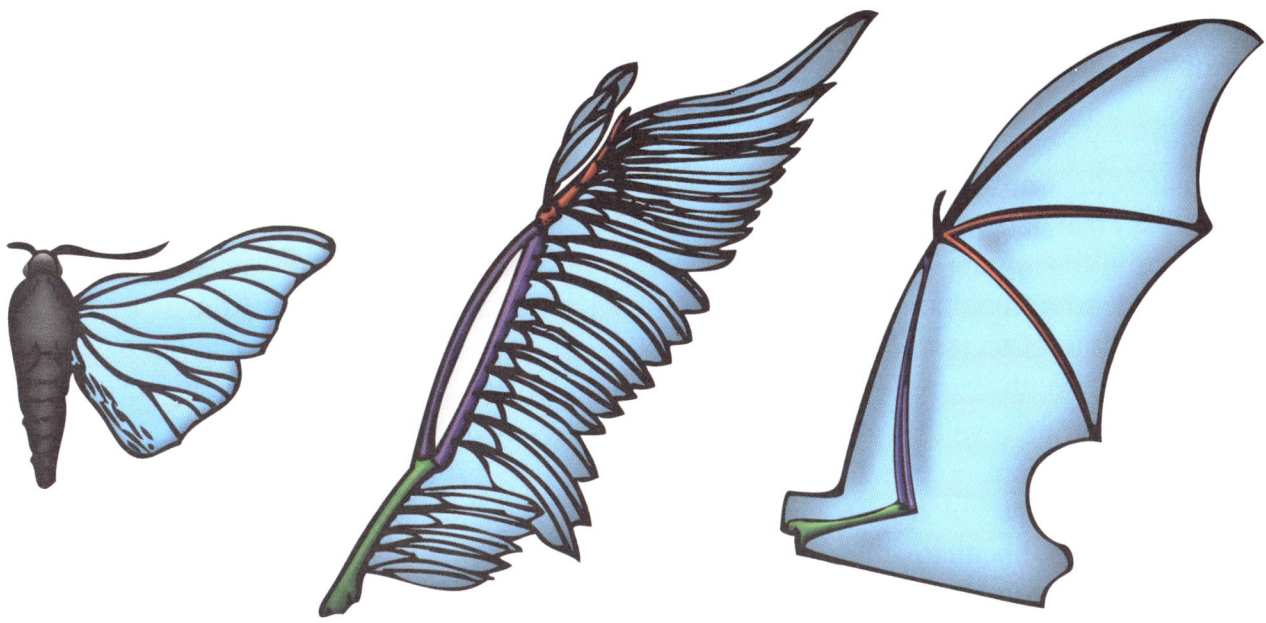

Figure IV.A.16.1: Analogous and homologous structures. The light blue wings represent analogous structures between different species: a flying insect, a bird and a bat, respectively. The bones are homologous structures. For example, green represents the humerus, purple represents the radius and ulna, red represents metacarpals and phalanges. Of course, insects have no bones. See the skeleton in BIO 11.3 to remind yourself of the meaning of some of these bony structures homologous in humans.

by sudden bursts of rapid evolution with long periods of inactivity in between. Punctuated equilibrium theorists point to the absence of fossils showing intermediate change as proof that evolution occurred in short time periods.

16.6.2 Basic Patterns for Changes in Macroevolution

1. Phyletic change (anagenesis): gradual change in an entire population that results in an eventual replacement of ancestral species by novel species and ancestral populations can be considered extinct.

2. Cladogenesis: one lineage gives rise to two or more lineages each forming a "clad". It leads to the development of a variety of sister species and often occurs when it is introduced to a new, distant environment.

3. Adaptive radiation: a formation of a number of lineages from a single ancestral species. A single species can diverge into a number of different species, which are able to exploit new environments.

4. Extinction: more than 99.9% of all species are no longer present.

THE BIOLOGICAL SCIENCES BIO-195

16.6.3 Eukaryotic Evolution

Eukaryotes evolved from primitive heterotrophic prokaryotes in the following manner:

1. Heterotrophs first formed in the primordial soup (mixture of organic material) present in the early Earth (BIO 16.4). As the cells reproduced, competition increased and natural selection favored those heterotrophs who were best suited to obtain food.
2. Heterotrophs evolved into autotrophs (capable of making own food) via mutation. The first autotrophs were highly successful because they were able to manufacture their own food supply using light energy or energy from inorganic substrates (i.e. cyanobacteria).
3. As a by-product of the photosynthetic activity of autotrophs, oxygen was released into the atmosphere. This lead to formation of the ozone layer which prevented UV light from reaching the earth's surface. The interference of this major autotrophic resource was caused by the increased blockage of light rays.
4. Mitochondria, chloroplasts, and possibly other organelles of eukaryotic cells, originate through the symbiosis between multiple microorganisms. According to this theory, certain organelles originated as free-living bacteria that were taken inside another cell as endosymbionts. Thus mitochondria developed from proteobacteria and chloroplasts from cyanobacteria. This is the belief of the endosymbiotic theory which counts the following as evidence that it bodes true:
   A. Mitochondria and chloroplasts possess their own unique DNA which is very similar to the DNA of prokaryotes (circular). Their ribosomes also resemble one another with respect to size and sequence.
   B. Mitochondria and chloroplasts reproduce independently of their eukaryotic host cell.
   C. The thylakoid membranes of chloroplasts resemble the photosynthetic membranes of cyanobacteria.

16.6.4 The Six-Kingdom, Three-Domain System

Genetic sequencing led to the replacement of the 'old' Five-Kingdom system of taxonomy (BIO 15.5). Under the current system, there are six kingdoms: Archaebacteria (ancient bacteria), Eubacteria (true bacteria; BIO 2.2), Protista (a diverse group of eukaryotic microorganisms), Fungi (BIO 2.3), Plantae ('plants'), and Animalia ('animals'). The Archaea and Bacteria domains contain prokaryotic organisms. The Eukarya domain includes eukaryotes and is subdivided into the kingdoms Protista, Fungi, Plantae, and Animalia.

BIOLOGY

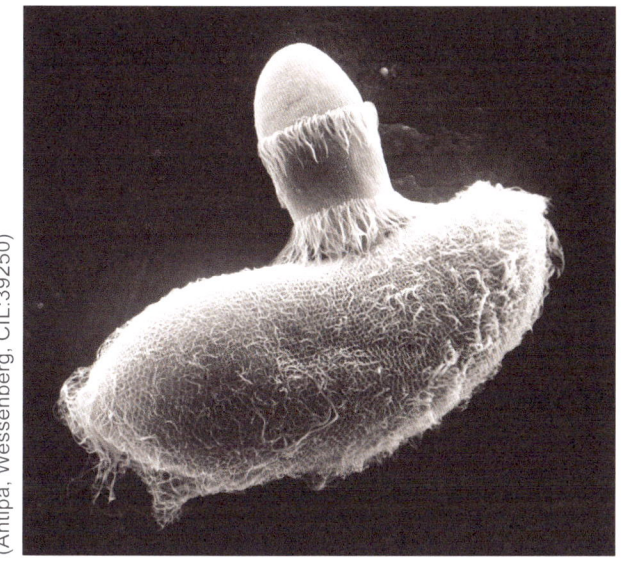

Figure IV.A.16.2: David and Golliath: Two animal-like unicellular, ciliated protists in an epic struggle. The larger of the two carnivores, Paramecium, is attacked from above by the smaller Didinium. In this case, the organisms were preserved for this SEM micrograph (BIO 1.5, 1.5.1) before the outcome could be determined. Like other ciliates (ciliaphora), they can reproduce asexually (binary fission) or sexually (conjugation); osmoregulation is via contractile vacuoles; and, they are also visible using a light microscope.

Six-Kingdom, Three-Domain System

- Archaea Domain
  Kingdom Archaebacteria

- Bacteria Domain
  Kingdom Eubacteria

- Eukarya Domain
  Kingdom Protista
  Kingdom Fungi
  Kingdom Plantae
  Kingdom Animalia

If your Section 3 review is now over, it's time to consolidate your Gold Notes and prepare for full-length (timed) GAMSAT practice exams! Good luck!

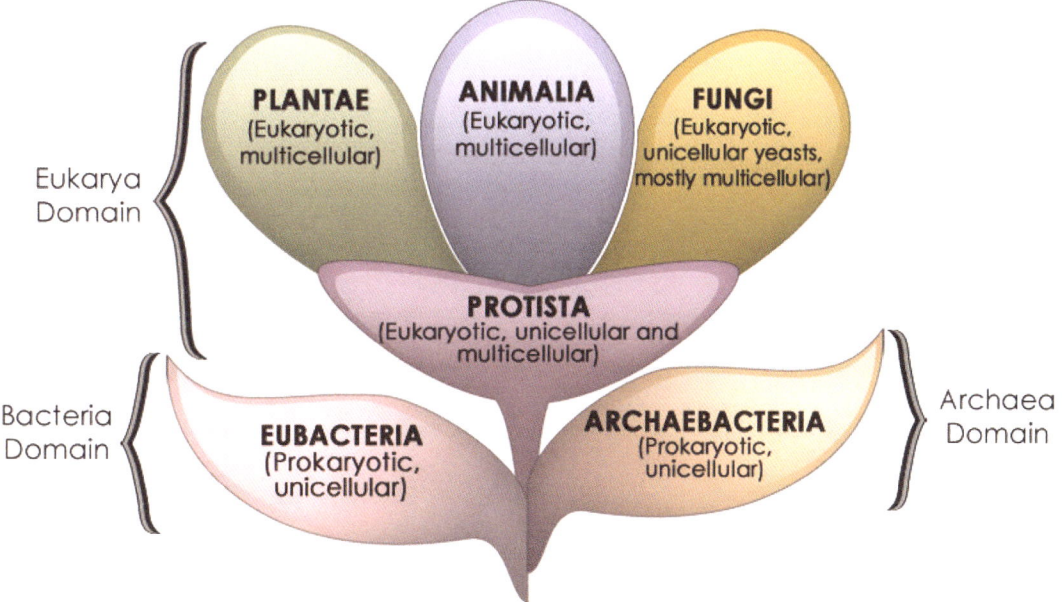

Figure IV.A.16.3: The Six-Kingdom, Three-Domain System.

Go online to GAMSAT-prep.com for additional chapter review Q&A and forum.

Gold Standard GAMSAT* Exam

Part V: The Gold Standard GAMSAT
* GAMSAT is administered by ACER which is not associated with this product.

THE GOLD STANDARD GAMSAT

Introduction

Prior to sitting this practice test, section 2.3 from Part II - Understanding the GAMSAT - should be reviewed.

The following full length practice Gold Standard (GS) GAMSAT is designed to challenge you and to teach you at a whole new level. You will need to take the tools you have learned and build new structures and create new paths to solving problems. The problems will range from very simple to very challenging, but they will all be very helpful for your GAMSAT preparation. Do not be afraid of making mistakes - it is part of the learning process. The student who makes the most mistakes has the greatest learning potential!

Timing is critical. Many students do not complete various sections of the exam. If you decide to do a few problems from time to time then you have never practiced for the GAMSAT. A full day exam is a rigorous event. It requires practice that simulates exam conditions. An important aspect of the latter is timing. Practice according to the prescribed exam schedule.

Upon finishing the exam, the next challenge is the equally important thorough review. Mistakes, and even correct answers for which some doubt existed, should be examined without time restrictions for maximum learning benefit.

Preparing the Tests

To sit the GAMSAT, you will need a watch or stopwatch, # 2 pencils, an eraser, and a pen with blue or black ink for Section II. During the actual administration, you will not be permitted a calculator for Section III. Calculations or notations must be made in the test booklet (scrap paper is not permitted).

For your GAMSAT test, you will find 3 test booklets and two answer documents. To create your test booklets tear your sheets out gently and systematically. Place the front of the book flat on a table and open to the pages just after the full length exam where you will find Answer Document 1 and Answer Document 2 for the exam you wish to write. Tear along the perforation.

The page numbers reflect the exam section to which the page belongs. For example, GS3-8 is the 8th page of Section III (3) of the GS GAMSAT. Begin pulling out pages while paying close attention to the page numbers. Once the complete exam is removed, you will require a stapler. Each of the 3 test sections has a cover page. Staple along the left margin of the cover page 5 times: the topmost and bottommost parts of the margin, once in between the two, and finally, staple once between the top and the middle staple, and again between the middle and the bottom staple. You should now have three test booklets.

Now you can use Answer Document 1 for multiple choice questions. Answer Document 2 will be used for Section II. Answer Document 2 should be stapled together forming a booklet similar to the other exam booklets.

Exam Schedule

You can expect to arrive at the designated exam center by 8 am, local time. Usually logistics are settled and students are sitting the exam by 9 am. About 7 hours later, the exam would have ended. Please see Section 1.2 in Part II of this textbook for your exam day schedule.

Answer Key Information

The answer key to Section III is cross-referenced. In other words, if you make a mistake, the answer key will direct you either to a specific area in a passage or to a specific section in the science review of this textbook. Alternatively, a key word, concept or equation might be written. If a problem strictly relies on reasoning skills, "deduce" may be written in the answer key without a cross-reference, or, with a cross-reference but only for background information. The hope is that you will find this new answer key informative and helpful as a quick reference. In addition, of course, the original owner of this textbook has 1 year of free online access to the explanations plus access to a Forum with a specific thread for each individual question.

Table 2: Identification of abbreviations and symbols for GS GAMSAT Answer Keys.

Ap	Appendix		PoE	Process of Elimination
B	Background Information		PT	Periodic Table
C	Concept		Q	Question
cf.	Compare		R	Reaction
D.A.	Dimensional Analysis (*see* Part II, 2.3, #16)		T	Table
			X.	Answer Choice X
E	Equation		X. = ba	emphasizes Choice X as being the *best* answer
EN	Electronegativity			
endo	Endothermic		X.:T/F	Choice X is true but does not answer Q
ESR	Electron Shell Repulsion		X. ↔ …	Choice X is wrong because...
exo	Exothermic			
F	Figure		Δ	Change, difference in
G	Graph		↑	Increase, higher
info	Information		↓	Decrease, lower
KS	Key Step		→	Proceeds to..., next step...
KW	Key Word		∴	Therefore
L	Line(s) where info can be found		*	Important!
			10.5–7	Section 10.5 to 10.7
P	Paragraph where info can be found		10.5/7	Section 10.5 and 10.7

CANDIDATE'S NAME _____   BOOKLET GS1-I

STUDENT ID _____

TEST GS-1

Section I:
Reasoning in Humanities and Social Sciences

Questions 1-75
Time : 100 Minutes

INSTRUCTIONS: Of the 75 questions in this test, many are organized into groups preceded by stimulus material. After evaluating the stimulus material, select the best answer to each question in the group. Some questions are independent of any descriptive passage or each other. Similarly, select the best answer to these questions. If you are unsure of an answer, eliminate the alternatives that you know to be incorrect and select an answer from the remaining alternatives. To indicate your selection, use a pencil to blacken the corresponding oval on Answer Document 1, GS-1. If you wish to make notes, it must be done ONLY in the test booklet. No scrap paper is permitted. No marks are deducted for wrong answers.

The Gold Standard GAMSAT* has been designed exclusively to test knowledge and thinking skills. The exam may contain hypothetical statements and/or express controversial ideas. Statements contained herein do not necessarily reflect the policy, position, or view of RuveneCo Inc.

OPEN BOOKLET ONLY WHEN TIMER IS READY.

Worked solutions are available to the original owner of this textbook at gamsat-prep.com.

GAMSAT is administered by ACER which is not associated with this product.
© RuveneCo Inc. All rights reserved. Reproduction without permission is illegal.

UNIT 1

The following two passages discuss different indigenous values.

Questions 1 – 2 refer to Passage I.

PASSAGE I

"Mitakuye Oyasin" is a Native American prayer and expression. Even though it only consists of two words in the Lakota Sioux language, the expression is considered the most powerful prayer when uttered. The phrase translates roughly as "all my relations" and "we are all-connected", within the same utterance.

The Lakota Sioux also honoured, respected, and can be said to have worshipped the Buffalo. Their ceremonies had rites and rituals and every part of the animal, after it was killed, was used for food, clothing, tools, and weapons.

In many ways, the Lakota Sioux exhibited wisdom in their views of the environment. Their prayer implies that all life deserves honour and respect, because all life is valued, and intertwined with each other. Their rituals also showed that from the smallest ant to the greatest and strongest creatures of the Earth, all are connected and useful in a biological system.

1. For the Lakota Sioux, "honour and respect" connotes:
   A   worship.
   B   interconnection.
   C   value.
   D   parity.

2. ". . . all life deserves honour and respect, because all life is valued, and intertwined with each other" is closest to which Native American proverb?
   A   Respect the gift and the giver.
   B   When we show our respect for other living things, they respond with respect for us.
   C   With all things and in all things, we are relatives.
   D   Treat the earth well: it was not given to you by your parents; it was loaned to you by your children. We do not inherit the Earth from our Ancestors; we borrow it from our Children.

Questions 3 – 6 relate to either Passage II or both passages.

PASSAGE II

For the Indigenous Australians, kinship to the land is a core spiritual value. While geographical boundaries such as lakes, rivers, and mountains distinguish each Aboriginal clan, these "traditional lands" bind the identity of its people to their territory. There are areas in a territory that certain clan members have a special connection with, like for example, the place where one's mother first conceived. This gives them a deeper affinity, respect and care for that locale and the lives surrounding it.

Understandably, an Aboriginal clan does not only possess the right to use their land and benefit from its returns; they also take on the duty to cultivate and preserve their own environment, including its animals. As one Kakadu elders, Bill Neidjie puts it, "Our story is in the land. . . it is written in those sacred places. . . My Children will look after those places, that's the law."

3. The phrase "Our story is in the land" connotes that:
   A   Aboriginal tribes are eternally bound to their land by tradition and history.
   B   among the Aborigines in Australia, the land and identity are inseparable.
   C   traditional lands embody the values and belief systems of the Aborigines.
   D   Aboriginal folklore is rich in stories about the origins of their land.

4. According to the Indigenous Australians, "respect and care" for the environment is an expression of:
   A   tribal worship.
   B   ancestral affinity.
   C   fiduciary duty.
   D   ethnic custom.

5. The Lakota Sioux and the Aborigines of Australia are only two of the native tribes which were labelled by 17th century European colonisers as "savages". However, the indigenous values presented in the two passages parallel much of today's principles about ecology. Which of the following statements would alter the old European perception regarding the culture of these native people?
   A   Indigenous people have always had a great sense of indebtedness and respect for the environment.
   B   The culture of the natives has always been guided by natural insights as compared to the highbrow rationalism of the Europeans.
   C   Native tribes have always had an advanced culture save for their unrefined wardrobe fashion.
   D   Indigenous people have long had a sophisticated code of conduct, which includes the preservation of and the harmonious co-existence with nature.

6. In both passages, the following is a common idea on the environment:
   A   both native cultures illustrate the interrelationships of all life.
   B   both cultures honour and respect ecosystems.
   C   indigenous tribes have a long history of worshipping nature.
   D   the two passages highlight indigenous spiritual orientation.

UNIT 2

Questions 7 - 16

*The following is an excerpt from **The Grapes of Wrath** by John Steinbeck.*

The owners of the land came onto the land, or more often a spokesman for the owners came. They came in closed cars, and they felt the dry earth with their fingers, and sometimes they drove big earth augers into the ground for soil tests. The tenants, from their sun-beaten dooryards, watched uneasily when the closed cars drove along the fields. And at last the owner men drove into the dooryards and sat in their cars to talk out of the windows. The tenant men stood beside the cars for awhile, and then squatted on their hams and   5
found sticks with which to mark the dust.
   In the open doors the women stood looking out, and behind them the children – corn headed children, with wide eyes, one bare foot on top of the other bare foot, and the toes working. The women and the children watched their men talking to the owner men.
   They were silent.   10
   Some of the owner men were kind because they hated what they had to do, and some of them were angry because they hated to be cruel, and some of them were cold because they had long ago found that one could not be an owner unless one were cold. And all of them were caught in something larger than themselves. Some of them hated the mathematics that drove them, and some were afraid, and some worshipped the mathematics because it provided a refuge from thought and from feeling. If a bank or   15
a finance company owned the land, the owner man said, The Bank – or the Company – needs – wants – insists – must have – as though the Bank or the Company were a monster, with thought and feeling, which had ensnared them. These last would take no responsibility for the banks or the companies because they were men and slaves, while the banks were machines and masters all at the same time. Some of the owner men were a little proud to be slaves to such cold and powerful masters.   20

The owner men sat in the cars and explained. "You know the land is poor. You've scrabbled at it long enough, God knows."

The squatting tenant men nodded and wondered and drew figures in the dust, and yes, they knew, God knows. If the dust only wouldn't fly. If the top would only stay on the soil, it might not be so bad.

The owner men went on leading to their point: "You know the land's getting poorer. You know what cotton does to the land; robs it, sucks all the blood out of it." 25

The squatters nodded – they knew, God knew. If they could only rotate the crops they might pump blood back into the land.

Well, it's too late. And the owner men explained the workings and the thinkings of the monster that was stronger than they were. "A man can hold land if he can just eat and pay taxes; he can do that." 30

"Yes, he can do that until his crops fail one day and he has to borrow money from the bank."

"But – you see, a bank or a company can't do that, because those creatures don't breathe air, don't eat side-meat. They breathe profits; they eat the interest on money. If they don't get it, they die the way you die without air, without side-meat. It is a sad thing, but it is so. It is just so."

7. The tenants are portrayed in the excerpt as:
   A   hard workers.
   B   poor and impoverished.
   C   well rewarded.
   D   lazy and incompetent.

8. "Monster" (line 17) in the passage refers to which of the following?
   A   The Dust
   B   The dying off of crops
   C   The banking system
   D   The owners of the land

9. The tone of the narrative in this passage suggests:
   A   perseverance.
   B   hopelessness.
   C   rage.
   D   anger.

10. The passage seems to describe a historical setting that took place during which American event listed below?
    A   The Great Depression
    B   World War 2
    C   The Dust Bowl
    D   The Great Immigration to the U.S.

11. "Scrabbled" (line 21) would mean:
    A   squandered.
    B   scrubbed away at.
    C   squatted on.
    D   tilled.

12. There are many references to "squatting" in the narrative. What would be the best definition listed below?
    A   Waiting for good soil
    B   Wasting time idly, not working
    C   Staying on the land, to own it
    D   Ready to get orders from the bosses

13. To some extent, the workers are portrayed as slaves in the excerpt. How are the bosses portrayed?
    A   Mean, cruel, and without conscience
    B   As slaves to the banks
    C   Supportive of the worker's rights
    D   As hard working farmers

14. Based on the excerpt, owners:
    A   are genuinely concerned about the squatters.
    B   are in cahoots with the banks.
    C   want the squatters to leave.
    D   have no interest in the squatters.

15. In this excerpt, the predominant image is:
    A   machinery.
    B   cotton.
    C   soil.
    D   dust.

16. In the colloquial phrase "cat side-meat" (lines 32-33), what does "cat" refer to?
    A   Stealing
    B   Eating
    C   Hording
    D   Portioning

UNIT 3

Questions 17 – 18

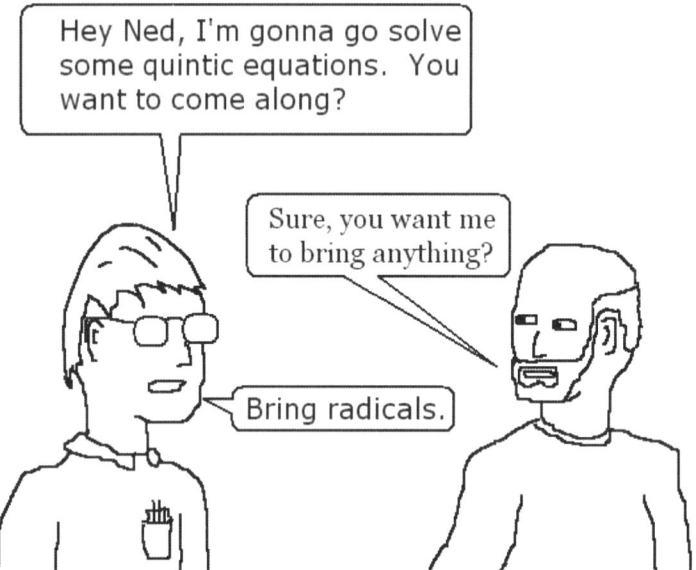

17. Even though we may not be familiar with quintic equations (which are polynomials as groups of 5, hence "quin"), the humour of this cartoon is due to which of the following?
    A   Math and geeks
    B   The diversity of meanings in language
    C   The unintended irony
    D   The logical fallacies presented

18. We can infer from the party or social get together context of the cartoon that:
    A   there is always somebody radical at an event.
    B   radicals are very significant in relation to quintic equations.
    C   the get together is for brainiacs and math whizzes.
    D   the author is not playing with language.

UNIT 4

Questions 19 – 21

The following is a short parable by the German philosopher Schopenhauer.

In a field of ripening corn I came to a place which had been trampled down by some ruthless foot; and as I glanced amongst the countless stalks, every one of them alike, standing there so erect and bearing the full weight of the ear, I saw a multitude of different flowers, red and blue and violet. How pretty they looked as they grew there so naturally with their little foliage! But, thought I, they are quite useless; they bear no fruit; they are mere weeds, suffered to remain only because there is no getting rid of them. And yet, but for these flowers, there would be nothing to charm the eye in that wilderness of stalks. They are emblematic of poetry and art, which, in civic life – so severe, but still useful and not without its fruit – play the same part as flowers in the corn.

19. The speaker in this parable regards the flowers as:
    A   symbolic of the colours and abundance of life.
    B   representative of the beautiful but useless in life.
    C   unnecessary splendour that makes life bearable.
    D   ideal symbols of poetic and artistic creations.

20. The parable suggests that the speaker regards poetry and art as:
    A   superfluous.
    B   purely ornamental.
    C   uplifting.
    D   purposive.

21. This parable could best be described as:
    A   comparing and contrasting useful corn and beautiful flowers.
    B   illustrating the functional aesthetics of poetry and art and nature.
    C   pointing out how diverse nature is.
    D   showing how poetry and flowers are like weeds.

UNIT 5

Questions 22 – 33

Extended Unit on Romanticism (in broken paragraphs)

PARAGRAPH I

The Romantic era, period, or movement, can be viewed as an artistic, political, and philosophical response to classical ideals and political dogma, the burgeoning paradigm of scientific rationalism, and the emergence of the industrial revolution. Within the historical context of the French and American Revolution, the individual was gaining new liberties over tyranny. The romantic hero emerged as a cultural icon becoming manifested in literary, philosophical, and historical stereotypes.

22. In Paragraph I, why would scientific rationalism, be considered a burgeoning paradigm?
    A   Because as a model of inquiry, it would be the dominant example to follow.
    B   Because the experimental method was beginning.
    C   Because technological innovations were at the forefront of culture.
    D   Because it was in direct opposition to poetic modes of thought.

PARAGRAPH II

Emphasizing subjective experience over objective agreement, as in Browning's phrase "the mind is a thousand times more beautiful than nature could ever be", the romantic hero became a common figure in lyrical poetry and theatre. This passionate, talented hero, rejects societal ideals and norms, yet is instilled with some tragic flaw, which leads to his demise. Imbued with the attainment of perfection, the romantic hero could easily utter Browning's remarks, "A man's reach must exceed his grasp, or what is a heaven for?"

23. In reference to one of Lord Byron's major works, he is often quoted as saying: "Man's greatest tragedy is that he can conceive of a perfection which he cannot attain." Lord Byron's statement and Browning's "A man's reach must exceed his grasp, or what is a heaven for":
    A   differ in their perceptions of a perfect society.
    B   differ in their outlook towards man's pursuit of achieving perfection.
    C   are similar in their positive views about obtaining a perfect world.
    D   are similar in their assumptions about the nature of worldly pursuits.

PARAGRAPH III

Such is the basic nature of Moliere and Lord Byron's "Don Juan", whose unattainable appetites and libertine excesses bring about his own downfall. During this era, William Blake, visionary poet, remarked "the road of excess leads to the palace of wisdom" as if predefining a Byronic type of hero. Byron's own exploits paralleled his literary creations, as well, as a kind of "unattainable excess". Keats would describe this affliction or obsession as "egotistical sublime", and we find it in different personae in this era. Goethe's Faust suffers from the same malady but also ultimately redeems himself.

24. Paragraph III implies that, for Keats, a typical Byronic hero:
    A   is a failed perfectionist.
    B   is an obsessive, soul-searching hero.
    C   has no defined identity.
    D   is an excessive pleasure-seeker.

PARAGRAPH IV

In history, we find this same overachieving ego-figure in Napoleon, releasing the serfs from oppression, insisting on equality, founding the Napoleonic code of law, extending his megalomaniacal military reaches across the globe, until he is turned away from Russia, and defeated at Waterloo. Finally Napoleon was exiled, like The Count of Monte Cristo, and brought down by his own lust for power.

25. When describing Napoleon's military reaches, the term "megalomaniacal" is used. This term roughly equates to:
    A   slovenliness.
    B   prestige.
    C   military-like.
    D   ego.

PARAGRAPH V

The maestro violinist, Niccolò Paganini, whose persecution by the Church, can be seen as a romantic hero. Undeterred in his efforts to compose and perform, many legends and myths surround him. Supposedly slowly poisoned by mercury used to treat his tertiary syphilis, he was believed to be a fiddling devil, being able to play virtuoso on one string, caricatured as the mad genius who sold his soul, much like Faust. Being that the romantic mind was fascinated with things distorted or beyond nature, in a word – grotesque, as evidenced in Mary Shelley's Frankenstein, the demonic character of Paganini was a perfect example of how romantic ideas could enter into popular folklore.

26. In Paragraph V, the association between a romantic mind and the characters of Frankenstein and Paganini suggests that:
    A   being experimental was a Romantic tendency.
    B   the Romantic Movement was preoccupied with the unconventional and bizarre.
    C   the duality of human nature polarized between the sinister and the extraordinary, between good and evil, was a typical characteristic of a Romantic hero.
    D   Romanticism was distorted.

PARAGRAPH VI

While the beginnings of the scientific method were being refined, many poets and philosophers stood in bleak contrast to the rational logico-deductive models, and also drifted away from the classical Apollonian muses. In fact, the concept of imagination was offered by the romantics as diametrically opposed. "We murder to dissect" was Wordsworth's herald and "contemplation of nature" was given the highest priority against reductionist forms of thought. By finding voice in Dionysian modes of expression, without the Hellenic order and restraint of tempered meter or rhyme, these romantics located truth in the individual. In philosophy, subjective idealism was finding its groundings in Leibniz and Berkeley, and later more radically, with Nietzsche. In Germany, the romantic virtuoso was Beethoven and later Wagner, whose operas portrayed the pinnacle of German Romanticism, with its excessive exuberance, reigniting Nordic myths into national epics.

27. Wordsworth's quote in Paragraph IV, "We murder to dissect" is a poetic response to:
    A   extreme egoism.
    B   the fatal flaw.
    C   fallacies of myth.
    D   the scientific method.

28. In Paragraph VI, an opposition between the classical Greek gods – Apollo and Dionysus – symbolizes which of the following?
    A   Truth and Illusion
    B   Order and Freedom
    C   Music and Poetry
    D   Ego and Pride

PARAGRAPH VII

Blake, Wordsworth, Keats, Shelley, et al. helped define poets "as unacknowledged legislators of the world, (Shelley)," who should break free of "the mind-forged manacles (Blake)" of contemporary thought through contemplation with and of nature. Keats' "Truth is Beauty, Beauty is Truth" is symptomatic of the romantic impulse to find an alternative to the reductive process of science, which many poets found "dissective" in its scope and process.

Perhaps the epitome and end of Romantic philosophers can be found in Nietzsche, who in virtual isolation from humanity, writes of a greater humanity, located in the 'Superman', beyond good and evil. Peering into the abyss and limits of philosophy, as such, brought about his own downfall in the form of madness.

29. According to Paragraph VII, which of the following is NOT true about the Romantic era?
    A   The Romantic era was concerned with individual experience.
    B   The Romantic era sought freedom from different constraints.
    C   The Romantic era was concerned with contemplation with Nature.
    D   The Romantic era was logical and scientific.

30. The description of Nietzsche "who in virtual isolation from humanity, writes of a greater humanity" is an example of what?
    A   Madness
    B   Contradiction
    C   Irony
    D   Metaphor

Questions 31 – 33 pertain to all paragraphs.

31. Which of the following statements does NOT describe the Romantic spirit implied in the preceding paragraphs?
    A   Do what you will, this world's a fiction and is made up of contradiction.
    B   Come forth into the light of things, let nature be your teacher.
    C   I have love in me the likes of which you can scarcely imagine. A rage, the likes of which you would not believe. If I cannot satisfy one, I will indulge in the other.
    D   I love you the more in that I believe you had liked me for my own sake and for nothing else.

32. A certain type of support in relation to the author's interpretation was extensively used in the paragraphs. Which of the following would be the best answer in defining this type of support?
    A   Historical examples
    B   Literary quotations
    C   Various juxtapositions
    D   Contrasting analogies

33. Based on the paragraphs, the term "subjective" in the Romantic context is:
    A   outside, verifiable.
    B   dependent upon.
    C   subject to.
    D   personal, individual.

UNIT 6

Questions 34 -37

The following is Graham's "Hierarchy of Disagreement".

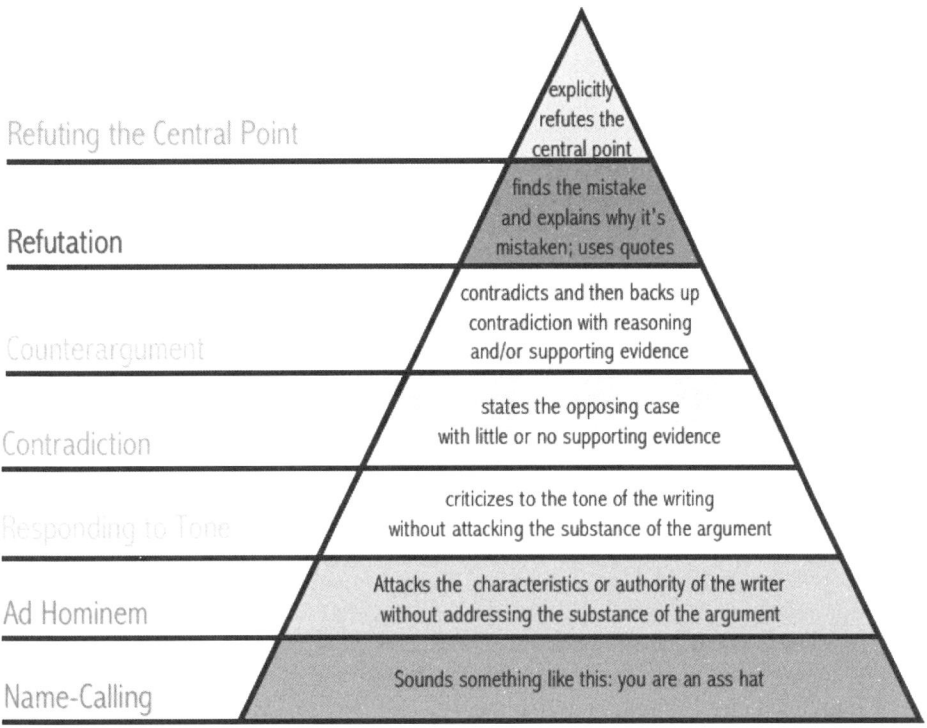

34. Based on the diagram, what makes "Responding to Tone" a weak form of disagreement?
    A   Tone is hard to judge.
    B   It overlooks the correctness of the writer's point.
    C   The response is still fundamentally a personal attack on the writer.
    D   It allows the critic to disagree without valid evidence.

35. This diagram shows that:
    A   it is necessary to differentiate between name-calling and Ad Hominem attacks.
    B   refuting the main point of an argument does not need supporting evidence.
    C   the tone of the argument is more important than the substance of the argument.
    D   the hierarchy moves from an emotional response to logical refutation.

36. Graham's "Hierarchy of Disagreement" seems to emphasize that:
    A   argumentation is inherently impassioned.
    B   anger makes argumentation personal.
    C   disagreeing essentially means arguing.
    D   it is possible to disagree without necessarily being angry.

37. The disagreement hierarchy is presented in the form of a pyramid in order to show that:
    A   disagreements occur in stages.
    B   forms of disagreement are arranged in an ascending manner.
    C   the more rational the disagreement, the less it is employed.
    D   rationality should govern disagreements.

UNIT 7

Questions 38 – 42

Afternoon in School - The Last Lesson

When will the bell ring, and end this weariness?
How long have they tugged the leash, and strained apart
My pack of unruly hounds: I cannot start
Them again on a quarry of knowledge they hate to hunt,
I can haul them and urge them no more.   5
No more can I endure to bear the brunt
Of the books that lie out on the desks: a full three score
Of several insults of blotted pages and scrawl
Of slovenly work that they have offered me.
I am sick, and tired more than any thrall   10
Upon the woodstacks working weariedly.

And shall I take
The last dear fuel and heap it on my soul
Till I rouse my will like a fire to consume
Their dross of indifference, and burn the scroll   15
Of their insults in punishment? - I will not!
I will not waste myself to embers for them,
Not all for them shall the fires of my life be hot,
For myself a heap of ashes of weariness, till sleep
Shall have raked the embers clear: I will keep   20
Some of my strength for myself, for if I should sell
It all for them, I should hate them -
- I will sit and wait for the bell.

D. H. Lawrence

38. The learning atmosphere depicted in the poem is:
    A   exhausting because of the healthy exchange of ideas.
    B   challenging.
    C   unruly and hateful.
    D   indifferent, therefore pointless.

39. What is meant by "slovenly work" (line 9)?
    A   Done obediently like a dog
    B   Repetitive and unnecessary
    C   Terse and unfocused
    D   Done in a hasty and sloppy fashion

40. The literary style of Lawrence's poem, with its series of rhetorical questions, theatrically most resembles a(n):
    A   dialogue.   B   soliloquy.
    C   imbrications.   D   aside.

41. Line 23 suggests that the attitude of the speaker is one of:
    A   impatience.
    B   detachment.
    C   resignation.
    D   frustration.

42. The ringing of the bell in this poem connotes:
    A   a relief from boredom.
    B   freedom from the burdens of teaching.
    C   a signal of opportunity for the speaker to channel his noble efforts to a more rewarding endeavour.
    D   hope for a better classroom situation the next day.

UNIT 8

Questions 43 – 47

From late 1950s to early 1960s, the issue of African-American Civil Rights was crucial in shaping the eventual structure of politics and image of democracy in America. The following are excerpts from speeches of two of the most influential advocate-leaders of the time.

Questions 43 – 44 pertain to Passage I.

PASSAGE I

The political philosophy of black nationalism means that the black man should control the politics and the politicians in his own community; no more. The black man in the black community has to be re-educated into the science of politics so he will know what politics is supposed to bring him in return. Don't be throwing out any ballots. A ballot is like a bullet. You don't throw your ballots until you see a target, and if that target is not within your reach, keep your ballot in your pocket.

The political philosophy of black nationalism is being taught in the Christian church. It's being taught in the NAACP. It's being taught in CORE meetings. It's being taught in SNCC Student Nonviolent Coordinating Committee meetings. It's being taught in Muslim meetings. It's being taught where nothing but atheists and agnostics come together. It's being taught everywhere.

Black people are fed up with the dillydallying, pussyfooting, compromising approach that we've been using toward getting our freedom. We want freedom now, but we're not going to get it saying "We Shall Overcome." We've got to fight until we overcome.

The economic philosophy of black nationalism is pure and simple. It only means that we should control the economy of our community. Why should white people be running all the stores in our community? Why should white people be running the banks of our community? Why should the economy of our community be in the hands of the white man? Why? If a black man can't move his store into a white community, you tell me why a white man should move his store into a black community. The philosophy of black nationalism involves a re-education program in the black community in regards to economics. Our people have to be made to see that any time you take your dollar out of your community and spend it in a community where you don't live, the community where you live will get poorer and poorer, and the community where you spend your money will get richer and richer.

"The Ballot or the Bullet" by Malcolm X
(Founder, Muslim Mosque Inc.)
April 3 1964

43. Based on the passage, Malcolm X associates the ballot with:
    A   wise decision-making.
    B   freedom to act out one's choice.
    C   a means for achieving advancement.
    D   civil rights.

44. Malcolm X proposes that the way for African-Americans to attain freedom is through:
    A   a drastic change in the national political system.
    B   the indoctrination of Black Nationalism.
    C   exigent measures.
    D   voting wisely.

PASSAGE II

Every American citizen must have an equal right to vote.

There is no reason which can excuse the denial of that right. There is no duty which weighs more heavily on us than the duty we have to ensure that right.

Yet the harsh fact is that in many places in this country men and women are kept from voting simply because they are Negroes. Every device of which human ingenuity is capable has been used to deny this right. The Negro citizen may go to register only to be told that the day is wrong, or the hour is late, or the official in charge is absent. And if he persists, and if he manages to present himself to the registrar, he may be disqualified because he did not spell out his middle name or because he abbreviated a word on the application. And if he manages to fill out an application, he is given a test. The registrar is the sole judge of whether he passes this test.

He may be asked to recite the entire Constitution, or explain the most complex provisions of State law. And even a college degree cannot be used to prove that he can read and write.

For the fact is that the only way to pass these barriers is to show a white skin. Experience has clearly shown that the existing process of law cannot overcome systematic and ingenious discrimination. No law that we now have on the books – and I have helped to put three of them there – can ensure the right to vote when local officials are determined to deny it. In such a case our duty must be clear to all of us. The Constitution says that no person shall be kept from voting because of his race or his colour. We have all sworn an oath before God to support and to defend that Constitution. We must now act in obedience to that oath.

from "We Shall Overcome" by Lyndon Baines Johnson
(Thirteenth President of the United States)
March 16 1965

Questions 45 – 47 apply to either Passage II or both passages.

45. Former U.S. President Johnson views equality in voting rights as a(n):
    A   social responsibility.
    B   constitutional right.
    C   political duty.
    D   affirmation of freedom.

46. In reference to the failure of granting equal rights to the African-Americans, both speakers assign the culpability to:
    A   the biased government system.
    B   segregation.
    C   cunning politicians.
    D   arbitrary legal provisions.

47. The two passages seem to suggest that:
    A   Malcolm X favours racial segregation while President Johnson favours integration.
    B   unlike Malcolm X, President Johnson maintains his confidence in the U.S. Constitution.
    C   both speakers claim that the government is responsible for racial inequities in America.
    D   Malcolm X views the act of voting as a choice while President Johnson views it as a must.

UNIT 9

Questions 48 – 54

Consider the following passage and comments in answering the questions.

Some aspects of postmodern art concern self-consciousness of the art act itself, the laying bare of the devices used to construct the illusion or representation, and blurring the divisions between the audience and the art. For example, John Cage, a pianist and to some extent experimentalist in art, recorded only audience noise for one of his compositions: the shuffling about in seats, coughs, whispers, etc... all to some extent, what would be considered noise. His most famous work is the 4'33", which he composed in 1952. This piece is performed in three movements without the musician hitting a single note for four minutes and thirty three seconds. The composition is supposed to consist of the sounds of the surroundings that the listener hears while it is performed.

The following remarks are quoted from Cage himself:

Comment I

Wherever we are, what we hear is mostly noise. When we ignore it, it disturbs us. When we listen to it, we find it fascinating.

Comment II

People who are not artists often feel that artists are inspired. But if you work at your art you don't have time to be inspired.

Comment III

Ideas are one thing and what happens is another.

Comment IV

The grand thing about the human mind is that it can turn its own tables and see meaninglessness as ultimate meaning.

Comment V

Art's purpose is to sober and quiet the mind so that it is in accord with what happens.

Comment VI

The first question I ask myself when something doesn't seem to be beautiful is why do I think it's not beautiful. And very shortly you discover that there is no reason.

Comment VII

The highest purpose is to have no purpose at all. This puts one in accord with nature, in her manner of operation.

48. In Comment I, which of the following could be reasonably inferred about John Cage's view of music?
    A   Music takes different forms.
    B   Music is an affirmation of life.
    C   Silence is music in itself.
    D   The appreciation of music depends on how you listen to it.

49. Comments V and VII support the notion that the purpose of music is to:
- A have no purpose at all.
- B bring about internal order out of chaos.
- C reveal the natural motion of life.
- D liberate the listeners from artificial conventions.

50. How many of the comments would contradict the concept that art should be an expression of the artist's inner state rather than his or her subject?
- A 4
- B 2
- C 3
- D 1

51. Which of Comments I to VII is closely similar to the idea of "art for art's sake"?
- A Comment II
- B Comment IV
- C Comment V
- D Comment VII

Questions 52 – 54 relate to the pictures or the comments, whichever is applicable.

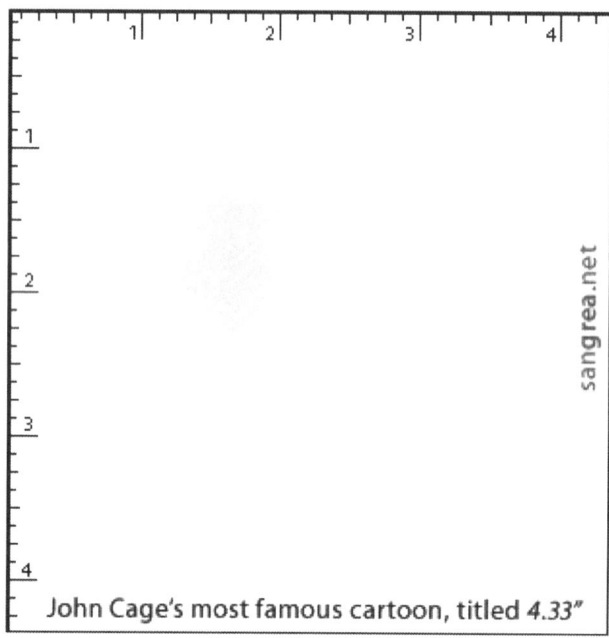

Picture 1

52. Which among Comments I to VII does Picture 1 relate with?
- A Comment III
- B Comment IV
- C Comment VI
- D Comment VII

53. In relation to the comments, what makes Picture 1 humorous?
- A Its self-referentiality
- B There is nothing there, except the two axes.
- C It mocks the pretensions of such notions.
- D All of the above

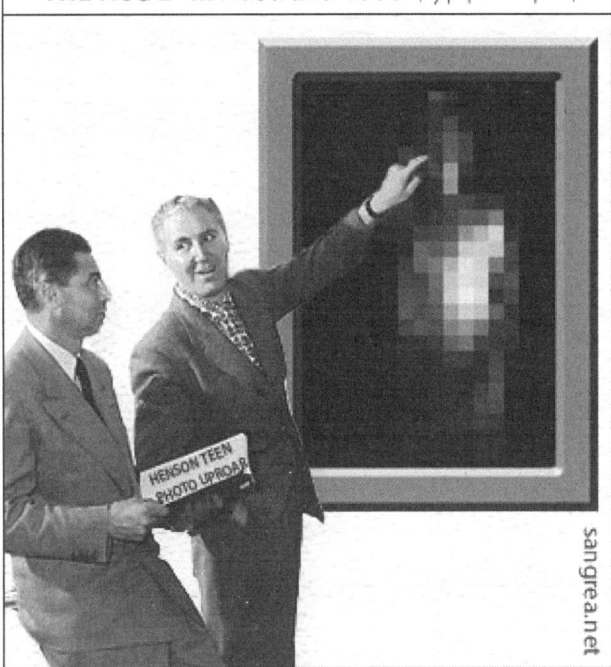

Picture 2

54. The humour in this picture is derived from the overbearing standards of:
    A   censorship.
    B   representation.
    C   traditional art.
    D   colour contrast to black and white.

UNIT 10

Questions 55 – 57

The following compilation of crime percentages were based on some Thailand research in relation to other countries of the Western world.

Table 1. Crimes Statistics: Thailand and selected Western Countries

Assaults (per thousand people)	Burglaries (per thousand people)
US 7.6	Australia 21.7
UK 7.5	UK 13.8
Canada 7.1	Canada 8.9
Australia 7.0	US 7.1
France 1.8	France 6.1
Germany 1.4	Japan 2.3
Thailand 0.3	Thailand 0.2
Japan 0.3	Germany N/A

Rapes (per hundred thousand people)	Gun Murders (per hundred thousand people)
Australia 79	Thailand 31
Canada 73	US 2.8
US 30	Canada 0.5
UK 14	Germany 0.5
France 14	Autraslia 0.1
Germany 9	UK 0.1
Thailand 6	Japan N/A
Japan 2	France N/A

55. The number of violent crimes (listed as Assaults, Rapes, and Murders) were committed in Australia and Thailand in this selected temporal frame. Which country had the LEAST amount of violent crimes listed?
    A   Japan
    B   Thailand
    C   France
    D   Germany

56. Which country would define the closest approximation to a mean or average of the crime of rape listed?
    A   Germany
    B   US
    C   UK
    D   France

57. The main purpose of the chart provided could be inferred to:
    A   assess Thailand's crime rates in relation to other countries.
    B   promote gun control measures or legislation in Thailand.
    C   provide statistics for analysis in Thailand's violent and non-violent crimes.
    D   compare and contrast the different crimes worldwide in relation to Thailand.

UNIT 11

Question 58

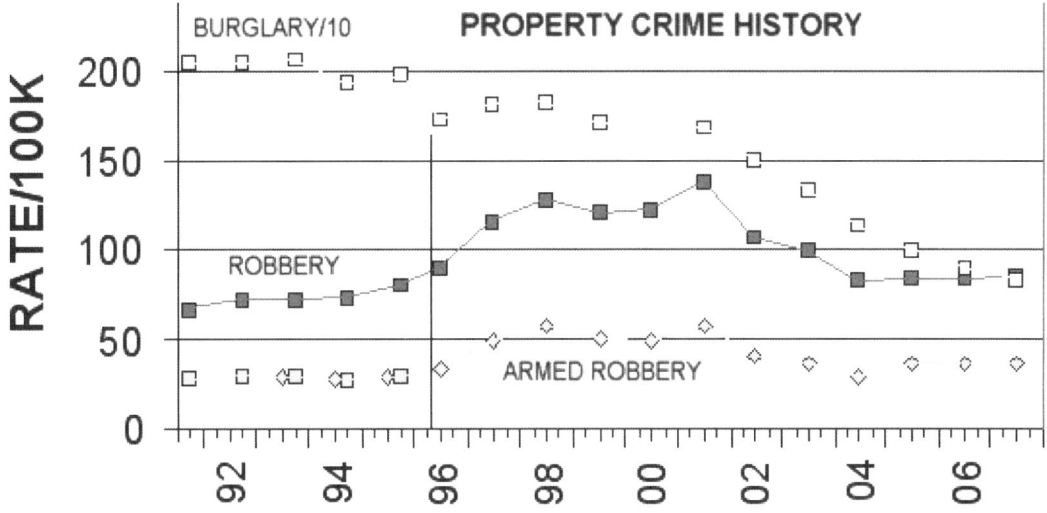

Figure 1. Property Crime History in Australia

58. Which of the following would make the best generalization concerning Australian crime rates based on Figure 1?
    A   The decline of burglary, over the years, corresponds to a rise in robbery.
    B   The rates for robbery and armed robbery rose faster after 1996, and stayed higher for a few years.
    C   All three types of crime do not decline after 1993.
    D   It appears that a short term increase in armed robbery occurred after 2002.

UNIT 12

Questions 59 – 65

The Englishman and Music

Englishmen have never cared for music as they care for football or film stars. They like singing, most of them, either making a noise themselves or listening to others. There is a long tradition both of religion and conviviality by which men and women who would not claim to be musical will gladly take part in a hymn or join in a chorus. There has been a tradition centuries old by which choral singing in parts has been a fairly widespread pastime. In Elizabethan times, it was something more: for about forty years it appears to have been a fashionable craze among cultivated people, and, though it is easy to overestimate the excellence of their performance, the singers of those days conferred an incalculable benefit upon the art of music and a rich heritage upon English musical life by their assiduous practice, thereby stimulating to activity a whole school of first-rate composers. Assuredly England has never been a "land without music", as the reproachful German phrase went a couple of generations ago. But music, musical affairs, musical politics, new compositions, the status of individual artists, have never in this country been "front page news": the bulk of the population does not really care how music gets along provided that on occasion it can obtain what it wants for ceremonial occasions, for occasional polite entertainment, for lubricating the wheels on which its theatrical or restaurant entertainment runs... Our festivals, our opera seasons, and the performance of our virtuosi, even our musical competitions, leave our national phlegm unmoved. The tantrums of a prima donna have a certain human interest for our popular newspapers, but by and large the great public does not care. Are we then a musical people?

... Are we a blue-eyed people? Some of us are blue-eyed and some of us are musical. The musical enthusiasts are a small minority, but the potentially musical are a much larger number. Perhaps five percent are definitely insusceptible to music... The rest are capable of having their interest, and perhaps ultimately their love, aroused for the art. There are many things in this beautiful world that compete for our attention, for our limited time, for our not unlimited mental energy, and for our pocket-money, and many will sacrifice music to fly-fishing or watching birds... many a gifted person with artistic abilities that run in several directions at once will devote himself to water-colours instead of the piano. But the coming of the wireless broadcasting has at least made numbers of people, running into the hundreds of thousands, aware of music as a factor in their experience of life.

The kind of satisfaction that comes from music... is one of the things that give value to life. Possibly it is the most perfect example of those higher disinterested values that give significance to life, in that it is unmixed with social, political and ethical purposes and so provides us with an instance of what is valuable in and for itself alone without further object. Not everyone will want this particular kind of satisfaction from music; some take a more hedonistic view of it and value it as just one more ingredient in the good life. Still others are content with the opiate of light music. But whichever of the many sorts of psychological satisfaction that can be getting from music may be found by any individual, it is so far a part of his life's experience, and more and more people are coming to be aware of it as such and to value it as an enrichment of their lives.

Adapted from Frank Howes, Fontana Guide to Orchestral Music, 8 1958 by Collins Clear Type Press

59. According to the passage, the attitude of the English during the Elizabethan era was most influential in resulting to:
   A   an interest in musical affairs which had never been there previously.
   B   increased participation in hymn and choir singing in churches.
   C   a revival in choral singing in parts.
   D   great musical compositions by a new era of composers.

60. The author rhetorically asks "Are we a blue-eyed people?" in order to:
   A   exemplify that nearly half of the population is, at least, partially musical.
   B   convey the irrelevance of questioning whether the English are musical or not.
   C   affirm that, as a whole, the English are a musical people.
   D   emphasize the contrasting attitudes towards music between the English, Germans and Russians.

61. The passage suggests that the English might be less interested than the Germans in news concerning:
   A   football and the newest developments in that sport.
   B   issues in musical entertainment that might affect business.
   C   outdoor hobbies.
   D   developments in the music and theatre industry.

62. According to the author, someone who is "insusceptible to music" is someone who:
   A   is uninterested in musical affairs, musical politics, and the state of individual artists.
   B   would rather not waste their time fly-fishing or bird-watching.
   C   is incapable of having their interest for music aroused.
   D   would rather devote their time to water-colours.

63. The passage indicates that the renewed musical awareness in England can in part be attributed to:
   A   the assiduous practicing of singers over the years.
   B   the introduction of wireless broadcasting into society.
   C   the emergence of a whole new school for talented composers.
   D   a decline of interest in football that has occurred over the years.

64. Based on the passage, one could conclude that the author believes that music's greatest value lies in the fact that:
   A   it has a great ability to bring joy.
   B   it is a form of expression which is detached from politics, social and cultural issues.
   C   it is a component of the good life.
   D   it has the power to enrich the life of every individual who becomes aware of it.

65. Which of the following would be the best reason why the English are NOT musically inclined as other Germanic countries?
   A   They are more interested in hobbies and sports.
   B   They have no great composers, in relation to Bach or Beethoven.
   C   Look at modern culture, such as the British invasion of Rock and Roll.
   D   Their musical proclivities are in the nascent stages of development.

UNIT 13

Questions 66 – 69

The following are two short passages from Shakespeare (Macbeth and King Lear).

Macbeth, after his queen's death, makes the following famous speech in Act 5, Scene 5, lines 17-28.

MACBETH: Wherefore was that cry?

SEYTON: The queen, my lord, is dead.

MACBETH: She should have died hereafter;
There would have been a time for such a word.
To-morrow, and to-morrow, and to-morrow,
Creeps in this petty pace from day to day
To the last syllable of recorded time,
And all our yesterdays have lighted fools
The way to dusty death. Out, out, brief candle!
Life's but a walking shadow, a poor player
That struts and frets his hour upon the stage
And then is heard no more: it is a tale
Told by an idiot, full of sound and fury,
Signifying nothing

Act III, Scene IV, during the terrible storm. While his fool takes shelter in a hovel, Lear, after learning of his daughter's treachery, throws himself into the wilderness, losing his sanity or so it seems. Here he remains standing for a moment in the rain and meditates on the poor citizens of his kingdom:

Poor naked wretches, whereso'er you are,
That bide the pelting of this pitiless storm,
How shall your houseless heads and unfed sides,
Your loop'd and window'd raggedness, defend you
From seasons such as these? O, I have ta'en
Too little care of this! Take physic, pomp;
Expose thyself to feel what wretches feel,
That thou mayst shake the superflux to them,
And show the heavens more just.

66. In the Macbeth passage, the tonality of Shakespeare suggests:
    A   remorse.
    B   despair.
    C   grief.
    D   anxiety.

67. In the King Lear passage, the tonality of Shakespeare suggests:
    A   shattered innocence.
    B   profound enlightenment.
    C   remorseful compassion.
    D   indignant defiance.

68. In the passage from King Lear "Take Physic, pomp" is a strange and anachronistic utterance. Based on the context of the passage, this would mean in modern day language:
   A   to understand the poor's suffering.
   B   to feel the elements of the storm arrogantly.
   C   to strive to make things just.
   D   pompous men take a taste of this medicine.

69. Which of the following generalizations could be inferred concerning both passages?
   A   Life is unjust.
   B   Life is meaningless.
   C   Life is constantly changing.
   D   Life is storm-like.

UNIT 14

Questions 70 – 73

The following are pictures from World War 1 and World War 2.

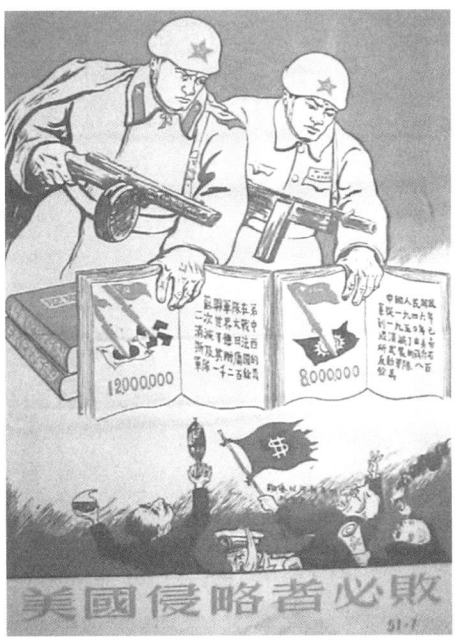

Picture 1–from China ("You will be defeated!" - translation)

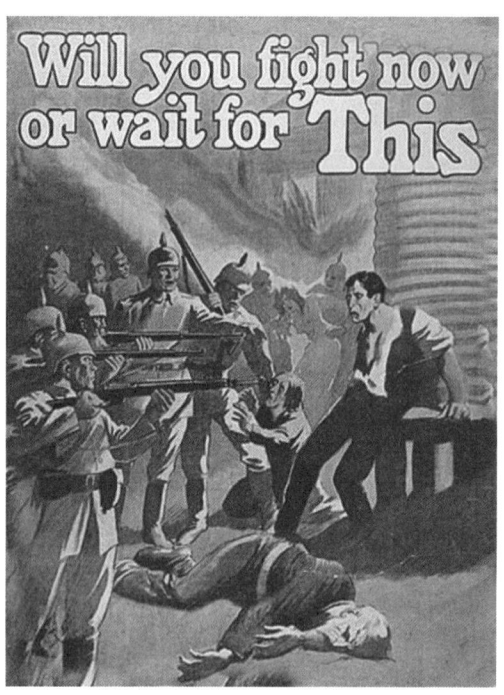
Picture 2–from Australia (WW1)

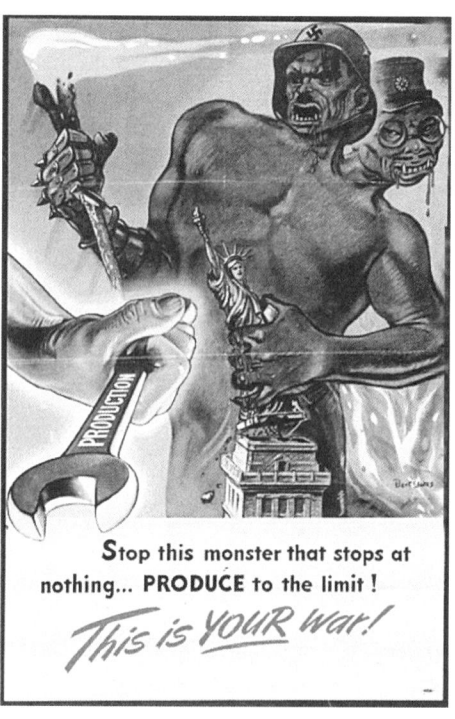
Picture 3–from the U.S.

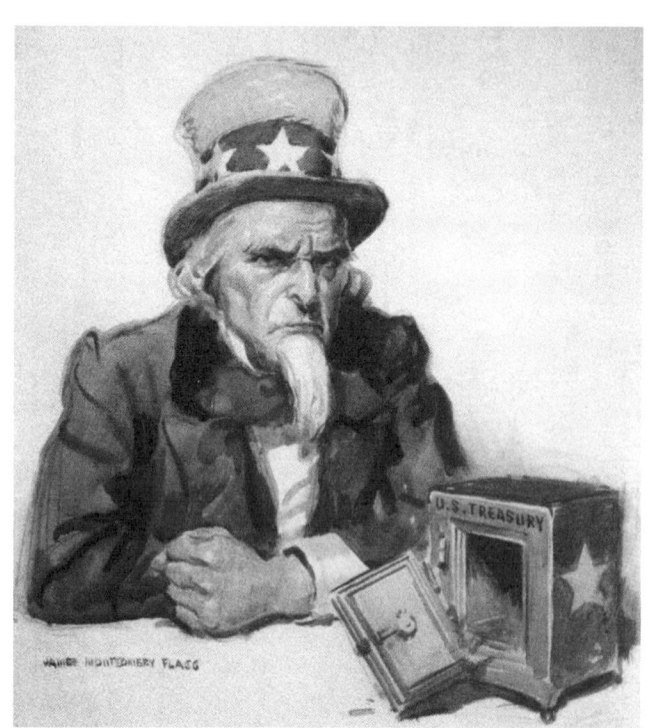
Picture 4–from the U.S.

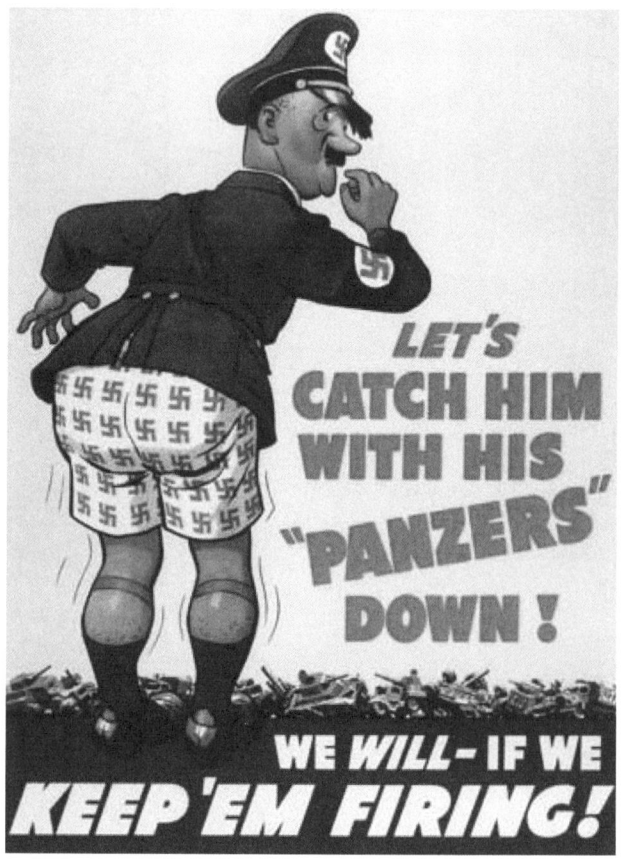
Picture 5–from the UK

It can be argued that all of the 5 pictures represent propaganda to at least some extent.

70. Which of the pictures appeals mostly to a "sense of patriotism and homeland"?
    A   1
    B   5
    C   3
    D   2

71. Which of the following ratios depict the representations' use of emotional appeals respectively (1-5)?
    A   Quantity, quality, labour, taxes, derision
    B   Rage, sentiment, workers, money, laughter
    C   Intimidation, fear, demonization, economic insecurity, humour
    D   Polarization, patriotism, caricatures, foolhardiness

72. Which picture is the most emotionally charged?
    A   3
    B   4
    C   1
    D   5

73. Which picture "polarizes"? (either/or thinking)
    A   2
    B   5
    C   1
    D   3

UNIT 15

Questions 74–75

How to Learn the Lost "Art of Memory"

Many scholars have claimed that "the art of memory" or lost art was due to the rise of the written word. The ancient Greeks and Romans supposedly had enormous memories, based on a few architectural tricks. Essentially, they would accomplish these by using mental rooms or diagrams, which were known as "loci". Even the internet has shown an increase of interest in such a lost art, with slogans, such as "memorize" by rooms of your house, or toolbox, or even building a mental palace which is compartmentalized to the extent that it can hold whatever you wish to remember! The pictures below were from Giordano Bruno, who tried to reinvent the art, in the late dark ages.

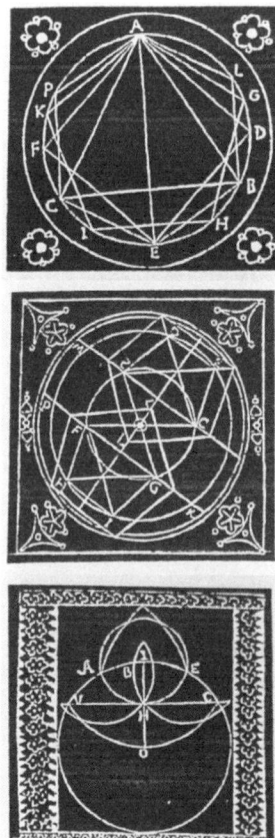

Even though orators such as Cicero and Quintilian have offered advice on how to do such an outrageous act of mental imagery, categorization, compartmentalization, and memory, below are some contemporaneous suggestions on how to start and accomplish this feat of mnemonics.

How to Build Your Memory Palace

At the World Memory Championships, top competitors memorize the order of 20 shuffled decks of cards in an hour and more than 500 random digits in 15 minutes, among other events. A Secret is to build a memory palace, an image in your mind.

- Decide on a blueprint for your palace. Real or imagined. You can use your home, if you wish, but it has to have route, and places of storage, for your items you need to memorize.

- Define a route. Take a walk through. If you need to remember items in sequence, it is important to do this, as imagery in your mind, walking through your home or palace.

- Identify specific storage locations in your palace or along your route. You can store things you need to remember, in specific rooms, closets, drawers, chests, and so forth. For example, if you wish to remember things you need to get at the store, store those items in the respective places, with a visual image–shampoo, toothpaste–bathroom, etc. Be Creative.

- Memorize your memory palace. Draw out your map, graphic or blueprint, with the rooms and items which you need to memorize–this will help you greatly by matching the visual image on paper, with the image in your mind.

- Place things to be remembered in your palace. Based on your route, place items you need to remember in select places.

- Use symbols. You may want to associate a symbol which is placed in a room, with something you need to remember–such as a musical note or staff, by the entertainment centre, indicating that new music you wish to purchase.

- Be creative. Associate rooms, objects, items, with each other in different ways. Experiment!

- Stock your palace with other mnemonics. You may have a special place where you keep old letters and pictures from your past, which trigger memories. Put such devices as the musical treble clef of "Every Good Boy Does Fine" (EGBDF) in this place.

- Explore your palace. Once you have stocked your palace with evocative images, you need to go through it and look at them. Visualize the walk through the rooms, the symbols and devices; if you cannot do this, write them out again on a pad.

- Use your palace. Try it out, see if it works. If not, rebuild sections, where there is a logical progression and association to assist your memory.

- Build new palaces. You can dump the current contents out, and start fresh on other things you need to remember such as parts of a speech, math formulas, birthdays, anything of importance which requires memory.

- Practice, Explore, Visualize, Associate.

74. According to the passage, such a memory device is based mainly on:
    A   visual and internal imagery.
    B   rigorous analysis and induction.
    C   hypnagogic dream states.
    D   associative synthesis.

75. Based on the passage, we do not have as much of a memory as the ancient Greeks and Romans due to:
    A   the blossoming of the scientific method.
    B   the rise of religion.
    C   the loss of instructional texts.
    D   the rise of literacy and the written word.

CANDIDATE'S NAME _____   BOOKLET GS1-II

STUDENT ID _____

TEST GS-1

Section II: Written Communication

2 Writing Tasks (A and B); 60 Minutes (total)
Two 30 Minute Prompts, Timed Separately

INSTRUCTIONS: This test is designed to evaluate your writing skills. There are two writing assignments. You will have 30 minutes to complete each part. Your answers for Section II should be written in ANSWER DOCUMENT 2. Your response to Writing Task A must be written only on answer sheets marked "A," and your response to Writing Task B should be written only on answer sheets marked "B." The first 30 minutes may be used to respond to Task A only. The second 30 minutes may be used to respond to Task B only. If you finish writing before time is up, you may review your work ONLY on the response you have just completed.

Use your time in an efficient manner. Prior to writing your response, read the assignment carefully. The empty space on the page with the writing assignment may be used to make notes in planning your response. Scratch paper is not permitted. Corrections or additions can be made neatly between the lines but there should be no writing in the margins of the answer booklet. You are not expected to use each page of your answer document but do not skip lines. Use a black or blue pen to write your response. Illegible essays cannot be scored.

OPEN BOOKLET ONLY WHEN TIMER IS READY.

* GAMSAT is administered by ACER which is not associated with this product.
© RuveneCo Inc. All rights reserved. Reproduction without permission is illegal.

WRITING TASK A

Read the following statements and write a response to any one or more of the ideas presented.

Your essay will be evaluated on the value of your thoughts on the theme, logical organization of content and effective articulation of your key points.

* * * * * * * * *

Comment 1

    Whoever said the pen is mightier than the sword obviously never encountered automatic weapons.

Gen. Douglas MacArthur

* * * * *

Comment 2

    Political power grows out of the barrel of a gun.

Chairman Mao Zedong

* * * * *

Comment 3

    A man of courage never wants weapons.

* * * * *

Comment 4

    Before a standing army can rule, the people must be disarmed, as they are in almost every country in Europe.

Noah Webster

* * * * *

Comment 5

    You can get more with a kind word and a gun than you can with just a kind word.

Al Capone

WRITING TASK B

Read the following statements and write a response to any one or more of the ideas presented.

Your essay will be evaluated on the value of your thoughts on the theme, logical organization of content and effective articulation of your key points.

* * * * * * * * *

Comment 1

Each friend represents a world in us, a world possibly not born until they arrive, and it is only by this meeting that a new world is born.

Anais Nin

* * * * *

Comment 2

A friend is one who walks in when the rest of the world walks out.

* * * * *

Comment 3

The best mirror is an old friend.

* * * * *

Comment 4

One friend in a lifetime is much; two are many; three are hardly possible. Friendship needs a certain parallelism of life, a community of thought, a rivalry of aim.

Henry Adams

* * * * *

Comment 5

Friendship is unnecessary, like philosophy, like art... It has no survival value; rather is one of those things that give value to survival.

C.S. Lewis

END OF WRITTEN COMMUNICATION.
DO NOT RETURN TO TASK A.

CANDIDATE'S NAME _____   BOOKLET GS1-III

STUDENT ID _____

TEST GS-1

Section III: Reasoning in Biological and Physical Sciences

Questions 1-110
Time : 170 Minutes

INSTRUCTIONS: Of the 110 questions in this test, many are organized into groups preceded by a passage. After evaluating the passage, select the best answer to each question in the group. Some questions are independent of any descriptive passage or each other. Similarly, select the best answer to these questions. If you are unsure of an answer, eliminate the alternatives that you know to be incorrect and select an answer from the remaining alternatives. To indicate your selection, use a pencil to blacken the corresponding oval on Answer Document 1, GS-1. Rough work is to be done ONLY in the test booklet. No scrap paper is permitted. No calculator is permitted. No marks are deducted for wrong answers.

The Gold Standard GAMSAT* has been designed exclusively to test knowledge and thinking skills. The exam may contain hypothetical statements and/or express controversial ideas. Statements contained herein do not necessarily reflect the policy, position, or view of RuveneCo Inc.

OPEN BOOKLET ONLY WHEN TIMER IS READY.

Worked solutions are available to the original owner of this textbook at gamsat-prep.com.

* GAMSAT is administered by ACER which is not associated with this product.
© RuveneCo Inc. All rights reserved. Reproduction without permission is illegal.

UNIT 1

Questions 1–6

The last step in translation involves the cleavage of the ester bond that joins the complete peptide chain to the tRNA corresponding to its C-terminal amino acid. This process of termination, in addition to the *termination* codon, requires release factors (RFs). The freeing of the ribosome from mRNA during this step requires the participation of a protein called ribosome releasing factor (RRF).

Cells usually do not contain tRNAs that can recognize the three termination codons. In *E. coli*, when these codons arrive on the ribosome they are recognized by one of three release factors. RF-1 recognizes UAA and UAG, while RF-2 recognizes UAA and UGA. The third release factor, RF-3, does not itself recognize termination codons but stimulates the activity of the other two factors.

The consequence of release factor recognition of a *termination* codon is to alter the peptidyl transferase center on the large ribosomal subunit so that it can accept water as the attacking nucleophile rather than requiring the normal substrate, aminoacyl-tRNA.

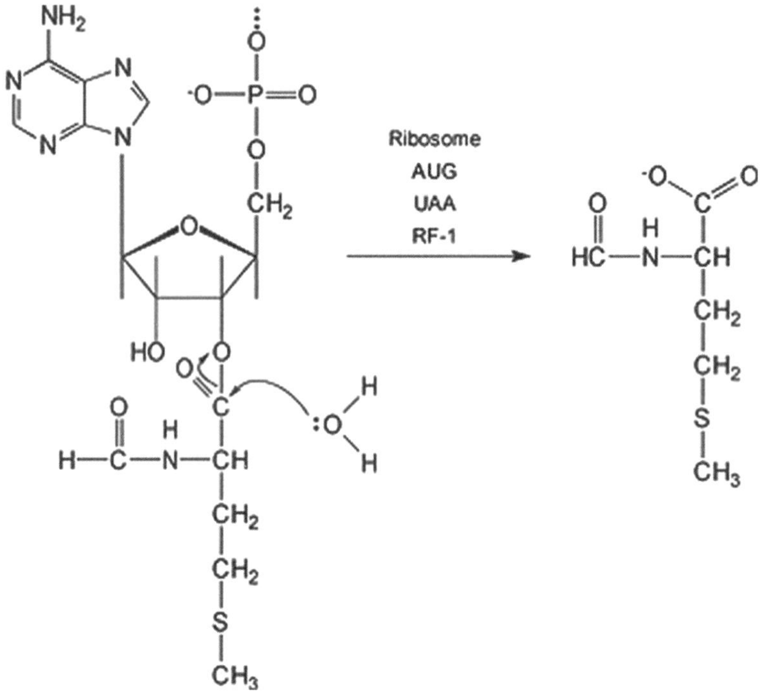

Figure 1

1. Where would the RFs be expected to be found in the cell?
   A   Within the nuclear membrane
   B   Floating in the cytosol
   C   In the matrix of the mitochondria
   D   Within the lumen of the smooth endoplasmic reticulum

2. The alteration to the peptidyl transferase center during the termination reaction serves to convert peptidyl transferase into a(n):
   A   exonuclease.
   B   lyase.
   C   esterase.
   D   ligase.

3. Sparsomycin is an antibiotic that inhibits peptidyl transferase activity. The effect of adding this compound to an in vitro reaction in which *E. coli* ribosomes are combined with methionine aminoacyl-tRNA complex, RF-1 and the nucleotide triplets, AUG and UAA, would be to:
A   inhibit hydrolysis of the amino acid, allowing polypeptide chain extension.
B   inhibit peptide bond formation causing the amino acid to be released.
C   induce hydrolysis of the aminoacyl-tRNA complex.
D   inhibit both hydrolysis of the aminoacyl-tRNA complex and peptide bond formation.

Figure 2 shows the kinetics of inhibition of rabbit red blood cell peptidyltransferase by Sparsomycin. The time plots shown were done using Sparsomycin concentrations of (∗) 0.1×10^{-6} M, (▲) 0.2×10^{-6} M, and (●) 0.4×10^{-6} M. The percentage (x′) of the remaining active peptidyltransferase is shown, as well as the percentage at equilibrium (x'_{eq}) for each curve which is indicated by the dashed --- lines.

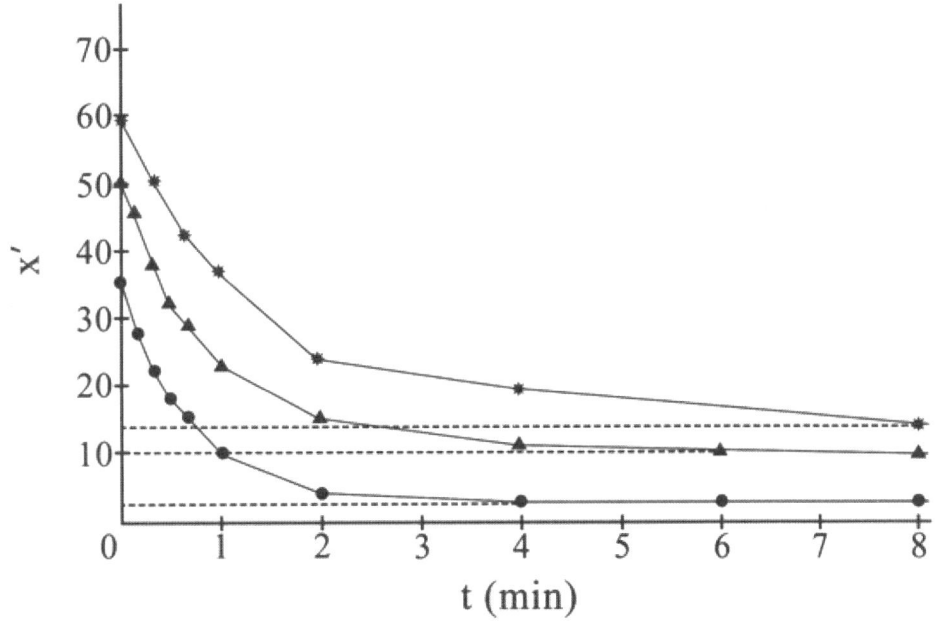

Figure 2
Adapted from D. Synetos, Molecular Pharmacology June 1, 1998 vol. 53 no. 6 1089-1096.

4. Which of the following is NOT true concerning the curves in Figure 2?
A   The equilibrium point of the curve using 0.4×10^{-6} M Sparsomycin is obtained at a point where more than 95% of the peptidyltransferase is not active.
B   The fact that the 3 plots are curved, does not in itself indicate if the reaction is first order or second order.
C   The curve where 0.2×10^{-6} M Sparsomycin is used is most consistent with a first-order reaction because the active concentration of peptidyltransferase decreases by approximately 50% at just under 1 minute, and then by another 50% (approximately) at just under 1 minute later.
D   If the curves were linear, they would be most consistent with zero-order and first-order reactions.

5. Which of the following graphs is consistent with the data in Figure 2?
   The following estimates may be of assistance: log 6 = 0.8, log 4 = 0.6.

A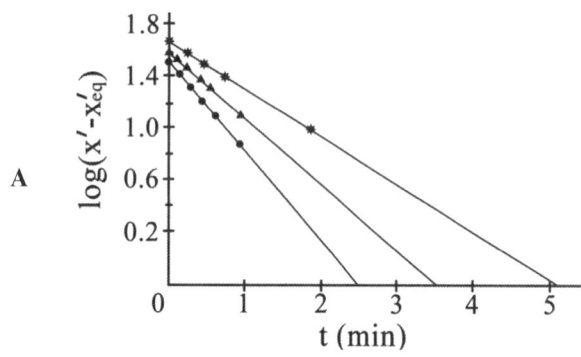

B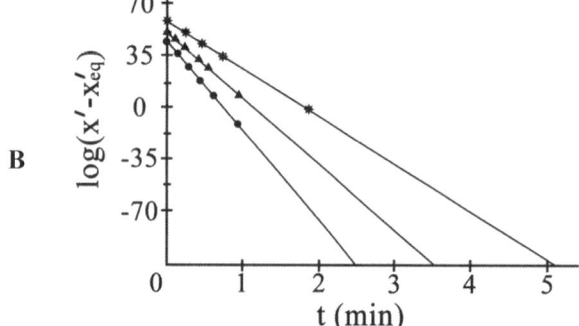

C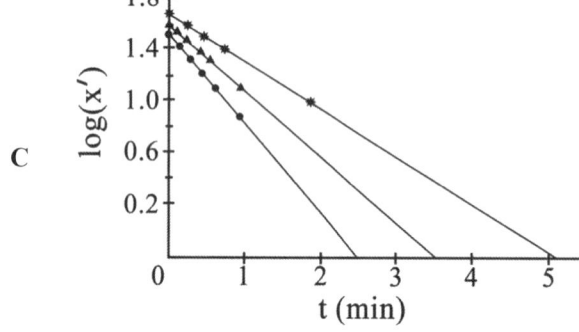

D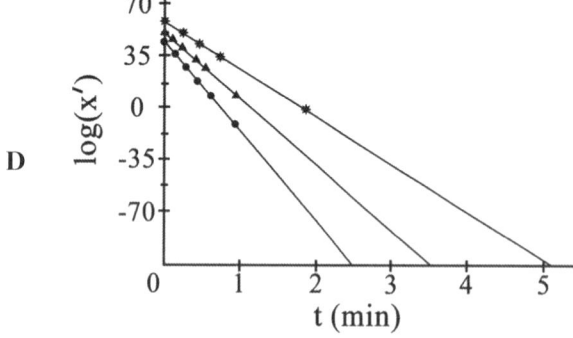

6. According to Figure 2, if 0.2×10^{-6} M of Sparsomycin is applied to 70 picograms of peptidyltransferase from rabbit red blood cells, estimate the rate of inhibition at t = 2 minutes.
   A 30 picograms/minute
   B 25 picograms/minute
   C 15 picograms/minute
   D 3.5 picograms/minute

UNIT 2

Questions 7-11

Reduction potentials (also referred to as *redox potentials*) reveal the tendency of a chemical species to acquire electrons and thus be reduced. Each species has its own intrinsic redox potential; the more positive the potential, the greater the species' affinity for electrons and tendency to be reduced.

A reduction potential is measured in volts (V). Because the true or absolute potentials are difficult to accurately measure, reduction potentials are defined relative to the standard hydrogen electrode (SHE) which is arbitrarily given a potential of 0.00 volts. Standard reduction potential is measured under standard conditions: 25 °C, a 1M concentration for each ion participating in the reaction, a partial pressure of 1 atm for each gas that is part of the reaction, and metals in their pure state.

Table 1: Standard State Reduction Potentials. Ions are in aqueous form.

Half-reactions	Standard reduction potential (E°)
$F_2 (g) + 2e^- \rightleftharpoons 2F^-$	2.87 V
$Cl_2 (g) + 2e^- \rightleftharpoons 2Cl^-$	1.36 V
$Br_2 (aq) + 2e^- \rightleftharpoons 2Br^-$	1.09 V
$Ag^+ + e^- \rightleftharpoons Ag (s)$	0.80 V
$Fe^{3+} + e^- \rightleftharpoons Fe^{2+}$	0.77 V
$Cu^{2+} + 2e^- \rightleftharpoons Cu (s)$	0.34 V
$2H^+ + 2e^- \rightleftharpoons H_2(g)$	0.00 V
$Pb^{2+} + 2e^- \rightleftharpoons Pb (s)$	–0.13 V
$Ni^{2+} + 2e^- \rightleftharpoons Ni (s)$	–0.41 V
$Zn^{2+} + 2e^- \rightleftharpoons Zn (s)$	–0.76 V
$Na^+ + e^- \rightleftharpoons Na (s)$	–2.71 V

7. What should happen when a piece of copper is placed in 1M HCl?
   A   The copper is completely dissolved by the acid.
   B   The copper is dissolved by the acid with the release of hydrogen gas.
   C   The copper bursts into greenish flames.
   D   Nothing happens.

8. What should happen when a piece of lead is placed in 1M HCl?
   A   The lead is completely dissolved by the acid.
   B   The lead begins to dissolve with the release of hydrogen gas.
   C   The lead bursts into flames.
   D   Nothing happens.

9. If standard state oxidation potentials are used instead of standard state reduction potentials and the half reactions are listed in descending order according to their standard state oxidation potentials, which one of the following would be true?
   A   The lead reaction would be above the silver reaction.
   B   The fluorine reaction would be above the chlorine reaction.
   C   The iron reaction would be above the nickel reaction.
   D   The hydrogen reaction would be below the copper reaction.

10. According to Table 1, which of the following species is the strongest reducing agent?
    A Fe^{3+}
    B Fe^{2+}
    C Zn^{2+}
    D   Zn (s)

11. Only considering the standard half-cell reactions of the species listed in Table 1, how many different voltaic cells with a voltage greater than 2V can be made?
    A   Fewer than 7
    B   7
    C   15
    D   More than 15

UNIT 3

Questions 12–16

The four forces that act on a plane are lift, weight, drag or air resistance, and thrust, the last of which is produced by the plane's engine.

Impact pressure produces 30% of the lift. It results from the fact that wings are given a *dihedral* angle where the distance from the tip of the wing to the ground is greater than that from the root of the wing to the ground.

The other 70% of lift can be accounted for by the Bernoulli effect. A cross-section of an airplane's wing reveals greater surface area above the wing compared to a flatter, lower surface. Thus air, moving in streamline flow, must move more rapidly over the top of the wing.

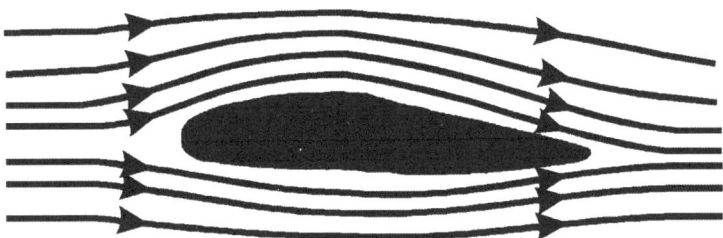

Bernoulli's equation, $P + 1/2\rho v^2 + \rho gh$ = constant, is often modified when discussing an airplane's wing. The "ρgh" component is usually left out since the difference in distance from the top of the wing to the ground compared to the bottom of the wing to the ground is usually negligible.

Note that:
- Streamline flow is governed by the continuity equation where $A_1v_1 = A_2v_2$
- For Bernoulli's and/or the continuity equation: P is pressure, ρ is density, v is velocity, g is gravity, h is the height and A is the cross-sectional area.

12. Newton's Third Law states that for every action there must be an equal and opposite reaction. This is applicable to lift and the dihedral angle because:
    A   the fast moving air above the wing increases the pressure.
    B   drag must be as low as possible to improve forward motion.
    C   there is a large pressure difference between the wings.
    D   the wing deflects the air downward and the air in turn deflects the wing upward.

13. Compared to the wing's upper surface, the air moving along the undersurface has:
    A   greater velocity, greater pressure.
    B   greater velocity, lower pressure.
    C   lower velocity, greater pressure.
    D   lower velocity, lower pressure.

14. An airplane is encircling an airport with DECREASING speed. When the airplane reaches point P, what is the general direction of its acceleration?

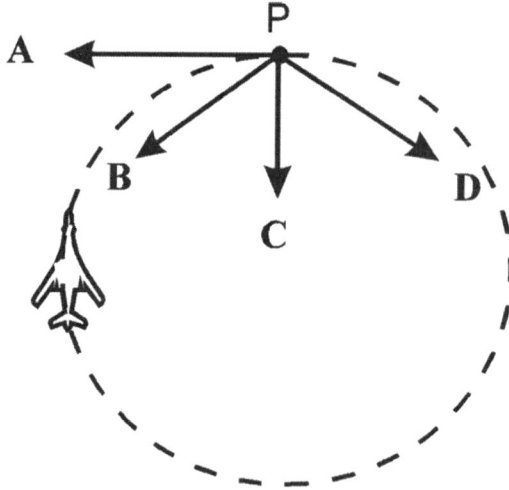

15. The following represents an incompressible fluid in laminar flow through pipes. Where is the pressure highest?

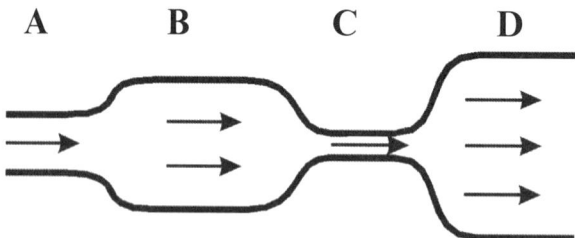

16. Flow is defined as volume per unit time. Concerning the preceding diagram, what can be determined regarding the flow?
    A   It is highest at C.
    B   It is highest at D.
    C   It cannot be determined.
    D   It is constant throughout.

UNIT 4

Question 17

17. What would be the expected change in terms of the solubility of a gas when a solution containing the gas is heated and when a solution containing the gas has the pressure over the solution decreased, respectively?
    A   Increase, increase
    B   Increase, decrease
    C   Decrease, increase
    D   Decrease, decrease

UNIT 5

Question 18

18. The structure of β-D-glucose is shown below in two different projection systems. The circled hydroxyl group in Fig. 1 would be located at which position in the modified Fischer projection depicted in Fig. 2?

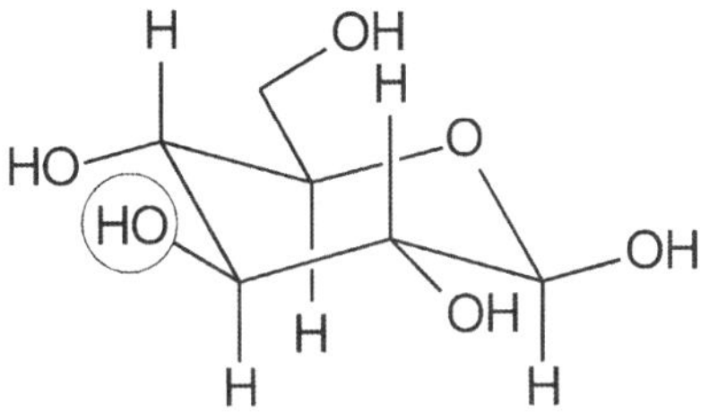

Figure 1 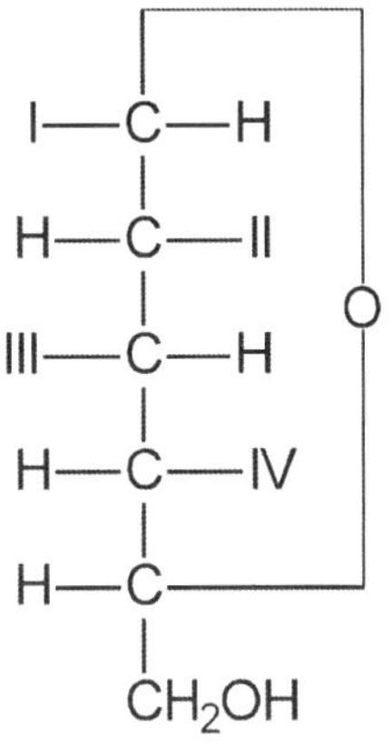   Figure 2

    A   I
    B   II
    C   III
    D   IV

UNIT 6

Questions 19–24

The essential stages in the manufacture of H_2SO_4 and H_2SO_3 involve the burning of sulfur or roasting of sulfide ores in air to produce SO_2. This is then mixed with air, purified and passed over a vanadium catalyst (either VO_3^- or V_2O_5) at 450 degrees Celsius. Thus the following reaction occurs.

$$2SO_2(g) + O_2(g) \rightleftharpoons 2SO_3(g) \qquad \Delta H = -197 \text{ kJ mol}^{-1}$$

Reaction I

If the SO_2 is very carefully dissolved in water, sulfurous acid (H_2SO_3) is obtained. The first proton of this acid ionizes as if from a strong acid while the second ionizes as if from a weak acid.

$$H_2SO_3 + H_2O \rightarrow H_3O^+ + HSO_3^-$$

Reaction II

$$HSO_3^- + H_2O \rightleftharpoons H_3O^+ + SO_3^{2-} \qquad K_a = 5.0 \times 10^{-6}$$

Reaction III

The concentration of H_2SO_3 in cleaning fluid was determined by titration with 0.10 M NaOH (strong base) as shown in Fig.1. Two equivalence points were determined using 30 ml and 60 ml of NaOH respectively:

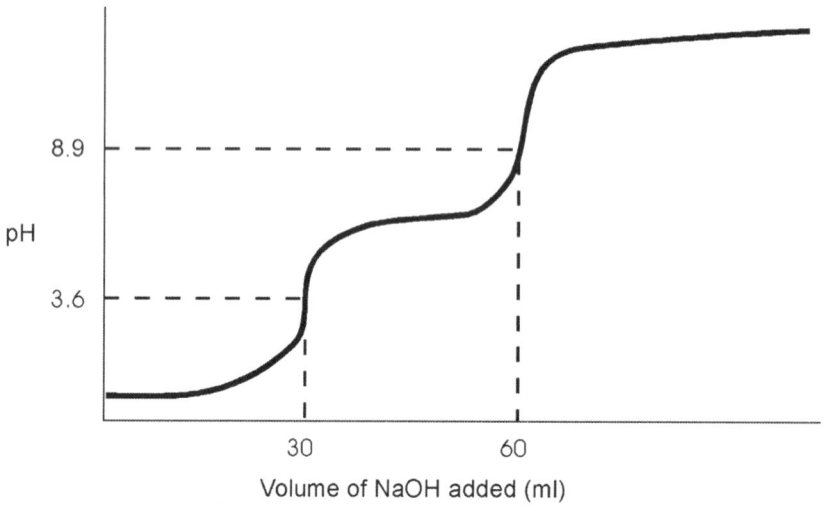

Figure 1

Note: You may find some of the following information helpful. Relative atomic masses: H = 1.0, N = 14.0, O = 16.0, S = 32, Cl = 35.5

19. What is the oxidation number of sulfur in sulfurous acid?
    A   +3
    B   +4
    C   +5
    D   +6

20. What is the percent by mass of oxygen in sulfurous acid?
    A   31.9%
    B   19.7%
    C   39.0%
    D   58.5%

21. Which of the following acid-base indicators is most suitable for the determination of the first end point of the titration shown in Figure 1?
    A   Cresol red (color change between pH = 0.2 and pH = 1.8)
    B   p-Xylenol blue (color change between pH = 1.2 and pH = 2.8)
    C   Bromophenol blue (color change between pH = 3.0 and pH = 4.6)
    D   Bromocresol green (color change between pH = 3.8 and pH = 5.4)

22. The equilibrium constant K_a is also called the acid dissociation constant and K_b is the base dissociation constant. The value of K_a given in Reaction III is relatively low which would mean that, relatively, its:
    A pK_a is low and the pK_b of its conjugate base is high.
    B pK_a is high and the pK_b of its conjugate base is low.
    C pK_a is low and the pK_b of its conjugate base is low.
    D pK_a is high and the pK_b of its conjugate base is high.

23. If no catalyst was used in Reaction I, which of the following would experience a change in its partial pressure when the same system reaches equilibrium?
    A   There will be no change in the partial pressure of any of the reactants
    B SO_3 (*g*)
    C SO_2 (*g*)
    D O_2 (*g*)

24. If the temperature was decreased in Reaction I, which of the following would experience an increase in its partial pressure when the same system reaches equilibrium?
    A   There will be no change in the partial pressure of any of the reactants
    B SO_3 (*g*)
    C SO_2 (*g*)
    D O_2 (*g*) and SO_2 (*g*)

UNIT 7

Question 25

25. The patella (i.e. kneecap) is a thick, mostly circular bone which articulates with the femur (thigh bone) and covers and protects the front (anterior) part of the knee joint. Approximate the rate of growth of the anterior surface area of the human patella from birth to age 20 years old.
    A 1.1×10^{-4} cm^2 per hour
    B 1.1×10^{-4} nm^2 per hour
    C 1.1×10^{-2} cm^2 per second
    D 1.1×10^{-2} nm^2 per second

UNIT 8

Questions 26–31

Much of the study of evolution of *interspecific* interactions had focused on the results rather than the process of coevolution. In only a few cases has the genetic bases of interspecific interactions been explored. One of the most intriguing results has been the description of "gene-for-gene" systems governing the interaction between certain parasites and their hosts. In several crop plants, dominant alleles at a number of loci have been described that confer resistance to a pathogenic fungus; for each such gene, the fungus appears to have a recessive allele for "virulence" that enables the fungus to attack the otherwise resistant host. Cases of character displacement among competing species are among the best evidence that interspecific interactions can result in genetic change.

Assuming that parasites and their hosts coevolve in an "arms race," we might deduce that the parasite is "ahead" if local populations are more capable of attacking the host population with which they are associated than other populations. Whereas the host may be "ahead" if local populations are more resistant to the local parasite than to other populations of the parasite.

Several studies have been done to evaluate coevolutionary interactions between parasites and hosts, or predators and prey. In one, the fluctuations in populations of houseflies and of a wasp that parasitized them were recorded. The results of the experiment are shown in Fig. 1.

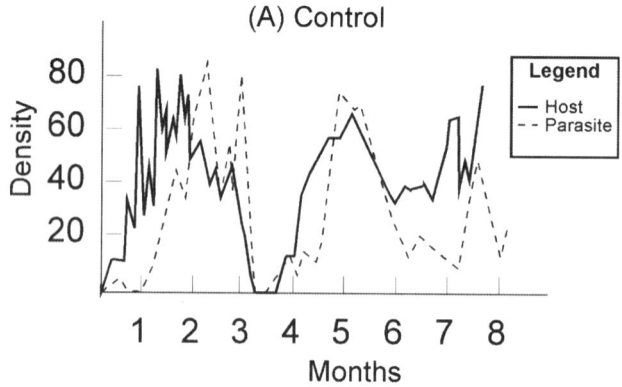

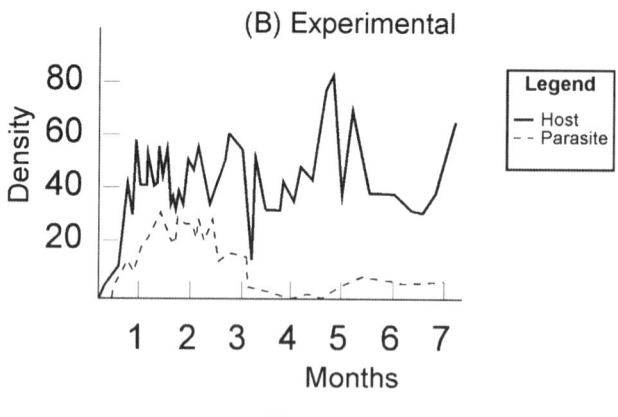

Figure 1

26. A pathogenic fungus is more capable of growth and reproduction on its native population of its sole host, the wild hog peanut, than on plants from other populations of the same species. It is reasonable to conclude that:
    A   the fungus, in this instance, was capable of more rapid adaptation to its host than vice versa.
    B   the fungus, in this instance, was capable of more rapid adaptation to all populations of the host species than vice versa.
    C   the host, in this instance, was capable of more rapid adaptation to the fungus than vice versa.
    D   all populations of the host species were capable of more rapid adaptation to the fungus than vice versa.

27. Allopatric refers to areas isolated geographically from one another whereas sympatric populations occupy the same or overlapping geographical areas. The passage suggests that one result of interspecific interactions might be:
    A   genetic drift within sympatric populations.
    B   genetic drift within allopatric populations.
    C   genetic mutations within sympatric populations.
    D   genetic mutations within allopatric populations.

28. According to Fig. 1, the experiment showed that over time:
    A   coevolution caused a decrease in both the host and parasite populations.
    B   coevolution caused both a decrease in fluctuation of the host and parasite populations, and a lowered density of the parasite population.
    C   coevolution caused a marked increase in the fluctuation of only the host population, and lowered the density of the parasite population.
    D   coevolution caused a decrease in the population density of the parasite population but caused a marked increase in the density of the host population.

29. The control in the experiment likely consisted of:
    A   members from different populations of the host and parasite species used in the experimental group, that had a short history of exposure to one another.
    B   members of the host and parasite species used in the experimental group, that had a long history of exposure to one another.
    C   members of the host and parasite species used in the experimental group that had no history of exposure to one another.
    D   members from different populations of the host and parasite species used in the experimental group, that had a long history of exposure to one another.

30. Which of the following is the least likely explanation of the results obtained for the control group in Fig. 1?
    A   A low parasite population results in a lowered host population by the sheer virulence of the parasite.
    B   A low host population can increase a parasite population by forcing the parasite to seek an alternate source for food.
    C   A high parasite population destroys the host population resulting in a lowered host population.
    D   A high host population creates a breeding ground for parasites thus increasing the parasite population.

31. Penicillin is an antibiotic which destroys bacteria by interfering with cell wall production. Could the development of bacterial resistance to Penicillin be considered similar to coevolution?
    A   Yes, a spontaneous mutation is likely to confer resistance to Penicillin.
    B   No, an organism can only evolve in response to another organism.
    C   Yes, as antibiotics continue to change there will be a selective pressure for bacterial genes which confer resistance.
    D   No, bacteria have plasma membranes and can survive without cell walls.

UNIT 9

Questions 32–37

The Diels–Alder reaction is a cycloaddition reaction that can occur between a conjugated diene (= 2 double bonds separated by a single bond) and a substituted alkene (= the dienophile) to form a substituted cyclohexene system.

Diene + dienophile = cyclohexene

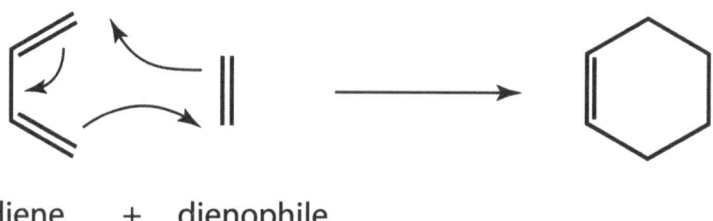

diene   +   dienophile

All Diels-Alder reactions have four common features: (1) the reaction is initiated by heat; (2) the reaction forms new six-membered rings; (3) three π bonds break and two new C-C σ bonds and one new C-C π bond are formed; (4) all bonds break and form in a single step.

The Diels-Alder diene must have the two double bonds on the same side of the single bond in one of the structures, which is called the *s-cis* conformation (= *cis* with respect to the single bond). If double bonds are on the opposite sides of the single bond in the Lewis structure, this is called the *s-trans* conformation (= *trans* with respect to the single bond).

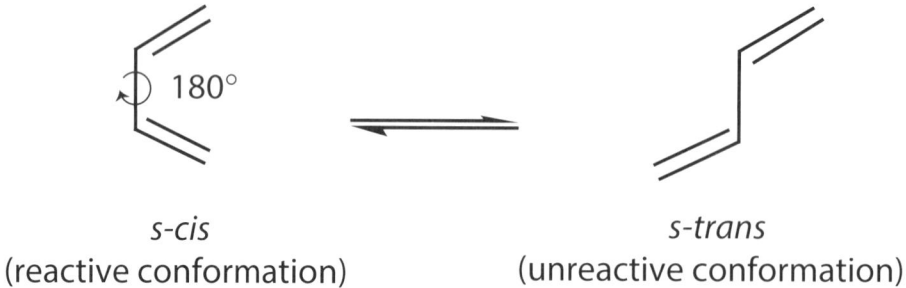

s-cis
(reactive conformation)

s-trans
(unreactive conformation)

32. All of the following are true regarding allene (C₃H₄) EXCEPT one. Which one is the EXCEPTION?
  A   The C-H bond angles are 120°.
  B   The hybridization of the carbon atoms are sp and sp².
  C   The bond angle formed by the three carbons is 180°
  D   Allene is a conjugated diene.

33. Which of the following would be the least reactive diene in a Diels-Alder reaction?

A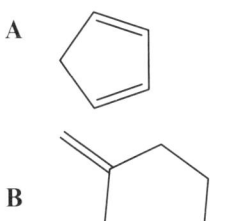

C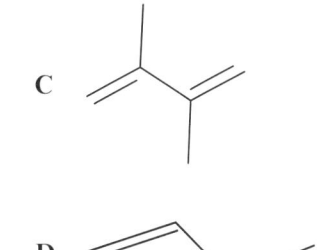

B

D

34. The number of conjugated dienes among the 5 structures below is:

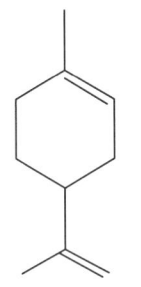 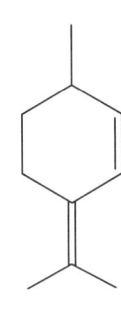 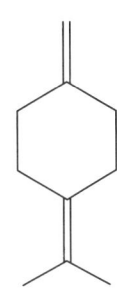 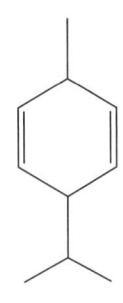 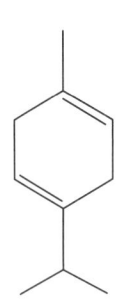

A 1 only. **B** 2 only. **C** 3 only. **D** more than 3.

35. Choose the diene and dienophile that could be used to produce the Diels-Alder product.

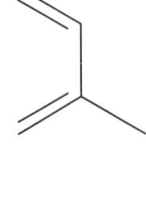 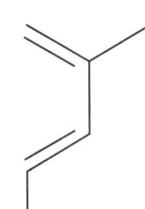 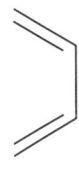 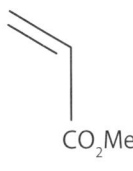 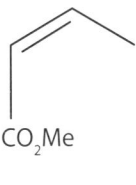

i ii iii iv v

A i and iv **C** iii and iv
B ii and iv **D** iii and v

36. Each of the following represents a pair of resonance structures EXCEPT:

I   [allyl cation structures] and [allyl cation structures]

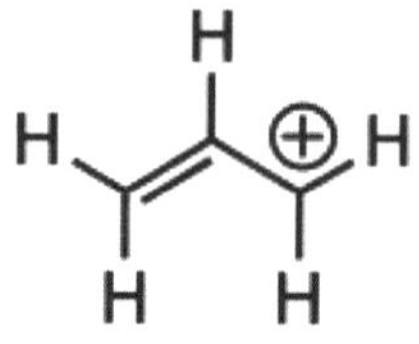

II [allyl radical structures] and [allyl radical structures]

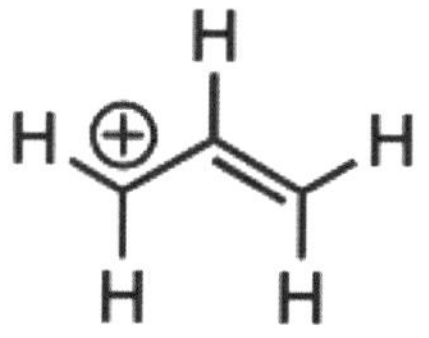

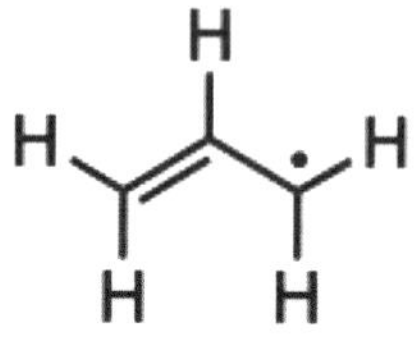

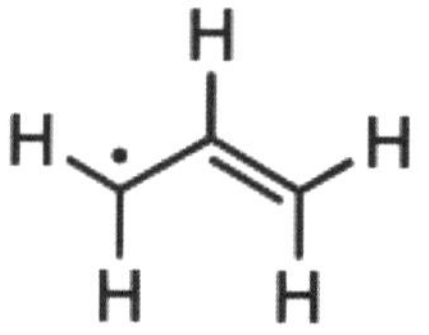

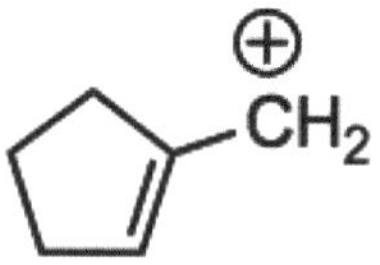

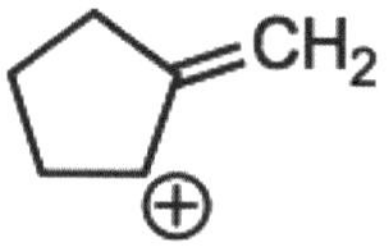

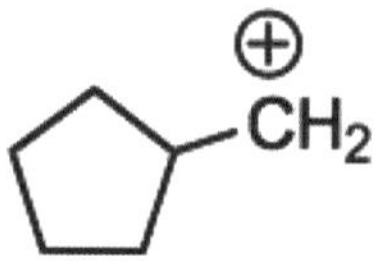

III [cyclopentenyl-CH2+] and [cyclopentane=CH2 with + on ring]

IV [cyclopentyl-CH2+] and [cyclopentyl(+)-CH3]

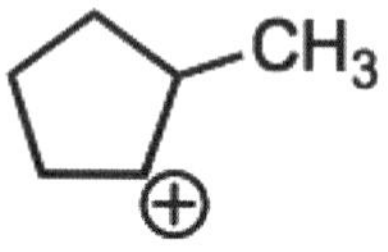

- A I
- B II
- C III
- D IV

37. How many possible structural isomers are there for C_4H_8?
- A 2
- B 4
- C 5
- D More than 5

UNIT 10

Questions 38–43

The phenomenon of refraction has long intrigued scientists and was actually used to corroborate one of the major mysteries of early science: the determination of the speed of light.

The refractive index of a transparent material is related to a number of the physical properties of light. In terms of velocity, the refractive index represents the ratio of the velocity of light in a vacuum to its velocity in the material. From this ratio, it can be seen that light is retarded when it passes through most types of matter. It is worth noting that prisms break up white light into the seven "colors of the rainbow" because each color has a slightly different velocity in the medium.

Snell's law allows one to follow the behavior of light in terms of its path when moving from a material of one refractive index to another with the same, or different refractive index. It is given by: $n_1 \sin\theta_1 = n_2 \sin\theta_2$, where "1" refers to the first medium through which the ray passes, "2" refers to the second medium, and the angles refer to the angle of incidence in the first medium (θ_1) and the angle of refraction in the second (θ_2).

A ship went out on a search for a sunken treasure chest. In order to locate the chest, they shone a beam of light down into the water using a high intensity white light source as shown in Fig.1. The refractive index for sea water is 1.33 while that for air is 1.00.

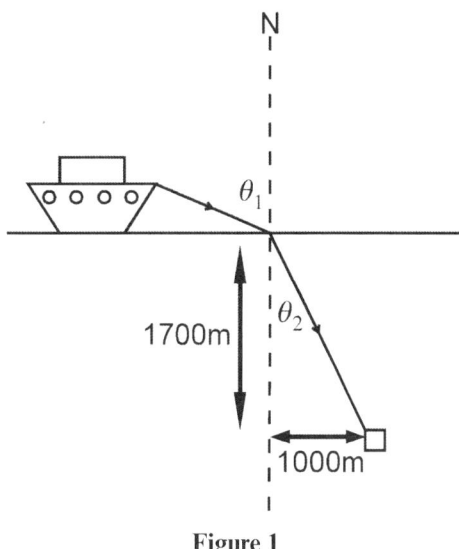

Figure 1

38. From the information in the passage, how would you expect the speed of light in air to compare with the speed of light in a vacuum (which is given by "c")?
   A   It would be approximately equal to c.
   B   It would be greater than c.
   C   It would be less than c.
   D   This cannot be determined from the information given.

39. Using the information in the passage, what must the approximate value of θ_2 be such that it hits the chest as shown in Figure 1?
   A   15°
   B   30°
   C   45°
   D   65°

40. How does the refractive index in water for violet light compare with that of red light given that violet light travels more slowly in water than red light?
  A $n_{violet} = n_{red}$
  B $n_{violet} < n_{red}$
  C $n_{violet} > n_{red}$
  D This depends on the relative speeds of the different colors in a vacuum.

41. Total internal reflection first occurs when a beam of light travels from one medium to another medium which has a smaller refractive index at such an angle of incidence that the angle of refraction is 90°. This angle of incidence is called the critical angle. What is the value of the sine of this angle when the ray moves from water towards air?
  A 2π
  B 0.75
  C 0.50
  D 0

42. What would happen to the critical angle, in the previous question, if the beam of light was travelling from water to a substance with a greater refractive index than air, but a lower refractive index than water?
  A It would increase.
  B It would decrease.
  C It would remain the same.
  D Total internal reflection would not be possible.

43. Which of the following would you expect to remain constant when light travels from one medium to another and the media differ in their refractive indices?
  A Velocity
  B Frequency
  C Wavelength
  D Intensity

UNIT 11

Questions 44-49

Aside from diabetes, thyroid disease is the most common glandular disorder. Millions of people are treated for thyroid conditions, often an underactive or overactive gland. Overwhelmingly, women between the ages of 20 and 60 are much more likely than men to succumb to these conditions. The etiology lies in the failure of the immune system to recognize the thyroid gland as part of the body and thus antibodies are sent to attack the gland.

The plasma proteins that bind thyroid hormones are albumin, a prealbumin called thyroxine-binding prealbumin (TBPA), and a globulin with an electrophoretic mobility, thyroxine-binding globulin (TBG). The free thyroid hormones in plasma are in equilibrium with the protein-bound thyroid hormones in the tissues. Free thyroid hormones are added to the circulating pool by the thyroid. It is the free thyroid hormones in plasma that are physiologically active (increasing the metabolic rate) and imbalances in these hormones result in thyroid disease. In thyroid storm, a form of hyperthyroidism, the normal body temperature of 37.5 °C may rise to over 40 °C.

In addition, in humans there are four small parathyroid glands that produce the hormone, parathormone, which is a peptide composed of 84 amino acids. Parathormone and the thyroid hormone calcitonin work antagonistically to regulate the plasma calcium and phosphate levels. Overactive parathyroid glands, *hyperparathyroidism*, can lead to an increase in the level of calcium in plasma and tissues.

Table 1: Different plasma proteins and their binding capacity and affinity for thyroxine.

Protein	Plasma Level (mg/dl)	Thyroxine Binding Capacity (µg/dl)	Affinity for thyroxine	Amount of thyroxine bound in normal plasma (µg/dl)
Thyroxine binding globulin (TBG)	1.0	20	High	7
Thyroxine binding prealbumin (TBPA)	30.0	250	Moderate	1
Albumin	...	1000	Low	None
Total protein-bound thyroxine in plasma	...	...	...	8

44. Is it reasonable to conclude that thyroid disease is sex-linked?
    A   No, because thyroid disease appears to be caused by a defect of the immune system and not a defective DNA sequence.
    B   No, because if the disease was sex-linked, there would be a high incidence in the male, rather than the female, population.
    C   Yes, because the high incidence of the disease in women suggests that a gene found on the X chromosome codes for the disease.
    D   Yes, because the same factor increases the risk of women getting the disease, regardless of familial background.

45. According to Table 1, it would be expected that:
    A   TBG has the highest binding capacity for thyroxine while TBPA has the highest affinity.
    B   TBG has the highest binding capacity for thyroxine while albumin has the lowest affinity.
    C   albumin has the highest binding capacity for thyroxine while TBPA has the highest affinity.
    D   albumin has the highest binding capacity for thyroxine while TBG has the highest affinity.

Question 46 refers to Fig. 1.

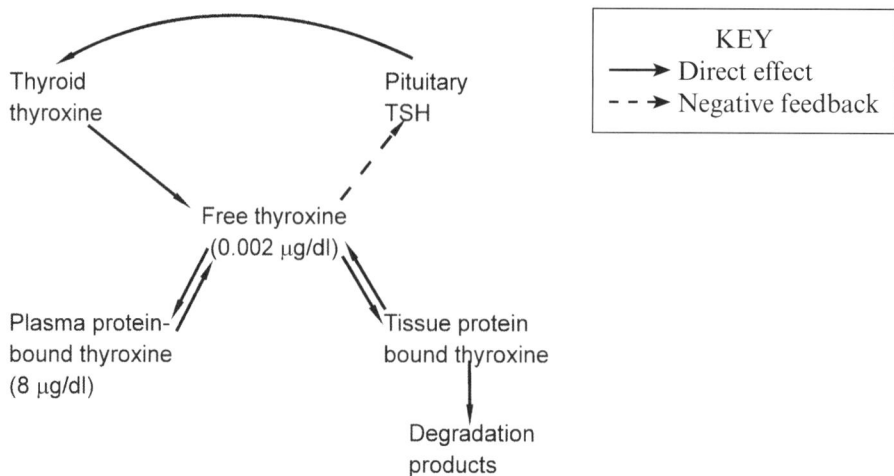

Figure 1

46. According to the equilibrium shown in Fig. 1, an elevation in the concentration of free thyroid hormone in the plasma is followed by:
    A   an increase in tissue protein-bound thyroxine.
    B   an increase in tissue protein-bound thyroxine and plasma protein-bound thyroxine.
    C   an increase in the amount of TSH secreted from the pituitary gland.
    D   an increase in both the amount of TSH secreted from the pituitary gland and the release of thyroxine from the thyroid gland.

47. Symptoms that can be inferred to be consistent with hypothyroidism and hyperthyroidism, respectively, include:
    A   a fine tremor and diminished concentration.
    B   brittle nails and kidney stones.
    C   rapid heart beat and increased irritability.
    D   lethargy and nervous agitation.

48. Which of the following is an example of positive feedback?
    A   A body temperature of 39 °C causes a further increase
    B   Elevated TSH results in elevated thyroxine
    C   Calcitonin and parathormone regulate calcium levels
    D   Increased TBG leads to an increase in TSH

49. Parathormone influences calcium homeostasis by reducing tubular reabsorption of PO_4^{3-} in the kidneys. Which of the following, if true, would clarify the adaptive significance of this process?
    A PO_4^{3-} and Ca^{2+} feedback positively on each other.
    B   Elevated levels of extracellular PO_4^{3-} result in calcification of bones and tissues.
    C   Increased PO_4^{3-} levels cause an increase in parathormone secretion.
    D   Decreased extracellular PO_4^{3-} levels cause a decrease in calcitonin production.

UNIT 12

Questions 50–54

The enthalpy of solution (ΔH_{soln}) of a salt depends on two other quantities: the energy released when free gaseous ions of the salt combine to give the solid salt (lattice energy: ΔH_{latt}) and the energy released when free gaseous ions of the salt dissolve in water via solute-solvent interactions to yield the solvated ions (enthalpy of hydration: ΔH_{solv}) where:

$$\Delta H_{soln} = \Delta H_{solv} - \Delta H_{latt} \qquad \text{Equation I}$$

From the formal definition of the quantities, it can be seen that both ΔH_{latt} and ΔH_{solv} are exothermic. Although these values seem to be in competition, the factors that affect ΔH_{latt} and ΔH_{solv} do so in the same way. Firstly, the smaller the ion, the closer the association of the ion with either other ions in the crystal lattice, or, with water molecules and thus the more negative ΔH_{latt} and ΔH_{solv} become. Also, the greater the charge on the ion, the greater the increase in electrostatic forces of attraction between itself and other ions or water molecules, and the more negative ΔH_{latt} and ΔH_{solv} become.

Although ΔH_{latt} and ΔH_{solv} undergo similar changes, the change in ΔH_{solv} up or down a group is much more profound than that of ΔH_{latt}. A good example of this is seen in the solubility changes of the Group II carbonates.

However, there is one exception to these general rules. If the cation of the salt is approximately the same size as the anion, the arrangement of ions in the crystal lattice is more uniform and hence the lattice is more stable and ΔH_{latt} is more negative.

Table 1: Note the order going down the periodic table is Mg, Ca, Sr, Ba.

Group II Carbonate	Solubility (mol L⁻¹ H₂O)
$MgCO_3$	1.30×10^{-3}
$CaCO_3$	0.13×10^{-3}
$SrCO_3$	0.07×10^{-3}
$BaCO_3$	0.09×10^{-3}

50. It is often useful to determine the solubility product (K_{sp}) of compounds that are sparingly soluble like those in Table 1. In this context, K_{sp} can be defined as the mathematical product of ion concentrations raised to the power of their stoichiometric coefficients. The solubility product for $MgCO_3$ is:
    A 1.3×10^{-4}
    B 2.6×10^{-4}
    C 1.7×10^{-6}
    D 6.7×10^{-8}

51. $Ca(OH)_2$ has approximately the same K_{sp} as $CaSO_4$. Which of them has the greater solubility in terms of mol L⁻¹?
    A   They both have the same solubility.
    B $Ca(OH)_2$
    C $CaSO_4$
    D   It depends on the temperature at the time.

52. Given the information in the passage, the CO_3^{2-} anion is approximately the same size as:
    A Mg^{2+}.   C Sr^{2+}.
    B Ca^{2+}.   D Ba^{2+}.

53. The ΔH$_{solv}$ for a doubly charged anion X^{2-} was found to be more negative than that for the carbonate anion. Given the information in the passage, which of the following is the most likely explanation?
    A   X^{2-} is the same size as the carbonate anion.
    B   X^{2-} is larger than the carbonate anion.
    C   X^{2-} is smaller than the carbonate anion.
    D   It depends on the H$_{latt}$ for the salt containing the anion.

54. A solution of SrCO$_3$ in water boils at a higher temperature than pure water. Why is this?
    A   SrCO$_3$ increases the density of water.
    B   SrCO$_3$ decreases the vapour pressure of the water.
    C   SrCO$_3$ has a low solubility in water.
    D   SrCO$_3$ decreases the surface tension of the water.

UNIT 13

Question 55

55. The following system includes a frictionless pulley and a cord of negligible mass. Since the system is at rest, what can be said about the force of friction between the platform and the large weight?

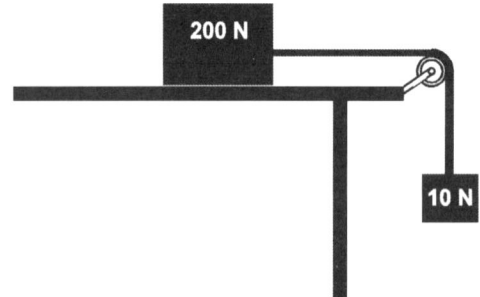

    A   It is 200 N.
    B   It is 10 N.
    C   It is 190 N.
    D   In this case, the force of friction is not necessarily present.

UNIT 14

Questions 56–61

In the simple model of a gas as described by the kinetic molecular theory, a gas is pictured as an assembly of particles travelling at high velocities in straight lines in all directions. The particles are constantly colliding, but they are supposed to be perfectly elastic so that no momentum is lost on impact. They are also supposed to be point masses, that is, they have mass but occupy no space. In addition, no attractive or repulsive forces are exerted between particles.

From this theory, and the work of other great scientists like Boyle and Charles, the ideal gas law was devised: PV = nRT where P = pressure of the gas, V = volume of the gas, n = number of moles of gas particles present, T = Kelvin temperature of the gas and R = universal gas constant.

However, no "real" gas conforms to this "ideal" gas theory, that is, no real gas obeys all of these laws at all temperatures and pressures. These deviations were investigated by the French physicist Amagat, who used pressures up to 320 atmospheres and a range of temperatures to investigate these deviations. The following diagram shows how the PV/nRT value varies with pressure for certain gases at 50 °C.

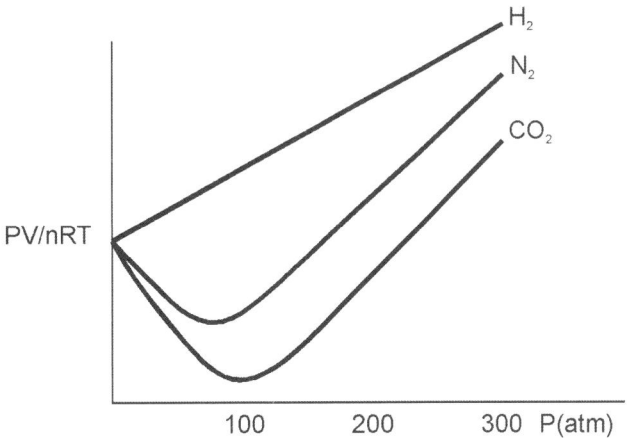

The deviations of real gases from ideality confers a number of properties on the gas which could not be explained by the kinetic molecular theory.

56. What would the PV/nRT versus P graph look like for an ideal gas?

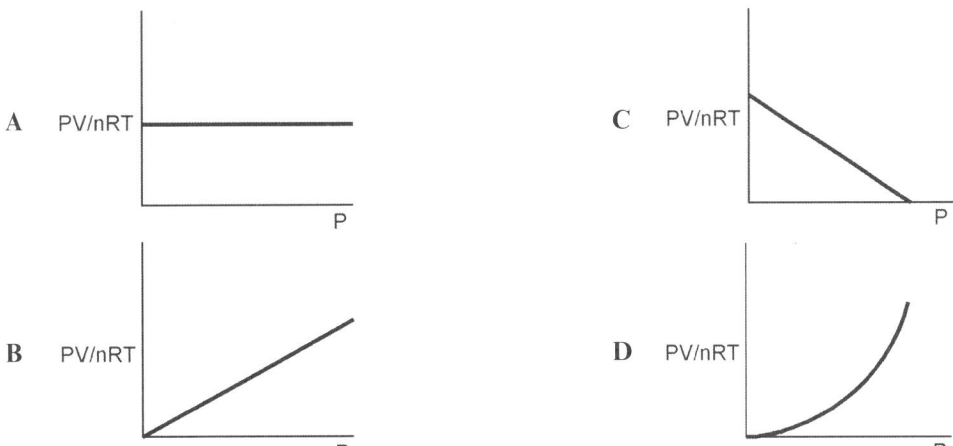

57. From the information in the passage, if 1 dm³ of H₂ gas initially at 50 atmospheres had its pressure increased to 100 atmospheres at a constant temperature, which of the following would be true?
    A   Volume = 500 cm³
    B   Volume > 500 cm³
    C   Volume < 500 cm³
    D   The change in volume will depend on the rate of increase of the external pressure.

58. Which of the following does not contribute to the explanation of the deviation of "real" gases from ideality?
    A   Gas particles occupy space.
    B   Gas particles have an attraction for each other.
    C   Gas particles possess mass.
    D   Gas particles do not undergo elastic collisions.

59. A sample of N₂, known to contain traces of water, occupied a volume of 200 dm³ at 25 °C and 1 atm. When passed over solid Na₂SO₄ (drying agent), the increase in mass of the salt was 35.0 grams. What was the partial pressure of the N₂ in the sample? (Assume ideality and molar volume at 25 °C = 24 dm³)
    A   0.1 atm
    B   0.2 atm
    C   0.4 atm
    D   0.8 atm

60. Which of the following would cause a gas to more closely resemble an ideal gas?
    A   Decreased pressure
    B   Decreased temperature
    C   Decreased volume
    D   None of the above

61. Consider the following graph illustrating the evolution of carbon dioxide gas under ideal conditions.

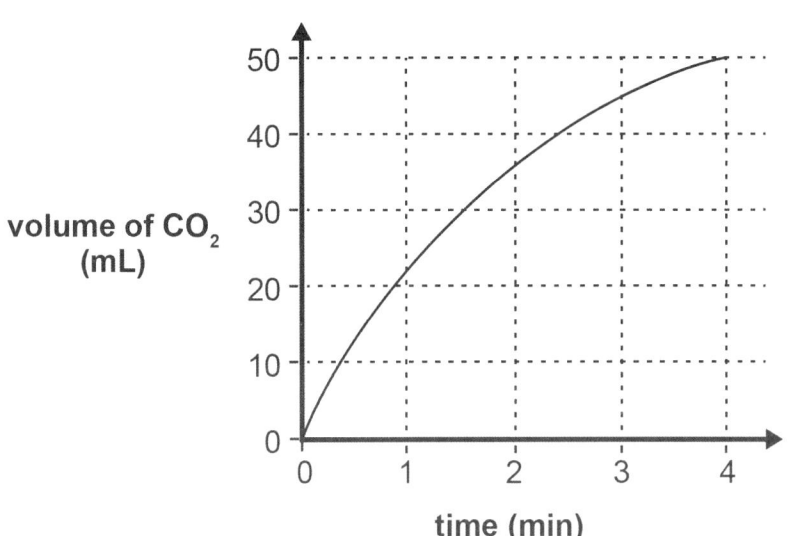

The average rate of reaction is greatest in which of the following time intervals?
A   0-30 seconds
B   30-60 seconds
C   0-1 minute
D   0-4 minutes

UNIT 15

Question 62

62. Von Willebrand's disease is an autosomal dominant bleeding disorder. A man who does not have the disease has two children with a woman who is heterozygous for the condition. If the first child expresses the bleeding disorder, what is the probability that the second child will have the disease?
A   0.25
B   0.50
C   0.75
D   1.00

UNIT 16

Questions 63–66

Ozone (O₃) reacts vigorously with alkenes. The reaction (= *ozonolysis*) leads to an oxidative cleavage of the double bond which can produce ketones, aldehydes or a combination thereof.

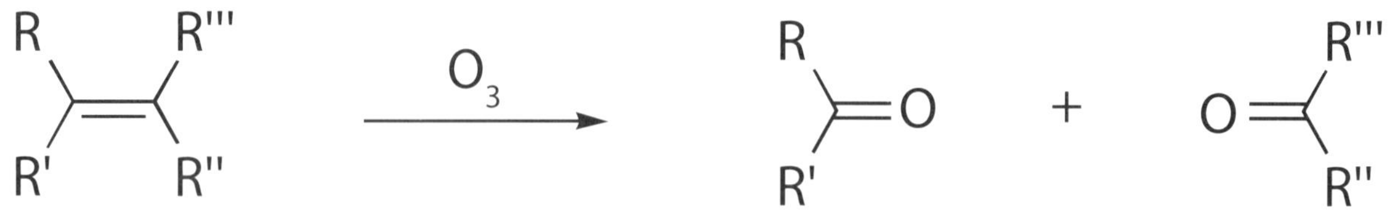

For the reaction above to occur, the second step must use a reducing agent such as zinc metal or dimethyl sulfide. Alternatively, an oxidative workup would oxidize any aldehydes to carboxylic acids.

Note: if the starting material is an alkyne, the result of ozonolysis with oxidative workup is oxidative cleavage and complete oxidation.

63. If the starting compound is a disubstituted alkene, which of the following must be true?
   A   Formaldehyde must be one of the 2 products
   B   At least one aldehyde must be one of the 2 products
   C   Two aldehydes must be the 2 products
   D   Both A and B are correct.

64. Ozonolysis of 5-chlorohexane-1-ene under reductive workup would be expected to produce 2 products. Which of the following would be one of those 2 products?
   A   Methanal
   B   Methanoic acid chloride
   C   Acetic acid
   D   Acetic acid chloride

65. Ozonolysis of cyclopentene under reductive workup would be expected to produce which of the following products?
   A   *cis*-Cyclopentane-1,2-diol
   B   *trans*-Cyclopentane-1,2-diol
   C   Pentane-2,4-dione
   D   Pentanedial

66. Ozonolysis of cyclodecyne under oxidative workup would be expected to produce which of the following products?
   A   *trans*-1,2-dihydroxycyclodecanene
   B   Decanedioic acid
   C   Decanone
   D   Decanedial

UNIT 17

Questions 67-69

Because of the symmetry of the benzene ring, if a monosubstituted benzene is evaluated, there could only be one such molecule. The one substituent, or ligand, replaces hydrogen at a carbon which would then be referred to as carbon-1.

However, when the benzene ring already has a substituent then substituted isomers are possible. Consider the following structure of toluene (methylbenzene).

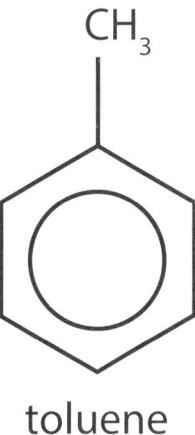

toluene

67. Consider the monosubstitution of toluene with fluorine. How many different fluorotoluenes are possible?
   A   2
   B   4
   C   5
   D   7

68. How many different difluorotoluenes are possible?
   A   4
   B   6
   C   8
   D   10

69. As compared to difluorotoluenes, how many different trifluorotoluenes are possible?
   A   Fewer
   B   Same
   C   An increase of 50%
   D   An increase greater than 50%

UNIT 18

Questions 70–71

70. The following equation is used to relate force and fluid viscosity η:

$$F = -2\pi r l \frac{v}{R}\eta$$

where F is force, r is radius, l is length, v is speed, R is distance and η is the viscosity. What are the dimensions of viscosity in the fundamental quantities of mass (M), length (L) and time (T)?
- A $M \cdot L^{3} \cdot T^{-3}$
- B $M \cdot L^{-1} \cdot T^{-1}$
- C $M \cdot L^{2} \cdot T^{-1}$
- D $M \cdot L^{-2} \cdot T^{-2}$

71. In the fundamental quantities described in the previous question, which of the following is equivalent to L^3?
- A (joules)/(pascals)
- B (joules)(pascals)
- C (volume)(joules)(pascals)
- D (volume)(joules)/(pascals)

UNIT 19

Questions 72-74

Viral hepatitis type B (serum hepatitis) is an infection of humans that primarily damages the liver. The causative agent is a virus called HBV, which is transmitted in much the same way as the HIV virus.

If HBV could be cultivated in the laboratory in unlimited amounts, it could be injected into humans as a vaccine to stimulate immunity against hepatitis type B. Unfortunately, it is not yet possible to grow HBV in laboratory culture. However, the blood of chronically infected people contains numerous particles of a harmless protein component of the virus. This protein, called HBsAg, can be extracted from the blood, purified, and treated chemically to destroy any live virus that might also be present. When HBsAg particles are injected into humans, they stimulate immunity against the complete infectious virus.

Of late, a new source of HBsAg particles have become available. Thanks to genetic engineering, a technique for cloning the gene for HBsAg into cells of the common bread yeast *Saccharomyces cerevisiae* has been developed. The yeast expresses the gene and makes HBsAg particles that can be extracted after the cells are broken. Since yeast cells are easy to propagate, it is now possible to obtain unlimited amounts of HBsAg particles.

72. Before being injected into humans, the HBV virus would first have to:
- A be cloned in yeast cells to ensure that enough of the virus had been injected to elicit an immune response.
- B have its protein coat removed.
- C be purified.
- D be inactivated.

73. The following graph shows the immune response for an initial injection of HBsAg and a subsequent injection of the HBV virus. Which of the following best explains the differences in the two responses?

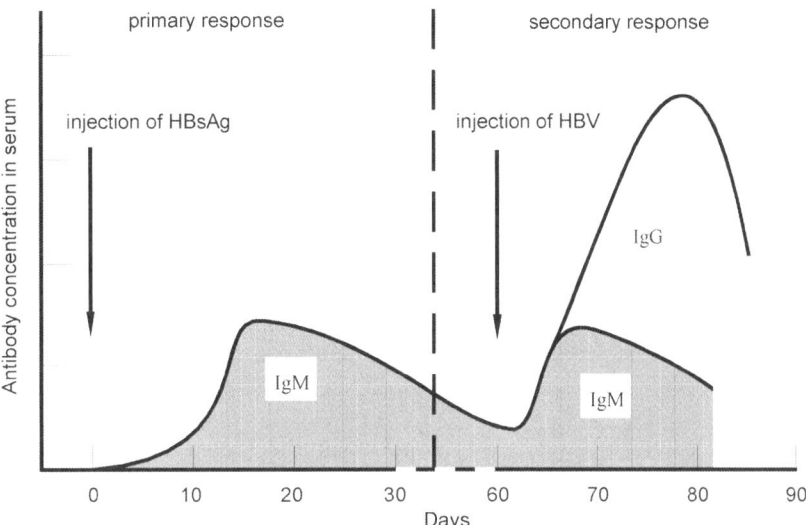

A   During the initial response, the immune response was carried out primarily by macrophages and B-lymphocytes.
B   During the secondary response, T-cells possessing membrane receptors, recognized and attacked the viral antigens.
C   Memory cells produced by T- and B-cells during the first exposure made the second response faster and more intense.
D   Memory cells produced by macrophages during the first infection recognized the viral antigens more quickly during the second infection, causing antibody production to be increased.

74. According to the preceding diagram, all of the following are correct EXCEPT:
A   if the slope of the curve was taken at any time t, the units could be in mg/day.
B   the time difference between the peak IgM and IgG secondary responses is less than the delay in the IgM primary response.
C   the peak IgM primary response has a delay similar in duration to the peak IgG secondary response.
D   the difference between peak IgG and peak IgM concentrations is greater than the peak IgM concentration.

UNIT 20

Question 75

75. A mass of 100 kg is placed on a uniform bar at a point 0.5 m to the left of a fulcrum. Where must a 75 kg mass be placed relative to the fulcrum in order to establish a state of equilibrium given that the bar was in equilibrium before any weights were applied?
A   0.66 m to the right of the fulcrum
B   0.66 m to the left of the fulcrum
C   0.38 m to the right of the fulcrum
D   0.38 m to the left of the fulcrum

UNIT 21

Questions 76–80

Sweat is a watery fluid containing between 0.1 and 0.4% sodium chloride, sodium lactate and urea. It is less concentrated than blood plasma and is secreted by the activity of sweat glands under the control of pseudomotor neurons. These neurons are part of the sympathetic nervous system and they relay impulses from the hypothalamus.

When sweat evaporates from the skin surface, energy as latent heat of evaporation is lost from the body and this reduces body temperature. Experiments have now confirmed that sweating only occurs as a result of a rise in core body temperature. Blood from the carotid vessels flows to the hypothalamus and these experiments have indicated its role in thermoregulation. Inserting a thermistor against the eardrum gives an acceptable estimate of hypothalamic temperature.

76. The transport of electrolytes in sweat from blood plasma to the sweat glands is best accounted for by which of the following processes?
   A   Osmosis
   B   Diffusion
   C   Active transport
   D   All of the above

77. Drinking iced water results in a lowering of core body temperature. Thus, a trial exposing the skin to heat while drinking iced water would result in which of the following according to the passage?
   A   If the person had been sweating prior to exposure to the trial then there would be an increase in sweating.
   B   If the person had been sweating prior to exposure to the trial then there would be a decrease in sweating.
   C   Irrespective of whether the person had been sweating prior to the trial, there would be an increase in sweating followed by a decrease in sweating.
   D   Irrespective of whether the person had been sweating prior to the trial, there would be no change in sweat production.

Questions 78-80 refer to Figure 1

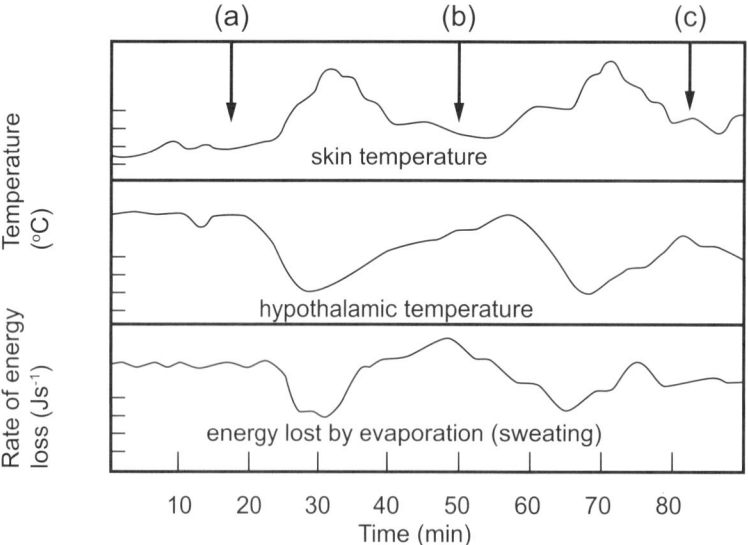

Figure 1: The relation between skin temperature, hypothalamic temperature and rate of evaporation for a human in a warm chamber (45 °C). Iced water is swallowed at points labeled (a), (b) and (c).

78. During the first 20 minutes the temperature and evaporation rate remain relatively constant because during this time:
    A   evaporation was at a minimum.
    B   the energy loss was not constant.
    C   the subject was allowed to equilibrate with his surroundings.
    D   45 °C was considerably higher than the mean body temperature.

79. The relationship between hypothalamic temperature and rate of sweating could be best described as:
    A   direct, suggesting that the rate of sweating is controlled by hypothalamic activity.
    B   direct, suggesting that hypothalamic activity is controlled by the rate of sweating.
    C   inverse, suggesting that changes in the rate of sweating occur in the opposite direction to changes in hypothalamic temperature.
    D   independent, suggesting that the rate of sweating and hypothalamic activity change independently of each other.

80. Shortly after ingestion of the iced water, skin temperature rises. This can best be explained by which of the following?
    A   As the evaporation rate falls, latent heat is no longer being lost from the skin, causing a rise in skin temperature.
    B   The unusually high temperature of the chamber over the 30 minute period caused the rise in temperature.
    C   The skin temperature rose to counteract the disturbance in body temperature caused by ingestion of the iced water.
    D   Change in skin temperature always occurs in the opposite direction to change in hypothalamic temperature.

C   IA, IIA, IIIA

UNIT 23

Questions 82–87

Active transport is the energy-consuming transport of molecules against a concentration gradient. Energy is required because the substance must be moved in the opposite direction of its natural tendency to diffuse. Movement is usually unidirectional, unlike diffusion which is reversible.

When movement of ions is considered, two factors will influence the direction in which they diffuse: one is concentration, the other is electrical charge. An ion will usually diffuse from a region of its high concentration to a region of its low concentration. It will also generally be attracted towards a region of opposite charge, and move away from a region of similar charge. Thus ions are said to move down *electrochemical gradients*, which are the combined effects of both electrical and concentration gradients. Strictly speaking, active transport of ions is their movement against an electrochemical gradient powered by an energy source.

Research has shown that the cell surface membranes of most cells possess sodium pumps. Usually, though not always, the sodium pump is coupled with a potassium pump. The combined pump is called the sodium-potassium pump. This pump is an excellent example of active transport.

Table 1: Concentration of Na^+, K^+, and Cl^- inside and outside mammalian motor neurons. The sign of the potential (mV) is inside relative to the outside of the cell.

Ion	Concentration (mmol/L H$_2$O) Inside cell	Concentration (mmol/L H$_2$O) Outside cell	Equilibrium potential (mV)
Na^+	15.0	150.0	+60
K^+	150.0	5.5	−90
Cl^-	9.0	125.0	−75

Resting membrane potential (Vm) = −70 mV

The value of the equilibrium potential for any ion depends upon the concentration gradient for that ion across the membrane. The equilibrium potential for any ion can be calculated using the Nernst equation. The following is an approximation of the equation for the equilibrium potential for potassium (E_k in mV) at room temperature:

$$E_k = 60 \log_{10} \frac{[K^+]_o}{[K^+]_i}$$

$[K^+]_o$ = extracellular K^+ concentration in mM
$[K^+]_i$ = intracellular K^+ concentration in mM

82. All of the following explain the ionic concentrations in Table 1 EXCEPT:
    A Na^+ and Cl^- ions passively diffuse more quickly into the extracellular fluid than K^+ ions.
    B Na^+ ions are actively pumped out of the intracellular fluid.
    C   the negative charge of the cell contents repels Cl^- ions from the cell.
    D   the cell membrane is more freely permeable to K^+ ions than to Na^+ and Cl^- ions.

83. If the concentration of potassium outside a mammalian motor neuron were changed to 0.55 mol/L, what would be the predicted change in the equilibrium potential?
    A   12 mV
    B   120 mV
    C   60 mV
    D   600 mV

84. A graph of E_k vs $\log_{10}[K^+]_o$ would be:
    A   a straight line.
    B   a logarithmic curve.
    C   an exponential curve.
    D   a sigmoidal curve.

85. In the process of osmosis, the net flow of water molecules into or out of the cell depends primarily on the differences in the:
    A   concentration of protein on either side of the cell membrane.
    B   concentration of water molecules inside and outside the cell.
    C   rate of molecular transport on either side of the cell membrane.
    D   rate of movement of ions inside the cell.

86. Active transport assumes particular importance in all but which of the following structures?
    A   Cells of the large intestine
    B   Alveoli
    C   Nerve and muscle cells
    D   Loop of Henle

87. At inhibitory synapses, a hyperpolarization of the membrane known as an inhibitory postsynaptic potential is produced rendering V_m more negative. This occurs as a result of:
    A   an increase in the postsynaptic membrane's permeability to Na^+ and K^+ ions.
    B   an increase in the permeability of the presynaptic membrane to Ca^{2+} ions.
    C   the entry of Cl^- ions into the synaptic knob.
    D   an increase in the permeability of the postsynaptic membrane to Cl^- ions.

UNIT 24

Questions 88

Infrared (IR) spectroscopy is an instrumental technique used to identify substances by keying in on functional groups. By measuring the absorption of infrared radiation over a range of frequencies and then comparing such data to tables for known substances, it is possible to reveal the underlying identity of the chemical.

Table 1: IR Absorptions

Functional Group	Characteristic Absorption(s) (cm^{-1})	Notes
Alkyl C-H Stretch	2950–2850	Alkane C-H bonds are fairly ubiquitous and therefore usually less useful in determining structure.
Alkenyl C-H Stretch Alkenyl C=C Stretch	3100–3010 1680–1620	Absorption peaks above 3000 cm^{-1} are frequently diagnostic of unsaturation
Alcohol/Phenol O-H Stretch	3550–3200	Specifity of the absorption is in part dependent on surrounding functional groups.
Carboxylic Acid O-H Stretch	3000–2500	
Amine N-H Stretch	3500–3300	Primary amines produce two N-H stretch absorptions, secondary amides only one, and tetriary none.
Aldehyde C=O Stretch Ketone C=O Stretch Ester C=O Stretch Carboxylic Acid C=O Stretch Amide C=O Stretch	1740–1690 1750–1680 1750–1735 1780–1710 1690–1630	The carbonyl stretching absorption is one of the strongest IR absorptions, and is very useful in structure determination as one can determine both the number of carbonyl groups (assuming peaks do not overlap) but also an estimation of which types.
Amide N-H Stretch	3700–3500	As with amines, an amide produces zero to two N-H absorptions depending on its type.

All figures are for the typical case only – signal positions and intensities may vary depending on the particular bond environment.

88. Consider the following reaction.

    The infrared spectrum of the product can be distinguished from that of the starting material by the:
    A   disappearance of IR absorption at 3360 cm^{-1}.
    B   disappearance of IR absorption at 2820 cm^{-1}.
    C   appearance of IR absorption at 3360 cm^{-1}.
    D   appearance of IR absorption at 1740 cm^{-1}.

UNIT 25

Questions 89–96

It is well known that there are two major forms of carbon, that is, carbon has two main allotropes: graphite and diamond. These differ greatly from each other with respect to their physical properties as shown in Table 1. The physical properties of silicon are also shown in Table 1 for comparison as carbon and silicon belong to the same group in the periodic table.

Table 1

Physical properties	Graphite	Diamond	Silicon
Density (g cm^{-3})	2.26	3.51	2.33
Enthalpy of combustion to yield oxide (ΔHc) kJ mol^{-1}	−393.3	−395.1	−910
Melting point (°C)	2820	3730	1410
Boiling point (°C)		4830	2680
Conductivity (electrical)	Fairly good	Non-conductor	Good
Conductivity (thermal)	Fairly good	Non-conductivity	Good

Graphite possesses what is commonly known as a layer structure: carbon atoms form three covalent bonds with each other to yield layers of carbon assemblies parallel with each other. These layers are held together via weak Van der Waals' forces which permit some movement of the layers relative to one another.

Both diamond and silicon (see Figure 1) form a diamond crystal lattice. The crystal lattice can be thought of as an array of 'small boxes', or cells, infinitely repeating in all three spatial directions: x, y and z. Continuing with the box analogy, consider that an atom in, for example, a top corner is shared by 3 other boxes at the same level plus another 4 boxes above. Fractions of atoms can be added to be equivalent to a full atom or atoms. There are 4 atoms completely within the lattice while all other atoms are shared between boxes to one degree or another. The length of one side of a crystal lattice for silicon is 0.543 nm.

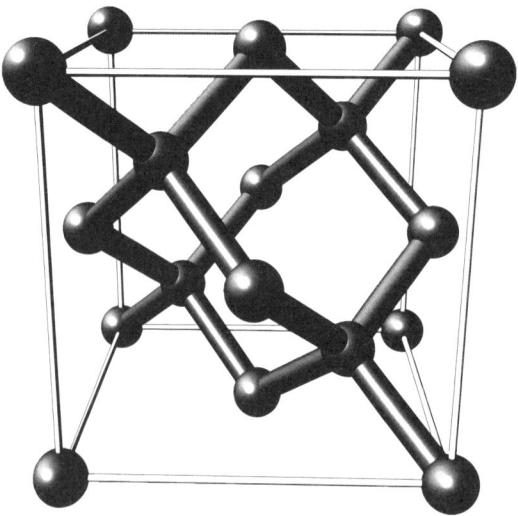

Figure 1: Diamond crystal lattice: Like a small box, or cell, that constitutes a repeating structure. Note that there is 1 atom centrally located on the surface of each face of the cubic cell.

A phase diagram is a graph that shows the relation between the solid, liquid and gaseous states. Any point in the graph is where 2 phases exist at equilibrium except the triple point where all 3 exist at equilibrium. Solid CO_2 is called "dry ice" because it can go directly from solid to vapour (sublimation) at room pressure (i.e. 101.3 kPa). The triple point of CO_2 occurs at 217 K and 515 kPa. A reduction in CO_2 pressure directly correlates with changes in its sublimation, melting and boiling points.

89. Which of the following is a correct representation of the phase diagram for carbon dioxide?

A 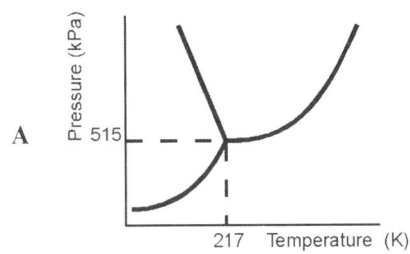   B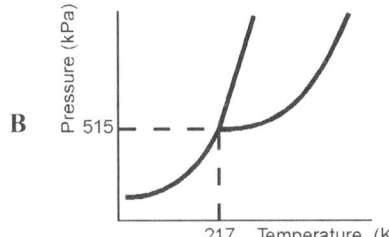

C 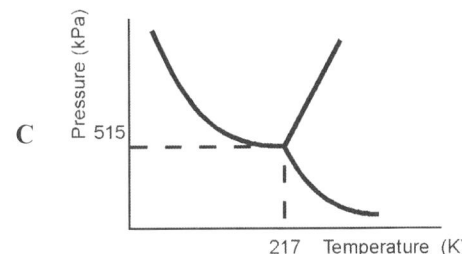   D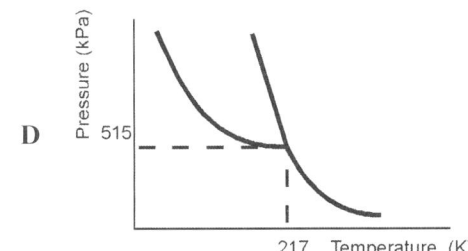

90. The properties of the layer-like structure of solid graphite stated in the passage would lend it to which of the following industrial uses?
    A   Insulator
    B   Structural
    C   Corrosive
    D   Lubricant

91. Using the information in the table, calculate the enthalpy change for the following process:

$$C_{graphite} \rightarrow C_{diamond}$$

    A   +1.8 kJ mol^{-1}
    B   −1.8 kJ mol^{-1}
    C   +1.0 kJ mol^{-1}
    D   −1.0 kJ mol^{-1}

92. It is possible to convert graphite into diamond via various chemical processes. Based on the information in the passage, which of the following would facilitate increased amounts of diamond assuming that the system is in equilibrium?
    A   Higher pressures
    B   Lower temperatures
    C   A catalyst
    D   None of the above

Questions 93 and 94 refer to the following additional information:

At a given temperature T in kelvin, the relationship between the three thermodynamic quantities including the change in Gibbs free energy (ΔG), the change in enthalpy (ΔH) and the change in entropy (ΔS), can be expressed as follows:

$$\Delta G = \Delta H - T\Delta S$$

93. The sublimation of carbon dioxide occurs quickly at room temperature. What might be predicted for the three thermodynamic quantities for the reverse reaction?
    A   Only ΔS would be positive.
    B   Only ΔS would be negative.
    C   Only ΔH would be negative.
    D   Only ΔG would be positive.

94. Which of the following statements is consistent with the triple point of carbon dioxide?
    A   The absolute temperature dominates the effect on Gibbs free energy.
    B   The reaction is spontaneous, Gibbs free energy is negative.
    C   The enthalpy change is equal to the effect of the entropy change.
    D   The entropy change is negative because there is more disorder overall.

95. To calculate the number of atoms per unit cell (crystal lattice), the degree to which atoms at the surface or corners are shared, as well as the number of whole atoms within the cell, must be taken into account. Considering the information in the passage and Figure 1, how many silicon atoms are there per unit cell (one crystal lattice)?
    A   4
    B   8
    C   16
    D   18

96. Given the information provided, which of the following is most consistent with an estimate of the number of silicon atoms per cm^{-3}?
    A 5×10^{22}
    B 5×10^{24}
    C 5×10^{26}
    D 5×10^{28}

UNIT 26

Questions 97–99

Hückel's Rule was developed to determine if a planar ring molecule, whether neutral or in ionic form, would have aromatic properties.

If a compound does not meet all the following criteria, it is likely not aromatic.
1. The molecule is cyclic.
2. The molecule is planar.
3. The molecule is fully conjugated (i.e. p orbitals at every atom in the ring).
4. The molecule has $4n + 2$ π electrons, where $n = 0, 1, 2, 3$, and so on.

If rules 1., 2. and/or 3. are broken, then the molecule is non-aromatic. If rule 4. is also broken then the molecule is antiaromatic.

Of course, benzene is aromatic (6 electrons, from 3 double bonds), but cyclobutadiene is antiaromatic, since the number of π delocalized electrons is 4.

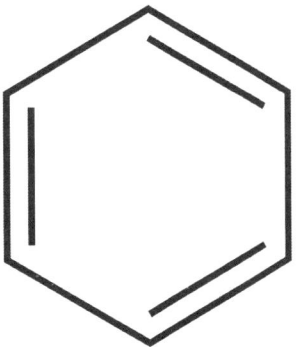

Note: All cyclic molecules among the following questions can be assumed to be planar except cyclodecapentaene which has many conformations including a boat-like conformation.

97. Which of the following would you expect to be aromatic?

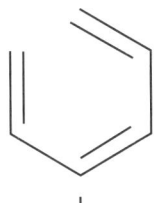   II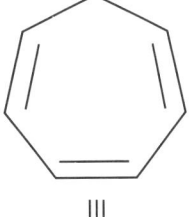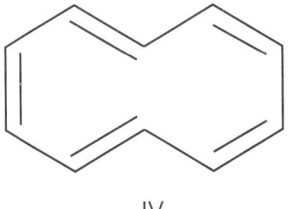

I   II   III   IV

- **A** None
- **B** I only
- **C** II and III only
- **D** I, II, III and IV

98. Which of the following is aromatic?

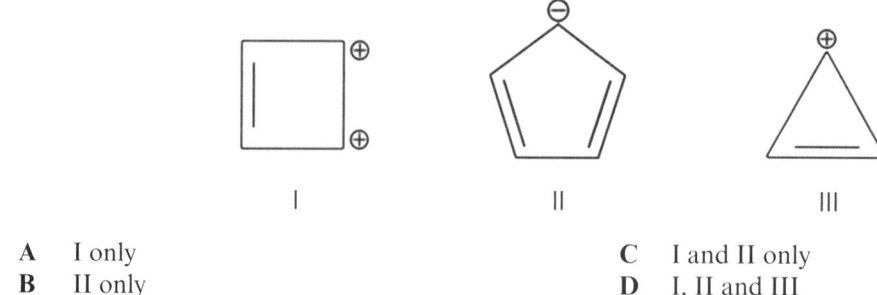

A   I only
B   II only
C   I and II only
D   I, II and III

99. Consider planar conformations of the following molecules. In that instance, which of the following would be considered anti-aromatic?

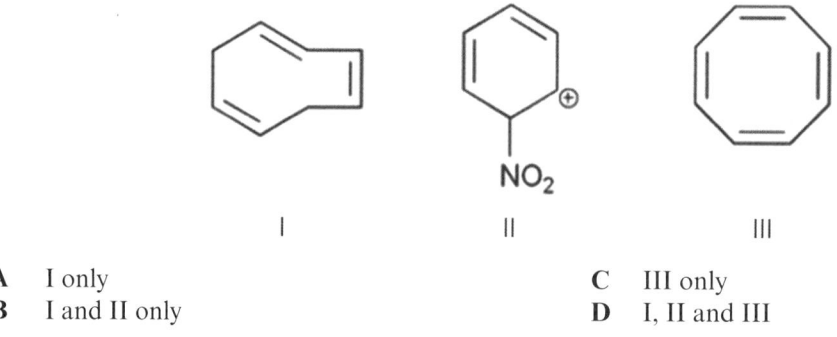

A   I only
B   I and II only
C   III only
D   I, II and III

UNIT 27

Question 100

Apoptosis is the process of programmed cell death that can occur in multicellular organisms. The proteins involved in apoptosis are associated with pathways for cell cycle arrest and DNA repair. These processes are mostly regulated through the interplay of various proteins involved in feedback loops including some of the ones shown in Figure 1.

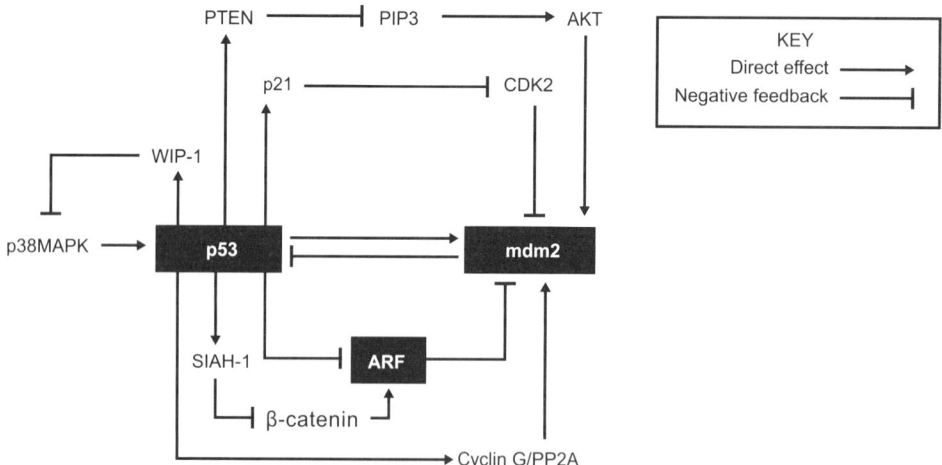

Figure 1: Feedback loops forming a regulatory network affecting apoptosis, cell cycle arrest and DNA repair. (Bioformatics Institute)

100. According to Figure 1, CDK2 activity would most reasonably increase due to all of the following EXCEPT:
   A   degradation of p21.
   B   high cyclin G concentrations.
   C   a mutation in the gene that produces PTEN.
   D   high p53 concentrations.

UNIT 28

Question 101

101. The data in Table 1 were collected for Reaction I:

$$2X + Y \to Z \qquad \text{Reaction I}$$

Table 1

Exp.	[X] in M	[Y] in M	Initial rate of reaction
1	0.050	0.100	8.5×10^{-6}
2	0.050	0.200	3.4×10^{-5}
3	0.200	0.100	3.4×10^{-5}

What is the rate law for the reaction?
   A   Rate = k[X]²[Y]
   B   Rate = k[X]²[Y]²
   C   Rate = k[X][Y]²
   D   Rate = k[X][Y]

UNIT 29

Questions 102–104

The following represents a summary of nucleophilic acyl substitution followed by nucleophilic addition:

- Carboxylic esters, R'CO$_2$R", react with 2 equivalents of organolithium or Grignard reagents to give tertiary alcohols.
- The tertiary alcohol that results contains 2 identical alkyl groups (R in the mechanism shown).
- The reaction proceeds via a ketone intermediate [Step (1)] which then reacts with the second equivalent of the organometallic reagent or Grignard reagent [Step (2)].
- Et = ethyl

102. Which of the following represents the product of the reaction between propyl ethanoate and 1 equivalent of 2-butyl lithium (*sec*-butyllithium)?
  A   2-hexanone
  B   3-methyl-2-pentanone
  C   4-methyl-3-hexanone
  D   3-heptanone

103. Given the mechanism provided, in order to produce a secondary alcohol, which of the following must be true?
  A   R' must be a hydrogen
  B   One R must be a hydrogen
  C   R' and R" must be hydrogens
  D   Either one R or R' must be hydrogen

104. Using 2 equivalents of the first and 1 equivalent of the second, respectively, which of the following pairs of compounds can be used to form the following tertiary alcohol?

A   Propyl lithium and methyl butanoate
B   Butyl magnesium bromide and propyl butanoate
C   Butyl lithium and pentyl pentanoate
D   Propyl magnesium bromide and hexyl pentanoate

UNIT 30

Questions 105-108

The viscosity of a fluid, that is, a gas, a pure liquid or a solution is an index of its resistance to flow. The viscosity of a fluid in a cylindrical tube of radius R and length L is given by:

$$n = \pi \Delta P R^4 t / (8VL) \qquad \text{Equation I}$$

where n = viscosity of fluid, ΔP = change in pressure, t = time, V = volume of fluid and V/t = rate of flow of fluid. This equation can be applied to the study of blood flow in our bodies. The heart pumps blood through the various vessels in our bodies to supply all of its tissues. At rest, the rate of blood flow is about 80 cm³ s⁻¹ and this is maintained in all blood vessels. However, the radii of the blood vessels decreases the further away blood moves from the heart. Therefore, in order to maintain the rate of blood flow, a pressure drop occurs as one moves from one blood vessel to another of smaller radius.

A great number of physiological conditions can be explained using Equation I, for example, hypertension.

105. What would be the pressure drop per cm of the blood in the first blood vessel leaving the heart if the blood vessel is of unit radius and the body is at rest?

$$n_{blood} = 0.04 \text{ dyn s cm}^{-3}$$

A $25.6/\pi$ dyn cm⁻³
B $16000/\pi$ dyn cm⁻³
C $\pi/25.6$ dyn cm⁻³
D $\pi/16000$ dyn cm⁻³

106. Which of the following has the greatest effect on the viscosity of a fluid per unit change in its value?
   A   Volume of the fluid
   B   Length of the tube
   C   Pressure of the fluid
   D   Radius of the tube

107. The equation for the rate of flow of a fluid (from Equation I) has often been compared to Ohm's law. Given that P can be likened to the voltage and flow rate can be likened to the current, which of the following can be likened to resistance?
   A πR^4
   B $\pi R^4/(8Ln)$
   C $8Ln/(\pi R^4)$
   D $8Ln$

108. Hypertension involves the decrease in the radius of certain blood vessels. If the radius of a blood vessel is halved, by what factor must the pressure increase to maintain the normal rate of blood flow, all other factors being constant?
   A   2
   B   4
   C   8
   D   16

UNIT 31

Questions 109–110

The red bread mold *Neurospora crassa* grows well on a cultural plate with "minimal" medium which is a fluid containing only a few simple sugars, inorganic salts, and vitamin. *Neurospora* that grows normally in nature (wild type) has enzymes that convert these simple substances into the amino acids necessary for growth. Mutating any one of the genes that makes an enzyme can produce a *Neurospora* strain that cannot grow on minimal medium. The mutant would only grow if the enzyme product were to be added as a supplement. On the other hand, if a "complete" medium is provided, containing all required amino acids, then *Neurospora* would grow, with or without mutation.

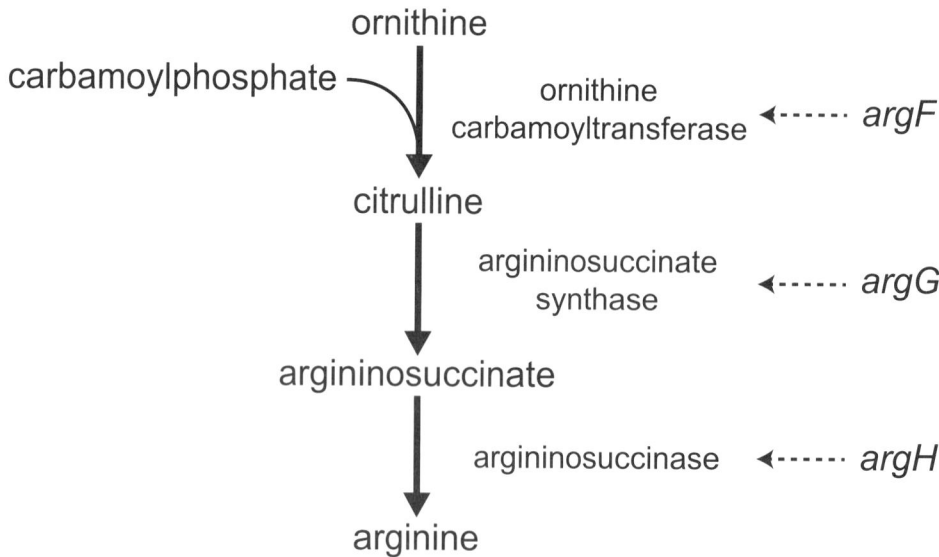

Figure 1: A synthesis pathway for the amino acid arginine. Each gene in italics in the diagram produces one enzyme necessary for the synthesis of this essential amino acid required for growth.

mutant strain	nothing	ornithine	citrulline	argininosuccinate	arginine
P	-	-	-	+	+
Q	-	-	-	+	+

Table 1: Growth response of mutant strains in "minimal" media with supplements as indicated. Growth is indicated by (+), and no growth is indicated by (−).

109. According to the information provided, a conclusion that can be made with certainty is that neither mutant strain P nor Q has the defective enzyme:
   A   carbamoyltransferase.
   B   argininosuccinate synthase.
   C   argininosuccinase.
   D   None of the above enzymes are defective in either mutant strain P nor Q.

110. Experiments using the two mutant strains P and Q, reveal that strain P accumulates citrulline, but strain Q does not. Which of the following statements is most consistent with the data provided?
   A   Strain Q has only one mutation.
   B   Strain P has a mutation in *argF* only.
   C   Strain P has mutations in *argF*, *argG* and *argH*.
   D   Strain P has a mutation in *argG* only.

END OF REASONING IN BIOLOGICAL AND PHYSICAL SCIENCES. IF TIME REMAINS, YOU MAY GO BACK AND CHECK YOUR WORK IN THIS TEST BOOKLET.

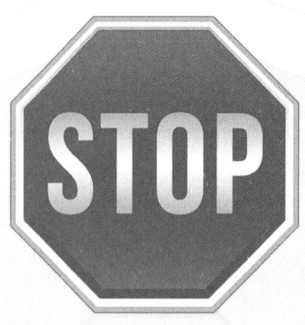

GAMSAT SCORE!

After you have completed test GS-1, you should spend the equivalent of a full day reviewing errors and guesses. Time must be taken to create "Gold Notes" which are high-density notes from your exam experience (preferably a maximum of 2 pages per exam section). By having a manageable number of pages, you can review all your exam experiences (ACER and GS tests) several times every week leading up to the real GAMSAT. This way you can always build on the progress you are making.

Worked solutions are available online for the original owner of this textbook by going to gamsat-prep.com, registering as an owner, clicking on Tests in the top Menu and scrolling down. Every question in the GS-1 exam also has a forum thread at gamsat-prep.com/forum so that if you do not understand the worked solution, we are happy to clarify any teaching points with you. There is no charge for this service.

We also have a free GS GAMSAT Score Calculator so that you can input your raw scores from this GS-1 exam to convert to scaled scores and a percentile rank.

The Gold Standard GAMSAT has put together a suite of home study materials, online courses, essay correction services and classroom lectures across Australia, Ireland and the UK. We recognize that everyone learns differently. Thus we created a multimedia integrated approach so you can choose the tools that help you study best. Good luck!

Gold Standard GAMSAT Practice Exams Summary

- GS-Free (1/3 length) available for free in all gamsat-prep.com accounts
- Full-length GS-1 which you have just completed; full solutions online
- Full-length GS-2, GS-3, and GS-4: available separately online only
- Full-length GS-5: available online or as an on-campus mock exam (paper)

All practice exams are revised every year to best reflect the current exam.

Answer Keys & Answer Documents

Answer Document

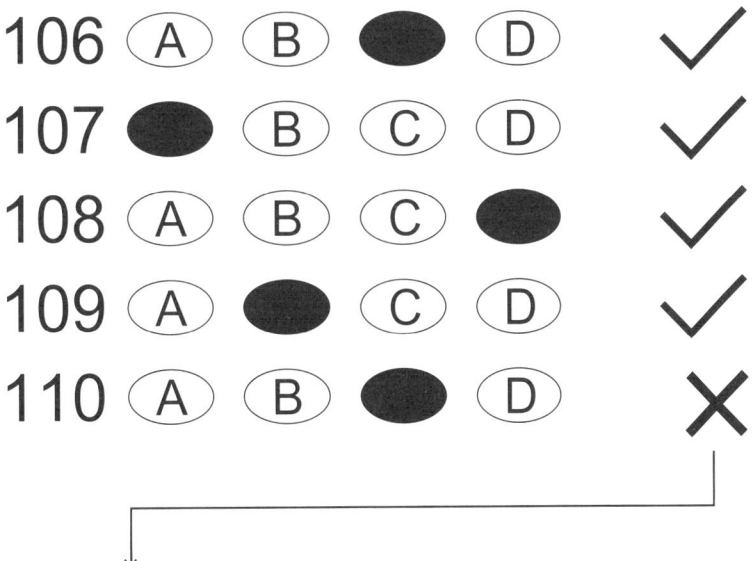

Answer Key

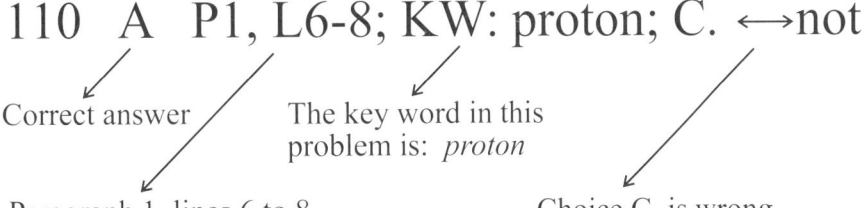

Correct answer: A

Paragraph 1, lines 6 to 8, is where the answer can be found

The key word in this problem is: *proton*

Choice C. is wrong because of the word "*not*"

The Gold Standard GAMSAT

GAMSAT is administered by ACER which is not associated with this product.

Test GS-1

You can use your Gold Standard Access Card to review worked solutions for all GS-1 problems. You will also be able to access a Forum to discuss any question as well as your exam experience. When you are logged in to your gamsat-prep.com account and click on Tests in the top Menu, you will also have access to a free GS Exam GAMSAT Score Calculator. You can use the calculator to input your raw scores from this GS-1 exam to convert to scaled scores and a percentile rank.

ANSWER KEY Section I

1.	D	20.	C	39.	D	58.	B
2.	A	21.	B	40.	B	59.	D
3.	B	22.	A	41.	C	60.	C
4.	B	23.	B	42.	C	61.	D
5.	D	24.	B	43.	C	62.	C
6.	B	25.	D	44.	C	63.	B
7.	B	26.	C	45.	A	64.	D
8.	C	27.	D	46.	C	65.	B
9.	B	28.	B	47.	D	66.	B
10.	C	29.	D	48.	B	67.	C
11.	B	30.	C	49.	C	68.	D
12.	C	31.	D	50.	A	69.	C
13.	B	32.	B	51.	A	70.	D
14.	C	33.	D	52.	A	71.	C
15.	D	34.	A	53.	D	72.	A
16.	B	35.	D	54.	A	73.	A
17.	B	36.	D	55.	A	74.	A
18.	B	37.	C	56.	B	75.	D
19.	C	38.	D	57.	B		

PHY = physics section; *KW = key word;* *G = graph;*
CHM = chemistry section; *T = table;* *L = line(s);*
BIO = biology section; *E = equation;* *P = paragraph;*
ORG = organic chemistry section; *F = figure;*
See **GS Part V**, **Table 2**, *for a complete list of symbols and abbreviations.*

ANSWER KEY SECTION III

Worked Solutions at GAMSAT-prep.com

Cross-reference

1.	B	BIO 1.2.1, 3.0
2.	C	BIO 4.1; ORG 9.4; P1; F
3.	D	ORG 12.2.1, BIO 3.0, 4.2
4.	D	GM 3.5.4; CHM 9.2, 9.2.1
5.	A	GM 3.7, 3.8
6.	D	GM 3.5.1, 3.5.4
7.	D	CHM 1.6, 10.1, 10.2
8.	B	CHM 1.6, 10.1, 10.2
9.	A	CHM 1.6, 10.1, 10.2
10.	D	CHM 1.6
11.	D	CHM 10.1, 10.2
12.	D	PHY 2.3
13.	C	P3, L5; PHY 6.1.3
14.	B	PHY 3.3; A + C = B
15.	D	PHY 6.1.3; Continuity then Bernoulli
16.	D	PHY 6.1.3
17.	D	CHM 5.3, 8.10, 9.10; BIO 12.4.2
18.	C	ORG 3.1, 12.3.2
19.	B	CHM 1.6
20.	D	CHM 1.4
21.	C	CHM 6.9
22.	B	CHM 6.1/2/3/7/8
23.	A	CHM 9.7, 9.8
24.	B	CHM 9.9
25.	A	Deduce; GM 2.1.3, 2.2
26.	A	P2; BIO 2.1, 2.3, 16.2
27.	B	P2; BIO 16.3; cf BIO 15.5
28.	B	F1 (B), cf (A); BIO 16.2 - 16.3
29.	C	BIO 2.5
30.	A	F1, deduce; BIO 2.5, 16.3
31.	C	deduce; P1-2; BIO 16.2; A. ↔ BIO 15.5
32.	D	CHM 3.5; ORG 1.2, 1.3, 4.1, 4.2
33.	B	ORG 4.1, 4.2, 4.2.4
34.	A	ORG 4.1, 4.2
35.	B	ORG 4.1, 4.2, 4.2.4
36.	D	ORG 1.4, 4.1
37.	C	ORG 2.1, 2.2, 2.3
38.	A	P2; P4; PHY 11.4
39.	B	PHY 1.1.1, 1.1.2
40.	C	PHY 11.4
41.	B	P4, L5; PHY 11.4
42.	A	PHY 11.4
43.	B	P2; PHY 11.4
44.	B	P1, S3; BIO 15.3
45.	D	T1
46.	B	F1; CHM 9.9, BIO 6.3.3, 6.3.6
47.	D	BIO 6.3.3
48.	A	P2, S4/5; F1; BIO 6.3.6/7
49.	B	deduce; BIO 5.4.4, 6.3.3
50.	C	CHM 5.3.2
51.	B	CHM 5.3.2; B → more moles
52.	C	P4, T; CHM 5.3.2
53.	C	P2, L4-7
54.	B	CHM 5.1.1/2
55.	B	PHY 3.2, 3.2.1, 3.4

Cross-reference

56.	A	PV/nRT = 1 = const. (ideal); CHM 4.1.6
57.	B	#1: F1; CHM 4.1.4/8
58.	C	CHM 4.1.2, 4.1.8
59.	D	CHM 1.3, 4.1.1/7
60.	A	CHM 4.1.2, 4.1.8
61.	A	GM 3.5; CHM 9.1
62.	B	BIO 15.3
63.	B	ORG 4.2, 7.2.1
64.	A	ORG 4.2, 7.2.1
65.	D	ORG 4.2, 7.2.1
66.	B	ORG 4.2, 4.3, 7.2.1
67.	B	ORG 2.1, 2.2, 2.3, 5.1
68.	D	ORG 2.1, 2.2, 2.3, 5.1
69.	D	ORG 2.1, 2.2, 2.3, 5.1
70.	B	GM 2.1.3, 2.2
71.	A	GM 2.1.3, 2.2; PHY 5.1, 6.1
72.	D	P2, S1, S4, deduce; BIO 2.1
73.	C	G; BIO 8.2
74.	A	G
75.	A	PHY 4.1, 4.1.1
76.	B	P1, S2; BIO 1.1.1, 1.1.2
77.	B	P2, S2; BIO 1.1.1, 1.1.2
78.	C	deduce
79.	A	F1; P1, S2-3
80.	A	deduce
81.	B	axial: ↑ESR; ORG 3.3, 12.3.2 Fig IV.B.12.1
82.	A	deduce; T1; P2, S2-3; BIO 1.1.2, 5.1.1 - 5.1.3
83.	B	T; E; CHM 6.5.1
84.	A	E; GM 3.7, 3.8
85.	B	BIO 1.1.1
86.	B	BIO 1.1.2, 12.3
87.	D	T1; BIO 5.1.1 - 5.1.3
88.	C	ORG 7.2.1, 8.2, 14.1
89.	B	P3; B: CHM 4.3.3
90.	D	P2, S2, deduce
91.	A	CHM 8.3, 1.4, ORG 3.2.1
92.	A	CHM 9.9
93.	D	E; CHM 8.10
94.	C	E; P3, S2; CHM 8.10
95.	B	P3; F1; deduce
96.	A	GM 1.5
97.	A	ORG 5.1, 5.1.1
98.	D	ORG 5.1, 5.1.1
99.	C	ORG 5.1, 5.1.1
100.	D	BIO 3.1, 4.4-4.10, 6.3.6, 6.3.7
101.	C	CHM 9.3
102.	B	ORG 1.6, 7.1, 8.1, 9.4
103.	A	ORG 1.6, 7.1, 8.1, 9.4
104.	D	ORG 1.6, 7.1, 8.1, 9.4
105.	A	E1
106.	D	E1; PHY 6.1.4
107.	C	E1; PHY 10.1
108.	D	E1; PHY 6.1.4
109.	C	BIO 3.1, 4.1-4.3
110.	D	BIO 3.1, 4.1-4.3

The Gold Standard GAMSAT

Answer Document 1

Test GS-1

CANDIDATE'S NAME ______________________________ STUDENT ID ____________________

Mark one and only one answer to each question. Be sure to use a soft lead pencil and completely fill in the space for your intended answer. If you erase, do so completely. Make no stray marks.

Section I

1	(A) (B) (C) (D)	39	(A) (B) (C) (D)
2	(A) (B) (C) (D)	40	(A) (B) (C) (D)
3	(A) (B) (C) (D)	41	(A) (B) (C) (D)
4	(A) (B) (C) (D)	42	(A) (B) (C) (D)
5	(A) (B) (C) (D)	43	(A) (B) (C) (D)
6	(A) (B) (C) (D)	44	(A) (B) (C) (D)
7	(A) (B) (C) (D)	45	(A) (B) (C) (D)
8	(A) (B) (C) (D)	46	(A) (B) (C) (D)
9	(A) (B) (C) (D)	47	(A) (B) (C) (D)
10	(A) (B) (C) (D)	48	(A) (B) (C) (D)
11	(A) (B) (C) (D)	49	(A) (B) (C) (D)
12	(A) (B) (C) (D)	50	(A) (B) (C) (D)
13	(A) (B) (C) (D)	51	(A) (B) (C) (D)
14	(A) (B) (C) (D)	52	(A) (B) (C) (D)
15	(A) (B) (C) (D)	53	(A) (B) (C) (D)
16	(A) (B) (C) (D)	54	(A) (B) (C) (D)
17	(A) (B) (C) (D)	55	(A) (B) (C) (D)
18	(A) (B) (C) (D)	56	(A) (B) (C) (D)
19	(A) (B) (C) (D)	57	(A) (B) (C) (D)
20	(A) (B) (C) (D)	58	(A) (B) (C) (D)
21	(A) (B) (C) (D)	59	(A) (B) (C) (D)
22	(A) (B) (C) (D)	60	(A) (B) (C) (D)
23	(A) (B) (C) (D)	61	(A) (B) (C) (D)
24	(A) (B) (C) (D)	62	(A) (B) (C) (D)
25	(A) (B) (C) (D)	63	(A) (B) (C) (D)
26	(A) (B) (C) (D)	64	(A) (B) (C) (D)
27	(A) (B) (C) (D)	65	(A) (B) (C) (D)
28	(A) (B) (C) (D)	66	(A) (B) (C) (D)
29	(A) (B) (C) (D)	67	(A) (B) (C) (D)
30	(A) (B) (C) (D)	68	(A) (B) (C) (D)
31	(A) (B) (C) (D)	69	(A) (B) (C) (D)
32	(A) (B) (C) (D)	70	(A) (B) (C) (D)
33	(A) (B) (C) (D)	71	(A) (B) (C) (D)
34	(A) (B) (C) (D)	72	(A) (B) (C) (D)
35	(A) (B) (C) (D)	73	(A) (B) (C) (D)
36	(A) (B) (C) (D)	74	(A) (B) (C) (D)
37	(A) (B) (C) (D)	75	(A) (B) (C) (D)
38	(A) (B) (C) (D)		

Section III

1	(A) (B) (C) (D)	38	(A) (B) (C) (D)	75	(A) (B) (C) (D)
2	(A) (B) (C) (D)	39	(A) (B) (C) (D)	76	(A) (B) (C) (D)
3	(A) (B) (C) (D)	40	(A) (B) (C) (D)	77	(A) (B) (C) (D)
4	(A) (B) (C) (D)	41	(A) (B) (C) (D)	78	(A) (B) (C) (D)
5	(A) (B) (C) (D)	42	(A) (B) (C) (D)	79	(A) (B) (C) (D)
6	(A) (B) (C) (D)	43	(A) (B) (C) (D)	80	(A) (B) (C) (D)
7	(A) (B) (C) (D)	44	(A) (B) (C) (D)	81	(A) (B) (C) (D)
8	(A) (B) (C) (D)	45	(A) (B) (C) (D)	82	(A) (B) (C) (D)
9	(A) (B) (C) (D)	46	(A) (B) (C) (D)	83	(A) (B) (C) (D)
10	(A) (B) (C) (D)	47	(A) (B) (C) (D)	84	(A) (B) (C) (D)
11	(A) (B) (C) (D)	48	(A) (B) (C) (D)	85	(A) (B) (C) (D)
12	(A) (B) (C) (D)	49	(A) (B) (C) (D)	86	(A) (B) (C) (D)
13	(A) (B) (C) (D)	50	(A) (B) (C) (D)	87	(A) (B) (C) (D)
14	(A) (B) (C) (D)	51	(A) (B) (C) (D)	88	(A) (B) (C) (D)
15	(A) (B) (C) (D)	52	(A) (B) (C) (D)	89	(A) (B) (C) (D)
16	(A) (B) (C) (D)	53	(A) (B) (C) (D)	90	(A) (B) (C) (D)
17	(A) (B) (C) (D)	54	(A) (B) (C) (D)	91	(A) (B) (C) (D)
18	(A) (B) (C) (D)	55	(A) (B) (C) (D)	92	(A) (B) (C) (D)
19	(A) (B) (C) (D)	56	(A) (B) (C) (D)	93	(A) (B) (C) (D)
20	(A) (B) (C) (D)	57	(A) (B) (C) (D)	94	(A) (B) (C) (D)
21	(A) (B) (C) (D)	58	(A) (B) (C) (D)	95	(A) (B) (C) (D)
22	(A) (B) (C) (D)	59	(A) (B) (C) (D)	96	(A) (B) (C) (D)
23	(A) (B) (C) (D)	60	(A) (B) (C) (D)	97	(A) (B) (C) (D)
24	(A) (B) (C) (D)	61	(A) (B) (C) (D)	98	(A) (B) (C) (D)
25	(A) (B) (C) (D)	62	(A) (B) (C) (D)	99	(A) (B) (C) (D)
26	(A) (B) (C) (D)	63	(A) (B) (C) (D)	100	(A) (B) (C) (D)
27	(A) (B) (C) (D)	64	(A) (B) (C) (D)	101	(A) (B) (C) (D)
28	(A) (B) (C) (D)	65	(A) (B) (C) (D)	102	(A) (B) (C) (D)
29	(A) (B) (C) (D)	66	(A) (B) (C) (D)	103	(A) (B) (C) (D)
30	(A) (B) (C) (D)	67	(A) (B) (C) (D)	104	(A) (B) (C) (D)
31	(A) (B) (C) (D)	68	(A) (B) (C) (D)	105	(A) (B) (C) (D)
32	(A) (B) (C) (D)	69	(A) (B) (C) (D)	106	(A) (B) (C) (D)
33	(A) (B) (C) (D)	70	(A) (B) (C) (D)	107	(A) (B) (C) (D)
34	(A) (B) (C) (D)	71	(A) (B) (C) (D)	108	(A) (B) (C) (D)
35	(A) (B) (C) (D)	72	(A) (B) (C) (D)	109	(A) (B) (C) (D)
36	(A) (B) (C) (D)	73	(A) (B) (C) (D)	110	(A) (B) (C) (D)
37	(A) (B) (C) (D)	74	(A) (B) (C) (D)		

The Gold Standard GAMSAT

Answer Document 2

Test GS-1 Section II

CANDIDATE'S NAME _____ STUDENT ID _____

When your timer is ready, you may turn the page and begin.

A A A A A

A A A A A

IF YOU NEED MORE SPACE, CONTINUE ON THE BACK OF THIS PAGE.

STOP HERE FOR WRITING TASK A.

B   B   B   B   B

IF YOU NEED MORE SPACE, CONTINUE ON THE BACK OF THIS PAGE.

B   B   B   B   B

IF YOU NEED MORE SPACE, CONTINUE ON THE NEXT PAGE.

STOP HERE FOR WRITING TASK B.

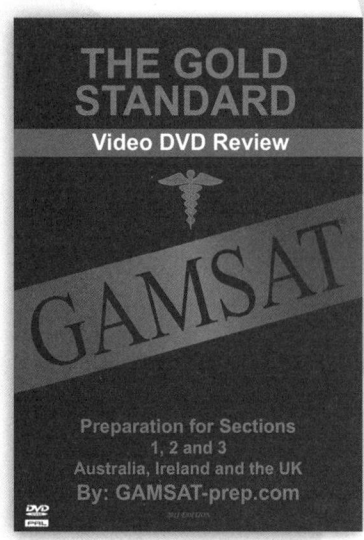
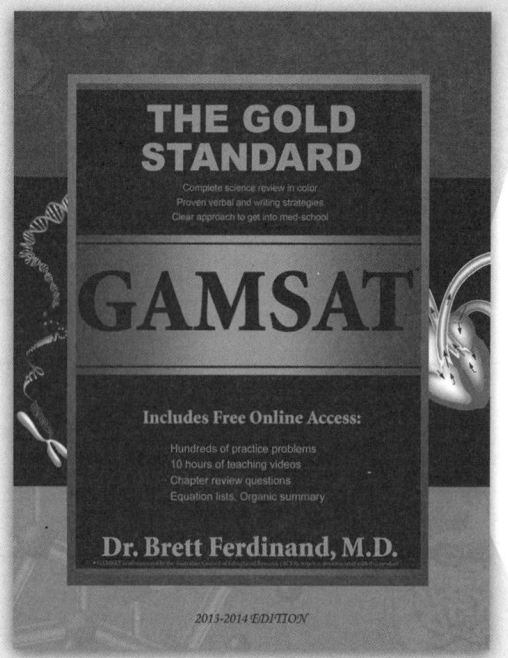
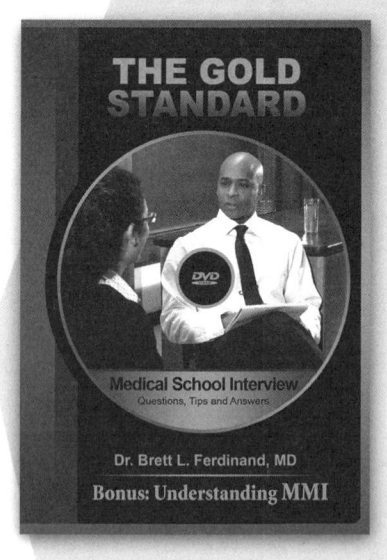

Gold Standard GAMSAT Preparation DVD for Section 1, 2, 3 (Australia, Ireland, UK)
ISBN: 978-1-927338-28-5

Gold Standard GAMSAT Textbook (Australia, Ireland, UK)
ISBN: 978-1-927338-28-5

The Medical School Interview DVD: Questions, Tips and Answer (The Gold Standard)
ISBN: 978-1-927338-28-5

You
Gold
Standard
GAMSAT textbook
·Cross-referenced & integrated·
MP3s·Smartphone Apps·Flashcards
Live GAMSAT Courses on campus in
Melbourne, Sydney, Brisbane, Perth, Adelaide,
London, Dublin·Mock Exams·Essay Correction Service
Online science teaching videos·DVDs·5 full-length practice tests with solutions·100+ YouTube videos: worked solutions to ACER's practice materials
·FREE GAMSAT Question of the Day FREE practice test

3000+ MCQs with worked solutions

Gold Standard GAMSAT. We can put **You** on top.

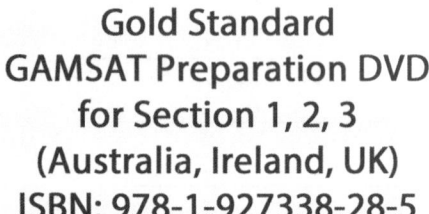

goldstandard-gamsat.com